Pharmacognosy

(Pharmacognosy & Phytochemistry)

Volume 1

Pharmacognosy

(Pharmacognosy & Phytochemistry)

Volume 1

Dr. Mohammad Ali
Professor and Former Dean
Faculty of Pharmacy, Jamia Hamdard
New Delhi-110 062

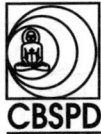

CBSPD

CBS Publishers & Distributors Pvt Ltd

New Delhi • Bengaluru • Chennai • Kochi • Kolkata • Lucknow • Mumbai
Hyderabad • Jharkhand • Nagpur • Patna • Pune • Uttarakhand

Pharmacognosy

(Pharmacognosy & Phytochemistry)
Volume 1

ISBN-13: 978-81-239-1438-1

First Edition: 2008

Reprint: 2009, 2011, 2012, 2016, 2018, 2019, 2020, 2022, **2024**, 2025

Published by **Satish Kumar Jain** and produced by **Varun Jain** for
CBS Publishers & Distributors Pvt Ltd
4819/XI Prahlad Street, 24 Ansari Road, Daryaganj, New Delhi 110 002, India
Ph: 011-23289259, 23266861   Website: www.cbspd.com
                                    e-mail: delhi@cbspd.com

Corporate Office: 204 FIE, Industrial Area, Patparganj, Delhi 110 092, India
Ph: 011-4934 4934   Fax: 011-4934 4935   e-mail: publishing@cbspd.com;
                                               publicity@cbspd.com

Branches

- **Bengaluru:** Seema House 2975, 17th Cross, KR Road, Banasankari 2nd Stage, Bengaluru 560 070, Karnataka, India
  Ph: +91-80-26771678/79   Fax: +91-80-26771680   e-mail: bangalore@cbspd.com
- **Chennai:** 7, Subbaraya Street, Shenoy Nagar, Chennai 600 030, Tamil Nadu, India
  Ph: +91-44-26680620, 26681266   Fax: +91-44-42032115   e-mail: chennai@cbspd.com
- **Kochi:** 42/1325, 1326, Power House Road, Opp KSEB, Power House, Ernakulum Kochi 682 018, Kerala, India
  Ph: +91-484-4059061-65,67   Fax: +91-484-4059065   e-mail: kochi@cbspd.com
- **Kolkata:** 147, Hind Ceramics Compound, 1st Floor, Nilgunj Road, Belghoria, Kolkata-700056, West Bengal, India
  Ph: +033-25633055, 033-25633056   e-mail: kolkata@cbspd.com
- **Lucknow:** Basement, Khushnuma Complex, 7 Meerabai Marg (Behind Jawahar Bhawan), Lucknow-226001, UP, India
  Ph: +91-522-4000032   e-mail: tiwari.lucknow@cbspd.com
- **Mumbai:** PWD Shed, Gala no 25/26, Ramchandra Bhatt Marg, Next to JJ Hospital Gate no. 2, Opp. Union Bank of India
  Noorbaug, Mumbai-400009, Maharashtra, India
  Ph: 022-66661880/89   e-mail: mumbai@cbspd.com

Representatives

- Hyderabad   0-9885175004
- Patna   0-9334159340
- Jharkhand   0-9811541605
- Pune   0-9664372571
- Nagpur   0-8692091830
- Uttarakhand   0-9716462459

Printed at Neekuni Print Process. Harvana. India

Preface

Through education, there has developed a public awareness that our health is not being fully served by conventional medicine. A remarkable development in the field of traditional medicine has attracted phytochemists, biologists and agriculturists. The natural wealth of medicinal plants has become a target for the search by multinational drug industries and research institutes for new drugs. There are large number of traditional plants, their extracts and phytoconstituents presently used in modern medicine. There is a world-wide majority of population that still relies on plants as a source of medicine. The western society has become interested in natural products with the general public acquiring herbal formulations. There is an introduction of laws to control the sale, quality and efficacy of such products. The students studying medicinal plants, including phytochemists and pharmacologists, expect in-depth studies of the subject.

Nature has been a source of medicinal agents for thousands of year, and an impressive number of modern phytoconstituents of therapeutical importance has been isolated from the natural sources. The majority of the isolated plant compounds are terpenoids, flavonoids and alkaloids and their structures are varied extremely and often very complex. They show a wide reactivity range and exert different physiological properties.

The purpose of this book is to provide pharmacognostical information of drugs, their classification, adulteration, quality control and pest control. The presence of the natural products found in trace amounts are also mentioned.

The pharmacological activities of the important drug constituents are included. It is hoped that new entries would add immensely to the usefulness of the book by highlighting the results of chemical and biological studies of the herbal drugs.

The source book is organized into 25 chapters. Each chapter covers general information. The drugs include information concerning biological sources, geographical distribution, morphology, histological characters, chemical constituents, chemical tests, medicinal uses, adulteration or substituents and pharmacological activities. The chapters offer a view over the enormous diversity of natural chemical molecules. The stereostructures of phytoconstituents are illustrated to introduce most of the concepts required for the study of natural products.

Since the nomenclatures of many plants have undergone revision in the preceeding decades, the names of plants and their families have been updated as far possible to provide currently accepted names.

A thorough understanding with an emphasis on the diagrams of the drugs, morphological characters and anatomical figures enable the readers to understand basic concepts of the drugs. Some of the data are presented in tabular forms. The length of this book, therefore, comes from metriculous explanations, chemical formulae, diagrams, chemical tests and pharmacological activities.

It is a pleasure to acknowledge the librarians of different libraries in Delhi for assisting me to afford relevant literature for compiling the book.

The author wishes to record his indebtedness to all the authors and publishers of various research papers, texts, monographs and reference sources for collecting important information included in the present manuscript whose works have been individually cited and duly acknowledged. I am happy to thank the assistance of Ms. Shaheen Sultana for checking the proofs. My greatest depth of gratitude is due to CBS Publishers and Distributors, Darya Ganj, New Delhi for continuous courtesy and full cooperation in bringing out the book to my satisfaction.

Finally, I express my deep gratitude to my family members for being supportive in times of stress in bring out this book. No major professional project can be completed without cooperation and encouragement of one's family.

Mohammad Ali

CONTENTS

Contents

Contents

Introduction

Pharmacognosy is concerned with the study of crude drugs of vegetable and animal origins. The term materia medica is used to refer to all substances used in medicine such as pure chemical compounds, herbal drugs, mineral substances, and biological preparations like vaccines and sera. Pharmacognosy involved a comprehensive study of individual drugs and elucidation of general principles. The word "Pharmacognosy" was used by C.A. Seydler in 1815 (Greek : *Pharmakon* = drug; *Gnosy* = knowledge). The subject deals with biological, biochemical, therapeutic, and economic features of natural drugs and their chemical constituents. At present pharmacognosy involves the study of crude drugs and their natural derivatives. Thus, Digitalis and its isolated glycoside, digoxin; Datura and its isolated alkaloid, atropine; Opium and its purified compound morphine, all are treated as the subject of pharmacognosy. For studying a drug, the following points must be considered :

1. **Biological source :** The biological source of a drug is mentioned in Latin language which also includes the family to which it belongs. After the Latin name, the name of the botanist responsible for the classification is mentioned in abbreviated form. The plant family to which the drug belongs determines certain of its characters.

2. **Habitat :** The principal areas of collection and routes of transport are considered under this head.

3. **Plant habit :** The general structure of the plant and morphology of crude drugs are studied.

4. **Cultivation, collection and preparation for market :** These factors require particular attention when they affect the appearance or quality of the product.

5. **Morphology and sensory characters :** A knowledge of the fine details of macroscopical sturcture is of vital importance in the examination of powdered drugs.

6. **Histology :** Microscopical characters such as cell structure and arrangement, starch granules, epidermal trichomes, calcium oxalate crystals and fibres are studied under this head.

7. **Commercial varieties, substitutes and adulteration :** With a knowledge of the diagnostic characters of official drugs, a critical examination may be made of commercial samples to determine their quality, substances known to be potential substitutes or adulterations.

8. **Chemical constituents :** The pharmacological active constituents, the percentage of the more potent components; constituents affecting the mode of action, the identity and the class of such compounds are considered.

9. **Evaluation of drugs :** The purity and quality of drugs are determined.

10. **Uses :** Various medicinal uses and toxic effects are studied.

PHARMACOGNOSY AND MODERN MEDICINE

Modern pharmacognosy has been developed rapidly due to improvement made in the technology of isolation processes which include the development of techniques such as column, paper, thin layer, gas-liquid, high performance liquid and droplet counter current chromatographic procedures. These methods have allowed the rapid isolation of compounds previously difficult to obtain by classical procedures. The most important factor has been the development of new spectroscopic techniques which are used to identify structures of the isolated compounds.

Simultaneous advancement in the fields of chemistry, biochemistry, biosynthesis and pharmacology has developed pharmacognosy. Various active compounds have been isolated from plants which are used in modern medicine. With the advancement of synthetic organic chemistry most of the active constituents of plants used in medicine have been synthesized. However, in spite of phenomenal progress in the area of development of new drugs from synthetic sources and appearance of antibiotics as major therapeutic agents, plants continue to provide basic raw material for some of the most important drugs. Although more than 100 plants are used in modern medicine in various parts of the world, the list of most important ones along with their pharma-cological properties is given in Table 1.1.

In addition to pure constituents the crude extracts of Belladonna, Ipecac, Opium, Henbane, Stramonium, Cascara sagrada, Glycyrrhiza, Rhubarb, Valerian, Podophyllum, Capsicum oleo-resin, Digitalis and Aloe are used in modern medicine. Besides these, the essential oils of Japanese mint, Peppermint, Eucalyptus, Anise seed, Clove, Cinnamon leaf, Lemongrass and Camphor are also utilized in modern medicine (Table 1.2).

Liver and stomach preparations of animals are used in therapy of pernicious anaemia. Bile secreted in liver is used in biliary secretion and parenterally as sodium salt to increase diuresis.

Approximately one-third of all pharmaceuticals are of plant origin. If fungi and bacteria are included, over 60% of the pharmaceutical preparations are plant based. However, in most modern pharmacopoeias the number of medicinal plants and preparations has declined and proportion of synthetic substances has increased due to changes in the use pattern of medicinal plants and new applications. Some are now offered to the public under manufacturers' brand names in the form of syrup, dragees, capsules and medicinal teas.

The National Prescription Audit (NPA) figures for 1973 for the USA indicate that 1.532 billion new and refilled prescriptions were dispensed from community pharmacies at an average cost of $ 6.32 billion for the market in that year. It has been estimated that 25.2% of these prescriptions contained one or more active constituents obtained from higher plants (seed plants). Furthermore, microbial products (such as antibiotics, ergot alkaloids and immunizing biologicals) accounted for 13.3% of all prescriptions, and animal derived prescriptions accounted for 2.7% of the total. A comparison with the year 1959 has shown that the percentage of natural products prescriptions had stayed constant, an indication that natural products represent an extremely stable market in the USA.

From the 1973 survey data, it was found that 99 different crude plant drugs or extracts from crude plant drugs, were found to be present in prescriptions analysed.

Emphasis of pharmaceutical research and development is on the creation of therapeutic, prophylactic and diagnostic substances with specific functions and minimum side effects in particular applications. Although, synthetic organic substances have achieved a substantial share in pharmaceutical applications, plant derived substances still remain a vital tool.

In modern medicine, *Vinca rosea* is used which contain some 70 alkaloids, the most important being vinblastine, vincristine and raubasine.

Medicinal plants as a whole appear to occupy a stable place in modern medicine; changes in respect of individual plants may be expected with the progress of scientific research. Industry is interested in synthesizing natural substances in order to combat supply shortages or reduce cost in comparison with the extraction of the active constituent(s) from natural raw materials. Certain products, natural or synthetic, may be found to be

Table 1.1. Important active constituents of plants used in modern medicine

Plants	Active constituents	Pharmacological activity
1. *Dioscorea* sp., *Agave* sp., *Solanum* sp.	Steroidal hormones	Anti-inflammatory, antiarthritic, hormonal
2. *Papaver somniferum*	Morphine, Codeine, Papaverine	Sedative, antitussive, smooth muscle relaxant
3. *Cinchona ledgeriana*	Quinine, Quinidine	Antimalarial, antiarrhythmic
4. *Datura* sp., *Hyoscyamus niger, Duboisia* sp.	Hyoscyamine, Hyoscine, Atropine	Parasympatholytic
5. *Digitalis lanata*	Digitoxin, Acetyldigoxin, Digoxin, Lanatosides	Cardiotonic
6. *Rauwolfia serpentina*	Reserpine, Ajmaline, Rescinamine, Deserpidine	Hypotensive, Vasodialator
7. *Catharanthus roseus*	Ajmalicine	Vasodialator
8. *C. roseus*	Vincristine, Vinblastine	Anticancer
9. *Camellia sinensis* (Tea)	Caffeine	CNS stimulant
10. *Erythroxylum coca*	Cocaine	Anaesthetic
11. *Ephedra* sp.	Ephedrine	Sympathomimetic
12. *Pilocarpus jaborandi*	Pilocarpine	Parasympathomimetic
13. *Cephaelis acuminata, C. ipecacuanha*	Emetine	Antiamoebic
14. *Claviceps purpurea*	Ergometrine, Ergotamine, Ergotoxine	Oxytocic, Vasoconstrictor, Vasodialator
15. *Plantago ovata*	Psyllium mucilage	Laxative
16. *Vinca minor, Voacanga africana*	Vincamine	Vasodialator
17. *Glycyrrhiza glabra*	Glycyrrhizinic acid, Glycyrrhetenic acid, Glycyrrhizin	Anti-inflammatory
18. *Cassia angustifolia, C. acutifolia*	Sennosides	Laxative
19. *Berberis aristata*	Berberine, Palmatine	Antidiarrhoeal, antiprotozoal
20. *Podophyllum peltatum*	Podophyllotoxin	Anticancer
21. *Colchicum autumnale*	Colchicine	Gout
22. *Theobroma cacao*	Theobromine	CNS stimulant, diuretic
23. *Coffea arabica*	Theophylline	CNS stimulant, diuretic
24. *Adonis vernalis*	Adoniside	Cardiotonic
25. *Aesculus hippocastanum*	Aescin	Anti-inflammatory, anti-exudative
26. *Aloe* species	Alloin	Purgative
27. *Anisodus tanguticus*	Anisodamine	Purgative
28. *Scopolia tangutica*	Anisodine	Sedative
29. *Areca catechu*	Arecoline	Anthelmintic
30. *Peumus boldus*	Boldine	Laxative, choleretics
31. *Ananas comosus*	Bromelain	Anti-inflammatory
32. *Brucea* species	Brucine	Central stimulant
33. *Cinnamomum camphora*	Camphor	Rubefacient
34. *Capsicum annuum*	Capsaicin	Counter-irritant

(Contd.)

Plants	Active constituents	Pharmacological activity
35. *Convallaria majalis*	Convallatoxin	Cardiotonic
36. *Curcuma longa*	Curcumin	Anti-inflammatory
37. *Mucuna pruriens*	L-Dopa	Anti-cholinergic, Anti-parkinsonian
38. *Erysimum canescens*	Erysimin (Helveticoside), Erysimoside	Cardiotonic
39. *Eugenia caryophyllata*	Eugenol	Analgesic
40. *Coleus forskohlii*	Forskolin	Heart diseases
41. *Commiphora mukul*	Guggul steroids	Anti-rheumatic
42. *Citrus* species	Hesperidine	Vitamin
43. *Hydrastis canadensis*	Hydrastine	Uterine haemorrhage
44. *Piper methysticum*	Kawain, Dihydrokawain	Stimulant
45. *Ammi visnaga*	Khellin	Vasodilator
46. *Nonnea macrosperma*	Linoleic acid	Vitamin F
47. *Scrophularia marilandica*	Linoleic acid	Vitamin F
48. *Lobelia inflata*	α-Lobeline	Anti-asthmatic
49. *Mentha* species	Menthol	Anti-pruritic
50. *Carica papaya*	Papain	Proteolytic enzyme
51. *Physostigma venenosum*	Physostigmine	Cholinergic
52. *Urginea maritima*	Procillaridin A, Scillarins A and B	Cardiotonic
53. *Veratrum album*	Protoveratrines A and B	Hypotensive
54. *Artemisia annua*	Artimissinin	Antimalarial
55. *Ruscus aculeatus*	Ruscogenins	Anti-inflammatory, Vasoconstructive
56. *Cassia* and *Fagopyrum* species	Rutin	Vitamin P
57. *Artemisia cina, A. maritima*	Santonin	Anthelmintic
58. *Datura metal, Scopolia tangutica*	Scopolamine	Mydriatic, cycloplegic
59. *Taxus brevifolia*	Taxol	Antitumor
60. *Silybum marianum*	Silybin, Silydianin, Silychristin	Hepatoprotective
61. *Strychnos nux-vomica*	Strychnine	Vermin killer
62. *Cannabis sativa*	Tetrahydrocannabinol	Euphoric
63. *Strychnos toxifera*	Tubocurarine	Skeletal muscle relaxant
64. *Vinca minor*	Vincamine	Vasodilator
65. *Valeriana officinalis, V. wallichii*	Valepotriates	Sedative
66. *Ammi majus*	Xanthotoxin	Photosensitizer
67. *Pausinystalia yohimbe*	Yohimbine	Aphrodisiac

more effective in certain other applications than those currently in use and the latter may, therefore, be abandoned. It is expected that medicinal plants and their derivatives would continue to play a major role in medicinal therapy.

Plants are a valuable source of therapeutic agents in the armory of modern medicine itself. Natural products that have come into modern therapy are the result of an approach that has been adopted during the past 50 years. Drug development in this way takes 8 to 18 years, and the cost of such a development programme has been variously estimated as being on the border of $ 15 to 50 million per drug, sometimes even more. This range of values

Table 1.2. Plant extracts used in modern medicine

Plants	Active constituents
1. *Aloe* species	Hydroxy anthraquinones (20%) calculated as aloin
2. *Atropa belladonna*	Hyoscyamine (1%)
3. *Cassia angustifolia*	Sennoside B (45%)
4. *Capsicum annuum*	Aloe resin containing capsaicin (8-10%)
5. *Centella asiatica*	Triterpenic acids (70%)
6. *Coriandrum sativum*	Total extract and oleoresin
7. *Cephaelis ipecacuanha*	Emetine (6%)
8. *Cynara scolymus*	Caffeylquinic acid (35%)
9. *Digitalis* species	Digitoxin
10. *Glycyrrhiza glabra*	Triterpene glycosides
11. *Harpagophytum procumbens*	Harpagoside (1.5%)
12. *Hamamelis virginiana*	Tannins (15%)
13. *Hyoscyamus niger*	Hyoscyamine (1%)
14. *Panax ginseng*	Ginsenoside Rg1 (10%)
15. *Passiflora incarnata*	Isovitexine (2.6%)
16. *Puemus boldus*	Boldine (0.04%)
17. *Polygala senega*	Tenuifolin (3.5%)
18. *Podophyllum peltatum, P. emodi*	Lignans
19. *Prunus africana*	Extract
20. *Rhamnus frangula*	Glucofrangulin (20%)
21. *Rheum officinale* and *R. palmatum*	Aloe-emodin (8%)
22. *Ruscus aculeatus*	Ruscogenin (10%)
23. *Ribes nigrum*	Anthocyanidins (25%)
24. *Serebia serrulata*	Fruit extract
25. *Silybum marianum*	Silybin, silydianin and silychristin (65%)
26. *Smilax* species	Saponins
27. *Vaccinium myrtillus*	Anthocyanidins (25%)
28. *Valeriana officinalis*	Valtrates (0.75%)
29. *Valeriana wallichii*	Valtrates (0.75%)
30. *Zingiber officinale*	Oleoresin and extract

is based on the experience of the development of pharmaceutical products in industrialized countries such as the U.S., the U.K. and Japan.

Many world's population can afford neither the money nor the time for drugs based on this existing strategy and pattern of development. Third World

Medical services are too poor to pay for a new drug even if it is discovered.

Between 50 to 80% of the developing world depends on traditional therapies for their health care. There is an effort toward improving these therapies as much as possible with the aid of modern science and technology. The factors that make these traditional remedies popular and acceptable should not be ignored.

Plants for industrial scale processing must be systematically cultivated after proper authentication of the correct species used. Gathering the plant material from the wild flora is unacceptable for a number of very important reasons. Each country must decide on the priority species to be cultivated and the choice of species must depend on factors such as the climatic conditions, the most abundantly used species, the species utilized for curing diseases which have no effective therapy in modern medicine, the species utilized for curing diseases for which modern therapy is disproportionately costly and species that have export potential.

The method of drug development from plant sources is based on a sequence of operations leading mainly toward the isolation of pure natural products. Organic chemists will tend to find such compounds which are easily isolated and purified into crystalline form for comparatively rapid structure determination. Compounds which by virtue of their structural characteristics have presented more formidable problems of isolation have in the past been missed and these may possessed the biological activity attributed to the plant. Isolation methods monitored by test for biological activity have only recently been adopted, but these can only be adopted if the nature of the bioactivity is known, and the test is suitable for repetitive application. In the standard strategy of drug development the costliest operations in time and money are those related to tests for toxicology, clinical research, and regulatory requirements. The process would generally be prohibitive for any developing country, even if the expertise were available; hence, new approaches must be considered for developing countries. The strategy that must be chosen should initiate some visible impact in minimum time without expenses. After assessment of the ethnomedical information, the plant species used in a preparation should be authenticated and then placed on a crop cultivation basis. Preparations based traditional medicines should be developed using modern methods of processing and subjected to clinical trials. Following indications of therapeutic potential, they should be formulated into modern dosage forms, and compared by clinical trials with these preparations. Simultaneously, methods of analysis and quality control should be developed, and after efficacy has been established, isolation procedures for chemical constituents could be initiated, while successful preparations are prepared and formulated in bulk for distribution to health programmes. This is now the considered approach recommended to Third World countries.

The chemical studies will bring up active chemical compounds with new structural features. They would enhance the development of quality control methods based on new analytical techniques such as are available today, and these methods may be extended for the quality control of extracts of multicomponent preparations as well. Such studies would also enable the development of standardized, internationally recognized techniques for the quality assessment of plant-derived product.

Herbal medicine

A herbal remedy is one in which the main therapeutic activity depends upon the plant or fungal metabolites which it contains. Some plants are purely dietary and are necessary for health (fresh vegetables, carrots, fruit, which we now know provide essential vitamins). Many plant products are consumed in reasonable quantity as foods but known to have medicinal effects (e.g., figs, prunes, and mucilages acting as mild laxatives). There are some purely medicinal plants, few apparently quite 'safe' and others more potent (e.g., containing cardioactive glycosides), which can be consumed only in small quantities but which at such dosage are suitable for the treatment of certain diseases.

In past, the cure of disease and the use of medicinal plants has been much influenced by religious practice and the exercise of magical rites.

From a pharmacognostical viewpoint the study of herbal medicines differs little from that for the allopathic medicinal plants. In practice, many herbal remedies have not been as extensively studied either

pharmacologically or phytochemically, a situation which must change for over-the-counter products as stricter licensing controls are implemented.

It is important also to distinguish between herbal medicine dispensed and supplied by a qualified medical herbalist as a result of a consultation, and those herbal remedies freely available to the public for self-medication at retail outlets.

In some countries the strict implementation of EC directives has caused problems and financial difficulties for those smaller companies unable to afford the licensing and research and development costs for the maintenance of existing, and the development of new products.

Supply of medicinal plants

Medicinal plants can be obtained through a medical herbalist or medical practitioner on prescription and as counter products from pharmacies and other retail outlets. In practice medical herbalists, who constitute a relatively small professional body, are not consulted by the majority of the public who purchase herbal preparations. General practitioners rarely prescribe herbal remedies.

A number of 'health' magazines, radio, television and wall advertisements, and brochures promote the use of vegetable diets and herbal remedies and bring to public attention the existence of such products. For example, jojoba (*Simmondsia chinensis*; Buxaceae) oil in tonic shampoos, evening primrose and borage oils, and the beneficial effects of ginseng, lal tail, cinchara, dashmool and turmeric creams are advertised.

The herbal medicine tradition in some European countries is strong. The quoted figures for herbalists is 16,000 for Germany and 4,000 for Denmark. In France, as a result of legislation enacted in 1941, the marketing of herbal products passed very much under the control of pharmacists, 65% of total sales being through pharmacies. Many physicians in Europe are now reportedly prescribing an increasing number of medicines based on plant sources, as distinct from synthetic ones. In the USA, there is a legal restraint on the general sale of herbal medicines, but this is to some extent circumvented by the use of 'Teas' which contain herbal constituents. In central London, the herbal teas are available in more than 100 varities on sale from pharmacies and involved 117 different herbs; they were mainly available as tea-bags containing either single or multi-herb components.

Legal control

In European countries, the supply of medicines is controlled by the Medicine Act,, 1968.

Few drugs, including Belladonna, Digitalis, Nux-vomica, Poppy capsules and Rauwolfia are obtainable only on the prescription of an appropriate practitioner; some 35 potent plants (e.g., Male fern and Strophanthus) are under pharmaceutical control; and a further 40 plants, including those containing tropane alkaloids, Cinchona and Colchicum, may be supplied by herbalists within certain specified limits. All these drugs represent about 550 herbs and their preparations which are in general use in herbal medicine. Some 341 herbal medicines are included in the General Sales List and, therefore, are freely available to the public without prescription. In Britain alone it has been estimated that 6,000-7,000 tons of herbs are extracted annually for use as ingredients of herbal remedies. For the health food market in 1983, it was estimated that the sale of herbal, homoeopathic and other remedies amounted to rupees 700 million. The manufacture of these products is carried out by relatively few companies. A product licence is required for their manufacture and sale.

Herbal physicians

A qualified herbal practitioner will diagnose particular symptoms and prescribe herbal treatment appropriate for the individual patient. Such treatment is directed towards restoring a state of homeostasis, or a normal physiological balance of the body, rather than directly attacking the symptoms of the disease. The extracts of the plants prescribed will contain a wide range of plant metabolites, of which some will be therapeutically active. This admixture, containing a spectrum of the constituents of the plant cell may give rise fewer side-effects than a single isolated principle. A number of constituents, which on their own may appear pharmacologically inactive, combine synergistically to produce therapeutic effects. Thus, *Convallaria majalis* (Lily of the

valley) is highly esteemed in the treatment of certain heart conditions. It contains glycosides similar to those of digitalis but having a different cardioactive effect. This treatment may be combined with, or followed by, according to the individual patient's requirements.

Many plants are available for the treatment of diseases of the digestive system, the respiratory system, the blood and blood-forming tissues, the locomotor system, the connective tissues and the endocrine system.

Efficacy of herbal drugs

Many of the plants used in herbal medicine contain active constituents whose effects can be demonstrated pharmacologically and the action of the whole plant extract can usually be related to that of the isolated constituents. However, for some herbal remedies the situation is complicated by the frequent use of a number of drugs in combination.

Valerian has long been used for its sedative properties, but the unreliability of its preparations and the lack of association of therapeutic activity with known constituents (essential oils, alkaloids) led to its decline in use in standard medical practice in the UK. The sedative action of the root resided in a group ot unstable, the epoxyiridoid esters (valepotriates) and these were marketed as a freeze-dried product to avoid decomposition. The valepotriates have cytotoxic activity, although no adverse reactions had been reported as a result of normal medication with the drug. The sesquiterpene valerenic acid derivatives of the root have a sedative action; these are not destroyed by the usual processing of the drug as are the valepotriates. Efforts have now been made to select plant producing high concentrations of these compounds but which are low in valepotriates.

The herbal remedies are inherently safer then the potent synthetic drugs, which often produce undesirable side effects. There are extremely toxic plants in the plant kingdom which produce carcinogens, teratogens and other compounds which cause disease and sensitization. Thus, Comfrey (*Symphytum officinale*), always considered a 'safe' herb, has been found to contain small quantities of pyrrolizidine alkaloids which are known to be hepatotoxic and which, when administered to rats, cause liver cancer.

Similarly reserpine, an alkaloid of *Rauwolfia serpentina*, has been associated with breast cancer, but no such cases have been reported as a result of administration of the root extract. A number of cases of toxicity arising from the over-consumption of herbal remedies have been reported, and the principal danger appears to be that arising from the uncontrolled supply and administration of these products.

Standardization

Precise methods for the evaluation of botanical drugs and their preparations have been devised and appropriate standards appear in the monographs. With herbal remedies, accurate methods of assay are often lacking. Where the active constituents are unknown there is no mean of assessing therapeutic potency except by the use of a biological assay. On the herbalist's contention that it is the effect of the complete extract of the plant that is most desirable, then, perhaps, the biological assay is the one which reflects the true activity of the drug most clearly.

Medical plants based drug industry

There are about 7,000 drug industries based on the Indian Systems of Medicine of which 551 are on loan licence and the remaining industries are on form D. There are also many small manufacturing units using medicinal plants and thousands of Vaidyas preparing their own drugs from various plants. Annual herbal drug production has been estimated at around Rs. 800 crores and is expected to reach Rs. 4,000 crores by the coming years. Medicinal plant based drug industry has three major segments.

1. Plant parts extract and galenicals

The direct plant material is used in traditional medicines not only in the developing world but also in Europe and the U.S.A., e.g., herbal formulations on health food shops. Preparations of decoctions, tinctures, galenicals and total extracts of plants also form a part of many pharmacopoeias of the world. The current trend of medicinal plants based drug industry is to procure standardized extracts of the plants as raw material.

2. Essential oils from plants

Since 1947, a number of industrial companies have been established for large scale production of essential oils, oleoresins and perfumes. The essential oils from plants being produced in India include ajowain oil, cedarwood oil, celery oil, citronella oil, davana oil, eucalyptus oil, geranium oil, lavender oil, lemongrass oil, Mentha oil, palmarosa oil, patchouli oil, rose oil, sandalwood oil, turpentine oil and vetiver oil. The manufacture of turpentine oil and resin from pines is a well established industry in India having 10,000-25,000 tonnes annual production of the oil. α-Pinene and δ-3 carene are the two vital components produced from the oil. α-Ionone from lemongrass oil for perfumery and β-ionone for vitamin A synthesis are produced in India. Before 1960, menthol was not produced in India but the introduction of Japanese mint, *Mentha arvensis* and subsequent improvements thereupon enabled India to produce over 500 tonnes of menthol and now tops the world market in export of natural menthol.

Annual world production of limonene is 50,000 tonnes and Brazil is the biggest producer in the world market. It is a by-product of citrus industry. Though turpentine oil and eucalyptus oil also yield limonene but the best economically cheap raw material is the discarded orange and lemon peel which is being used by Brazilian phytochemical industry. India has not yet tapped this source for limonene production.

3. Phytopharmaceuticals

Before 1947, there was production of quinine from *Cinchona* as a plant based modern drugs in India. After 1965, bulk production of plant-based modern drugs has become an important segment of Indian pharmaceutical industry. Some of the phytopharmaceuticals produced in India at present include morphine, codeine, papaverine, thebaine, emetine, quinine, quinidine, digoxin, caffeine, hyoscine, hyoscyamine, xanthotoxin, psoralen, colchicine, rutin, berberine, vinblastine, vincristine, nicotine, strychnine, brucine, ergot alkaloids, senna glycosides, pyrethroids and podophyllotoxin resin.

Phytopharmaceuticals for which technology has been developed for undertaking large scale production include L-dopa from *Mucuna* beans, ajmaline and ajmalicine from *Rauwolfia serpentina* and *Catharanthus* roots, respectively, and 18 β-acetyl glycyrrhetic acid from *Glycyrrhiza glabra.*

Indian Institute of Chemical Technology (IICT), Hyderabad has developed methods for etoposide and tenoposide production and CIPLA is now producing it on commercial basis. At present 100 mg of etoposide is sold at Rs. 400 per vial. National Chemical Laboratory, Pune, developed the method of vincristine and vinblastine production. CIPLA has further improved the process and now they are the third largest manufacturer of these alkaloids in the world.

Medicinal plants based drug industry is progressing very fast in India, but it faces a number of problems. Most alarming problem is the scare supply of plant material from natural resources. A national policy on medicinal plants with a view to preserve endangered species and promoting cultivation of plants which are being extensively used by industry will help in solving the major problem of the industry. Special attention is required on medicinal plants on which significant research leads have been obtained (Table 1.3), medicinal plants which are being imported, medicinal plants having export potential and the threatened medicinal plants.

Table 1.3. Medicinal plants with significant research leads

Commiphora mukul	Antihypercholesterolaemic
Boswellia serrata	Antiarthritic
Picrorhiza kurroa	Antihepatotoxic
Phyllanthus amarus	Antihepatotoxic
Centella asiatica	Brain tonic
Curcuma longa	Antiinflammatory
Andrographis paniculata	Antihepatotoxic
Withania somnifera	Adaptogen
Coleus forskohlii	Cardiotonic
Acorus calamus	Tranquillizer
Sida rhombifolia	Anabolic
Albizzia lebbeck	Immunomodulator
Valeriana wallichii	Tranquilizer

Trade in medicinal plants is largely unorganised and uncertain, both in demand and price structure.

There is a need to have an organisation which could interact with the growers and user industry to bring stability in their production, demand, price, quality and also to help in international trade.

The development of a medicinal plant industry becomes for many countries of the Third World both a health and an economic necessity. The benefits of such an industry can be as follows :

(a) Crop diversification and increase of agro-production.

(b) More productive use of available land resources particularly in the case of lands which are only marginally suitable for other types of economic crops such as food grains, fruits, tea, rubber, coconut, cocoa, and spice crops.

(c) Stimulation of rural-based industrial efforts and offering greater stability to farmers.

(d) Generating employment in area where there is unemployment; the opportunity that such an industry offers for self-employment of educated youth in developing countries is also significant.

(e) Creating new export opportunities and providing existing industries with alternative locally produced raw material, e.g., oils and fats, essential oils, pigments, gums, tannins, and other phytochemicals which may result as by-products of a medicinal plant industry and be gainfully utilized in the cosmetics, paints, and leather industries, in place of imported materials.

(f) Therapeutic preparations specific to maladies that are localized or prevalent within a particular region.

(g) Plant-derived biocides and pest repellents which are relatively inexpensive, and are biodegradable, and would cause little long-term ecological damage, and hence would serve as alternatives to hazardous synthetic pesticides.

The industry would also increase the local, regional, or national self-sufficiency with respect to therapeutic and related pharmaceutical products.

In developing a medicinal plant industry in Third World countries, the regions of the world that most require such as industry, certain constraints will have to be overcome. Some of these are of a general nature, i.e., the need for systematic programmes for cropwise cultivation of medicinal plant. An industry cannot draw on spontaneously growing plant species for reasons of species depletion and the fact that the raw materials for processing will vary with regard to quality. Cultivation on a cropwise basis involves a long research and development effort consisting of the following elements:

(a) Selection of plant species based on ethno-medical usage, modern assessments and chemical and biological characteristics of the species.

(b) Crop development, including genetic improvement of species, agronomic research, harvesting techniques, and postharvest methods.

(c) Farm and estate management, methods of transport, storage, marketing and distribution to central authorities.

(d) Technology, which would include basic processing, quality assessment of raw materials, and the first stage products, such as essential oils, extracts, or formulated drug delivery forms.

The major constraint for almost every developing country is the shortage of funds. Entrepreneurship is based on the visibility of the profit prospect. State entrepreneurship is sometimes the only possibility, but here too, foreign exchange is scarce and this is a barrier to the acquisition of equipment, expertise, and training. Research and development efforts, therefore, cannot be productively initiated and sustained. Often the lack of local capital hinders all efforts directed toward the necessary research and development. The lack of expertise in developing countries is a serious barrier to technology transfer in all areas such as agronomy, processing, and quality control. In the attempts to initiate such technology transfer one frequently faces the lack of infrastructural necessities such as ongoing relevant research programmes at local institutions, universities, polytechnics, or technical schools graduating quality personnel to staff a developing industry, and managerial expertise at all levels. Finally, one of the most important considerations is a political vision to develop a medicinal plant industry in a

given situation. The presence of such a political manifest must be translated into state policy responses favourable to the industry, protective acts for products and operations, and above all the availability of investment incentives, without which the industry, even if initiated satisfactorily, will soon cease to exist. In China, all the research activities on herbal drugs have been carried out under one organisation resulting in remarkable contribution in phytotherapeutics. Therefore, Chinese herbal drugs are accepted in developed countries. In India, research activities in phytomedicines are conducted under supervision of many councils and in different ministries without any co-ordination and no conclusive result has been drawn.

Drug designing technology

Research is vital to the successful transfer of technology in the medicinal plant industry. Initiation of research activity has its own set of problems.

The medicinal plant industry utilizes plant materials with such a diversity of physical properties, e.g., delicate flowers, soft leaves, succulent fruits, fibrous materials and grasses, hard woods, brittle barks, oily seeds and nuts, and so on. The processing of such material imposes a wide range of requirements due to both physical diversity and chemical variety.

There is also a wide range of agronomic requirements and thus the research necessities become accordingly complex and multidimensional. A concerted research programme should involve the disciplines of botany, plant genetics, agronomy, entomology, phytochemistry, pharmacology, chemical engineering, pharmacy, and clinical and marketing studies oriented toward the common goal of product development. The research, therefore, complements the scientific functions of the industry.

For the development of technology to be accomplished and sustained, research expertise has to be built up over several years—involving a number of existing institutions and with the collaboration of one or more funding agencies. The competence of the national institutions has to be slowly developed to enable them to undertake indigenous goal-oriented research. The institutions may be universities, research institutes, or private sector research organizations.

Several problems are encountered in developing indigenous research competence and not all of these problems are peculiar to the medicinal plant industry. Much effort in planning is needed and even normal interinstitutional links must be forged to ensure the coordination research activities to enable goal-directed priorities to be maintained. For example, agronomic research expertise as generally available in developing countries is more often that not related to the major crops such as rice, coffee, tea, rubber, and cocoa and located in departments or institutions that are responsible for the development of these crops; botanical expertise is usually located in established botanical gardens, universities, and forestry institutions; chemical expertise will be found in university chemistry departments, industrial or technological research institutions, and pharmacological and pharmaceutical expertise is found within medical and pharmaceutical research organizations and universities.

The source of personnel, funds, and equipments which may be utilized for an industry-oriented research exercise on medicinal plants would be divided between several institutions. This makes coordination of research activities a goal common to all, but of lesser priority to each. Yet, coordination of activities within an existing infrastructure is the most economical way open to developing countries, given the constraints of time and funds. Furthermore, the public sector must shoulder the burden of laying the foundations of basic research and provide the leadership for the development of research to initiate and sustain an endogenous crop-oriented medicinal plant industry. Most often, the private sector tends to wait until sufficient basic and applied research has been done to demonstrate profit potential before they invest in further research. New products have to be conceived based on laboratory research activity. They must be formulated, tested, manufactured, first in pilot scale amounts on a trial basis, then in bulk, clinically evaluated, launched, and marketed. This activity can be the responsibility of the private sector. Governments of developing countries could commit such activity to the private

sector on pre-arranged terms and even stimulate private sector involvement by legislative and policy incentives, tax benefits, low interest loans and market safeguards against imported competitor products. Bridging the vast gap between basic research, in many instances just phytochemical or pharmacological screening, and product development is the problem of developing countries within the medicinal plant sector.

Product processing methods at the laboratory level must be tested on a pilot scale for process suitability and to ensure some measure of economic feasibility. Acquisition of such pilot plants is generally the major problem for research and development institutions in developing countries. Versatile pilot plants that can be used for solvent extraction, percolation, steam distillation and concentration of extract with recovery of solvent are generally produced in developing countries. International funding agencies can fill a major need. Some developing countries are now able to construct such prototype pilot plants themselves, which can be equally effective for product quality, though perhaps not product economy. Sometimes processing technologies that appear feasible at the pilot plant level may encounter difficulties on scaling up to commercial production. Problems of magni-tude, such as handling large quantities of plant material, waste material disposal, solvent recovery, product drying, etc., can become disproportionately large when moving from pilot scale to commercial levels. It is also necessary at the commercial level to match processing with the availability of plant material to ensure economic operation.

Marketing facilities are necessary for the industry to sustain itself in a Third World context. Investors always seek existing or potential market availability before investing in research and development ventures, and in the medicinal plant industry it is not often easy to possess such availability. Development of a market depends on the production of a quality product on a viable commercial scale. Research and development is, however, a necessary pre-requisite to produce a quality product which will stimulate market interest. For products based on medicinal plants several formidable regulatory barriers are to be removed.

The legal and ethical requirements for products

include ensuring that products are safe when taken within the dosage stipulations by large sections of people. Such insurance involves quality assessment of drugs. It also faces another barrier in the form of uncertainty of patent protection, due both to the complexities of obtaining such protection and the costs.

The transfer of technology to Third World countries must in reality recognize marketing and regulatory aspects as well. A new strategy must be adopted toward developing the medicinal plant industry. This strategy must address itself to the contingency situation existing in Third World countries and should have the following approach:

1. The generation of factory produced traditio-nal medicines with attendant standardization, quality control and acceptable manufacturing practices.

2. The formulation of new products based on traditional remedies, including modern dosage forms, and at economic prices in the Third World context.

3. Natural product drug development.

The strategy should be designed to draw support from all interested, on humanitarian grounds, concern for the health of the underprivileged, the need to develop appropriate industries in the poorer parts of the world, and the global benefits that can be obtained by sharing a research and development enterprise.

It is well established that plants both terrestrial and marine could continue to provide mankind with valuable therapeutic agents for a long time to come. The use of plant species in cultures where such therapies were developed should be scientifically examined and the theories on which they are based. There are numerous scientific instances when the dosage regimen or preparative methods are prescribed in old texts.

AYURVEDA AND DRUG DEVELOPMENT

Ayurveda is an ancient Indian system of health-care, both physical and mental, and literally means, science of life. Health in Ayurveda has been defined as a well balanced metabolism plus a happy state of being . Disease has been considered four fold :

1. body,
2. mind,
3. external factors and
4. natural intrinsic causes.

In Ayurveda treatment is done by a salubrious use of drugs, diets and practices.

Pharmaceutics occupies an important place in Ayurveda. Medicinal preparations are invariably complex mixtures, being derived from plant and animal products as well from minerals and metals.

Utilization of plants is mentioned in *Rigveda* and *Atharvaveda*. *Charaka Samhita* (900 B.C.) is the first recorded treatise on Ayurveda. It consists of eight sections divided into 150 chapters, and describes 341 plants used in medicine. The other treatise on Ayurveda is *Sushruta samhita* (600 B.C.) with special emphasis on surgery. It has six sections covering 186 chapters and describes 395 medicinal plants, 57 drugs of animal origin, and 64 minerals and metals as drugs. The next important authorty in Ayurveda was Vagabhatta of Sind, who practised during about 7th century A.D. His manuscript entitled *'Astanga Hridaya'*, is considered unrivalled for principles and practice of medicine. The manuscript is divided into six sections covering 120 chapters and contains 7444 verses. Madhava of Vijayanagar (12th century A.D.) comprised *Madhava Nidana* which consisted 69 chapters and 1552 verses. Sarangdhara (14th century), the author of *Sarangdhara Samhita,* systematized Ayurvedic *Materia media.* This book consists of three parts, 32 chapters, and 2500 verses. Bhava Mishra of Magadha wrote his treatise *Bhava Prakashan* in 1550 A.D. which contained 10,831 verses; nearly 470 medicinal plants are mentioned. In addition, about 70 pharmacy chapters have been written. *'Raja Nighantu'* by Narhari Pandita and *'Madanpala Nighantu'* by Madanpala are considered as masterpieces on medicinal herbs.

Kashmir-born Dridhobala (9th century A.D.), a well known physician of India, re-constructed and re-edited the great Ayurvedic medical treatise *Charaka Samhita.* Another famous scholar of 9th century A.D. was Ugraditya Charya Jain, a native of Deccon, who wrote a treatise under the title *Kalyana Karaka.* He has described the use of mercury and many other compounds. Vrinda (1000 A.D.) composed a book of medicinal chemistry called *Siddhayoga*. The book describes methods for the preparation of various metallic drugs. Chakarapanidatta (1066 A.D.) wrote *Chikitsa Sarsamgraha* which described uses of more metals for curing diseases. A treatise called *Chikitsa Sarsamgraha* was written by Vangasena in 1200 A.D. The book describes uses of mica, iron, mercury, sulphur and copper.

Ayurvedic medicinal system

Like all systems of Indian sciences, the origin of Ayurveda has been taken from the gods. Ayurveda was first perceived by Brahma, and he taught this science to Daksa - Prajapati, who taught it to the Aswni-Kumaras, and they taught it to Indra and so on. All the four Vedas are replete with references to various aspects of medicine. Many miraculous achievements in the field of medicine and surgery are mentioned in Vedas. The concept of digestion, metabolism, anatomical descriptions and discussion about several diseases are available. Different types of bacteria causing diseases are also described. The process of delivery, cauterization, toxins, control of evil sprites, rejuvenation therapies and aphrodisiacs have been mentioned. Medicinal plants, the different parts and their therapeutic effects are also described. Ayurveda believes in the existence of soul in the individual's body and in the unity of the body and the mind. Mental perversions affect the physical functions, and morbidity of the body affects the mental activities. Intellectual blasphemy, unwholesome conjunction of sense organs with their objects and vagaries of weather and time are causative factors of diseases. Forcible stimulation of natural strength, negligence in treatment, loss of good conduct, avoidance of health activities, malice, fear and anger are some examples of intellectual blasphemy. Unwholesome conjunction of sense organs include vision, sound, smell, taste and touch. Cold, heat and rain are characteristic features of seasonal diseases. *Rasa, rakta, mamsa, medas, asthi, majja* and *sukra* are the seven basic tissue elements. There are thirteen groups of enzymes which are responsible for digestion and metabolism in the body.

Principles of Ayurveda

Life in the purview of Ayurveda connotes a combination of body, sense organs, mind and soul. It is a system of health care which treats each person. The "Tridoshic" concept is the fundamental principle in Ayurveda.

There are three basic constituents of the physiological systems according to this concept. These constituents are called "Doshas". They are the ultimate irreducible basic metabolic elements constituting the body and mind of the living organism. They are classified into Vata, Pitta and Kapha. They correspond primarily to elements of air, fire and water. They determine the life processes of growth and decay.

Vata

The biological air humour is called "Vata" (air). It is primarily dry, cold and light. It is most important, or primary, of the three biological humours. It governs the other two and is responsible for all physical processes in general. It sustains effort, exhalation, movement and the discharge in impulses, the equilibrium of tissues and the coordination of senses. When aggravated, Vata (air) causes emaciation, debility, liking of warmth, tremors, distension, constipation, insomnia, sensory disorientation and incoherent speech. Vata is located in the colon, thighs, hips, ears, bones and organ of tough.

Pitta

The biological fire humour is called Pitta, sometimes also translated as bile. It is responsible for all chemical and metabolic transformation in the body. Pitta exists mainly in the acid form as fire and cannot exist directly in the body without destroying it. Pitta is primarily hot, moist and light. It governs digestion, heat, visual perception, hunger, thirst, lustre, complexion, understanding, intelligence, courage and softness of the body. Pitta in excess causes yellow colour of stool, urine, eyes and skin, hunger, thirst, burning sensation and difficulty in sleeping. High Pitta results in accumulation of internal heat or fever with inflammation and infections. Pitta is located in small intestine, stomach, sebacious glands, blood, lymph, organs and vision. Its primary site is in small intestine.

Kapha

The biological water humour is called Kapha, sometimes also translated as phlegm. Etymologically it means 'that which holds things together'. It provides substance, gives support and makes up the bulk of our bodily tissues. It also governs emotional traits as love, compassion, modesty, patience and forgiveness. Kapha is primarily cold, moist and heavy. It gives stability, lubrication, holding together of the joints and such qualities as patience. Kapha is the material substratum and support of the other two humours and also gives stability to the emotional nature. Excessive Kapha causes depression of the digestive fire, nausea, lethargy, heaviness, white colour, chills, looseness of the limbs, cough, difficult breathing and excessive sleeping. High Kapha results in the accumulation of weight and gravity in the body, inhibits normal function and causes hypoactivity through excessive tissue accumulation.

Treatment

Vata is treated by mild application of oils, mild sweating and purification methods. Pitta is treated with the ingestion of ghee (clarified butter), by purgation with sweet and cold herbs, by sweet, bitter and astringent foods and herbs, by applying cool, delightful and fragrant essential oils, by amounting the heat with Camphor, Sandalwood, Vetivert oils, etc. Kapha is treated by strong emetic and purgation methods according to the rules by all kinds of exercises, by smoking of herbs and by doing physical hard work.

Thus herbal medicine plays a major role in the treatment of Vata, Pitta and Kapha.

Ayurvedic therapies

There are many different therapies applied in Ayurveda. They can all be defined in two groups, viz :

(i) Tonification (supplementation–make heavy).

(ii) Reduction (elimination–to lighten)

Reduction therapies decrease body weight and are indicated for overweight accumulation of toxins and aggravated humours. It is indicated in acute stage of disease, when the attack is strong, and primarily for Kapha.

Tonification methods nourish deficiencies in body and are indicated in underweight, debility or tissue weakness. They are indicated in chronic diseases, in convalescence or after reduction methods have been used, and primarily for Vata. A mixed therapy is required for Pitta.

Ayurvedic methods of diagnosis are extremely simple. Stress is given on urine, stool, semen, flatus, vomiting, sneezing, eructation, yawning, hunger, thirst, tears, sleep and heavy breathing for diagnosis of a disease. Ayurveda also stresses upon the use of a wholesome diet along with the use of drugs for the successful treatment of diseases. Knowledge of the site of manifestation of the disease is essential for successful treatment. Pulse is examined in the early morning when the patient is in empty stomach. Pulse examination is carried out through the help of the radial artery.

In Ayurveda drugs are classified depending on their taste, attributes, potency, taste after digestion, and therapeutic effect. Four types of therapies - elimination therapy, alleviation therapy, psychic therapy and surgery, are used for the treatment of diseases. In addition to single drugs, compound formulations are generally used by Ayurvedic physicians in the form of pills, powders, decoctions, infusions, linctus, alcoholic preparations, medicated ghee, fractional distillation and collyrium. Several pharmaceutical processes are followed for the preparation of medicines for easily administration; making the products delicious to the taste, easily digestable and assimilatable, therapeutically more effica-cious, rendering them non-toxic and more tolerable and for preservation of medicines for a longer time. Ayurvedic drugs are administered both externally in the form of ointment, dusting powder, collyrium, ear drops and eye drops, and internally as tablets, pills, powder, syrups, etc. Along with medicines some regimens like sleep, walk, rest and physical exertion are also prescribed to the patients.

Asava and arista

Asavas and Aristas are medicinal preparations made by soaking the drugs, either in powder form or in the form of decoction (Ksaya), in a solution of sugar or jaggery, as the case may be, for a specified period of time, during which it undergoes a process of fermentation generating alcohol, thus facilitating the extraction of the active principles contained in the drugs. The alcohol so generated also serves as a preservative.

Preparation of arista

The drugs are coarsely powdered and decoction is prepared. The decoction is strained and kept in the fermentation pot, vessel or barrel. Sugar, jaggery or honey, according to the formula, is dissolved, boiled and added. Drugs mentioned as *praksepa dravyas* are finely powdered and added. At the end, *dhataki puspa*, if included in the formula, should be properly cleaned and added. The mouth of the pot, vessel or barrel is covered with a lid and the edges sealed with clay-smeared cloth. The container is kept either in a special room, in an underground cellar or in a heap of pady, so as to ensure that for the duration of fermentation and a constant temperature is maintained, since varying temperatures may impede or accelerate the fermentation.

After the specified period, the lid is removed, and the contents examined to ascertain whether the process of fermentation has been completed. The fluid is first decanted and then strained after two or three days. When the fine suspended particles settle down, it is again strained and bottled.

Preparation of asava

The required quantity of water, to which jaggery or sugar as prescribed in the formula, is added, boiled and cooled. This is poured into the fermentation pot, vessel or barrel. Fine power of the drugs mentioned in the formula are added. The container is covered with a lid and the edges are sealed with clay-smeared cloth. The rest of the process is as in the case of Arista.

If the fermentation is to be carried on in an earthen vessel, it should not be new. Water should be boiled first in the vessel, absolute cleanliness is required during the process. Each time, the inner surface of the fermentation vessel should be fumigated with pipali curna and smeared with ghrta before the liquids are poured into it. In large scale manufacture, woodenvats, porcelain-jars or metal vessels are used in place of earthen vessels.

Arka

Arka is a liquid preparation obtained by distillation of certain liquids or of drugs soaked in water using the *Arkayantra* or any convenient modern distillation apparatus.

Preparation of arka

The drugs are cleaned and coarsely powdered. Some quantity of water is added to the drugs for soaking and kept over-night. This makes the drugs soft and when boiled releases the essential volatile principles easily. In the following morning it is poured into the Arka yantra and the remaining water is added and boiled. The vapour is condensed and collected in a receiver. In the beginning, the vapour consists of only steam and may not contain the essential principles of the drugs. It should, therefore, be discarded. The last portion also may not contain therapeutically essential substance and should be discarded. The aliquots collected in between contain the active ingredients and may be mixed together to ensure uniformity of the arka.

Arka is a suspension of the distillate in water having slight turbidity and colour according to the nature of the drug is used.

Avaleha or lehya and paka

Avaleha or Lehya is a semi-solid preparation of drugs, prepared with the addition of jaggery, sugar or sugar-candy and boiled with prescribed drug juice or decoction.

Preparation of avaleha

Those preparations generally have (1) decoction or other liquids, (2) jaggery, sugar or sugar-candy, (3) powders or pulps of certain drugs, and (4) ghee, or oil and honey, jaggery, sugar or sugar candy is dissolved in the liquid and strained to remove the foreign particles. This solution is boiled over a moderate fire. When paka (Phanita) is thready (tantument) on pressing between two fingers or if it sinks in water without getting easily dissolved, it should be removed from the fire. Fine powders of drugs are then added in small quantities and stirred continuously and vigorously to form a homogenous mixture. Ghee or oil, if mentioned, is added while the preparation is still hot and mixed well. Honey, if mentioned, is added when the preparation is cool and mixed well.

The Lehya should be kept in glass or porcelain jars. It can also be kept in a metal container which does not react with it. Normally, Lehyas should be used within one year.

Ghrta

Ghrtas are preparations in which ghee is boiled with prescribed decoction and *Kaikas* of drugs according to the formulae. This process ensures absorption of the active therapeutic principles of the ingredients used in fat.

Preparation of ghrta

There are generally three essential components for the preparation of sneha (ghrta or taila), viz :

(i) A liquid which may be one or more as *Kasaya, Svarasa, dugdha* and *mastu*.

(ii) A fine paste of the drug.

(iii) Ghrta and taila.

Generally, if *kalka* is one part by weight, *sneha* should be four parts and the *drava dravya* should be sixteen parts. Exceptions are as follows:

(i) where no liquid is prescribed, four parts of water is added to one part of *sneha*, the paste is one fourth the weight of the *sneha*.

(ii) where *drava, dravya* is either *kvatha* or *svarasa, kalka* should be one-sixth and one-eighth, respectively, of *sneha*.

(iii) where is number of *drava dravya* is four or less than four, each *drava* has to be taken four times the weight of *sneha*.

(iv) where the *drava dravyas* are more than four, each *drava* will be equal in weight to the *sneha*.

(v) if in a preparation, no *kalka dravya* is prescribed, then the drugs of the kasaya may be used as *kalka*.

The paste and the liquid are mixed together, *sneha* is then added, boiled and stirred well continuously so that the paste is not allowed to adhere to the vessel. Sometimes, the *drava dravya* are directed to be added one after another as the process of boiling is continued till the liquid added earlier has evaporated.

When all the *drava dravya* have evaporated, the moisture in the paste will also begin to evaporate at this stage, it has to be stirred more often and carefully to ensure that the paste does not stick to the bottom of the vessel. The paste is taken out of the ladle and tested from time to time to know the condition and stage of the *paka*.

Patrapaka

Patrapaka is the process by which the *sneha* is flavoured or augmented by certain soluble or insoluble substances. The powders of the drug is placed in the vessel into which fairly warm *sneha* is filtered.

Mrdupaka sneha is used for nasya; *madhyama-paka sneha* is used for pana and vasti, *kharapaka sneha* is used only for *abhyanga*.

In the beginning the boiling should be on mild fire and in the end also it should be only on mild fire.

Whenever *lavanas* and *ksaras* are used in these preparations, they are added to the *sneha* and then strained.

The *Ghrta* will generally solidify when cooled. It will have the colour, odour and taste of the drug(s) used.

Ghrta are preserved in glass, polythene or aluminium containers. Ghrta preparations for internal use keep their potency for sixteen months.

Churna

Churna is a fine powder of drug or drugs.

Preparation of churna

Drugs mentioned in the Yoga are cleaned and dried properly. They are finely powdered and sieved. Whether there are a number of drugs in a yoga, the drugs are separately powdered and sieved. Each one of them (powder) is weighed separately, and well mixed together. As some of the drugs contain more fibrous matter than others, this method of powdering and weighing them separately, according to the Yoga, and then mixing them together is preferred.

In industry, however, all the drugs are cleaned, dried and powdered together by disintegrators. Mechanical sifters are also used. Salt, sugar, camphor etc., when mentioned are separately powdered and mixed with the rest at the end.

Asafoetida (hingu) and salt may also be roasted, powdered and then added. Drugs like satavari, guduci, etc., which are to be taken fresh, made into a paste, dried and then added.

The powder is fine of at least 80 mesh sieve. It should be free from moisture. The finer the powder, the better its therapeutic value. They retain potency for one year and should be kept in air tight containers.

Kvatha churna

Certain drugs or combination of drugs are made into coarse powder (Javkut) and kept for preparation of Kasaya. Such powders are called Kavtha Churna.

Preparation

Drugs are cleaned and dried. They are coarsely powdered (Javkut), weighed as per formula, and then mixed well.

Taila

Tailas are preparations in which taila is boiled with prescribed decoction and Kalkas of drugs according to the formulae. This process assures absorption of the active therapeutic properties of the ingredients used.

Preparation of taila

There are generally three essential components for the preparation of taila, viz :

(i) drava (a liquid which may be one or more as kasaya, svarasa, dugdha, mastu, etc.).

(ii) kalka (a fine paste of the drug(s).

(iii) sneha dravya (ghrta, taila, etc.).

Generally if paste is one part by weight, snena should be four parts and the drava-dravya should be sixteen parts. Exceptions are as follows:

(i) where no liquid is prescribed, four parts of water is added to one part of sneha; the paste is one fourth the weight of the sneha.

(ii) where liquid is either kvatha or svarasa, paste should be one-sixth and one-eighth, respectively of sneha.

(iii) where the number of liquid is four or less than four, each liquid has to be taken four times the weight of sneha.

(iv) where the drava dravyas are more than four, each drava will be equal in weight to the sneha.

(v) if in a preparation, no kalka dravya is prescribed, then the drugs of the kasaya may be used as kalka.

The paste and the liquid are mixed together, sneha is then added, boiled and stirred well continuously so that the kalka is not allowed to adheres to the vessel. Sometimes, the drava dravyas are directed to be added one after another as the process of boiling is continued till the drava-dravyas added earlier has evaporated.

When all the drava-dravyas have evaporated, the moisture in the paste will also begin to evaporate; at this stage, it has to be stirred more often and carefully to ensure that the paste does not stick to the bottom of the vessel. The paste is taken out of the ladle and tested from time to time to know the condition and stage of the *paka*.

There are three stages of paka :

(i) mrdu paka

(ii) madhyama paka and

(iii) khara paka

In mrdu paka, paste is waxy and when rolled between the fingers rolls like lac without sticking. In madhyama paka, paste is harder and when put in fire burns without any cracking noise. A further degree of heating leads to khara paka. Any further heating will lead to dagdha paka and the sneha becomes unfit for use. When the taila attains the correct paka stage froth comes out.

In the sneha group sarkara, if mentioned, is added to the final product when cool.

Where the paka is to be done with kvatha, svarasa, dugdha and mamsarasa, etc., the paka is to be done with these dravyas separately in the above order. The period of paka with various dravyas should be below :

(i) kvatha, aranala, takra, etc.   5 days

(ii) svarasa   3 days

(iii) dugdha   2 days

(iv) mamsa rasa   1 day

Taila will generally have the colour, odour and taste of the drugs used and have the consistency of oil. When considerable quantity of milk is used in the preparation, the oil becomes thick due to ghrta and in cold season may solidify further.

Tailas are preserved in glass, polythene or aluminium containers. Preparations for internal use keep their potency for about sixteen months.

Tailas are generally used for abhyanga. Some of them are used internally and in Ayurvedic texts various types of anupanas are described for this purpose. When no such anupana is mentioned it should be taken with warm water or warm milk.

Lepa

Medicines in the form of a paste used for external application are called lepas.

Preparation of lepa

The drugs are made into a fine powder. Before use on the body, it is mixed with some liquid or other medium indicated in each preparation and made into a soft paste. Water, cow's urine, oil and ghee are some of the media used for mixing.

Vegetable lepa churna will preserve their potency for 30 days if kept in air tight containers. Mineral and metallic preparations last indefinitely.

Vati and gutika

Medicines prepared in the form of tablets or pills are known as Vati and Gutika. These are made of one or more drugs of plant, animal or mineral origin.

Preparation of vati and gutika

The drugs of plant origin are dried and made into fine powder separately. The minerals are made into *bhasma* or *sindura*, unless otherwise mentioned. In cases where *parada* and *gandhaka* are mentioned, *kajjali* is made first and other drugs added, one by one, according to the formula. These are put into a *khalva* and ground to a soft paste with the prescribed fluids. When more than one liquid is mentioned for grinding, they are used in succession. When the mass is properly ground and is in a condition to be made into pills *sugandha dravyas*, like kasturi, karpura, which are included in the formula, are added and ground again. The criterion to determine the final stage of the formulation before making pills is that it should not stick to the fingers when rolled. Pills

may be dried in shade or in sun as specified in the texts. In cases where sugar or jaggery (guda) is mentioned, paka of these should be made on mild fire and removed from the oven. The powder of the ingredients are added to the paka and briskly mixed. When still worm, *vatakas* should be rolled and dried in shade.

Pills made of plant drugs when kept in air tight containers can be used for two years. Pills containing minerals can be used for an indefinite period.

Pills and vatis should not lose their original colour, smell, taste and form. The pills should be kept away from moisture.

Vartti-netrabindu and anjana

Medicines used externally for the eye come under the category of Vartti, netrabindu and Anjana. Vartties are made by grinding the fine powders of the drugs with the fluids specified in the formula to form a soft paste. This is then made into thin sticks of about 2 centimeters in length and dried in shade. Netrabindu is prepared by dissolving the specified drugs in water or kasaya and used as eye drops.

Anjanas are very fine powders of drugs to be applied with netra salaka.

Colour and smell depend on the drugs used. These can be preserved for one year if kept in air tight container. In case of formulation in which minerals are used, the drugs are preserved indefinitely.

Parpati

Parpati is a rasa preparation. The name is derived from the method by which flakes of the compound are obtained.

Kajjali is prepared first with purified mercury (parada) and sulpaur (gandhaka). Other drugs mentioned in the formula are added one by one and mixed well by trituration in a khalva. The powder is put in an iron vessel and kept over fire in the sikatayantra. A shallow pit in fresh cow dung is made and a kadali leaf or an eranda leaf is spread over the pit. When the medicine melts and becomes liquid it is poured on the leaf carefully. This is covered with another leaf and fresh cow dung is spread and gently pressed. After it is allowed to cool the flakes of the medicine are removed and powdered.

Parpaties are dark in colour. They preserve their potency indefinitely and are kept in glass bottles.

Pisti

Pisties are prepared by triturating the drug with the specified liquids and exposing to sun or moon. These are termed anagnitapta bhasma (bhasma prepared without the medium of fire).

Preparation of Pisti

After purification (sodhana) the drug is put in a khalva and triturated generally with rose water, unless otherwise mentioned. It is triturated with the liquid for a day and dried in the sun for another day. This process is generally continued for seven days or more till fine pisti in powder form is obtained.

Depending upon the colour of the drug pisties are of different colours. They are as fine as bhasma and have the characteristics of bhasma. They preserve their potency indefinitely. They are stored in glass stoppered bottles.

Bhasma

Powder of a substance obtained by calcination is called Bhasma. In this section, it is applied to the metals and minerals and animal products which are, by special process, calcined in closed crucibles in pits and with cow dung cakes (Puta).

Preparation of bhasma

First stage (Sodhana) : Bhasmas are prepared from purified minerals, metals, marine and animal products. In Ayurveda, the process of purification is called Sodhana. Chemical purification is different from medicinal purification. In chemical purification it is only elimination of foreign matters. In medicinal purification, the objects aimed at are (a) elimination of harmful matter from the drug; (b) modification of undesirable physical properties of the drug; (c) conversion of some of the characteristics of the drugs; (d) the enhancement of the therapeutic action, thereby potentizing the drug.

Second stage (Marana) : The second stage is the preparation of Bhasma. The purified drug is put into a Khalva (stone mortar and pestle) and ground with juices of the specified plants or kasayas of drugs mentioned for a particular mineral or metal. It is ground for the specified period of time. Then small cakes (cakrikas) are made. The size and thickness of the cakes depend on the heaviness of the drug. The heavier the drug, the thinner are the cakes. These cakes are dried well under sunlight and placed in one single layer in a shallow earthen plate (sarava) and closed with another plate. The edge is sealed with clay-smeared cloth in seven consecutive layers and dried.

A pit is dug in an open space. The diameter and the depth of the pit depends on the metal or mineral that is to be calcined. Half the pit is filled with cow dung cakes. The sealed earthen container is placed in it and the remaining space is filled with more cow dung cakes. Fire is put in all four sides and the middle of the pit. When the burning is over, it is allowed to cool completely. The earthen container is removed. The seal is opened and the contents taken out. The medicine is ground into a fine powder in a khalva. This process of triturating with the juice, making cakrika and giving putas, is repeated as many times as prescribed in the texts or till the proper fineness and quality are obtained.

The putas are described under different names to indicate the size of the pit and the number of cow dung cakes to be used. They also indicate the amount of heat required and the period of burning. Maha puta, Gaja puta, Varaha puta, Kukkuta puta, Kapota puta, and Bhanda puta are commonly used in the preparation of Bhasmas.

The tests for properly prepared Bhasma are (1) there should be no chandrika (metallic lustre) (nischandrika); (2) when taken between the index finger and thumb and spread, it should be so fine as to get easily into the finger lines (rekha purita); (3) when a small quantity is spread on cold and still water, it should float on the surface (varitara); and (4) the bhasma should not revert to the original state (apunarbhava).

Bhasma are, unless otherwise specified in individual formulations, generally yellowish, black, dark white, grey, reddish black and red; depending upon the predominant drug as well as the other drugs used in the process of marana.

Bhasmas are preserved in air tight glass or earthen containers. They maintain their potency indefinitely. They have no characteristic taste.

Rasa yoga

Preparations containing mineral drugs as main ingredients are called Rasa Yogas. They may be in pill form or in powder form. They are mixed and triturated together.

Preparation of Rasa yoga

Drugs such as abhraka, maksika, svama, rajata, tamra, kamsya etc., are used only in bhasma form in these preparations. Drugs such as gandhaka, manahisila, etc. are used in purified form. Where rasa and gandhaka are drugs, kajjali is prepared first with these two and only then other drugs are added in small quantities and ground in the khalva itself and mixed well.

Bhavana with the prescribed svarasa, kvatha, etc. should be given to this for a prescribed period.

The colour and smell depend on the drugs in the Yogas. They keep their potency indifinitely unless otherwise prescribed.

Lauha

Lauha kalpas are preparations of Loha Bhasma as main ingredient added to other drugs.

Preparation of lauha

The drugs are reduced to fine powder and mixed with loha bhasma. Bhavana is given with prescribed liquids if mentioned.

The powder should be very fine and the bhasma used should be well prepared. When well protected from moisture and heat, they keep their potency for a period of two years. Preparations containing mercury or its compounds keep their potency indefinitely.

CONTRIBUTION OF UNANI MEDICINAL SYSTEM TO PHARMACY

In the seventh and eighth centuries the Arabs conquered a great part of the ancient civilized world and extended their empire from Spain to India. Like the Romans, they respected the cultures of the conquered people. During the reign of Abbasid Caliph Harun al-Rashid (786-814 A.D.) Baghdad achieved fame as a city of learning. Some Indian physicians were invited to Baghdad, received the favours of the Caliph and settled there.

Juhanna ibn Masawaih (777-857 A.D.) translated the Greek manuscripts into Arabic and wrote a medical book. He modified the effects of certain remedies recommended as mixtures. The first London Pharmacopoeia was largely based on his formulae.

Manaka, a popular Indian physician at Baghdad, translated some books from Sanskrit into Arabic or Persian and composed *Kitab tafsir isma al-Aqaqir* which included a list of drugs and herbs of Indian origin.

The work of Persian born Abu Bekr Muhammad Ibn Zakaria or Rhaze (841-926) has been very much used in the European world. He wrote about one hundred medical books. His book, *Kitab al-Hawi*, has been used as a medical encyclopaedia. Abu'l Qasim al-Zahrawi or Albucasis, born in Spain in 936 A.D., practised as physician - pharmacist - surgeon and wrote on surgery and pharmaceutical subjects. Abu Mansur (C.970), a Persian pharmacologist, was the author of Arab Pharmacopoeia in which he described 466 vegetable drugs, 75 meneral drugs and 44 animal drugs. Al-Biruni (973-1050) of Khwarizm made great contribution towards the development of pharmacy. He defined pharmacognosy and pharmacology first of all, studied the natural products and their sources and mentioned 720 drugs in an alphabetical order in his book *al - Saidana fil tibb*.

Abu Ali al-Husain bin Abdallah or Avicenna (980 - 1037), born in Bukhara, was called as the "Prince of Physicians". His book, '*Qanun fil Tibb*'. was used as a guide and authority up to 17th century. Ali ibn Abbas (994 A.D.), a persian medical author, wrote a medical encyclopaedia, *Kitab al Maliki*. Seville–born Abu Mervan or Ibn Zuhr or Avenzoar (1113-1199) was a medical botanist and pharmacist. His main work was on diet, which is incorporated in the book *al-Aghdhiya*. Abu'l–Walid Muhammad ibn Ahmad or Ibn Rushd, born in 1126 A.D. at Cardova in Spain, composed a medical book *Kitab al-Kulliyat*. Rabbi Moses (1135 - 1208) was a Jewish scholar and physician who wrote dietetic rules in a book. It describes diet and regimen including Rhubarb and tamarind pills. The publications of Spanish-born Ibn al-Baytar (1197-1248) gave the most comprehensive list of drugs. He mentioned detailed outlines for the preparation of rose water and recommended the use of Colocynth, Croton oil, Nutmeg and Pyrethrum. Ibn Serabi, an important pharmacist of the Muslim world, was famous for writing on medieval pharmacy. Abu'l Qasim-al-Iraqi (1300 A.D.) deseribed the preparation and properties of an anaesthetic powder in his book *Uyun al-Haqaiq*.

The Arabs greatly improved pharmaceutical products and made them more elegant and palatable. Their pharmacy and Materia Medica were followed for a long time. The use of sugar is a chracteristic of Arab Pharmacy. Many drugs of India or of the East, such as Musk, Cloves, Cubebs, Dragon's blood, Galanga root, Betel nut, Sandalwood, Rhubarb, Nutmeg, Tamarind, Cassia bark, Croton oil, and Nux vomica were introduced by Arabs into Egypt. Alcohol, Jalap, Syrup, Aloe, Cinnamon, Camphor (Kafur), Anise, Zingiber, Myrrh, Styrax, Coffea, etc. are the Arabic names which are common in English. In the 7th century A.D. Arabs founded trading centres on the Malabar coast of South India. Through these centres they purchased spices, dyes, drugs and perfumes and introduced these articles in Iran, Turkey, Egypt, Saudi Arabia and other countries.

It was in the 8th century that Arab Pharmacy and Medicine became two separate branches. This separation was made compulsory by law in 11th century and governmentally supervised stores were established in Baghdad. An inspector was appointed to check and ensure the supply of genuine herbs, and for inspecting the preparation of formulations for patients. There was deterrent punishment for adulteration of medicines and fake prescriptions. In Middle Ages schools of pharmacy were established for a regular pharmaceutical education. They discovered new and potent medicaments. If the new drugs proved bitter in taste, the ingenious Arab pharmacists devised chemical and mechanical methods to make them tolerable. The candy-coated pills were first employed by Avicenna who always tried to keep his patients cheerful. Arab pharmacists

mixed rose-water and perfumes with medicines. They invented tinctures, confections, syrups, pomades, plasters, and ointments to ease the physicians task. The use of hashish and bhang *(Cannabis sativa)* and the behaviour of addicts of these drugs are described in the *Arabian Nights*. They invented the apothe cary, which they called 'Saidala'. Ibn al-Attar, the son of a druggist, referred to the Sandalwood for therapeutic uses. In the reign of al-Mansur's son the drug shops were run by educated and morally responsible apothe caries.

Alchemy was developed along with medicine. The idea of "elixir of life", an "all-cure" was developed. The Arab pharmacists from the 9th century invented valuable techniques and apparatuses and included in their stock many of the commodities required in different branches of technology. Their pharmaceutical preparations consisted of powders, suspensions, syrups, electuaries, distilled medicinal waters and many other forms exceeding seventy in number. Some typical apparatuses were designed for manufacturing the medicines. Akbar the Great sent many Unani physicians all over India and paid attention to the profession of pharmacy. Most of the physicians were interested in medicinal plants and mentioned their preparations, properties, therapeutic effects, mode of administration and reactions in their books. Ilyas bin Shehab described many Indian drugs and herbs in his book *Rahat al - insan* during the rule of Firoz Shah Tughlaq (1351-1368 A.D.).

Unani system of medicine

Like Ayruveda, the Unani system of medicine is based on ancient principle. So there is a similarity between *Ayurveda* and *Tibb* regarding the contemplation of the same dogmatisms and traditionalism. The most important similarity is the principle of four elements which is identical to *Ayruveda's Panchbhuta* principle. According to four elemental principles of *Tibbi* discipline all the universal inanimate and animate things are produced from *Al-Nar* (Fire), *Al'- hawa* (Air), *Al-ma* (Water) and *Al-ardh* (Earth). According to Ayruveda, all of the universal objects are made of *Panchbhuta* and body has its root and support of Doshas (*Tridosha*, i.e., *Vata, Pitta* and *Kapha*), Dhatus (seven metals : *Rasa,*

Rakta, Mansa, Meda, Asthi, Majja and Sukra) and Mala (*Sweda, Mutra,* and *Purisha*). When these remain in the equilibrium and in normal functioning, then the health of an individual is maintained. In the same manner *Tibb* also maintains this view that the human body is composed of seven natural principles or components of the body known as *Al-umur Al-tabiyah.* The loss of the any one of these components may lead to diseases, or even death of the individual. These are as follows:

1. *Al - arkan* or *al - anasir* (Elements)
2. *Al - mizaj* (Temperament)
3. *Al - akhalt* (Humours - body fluids)
4. *Al a'za'* (Organs or members)
5. *Al - arwah* (Pneuma or vital spirit)
6. *Al - quwa* (Faculties or Powers)
7. *Al - at'al* (Functions)

In addition to these seven components, the essential causes influencing the human body are:

1. Atmospheric air
2. Foods and drinks
3. Physical or bodily movement and repose
4. Mental or Psychic movement and repose
5. Sleep and wakefulness
6. Evacuation and retention.

These factors essentially influence each and every body. Nobody could escape from these factors so long he is alive.

Some of the non-essential causes are not concerned with everybody and do not necessarily influence each and every human body. These are habit, habitat, profession, sex, temperament, other social factors, cosmic and terrestrial influences, etc. These factors influence to those only who come across them, therefore, they are considered non-essential. These are as :

1. Geographical conditions of the country and town and other related matters,
2. Residential conditions and related matters,
3. Occupation and related matters
4. Habits and related matters
5. Age and related matters
6. Sex and related matters
7. Any other factor antagonistic to nature and bodily health, e.g., micro-organisms, ion-

izing radiations, electricity and other natural forces.

The temperaments of persons are accordingly expressed by the words sanguine, phlegmatic, choleric and melancholic according to the preponderance in them of humours – blood, phlegm, yellow bile and black bile, respectively. The humours themselves are assigned tempera-ments – blood is hot and moist; phlegm cold and moist; yellow bile hot and dry; and black bile cold and dry.

Every person is supposed to have a unique humoral constitution which represents his healthy state. To maintain the correct humoral balance there is power of self preservation of adjustment called *Quwwat-e-Mudabbira* (Medicatrix naturae) in the body. If this power weakens, imbalance in the humoral composition occurs, and this causes disease. In Unani medicine great reliance is placed on this power. The medicines used in this system, in fact, help the body to regain this power on the optimum level and thereby restore humoral balance, thus retaining health. The correct diet and digestion are also considered to maintain humoral balance.

Therapeutics

In Unani system of medicine various types of treatment are employed, such as Ilaj bit - Tadbeer (regimental therepy), Ilaj bil-Ghiza (dietotherapy), Ilaj bid-Dawa (pharmacotherapy) and jarahat (surgery).

The regimental therapy includes venesection, cupping, diaphoresis, diuresis, Turkish bath, massage, metastasis, cauterization, purging, emesis, exercise and leeching. Dietotherapy aims at treating certain ailments by administration of specific diets or by regulating the quantity and quality of food, whereas pharmacotherapy deals with the use of naturally occurring drugs of herbal, animal and mineral origin. Similarly, surgery has also been in use in this system for quite long. The naturally occurring drugs used in this system are symbolic of life and are generally free from side-effect. If such drugs are toxic in crude form, then they are processed and purified in many ways before use. In Unani medicine although general preference is for a single drug, compound formulations are also employed in the treatment of various complex and chronic disorders. Since in this system, stress is laid on a particular temperament of an individual, the medicines administered are such as go well with the temperament of the patient, thus accelerating the process of recovery and also eliminating the risk of drug reaction.

Unani medicine aims of combating disease and preservation and promotion of health through curative, preventive, and promotive measures. For the treatment of various common and stubborn diseases, medicines obtained from natural sources, *e.g.*, plants, animals and minerals, are used in this sysem. Unani medicines are not only cheap and easily available, but are also effective and free from side effects.

Unani system of medicine has grown by experiences of nations and countries like Egypt, Iraq, India and China. Diagnosis of a disease is carried out by knowing past history of the patient and examination of pulse and other body organs. The Unani pharmaceutical preparations consist of powder, suspension, syrups, electuries, distilled medicinal waters and many other forms exceeding seventy in number.

The important Unani preparations are as follows:

Jawarishat

A *Jawarish* is a pleasant tasting stomachic and digestive formulation. Its ingredients are so incorporated as to be neither too coarse or large or small. They are all ground to medium size in the powder, so that the action of a *Jawarish* is prolonged.

Habub (Pills)

They are prepared by mixing one or more constituent in water or a liquid in appropriate quantities. For their preparation, the powder should be very fine. If the pills contain pearls or minerals, these should be triturated separately and added to the powder. The mixture should be triturated again and mixed with a liquid to prepare pills. If fragrant and saffron are to be added to a particular pill, they should be triturated separately in an extract and added to the powder prepared from other constituents. Very fine powders may be so kneaded with gum to prepare pills. For preparing pills from *Berberis aristata,* guggul and opium, they should be first

soaked in water and heated till they dissolve. Then powder prepared from other constituents is added to them and the mixture is kneaded to prepare pills. In case of viscous and sticky constituents, *ghee* should be rubbed on the hands or starch is kneaded. Oily drugs should be finely ground to prepare pills. Large quantities of pills are prepared from machines. Before packing, pills should be dried in the sun. Pills may be decorated by coating with gold or silver foils. The taste of bitter pills can be masked by coating them with sugar.

Khamira

A *khamira* is prepared from a decoction of one or several drug ingredients in a white sugar syrup. The syrup is thicker and more concentrated than that of a juice. When the *khamira* is stirred, carbon dioxide from the air reacts with it and it swells like yeast. Each *khamira* is named on the basis of its main ingredient.

Rub (Extract)

An extract is obtained by regulated concentration of a fruit or vegetable juice with or without addition of sugar. The fruit juice is heated till the volume is halved or less than halved followed by incorporation of sugar. In this way, the ingredients of fruits and vegetables are available in off-season also.

Safuf (Powder)

It is a dry medicament or a mixture of several drugs which have been ground or triturated and sieved. A churan is a form of *safuf* which is digestive and has its principal ingredients as inorganic salts. Powders used for detrificial purposes are called *sumunat* and those used in occulistics are *surma* (collyrium).

Sikanjbin

It is a honey-based vinegar preparation.

Sharbat

It is a soft drink or liquor that incorporates white sugar, *misri*, honey and *gur* which have been dissolved in water. In Unani medicine, it is a concentrated liquor which is prepared from decoctions or fruit juices by adding sugar to yield a syrup. The incorporation of various ingredients into a sharbat prolongs the life of medicinal ingredients incorporated into it.

Shaf (Suppository)

It is applied to external cavities of the body, *i.e.*, nostrils, ears, rectum, urinogenital tract, womb and eyes. A suppository used for eyes is of conical shaped grain-like in size.

Zimad (Paste, Poultice)

It is a thick, viscous liquid which is applied to external organs or on the affected internal spots.

Tila

It is a viscous liquid preparation applied on male genital organs.

Arq

It is a distillate obtained from one or more medicinal ingredients with or without previous dilution with water. A distillate postulates the condensations of vapours.

Qurs (Tablets)

They are flat and round composed of different ingredients.

Kuhl (Collyriums)

These are fine powders meant for ocular treatment. They are applied to the eyes by means of a stick.

Kushta

It is a blend of metals, metallic oxides, non-metals and their compounds or minerals. The ingredients are oxidized through the action of heat. It is used in small quantities and it has immediate effect. *Kushta* tablets are prepared by incorporation of magnesium carbonate to the *kushta* followed by addition of arrowroot and gelatin pastes and then drying the tablets in the sun or an electric heater.

Gulqands

These are palatable preparations in which sugar is incorporated into flower petals which have been thoroughly rubbed followed by keeping in a glass jar till both mix well. They are generally taken with an excipient.

Laooq (Electuary)

It is a kind of *majun* that is taken orally with the tongue. It is prescribed to treat lung and throat infections.

Murabba (Preserve)

It is prepared from fresh fruits and roots which has been preserved in the white sugar syrup or honey. Preserves are good substitutes for fresh fruits and used in off-seasons.

Marham (Ointment)

It is a semi-solid substance prepared from the powders of more than one ingredient, wax and oil. It is applied externally to inflammation, abrasions, wounds, cuts, boils and pustules.

Majuns

These are semi-solids prepared from the syrup of white sugar or honey and a drug powder.

Muffareh

It is a kind of majun used as exhilirant, prescribed as a cardiac stimulant and general tonic.

HOMOEOPATHIC MEDICINAL SYSTEM

Homoeopathic medicinal system was started by the chemist, physician and pharmacist Samuel Hahnemann (1755-1843) of Germany who was dissatisfied with the side effects of the then current regimens of medication. He initiated the treatment of a disease with a low dose of those drugs which themselves produced similar symptoms of the disease in normal individuals. A medicine produces some symptoms in healthy state and if the identical symptoms are present in a sick person, then the patient will get relief with a minor dose of the medicine. According to Hahnemann, there is no any normal and natural method for diagnosis of a disease except its symptoms. This principle of the treatment of 'like with like' is quite the reverse of the allopathic system.

In any medicinal system there is no co-relation between the cause of the disease and human potency. According to homoeopathic medicinal system until the potency governing on the body of a human being is powerful and controls the functions of all organs, then the person will not be affected by a disease. A disease produced in the body and brain will effect other body organs. The habits of telling lie, theft, deceit, evil, narcosis, under diet, anger, etc. are symptoms of mental diseases. After collecting the information about a disease, stress is given on mental disorders. Any symptom of a disease can not be completed without the governing power of the body.

Homoeopathy relies most on the patient's description of his symptoms. By administering a medicine 'tailored' precisely to the symptoms specific to each patient and his complaint, the Homoeopath encourages the body's own innate healing response; he stimulates the 'vital' force.

Hahnemann believed that symptoms are no more than an outward reflection of the body's inner fight to overcome illness; not a manifestation of the illness itself. The medicine given to cure should reinforce these symptoms rather than counteract them. In other words, let like be cured by like. This is the Law of Similars and is the single most fundamental tenet of Homoeopathy. With this concept in mind he set about examining the effects produced by the ingestion of various extracts. He began with Cinchona.

Hahnemann's original observation involved Cinchona, which produced, in normal individuals, symptoms similar to those of malaria, for which the drug was used. In the same way, Belladonna on administration produced symptoms associated with Scarlet fever. If the symptoms of a disease are considered a manifestation of the body's own defence mechanism against the disease, then the Homoeopathic treatment serves to stimulate such inherent defensive and curative processes. Hahnemann prepared a list of drugs with their effects on healthy individuals. A patient's symptoms could then be matched as closely as possible against the drug pictures and the appropriate treatment prescribed. In this way Nux vomica and Gelsemium root (yellow jasmine) became drugs for the treatment of influenza and the common cold.

When an onion is peeled it causes a watery discharge from the eyes and, if continued, a discharge from the nose—symptoms not far removed from those of the common cold. An extract of *Allium cepa* (red onion) is used homoeopathically to treat the common cold on the basis of like for like.

In Homoeopathy, the process whereby a healthy individual takes doses of an extract to assess the symptoms it induces is known as *Proving*. The person *proving* the drug, the *prover*, maintains a precise, detailed and accurate record of the physical, mental and emotional changes various doses induce over a period of time. A drug picture of an extract is built up which enables it to be matched precisely to similar symptoms produced by an illness in the individual being treated. The drug is tailored to the individual. Thus, one patient suffering from depression may feel tired and restless whilst another may be irritable and agitated. Different remedies would be found to match the different symptoms of what is essentially the same condition. Similarly, different conditions presenting with similar symptoms may be treated with the same remedy. Inflammation for a skin rash and inflammation from a burn are both inflammation as far as Homoeopathy is concerned. In both cases the treatment would be designed to fit the patient's symptoms, not the causal condition.

At 'normal' doses the symptoms of the illness for which they were prescribed became significantly worse. This led to the second feature of Homoeopathy. More the drug is diluted, or *potentized*, the greater is its ability to cure.

Hahnemann observed that in the initial stages of treatment with the appropriate drugs at normal dosage rates, the illness appeared to be worsen in the beginning as the symptoms are inhanced by the drug. Therefore, subsequent doses are lowered. He observed that as the dose of a drug was reduced, its potency was enhanced. Thus, this process was no longer referred to as dilution but as potentiation. Thus, the Homoeopathic treatment arrived at in conjunction with the patient's very detailed case history and constitutes the use of often very active drugs in extremely low doses. For the higher potencies of Homoeopathic drugs the possibility of a current scientific explanation becomes non-existent, because individual doses at the dilution of the sixth or eight decimal may no longer contain a single molecule of the drug. Homoeopathic remedies have the distinct advantage that they are without side-effects.

Homoeopathic medicines are used in the form of mother tinctures, small pills, powder and distilled water. The patient should not take any kind of food or drink prior or after one hour of the dose.

Diagnosis

The process of diagnosis and the determination of the appropriate remedy are lengthy.

The homoeopath tries to know every aspect of the patient's health, life style, complete history of problems and symptoms, food habit, dressing, body weight, height, colour, family health, temperament, sleep, dreaming, etc.

After much deliberation, he selects a remedy corresponding precisely to the 'totality' of the patient's symptoms.

A simplified approach to diagnosis can be employed in appropriate circumstances. For the treatment of acute conditions a suitable remedy could be determined with the presence of only three good symptoms.

In headache, if the patient reports that the headache is in one part of the head and is associated with visual disturbance as well as nausea then a remedy could be selected.

For prescribing the medicine it is essential that information about characteristics of elements, mental symptoms and other symptoms should be collected. The medicine with more pronounced characters should be prescribed. If there is no relief then according to elements any medicine belonging to anti-soric, anti-cycotic and anti-syphilic category should be prescribed in one or two doses prior to the earlier medicine. Sora, syphilic and cycosis are related with the production of air, bile and cough as mentioned in Ayurveda. Diseases produced by air are identical to those which are produced by entering *sora*, e.g., mental exitement by bile and of syphilic and cycosis, respectively. These disorders are sometimes combined with each other. In some diseases the air and bile predominate and in others, cough and bile are in excess. In Homoeopathy, diseases are not produced by the attack of micro-

organisms. Weak body potency is responsible for a disease. This body potency becomes weak due to sora, syphilic and cycosis. Therefore, they are searched in the body.

Hahnemann's fundamental propositions peculiar to Homoeopathy may be said, as :
  (a) that the action of drugs are demonstrable by observing the subjective symptoms, objective symptoms and pathological changes that occur when they are administered to healthy human subject.
  (b) that the action of drugs so observed in a healthy human being constitutes their therapeutic potentiality with respect to the sick individual.
  (c) that a similarity between disease processes in a particular individual and the known effects of a particular drug in healthy human being (known as drug proving of Homoeopathy) will lead to its successful application in the treatment of diseased individual (*i.e.,* to bring a change in the altered dynamis).
  (d) the conception of dynamis (vital force-active-driving force) is applicable in respect of health, disease and cure.

Potentization

There are three essential processes involved in preparation of remedies: (a) Serial dilution (b) Succession (c) Trituration. Dilution is the meant by which we reduce the toxicity of the original crude drug. Serial dilution means that each dilution is prepared from the dilution that immediately proceeded it. Succession and trituration are the methods by which mechanical energy is delivered to our preparations in order to imprint the pharmacological message of the original drug upon the molecules of the diluent.

An initial extraction is prepared from freshly gathered material. Usually, the process involves washing the plant to remove dust, macerating in a mincer, soaking in pure alcohol for several days before finally filtering and collecting the resulting solution. The solution is termed the *mother tincture*. One drop of this mother tincture is then diluted.

There are various scales of serial dilution. If it is added to 99 drops of an inert solvent such as water, alcohol or lactose, it commences in the 1 in 100 dilution series. The result is known as the first *centesimal* potency and is denoted by the symbol lc. The solution is then vigorously shaken and tapped on a resilient surface. This process is known as *succession*. This 'rubbing and shaking' developed the action of the drug and 'released the power to heal', so that 'even a totally inert substance can come to influence the vital force'. Thus, one drop of the first centesimal potency is then added to a further 99 drops of solvent, succussed, and produces the second centesimal (2c) potency. The process may be repeated up to a potency of 10 M, equivalent to a 10000th centesimal potency. Typically potencies of 6c, 12c, 30c, 200c and 1000c are used by the Homoeopath to treat his patients.

Alternatively, *decimal* potencies in the dilution series of 1 in 10 are made using one part of mother tincture of 9 parts diluent. These are denoted by the symbol D2, D10, D30, etc.

The process of serial dilution with succussion at each stage results in a Homoeopathic mixture. Single dilution to the final concentration without succession at each stage would not result in a Homoeopathic solution. Each dilution is claimed to increase the power of the drug to heal.

From the pharmaceutical point of view there are two main classes of original substance : (a) Soluble (b) Insoluble.

In the class of soluble substances mother tinctures (alcohol or water extraction) of the plant material are used. The symbol is used to denote the mother tincture of any soluble substance. For soluble substance alcohol and water are applied. At each stage rhythmical violent agitations are carried out, either by hand or machine, and this is known as "Succession". Insoluble natural substances are prepared in a different way. The diluent in one sense is lactose. The physical process applied at each stage is known as 'Trituration', it is a prolonged circular grinding with mortar and pestle. Once this trituration has obtained 6 x or 1/10, this be dispersed into alcohol water diluent. Thereafter, it is treated like a soluble substance.

These two major scales of preparing medicine are denoted as '*c*' for centesimal scale and '*x*' for decimal scale.

Centesimal scale involves a serial dilution 1/100, whereas decimal involves a serial trituration 1/10.

For the preparation of the Homoeopathic potencies of a liquid drug substance three scales are in use, i.e. (a) Decimal (b) Centesimal and (c) Millesimal.

For the preparation of potencies from solid drug substances, (a) Decimal and (b) Centesimal scales are in use. When trituration attains the 6 x potency, then only it will be fit to be converted into liquid potency.

Prescription

There are now some 2500 provings available to the Homoeopath. For these he must search through the massive tomes of the materia medica to match precisely, by a process known as *repertoirizing*, the patient's description of his symptoms to the drug picture. Today, some Homoeopaths use computers to assist in this process.

The quinine alkaloid derived from Cinchona has a distinguished record in the treatment of malaria. The Arnica extract from *Arnica montana* has been used extensively as an orthodox remedy for bruising and local trauma treatment. It is applied similarly in Homoeopathic strengths of 30c or 20c. However, its provings include lethargy, irritability and an aversion to being touched. Because of this it is also used by the Homoeopath, in dose strengths of 6c or 30c, in the treatment of trauma such as surgical operations and accidents which have occurred a number of years past. *Atropa belladonna* clearly fits this category. Ingestion by adult or child of just a few of its attractive berries rapidly produces symptoms of severe poisoning: dry mouth, excessive thirst, flushed countenance and restlessness, symptoms which are also characteristic of a febrile, infectious illness. Consequently, belladonna has been used homoeopathically in suitable dilutions for the treatment of feverish illnesses. Historically, it is reputed to have been successfully employed in the control of scarlet fever.

Mercury, a metal well known for its toxicity,

giving rise to severe gastric disturbance, vomiting and diarrhoea, among other symptoms, has been used homoeopathically to treat rectal bleeding and stomach disorders leading to diarrhoea. Similarly, arsenic is another well known poison, used for anxiety, stomach ulceration and gastro-enteritis, again employing precisely the like for like principle.

Aconitum napellus (pain reliever), *Cactus grandiflorus*, flowers and tender stems (cardiac problems), *Cannabis indica* (psychotic states), *Colchicum autumnale* (gout), Colocynth (emotional disturbance and facial neuralgia), *Ledum palustre* (respiratory and rheumatic problems), *Lycopodium clavatum* spores (various conditions), Opium (typhoid fever, fright, etc.) and *Thuja occidentalis* (varies infections) are also used in Homoeopathy.

The sources of homoeopathic remedies are many and varied. Botanical substances, flowers, leaves, roots, seeds, berries and barks, are the most important. Mineral extracts are also pres-cribed : the metals, gold, silver and platinum; compounds such as calcium phosphate and sodium chloride, and elements such as sulphur. Remedies from animal sources include venoms and stings, oyster shell, cow's milk and cuttlefish dye. A source of extract may be a disease tissue, e.g., *Tuberculinum* or an extract of pus from a tubercular abscess. Such substances are known as *nosodes* and used in the treatment of illnesses which present with similar symptoms to the disease from which the extract originated. Thus, tuberculinum was used in the treatment of chest and throat infections. Other nosodes include measles and glandular fever. Typical potencies are 30c and 200c.

A relatively recent development has been the use of extracts of allopathic drugs. It is not uncommon for such medicines to induce side-effects. What the Homoeopath does is to use these side-effects to advantage by using them to treat illness which themselves present with a similar clinical picture. Thus, penicillin can cause a skin rash to develop in a sensitive patient. Homoeopathy uses this fact to use an extract of penicillin in the treatment of certain skin conditions.

Extracts of allergens are used to increase an individual resistance to the material to which he or she is allergic. Thus, for patients suffering from hay fever and asthma, an extract of grass pollen or house dust may be prescribed. Once the remedy has been chosen, it has then to be made into a form suitable for use by the patient.

Dispensing

The preparation and dispensing of homoeopathic remedies is governed by the Medicines Act. The same standards of quality control and assurance in manufacture apply as for any allopathic product. The above procedures are, therefore, carried out with meticulous care. Once the appropriate potency has been achieved, the material must be *medicated*, that is, made into a form suitable for dispensing.

Generally, the oral route is favoured although administration as a cream or ointment is more common with some preparations. One such example is *Calendula* extract used in the treatment of eczema and as a first aid ointment for minor abrasions.

To avoid contamination, glass is used for long-term storage of all homoeopathic remedies. For similar reasons, it is also recommended that they are not taken by the patient before or after a cup of tea or coffee. Some Homoeopaths recommend that coffee and tea are avoided completely whilst taking their remedies.

Materia medica

Homoeopathy can be used to complement allopathic treatments in a number of reversible chronic or acute illnesses. The use of antibiotics for infection control can be supplemented by homoeopathic remedies during convalescence as an aid to recovery. Patients have reported a successful outcome when Homoeopathy has been used to treat allergies such as hay fever, allergic rhinitis and eczema which may have an environmental or food origin. Such homoeopathic remedies have also found favour in relieving conditions which may have been stress induced, for example, digestive problems, migraine and headaches.

In the absence of scientific justification for many processes of Homoeopathy, successful cures have been achieved through its use. Its practice in Asia is

Table 1.4. Homoeopathic natural products

Natural source	Common name	Homoeopathic uses
Aconitum napellus (Ranunculacene)	Monk's Hood, Wolf's Bane	Effect of fear, facial neuralgia, throats and colds
Allium cepa (Liliaceae)	Onion	Common colds and related symptoms
Apis mellifica (Apidae)	Honey Bee	Insect stings, surburn and to ease burning and stinging pains. The whole bee is used in the preparation of the mother tincture
Arnica montana (Asteraceae)	Leopard's Bane	Bruising, contusions and in mental and physical shock
Atropa belladonna (Solanaceae)	Belladonna, Deadly Nightshade	CNS stimulant, earache, neuralgia, headache, spasms and to control chicken pox and measles.
Berberis vulgaris (Berberidaceae)	Barberry	Renal colic.
Bryonia dioica, B. alba (Cucurbitaceae)	White Bryony	Coughs, colds and muscular pain.
Calcium carbonate	Carbonate of lime	Cramp, acne rosacea and control of period bleeding in young girls
Calcium fluoride	Fluorspar	Dental caries, for varicose veins, piles and catarrh
Calcium sulphide	Hepar sulphuris	Boils, abscesses and upper respiratory tract infections.
Calendula officinalis (Asteraceae)	Marigold	Sores and wounds
Cephaelis ipecacuanha, C. acuminata (Rubiaceae)	Ipecac	Nausea and morning sickness in pregnancy, applied for nose bleeds and in depression
Chamaemelum nobile (Anthemis nobilis) (Asteraceae)	Chamomile	Nausea and migraine and to ease teething pains in young infants
Cinchona spp. and hybrids (Rubiaceae)	Peruvian bark	Malaria and as a curative for digestive disorders during convalescence
Copper metal		Circulatory disorders, cramp and stomach pains
Drosera rotundifolia (Droseraceae)	Sundew, Red Rot	Coughs due to upper respiratory tract infections and in whooping cough
Euphrasia officinalis (Scrophulariaceae)	Eyebright	Conjunctivitis, hay fever and German measles
Gelsemium sempervirens	Yellow jasmine	Cold symptoms and stress related effects, headache, migraine.
Lycopodium clavatum (Lycopodiaceae)	Club moss, Foxtail	Digestive imbalances derived from emotional and stressed states
Potassium phosphate		Indigestion and as an aid in the recovery of strength during convalescence after illness
Rhus toxicodendron (Anacardiaceae)	Poison ivy	Sprains, strains, lumbago, rheumatism, shingles, herpes of the lip and other illnesses.
Thuja occidentalis	Tree of life	Headaches, warts and cystitis.
Urtica urens (Urticaceae) Metallic zinc	Stinging nettle	Burns, scalds, insect bites, stings, convulsions and fits

flourishing. Within Europe, particularly in Germany and France, it is employed along side allopathic medicine. In Britain, it is unique among alternative medicines in having six of its own hospitals where patients may be treated under the NHS.

SIDDHA SYSTEM OF MEDICINE

Siddha is extensively practised in the southern parts of Tamil Nadu and in the neighbouring states.

Siddha is an ancient system of medicine. In treatment it uses minerals and metals mainly, but some products of vegetable and/or animal origin are also used. Work relative to Siddha contained atleast 3500 formulae written in Tamil initially on palm leaves.

Siddha medicine is essentially a psychosomatic system of medicine. Unlike Ayurveda importance is given more to minerals and metals rather than herbs in pharmaceutics. Herbs are used only to triturate and calcinate the metals into their basmam and sindooram.

As the world is made up of five elements or panchabutas, so also the human body. The human body is composed of earth and water, the soul is made up of air and ether and heat and fire combine them and make them to live together.

Hence, medicines for the human body are prepared based on the theory of panchabutas (metals of gold, lead, copper, iron and zinc). Gold and lead are used for the maintenance of the body. Iron, the only metal attracted by the electric power of magnet, and zinc, used for generating electricity, are employed in the medicine which are administered for the extension of life. Copper is used for the preservation of heat in the body. All the metals are used only after proper detoxification.

Siddha gives more attention to the disorders of the elements of the intrinsic factors of body than to the extrinsic ones.

The materia medica of Siddha science contains vegetables, minerals and marine elements and the three cordinal humours. All the drugs contain one or more of these humours.

The raw drugs are used either individually or in combination with other drugs. They are subjected to specific processes and the products are administered after purification methods which include detoxification. A preparation contains several crude drugs.

SCOPE OF PHARMACOGNOSY AND PHYTOCHEMICAL INDUSTRY IN INDIA

Since indiscriminate use of synthetic drugs and antibiotics have resulted into serious symptoms all over the world, the demand of plant based raw materials for pharmaceuticals has increased enormously. Moreover, the synthetic drugs and intermediary chemicals are extremely expensive. The World Health Organization has emphasized the utilization of indigenous systems of medicines based on the locally available raw materials, *i.e.*, medicinal plants. Furthermore, approximate one third of all drugs are plant-based and if bacteria and fungi are also included, nearly sixty per cent of pharmaceuticals are of plant origin. Our country is rich in large number of such plants that either be used directly or as the source of active principles in formulaion of drugs curing dreaded diseases. India as a whole is the richest source of medicinal plants which are distributed in almost all parts of the country. The herb collectors and small traders collect the drugs for the manufacturers of Ayurvedic and Unani medicines. But there is a shortage of these materials for maintaining the sustained supply to the plant based drug industries. It is also not proper under the present situation to be dependent only on natural resources to keep the wheel of the industries running all the time in view of the fast depleting natural wealth. This calls for the domestication and cultivation of these plants as well as increment of the drug production with uniformly high potency. At the same time increased demand of plant raw materials has led to over exploitation of wild plants resulting into serious hazard. This necessiates the urgent need of their systematic cultivation for constant supply to the user industries.

Domestication and cultivation of some of the important plants are necessary to cope up the demand of constant supply for the phytochemical industries. These plants include *Adhatoda vasica, Claviceps purpurea, Costus speciosus, Digitalis lanata, Dioscorea deltoidea, Hyoscyamus niger, Mentha piperita, Ruta graveolens, Santalum album, Solanum khasianum, S. lancinatum* and *Eucalyptus* species.

Plants are popularized due to their effectiveness, easy availability, low cost and comparatively being devoid of serious toxic effects. Some herbal drugs like *Achyranthes aspera* (diuretic), *Acorus calamus* (tranquilizer), *Artemisia vulgaris* (cardiac tonic), *Butea frondosa* (anthelmintic), *Bacopa monnieri* (memory), *Boerhaavia diffusa* (anti-inflammatory), *Cassia fistula* (cathartic), *Centella asiatica* (intelligence), *Curcuma longa* (anti-inflammatory), *Syzygium cumini* (hypoglycemic), *Euphorbia thymifolia* (antiasthmatic) and *Sida rhombifolia* (anabolic) have been proven to exhibit the respective pharmacological actions. A derivative of artemisinin, prepared from *Artemisia annua*, is effective against resistant strains of *Plasmodium falciparum* where synthetic anti-malarials fail to cure the disease. A derivative of podophyllotoxin obtained from *Podophyllum hexandrum* and *P. emodi* and taxol isolated from *Taxus baccata* have been approved as an anticancer agents in USA. A flavonoid, isolated from *Silybum marianum*, has been approved as drug against various liver disorders in Germany and other western countries. Iridoid glycosides, called valepotriates, obtained from *Valeriana* species, have been used as tranquilizer and sedative in Germany and other European countries. Total saponins from the Indian plant *Commiphora mukul*, often referred as guggulipid, have been approved as hypolipidaemic agent for lowering blood cholesterol.

There are many drugs which are imported to India. These include Balsam of Tolu, Peru Balsam, Benzoin, Storax, Copaiba, Asafoetida, Ipomoea, Colocynth, etc. If the cultivation of these drugs producing plants is carried out in India, sufficient foreign exchange can be saved.

As mentioned earlier, a derivative of artimisinin from *Artemisia annua*, podophyllotoxin obtained from *Podophyllum hexandrum (P. emodi)*, silymarine flavanoid isolated from *Silybum marianum* seeds and total saponins from the Indian plant *Commiphora mukul* have been approved as drugs in various countries.

One of the new areas in medicine during the recent years has been the use of adaptogenic drugs from plants. Most of these drugs are used as general tonic and stimulants to improve the defence mechanism of the body and to protect the body against stress and infection. These drugs also help the body to improve and tone up metabolism in old age and in persons weakened by serious diseases. These drugs, although not accepted in modern medicine, are now sold widely in Europe, USA and Asia mostly as health foods. Ginseng (*Panax* sp.), and Siberian Ginseng *(Eleutherococcus senticosus)*, Korean ginseng *(Panax ginseng)*, American Ginseng *(P. quin-quefolium)*, Ashwagandha *(Withania somnifera)*, Brahmi *(Centella asiatica* and *Bacopa monnieri)* and Satwar *(Asparagus racemosus)* are used as adaptogenic drugs.

In spite of the tremendous advance in medicine, there is a number of diseases for which modern medicine has no cure. In such cases it treats only symptoms to provide relief to patients. These include viral diseases, such as herpes (genitalis, simplex, zoster, etc.), muscular dystropy, parkinsonism, diabetes, alcoholism, obesity, smoking, stress, genetic diseases, arthritic diseases, liver disorders, cancer, AIDS, etc. Recent trends have shown that plant drugs have the answer to such cases. Recently, a number of formulations based on Ayurvedic medicine have come to the market for control of liver disorders and some of these have been found effective against these diseases. There is a considerable scope to screen such plants for active constituents which may be used in future for treatment of such incurable diseases.

Medicinal plant can be considered to include all plant materials such as foliage, root, flower, fruit, and seed which may be used as such or in the form of their extracts and chemical compounds isolated from them to produce drugs for human and veterinary medicine. These plants are closely related to those that produce stimulants, condi-ments, spices, essential oils, and such other higher forms of plant life that produce specific influences on cell metabolism. Medicinal plants were among the first from the vegetable kingdom to be used by man. The oriental countries were known to be particularly rich in diversity of plants found in their flora and the knowledge on their utilization in medicine. The World Health Organization (WHO) has complied a list of over 20,000 common medicinal plant used in different parts of the globe. Over 100 botanicals enter into regular trade and these have a consistently large demand in the organized sector of the plant-based pharmaceutical industry. However, the list of major medicinal plants in the international trade has always remained fluid, since some of these lose their relative importance to others, whereas as new ones are discovered, their contents are identified and efficacy established. The plant-based recipes are still very popular and largely used in most developing countries of the Old World. About 95% of the drugs manufactured in the African continent are derived from plants. In the industrialized countries also the plant-based drugs are becoming important sources of medicaments. In these countries compound galenical preparations are now increasingly used in domestic medicines.

PHYTOCHEMISTRY

The subject phytochemistry (Greek words: phyton = plant; chemeia = chemistry) deals with the knowledge of bioactive natural products or phytochemicals isolated from natural products. Phytochemicals are not required for functioning of the body, but they have a beneficial effect on health or active role in the treatment of diseases. They differ from phytonutrients in that they are not a necessity for normal metabolism and their absence will not result in a deficiency disease. The phytonutrients have many healthy functions in the body. For example, they may promote the function of the immune system, act directly against microorganisms, reduce inflammation and used to treat or prevent cancer, cardiovascular diseases or any other malady affecting the health of an individual. The phytochemicals are secondary metabolites derived from plants. These phytoconstituents are marketed as fluid extracts, herbal teas, tablets and capsules. They exhibit a number of protective functions in human consumers.

Traditional Pharmacognosy was focused on morphological studies, but the modern Pharmacognosy is specially devoted to the bioactive natural compounds. Modern phytochemistry or pharmaceutical biology is an interdisciplinary science including three primary roles : (1) drug discovery, (2) usefulness of plant extracts in disease treatment and (3) development of plant products as chemopreventive agents. Studies on phytochemistry involve biodiversity of phytoconstituents, biosynthesis, extraction, isolation, analysis, bioactivities and synthesis of the natural compounds. Phytochemistry also includes basic concept of phytochemicals, novel structures, biologically significant secondary metabolites, new drugs, quality control, efficient utilization of plant resources and cultivation of plant drugs. The preparation of herbal drug extracts involves the techniques like liquid-liquid distribution, supercritical fluids, solid phases and microwave extractions. The natural products are isolated from the extracts by chromatographical techniques. The isolated chemical compounds are identified by using spectroscopic techniques and chemical reactions. The bioactivity of the plant products is determined by *in vitro* and *in vivo* bioassays. Expertization in phytochemistry required a thorough knowledge of the above-mentioned techniques in their most sophisticated forms, e.g., MS ionization studies and multidimensional NMR techniques.

Phytochemicals have made a major impact on modern pharmaceutical industry. About 40% drugs approved between 1983 and 1994 were derived from natural products. Nearly 50% all drugs sold in the developed world have their origins from natural sources. Nine out of top 20 selling drugs were derived from natural sources and generated more $ 16 billion (US) in 1998. Up to 80% of all anti-cancer and anti-bacterial drugs have come from natural sources. For example, drugs that are derived from nature include : anti-infectives, anti-cancer agents (taxol), CNS drugs (cannabis), cardiovascular drugs (digoxin), analgesics (opioids, aspirin) and cholesterol lowering drugs (pravastatin).

Paclitaxal, derived from *Taxus brevifolia*, is the drug of choice in several cancers including breast cancer. Vinblastine and vincristine are chemicals discovered in Vinca in 1950s. Vinblastine is the first drug of choice in many forms of leukemia and since the 1950s it has increased the survival rate of childhood leukemias by 80%.

2

Classification of Crude Drugs

Higher plants, microbes and animals are the main sources of crude drugs. However, enzymes and antibiotics used in modern medicine are obtained from animals and microbes. For the study of crude drugs, they may be classified mainly according to morphological, taxonomical, chemical and pharmacological characters. Each of these systems has its own merits and demerits. Morphological classification is more helpful to identify and detect adulteration. For studying evaluationary developments, the drugs are classified according to taxonomical classification. The activity of a drug is due to its chemical constituents and, therefore, the drugs are divided according to the presence of chemical components in chemical classification of drugs. Pharmacological classification of drugs is more relevant to study therapeutic utility of the drugs.

MORPHOLOGICAL CLASSIFICATION

Under morphological classification the drugs are arranged according to the part of the plant used such as leaves, stems, roots, barks, flowers and seeds. The drugs obtained from the direct parts of the plants and containing cellular tissues are called as organized drugs, *e.g.*, rhizomes, barks, leaves, fruits, entire plants, hair and fibres. The drugs which are prepared from plants by some intermediate physical processes such as incision, drying, or extraction with a solvent and not containing any cellular plant tissues are called as unorganized drugs, *e.g.*, Aloe juice, Opium latex, Agar, Gambier, Gelatin, Traga-

canth, Benzoin, Honey, Beeswax and Lemongrass oil (Table 2.1).

Table 2.1. Gross classification of drugs on the basis of morphological characters

Plant Parts	Drugs
1. ORGANIZED DRUGS	
Wood	Quassia, Sandalwood, Red Sandalwood.
Leaves	Digitalis, Eucalyptus, Gurmar, Pudina, Senna, Spearmint, Squill, Tulsi, Vasaka, Coca, Buchu, Hamamelis, Hyoscyamus, Belladonna, Tea.
Barks	Arjuna, Ashoka, Cascara, Cassia, Cinchona, Cinnamon, Kurchi, Quillaia, Wild Cherry.
Flowering Parts	Clove, Pyrethrum, Saffron, Santonica, Chamomile.
Fruits	Amla, Anise, Bael, Bahera, Bitter Orange peel, Capsicum, Caraway, Cardamom, Cassia, Colocynth, Coriander, Cumin, Dill, Fennel, Gokhru, Hirda, Lemon peel, Psoralea, Senna pod, Star anise, Tamarind, Vidang.
Seeds	Bitter Almond, Black Mustard, Cardamom, Colchicum, Ispaghula, Kaladana, Linseed, Neem, Nutmeg,
	Nux vomica, Physostigma, Psyllium, Strophanthus, White Mustard.
Roots and Rhizomes	Aconite, Ashwagandha, Calamus, Calumba, Colchicum corm, Dioscorea, scorea, Galanga, Garlic, Gentian,

(Contd.)

33

Plant Parts	Drugs
	Ginger, Ginseng, Glycyrrhiza, Podophyllum, Ipecac, Ipomoea, Jalap, Jatamansi, Male fern, Picrorhiza, Piplamul, Rauwolfia, Rhubarb, Sassurea, Senega, Shatavari, Turmeric, Valerian, Squill, Serpentary, Indian Podophyllum, Krameria, Derris, Indian Valerian.
Plants and Herbs	Andrographis, Bacopa, Banafsha, Belladonna, Cannabis, Centella, Chirata, Chondrus, Datura, Ephedra, Ergot, Hyoscyamus, Kalmegh, Lobelia, Punarnava, Shankhpushpi, Stramonium, Vinca, Yeast.
Hair and Fibres	Cotton, Hemp, Jute, Silk, Flax.

2. UNORGANIZED DRUGS

Dried Latex	Opium, Papain.
Dried Juice	Aloe, Kino.
Dried Extracts	Agar, Alginate, Black Catechu, Pale Catechu, Pectin.
Gums	Acacia, Guar gum, Indian gum, Sterculia, Tragacanth.
Resins	Asafoetida, Benzoin, Colophony, Copaiba, Guaiacum, Guggal, Mastic, Myrrh, Peru Balsam, Sandarac, Storax, Tolu Balsam, Tar, Coal Tar.
Fixed Oils and Fats	Arachis, Castor, Chaulmoogra, Coconut, Cottonseed, Linseed, Olive, Sesame, Almond, Theobroma, Lard, Cod-liver, Halibut liver, Kokum butter.
Waxes	Beeswax, Spermaceti, Carnauba wax.
Volatile Oil	Turpentine, Anise, Coriander, Peppermint, Rosemary, Sandalwood, Cinnamon, Lemon, Caraway, Dill, Clove, Eucalyptus, Nutmeg, Camphor.
Animal Products	Beeswax, Cantharides, Cod liver oil, Gelatin, Halibut liver oil, Honey, Shark-liver oil, Shellac, Spermaceti wax, Wool fat, Musk, Mylabris, Lactose.
Fossil Organisms and Minerals	Bentonite, Kaolin, Kiesselguhr, Talc.

The main drawback of morphological classification is that there is no co-relation of chemical constituents with the therapeutic actions. Usually this classification is adopted in the practical classes.

TAXONOMICAL CLASSIFICATION

Taxonomical classification is based on the principles of natural relationship and evolutionary development. They are grouped in phyllum order, family, genus and species. As all the entire plants are not used as drugs, therefore, it is of no significance of this division from identification point of view. This system also does not co-relate in between the chemical constituents and biological activity of the drugs. The taxonomical classification is summerized in Table 2.2.

CHEMICAL CLASSIFICATION

The biological activity of a drug is due to the presence of certain chemical constituents in the drug. Plants and animals synthesize chemical compounds such as fats, carbohydrates, proteins, volatile oils, alkaloids, resins etc. and some of these are pharmacologically active constituents. A single active constituent may be isolated from the crude drug and used as a medicinal agent. More than 100 pure compounds derived from higher plants find their place in modern medicine. For example, the important traditional active plant principles are codeine, atropine, ψ-ephedrine, hyoscyamine, digoxin, hyoscine, digitoxin, pilocarpine, theobromine, theophylline, quinidine, quinine, emetine, caffeine, papaverine and colchicine. These active constituents are differentiated from the inert compounds like starch, cellulose, lignin and cutin. The active constituent may be present in a very low concentration in the drug. The chemical classification of drugs is dependent upon the grouping of drugs with identical chemical constituents as shown in Table 2.3.

PHARMACOLOGICAL CLASSIFICATION

In Pharmacological classification the drugs are grouped according to their therapeutic uses. Thus cardiotonic drugs include Digitalis, Squill and Strophanthus. Senna leaves and Castor oil are termed as purgative drugs. A particular drug containing known chemical constituents can be grouped according to its therapeutic use. The main drawback of this classification is that a drug can be placed in various classes according to its thera-

Table 2.2. Taxonomical classification of drugs

Phyllum	Order	Family	Drugs
Angiosperms (Monocotyledons)	Liliflorae	Liliaceae	Scilla, Colchicum, Asparagus
		Dioscoreaceae	Dioscorea
	Microspermae	Orchidaceae	Vanilla
Angiosperms (Dicotyledons)	Papaverales,	Papaveraceae	Opium,
	Rosales	Rosaceae	Almond, Quillaia, Rose oil
		Papilionaceae	Balsam of Tolu, Glycyrrhiza
		Caesalpiniaceae	Senna
	Rutales	Rutaceae	Bael, Lemon, Orange peel
	Rhamnales	Rhamnaceae	Cascara bark
	Malvales	Malvaceae	Sida
	Umbelliflorae	Apiaceae	Coriander, Caraway, Dill, Fennel
	Gentianales	Loganiaceae	Nux-vomica
		Gentianaceae	Chirata
		Apocynaceae	Kurchi, Rauwolfia, Strophanthus
	Tubiflorae	Convolvulaceae	Shankhpushpi
		Lamiaceae	Mentha, Ocimum
		Solanaceae	Belladonna, Capsicum, Datura, Hyoscyamus
		Scrophulariaceae	Digitalis
	Plantaginales	Plantaginaceae	Plantago
	Dipsacales	Valerinaceae	Valerian
	Companulales	Lobeliaceae	Lobelia
		Asteraceae	Artemisia, Kuth
Bryophyta and Pteridophyta (Liverworts, Mosses and Ferns)	Filicales	Polypodiaceae	Male Fern
Gymnosperms	Genetales	Ephedraceae	Ephedra
	Coniferae	Pinaceae	Colophony
Thallophyta (Bacteria, Fungi, Lichens) Rhodophyta	Gelidiales	Gelidaceae	Agar

Table 2.3. Chemical classification of drugs

Chemical constituents	Drugs
1. Carbohydrates	
Gum	Acacia, Tragacanth, Guar gum, Sterculia
Mucilages	Plantago seed
Others	Starch, Honey, Agar, Pectin, Bael, Cotton
2. Glycosides	
Anthraquinone	Aloe, Cascara, Rhubarb, Senna,
Saponins	Quillaia, Arjuna, Glycyrrhiza, Dioscorea
Cyanophore	Wild Cherry bark
Isothiocyanate	Mustard
Cardiac (Steroidal)	Digitalis, Strophanthus, Scilia
Bitter	Gentian, Calumba, Quassia, Chirata, Picrorhiza, Kalmegh

(Contd.)

Chemical constituents	Drugs
3. **Tannins**	Pale Catechu, Black Catechu, Ashoka bark, Galls, Myrobalan, Bahera, Amla
4. **Volatile oils**	Cinnamon, Nutmeg, Fennel, Dill, Caraway, Coriander, Cardamom, Orange peel, Mint, Clove, Ginger, Valerian, Saffron, Banafsha, Tulsi, Anise, Lemon grass and Jatamansi
5. **Lipids**	
Fixed oils	Castor, Olive, Peanut, Cottonseed, Almond, Shark liver,
Fats	Theobroma, Lanolin
Waxes	Beeswax, Spermaceti
6. **Resins**	Colophony, Podophyllum, Jalap, Cannabis, Capsicum, Turmeric, Ginger, Myrrh, Asafoetida, Storax, Balsam of Tolu, Balsam of Peru, Benzoin
7. **Alkaloids**	
Pyridine and piperidine	Lobelia, Nicotiana, Areca nut
Tropane	Coca, Belladonna, Datura, Hyoscyamus, Stramonium, Henbane
Quinoline	Cinchona
Isoquinoline	Opium, Ipecac, Calumba
Indole	Ergot, Nux vomica, Rauwolfia, Catharanthus, Physostigma,
Amines	Ephedra
Steroidal	Kurchi, Veratrums
Purine	Tea, Coffee
Diterpene	Aconite
8. **Proteins**	Gelatin, Ficin, Papain
9. **Vitamins**	Yeast
10. **Triterpenes**	Rasna, Colocynth

peutic use. Thus Cinchona can be grouped in antimalarial and antiarrhythmic catagories. The classification of drugs based on pharmacological action or therapeutic uses is given in Table 2.4.

Table 2.4. Classification of drugs based on pharmacological action

Pharmacological Action	Drugs
Anticancer	Vinca, Podophyllum, Taxus
Anti-inflammatory	Colchicum corm and seed, Turmeric
Antiamoebic	Ipecac root, Kurchi bark
Anthelmintic	Artemisia, Male Fern, Quassia wood, Vidang, Chenopodium oil
Antiasthmatic	Ephedra, Lobelia, Vasaka, Tylophora
Antispasmodic	Belladonna, Datura, Hyoscyamus
Astringent	Catechu, Tannic acid, Myrrh, Myrobalan, Ashoka bark
Analgesic	Opium, Cannabis
Bitter tonics	Quassia wood, Nux-vomica, Gentian, Picrorhiza, Chirata, Kalmegh
Carminatives	Cinnamon bark, Cardamom seed
Flavours	Nutmeg fruit, Clove, Umbelliferous fruits, Peppermint, Saffron, Asafoetida, Oleo-gum resin, Mint, Tulsi, Ginger, Vanilla
Purgatives	Cascara bark, Senna, Rhubarb, Aloe, Castor oil, Plantago seed husk
Expectorant	Benzoin, Balsam of Tolu, Glycyrrhiza, Vasaka
Cardiotonic	Digitalis, Squill, Strophanthus
CNS Action	Ergot, Belladonna, Stramonium, Hyoscyamus, Ephedra, Physostigma
Hallucinogens	Cocaine, Cannabis
Tranquilliser	Rauwolfia roots.

ALPHABETICAL CLASSIFICATION

In this classification the drugs are arranged in alphabetical order from A, B, C to X, Y and Z according to their names in a particular language. In European Pharmacopoea the drugs are arranged according to their names in Latin. In United States Pharmacopoea, British Pharmacopoeia, European Pharmacopoeia and Indian Pharmacopoeia, the drugs are arranged in English.

This system of classification does not provide information about chemical nature, biological activity or medicinal uses of the drugs. Location, tracing and addition of a drug is easy in this system and it is suitable for quick reference. It gives no indication of inter-relationship between drugs.

CHEMOTAXONOMICAL CLASSIFICATION

Some chemical constituents are characteristic of certain classes of plants. For example, tropane alkaloids are generally present in the drugs of Solanaceae family. Volatile oils are present in the plants of Apiaceae, Asteraceae, Rutaceae, Lamiaceae, Lauraceae, Pinaceae, Myristicaceae, Araceae, Myrtaceae, Zingiberaceae and Santalaceae. This is a relationship between chemical constituents and taxonomical status of plants.

3

Plant Description and Morphology

Plant form varies from unicellular plants, *e.g.*, yeasts and green algae, to the higher plants. The higher plants consist in the vegetative phase of roots, stems and leaves with flowers, fruits and seeds forming stages in the reproductive cycle. Modifications of the above structures are rhizomes (underground stems), stolons (runners with a stem structure), stipules, bracts (modified leaves), tendrils (modified stems), etc. Certain organs may be missing or much reduced, *e.g.*, the reduction of leaves in some xerophytic plants.

AERIAL PARTS

These consist of stems and leaves often associated with flowers and young fruits. All portions of such drugs are to be mentioned.

Herbs include drugs consisting of the entire plant, such as Irish moss and also drugs derived from flowering plants and consisting of flowering tops which include smaller stems, leaves, flowers and fruits, as well as others consisting of all parts of the plant growing above the ground level, such as Lobelia, and in some instances also the root and rhizome.

The type of stem is that known as a herbaceous stem, of which there are two main types, *viz.*, (1) the stems of annual plants such as Stramonium, and (2) the stems of second year plants of biennials such as Digitalis and of herbaceous perennials, which have perennial root-stocks and throw up aerial shoots annually, as does Belladonna. In all cases the stems lie down at the end of the season and

consequently, if they are dicotyledonous, cambial activity is limited to one season or part of a season. In some herbaceous stems, the vascular tissues are ill-developed.

Herbaceous stems afford many useful characters for the identification of the drugs to which they belong. The shape may be *terete* or nearly cylindrical as in Chiretta; pentagonal or five-sided as in Broom; collapsed and grooved due to shrinkage during drying as in Belladonna and Henbane. The colour may be green as in Broom; pale green with purple patches as in Lobelia; brownish with purple patches as in *Euphorbia pilulifera*. The surface may be glabrous as in Chiretta or hairy as in Lobelia and *Euphorbia pilulifera*. The transversely cut surface and the pitch both give diagnostic characters. The transverse surface is always studied in the internodes and shows a characteristic outline, *e.g.*, circular in Chiretta; pentagonal in Broom. The pitch may be solid as in Chiretta, or have a central hollow as in Belladonna and Henbane.

The root, when present, is usually a tap root and may be vertical as in Lobelia or oblique as in Chiretta.

The characters of the pollen grains, present in all herbs and their powders, are also studied.

Aerial stem

Observe dimensions, shape, colour, whether herbaceous or woody, upright or creeping, smooth or ridged, hairs present or not and if so whether of the glandular or covering form. Note arrangement of tissues as seen in transverse section.

Microscopically, the herbaceous stem consists of a ground tissue in which conducting vascular strands or bundles are embedded. The main axial bundles run vertically through the internodes in many dicotyledonous stems, such as Cannabis and Grindelia. The vascular tissue being developed as a cylinder of xylem surrounded by a cylinder of phloem as in Digitalis and Belladonna. In the case of dicotyledons, either separate procambial strands arise and develop into a ring of discrete bundles or a complete cylinder of conducting tissue is developed as the primary formation. In the majority of stems having separate or discrete bundles, these eventually become united into a continuous cylinder by the formation and activity of interfascicular cambium, as in Lobelia, Grindelia and Cannabis. In a few plants, such as Ranunculus and Podophyllum, the bundles are permanently separate. The main axial strands or cylinder is surrounded externally by a pericycle and an endodermis. The pericycle and all tissues within it are known collectively as the *stele* and the tissues external to the pericycle constitute the cortex, the innermost layer of which, termed the *endodermis*, is differentiated. In stems, the xylem does not reach to the centre, which is occupied by a region of fundamental tissue, of greater or less extent, termed the pith or medulla. At or near the nodes, opening or gaps are formed in the stelar cylinder to allow branches of the conducting tissue to be separated and to become united across the cortex with the foliar strands developed in the leaves and petioles. The gaps in the vascular cylinder are termed foliar-gaps and the small branches passing into the leaves are the leaf-trace bundles.

Monocotyledonous stems have a less regular arrangement of vascular strands. The leaf-trace bundles pass independently into the stem in a slightly downward sloping direction and cross the endodermis into the pith, then they turn slowly outwards and downwards in steeply sloping lines, fusing eventually near the endodermis with other bundles much lower down the stem. One, therefore, finds bundles in both the cortex and pith and much crowded in the region just within the endodermis.

Transverse sections of the internodes of herbaceous stems show in dicotyledons either a circle of separate open collateral bundles, usually connected by interfascicular cambium, or a continuous xylem and phloem or a band of xylem and phloem having projections of xylem—that of the primary bundles—into the pith. In monocotyledons, transverse sections usually show vascular bundles in large numbers in the periphery of the stele just within the endodermis and also scattered bundles in both the cortex and pith, these bundles being usually larger in transverse section than the more numerous bundles near the endodermis.

The vascular bundles of the dictyostele are usually collateral, or bicollateral (Cucurbitaceae, Solanaceae, Convolvulaceae). The xylem is differentiated centrifugally and the protoxylem is endarch; the phloem is differentiated centripetally and the protophloem is exarch (cf. the root). The differentiation, in dicotyledons, is usually incomplete. A zone of meristematic cells (the intrafascicular cambium) separates the primary vascular tissues. Such a bundle is described as open, in contrast to the closed bundle typical of monocotyledons. In the bicollateral bundle the intrafascicular cambium occurs between the xylem and the outer phloem group.

Secondary thickening is initiated by tangenital divisions in the cambium. The daughter cells cut off on the inner side differentiate into xylem and those cut off to the outside into phloem. The amount of secondary xylem produced in both stems and roots, in general, exceeds the amount of secondary phloem. As the process of secondary thickening of the stem proceeds, its dictyostele is converted into a solid cylinder of secondary tissues. The intrafascicular cambia become linked to form a continuous cambial cylinder by the development of interfascicular cambia in the ray tissue. The cambial activity may spread out from the intrafascicular cambia across the rays.

In woody perennials the cambial divisions are arrested during the winter but are renewed each spring. The xylem produced at different seasons varies in texture. The spring wood is characterized by abundance of relatively thin-walled large conducting elements; the autumn wood, by a high proportion of thick-walled mechanical elements such as wood fibres. A similar alteration between sieve tissue and phloem fibres may occur in the secondary phloem. With increase in girth the central core of xylem may become nonfunctional, dark in colour and packed with metabolic byproducts forming a heartwood or duramen. Sandalwood is the heartwood of *Santalum album* and is packed with volatile oil. The blocking of the vessels in the formation of heartwood occurs by the development of tyloses.

The secondary increase in diameter of the vascular cylinder is accompanied by changes in the outer tissues. The epidermis and part or all of the primary cortex may be shed. A phellogen may arise in the epidermis, cortex or pericycle and give rise externally to cork and internally to a variable amount of phelloderm.

The structures constantly present in powdered stems are cork and vascular tissues in varying amount, abundant parenchyma often containing starch. Calcium oxalate and other cell inclusions may be present. Aleurone grains are absent.

The endodermis is not always evident as a distinctly differentiated layer, but in most dicotyledons it can be recognised by the peculiar thickening of its walls and frequently also by the contents of its cells. The shape of the endodermal cells is greatly elongated like rectangular prism, the shortest dimension being the radial one. Each cell has, therefore, two parallel tangential walls and four radial walls, *viz.*, two longitudinal and two transverse. The radial walls are usually thickened by a band of cuticularised, and often also lignified material, which extends round the four radial walls; this band is known as the casparian strip. In transverse sections the casparian strip appears as a bright spot upon the radial walls and responds to the tests for suberin and often also to those for lignin. In many plants the endodermal cells contain numerous small starch grains, which may disappear if a freshly cut specimen is kept for some hours before examination. The presence of starch has given rise to the name starch-sheath often applied to this layer of cells.

The pith or medulla is the tissue at the centre of the stem and is parenchymatous, being cellulosic in young stems, but usually lignified in mature stems. The pith of the stems of Lobelia, Chiretta,

Andrographis, and many similar stems is thin-walled and lignified with very fine pits on the walls. Sometimes the cell-walls are strongly thickened throughout as in *Berberis aquifolium*.

Another peculiarity of the pith, characteristic of certain families, is the presence in its periphery of small groups of phloem or sieve-tissue.

The cells of the pith often contain characteristic cell-contents, such as starch, mucilage, calcium oxalate and tannin. Starch is found in the pith of the stem of Senna; calcium oxalate occurs in microsphenoidal crystals in idioblasts in the pith of Belladonna stem, in cluster crystals in the pith of Cannabis and in prisms in the pith of Andrographis.

BARKS

Bark consist of all tissues outside the cambium removed by peeling them after making suitable incisions through the outer layers.

The inner surface of a bark corresponds to the position of the cambiform tissue, which has been torn during the removal of the bark. The external tissues of older barks often have a rugged and scaly appearance, due to the splitting away, or exfoliation, of some of the outer tissues, a condition brought about by the formation of phellogens of local extent and often concave in form, which cut out lenticular masses of cells. Layers of dead phloem alternating with bands of cork frequently form a massive external covering of a bark and a composite dead tissue of this type is termed a *rhytidoma*.

The time of collection is usually spring or elderly summer, when the sap is rising in the stem and the cambium is active and, therefore, more easily torn than at other seasons. If there is a rainy season, it is during that period that the bark is most easily collected, as is done with Cinnamon. Wild cherry bark, from *Prunus serotina*, is removed in the autumn because at that season the amount of active principle present is greatest. For the removal of the bark longitudinal incisions are made at intervals round the circumstance of the stem and the bark is stripped off in long pieces, as is done with Cascara sagrada, or longitudinal incisions are made and also horizontal ones at intervals of about 30 cm and the pieces removed as for Cinnamon. Bark is also sometimes whittled off with a knife, such as a draw-knife, producing pieces of fairly small size and often showing adherent wood on the inner surface. Drying of barks is nearly always effected by the sun heat in open air, or sometimes, after a preliminary drying in the open, the operation is completed by some kind of artificial heat.

Barks are characterised by certain peculiar structural features. The shape of the pieces depends upon the type of incisions made in removing it and also upon the extent and nature of the shrinkage which occurs during drying. Very large heavy pieces of bark from old tree trunks are often dried under pressure, so that the finished product consists of large flat pieces of considerable thickness, and these are generally referred to as flats, they are found in both Cinchona and Quillaia. More usually the commercial bark is that removed from the smaller branches and it becomes curved during drying owing to the unequal shrinkage of its constituent parts. Pieces of bark usually remain straight longitudinally because the stronger and less shrinkable elements, such as the fibres, lie in a longitudinal direction; curvature mostly takes place transversely, and since the inner tissues are softer than the outer ones and occur in considerable masses between the strands of fibres, there is a greater shrinkage in the inner than in the outer tissues, resulting in curvature of the bark with the inner part of the concave surface. According to the extent of this curvature different characteristic shapes are assumed and special terms are used to describe them. When only slightly concave on the inside, the pieces are termed curved, and if the concavity is on the outside, recurved. When the curvature on the inside is so great as to form a deep trough, the piece is said to be channelled; when still more curvature is present and one edge overlaps the other, a quill is formed, and is a double quill. When quills are packed one inside the other, as is done with Cinnamon and sometimes with Cinchona, compound quills result.

The colour and condition of the outer surface afford useful characters when the cork is evenly developed, a smooth surface results, and this is marked by lenticels which are commonly elongated and placed transversely to the long axis of the bark, as in Cascara and Wild cherry bark. The presence of rhytidoma gives a scaly appearance, though this is often absent in such barks as Quillaia because the outer dead tissues are removed during the preparation of the bark. The corky layer frequently flakes off, or exfoliates in large pieces, exposing the cortical layer beneath; this happens in the calisaya variety of Cinchona, where the exposed surface is dark brown and in Wild cherry bark where the exposed layer is green or in older specimens Cinnamon brown. Cracks and fissures of characteristic type arise in the outer surface owing to the lack of elasticity in the dead tissues and the continued increase in girth of the tree; these cracks are often characteristic, having, for example, clean cut edges in *Cinchona succirubra*, but thickened, recurved edges in *Cinchona officinalis*. On older barks small circular dusty patches frequently develop in the cork, and these are described as corky warts; a good example is the older bark of *Cinchona succirubra*. The shrinkage of barks during drying occurs transversely, because the longitudinally directed fibres tend to prevent extensive shrinking in length and the greater shrinkage of the softer tissues results in the formation of wrinkles externally; if the troughs between the wrinkles are very wide, they are termed furrows. An additional character is sometimes provided by the presence of *epiphytes* upon the outer surface, most commonly lichens or bryophytes, including both liverworts and mosses.

Lichens are recognised by their greyish colour and thalloid structure or, if they are of the crustaceous type, by the general smooth grey surface they give to the bark and by the presence of small scattered dark points, which are the apothecia or fructifications of the lichens.

Liverworts on barks are usually foliaceous and consist of very slender stems to which small leaves are attached so as to lie all in one plane, giving the plants a dorsiventral structure. The leaves are only one cell in thickness and show no central thickening or midrib.

Mosses have a slender stem bearing spirally arranged leaves, which possess a midrib and have a lamina one cell thick; the margins of the leaves sometimes bear characteristic teeth.

The inner surface of pieces of bark also shows features of colour and condition which are of diagnostic value. The shrinkage results in the production of parallel longitudinal ridges, which are sometimes very fine and in other cases quite coarse; they are termed striations. Occasionally also, as in Cascara, longitudinal shrinkage produces parallel transverse wrinkles, known as corrugations.

The behaviour of barks when broken across transversely and the appearance of the exposed surfaces are known as the fracture, and this provides one of the most useful diagnostic characters. When the fractured surfaces are smooth, the fracture is described as short; if the surfaces exhibit small rounded prominences, it is granular; if jagged projecting points are formed, the fracture is splintery; if fine fibrous threads extend from the broken surfaces, it is fibrous; and if the fractured region breaks into a tangentially arranged layers, as in Quillaia, it is laminated. The arrangement of the tissues in barks is largely responsible for the type of fracture, and the arrangement can be best seen in the smoothed transversely cut surface, which affords a further valuable diagnostic character for most barks.

A young bark is composed of :

(1) *Epidermis* : A layer of closely fitting cuticularized cells with occasional stomata. It is absent in commercial samples.

(2) *Primary cortex* : A zone usually consisting of chlorophyll-containing collenchyma and parenchyma.

(3) *Endodermis* or inner layer of the cortex, which frequently contains starch.

(4) *Pericycle* which may be composed of parenchyma or of fibres. Groups of fibres often occur opposite each group of phloem.

(5) *Phloem* which consists of sieve tubes, companion cells and phloem parenchyma separated by radially arranged medullary rays.

In some barks the above structures have been modified by the activity of the cambium and the cork cambium or phellogen. Growth of the new tissues produced by the cambium causes the tissues of the primary bark to be tangentially stretched, compressed or torn. As these cells are stretched tangentially they may be divided by radial walls as in the medullary rays. During this dilatation groups of parenchymatous cells in the cortex and phloem may be thickened into sclerenchymatous cells. The cambium produces secondary phloem, which often consists of alternating zones of sieve elements and phloem fibres. The pericycle is frequently ruptured, and parenchymatous cells which grow into the spaces may develop into sclerenchyma.

The cork cambium or phellogen may arise in the epidermis (e.g., willow), primary cortex or pericycle. The phellogen produces on its outer side cork, and on its inner side chlorophyll containing suberized cells which form the secondary cortex or phelloderm. These three layers are known as the periderm. If the cork cambium develops in or near the pericycle, a part or the whole of the primary cortex will lie outside the cork and will be gradually thrown off. Lenticels replace stomata for purposes of gaseous exchange; and as the cork increases, the amount of chlorophyll-containing tissue decreases.

Sieve-tubes constitute the most characteristic element of the phloem, and as a type of this one may use the well-developed sieve-tube of Cucurbita. The sieve-tube is a vessel or long tube formed by several large prismatic or cylindrical cells united end to end. The walls are cellulosic and the cross-walls are at right angles to the tube and are perforated by comparatively large holes, eaten away by the action of enzymes, thus forming the sieve-plates which give the name sieve-tube to this type of vessel. Through the perforations of the plates pass strands of stringy material of a nitrogenous nature, known as slime-strings. The fully developed tubes do not contain nuclei and the protoplasm exists as a thin layer lining the walls; the vacuoles are filled with a thin nitrogenous mucilage; in the living protoplasmic layer there are embedded leucoplasts with minute starch grains. After reaching a certain age, sieve-tubes become blocked by the formation of plugs of a hemi-cellulosic substance, termed callus or callose, which is formed by the protoplasm and is deposited upon the sieve-plates. In the majority of plants this permanently closes the tubes; the lining layer of protoplasm then disappears and they finally become collapsed owing to the pressure due to the continued formation of new layers of secondary tissues internal to them. In a few plants, the sieve-tubes may function for several seasons, the callose forming in the autumn and being dissolved away by enzyme action in the spring, so reopening the sieve-tubes; this happens in the grape vine and the barberry. After a few years these exceptional tubes become permanently closed, empty and dead. The callus of sieve-tubes is insoluble in dilute acids, in dilute alkali, and in cuoxam, and is stained a bright pink by corallin-soda, which is a reagent made by adding one volume of a 5 per cent solution of corallin in alcohol to 20 volumes of a 25 per cent solution of crystalline sodium carbonate. This reagent also stains lignified tissue, starch grains and some forms of resin and mucilage. Sieve-tubes commonly occur in tangential bands so that the walls of a number of collapsed tubes form an irregular hyaline band, and this modified tissue is described as ceratenchyma because of its translucent horny appearance. Sieve-tubes of the type described are accompanied by long narrow cells with dense cytoplasm and large nuclei; these are named companion cells, and their end walls usually coincide with the ends of the segments of the sieve-tubes, a condition owing to their formation from the same initial cells as the sieve-tube segments. They are connected by pits with the sieve-tubes, but their other walls are unpitted. In transverse section they are triangular in shape and are situated in the angles of the large sieve-tube elements, which are polygonal in shape.

Phloem parenchyma consists of cellulosed-walled cells which are more or less rectangular in transverse section and somewhat elongated axially; they have large nuclei, abundant cytoplasm and usually contain small starch grains. These cells are arranged in vertical files very similarly to xylem parenchyma. When bundles of phloem fibres are present, the parenchymatous cells adjacent to them are commonly subdivided into smaller cells each of which contains a prism of calcium oxalate. Phloem fibres closely resemble xylem fibres; they are usually very heavily thickened and possess a narrow lumen; their walls may be cellulosic as in mezereon bark and slippery elm bark, where however, the middle lamella is lignified, or they may be strongly lignified as in Cinchona and Cascara. These fibres are present in the majority of barks, but are absent from a few, such as canella bark, viburnum bark, pomegranate root bark and euonymus bark. They vary much in size and their dimensions afford useful characters for the identification of barks.

Sclereids, stone cells or sclerenchymatous cells occur in the parenchyma of many barks. These cells are parenchymatous elements and may be rounded,

polyhedral or prismatic; they have thick lignified walls and the lumen may vary from a narrow, branching, slit-like hollow to a fairly large, sub-rectangular cavity. The walls commonly show striations and are perforated by tubular pits, which are often branched. The external openings of the pits appear as small circular or irregular pores dotted over the surface of the cells seen in surface view. They are absent from Frangula bark, but present in the very similar Cascara bark; they are few in Quillaia and very numerous in Cinnamon and Cassia.

The medullary rays are composed of parenchymatous cells which tend to be elongated radially, and generally have cellulose walls. In some plants, such as *Coscinium*, the primary rays become sclerotic and lignified, while in others, such as Cascara and Hamamelis, groups of sclereids appear as the rays become older, particularly in the outer part. The primary medullary rays, continuous with those of the xylem which penetrate to the pith, widen as they approach the cortex, the increase being brought about by tangential and radial division of the cells of the original rays, thus enabling them to keep pace with the extension of the outer region in circumference as secondary growth proceeds. The secondary rays are more numerous towards the cambium and the outer rays of each group often bend towards the central line as they approach the cortex, forming roughly triangular groups. At the apex of such triangular groups one may find the primary phloem consisting of collapsed sieve-tubes and parenchyma.

Beyond the phloem is the pericycle, the outermost stelar tissue; this varies in extent, being sometimes a cylindrical sheath one layer of cells in thickness, as in *Lobelia*, while in other plants the sheath may be many cells thick as in Cinnamon, Hamamelis and Barberry. The pericycle may be parenchymatous and thin-walled throughout, but frequently it includes sclerenchymatous elements; in Cinnomon and Hamamelis the tissue consists of a band of several rows of sclereids external to which are fibres in small isolated groups. These pericyclic fibres are often less lignified than phloem fibres, and, in transverse section, the lumen is more rounded in outline and the walls highly refractive.

Cortex is often entirely absent from commercial barks, either because it has been cut away, as in Cinnamon and Quillaia, during the preparation or because it has exfoliated after the formation of a layer of cork. When present, the cortex consists of parenchyma which is often divisible into an outer collenchymatous region and an inner thin-walled region. The cortex usually contains starch and frequently also calcium oxalate, most commonly in cluster crystals, and secretory structures. Secretory structures also often occur in the phloem, for example, oil cells in Cinnamon and Cassia, mucilage cells in slippery elm, latex tubes in Alstonia and Cascarilla, latex vessels in Lobelia.

Phellogen or cork-cambium arises in stems, either in the outer epidermis, as in *Salix alba*, *Solanum dulcamara* and *Viburnum prunifolium* or in the sub-epidermal layer, as in *Quillaia saponaria*, *Cinnamomum zeylanicum*, *Cinchona*, Cascara and Alstonia, or occasionally in the pericycle as in *Berberis*. The phellogen cuts off cells on the outside, the walls of which become suberised and form the tissue known as cork or phellem. Cork cells are, therefore, in regular radial rows and are usually thin-walled; sometimes they become lignified or both lignified and thickened as in Cassia bark. In Cascarilla bark the walls are lignified and the inner walls are encrusted with small prisms of calcium oxalate. On the inside the phellogen gives rise to rows of cells which are added to the cortex and form a tissue termed phelloderm; this tissue may consist of one or two rows only, or it may form a fairly wide band, the cells of which are sometimes sclerotic as in Canella bark. The whole of the tissues, cork, phellogen and phelloderm constitute collectively the periderm. In older barks the earliest phellogen ceases to divide and new phellogens are formed in the deeper layers, leading to the death and exfoliation of the cortical tissues, and, finally, when the phellogens dip into the secondary phloem, masses of phloem are cut out and die. There thus arises a dead tissue consisting of alternate layers of dead phloem and cork, a tissue which is termed rhytidoma and is found in thicker barks such as Cinchona and Quillaia.

The walls of the cork cells are said to be suberised, a change which is brought about by the deposition in the wall of fatty matter, which to a large extent undergoes a change rendering it insoluble in the usual fat solvents such as chloro-form; this substance is known as suberin. The acids present in the suberin are named suberogenic acids. Corky cell-walls, therefore, always contain a small amount of fatty matter, soluble in chloroform, amounting to form 1.5 to 3.5 per cent of the cork, and it is to this unchanged fatty matter that the cork owes its characteristic behaviour towards staining reagents, the reagents which stain cork being those which are used for staining fats and oils, *viz.*, tincture of alkaline, soudan red III and scharlach R. Suberised walls may also be recognised by their insolubility in strong sulphuric acid and by their saponification by a 20 per cent aqueous solution of caustic potash, the soap appearing as globules when cork cells are warmed with the reagent. Suberised walls are easily oxidised by nitric acid, by a mixture of potassium chlorate and hydrochloric acid or by chromic acid. Suberised walls resemble lignified walls by giving a yellow colour with iodine and sulphuric acid, but they differ in remaining colourless with phloroglucin and hydrochloric acid.

Middle lamella

The greater part of most barks consists of cellulose-walled tissue. The middle lamella is pectic in nature; pectose, pectin and pectic acid are all apparently present. Pectic acid is an aldobionic acid yielding on hydrolysis galacturonic acid, arabinose and galactose and possibly also methyl pentose. Pectin, which is soluble in water, is a neutral methoxy ester of pectic acid and is hydrolysed by pectase or by dilute caustic soda to give pectic acid and methyl alcohol. Pectose is a glycosidal compound of pectin and cellulose and is insoluble in water. Intermediate between pectin and pectic acid is a group of acids containing different proportions of unchanged methoxy groups; these are termed pectinic acids. Alkaline hydrolysis converts pectose into pectin and cellulose and converts pectin into pectic acids or pectinic acids. All the products of the hydrolysis are present in the form of soluble sodium salts, hence by digestion with a 5 per cent, aqueous solution of caustic alkali, the cellulose tissues of barks may be disintegrated for the study of their constituent cells. If lignified tissues also are present, they may be removed from the alkaline macerate and treated with an oxidizing agent.

Barks may be described under the following headings :

Origin and preparation

From trunk branches or roots. Whole or inner bark.

Size and shape

Outer surface

Lichens, mosses, lenticels, cracks or furrows, colour before and after scraping.

Inner surface

Colour, striations, furrows.

Fracture

Short, fibrous, splintery and granular. The fracture depends largely on the number and distribution of scleroids and fibres. A bark frequently breaks with a short fracture in the outer part and a fibrous fracture in the phloem.

Transverse surface

A smoothed transverse surface, especially if stained with phloroglucinol and hydrochloric acid, will usually show the general arrangement of the lignified elements, medullary rays and cork.

Anatomy

In transverse section the cork cells are often tangentially elongated and arranged in regular radial rows. In surface view they are frequently polygonal. The cell walls give a suberin reaction; the cell contents give a positive tannin reaction. The cortex is usually composed of a ground mass of parenchyma. An outer band of collenchyma often occurs. Secretion cells, scleroids and pericyclic fibres may occur scattered or in groups in the cortex. The cortical cells often contain starch or other typical cell inclusions such as calcium oxalate.

Phloem contains sieve tubes, companion cells, phloem parenchyma and medullary ray cells, but these soft tissues may not be well-preserved in medicinal barks. The sieve tubes, unless well-developed, are observed only after special treatment. Secretion cells, phloem fibres and scleroids may or may not be present in the phloem.

Xylem tissue is usually absent but may be present in small amount on the inner surface of the bark.

In the anatomical examination of barks there may be the presence or absence of outer bark (cork, phellogen, phelloderm); cell structure and cell contents of the cortex; the presence or absence and, if present, the distribution, size and form of scleroids, phloem fibres and secretion cells; and the width, height, distribution and cell structure and contents of the medullary rays. When calcium oxalate is present, its crystalline forms and their distribution should be studied.

Transverse and longitudinal sections should be prepared. The size and form of scleroids and phloem fibres are best studied in disintegrated material. Preparations treated with cellulose, lignin, starch, callus, oil, suberin and tannin stains should be examined.

Powdered barks

Powdered barks always possess sieve tubes and cellulose parenchyma. Cork, fibres, scleroids, starch, calcium oxalate and secretory tissues are present. Xylem tissues are absent or only present in very small amount. Chlorophyll and aleurone grains are absent.

WOODS

Wood consists of the secondary tissues produced by the cambium on its inner surface. The cells composing these tissues are the vessels, tracheids, wood fibres and parenchyma which may not be lignified. In some cases (e.g., the wood of Belladonna root) non-lignified elements predominate. The distribution of the lignified elements may be ascertained by treating surfaces or sections with phloroglucinol and hydrochloric acid. In trees, the cells of the old wood frequently become coloured as they fill with waste products such as resins, tannins and colouring matters. This central region is called the heartwood, while the outer wood, which still retains its normal appearance and functions, is called the sapwood. Commercial guaiacum wood and logwood consist of heartwood.

Woods used pharmaceutically consist almost entirely of the tissue named xylem and the great bulk is secondary xylem formed by the activity of the cambium. At the centre of a log a very small amount of other tissues is present, for example, a log of Quassia wood includes the pith which was present in the primary stem; a very small amount also of primary xylem abuts upon the periphery of the pith.

The density of the cell walls of which wood is composed is about 1.5, so that all woods, on becoming waterlogged, *i.e.*, the cell cavities filled with water, will sink in water. Ordinarily woods float on water because air is present in the cell cavities and, in the air-dry condition, they are dense according to the thickness of the cell walls of the constituent cells and to the extent to which resin, oil, tannin or other contents fill the cell cavities. The term density is usually applied to the air-dry wood, containing about 12 per cent of moisture.

The external characters of a wood are observed on surfaces exposed by cutting the wood in three specified directions at right angles to one another, *viz.*, a transverse surface, a radial surface and a tangential surface, the two latter being longitudinal.

Annual rings are evident as bands crossing the piece of wood from one radial surface to the other. Each ring consists of spring wood and summer wood, the latter being much darker in appearance, owing to the smaller lumina of the cells, and forming a dark line on the outer edge of each annual ring. These rings are usually well marked in woods of temperate regions, but are often absent from tropical woods because there is not sufficient seasonal variation to materially affect the size of the xylem elements. Guaiacum and sappan woods show annual rings, but Quassia and logwood have none. Crossing the annual rings at right angles are fine parallel lines; these are the medullary rays. The medullary rays usually appear lighter in colour than the remainder of the wood, and the number of rays per unit of arc varies in different woods and frequently supplies a useful diagnostic feature. In the substance of the wood between the rays, small holes or pores are evident; these are the vessels of the xylem and terms are used to describe their arrangement. A wood or timber is said to be diffuse porous when the vessels or pores, which occur either isolated or in small groups, are scattered uniformly throughout the wood as in Quassia, Guaiacum and logwood.

A wood is described as ring porous when the vessels or pores, which occur either isolated or in small groups, are scattered uniformly throughout the wood as in Quassia, guaiacum and logwood. A wood is described as ring porous when the vessels occur chiefly in the earliest formed spring wood and thus form well-marked concentric rings as in oak and ash. Associated with the vessels there are usually small patches or bands of tissue, rather paler in colour than the remainder of the xylem. These patches and bands are the xylem parenchyma and it is described as diffuse when scattered throughout the wood. Parenchyma which occurs in tangential bands of varying extent is named metatracheal; that which occurs adjacent to the vessels, but not completely surrounding them in paratracheal and that completely surrounding a vessel is vasicentric. The remainder of the wood consists of fibres upon which the strength and hardness of the wood mainly depends. A wood with straight fibres arranged parallel to one another will split easily, leaving smooth longitudinal surfaces, and is called straight-grained, as in Quassia and sappan. A wood having wavy fibres crossing one another at an angle of about 30 degrees splits with great difficulty, leaving rough and irregular longitudinal surfaces, and is said to possess an interlocked grain, *e.g.*, Guaiacum wood.

The radial surface shows the vessels as coarse lines running vertically down the surface and the medullary rays appear as narrow horizontal bands crossing the direction of the vessels. On a tangential surface, the vessels appear as on a radial surface, but the medullary rays are now seen as small lenticular areas. In many tropical woods, such as Quassia, an appearance known as ripple marks is evident on this surface and is due to the occurrence of the medullary rays in horizontal rows, all the rays being equal in height, so that the wood is divided into a number of narrow layers or storeys.

In transverse section woods usually show annual rings each of which normally represents a seasons growth. In some tropical species the annual rings are not well-marked, owing to the absence of a seasonal interruption in growth. The so-called false annual rings found in Quassia are irregular rings formed by alternating zones of wood parenchyma and fibres. The width and height of medullary rays are of diagnostic importance in the case of Jamaica and Surinam Quassias and Rhubarbs. The grain of wood primarily results from the arrangement of the annual rings and medullary rays, but is modified by the wavy course of the wood elements which causes the wood to split irregularly. Irregular splitting is largely dependent on the number of lateral branches which cause knots in the wood.

Vessels, like tracheids, are conducting elements, but whereas tracheids are single cells, vessels are cell-fusions. The individual cells, or vessel-segments, are from one to seven or eight times as long as they are wide, and in monocotyledons and most dicotyledons the end walls are flat and at right angles to the side walls and the perforation is a single large opening occupying practically the entire width of the vessel. The side walls of vessels often bear numerous pits, which are usually bordered, but vary in form and distribution in different parts in a manner similar to that found in tracheids. The vessels of the protoxylem are more simply constructed than other vessels and either possess thickened rings at intervals, forming an annular vessel, or are strengthened by a spiral line of thickening, forming a spiral vessel. The bordered pits on the walls of vessels are usually in rows and may be spaced. In many vessels the pits are closely arranged and the margins of the pit membranes become hexagonal, owing to mutual pressure; the pit pore is sometimes circular, but is frequently elongated or slit-shaped; such vessels are termed pitted vessels. The pits are sometimes very much elongated, extending entirely across each of the flat faces of a prismatic vessel-segment, and they are regularly arranged in vertical rows down each face so as to give rise to a ladder-like appearance; such vessels are named scalariform. In other examples the pits are much elongated transversely and are irregularly placed so that the thickening resembles a network with narrow elongated meshes and the vessel is termed reticulate. In the older parts of the xylem, the heartwood, the majority of the vessels are closed by the development of tyloses, *i.e.*, the parenchymatous cells surrounding the vessels grow through the pit openings of the vessel and form bladder-like expansions, each of which is a tylose, within the cavity of the vessel. These intrusions usually remain thin-walled, but may become heavily thickened like scleroids. Tylosis is well exhibited in sassafras wood.

Fibres of the xylem are mechanical or supporting elements, and each consists of a single prosenchymatous cell. They are polygonal in transverse section and are from thirty to fifty times as long as wide with very long tapering ends. The cavity is narrow, the walls thick and the pits simple and slit-shaped. Fibres sometimes have delicate transverse partitions formed of cellulosic or pectic material and are then called septate fibres; such fibres occur in teak wood and also in the fibrous bundle sheath of ginger. Cell forms, intermediate between tracheids and fibres, occur in ephedra and in calumba root; they have walls thicker than those of the ordinary tracheid, while the pits are larger than those of the typical fibre and the ends are less tapering. These fibre tracheids do not contain protoplasm or starch.

Xylem parenchyma consists chiefly of square-ended cells arising by the segmentation of cambial cells by transverse walls. They are arranged in vertical files of about three to five cells, the end cells of each file being somewhat pointed at one end. In the living wood, these cells contain protoplasm, a nucleus and storage material, such as starch. The starch is present in the Quassia wood. The walls of xylem parenchyma are usually pitted with simple, circular pits, but the form of pitting may vary according to the type of adjoining element. Crystals of calcium oxalate, prisms, may occur in the xylem parenchyma especially that adjacent to the fibres, and such cells are usually subdivided into small approximately cubical cells each containing one prism of calcium oxalate.

Medullary rays

The cells of the medullary rays are parenchymatous with square ends and simple pits; their function is mainly that of storage and they often contain starch grains and sometimes calcium oxalate crystals. If the cells of a medullary ray are all similar, the ray is termed homogeneous, but if some of the cells differ morphologically from the remainder, as is the case in Pinus, the ray is termed heterogeneous.

The middle lamella of woody tissues is the most highly lignified part of the cell walls; the remainder of the walls contains a lower proportion of lignin. The chemical structure of lignin is regarded as an aromatic aldehydic substance. Lignin is readily decomposed by oxidising reagents such as a mixture of nitric and chromic acids.

Lignified walls are permeable to water, but do not retain any appreciable amount as do cellulose walls; they are completely soluble in 80 per cent v/v sulphuric acid and are insoluble in cuoxam. Dilute aqueous iodine (N/50) followed by a dehydrating agent such as zinc chloride or sulphuric acid gives a yellow colour; aniline salts stain them yellow; phloroglucin 1 per cent in alcohol followed by strong hydrochloric acid colours them red.

Woods may be described under the following headings.

Size and colour

Note any differentiation into sapwood and heartwood. The latter may not be coloured uniformly (e.g., logwood).

Relative density

Woods vary considerably in this respect (e.g., Guaiacum has a relative density of 1.33 and poplar one of 0.38).

Transverse surface

The lignified elements may show a markedly radiate arrangement or they may be irregular scattered. Note distribution of wood fibres and wood parenchyma and of true and false annual rings. Measure the distances between medullary rays and between annual rings.

LEAVES AND LEAFLETS

Leaves are appendages to the stem, which show a great variation of external form. There are two constant features: (1) leaves possess neither nodes nor internodes and (2) branches arise in their axils. In most of the plants, leaves may be recognised by four well-marked characters: (1) their flattened form, (2) their thinness, (3) the presence of chlorophyll and (4) the presence of supporting and conducting strands—the veins.

The expanded blade or lamina is not always the whole of the leaf; frequently the blade is attached to the stem by a stalk—the *petiole*; if there is no stalk, the leaf is termed *sessile*. Leaves of commerce are not all of them leaves in the botanical sense, *e.g.*, Jaborandi and Senna consist of leaflets. If senna is examined two kinds of leaflets in equal numbers will be found, one type having the left-hand portion of the lamina smaller and the other having the right-hand portion smaller; this condition indicates a paripinnate leaf. Jaborandi consists of two types of asymmetric leaflet in equal numbers and a third type of leaflet which is symmetrical and is present in a smaller number; this condition indicates an imparipinnate leaf and the number of symmetrical leaflets in the sample is the number of leaves present. Leaves such as Coca, Belladonna and Bearberry, which have undivided laminae, are termed simple.

The usual time for the collection of leaves is when the flowers are just beginning to expand, or the flowering is just arriving at its height. At this time it is reasonable to assume that the whole plant has arrived at its condition of maximum vigour and that the leaves are in the most healthy state and contain an optimum of the products of the plant's metabolism and, therefore, should be at this period of their development suited to exert the most desirable therapeutic action. The actual collection should be made in dry weather, since leaves collected in wet weather deteriorate in quality and are apt to become discoloured during drying.

The time of collection is sometimes varied for special reasons; for example, for the more highly prized varieties of Tea, the leaves are collected when still unfolded in the bud; Cherrylaurel leaves are gathered while still young, but fully formed and in the first year of their duration; Coca leaves are collected when they are nearly ready to fall from the stem; Bearberry leaves may be collected at any time of the year.

The method of collection differs for different drugs. In collecting Tea, the terminal bud and the three or four leaves immediately below it are cut off separately and kept in distinct groups each of which produces a particular grade of tea; Coca, Digitalis and Hamamelis leaves are removed individually from the plant; in collecting Senna, the entire plants are cut down and the leaves are picked off after drying the plants in the sun; in the case of Buchu, the leafy stems are cut off and dried, after which the leaves are removed by beating the heaped twigs with a flexible rod; Belladonna, Hyoscyamus and Stramonium are collected by cutting down the flowering tops and drying the leaves on the stems with the flowers and young fruits without further treatment. They may be fresh as for cherrylaurel or they may be dry and whole or broken or shrivelled or flat or matted, etc.

Leaves must be dried carefully so as to retain their fresh green colour and prevent factors are to use as low a temperature as possible and to carry out the operation as rapidly as possible. Ordinarily leaves should be protected from direct sunlight and be taken under cover at night. Drying in sheds at the air temperature is frequently adopted, especially for leaves containing essential oil. Buchu leaves are dried by spreading the leafy twigs in a thick layer on the floors of sheds with corrugated iron roofs. Drying in specially constructed heated sheds or drying chambers is now one of the common methods of drying leaves. Leaves are most commonly packed in sacks or bales.

Storage of dried leaves should be in a cool dry place, protected from the light; before packing they are commonly stored loose in barrels or sacks in the drying rooms.

The following features can be used to describe leaves.

Duration : Deciduous or evergreen.

Leaf base : Stipulate or exstipulate.

Petiole : Petiolate or sessile. If present, describe size, shape, colour, hairs, etc.

Lamina

1. *Composition* : If simple, whether pinnate or palmate. If compound, whether paripinnate (with an equal number of leaflets) or imparipinnate.
2. *Incision* : The leaf may be more or less cleft, the amount being indicated by adding -fid, -partite or -sect to a prefix denoting whether the leaf is of a pinnate or a palmate type.
3. *Shape* : If the shape is obscured by drying, soak the leaf in warm water and spread it on a tile.

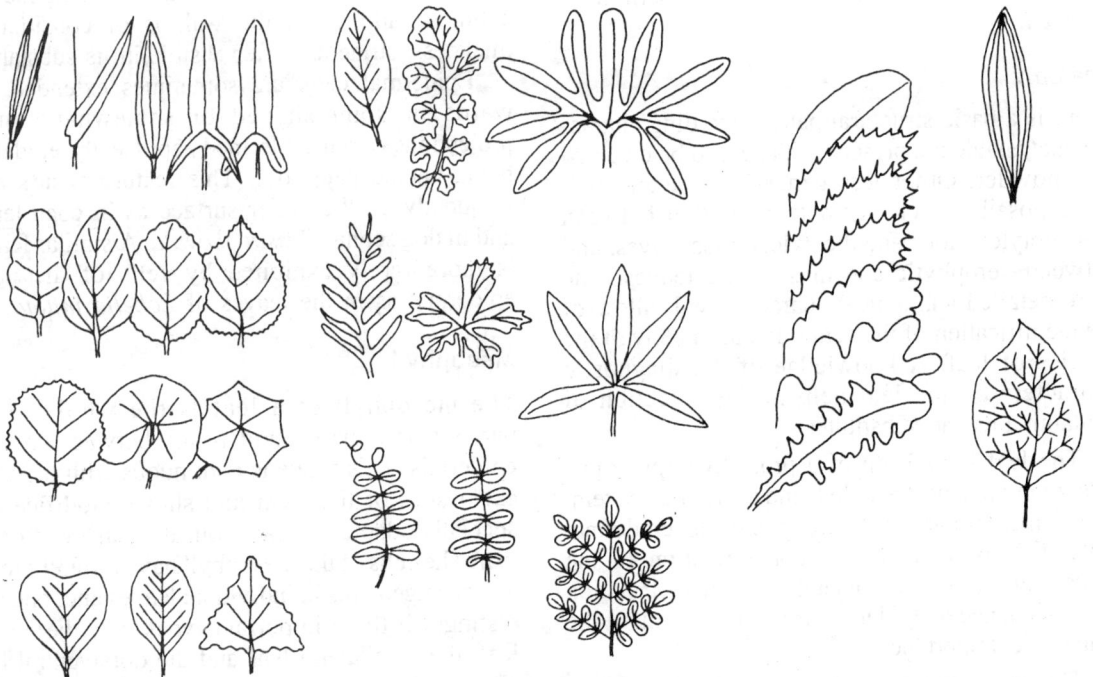

Fig. 3.1. Different types of leaves.

4. *Venation* : Parallel, pinnate (feather-like), palmate, reticulate (net-veined).

5. *Margin*.

6. *Apex*.

7. *Base* : Symmetrical or asymmetrical; cordate and reniform.

8. *Surface* : Colour; glabrous (free from hairs) or pubescent (hairy); if the latter, whether hispid (with rough hairs), hirsute (with long distinct hairs) or with glandular hairs; punctate (dotted with oil glands). Note lines on surface of Coca leaves, raised points on Belladonna, press marks on Tinnevelly senna, etc. Note any differences between the upper and the lower surfaces.

9. *Texture* : Brittle, coriaceous, papery and fleshy.

Arrangement of leaves

Radical (arising from the crown of the root) or *cauline* (arising from the aerial stem). In the Solanaceae note *adnation* (the fusion of part of the leaf with the stem). The arrangement may be *alternate* (e.g., Lobelia), *opposite*, *decussate* (in pairs alternately at right angles; *e.g.*, Peppermint or *whorled*.

Anatomy

There is a basic structural pattern yielding characters that enable the presence of a leaf to be detected in a powder. Other less general characters will make possible such distinctions as that between monocotyledonous and dicotyledonous leaves, and between xerophytic and mesophytic leaves. The more detailed anatomical characters will allow of the identification of the genus and ultimately of the species of leaf. A knowledge of the diagnostic characters of any leaf help in the detection of contaminants and substitutes.

The leaf is built up of a protective epidermis, a parenchymatous mesophyll and a vascular system. The shape, size and wall structure of the epidermal cells; the form, distribution and relation to the epidermal cells of the stomata; the form, distribution and abundance of epidermal trichomes are all of diagnostic importance.

The epidermis is continuous with that of the stem and is the tissue derived from the dermatogen

of the growing point. Usually it consists of a single layer of cells. Many-layered epidermises are seen in *Piper betle* (Betal leaf), *Piper angustifolium* (Matico) and *Ficus elastica* (Indian rubber plant). A many-layered epidermis often acts as water storage tissue as in *Piper betle* and the inner layer is often described as a hypodermia, although a true hypodermis is formed from the cortical tissue—the mesophyll—and not from the dermatogen. The epidermal cells are tabular or lenticular and show a complete absence of intercellular spaces, except where the pores of the stomata occur. The cells, with the exception of the guard cells of the stomata, are all of one kind and in dicotyledons are approximately isodiametric, the depth being usually smaller than the length and breadth; in many monocotyledons, which have long, narrow leaves, the cells are axially elongated and in grasses dwarf cells alternate with others which are many times their length. The outer walls of epidermal cells are usually differentiated into layers; externally is a layer which reacts to the stains for fats and is quite impervious to water; this is the cuticle.

Within the cuticle the wall is composed of cellulose and when the wall is of considerable thickness, striae are often visible in its substances.

Epidermal cells are sometimes extended outwards in dome-shaped or somewhat conical projections which are termed papillae, the epidermis being named pappilose. This feature occurs most frequently on the under surface as in coca leaves and in dog senna, *Cassia obovata*. A similar feature is more rarely exhibited by cells of the upper epidermis as in the leaves of *Lobelia inflata*,

Mesophyll

The mesophyll of a leaf is the whole of the parenchymatous ground tissue between the two epidermis. This tissue is continuous with the cortical tissues of the stem and shows modifications specially adapted to carry out the functions of the leaf. The cells of the mesophyll have different forms and arrangements in individual leaves and, one may distinguish three important types, *viz,* the centric leaf, the isobilateral leaf and the dorsiventral leaf. The centric leaf is approximately cylindrical in shape and the mesophyll shows a radial symmetry. Such leaves have a single axially placed vein, completely surrounded by the mesophyll, which is similar in construction on all sides; examples are the leaves of *Pinus* and of the *Hakea*. The isobilateral leaf is flat and has a layer of one or more rows of palisade cells under each epidermis, as in Senna. The palisade cells are cylindrical and closely packed with their long axes at right angles to the epidermis. Between the cells there are small spaces parallel to the long axes of the cells. Examples of isobilateral leaves are Eucalyptus, in which there are from three to five rows of palisade under each epidermis, and Senna in which there is a single row above and below. The dorsiventral leaf is flat and has a distinct upper and under surface; the upper surface is usually darker in colour than the lower. The mesophyll is divided into a palisade layer of one or more rows of cells under the upper epidermis, and a loose tissue of irregular cells with short projecting arms enclosing abundant intercellular spaces and known as "spongy" parenchyma. The number of layers of cells in the palisade may vary in the same plant according to the degree of exposure to light; this has been demonstrated in the leaves of the beech tree.

The number of layers of palisade is, however, useful in certain plants, *e.g.*, *Cassia montana*, sometimes found as an adulterant of Senna, has 3 or 4 layers of cells in the palisade tissue, whereas Senna has only one layer of palisade cells. Sometimes, the palisade tissue may be absent, as in some leaves of *Digitalis purpurea* and of *Taraxacum officinale*, which then have undifferentiated mesophyll; these leaves are those which have grown in the shade.

In certain leaves the layer of cells immediately beneath the palisade are somewhat funnel-shaped and two or more palisade cells converge at their lower ends and rest upon each funnel-shaped cell, which is known as a collecting-cell.

Idioblasts are cells which differ markedly from the ordinary cells of a tissue in either form, size or contents. Such cells are often present in the mesophyll of leaves; in tea, and hamamelis.

The palisade cells of the mesophyll bear a definite relation to the epidermal cells. Palisade ratio is the average number of palisade cells beneath one epidermal cell, using four contiguous epidermal cells for the count. This ratio has been shown to be sufficiently constant to serve as a diagnostic character of species belonging to the same genus in certain instances, such as the genus *Barosma* and several genera of the Asteraceae.

The mesophyll is divided into small portions by the branching and anastomosis of the veins throughout the tissue. The small areas of green tissue outlined by the veinlets are termed vein-islets and frequently a small vein-tip runs out from the surrounding veinlets into the centre of each islet. The shape of the vein-islets is frequently characteristic and will often enable one to sort out a mixture of leaves which have been broken into small fragments. The number of vein-islets per unit area of leaf surface is constant for any given species of plant and can be used as a character for the identification of species. The *vein-islet number* is the number of vein-islets per square millimetre, and this number is independent of the size of the leaf and does not alter with the age of the plant. The following examples illustrate the value of this character :

Around the veins and midrib the cortical tissues are usually less specialised. In many leaves the palisade is not continued over the veins, which are sometimes associated with colourless collenchyma both above and below and are then said to be transcurrent; in other leaves the palisade is continuous over the veins which are then said to be embedded. Collenchyma is usually present in the midribs and larger veins of most leaves, forming the layer of mechanical elements which supports the projecting tissue of the midrib and large veins; the remaining cortical tissue of these veins consists of round-celled parenchyma.

Stelar tissues

The meristele, in a transverse section of the midrib is usually in the form of an arc having the xylem towards the upper surface arranged in radiating bands spreading towards the lower surface. The phloem forms a band between the xylem and the cortical parenchyma on the lower side. Medullary rays traverse the xylem and phloem in radiating lines. The pericycle lying between the phloem and the cortex is sometimes developed as a band of collenchyma as in *Digitalis purpurea* or, more usually, as an arc of pericyclic fibres as in Senna.

The vascular systems of leaves fall into two main classes : the reticulate venation typical of dicotyledons and the parallel venation of monocotyledons. The midrib bundle of the dicotyledonous leaf may be differentiated. In leaves with a well-differentiated midrib the palisade tissue is usually interrupted in the midrib region and collenchyma frequently occurs above and below the midrib bundle. The main veins, in dicotyledonous leaves, are open and usually collateral. The xylem faces towards the upper surface. The lateral veins are almost entirely collateral even in cases where the midrib bundle is bicollateral. The smallest veins often consist of xylem only. The veins of monocotyledonous leaves are closed bundles.

The midrib bundle is often, as in the Solanaceae, enclosed in an endodermis which may take the form of a starch sheath. The development of the pericycle is variable, in some cases being parenchymatous and containing secretion cells, in some cases consisting of a sheath of pericyclic fibres with their long axes parallel to the vein.

The lateral branches from the midrib sometimes terminate in the apices of the marginal teeth, as in raspberry, and in mulberry, or they may anastomose near the margin and ultimate veinlets from the anastomosis may enter the area of the tooth (serration) and give a characteristic arrangement, as in *Digitalis*, and *Mentha*. These features together with the shape of the outline of the teeth often provide useful diagnostic characters.

Cell contents

All the cells of the mesophyll and the epidermis contain protoplasm, cell-sap and a nucleus; in addition chlorophyll is present in plastids in the cells of the palisade and spongy parenchyma. The chloroplasts are most abundant in the palisade and numerous very small starch grains, frequently somewhat needle-shaped, often occur embedded in the chloroplasts. The epidermal cells of the fronds of ferns normally contain chloroplasts, but the epidermis of angiospermous leaves is generally without them. Many shade plants, however, such as Foxglove, Stramonium and Belladonna, show the presence of small numbers of chloroplasts in the epidermis. Calcium oxalate is an important cell-content and is sometimes, present in the epidermis; the examples are Coca leaves, Savin, *Cupressus sempervirens* and *Globularia alypum*. When calcium oxalate occurs in the palisade tissue, it is usually in the form of cluster crystals, as in Senna. Idioblasts containing microsphenoidal crystals are found scattered throughout the mesophyll of Belladonna. Calcium carbonate occurs as a concretionary deposit encrusted upon cellulose outgrowths from the walls of certain trichomes of *Cannabis sativa* and of unusually large cells of the epidermis of *Ficus elastica*. Cystoliths of an ovoid or elongated cylindrical-ovoid form occur in the epidermis of *Andrographis*, family Acanthaceae. *Diosmin*, $C_{34}H_{44}O_{21}2H_2O$, is another crystalline substance occurring in the epidermis of some leaves such as Buchu and Hemlock. Diosmin occurs in yellowish-grey crystalline masses of various forms and is insoluble in solution of ammonia and in the ordinary microscopical reagents, including solution of chloral hydrate. *Volatile oil* occurs in idioblasts in the leaves of plants belonging to the Lauraceae and to the Piperaceae, such as *Piper betle*. More rarely crystals of *fat* are present in the mesophyll as in *Ilex aquifolium* and Lobelia.

Powdered leaves

The following are consistently present; epidermis with stomata; cellulose parenchyma; not very abundant small-sized vascular elements and chlorophyll. Structures frequently present are epidermal trichomes, glands, palisade cells, crystals of calcium oxalate, collenchyma and pericyclic fibres.

For the differentiations of closely allied leaves it may be necessary to make determinations of such differential characters as vein-islet number, stomatal number, stomatal index and palisade radio.

FLOWERS

The flowers include a number of influorescences.

Convallaria flowers (Lily of the valley) are simple racemose inflorescences, other examples of which are found in Lobelia, Aconite and Foxglove. There is an elongated axis or *rachis*, bearing flowers on *pedicels*, which arise in the axils of the leaves, usually termed *bracts*, the youngest bracts and flowers being nearest to the apex or growing point of the rachis. Other types of recemose inflorescence are the capitula of Chamomile, insect flower, Santonica or wormseed, etc., in which the axis is shortened to form a disc-shaped structure, the receptacle, upon which the flowers or florets are arranged in crossing spiral lines, the youngest florets being at the centre where is the apex of the receptacle. Frequently in a capitulum, the outermost florets possess a corolla elongated to form a strap or ligule, as in Chamomile and insect flowers, such florets being termed ligulate florets have a tubular corolla and constitute the *disc* of the inflorescence. The bracts of a capitulum are partly grouped as an involucre below the inflorescence, when they are barren, *i.e.*, having no flowers in their axils, and they partly occur with the florets as delicate scale-like structures named palece, a floret arising in the axil of each palea.

An umbel having the youngest flower in the centre is an example of a recemose inflorescence in which the internodes of the main axis have not developed and the pedicles of the flowers appear to arise from a common point. Umbels are most usually compound, that is, a number of small umbels arise from the ends of the stems which are themselves arranged in an umbel; this type of inflorescence is found in the drug Kousso, which is an example of a panicle and consists of a number of small recemes arranged in the recemose manner upon a primary axis. Cloves are also arranged in panicles, but the arrangement of the branches is opposite and decussate instead of alternate as in kousso.

A cymose inflorescence is formed when the axis ends in a flower and further flowers must arise upon branches borne laterally upon the first axis. The oldest flower is, therefore, found at the centre of a cymose inflorescence. Stramonium has a dichasial cyme because two lateral axes arise below each flower as it is formed. In Belladonna, one lateral branch only is formed each time, first on one side and then on the other, giving rise to a monochasial cyme, termed a cincinnus. In the Elder, *Sambucus nigra*, several branches arise below the terminal flower and produce a polychasial cyme.

The inflorescences of Lavender, Rosemary and other Lamiaceae plants are good examples of mixed inflorescences, where a number of small cymes are arranged upon a parent axis in a recemose manner.

Individual flowers have the general arrangement of parts found in a leaf-bud, the short axis with undeveloped internodes being termed the thalamus or torus, and the floral leaves are generally arranged in whorls named from below upwards, the calyx, corolla, and androecium and gynoecium or pistil. The individual members of the calyx are sepals which are usually green and most nearly approach foliage leaves in their general character. The petals of the corolla are often white or brightly coloured and of a delicate texture with slender veins and a velvety upper surface. The androecium consists of stamens, each of which has a stalk-like portion or filament and a head or anther within which the pollen is found. The members of the gynoecium are termed carpels and are leaves greatly modified to form one or more closed chambers, called the ovaries, within which the ovules are borne upon a placenta; the ovary is surmounted by a style or styles and stigma.

Amongst common drugs, Saffron and Corn-silk consist of styles and stigmas only; Red poppy, Red rose and Marigold of petals only; elder flowers of petals and stamens.

Collection and drying

Collection of flowers must always be made in fine, dry weather, because petals which are damp when gathered become badly discoloured during drying. Since flowers must be obtained in good condition, they must be gathered at precisely the correct time and consequently the process of collection may extend over several days or in some cases weeks, so that the flowers may be taken as they come to the proper condition upon the inflorescences. The collection is usually made by picking or cutting the flowers by hand.

Cloves, Red rose and Wormseed are collected when in bud; Arnica, Chamomile, Elder and insect flowers when just fully expanded, while Kousso is collected after pollination and fertilisation.

Drying must be done carefully and rapidly, otherwise the colours are spoilt. Most flowers and floral members contain volatile oil, upon which their pharmaceutical value depends and are, therefore, dried at low a temperature. Large airy lofts or barns are often used and the flowers are spread on canvas stretched on frames so that air may get to both sides of the flowers. The flowers or petals are put in a thin layer on the canvas and are turned two or three times a day, the drying being effected at ordinary temperatures and usually in the dark. The drying room should be without windows because light tends to bleach the delicate colours of petals. In an unfavourable climate, petals are sometimes dried by gentle artificial heat in special drying sheds similar to those used for drying leaves.

Flowers and floral parts should be packed and stored in air-tight containers and kept in a cool place away from the light.

The following features are used to describe the complex structure of flowers.

Type of inflorescence

Racemose, cymose or mixed (*e.g.*, racemes of cymes in clove).

Axis or receptacle of inflorescence

The main axis of an inflorescence is called the rachis, while the branches bearing flower clusters and individual flowers are termed peduncles and pedicels, respectively.

Types of flower

Monocotyledon or dicotyledon. Unisexual or hermaphrodite. Regular or zygomorphic. Hypogynous, perigynous or epigynous.

Receptacle of the flower (thalamus or torus)

It is the extremity of the penduncle on which the calyx, corolla, etc. are inserted. When the receptacle is elongated below the calyx, it is called a hypanthium, or if below the ovary, a *gynophore* or stalk of the ovary (Clove).

Calyx

Polysepalous or gamosepalous. Caducous (e.g., poppy) or *persistent* (e.g., belladonna). Describe colour, shape and hairs as for a leaf.

Corolla

Polypetalous or gamopetalous. Observe venation (henbane) and oil glands (clove petals).

Androecium

Note number of stamens; whether free or joined (monadelphous and diadelphous), didynamous or tetradynamous and epipetalous. Dehiscence of anthers (valves, pores or slits).

Gynaecium

Note number of carpels; apocarpous or syncarpous; superior or inferior. Sizes and shapes of stigma, style and ovary. The enlarged base of the styles in the Apiaceae is called a stylopod. Number of loculi, placentation (parietal, axile and free-central).

Ovules

Note number in each loculus; orthotropous, campylotropous, anatropous.

Anatomy

The flower stalk or pedicel has a stem structure. The bracts, calyx and corolla have a leaf structure and will yield such elements as epidemris with stomata, glandular and covering hair, mesophyll cells, oil glands and crystals. The epidermal cells of the corolla often have a papillose or striated cuticle. Delicate coloured fragments of the corolla can often be distinguished in coarsely powdered drugs. The gynaecium sometimes yields from the stigmas a characteristic papillose epidermis. Characteristic fragments of the anther wall are diagnostic of the presence of flowers. The occurrence, size, shape and wall structure of pollen grains are studied.

The sepals commonly possess upper and lower (inner and outer) epidermises which closely resemble those of the leaves and stem of the same plant. Stomata are present and frequently also covering trichomes; when glandular trichomes are present they are often of diagnostic value. The mesophyll is usually undifferentiated and resembles the spongy tissue of a foliage leaf, chloroplasts being present in most of the cells. Petals are much more specialised than the sepals. The upper or inner epidermis is frequently papillose, a condition which gives the velvety appearance to petals. The lower or outer epidermis is without papillae and stomata are often present, but in small numbers. The mesophyll is thin and frequently consists of three or four rows of cells with large intercellular spaces. The colour of petals is due either to a coloured cell-sap or to coloured plastids. Blue and red colours result from the presence of anthocyanin dissolved in the cell-sap and they give red colours with acids and blue or green with alkalies, as in Lavender and Red rose. Yellow pigments may be dissolved in the sap, when they are flavonol derivatives. More commonly yellows are due to the presence of plastids containing carotin and xanthophyll, as in Arnica and Hyoscyamus. Typical glands and trichomes are also common on petals. The vascular system is much reduced, the delicate veins usually consisting of a few very narrow spiral vessels. The anthers of the stamens provide two of the most easily identified structures found in flowers. These are the fibrous layer or endothecium of the pollen sacs and the pollen-grains. The pollen grains are often characteristic either of the plant or of the family, their chief features being the size, shape, sculpturing and markings of the exine, the germinal furrows and germ-pores. The germinal flowers are narrow lanceolate areas where the exine is thinner and their function is to accommodate the expansion and shrinkage of the grain due to changes in humidity.

FRUITS

With the development of the seed from the ovule, the ovary wall develops to form a case, named the pericarp, for the seeds, thus forming a fruit. The wall of the pericarp is usually divisible into three regions, *viz.*, the epicarp on the outside, the endocarp on the inside and the mesocarp between them. The epicarp is usually the outer epidermis only, as in prunes, Lobelia and *Capsicum minimum*. The endocarp similarly may be the inner epidermis only, as in Fennel, or it may consist of several modified layers as in the prune and Olive, where it is developed as a thick woody structure forming the "stone" or casing of the seed. The mesocarp may be succulent as in the prune and Tamarinds, or pithy as in Colocynth or it may consist of several layers of different types, or may be composed of a spongy parenchyma similar to that of foliage leaves, as in

Lobelia; in all cases the vascular strands ramify in the tissues of the mesocarp. When the ovary has two or more loculi, these are found in the fruit and are separated by a septum or septa which are often membranous.

In a superior fruit the pericarp shows at the apex a small point-like scar where the style was attached, a strongly developed persistent stigma as in the capsule of a Poppy. At the base of a superior fruit is found either the persistent calyx, or scars left by the fall of the perianth parts from the thalamus, as in the Poppy. In an inferior fruit the pericarp is surmounted by the persistent calyx and other remains of the perianth as in Lobelia and Pimento, or the scars left by the fall of the perianth parts as in Vanilla. At the base an inferior fruit tapers directly into the pedicel.

Sometimes other floral members such as the thalamus or sepals or other parts of the inflorescence, such as bracts or the inflorescence axis also undergo development and become enlarged or succulent and take part in the formation of fruits.

A simple fruit is formed from a single carpel or from a syncarpous gynaecium, as the prune, olive and quince. An aggregate fruit is formed from an apocarpous gynaecium, examples are Star anise, Aconite and the Raspberry. A compound fruit is formed from a number of flowers closely grouped together, often from an entire inflorescence, examples are the fig, mulberry, long pepper and hops.

The fruits are classified as :

A. Simple (i.e., formed from a gynaeceum with one pistil).

B. Aggregate (i.e., formed from more than one pistil, *e.g.*, Aconite).

C. Collective (i.e., formed not from one flower but from an inflorescence, *e.g.* fig).

1. Simple, dry, indehiscent fruits

1. *Achene* : A small hard indehiscent fruit, formed from one carpel or from two carpels (*e.g.*, the fruit of the Asteraceae). The latter is better termed a cypsela.

2. *Nut* : This is similar to an achene, formed from two or three carpels (*e.g.*, dock fruit).

3. *Caryopis* : This is the type of fruit in which the testa and pericarp are fused (found in the cereals).

2. Simple, dry, dehiscent fruits

1. *Legume* : A fruit formed from one carpel which splits along both dorsal and ventral sultures (*e.g.*, Senna).
2. *Follicle* : A fruit from one carpel which dehisces by the inner suture only; found in aggregates or etaerios (*e.g.*, Aconite and Strophanthus).
3. *Capsules* : Capsules are dry dehiscent fruits formed from two or more carpels. Some bear special names (*e.g.*, the *siliqua* and *silicula* of the Brassicaceae, and the pyxis or pyxidium found in Henbane). The latter is a capsule which opens by means of a lid.

3. Schizocarpic or splitting fruits

A cremocarp, the bicarpellary fruit of the Apiaceae, which splits into two mericarps.

4. Succulent fruits

1. *Drupe* : This is formed from one superior carpel (*e.g.*, Almond and Prune). The inner part of the pericarp, which is called the endocarp, is hard and woody and encloses one seed.
2. *Berry* : This fruit is formed from one or more carpels and the pericarp is entirely fleshy. It is usually many-seeded, *e.g.*, Nux vomica, Colocynth, Orange, Lemon, Capsicum. *Pepo* is the berry of the Cucurbitaceae and hesperidium that of the Orange and similar rutaceous fruits.

Shape and dimensions

Adhesion

Superior or inferior : Fruits from inferior ovaries show floral remains at the apex (*e.g.*, Cardamom, Fennel, unpeeled Colocynth and Lobelia).

Dehiscence

Different types of dehiscence are shown by the legume, follicle, siliqua and the pyxidium and other capsules. Most capsules split longitudinally into valves which are usually equal in number to or double those of the loculi or placentae. Dehiscence is termed septicidal if the valves separate at the line of junction of the carpels or loculicidal if the valves separate between the placentae or dissepiment. In the latter case the placentae or dissepiment may remain attached either to the axis or to the valves.

Pericarp

Colour, texture, markings, number of sutures uniform throughout or modified into epicarp, mesocarp and endocarp.

Placentation

Placentation (*e.g.*, marginal in Senna, parietal in Poppy and axile in Cardamom).

Seeds

Number, shape, colour and size.

Other characters

Odour, taste, food reserves.

Anatomy

The pericarp is bounded by inner and outer epidermal which resemble those of leaves. The outer epidermis may bear stomata and hairs. In fleshy fruits the internal tissue is mainly parenchymatous, resembling the mesophyll of leaves. In dry fruits and fleshy dry fruits it usually contains fibres or sclereids. Secretory tissues such as vittae, oil ducts or cells, and latex tissue are commonly present in the pericarp of medicinal fruits. Husk of cardamoms can be detected by the presence of pitted fibres, spiral vessels and abundant empty parenchymatous cells. The endocarp of almond, used as an adulterant, consists mainly of sclereids.

Portions of receptacle (*e.g.*, the rind of Colocynth), persistent sepals and flower stalk may be present.

The epidermises of the pericarp have the characters of epidermal structures in general and possess stomata, usually in small numbers.

In Coriander certain cells of the outer epidermis contain well-formed solitary crystals of calcium oxalate; in Pepper and Cubeb each epidermal cell contains numerous small rectangular prisms. The epicarp of Pepper and of Cubeb consists of the epidermis and a hypodermal layer of sclereids and parenchyma. Colocynth has a more complex epicarp composed of the epidermis, a few layers of parenchyma and then several layers of lignified sclereids. The inner epidermis of the pericarp. In the fruits of *Capsicum* it consists of parenchyma containing numerous large islands of lignified sclerenchyma, each island corresponding in extent to a giant cell in the hypodermal layer. In *Piper nigrum* the inner epidermis is entirely lignified, the thickening forming beaker-shaped cells and appearing in sections as horse-shoe thickening. In Fennel this epidermis is developed as a lignified parquetry layer, that is, the cells are elongated and arranged in groups of about five to eight parallel cells, each group having arisen from a single mother-cell; these groups are often arranged with the long axes of their cells orientated in different directions as are the blocks of a parquetry flooring. In many fruits a hard endocarp is produced by the formation of one or more layers of sclereids in the hypodermal region; when the layers are very thick a stone results as in the Prune and the Olive. In Cubeb the sclereids are chiefly in a single layer; but in apples and currants there are several layers of elongated fusiform sclereids, the cells of successive layers crossing at a wide angle those of the layers above and below them, the whole forming a strong cartilaginous membrane. The mesocarp may be parenchymatous throughout excepting for the slender vascular strands present in its middle region; this condition is found in the prune and many other fruits. Sometimes lignified idioblasts occur in the parenchyma of the mesocarp as in Lobelia. Frequently the mesocarp contains oil-cells as in Laurel berries, Cubeb and Pepper, or oil-glands as in Pimento, or oil-ducts as in many Apiaceae fruits such as Fennel and Dill. Associated with the vascular bundles laticiferous tissue sometimes occurs as in the capsule wall of *Papaver*, and in many fruits the cells of the mesocarp contain starch grains as in pepper.

SEEDS

A seed is a plant member derived from a fertilised ovule; it contains an embryo and is constructed so as to facilitate its transportation. Structurally a seed is developed from an ovule as a result of growth stimulated by the formation of a zygote from the ovum and of the primary endosperm nucleus from the central fusion nucleus of the embryo-sac. These developments result in the growth of an embryo from the zygote and of food-storage tissues from the embryo-sac and nucellus.

A fertilised ovule is usually protected externally by one or two coverings or coats from which the testa of the seed is developed. When two coats, outer and inner, are present in a seed they are termed the *testa* and tegmen, respectively. Testa is the single coat of seeds having only one coat or to signify the two coats considered as one protective coverings. In the ovule, the coats are not quite complete at the apex, a small hole, the micropyle, being left through which the pollen-tube may pass on its way to embryo-sac; this micropyle persists in the seed and forms a character of the testa.

Within the coats of an ovule is a mass of parenchymatous tissue known as the nucellus. The nucellus is absorbed by the rapidly developing embryo or endosperm and is then represented in the seed by a layer of collapsed cells usually only to be observed in microscopical preparations. In certain seeds, as Cardamom and Pepper, the nucellus increases in bulk as the seed matures and forms a massive storage-tissue, called the perisperm.

Embedded in the nucellus of the ovule is a very large cell, the embryo-sac or megaspore and after fertilisation one finds inside the embryo-sac a zygote, a primary endosperm nucleus and three antipodal cells. The zygote develops by cell-division and becomes the embryo with its cotyledons and a radicle and stem growing point, sometimes developed as a plumule. This development may be so rapid and vigorous that the embryo absorbs the other contents of the embryo-sac and also the contents of the nucellus so that in the seed there is a large embryo surrounded only by the testa, thus forming a non-endospermic or exalbuminous seed.

In other plants the endosperm nucleus rapidly divides and walls form between the protoplasts resulting in a mass of tissue, called endosperm, surrounding the embryo which has developed less vigorously than in exalbuminous seeds. The nucellus is absorbed by the developing endosperm so that the ripe seed consists of an embryo embedded in an endosperm, the whole being surrounded by the testa. These are endospermic or albuminous seeds, containing an embryo surrounded by endosperm.

A third type of development occurs when the endosperm nucleus forms an endosperm and the embryo develops only moderately, but at the same time the cells of the nucellus are stimulated into activity and multiply to form a tissue outside the embryo-sac and surrounding the endosperm. This tissue is the perisperm and the albuminous or endospermic seed which results, consists of an embryo enclosed in an endosperm which is itself surrounded by a perisperm, the whole being enclosed by the testa.

On the surface of the testa some markings can be observed in addition to any mottling or variations in the colouring of the general surface. These markings are the hilum, the raphe, the micropyle and the chalaza, the relative positions of which vary with the type of ovule. The *hilum* is the scar left by the removal of the seed from its funiculus or stalk. The chalaza is the position at the base of the nucellus where the vascular strand from the funiculus branches to enter the different parts of the ovule. The four types of ovule arise by the variation in the extent to which ovules are turned upon their stalks. In the orthotropous or atropous ovule, the nucellus is in a straight line with the funiculus and the micropyle is at the end of the ovule opposite to the hilum; the chalaza at the base of the nucellus is immediately above the hilum; there is no raphe. The most common type of ovule is the anatropous one in which the stalk has grown adherent to one side of the ovule and has also grown so rapidly as to completely invert the ovule on its stalk, thus bringing the micropyle adjacent to the hilum and the chalaza to the distal end of the ovule. In most common seeds, the raphe and chalaza can be observed as markings on the testa and the micropyle is found adjacent to the hilum. Sometimes the rotation of the ovule on its stalk is through an angle of 90 degrees instead of 180 degrees as in the anatropous ovule. When this more limited turning occurs the ovule is termed amphitropous. In such ovules the nucellus is straight with its axis at right angles to the direction of the stalk, which enters the ovule at the middle of one side. There is a short raphe as far as the chalaza at one end of the nucellus; at the other end is the micropyle. In this type, the hilum, chalaza and micropyle are widely separated; an example is the seed of Colchicum. The fourth type of ovule has a curved nucellus produced by a rapid growth of one side of the nucellus and of the coats on the same side, development on the other side being almost arrested. As a result the micropyle is brought adjacent to the chalaza as well as the hilum; there is no raphe. Examples of this type are Stramonium, Henbane and other Solanaceous seeds; they are developed from campylotropous ovules.

An *aril* is a fleshy covering arising from the hilum and almost completely enveloping the seed; *e.g.*, the seed of yew, *Taxus baccata*, and seeds of the Nymphaceae. An *arillode* is a covering similar to an aril, but arising from the micropylar edge as in Cardamom and Euonymus. A caruncle is a localised fleshy growth arising from the micropyle as in seeds of the Euphorbiaceae, such as Castor oil and Croton. A strophiole is a wing-like or barrel-shaped outgrowth along the line of raphe, due to an increase in the amount of parenchyma around the vascular strand of the raphe; such a growth is found in the seed of Colchicum. A *wing* is an extension of the testa in the form of a membranous fold as in the seed of Honesty.

All seeds contain reserve foods for the nourishment of the embryo during germination. These foods may be present in the endosperm or the perisperm or in both, or they may be stored in the embryo itself either in the cotyledons or in the axis. Sometimes, as in Linseed, the food is found in both endosperm and cotyledons. The reserve foods present are usually of two types, *viz.*, carbohydrates and fixed oils which supply the elements carbon, hydrogen and oxygen, and proteins which supply nitrogen, sulphur and phosphorus in addition to the other three elements. The commonest carbohydrate is starch; others are cellulose, hemicellulose and sugar. Starches, sugars, fixed oils and proteins are stored in the cell-cavities, whereas the celluloses are present as heavily thickened cell walls. This gives rise to starchy seeds, such as Wheat and Calabar bean, oily seeds, such as Linseed and the Apiaceae seeds, and very hard horny seeds such as Nux vomica, Ignatius bean and Date stones.

Seeds may be produced from orthotropous, campylotropous or anatropous ovules. The seed consists of a kernel surrounded by one, two or three seed coats. Most seeds have two seed coats, an outer testa and an inner tegmen. The seed is attached to the placenta by a stalk or funicle. The hilum is the scar left on the seed where it separates from the funicle. The raphe is a ridge of fibrovascular tissue formed in more or less anatropous ovules by the adhesion of funicle and testa. The micropyle is the opening in the seed coats which usually marks the position of the radicle. An expansion of the funicle or placenta extending over the surface of the seed like a bag is known as an aril or arillus. A false aril or arillode resembles an aril, but is a seed coat. A caruncle or strophiole is a protuberance arising from the testa near the hilum.

The kernel may consist of the embryo plant only (exalbuminous seeds), or of the embryo surrounded by endosperm or perisperm or both (albuminous seeds). Endosperm and perisperm are tissues containing food reserves and are formed, respectively, inside and outside the embryo sac.

The description of a seed may be arranged as follows :

Size, shape and colour

Funicle, raphe and aril.

Hilum and micropyle

Size and positions.

Seed coats

Number, arillode, caruncle or strophiole. Thickness and texture of testa; whether uniform in colour or not; smooth, pitted or reticulate. If hairs are present, describe their length, texture and arrangement. Mechanism for dispersal (e.g., awn of strophanthus).

Perisperm

Present or absent. Nature of food reserves.

Endosperm

Present or absent. Nature of food reserves.

Embryo

Size and position (e.g., straight in Strophanthus, curved in Stramonium, folded in Mustard). Size, shape, number and venation of cotyledons. Size and shape of radicle.

Anatomy

A highly diagnostic sclerenchymatous layer is often present. The number of cell layers, and their structure, arrangement, colour and cell contents are varied. The epidermis of the testa is often composed of highly characteristic, thick-walled cells. It may bear typical hairs.

The *epidermis* is variously developed in different seeds and may take the following forms:

(a) A palisade layer, which consists of cells having the form of polygonal prisms, the length being from three to eight times the breadth. In the Leguminosae, such as calabar bean, soy bean and peas, the lumen is enlarged at the base of each cell and then suddenly narrow to a fine pore for the greater part of its length, the wall being very thick and usually cellulosic.

(b) A layer of sclereids is present in Stramonium, Capsicum, Henbane and Nux vomica. In the Solanaceous seeds the thickening is usually on the radial walls and the base giving beaker-shaped cells and they are usually lignified. In Lobelia the elongated polygonal cells are lignified and thickened strongly on the anticlinical walls and in Strophanthus the cells are similar.

(c) A layer containing scattered scleroids either singly or in groups as in Almond and Peach kernel.

(d) A *mucilaginous* layer is present in Linseed, Mustard, Psyllium, Ispaghula, Cress, etc. Mucilage fills the lumina of the cells, having been laid down by the protoplasm as a deposit on the walls. Before the appearance of the mucilage, the cells are usually filled with starch granules and as these disappear the mucilage accumulates.

(e) A layer bearing trichomes. The trichomes are generally unicellular, but vary much in number, size, form and thickening. In *Strophanthus gratus* the trichomes are scattered and are only slightly larger than conical papillae. In Kaladana, *Ipomoea hederacea*, the trichomes are erect, conical, unicellular and scattered; to the naked eye these seeds also appear glabrous. In Nux vomica and *Strophanthus kombe* nearly every cell is prolonged into an appressed trichome, about 1 mm long, giving a silky appearance to the seeds. In species of *Gossypium* the trichomes are very long—about 20 to 40 mm—and slender—about 16 to 21 μ wide—and are unicellular and arranged at right angles to the seed epidermis to form a woolly covering.

(f) In Cardamom the epidermis consists of a layer of thin-walled *prosenchyma*.

(g) Stomata occur in the epidermis. In the seed of *Gossypium spp.*, stomata are present both singly and in pairs.

The pigment layer

In all coloured seeds pigment is deposited in one of the layers of the testa. In Linseed and Mustard, the cell-contents of a layer of the inner seed-coat are deeply coloured, and in Cardamom, the cell-walls of the outer epidermis of the inner seed-coat contain the pigment. In Ispaghula seeds the inner epidermis of the testa contains the colouring matter.

The storage tissues perisperm, endosperm, and cotyledons, are composed of uniform cells often containing characteristic cell contents (*e.g.*, aleurone, starch, calcium oxalate, fixed oil, volatile oil).

The radicle, plumule and leaf-like cotyledons yield little of diagnostic significance to the powdered drug.

Aleurone grains, carbohydrate reserves and a little vascular tissue are constantly present in seeds. Fruits yield similar characters, except that the amount of vascular tissue is greater and lignified elements of the pericarp are often present.

When perisperm is present as a well-developed tissue, it is usually composed of a thin-walled parenchyma containing abundant starch, as in Cardamom, Pepper and Grains of paradise (*Amomum melegueta*).

In the castor seed (*Ricinus communis*) the perisperm appears as a very narrow film surrounding the endosperm and is often described as a tegmen.

Endosperm which is present in many seeds is composed of a cellulose-walled parenchyma containing food reserves. The walls are usually thin, but in some seeds such as Nux vomica and Ignatius bean, the walls become very thick, being largely composed of hemi-celluloses; in other seeds, such as the date (*Phoenix dactylifera*) they are so heavily thickened that they resemble stone-cells. The cells contain protoplasm and various reserve foods. The cotyledons frequently show an approach to a typical leaf structure with a palisade layer beneath the upper epidermis.

Of the reserve foods found in seeds, the most characteristic are the protein reserves, which may be present as an amorphous mass completely filling the cells as in the endosperm of cardamoms, or may take the form of definite grains named aleurone grains. Seeds are the only plant members in which aleurone grains occur and hence a powder containing these grains may be known to have been derived from a seed. The aleurone may be segregated in a particular tissue or part of a tissue or it may be distributed throughout the tissues in association with other reserves. In Cardamom it is present in the endosperm and starch is stored separately in the much larger perisperm. In many cereals, such as wheat and maize, the aleurone is confined to the outermost layer of the endosperm; in *Ricinus communis*, Linseed and Strophanthus it is stored in both embryo and endosperm in association with fixed oil and in peas and beans it is stored in the cotyledons in association with starch; in Nutmeg, *Myristica fragrans*, fat, aleurone and starch all occur together in the cells of the endosperm.

RHIZOMES AND ROOTS (Subterranean organs)

Rhizomes are stem structures growing horizontally, vertically or in an oblique direction at the surface of the ground in which much of the lower part is embedded. The surface bears scale-leaves with occasional buds in their axils and is often marked with the encircling scars of fallen aerial leaves. The lower surface of horizontal rhizomes and the whole surface of vertical and oblique rhizomes bear the *roots* which are usually slender and are adventitious. Scars of fallen roots appear as small circular marks.

The growth of the rhizome may proceed monopodially as in Male fern, when the same growing point persists from year to year and produces the successive yearly portions of the rhizome. In other plants such as Podophyllum, the rhizome develops sympodially, each season's growth ending in a flowering stem, while the rhizome is carried forward by the development of a bud in the axil of one of the basal leaves of the stem. Each flowering aerial axis has its scar on the upper surface of the rhizome. A vertical rhizome is often termed a rootstock and is usually not much greater in diameter than the main tap-root; the internodes are short and the surface has ring-shaped leaf-scars and often transverse wrinklings due to shortening to keep the crown at the ground level, as in Gentian. A stolon is an underground stem similar in function to a runner, like that of a Strawberry, but is much thicker and travels near or below the surface of the soil and roots at its extremity. Stolons form the bulk of the so-called root of liquorice.

If a number of separate steles are present, the drug is cryptogamic in origin; if a circle of bundles and a central pith, it is dicotyledonous, and if bundles are scattered uniformly throughout stele and cortex and an endodermis is evident, the drug is monocotyledonous in origin. In rhizomes, the transverse surface never shows a central solid mass of xylem, a useful character which helps to distinguish rhizomes from roots.

Functionally rhizomes are organs of parennation and contain reserves in the parenchyma, most commonly starch as in Rhubarb and Valerian. Inulin, sugar and other reserves also occur and afford characteristic appearances and tests.

A corm, being an underground axis, is closely related to a rhizome. It differs from a rhizome since one season's development only is usually present, the axis of the previous season having entirely disappeared. In a few plants, such as *Tritonia* (= *Montbretia*), the corms of successive seasons remain attached in a vertical row, forming a kind of rhizome and indicating the close relationship of corm and rhizome.

Roots

The root is that portion of the plant axis, which, in seedlings, grows vertically downwards into the soil. When the primary root persists and is much more strongly developed than its branches, it is named a tap-root, as in Aconite, Belladonna and Dandelion. Roots bear only one kind of lateral appendage, namely, branches, which are similar in construction to the main root. The origin of the branches is described as endogenous, because the growing point arises in the outermost layer of the stele, in the pericycle. The branches are arranged in regular vertical lines, since they arise opposite to the protoxylem groups of the vascular system. There are as many rows of lateral branches as there are protoxylem groups in the stele. Sometimes two rows of lateral roots arise opposite each protoxylem mass thus giving double rows of lateral roots. As the young root descends into the soil, it meets with obstacles and turns aside to avoid them; as a result roots are rarely straight, and most drugs consisting of roots are, therefore, tortuous.

The appearance of the smoothed transversely cut surface of a root differs in dicotyledons and monocotyledons. In dicotyledons, to which the majority of drugs occurring as roots belong, there is a central woody core surrounded by the cambium, a cylinder of secondary phloem and covered externally by a layer of cork. After secondary growth has commenced, the phellogen arises in the pericycle so that in all dicotyledonous roots of any size, the whole of the cortex is exfoliated and most commercial roots show neither pith nor cortex. The root of Aconite is an exception in both of these respects, because no phellogen is formed and there is a large pith which increases in bulk as the root matures.

In monocotyledonous roots, a pith is usually present and is often composed of thick-walled lignified cells; the xylem is porous and a cortex is present and frequently also root-hairs, as in the sarsaparillas.

Collection and drying

Roots and rhizomes are usually collected when their tissues are fully stored with reserve foods, it being assumed that medicinal constituents will also be most abundant at this season. In Britain and other temperate regions autumn is, therefore, the season for collection. Large roots and rhizomes are generally sliced transversely or longitudinally or in both directions to facilitate drying. They are usually spread out on a floor or shelves, which in suitable weather may be arranged out of doors under a roof so that the warm air may blow through them. In cold places some artificial heating must almost always be employed and a quite gentle heat is used at first to avoid gelatinisation of starch. After partial drying, the temperature is raised as drying approaches completion. Care must be taken that the finished drug is completely dry to the centre as evidenced by its breaking with a short, crisp fracture; carelessness in this operation leads to the appearance of moulds during storage. Most roots and rhizomes require from ten days to three weeks to dry thoroughly. Some roots develop their important constituents as a result of fermentation during drying, which is then a prolonged operation carried out at a low temperature. In tropical and subtropical countries the heat of the sun is commonly used for drying operations.

Roots and rhizomes, which are transversely sliced preparatory to drying, are Calumba, Ipomoea (Orizaba jalap), Colchicum, Rhubarb (in very thick slices), Bryony, Gentian (rarely), Jalap (rarely), Aconite when dried in China. Those which are usually sliced longitudinally are Male fern, Valerian, Belladonna, green Hellebore, Rhubarb and Marshmallow.

The following scheme may be used with suitable modifications for the description of most subterranean organs.

Morphological nature

Rhizome and root.

Condition

Fresh or dry; whole or sliced; peeled or unpeeled.

Subaerial stems

Remains of subaerial stems occur in Aconite and Serpentary. They may be present in sufficient amount to constitute an adulteration.

Subterranea stems

1. Size and shape.
2. Direction of growth and branching.
3. Surface characters : Colour, stem scars, buds, cataphyllary leaves, roots or root scars, lenticels, cracks, wrinkles, surface crystals, evidence of insect attack and peeling.

4. Fracture and texture : Flexible, brittle, hard, horny, mealy and splintery.
5. Transverse section : Colour, distribution of lignified and secretory elements (*e.g.*, in Ginger); relative sizes of bark, wood and pith; any abnormalities such as the star spots and absence of a lignin reaction in rhubarb.

Roots

1. Kind : True (*i.e.*, developed from the radicle or its branches) or adventitious.
2. Size and shape : Tuberous, conical and cylindrical.
3. Surface characters : Colour, cracks, wrinkles, annulations and lenticels.
4. Fracture and texture.
5. Transverse section : Note absence of pith, whether the wood is markedly radiate or not, and any abnormalities such as are found in Jalap and Senega.
6. Food reserves and chemical tests
7. Odour and taste

Anatomy of rhizomes

Rhizomes, being modified stems, possess a structure having a general resemblance to that of aerial stems. Since, rhizomes grow at or below the ground level, they have no need to develop a structure which could enable them to support themselves in a rare medium, like air, or to resist lateral stresses such as result from violent winds. The supporting tissues in rhizomes are, therefore, ill-developed and an arrangement of either xylem or sclerenchyma in the form of a tube, as is so frequent in aerial stems, is rarely seen.

Tegumentary tissues are not very extensive, usually either an epidermis as in Podophyllum or a few layers of thin-walled cork as in Ginger and Liquorice. Nothing in the nature of rhytidoma is developed. Cork is sometimes replaced by a modification of the outer layers of the cortex. The walls of these cortical cells become suberised and form a protective tissue named metaderm, as in Veratrum rhizome. The metaderm is easily distinguished from cork because its cells are rounded and are not arranged in radial rows.

The cortex usually consists of thin-walled parenchyma containing reserves, such as starch.

The endodermis is not always differentiated and there is an absence of sclerenchyma and supporting tissues in all large bulky rhizomes, such as Rhubarb and Ginger.

The *stele* in rhizomes shows the arrangement characteristic of the group of plants to which the rhizome belongs. For this reason, the transversely cut surface of a rhizome affords a useful character of identification. The Male fern has a characteristic dictyostele; some dicotyledons, such as Podophyllum, have a circle of separate bundles and show an absence of interfascicular cambium. In other dicotyledons, such as Liquorice and Ipecacuanha, a complete cambium ring is formed and secondary xylem and phloem are developed as in aerial stems. Monocotyledonous rhizomes usually possess a definite endodermis, near which numerous smaller vascular bundles occur, while larger bundles are found towards the centre, scattered throughout the ground tissue, and leaf-trace bundles are fairly numerous in the cortex. The tegumentary tissue may be cork as in Ginger, or metaderm as in Veratrum, or epidermis as in Couch grass.

Anatomy of roots

Roots of vascular plants belonging to different groups shows a close similarity in their primary structure. Externally there is a piliferous layer, covering the parenchymatous cortex. The endodermis is generally well-marked and has either a strongly developed casparian strip or some special form of thickening. The stele is surrounded by a single layer of pericycle and has bundles of xylem and phloem arranged in a circle, alternating in position so that each lies on a different radius. The bundles are all centripetal in development, and the xylem bundles frequently develop until they meet at the centre of the root, forming a rod-shaped mass of xylem.

Pteridophyte roots are usually very simple and slender and they permanently retain the primary structure; the roots of *Dryopteris filix-mas* are diarch. The slender roots of many rhizomes also show a well-marked primary structure, which is dicotyledonous plants, such as *Helleborus niger*, which is four- to five-arch, and *Podophyllum peltatum* which is four- to nine-arch, may show a slight amount of secondary development in the older parts, which are the portions of the roots nearest to the rhizome.

Other dicotyledonous roots, which grow to a large size, such as Belladonna and Gentian, develop a cambium on the inside of the primary phloem bundles and outside the protoxylem groups. The greater activity of the cambium on the inside of the phloem bundles forms wedges of secondary xylem and the cambium and phloem are carried outwards until they are equidistant radially with the cambium outside the protoxylem groups. Opposite each protoxylem group the cambium usually forms parenchyma only, thus giving rise to the largest medullary rays which can be easily observed in the transverse section of almost any dicotyledonous root.

Cork formation usually takes place at a deeper layer than in stems, the phellogen arising in the pericycle. This formation of cork results in the death of the endodermis, cortex and piliferous layer, all of which are ultimately rubbed off. Large dicotyledonous roots, such as Belladonna, Gentian and Ipecacuanha, therefore, show a complete absence of cortical tissues. The phellogen cuts off cells on the inner side and these constitute a phelloderm, which is often largely developed, as in Ipecacuanha, and becomes stored with reserves such as starch.

Monocotyledonous rhizomes can be distinguished from dicotyledonous rhizomes by the scattered arrangement of their vascular bundles. Stem structures may usually be distinguished from roots by the fact that they bear buds and possess a well-marked pith. In underground organs chlorophyll is absent, and starch, when present, is usually abundant and in the form of the large grains of reserve starch.

The primary root shows the following structures : a piliferous layer composed of a single layer of thin-walled cells, devoid of cuticle and bearing root hairs formed as lateral outgrowths of the cells; a parenchymatous cortex, the innermost layer of which is differentiated into an endodermis; and a vascular cylinder or stele taking the form of a radial protostele or less frequently of a medullated protostele. The vascular tissues of the stele are enclosed in a single or many-layered pericycle. The protostele is composed of a central mass of xylem tissue with two or more radiating arms and of phloem groups located between the xylem arms. The xylem is differentiated in a centripetal direction, so that the protoxylem groups occupy the ends of the xylem arms and the metaxylem makes up the inner xylem mass. The number of protoxylem groups is usually fairly constant for a given species. The xylem is described as diarch (*Solanum* spp.), triarch (Alfalfa), tetrarch (Liquorice, *Ipomoea* spp.) or polyarch, according to the number of protoxylem groups present. The central xylem cylinder is medullated in some cases (e.g., Valerian). The phloem groups are usually separated from the xylem cylinder by a narrow zone of parenchyma ('fundamental parenchyma').

In many roots size of the axis is accomplished by secondary thickening. Secondary thickening is initiated in the zone of 'fundamental parenchyma', the whole or part of which becomes meristematic. The derived cells mature as secondary phloem centrifugally and as secondary xylem centripetally. From the point of initial cambial activity there is a progressive tangential development, the cambia extending laterally until they reach the points where the protoxylem groups abut on to the pericycle. The pericycle opposite the protoxylem groups becomes meristematic and thus a continuous cambial cylinder is formed. The activity of the cambium opposite the protoxylem groups gives rise to the broad primary rays.

With the development of the secondary vascular tissues, the primary phloem groups are forced outwards and gradually obliterated. Divisions take place in the pericycle, so that it increases in diameter with the expansion of the vascular cylinder. Often the pericycle also increases in thickness, becoming many layers, and forms a 'secondary cortex'. The piliferous layer, cortex and endodermis become fractured and are cut off by the formation of a phellogen in the outermost layer of cells derived from the pericycle. At a still later stage a new phellogen may arise in the secondary phloem, with a consequent disintegration of the pericycle.

Monocotyledons characteristically exhibit no secondary thickening. Jalap shows anomalous secondary thickening.

UNORGANIZED DRUGS

Unorganized drugs have no uniform structure throughout and are not composed of cells built up into definite plant or animal members or organs. They are usually derived from parts of plants or animals by some process of extraction, such as incision, e.g., Opium, decoction, e.g., Agar, expression, e.g., Olive oil, or are natural secretions such as Beeswax and Myrrh.

Unorganized drugs can be classified under headings based upon their origin and nature, giving well-characterised groups, such as dried latex (Opium), dried juice (Aloes), extracts (Catechu), gums (Acacia), resin (Colophony), gum-resins (Myrrh), oleo-resins (Copaiba), waxes (Beeswax), saccharine substances (Honey), oils and fats (Castor oil, Lard), volatile oils (oil of Cloves) and balsams.

The commercial articles so obtained are frequently solids, but some, such as oils and balsams, are fluids. In describing them various physical characters of form, colour, fracture, etc; solubilities in common solvents, and chemical tests are used. These characters and tests enable one to identify and distinguish the drugs included in this category.

The following scheme may be used in their examination.

Physical state

Solid, semisolid or liquid.
1. If solid :
   (a) Size and form : Tears, lumps, etc., and their approximate size and weight.
   (b) Packing : Paper, skins, leaves, plastic, etc.
   (c) External appearance : Colour, shiny or dusty; opaque or translucent; presence of vegetable fragments.
   (d) Hardness and fracture : Conchoidal and porous.
   (e) Solubility in water and organic solvents.
   (f) Vegetable debris, if any, remaining insoluble (e.g., in Myrrh and Asafoetida).
   (g) Effect of heat : Melting, charring, sublime or burn without leaving appreciable ash.
   (h) Microscopical appearance of powder, sublimate (e.g., Balsams) or insoluble matter (e.g., Opium and Catechu).
2. If liquid : Colour, fluorescence, viscosity, density, optical rotation, solubility.

Odour and taste

Chemical tests, chromatographic and spectroscopic characteristics.

Plant Identification

Identification of an unknown plant is an important taxonomic activity. A plant specimen is identified by comparison with already known herbarium specimens in a herbarium, and by utilising available literature. Many plants grow in areas far removed from the centres of botanical research and training. Therefore, a large number of specimens are collected. For proper description and documentation of these specimens, these have to be suitably prepared for incorporation and permanent storage in a herbarium.

There are various other methods employed for identification, and their choice largely depends on the nature of problem being handled. Since the activity of plant identification and nomenclature is carried out with the help of herbaria, botanic gardens, taxonomic literature and information in respect of these are essential.

HERBARIUM

A herbarium is a place where plant material is preserved using various techniques and arranged in the sequence of an accepted classification. Mostly this preservation includes drying and pressing of the plant material. Certain plants, which are either succulent or otherwise unsuitable for pressing and drying technique, may be fixed in suitable liquid preservations such as formaldehyde (2-5%) - acetic acid - alcohol or FAA (5 : 5 : 90).

Herbarium techniques involve : (i) collection, (ii) drying, (iii) poisoning, (iv) mounting, (v) stitching, (vi) labelling and (vii) deposition.

Specimens, properly prepared, can retain their essential features for a very long period. Such specimens can prove immensely useful for future scientific studies including compilation of floras, taxonomic monographs and, in some cases, even experimental studies, since the seeds of several species can remain viable for many years even in dry herbarium specimens.

Collection

Collection of plant material for the herbarium should be done using aesthetic sense and scientific mind. One who collects must know what is to be collected. Indiscriminate collection may often prove to be worthless.

Angiospermic material must be so chosen that it is perfect and complete for determination, *i.e.*, it must have fully grown leaves, complete inflorescence, flowers and fruits as far as possible. In forests with deciduous elements this may not be possible and satisfactory material may be obtained by repeated visits to the locality. Size of the material depends upon the requirement and availability. The woody elements can well be represented by flowering twigs 30-40 cm in length while herbaceous forms may be suitably collected along with the underground parts. There is no fixed rule for the number of specimens required but normally 4 to 6 twigs or complete plants may be enough for routine collections. Tiny herbaceous plants may be collected in large numbers since many can be made into a single herbarium sheet.

Diseased plants, depauperate specimens and infected twigs and should be avoided as far as practicable. All such collections should be given field numbers, roughly one field number per species with about 4-6 duplicates. Relevant information in respect of all those aspects needed for determination must be noted in a field notebook. This should include notes on habit, habitat, flower colour, locality, altitude and other interesting features which cannot be preserved on herbarium sheets.

The plants are collected for various purposes: building new herbaria or enriching older ones, compilation of floras, material for museums and classwork, ethnobotanical studies, and introduction of plants in gardens. In addition, bulk collections are done for trade and drug manufacture. Depending on the purpose, resources, proxi-mity of the area and duration of studies, fieldwork may be undertaken in different ways :

(i) *Collection trip* : Of short duration, usually one or two days, to a nearby place, for brief training in fieldwork, vegetation study and plant collection by groups of students.

(ii) *Exploration* : Repeated visits to an area in different seasons, for a period of a few years, for intensive collection and study, aimed at compilation of floristic accounts.

(iii) *Expedition* : Undertaken to remote and difficult areas, to study the flora and fauna, and usually takes several months. Most of our early information on Himalayan flora and fauna has been the result of European and Japanese expeditions.

Equipment

The equipment for fieldwork may involve a long list, but the items essential for collection include plant press, field notebook, bags, vasculum, pencil, cutter, pruning shears, knife and a digging tool such as trowel or pickaxe.

(i) Plant press

A plant press consists of two wooden, plywood or wire mesh planks, each 12 inches × 18 inches (30 cm × 45 cm), between which are placed corrugated sheets, blotters and newspaper sheets. Two straps, chains or belts are used to tighten the press. Corrugated sheets or ventilators are made of cardboard, and help ventilation and the consequent drying of specimens. The ducts of the corrugated sheet run across and not lengthwise to afford shorter distance and larger number of ducts.

The plant press carried in the field and called a field press is light weight and generally has one corrugated sheet alternating with one folded blotter containing ten folded newspaper sheets, one meant for each specimen.

The plant press used for subsequent pressing and drying of specimens is called the drying press. It is much heavier and has an increased number of corrugated sheets, one alternating each folded blotter containing one folded newspaper. In countries such as India which use thick coarse paper for newsprint, blotters can be dispensed with, in at least subsequent changes, as the paper soaks sufficient moisture and serves the purpose of blotters as well.

(ii) Field notebook

Field notebook or field diary is an important item for a collector. A well-designed field notebook (Fig. 4.1) has numbered sheets with printed proforma for entering field notes such as scientific name, family, vernacular name, locality, altitude, date of collection and for recording any additional data collected in the field. The multiple detachable slips at the lower end of the sheet, separated by perforated lines

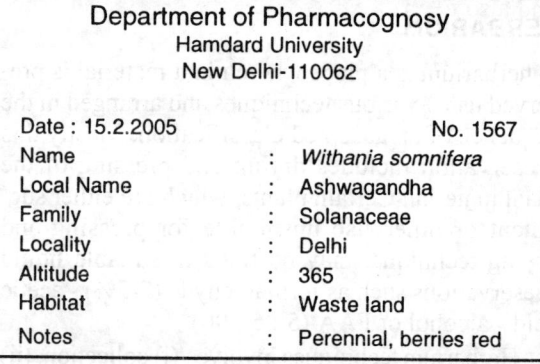

Department of Pharmacognosy
Hamdard University
New Delhi-110062

Date : 15.2.2005		No. 1567
Name	:	*Withania somnifera*
Local Name	:	Ashwagandha
Family	:	Solanaceae
Locality	:	Delhi
Altitude	:	365
Habitat	:	Waste land
Notes	:	Perennial, berries red

Fig. 4.1. A sheet from the field notebook with relevant entries.

and bearing the serial number of the sheet, can be used as tags for multiple specimens of a species collected from a site, and serve as ready reference to the information recorded in the field notebook. The number also serves as the collection number for the collector.

(iii) Vasculum

This is a metallic box with a tightly fitted lid and with a shoulder sling. It is used to store specimens temporarily before pressing, and also to store bulky parts and fruits. It is generally painted white to deflect heat and affords easy detection when left in the field. Being bulky, the vasculum is commonly substituted by a polythene bag, which is almost weightless. A number of polythene bags can be carried for easy storage, as these can be readily made airtight using a rubber band and, as such the plants retain freshness for many hours.

Collection

The specimen collected should be as complete as possible. Herbs, very small shrubs, as far as possible should be collected complete, in flowering condition, along with leaves and roots. Trees and shrubs should be collected with both vegetative and flowering shoots, to enable the representation of both leaves and flowers. All information concerning the plant should be recorded in the field notebook and a tag from the sheet attached to the concerned specimen. It is advisable to collect a few specimens of each species from the site, to ensure that reserve specimens are available if one or more get destroyed, and also to ensure that duplicates can be deposited in different herbaria, when finally mounted on sheets.

Pressing

The specimens should be placed in the field press at the first opportunity, either directly after collection, or sometimes after temporary storage in a vasculum or a polythene bag. A specimen shorter than 15 inches (38 cm) should be kept directly in the folded newspaper after loosely spreading the leaves and branches. Herbs, which are generally collected along with the roots, if longer than 15 inches, can be folded in the form of a V, N or W,

always ensuring that the terminal part of the plant with leaves, flowers and fruits is erect, and when finally mounted, the specimens can be easily studied, without having to invert the herbarium sheet. Specimens of grasses and some other groups, which show considerable elasticity, are difficult to hold in a folded condition. These specimens can be managed by using flexostat (a strip of stiff paper or card with 2.5 cm long slit). One flexostat inserted at each corner holds the specimen in place.

To press bulky fruits, these may be thinly sliced. Large leaves can be trimmed to retain any lateral half. It is useful to invert some leaves so that the undersurface of the leaves can also be studied from a pressed leaf.

Collection and pressing of special groups

A few groups of plants such as conifers, water plants, succulents and mucilaginous plants pose problems during collection and need special methods.

Conifers, although easy to collect and press, pose problems during drying. The tissues of conifers remain living for a long time and progressive desiccation during pressing and drying initiates an abscission layer at the base of leaves and sporophylls. As such a dry twig readily disintegrates, losing its leaves with a slight touch, a problem occasionally encountered in *Abies, Picea, Cedrus* and several other genera. Before pressing, such twigs should be immersed in boiling water for one minute, a pretreatment that kills tissue and prevents the abscission formation during drying. A pretreatment method involves immersion in 70% ethyl alcohol for 10 minutes followed by immersion in 50% aqueous glycerine solution for four days. Since the pretreatment removes the bloom and waxes, and results in a slight colour change, an untreated portion of the plant should be preserved, kept in a small pouch and attached to the herbarium sheet along with the pretreated specimen for reference.

Water plants, especially with submerged leaves and Aloe readily collapse due to the absence of cuticle and are difficult to press normally. Such specimens are collected in bags and made to float in a tray filled with water, at the bottom of which a white sheet of paper is placed. The paper is lifted gently, carrying the specimen along, placed in a blotter and pressed. As the slender water plant sticks to the paper, the sheet along with the specimen is shifted from one blotter to another during the process of drying, and finally pasted on the herbarium sheet as such.

Succulents and cacti have a large amount of proliferated parenchyma storing water and, unless special care is taken, these plants readily rot and fungal infection sets in. Such plants are handled by giving slits on thick organs and scooping out the succulent tissue or, alternatively, salt is sprinkled on slits to drive out the moisture. The plants may also be killed by pretreatment with ethyl alcohol or formaldehyde.

Mucilaginous plants such as members of the family Malvaceae stick to the blotters and are difficult to process. These plants should be placed between waxed or tissue paper or else folds of muslin cloth. Only the blotter should be changed every time and the specimen separated from the tissue paper or muslin when fully dry.

Aroids and bulbous plants continue to grow even in a press and should be killed with ethyl alcohol and formaldehyde before pressing.

Drying

Drying of pressed plant specimens is a slow process if no artificial heat is used.

(i) Natural drying

A slow process, which may take up to one month for complete dessication. The plants, freshly collected are placed in a press without corrugated sheets and the press locked for 24 hours. During this sweating period, plants lose some moisture, become flaccid and can be easily rearranged. The folded sheet containing the specimen is lifted and placed in a fresh dry folded blotter. In countries using thick coarse newsprint, changing the newspaper is also necessary, and the plant should be carefully transferred from one newspaper to another. The use of a blotter in such a case can be dispensed with, especially after one or two changes. The change of blotters or newspaper sheets is repeated every few days, increasing the interval between the change successively until the specimens are fully dry. The whole process of drying may take about 10 days to one month, depending on the specimens and the climate of the area.

(ii) Drying with artificial heat

Drying with the help of artificial heat takes 12 hours to two days. The specimens after the initial sweating period in the field press are transferred to a drying press, with an ample number of corrugated sheets, usually one alternating every folded blotter containing one specimen. The press is kept in a drier, a cabinet in which a kerosene lamp or electric bulb warms the air, which dries the specimens by movement through the corrugates. Use of a hot air blower in the cabinet speeds up circulation of the hot air and consequently faster drying is achieved. A solar-powered drier is capable of drying 100 specimens on a sunny day, and attaining a temperature of up to 60°C in the centre of the press. The unit consists of a flat plate collector and a drying box to hold the press. The collector is composed of a wooden frame, a blackened aluminium absorber plate, insulation and a glass or Plexiglas glazing to retain and channel heat into the drying box. One-inch space is provided between the glazing and the absorber plate. The air enters the collector at the open bottom of the collector panel, is heated by conduction from the absorber, rises by convection into the drying box, moves through the corrugates and finally exits from the uncovered top of the drying box, taking with it moisture from the plant specimens. Drying is accomplished in a single day, occasionally two days for complete drying. This solar drier, with practically no operational cost, should provide a right step towards energy conservation.

The rapid drying of specimens using artificial heat has, however, inherent limitations of rendering plants brittle, loss of bloom and some colour change in leaves.

In arid regions the plants can be dried partially during travel by placing the press horizontally on the luggage rack of the vehicle, with the corrugation ducts facing front, forcing the dry wind through the corrugates as the vehicle moves forward.

Specimens pressed and dried are next mounted on herbarium sheets and properly labelled before these can be incorporated in a herbarium.

Important herbaria

Plant specimens collected over the years have been preserved with great care in herbaria throughout the world and are available for reference and study. The herbaria were established as early as the eighteenth century but gradually there have been great many improvement and modern herbaria are very much different from those of say, Linnaeus in Sweden in the eighteenth century or Roxburgh's in India in the early nineteenth century.

Now there are many herbaria located throughout the world that are of great value to botanists and other workers who need information regarding plants. A detailed index of the world herbaria has been compiled wherein about 850 institutions including 50 major herbaria have been reported. Most of these have long names and for the sake of brevity and convenience their names have been abbreviated. Some of the more important herbaria are listed here. Figures on the right-hand side indicate the approximate number of specimens.

Royal Botanic Gardens, Kew	over 6,000,000
British Museum of Natural History	6,000,000
Museum of Natural History, Paris	6,000,000
V.L. Komarov Botanical Institute of Azerbaijan Academy of Science of Baku, Russia	4,000,000
Conservatoire at Jardin Botaniques de Geneve	5,000,000
Royal Botanic Garden, Edinburgh	1,500,000
National Herbarium of Victoria, Melbourne, Australia	1,500,000
US National Herbarium, Washington D.C.	3,860,000
New York Botanical Garden	4,000,000
Herbarium of Missouri Botanical Garden, St. Louis	2,357,000
Gray Herbarium of Harvard University, Cambridge Mass	1,694,206
Central National Herbarium, Kolkata (W.B.)	2,000,000
Herbarium of the Forest Research Institute, Dehradun	300,000
Madras Herbarium, Coimbatore	150,000
Herbarium of the National Botanical Research Institute, Lucknow	80,000
Herbarium of the Botanical Survey of India, Central Circle, Allahabad	26,440
Regional Herbarium of the Botanical Survey of India, Shillong (Meghalaya)	86,400
Dehradun	42,000
Pune	120,000
Industrial Section, Botanical Survey of India, Indian Museum, Kolkata (W.B.)	40,000

Functions of a herbarium

There are two primary functions served by a herbarium, namely, accurate identification and alpha taxonomic research, both monographic and floristic. There are secondary functions which include a closer interaction between the student of general systematics and the herbarium.

The major herbaria or national institutes with large herbaria adequately cover the flora of the world. They serve the dual purpose of research and identification, *i.e.*, (i) research programmes; (ii) service as repositories of type and other historical plant materials; (iii) the loan of specimens for study at other institutions; and (iv) the training of graduate students. There is a close co-operation between them and thus overlapping of work has been greatly avoided. The national herbaria were brought into existence primarily to fulfil public needs, since they are supported by public funds. This service must take a high place among other functions. The public interests embrace a wide range of people and bodies such as private ordinary members, amateurs of botany, research institutes and government departments.

The functions of national herbaria are as follows:

1. To fulfil public needs by way of supplying materials and scientific information in respect of medicinal plants, by arranging training courses and exhibitions on plant science and by providing research facilities and job opportunities to young workers.
2. To carry out their own research program-mes of fundamental as well as applied value.
3. To preserve national plant wealth including type material and palaeobotanical collections.
4. To facilitate exchange and loan of preserved plant material for various purposes including research in pharmacognosy and other branches, exhibitions, etc.

Most of the developed and developing countries have smaller herbaria built up by private or government agencies. These can be classified into three main categories : (i) regional herbaria; (ii) local herbaria including personal collections; and (iii) herbaria of the educational institutions such as the universities, colleges and schools.

Regional herbaria mainly cover the above mentioned functions on the regional level and in most cases they are supported by government aid. In India, the Botanical Survey of India has established seven such regional herbaria in addition to the national herbarium. Local herbaria serve the purpose of a small area like that of a district and mainly represent the flora to that area. Thus, collectively, they serve to provide data for distributional studies. University or college herbaria are primarily used for teaching and post-graduate research in taxonomy. They also can help in the dissemination of scientific information to the needy public. In India, only a few universities have maintained herbaria with proper care. In some instances, herbaria maintained by colleges and schools are much more satisfactory than those maintained by the universities, *e.g.*, in Bangalore, Baroda, Calicut, Delhi, Marathwada, Mysore, Trivandrum, Utkal and a few other universities where herbaria of some kind have been maintained.

From a safe place for storing pressed specimens, especially type material, herbaria have become major centres of taxonomic research. Additionally, herbaria also form an important link for research in other fields of study. Classification of the world flora is primarily based on herbarium material and associated literature. More recently, herbaria have gained importance as sources of information on endangered species and are of primary interest to conservation groups. The major roles played by a herbarium include :

1. *Repository of plant specimens* : To store dried plant specimens, safeguard these against loss and destruction by insects, and make them available for study.

2. *Safe custody of type specimens* : Type specimens are the principal proof of the existence of a species or an infraspecific taxon. These are kept in safe custody, often in rooms with restricted access, in several major herbaria.

3. *Compilation of floras, manuals and monographs* : Herbarium specimens are the authenticated documents upon which the knowledge of taxonomy, evolution and plant distribution is dependent. Floras,

manuals and monographs are largely based on herbarium resources.

4. *Training in herbarium methods* : Many herbaria carry facilities for training graduates and undergraduates in herbarium practices, organising field trips and even expeditions to remote areas.

5. *Identification of specimens* : The majority of herbaria have a wide-ranging collection of specimens and offer facilities for on-site identification or having the specimens sent to the herbarium identified by experts. Researchers can personally identify their collection by comparison with the duly identified herbarium specimens.

6. *Information on geographical distribution* : Major herbaria have collections from different parts of the world and thus scrutiny of the specimens can provide information on geographical distribution of a taxon.

7. *Preservation of voucher specimens* : Voucher specimens preserved in various herbaria provide an index of specimens on which a chromosomal, phytochemical, ultrastructural, micro-morphological or any specialised study has been undertaken. In the case of a contradictory or doubtful report, the voucher specimens can be critically examined to arrive at a more satisfactory conclusion.

Mounting of specimens

Pressed and dried specimens are finally mounted on herbarium sheets. A standard herbarium sheet is 29 by 41.5 cm (11½ by 16½ inches), made of thick handmade paper or a card sheet. The sheet should be relatively stiff to prevent damage during handling of specimens. It should have a high rag content (preferable 100 per cent) with fibres running lengthwise.

The specimens are attached to the sheet in a number of ways. Many older specimens in the herbaria are frequently found to have been sewn on the sheets. Use of adhesive linen, paper or cellophane strips is an easier and faster methods of fixing specimens. Most of the contemporary specimens are fixed using liquid paste or glue in one of ways, however:

(i) Paste or glue is applied to the backside of the specimen, which is later pressed onto the mounting sheet and allowed to dry in pressed condition for a few hours. This method is slower but more economical.

(ii) Paste or glue is smeared on a glass or plastic sheet, the specimen placed on the sheet and the glued specimen transferred to a mounting sheet. The method is more efficient but expensive.

The stem and bulky parts may often require adhesive strips or even sewing for secure fixing of specimens. Small paper envelops called fragment packets are often attached to the herbarium sheet to hold seeds, extra flowers or loose plant parts.

Labelling

An herbarium label is an essential part of a permanent plant specimen. It primarily contains the information recorded in the field diary at the time of collection, as also the results of any subsequent identification process. The label is located on the lower right corner of the herbarium sheet, with information recorded on the preprinted proforma, printed directly on the sheet or on the paper slips which are pasted on the sheets. It is ideal to type the information. If handwritten, it should be in permanent ink. Ball pens should never be used as the ink often spreads after some years.

The size of a herbarium label is recommended as diverse as $2^3/_4$ by $4\frac{1}{4}$ inches and 4 by 6 inches. The information commonly recorded on the herbarium label includes :

(i) Name of the Institution
(ii) Scientific name
(iii) Common or vernacular name
(iv) Family
(v) Locality
(vi) Date of collection
(vii) Collection number
(viii) Name of the collector
(ix) Habit and habitat including field notes.

An expert visiting a herbarium may want to correct an identification or record a name change. Such correction is never done on the original label but on a small annotation label or determination label, usually 2 by 11 cm and appended left of the original label. Such a label, in addition to the correction, records the name of the person and the date on which the change was recorded. Such information is useful, especially when more than one annotation label is appended by different persons. The last label is likely to be the correct one.

Voucher herbarium specimens of a research study often have authentic information about the specimens recorded in the form of a *voucher label*.

Filling of specimens

Mounted, labelled and treated (to kill insect pests) specimens are finally incorporated in a herbarium, where they are properly stored and looked after. Small herbaria arrange specimens alphabetically according to family, genus and species. Larger herbaria, however, follow a particular system of classification. Many herbaria follow the number code of families and genera.

The specimens belonging to a species are placed in a folder made of thin strong paper, termed species cover. The species covers belonging to a particular genus are often arranged alphabetically and placed inside a genus cover made of a thicker paper. More than one genus cover may be used if the number of species are more, or if the specimens are to be arranged geographically. The genus covers of a family are arranged according to the system of classification being followed. The demarcation between the two families (last genus of a family and first genus of the next family) is done using a sheet of paper with a front-hanging label indicating the name of the next family. The folders are stacked in pigeonholes of the herbarium cases and the arrangement is suitable for shifting of folders as the number of specimens increase with time. Unknown specimens are kept in separate folders marked dubia, placed towards the end of a genus (when the genus is identified) or a family (when the family is identified but not the genus), as the case may be, so that an expert can examine them conveniently. Standard herbarium cases are insect and dustproof with two tiers of pigeonholes, each 19 in. deep, 13 in. wide and 8 in. high.

Type specimens are usually kept separately in distinct folders or often in separate herbarium cases, sometimes even separate rooms, for better case and safety.

A herbarium commonly maintains an index register in which all the genera in the herbarium are listed alphabetically and against each genus is indicated the family number and the genus number, the two helping for convenient incorporation and retrieval of specimens in a herbarium.

Pest control

Herbarium specimens are generally sufficiently dry and as such not attacked by bacteria or fungi. They are, however, easily attacked by pests such as silverfish, dermestid beetles (cigarette beetle, drugstore beetle and black carpel beetle). Control measures include :

1. *Treating incoming specimens* : Specimens have to be pest free before they can be incorporated into a herbarium. This is achieved in three ways :

   (i) *Heating* at temperatures up to 60°C for 4-8 hours in a heating cabinet. The method is effective but the specimens become brittle.

   (ii) *Deep-freezers* have now replaced heating cabinets in most herbaria of the world. A temperature of –20 to –60°C is maintained in most herbaria.

   (iii) *Microwave ovens* have been used by some herbaria, the use of microwave ovens has some serious shortcomings including :

      (a) Stems containing moisture burst due to sudden vaporisation of water inside.

      (b) Metal clip staples on the sheets get overheated and may char the sheet.

      (c) The embryo in the seeds gets killed, thus destroying a valuable source of experimental research, as seeds from herbarium specimens are often used for growing new plants for research projects.

2. *Use of repellents* : Chemicals with an offensive odour or taste are kept in herbarium cases to keep pests away from specimens. Naphthalene and para-dichlorobenzene (PDB) are commonly used as repellents, usually powdered and put in small muslin bags kept in pigeonholes. PDB is more toxic and as such prolonged exposure of workers should be avoided. For people working 8 hours a day in a 5-day per week schedule, the upper exposure level for naphthalene is 75 PPM and for PDB 10 PPM.

3. Fumigation : In spite of pretreatment of specimens and use of repellents, the use of fumigants is necessary for proper herbarium management. Fumigation involves exposing specimens to the vapours of certain volatile substances. A mixture of ethylene dichloride (3 parts) and carbon tetrachloride (1 part) was once commonly used for fumigation. Ethylene dichloride is explosive without cabron tetrachloride, but the latter is extremely toxic to humans, causing liver damage, and as such the use of this fumigant has been banned. Dowfume-75 has been cleared by the Environmental Protection Agency for use in herbaria. Under controlled conditions Vapona resin strips (Rapid strips) are suitable for herbarium cases. One-third of a strip is placed in each herbarium case for seven to ten days twice a year. The cases should not be opened during the period of fumigation.

IDENTIFICATION METHODS

Identification of an unknown specimen is a common taxonomic activity, and often combined with determination of a correct name. The combined activity is appropriately referred as specimen determination. The identification of an unknown plant may be achieved by comparison with identified herbarium specimens or through the help of taxonomic literature. Both methods may be combined for a more reliable identification.

The unknown specimen meant for identification is sent to a herbarium, where an expert on the plant group examines and identifies it by comparison with duly identified specimens. The user can also visit a herbarium and personally compare and identify his specimens.

Computers have entered in a big way into solving identification problems. Electronic revolution in recent years has opened up a new, faster and more reliable method of identification. The photograph, description or illustration of parts can be put up on a web site, with information to a relevant e-mail list, whose members can help in achieving identification without hours.

TAXONOMIC LITERATURE

Various forms of literature incorporating description, illustrations and identification keys are useful for proper identification of unknown plants. The library is, therefore, as important in taxonomic work as a herbarium and a knowledge of taxonomy is one of the oldest and most complicated literatures of science. Several bibliographic references, indexes and guides are available to help taxonomists to locate relevant literature concerning a taxonomic group or a geographical region. The major forms of literature helpful in identification are described below.

Floras

A Flora is an inventory of the plants of a defined geographical region. A Flora may be fairly exhaustive or simply synoptic. Lists of the Floras may be found in the *Geographical Guide to the Floras of the World* by S.F. Blake (Part I, 1941; Part II, 1961) and *Guide to the Standard Floras of the World* by Frodin (1984). Depending on the scope and the area covered the Floras are categorised as :

1. *Local Flora* covers a limited geographical area, usually a state, city, a valley or a small mountain range. Examples : *Flora of Delhi* by J.K. Maheshwari (1963), *Flora Simlensis* by H. Collet (1921), *Flora of Tamil Nadu* by K.M. Mathew (1983), and *Flora of Central Texas* by R.G. Reeves (1972).

2. Regional Flora includes a larger geographical area, usually a large country or a botanical region. Examples : *Flora of British India* by Sir J.D. Hooker (1872-97), *Flora Malesiana* by C.G. Steenis (1948), *Flora Iranica* by K.H. Rechinger (1963), and *Flora SSSR* by V.L. Komarov and B.K. Shishkin (1934-64). A Flora covering a country is more appropriately known as a *National Flora*.

3. Continental Flora covers the entire continent. Examples : *Flora Europaea* by T.G. Tutin *et al.* (1964-80) and *Flora Australiensis* by G. Bentham (1863-78).

4. Comprehensive Treatments have a much broader scope. Although no World Flora has ever been written, several important works have attempted a worldwide view. Examples: *Genera plantarum* of G. Bentham and J.D. Hooker (1862-83), *Die Naturlichen pflanzenfamilien* of A. Engler and K.A. Prantl (1887-1915) and *Das Pflanzenreich* of A. Engler (1900-54).

Manuals

A *manual* is a more exhaustive treatment than a Flora, always having key for identification, description and glossary but generally covering specialised groups of plants. Examples : *Manual of Cultivated Plant* by L.H. Bailey (1949), *Manual of Cultivated Trees and Shrubs Hardy in North America* by A. Rehder (1940) and *Manual of Aquatic Plants* by N.C. Fassett (1957).

A manual differs from a monograph in that the latter is a detailed taxonomic treatment of a taxonomic group.

Monographs

A *monograph* is a comprehensive taxonomic treatment of a taxonomic group, generally a genus or a family, providing all taxonomic data relating to that group. Usually the geographical scope is worldwide since it is impossible to discuss a taxon without including all its members, and often all its species, subspecies, varieties and forms are discussed. The monograph also includes an exhaustive review of literature, as also a report on author's research work. A monograph includes all information related to nomenclature, designated types, keys, exhaustive description, full synonymy and citation of specimens examined.

A *revision* is less comprehensive than a monograph, incorporating less introductory material and including a synoptic literary review. A revision includes a complete synonymy but the descriptions are shorter and often confined to diagnostic characters.

A *conspectus* is an effective outline of a revision, listing all the taxa, with all or major synonyms, with or without short diagnosis and with brief mention of the geographical range.

A *synopsis* is a list of taxa with very abbreviated diagnostic distinguishing statements, often in the form of keys.

Journals

Whereas floras, manuals and monographs are published after a lot of taxonomic input and it may take several decades before they are revised. Taxonomic journals provide information on the results of ongoing research. A continuous update on additional taxa described or reported from a region, nomenclature changes and other taxonomic information are essential for continuing taxonomic activity. Reference to a publication in a journal includes volume number (all issues within a year bear the same volume number), issue number (numbered within a volume, a monthly journal would have 12 issues, quarterly 4 issues and so on) and page numbers on which a particular article appears. Common journals devoted largely to taxonomic research include : *Taxon* (International Association of Plant Taxonomy, Berlin), *Kew Bulletin* (Royal Botanic Gardens, Kew), *Plant Systematics and Evolution* (Denmark), *Botanical Journal of Linnaean Society* (London), *Journal of the Arnold Arboretum* (Harvard), *Bulletin Botanical Survey of India* (Calcutta), *Botanical Magazine* (Tokyo) and *Systematic Botany* (New York).

Supporting literature

With a large amount of research material being published throughout the world, there is always need for supporting literature to give consolidated information about the works published world over. They also help in tracking down material concerning a particular taxon and a certain period. Taxonomic Literature, an exhaustive series of *Regnum vegetabile*, covers full bibliographical details of literature very helpful in searching type material, priority of names, dates of publication and biographic data on authors.

Abstracts or Abstracting journals provide a summary of various articles published in various journals throughout the world. Biological Abstracts and Current Advances in Plant Science are more general in approach. Kew Record of Taxonomic Literature covers all articles relevant to taxonomy.

An *Index* provides an alphabetic listing of taxa with reference to their publication. *Index Kewensis* is the most important reference tool, first published in 2 volumes from Royal Botanic Gardens, Kew (1893-1895), covering names of species and genera of seed plants published between 1753 and 1885. Regular *Supplements* used to be published every 5 years and 18 *Supplements* appeared up to 1985. Since then the listing has been published annually under the title *Kew Index*.

Index Kewensis is a list of new and changed names of seed-bearing plants with bibliographic references to the place of first publication. Supplement 19 was published in 1991 covering the years 1986 to 1990. At the beginning of the nineteen eighties the data were transferred to a computer database which continues to expand at the rate of approximately 6000 records per year. To make this data generally available it was decided to publish the whole *Index Kewensis* as a CD-ROM in 1993. This contains almost 968,000 records.

Illustrations of vascular plants can be located through *Index Londinensis*, which contains information up to 1935. More recent information can be found in the 2-volume work *Flowering Plant Index of Illustrations and Information* compiled by R.T. Isaacson (1979). A listing of all generic names can be found in *Index nominum genericorum* (ING) a 3-volume work published in 1979 under the series *Regnum Vegetabile*. The first supplement appeared in 1986. It has now been put on the database and can be directly accessed through the Internet. *Index holmiensis* (earlier *Index holmensis*) is an alphabetic listing of distribution maps found in taxonomic literature of vascular plants. It started publication in 1969. *Gray Herbarium Card Index* is information on cards, which has now been set up on a database. Usually on the same pattern as *Index Kewensis*, the Index has been published in 10 volumes between 1893 to 1967. A 2-volume *supplement* was published by G.K. Hall in 1978. The *Gray Herbarium Index* database currently includes 287,225 records (in 1998) of New World vascular plant taxa at the level of species and below. The Index includes from its 1886 starting point, the names of plant genera, species and all taxa of infraspecific rank. The *Grey Index* covers vascular plants of the Americas, *Index Kewensis* includes seed plants worldwide. Only the

Gray Index has nomenclatural synonyms cross-referenced to basionyms. The information is now accessible over the Internet via keyword searches from the E-mail Data Server and through the Biodiversity and Biological Collections Gopher. Indices covering other groups of plants have also been published : *Index Filicum* for Pteridophytes, and *Index Muscorum* for Bryophytes.

Numerous valuable Dictionaries have been published but by far the most useful is Dictionary of Flowering Plants and Ferns published by J.C. Willis. The 8th edition revised by Airy Shaw appeared in 1973. The book contains valuable information concerning genera and families, providing name of the author, distribution, family and number of species in the genus.

PREPARATION AND USE OF KEYS

A large collection meant for deposition in the herbarium needs identification and proper labelling. Initial identification has to be at the family level and subsequently into genera, species, varieties and so on. As stated earlier, in most cases this is done by comparison with the predetermined material but specimens from newly explored areas need careful observation. Usually, identification of such material is done with the help of keys provided in the floras and manuals. There are a few keys prepared specially for this purpose. These are prepared in such a way that any one possessing working knowledge of morphological terms can be able to use them profitably.

The first aim of the key is to provide ease and certainty of identification. Obviously, it is often difficult to arrange taxa according to their natural relationship, and for the sake of convenience, it is many a times profitable to employ artificial separation of groups using one or two easily observable characters.

Keys are of two types : punched cards keys and dichotomous keys. The former can be tackled by school or college students who find it a most interesting exercise in taxonomic practice. The latter can be found in most of the floras and are of two types : indented and bracketed.

Punched cards keys consist of cards of suitable size with names of all the taxa (all families, genera or species for which the key is meant) printed on each one of them. Each card also has a number and any one character printed near one of the corners. All the taxa showing this character are indicated by a perforation in front of their names, while those lacking this character are without any perforation. There are as many cards as there are characters chosen for the purpose. With a plant specimen to be identified in hand, only those cards showing characters possessed by the specimen, are selected. Character combination exhibited by the specimen is then referred to that family to which the card indicates this perforation.

Dichotomous keys consist of pairs of contrasting characters (couplets) each statement of which is a lead. The leads are numbered and both begin with the same word as far as possible. The characters to be used for this purpose should be easily observable, constant and thus dependable. Quantitative characters should usually be preferred to qualitative ones. In closely related taxa with overlapping characters, it is profitable to employ more than one contrasting characters so that the combination of characters is taken to decide the similarity or difference between the taxa.

Bracket key

1. Gynoecium of free carpels; carpels usually many
   Gynoecium of united carpels or carpel solitary
2. Plants terrestrial
   Plants aquatic
   Nelumbonaceae
3. Leaves simple
   Leaves pinnately compound
   Rosaceae
4. Leaves stipulate; sepals and petals often coloured and imbricate; fruit dry
   Magnoliaceae
5. Leaves exstipulate; sepals and petals usually green and valvate; fruit fleshy
   Annonaceae

Indented key

1. Gynoecium of free carpels; carpels usually many :

2. Plant terrestrial
3. Leaves simple
4. Leaves stipulate; sepals and petals usually coloured and imbricate; fruit dry
   Magnoliaceae
5. Leaves exstipulate; sepals and petals usually green and valvate; fruit fleshy
   Annonaceae
6. Leaves pinnately compound
   Rosaceae
7. Gynoecium of united carpels or carpel solitary
   Nelumbonaceae

The punched cards keys are fascinating to handle and create much interest in the identi-fication exercise but are very costly, at least ten times (if not more) costlier than the dichotomous keys. Further, the printed matter on the cards becomes obscure due to constant handling. Thus they are relatively short-lived. Dichotomous keys, on the other hand, are most suitable for practicing taxonomists and can be carried in the field. Most of the floras adopt either indented or bracket keys. The former have advantage of giving a visual presentation of the group so that the user can readily obtain a picture of the taxon. However, if these are too large, the individual leads in the couplets get widely separated from each other while these occur in pairs in the bracket keys.

Construction of key requires sound knowledge of the character differences and a good familiarity of the flora. Many a times, distinct taxa which can be readily distinguished in the field by their stature and general appearance, are difficult to separate out by key characters. Similarly, certain polymorphic taxa cannot be distinguished by one or two characters and have to be repeated twice or many more times in the key. In short, it can be said that the author of the group has to accept the challenge of crystallising the essence of his work in constructing a key which can be used profitably to distinguish taxa in a given area.

In practice herbarium is a name given to a place owned by an Institution, which maintains this orderly collection of plant specimens. Most of the well-known herbaria of the world made their beginning from *botanical gardens*.

BOTANICAL GARDENS

Although gardens existed in ancient China, India, Egypt and Mesopotamia, these gardens were not botanical gardens in the true sense. They existed for growing food plants, herbs and ornamentals for aesthetic, religious and status reasons. The famous 'hanging gardens' of Babylon in Mesopotamia is a typical example. The first garden for the purpose of science and education was maintained by Theophrastus in his Lyceum at Athens. Although the majority of the botanical gardens house plant species which the climate of the area can support, several well-known botanical gardens have controlled enclosures to support specific plants. Tropical gardens often need indoor growing space— *screen houses* for most plants and *glasshouses* for the majority of cacti and succulents in wet tropical and temperate gardens. Glasshouses in temperate gardens often require winter heating. Botanical gardens play the following important roles :

(i) *Aesthetic appeal* : Botanical gardens have an aesthetic appeal and attract a large number of visitors for observation of general plant diversity as also the curious plants, as for example the Great Banyan Tree (*Ficus benghalensis*) in the Indian Botanical Garden at Calcutta.

(ii) *Material for botanical research* : Botanical gardens generally have a wide range of species growing together and offer ready material for botanical research, while can go a long way in understanding taxonomic affinities.

(iii) *On-site teaching* : Collection of plants is often displayed according to families, genera or habitats, and can be used for self-instruction or demonstration purposes.

(iv) *Integrated research projects* : Botanical gardens with rich living material can support broad-based research projects which can integrate information from such diverse fields as anatomy, embryology, phytochemistry, cytology, physiology and ecology.

(v) *Conservation* : Botanical gardens are now gaining increased importance for their role in conserving genetic diversity, as also in conserving rare and endangered species.

The proceedings of the Symposium on Threatened and Endangered Species, sponsored by the New York Botanical Garden in 1976, published as *Extinction in Forever*, and the conference on the practical role of botanical gardens in conservation of rare and threatened species sponsored by the Royal Botanical Gardens, Kew and published as *Survival and Extinction*, are among the major examples of the role of botanical gardens in conservation.

(vi) *Seed exchange* : More than 500 botanical gardens of the world operate an informal seed exchange scheme, offering annual lists of available species and a free exchange of seeds.

(vii) *Herbarium and library* : Several major botanical gardens of the world have herbaria and libraries as an integral part of their facilities, and offer taxonomic material for research at a single place.

(viii) *Public services* : Botanical gardens provide information to the general public on identification of native and exotic species, methods of propagation and also supply plant material through sale or exchange.

Plant Anatomy : Cell Differentiation and Ergastic Cell Contents

Cell is a fundamental unit of a living organism. The cell contains a cell wall and consists of the protoplasmic components and nonprotoplasmic materials.

A group of cells with the identical form and function is known a tissue in which the cell mem-branes are connected with a pectin layer called middle lamella. The cytoplasmic threads, called plasmodesmata, are consisted of cell wall, cell membrane, protoplasm and middle lamella. They interconnect the protoplasm of different cells and assist to conduct food and communicate stimuli.

CELL WALL

The original cell wall may undergo various chemical modifications that profoundly change its physical properties, *e.g.*, the deposition of further cellulose or hemicellulose and incrustation of the wall by lignin, cutin or suberin. Algae cell walls contain pectin mixed with cellulose, xylose, mannose or silica, hemicellulose, alginic acid, fucoidin and fucin (Phaeophyta), geloses (Rhodophyta) and chitin.

Cellulose walls

Some colour reactions are used for the recognition of cellulose cell walls which vary with differences in the relative proportions of cellulose, hemicellulose and pectin present.

1. Chlor-zinc-iodine yields a blue colour with celluloses and a yellow colour with pectic substances. Walls containing these in different proportions stain blue, violet, brownish-violet or brown. Similar colours are obtained with iodine followed by concentrated acids.

2. Iodine gives no colour with true celluloses but may give a blue if hemicelluloses are present.

3. Ammoniacal solution of copper oxide, dissolves celluloses, and on adding dilute sulphuric acid the cellulose is precipitated. Walls containing hemicelluloses are incompletely soluble in this reagent.

4. Phloroglucinol and hydrochloric acid forms no pink or red colour with cellulose walls.

Lignified walls

Lignin is a strengthening material. It impregnates the cell walls of tracheids, vessels, fibres and scleroids of vascular plants. It constitutes 22-34% of woods. Lignin is a complex phenylpropanoid (C_6-C_3) polymer which differs according to its source. In the wall, it is combined with hemicellulose and built up in high concentration in the middle lamellae and in the primary walls. Lignified cell walls on treatment with Schultze's macerating fluid will show cellulose reactions.

The colour tests of lignin are:

1. On treatment with 'acid aniline sulphate' the walls turn bright yellow.

2. Phloroglucinol and hydrochloric acid stain lignified walls pink or red. Pentose sugars when warmed with this reagent, give a similar colour.

3. Chlor-zinc-iodine stains lignified walls yellow.

Suberized and cutinized walls

Suberin and cutin are highly polymerized different fatty acids such as suberic acid, $COOH[CH_2]_6$ COOH. These materials make waterproof the cells. Suberin thickenings are found in cork cells and endodermal cells, which are carbohydrate-free suberin lamellae. Cutin forms a secondary deposit on or in a cellulose wall. Leaves contain a deposit of cutin which may show characteristic papillae, ridges or striations. Beneath the cuticle, the cellulose wall may be cutinized. Waxes, the esters of higher monohydric alcohols and fatty acids, occur with suberin and cutin. They readily melt on warming and are extractable with fat solvents. Such waxes in the form of minute rods or particles give a glaucous effect to the structures which they cover. Wax is found in larger amounts on the leaves of *Myrica*, and in the wax palms, *Copernicia*, it coats the leaves heavily (Carnauba wax).

The colour reactions of suberin and cutin are almost identical.

1. Chlor-zinc-iodine gives a yellow to brown colour.
2. Sudan-glycerin stains both suberin and cutin red, on warming. The reagent is prepared by dissolving 0.01 g of Sudan III in 5 ml of alcohol and adding glycerin (5 ml).
3. Strong solution of potash gives yellow colour with both suberin and cutin. On warming suberin with a 20% solution of potash, yellowish droplets exude, but cutin is more resistant.
4. Diluted tincture of alkanna colours the walls red.
5. Concentrated sulphuric acid does not dissolve suberin or cutin.
6. *Oxidizing agents* : When heated with potassium chlorate and nitric acid, the walls change into droplets, which are soluble in organic solvents or in dilute potash. At ordinary temperatures concentrated chromic acid solution has little effect.

Mucilaginous cell walls

Some cell walls may be converted into gums and mucilages as in the stems of species of *Prunus, Citrus* and *Astragalus*, in testas of many seeds (*e.g.*, Linseed and Mustard) and in the outer layers of many aquatic plants. In *Astragalus*, gummosis commences near the centre of the pith and spreads outwards through the primary medullary rays. The polysaccharide walls swell and are converted into gum, the lumen, which frequently contains starch, becoming very small. When the stem is incised, whole tissues are pushed out by the pressure set up by the swelling of the gum.

Chitinous walls

Chitin $(C_8H_{13}O_5N)_n$, a polyacetylaminohexose, is present in the cell walls of crustaceans, insects and many fungi (*e.g.*, ergot). It gives no reactions for cellulose or lignin. When heated with 50% potash at 160-170°C for 1 hour, it is converted into chitosan, $C_{14}H_{26}O_{16}N_2$, ammonia and acids such as acetic and oxalic. The mass dissolved in 3% acetic acid and the chitosan is reprecipitated by the addition of an alkali. Chitosan gives a violet colour when treated first with a 0.5% solution of iodine in potassium iodide, and then with 1% sulphuric acid.

PARENCHYMATOUS TISSUE

Meristematic tissue is composed of isodiametric form of cells by possessing a protoplast capable of division and a primary cell wall of cellulose. The fundamental parenchyma in various parts of the plant is meristematic. The pith, cortex and rays of the plant axis and the mesophyll of the leaves are composed of such parenchyma. The mesophyll cells contain chloroplasts, and may be differentiated into palisade and spongy mesophyll. The lignified pitted parenchyma constituting the pith of the stems of *Lobelia inflata* and *Cephaelis ipecacuanha* differs from the pitted cellulose parenchyma of the pulp of *Citrullus colocynthis*.

Dermal tissues

These tissues consist of outer protective coverings such as epidermis, periderm, trichomes and stomata.

(i) Epidermis

Epidermis is the outermost protective single layer of young plant body. The epidermal cells are narrowly placed with no intercellular spaces. They show wide variation in shape, size and arrangement. A cuticle layer, containing cutin, is usually present on the outer surface. The cuticle layer is not present in root epidermal tissues.

The epidermis of the root constitutes the piliferous layer and that of the shoot is a highly differentiated and compact layer of cells. The epidermal cells are often devoid of chloroplasts. Epidermal cells give characteristic patterns when seen in surface view. In transection they are flattened parallel to the surface, and square or rectangular in shape. The outer walls are often convex and thickened.

The epidermis of the stems of trees and shrubs is usually obliterated early by the development of a cork cambium, but on the stems of herbaceous plants and in leaves, fruits and seeds the epidermis persists.

For leaves, the shape of the epidermal cells, the nature and distribution of the wall thickening, the presence or absence of cuticle and its form, the distribution and structure of the stomata, the presence or absence of subsidiary cells to the stomata, characteristic cell inclusions such as cystoliths and water-pores should all be carefully noted in describing the characters of an epidermis.

Characteristic cells with thickened pitted walls are present in the outer epidermis of the pericarp in Vanilla, Jupiter and Capsicum. The outer epidermis of the pericarps of Coriander and Vanilla contain prisms of calcium oxalate. A striated cuticle is present in Aniseed, Caraway and Star anise fruits. Thickened palisade-like cells exist in the epidermis of the testa of Colocynth and Fenugreek seeds. Elongated tapering cells are present in the epidermis of Cardamoms. Thickened lignified cells are seen in the epidermis of Lobelia seed, and mucilage cells that of Linseed and of white and black Mustard.

The structures of the epidermis and stomata are helpful in the identification of leaves. Straight-walled epidermal cells are present in Coca and Senna leaves, wavy-walled epidermal cells in Stramonium, Hyoscyamus and Belladonna; beaded walls in Lobelia and Digitalis species; a papillose epidermis in Coca Leaf. A thick cuticle is developed in *Aloe* leaf and bearberry leaf; a striated cuticle in belladonna, jaborandi, *Digitalis lutea* and *D. thapsi*. Mucilage is present in the epidermis of senna and buchu leaves. Cystoliths of calcium carbonate occur in the epidermal cells of Urticaceae and Cannabinaceae; sphaero-crystals of diosmin occur in buchu epidermis.

(ii) Stomata

A stomata is made of a pair of similar cells, called guards cells, placed parallel to each other. It contains a pore in the centre through which gaseous exchange takes place. The epidermal cells surrounding the stomata are called subsidiary cells and they are different in shape. On the basis of arrangement with the subsidiary cells, the stomata are divided into five different classes (Fig. 5.1) :

(a) *Anomocytic or Ranunculaceous type (irregular type)* : The cells surrounding the stomatal pore are irregularly arranged and cannot be distinguished from the other epidermal cells, *e.g.*, Lobelia, Digitalis, Buchu.

(b) *Cruciferous or Anisocytic (unequal celled)* : The stomatal pore is surrounded by three or four subsidiary cells, one of which is markedly smaller than the others, *e.g.*, Belladonna, Stramonium.

(c) *Rubiaceous or Paracytic type (parallel-celled)* : Two subsidiary cells with their long axis are parallel to the pore, *e.g.*, Senna, Coca.

(d) *Diacytic or Caryophyllaceous type (crossed celled)* : The stomata is accompanied by two subsidiary cells, with their long axis at right angles to the pore of the stomata, *e.g.*, Spearmint, Peppermint, Thyme, etc.

(e) *Actinocytic (radiate-celled)* : This stomata is surrounded by a circle of radiating cells, *e.g.*, Ursi.

The distribution of stomata between the upper and lower epidermis is different. The stomata may be entirely confined to the lower epidermis, as in *Ficus* species, bearberry, buchu, coca, jaborandi and mate leaves. The leaves of savin shown stomata confined to two localized areas of the lower surface.

The floating leaves of aquatics have stomata confined to the upper epidermis. Sometimes they are distributed on both surfaces; most commonly they are more numerous on the lower surface.

The *Stomatal Index* is the percentage which the number of stomata form of the total number of epidermal cells, each stoma being counted as one cell. Thus, if S represent the number of stomata per unit area and E the number of epidermal cells in the same unit area, the stomatal index is S × 100 ÷ (E + S). The figure so obtained is fairly constant for any species and can be used as a specific character, which has proved useful for distinguishing leaflets of Indian from those of Alexandrian senna and also leaves of *Atropa belladonna* from those of *A. acuminata*. Recorded values are as follows :

Atropa belladonna lower surface 19.5–23.9

Atropa acuminata lower surface	16.7–18.8
Cassia acutifolia both surfaces	11.4–13.0
Cassia angustifolia both surfaces	17.1–20.0
Cassia auriculata both surfaces	7.1–14.5
Erythroxylum coca lower surface	12.0–15.4
Erythroxylum truxillense lower surface	8.4–11.5

(iii) Epidermal trichomes

Trichomes are present on many leaves, herbaceous stems, flowers, fruits and seeds. A trichome may be differentiated into a base embedded in the epidermal cell and a tube like projecting body. Trichomes may be classified into two groups :

(a) *Covering trichomes* : They have protective function.

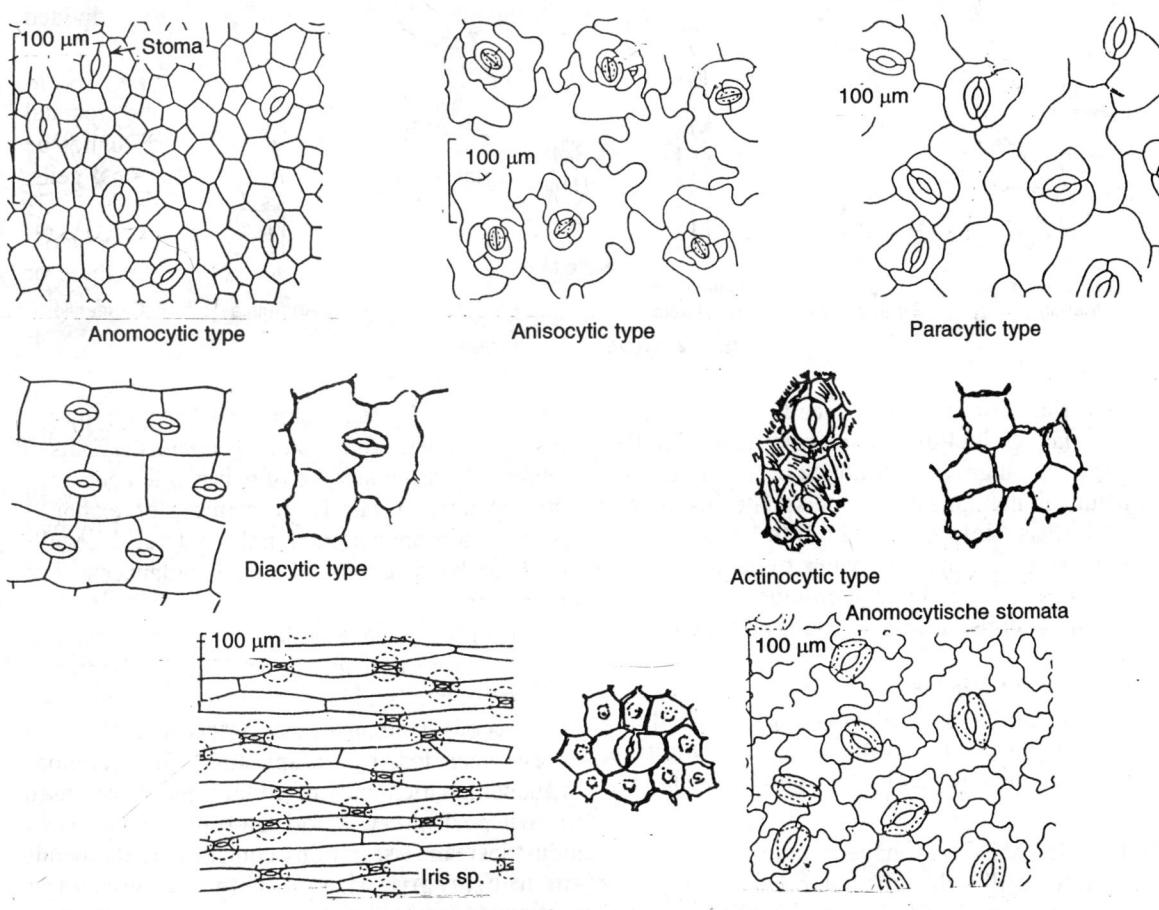

Fig. 5.1. Different kinds of stomata.

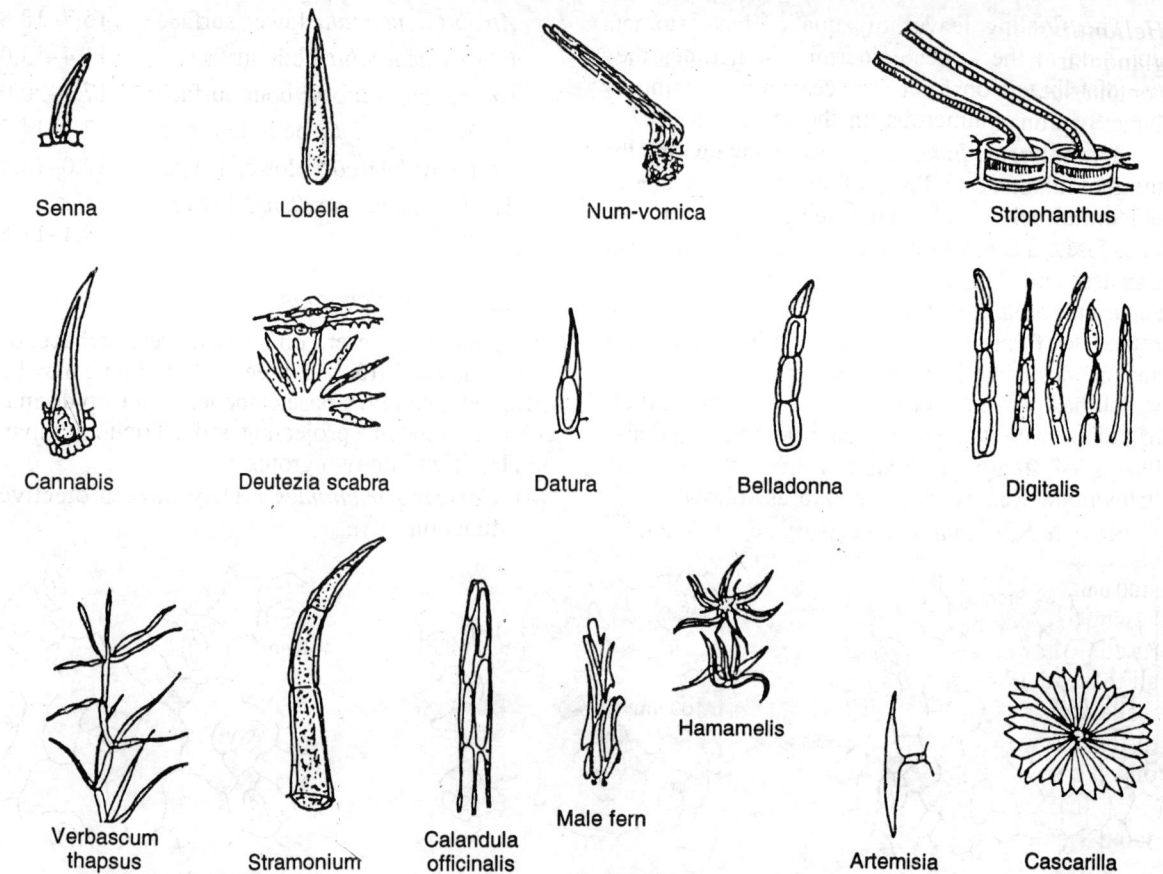

Senna   Lobella   Num-vomica   Strophanthus

Cannabis   Deutezia scabra   Datura   Belladonna   Digitalis

Verbascum thapsus   Stramonium   Calandula officinalis   Male fern   Hamamelis   Artemisia   Cascarilla

Fig. 5.2. Covering trichomes.

Covering hairs may be unicellular or multi-cellular. Unicellular hairs vary from small papillose outgrowths to large robust structures. Multicellular hairs may be uniseriate, biseriate or multiseriate or complicated branched structures. The chemical nature of the cell wall, and the presence of pits or protuberances or of cell inclusions, such as cystoliths, should be noted.

(b) *Glandular trichomes* : They secrete essential oils or oleo-resins. Both covering and glandular trichomes may be unicellular or multi-cellular, uniseriate or multiseriate and stalk or sessile.

Glandular hairs may have a unicellular or a multi-seriate stalk; the glandular head may be unicellular or multicellular. The cuticle of the gland may be raised by the secretion. In peppermint the oil secretion beneath the cuticle contains crystals of menthol. A particular type of hair is often characteristic of a plant family or genus—for example, biseriate hairs are common in the Asteraceae, while glandular hairs are found in the Solanaceae and Lamiaceae.

Trichomes have functions, *e.g.*, physical and chemical protection for the leaf against microbial organisms, aphids and insects, and the maintenance of a layer of still air on the leaf surface, thus checking excess water loss by transpiration. The secretions of glandular trichomes of certain genera are used in the perfumery, food and pharmaceutical industries; some secretions contain narcotic resins and others give rise to skin allergies. The sesquiterpenes of the glandular trichomes of

Helianthus annuus are antimicrobial and the glandular trichomes of some *Solanum* species contain sucrose esters of carboxylic acids such as 2-methylpropanoic and 2-methylbutyric acids, which are aphid deterrents. The isolated secretory cells of the glandular trichomes of *Mentha piperita* can carry out the synthesis of monoterpenes.

Most glandular trichomes are pluricellular, the simplest type having a uniseriate stalk with a single spherical secreting cell at the apex; in *Digitalis purpurea* a few such trichomes have a unicellular stalk, in *Digitalis thapsi* the stalk is usually three- to four-celled; belladonna leaves also bear similar trichomes. Most glandular trichomes of *D. purpurea* have a unicellular stalk and a bicellular head. In henbane the stalk is uniseriate and the secreting head ovoid and pluricellular. The glandular trichome characteristic of the Asteraceae has a short biseriate stalk and a biseriate secreting head. Trichomes having a multiseriate cylindrical stalk and a capitate rosette of secreting cells are found in cannabis. In all these glands the secretion is formed in the outer walls of the cells beneath the cuticle, which is raised to form a delicate bladdery envelope enclosing the oil or oleo-resin.

A leaf bearing trichomes is *Piper betle*, where some trichomes are developed for the absorption or secretion of water.

Frequently, in dried leaves, many of the trichomes have fallen or been rubbed off, leaving a scar or *cicatrix*, which is usually surrounded by epidermal cells showing a characteristic arrange-ment, often radiating from the cicatrix; this is well seen in Senna and Stramonium.

(iv) Endodermis (periderm)

The endodermis is a specialized layer of cells making the inner layer of the cortex. In mature plants the epidermis is replaced by endodermis due to the activity of the meristematic tissue called phellogen or cork cambium. The cells of the endodermis appear in transverse section four sided, oval or elliptical and often extended in the tangenital direction. The cells are longitudinally elongated.

Endodermis is generally found in roots, in aquatic and subterranean stems and in the aerial stems of certain families (*e.g.*, Lamiaceae and Brassicaceae). Leaves and aerial stems often contain a starch sheath which is a modified endodermis.

The cells of the endodermis appear in transverse section four-sided, oval or elliptical. They are extended in the tangential direction. The cells are longitudinally elongated, with the end walls often transverse. A primary endodermis, as in Lobelia stem, is characterized by the deposition, in the radial walls, of special modified material (resembling

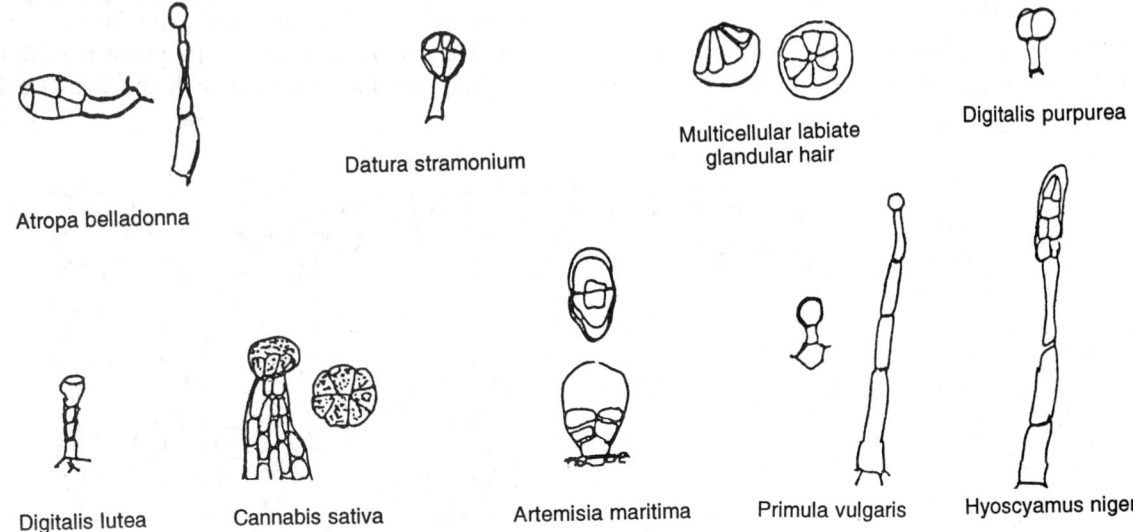

Fig. 5.3. Grandular hairs.

cutin). Subsequently, a suberin lamella is formed within the primary wall, giving a secondary endodermis. This may be followed by the deposition of a secondary wall of lignocellulose, giving a tertiary endodermis, as in *Aletris* and *Smilax*.

In periderm lenticels are present which are pores identical to stomata in function. In lenticels, there are no guard cells and they remain always open. The lenticels are larger in size and smaller in number than the stomata they replace. The simplest form of lenticel consists of a mass of unsuberized thin-walled cells which become rounded off and are known as complementary tissue.

FUNDAMENTAL OR GROUND TISSUES

Fundamental tissues include hypodermis, cortex, pith, mesophyll and midrib region.

(i) Parenchyma

Parenchyma contains living and thin walled cells with intercellular spaces. These cells vary in shape and are present in the cortex of root, cortex and pith of stem and mesophyll of leaves. Some parenchyma cells are pitted and contained reticulated thickening. Aerenchyma is parenchyma with large intercellular spaces. Chlorenchyma is parenchyma containing chloroplasts. The main functions of parenchyma are storage and photosynthesis.

(ii) Collenchyma

Collenchyma is a living tissue derived from parenchyma and has greater mechanical strength. The walls are thickened due to deposition of cellulose. These cells are usually present in cortical region of stem, petiole, bark and midrib of a leaf. The cells are usually 4 to 6 sided in transverse section, and axially elongated.

Their walls are composed of cellulose and have considerable plasticity. Collenchyma consti-tutes the typical mechanical tissue of herbaceous stems and of the petioles and midribs of leaves. Collenchyma is present above and below the midrib bundle in many leaves (*e.g.*, Senna, Stramonium, Hyoscyamus, Belladonna, Digitalis and Lobelia); in the wings of Lobelia stem; in the cortex of Cascara bark; and in the pericarp of Colocynth and Capsicum.

(iii) Cork tissue

A cork cambium or phellogen usually arises as the plant axis increases in diameter. The plant, by its activity, produces new protective tissues, known collectively as periderm, which replace the epidermis and part or all of the primary cortex. The cells of the cork cambium undergo tangential divisions giving rise externally to cork tissue and internally to phelloderm or secondary cortex. Usually, a limited production of phelloderm occurs, so that the number of cork layers greatly exceed the number of phelloderm layers.

In roots the cork cambium is formed in the pericyle; in stems it may form in the epidermis or the subepidermal layers. The first-formed cork cambium may be functional throughout the life of the plant and may increase with the increase in

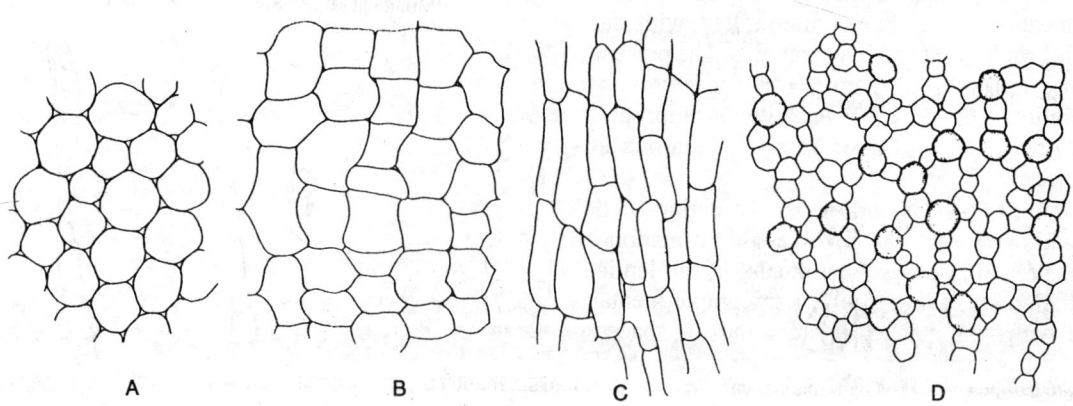

Fig. 5.4. Parenchyma (A, B, C) and aerenchyma cells (D).

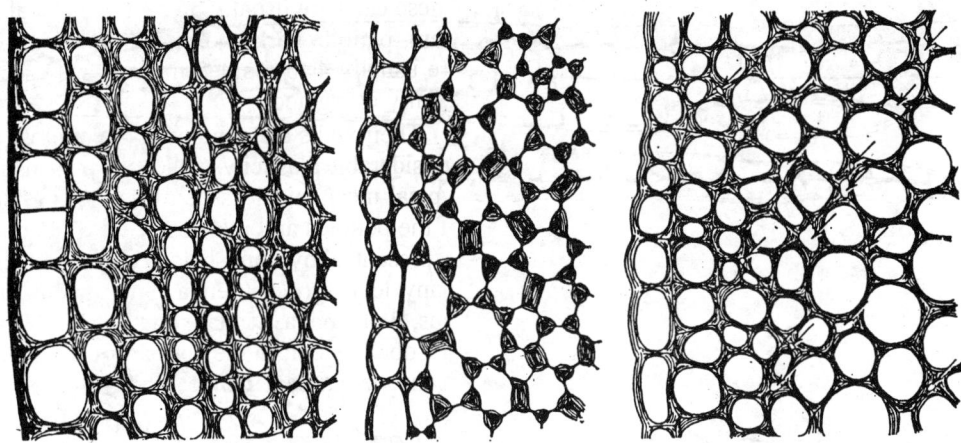

Fig. 5.5. Collenchymatous tissue

girth, giving rise to an even smooth bark. A persistent cork cambium gives rise to the fissured bark of the cork oak and cork elm. The first-formed cork cambium has only a limited period of activity and is replaced by secondary cambia of more deep-seated origin; this process may be repeated again and again.

Cork tissue contains a compact mass of cell, rectangular in transverse sections five- or six-sided in surface view and often arranged in regular radial rows. The cell wall is composed of inner and outer cellulose layers and a median suberin lamella, or of a suberin lamella laid down upon the primary cellulose wall. The cellulose layers may be lignified, as in Cassia bark. The mature cork cell is dead, impermeable to water and often filled with dark reddish-brown contents rich in tannins. The presence of cork cells in powdered drugs may show adulteration or use of low-quality or improperly peeled drug (*e.g.*, Cinnamon, Ginger, Liquorice and Turmeric).

The formation of cork stops the action of the stromatal apparatus, and involves the formation of special breathing pores or lenticels. In the lenticel area, the cork cambium gives rise comple-mentary tissue, with well-marked intercellular air spaces.

(iv) Sclerenchyma

Sclerenchyma cells are the dead and lignified tissues. The cell walls are heavily thickened with lignin. They occur in all parts of the plant body and give mechanical strength. These cells may occur as stone cells or fibres showing well-marked stratification and traversed by pit-canals which are funnel-shaped or branched. The cell lumen is small, sometimes obliterated. Cell contents may be present (*e.g.*, prisms of calcium oxalate in Calumba, Starch grains in Cinnamon).

Sclereids commonly occur in the hard outer coats of seeds and fruits and in the bark and pericyclic regions of woody stems. They occur isolated or in small groups in Quillaia and Calumba, in larger groups in Cascara and Wild Cherry bark or in definite sclereid layers, as in Cinnamon and Cassia bark. Sclereids are absent in Frangula and Cinchona barks. The presence of elongated sclereids in powdered Ipecacuanha is diagnostic of the presence of stem. Lignified sclereids are present in Clove stalk which should be almost absent from powdered cloves. Characteristic sclereids are present in the rind and seed coat of Colocynth. The stone cells or sclereids are isodiametrical or irregular in shape. Their walls are thick, lignified. Sclerenchymatous fibres are narrow, usually elongated with pointed ends. The tissue is composed of spindle-shaped or elongated cells with pointed ends and known as prosenchyma. The cell wall may be composed of pure cellulose and is usually lignified. Most mature fibres are unicellular and give mechanical support to the plant.

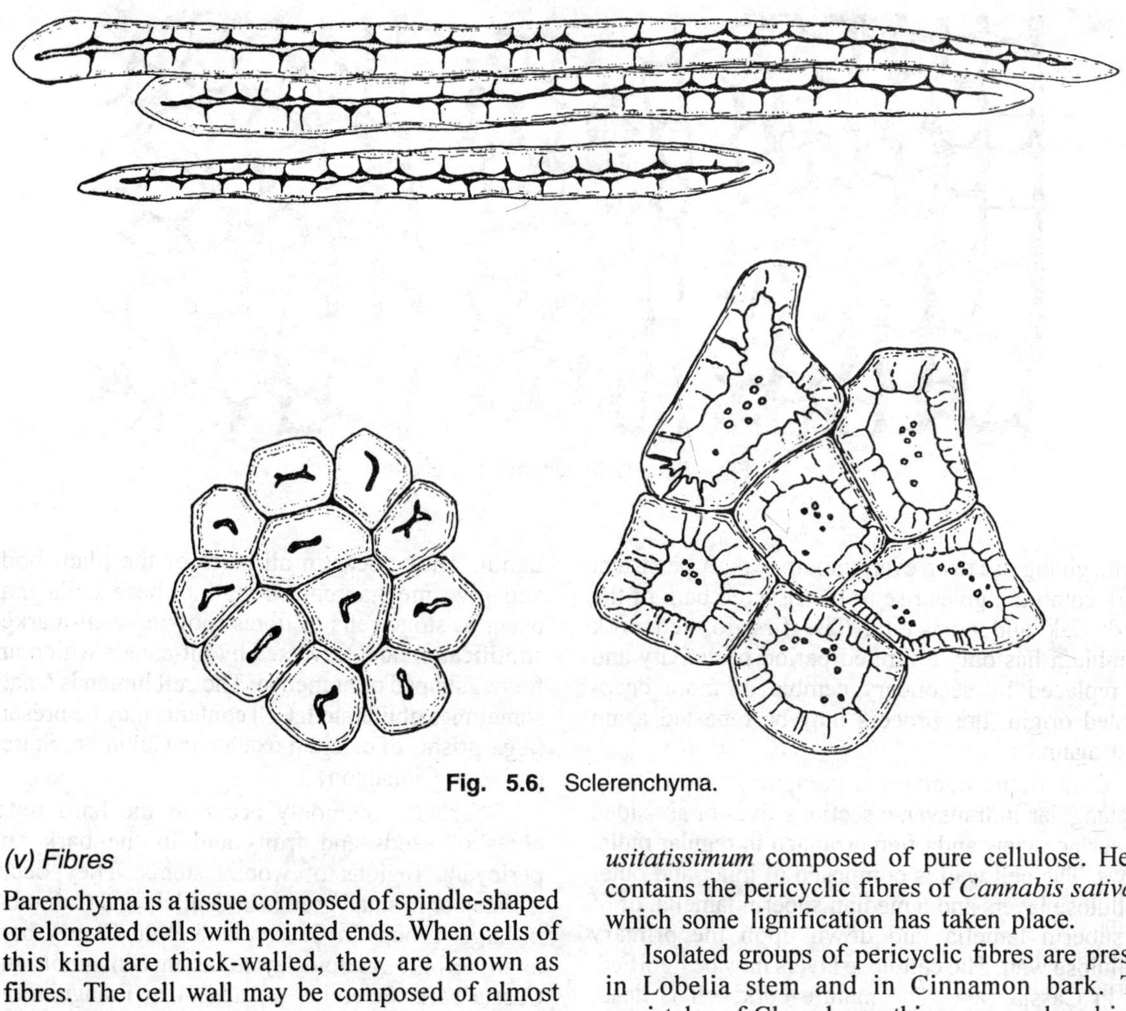

Fig. 5.6. Sclerenchyma.

(v) Fibres

Parenchyma is a tissue composed of spindle-shaped or elongated cells with pointed ends. When cells of this kind are thick-walled, they are known as fibres. The cell wall may be composed of almost pure cellulose or may show various degrees of lignification in the form of sclerotic or sclerenchymatous fibres.

Fibres are produced from a single cell which during its development grows rapidly in the axial direction. During growth the tips of the elongating cells may push past one another, a process known as 'gliding growth'. Most mature fibres are unicellular, but occasionally transverse septa develop (*e.g.*, ginger). Fibres are differentiated on the basis of the tissue in which they occur (*i.e.*, as cortical fibres, pericyclic fibres, xylem fibres or phloem fibres).

Flax consists of the *pericyclic fibres* of *Linum usitatissimum* composed of pure cellulose. Hemp contains the pericyclic fibres of *Cannabis sativa* in which some lignification has taken place.

Isolated groups of pericyclic fibres are present in Lobelia stem and in Cinnamon bark. The meristeles of Clove hypanthium are enclosed in an incomplete sheath of pericyclic fibres. The lignified, moderately thick-walled pericyclic fibres, with a parenchymatous sheath of cells containing prisms of calcium oxalate, are only present in Senna leaf. The pericyclic fibres are present in the midrib of the leaves of *Digitalis lutea* and *D. thapsi*. But they are absent in *D. purpurea* and *D. lanata*.

Xylem fibres may be directly derived from tracheids. The intermediate forms, having a limited conducting function, are known as fibre-tracheids. The fibre-tracheid has smaller pits, thicker walls and usually more tapering ends than the typical tracheid. Wood fibres have thicker walls and pits reduced to minute canals. Occasionally, wood fibres are septate. Cells having a fibre-like form with living contents and simple pits are fusiform xylem parenchyma cells and termed 'substitute fibres'. The mature wood fibre is a dead lignified element. The autumn wood is usually characterized by containing a higher proportion of wood fibres than the spring wood. The secondary xylem of Liquorice contains wood fibres arranged in bundles, which alternate with the small groups of vessels and are enclosed in a sheath of xylem parenchyma containing prisms of calcium oxalate. The secondary xylem in Gentian, Rhubarb and Jalap is free from fibres.

Phloem fibres are present in both primary and secondary phloem; they may or may not be lignified. Their thickened walls are traversed by simple pits. Phloem fibres are also known as the 'hard bast'. Jute consists of the phloem fibres from the stems of various species of *Corchorus*. The distribution, abundance, size and shape of the phloem fibres constitute important characters for the differentiation of medicinal barks. Phloem fibres occur singly or in irregular rows in the barks of Cinnamon, Cassia and Cinchona. The phloem fibres of Cinnamon can be differentiated from those of Cassia by their smaller diameter. In barks the fibres occur isolated or in rows. The area of fibres per gram of powdered bark can be made a criterion for determining the amount present in mixtures. The phloem fibres of Cinchona are large (80-90 μm in diameter), fusiform in shape and have very thick walls, conspicuously striated and traversed by funnel-shaped pits. The secondary phloem of Cascara, Frangula and Quillaia is composed of alternating zones of hard and soft phloem. The phloem fibres of Cascara are accompanied by a crystal sheath. The phloem fibres of Quillaia are characterized by their tortuous, irregular outline and often exhibit enlarged and forked apices. Fibres are absent from the phloem of Gentian and Ipecacuanha.

VASCULAR TISSUES

Vascular tissue system conducts food material and water. Phloem is a living tissue and conducts food material from leaves to the different parts of the plant. Xylem is a dead tissue and conducts water from roots to the leaves.

(i) Phloem

Phloem consists of sieve-tubes, companion cells, phloem parenchyma and secretory cells.

The sieve tube is the conducting element of the phloem. It has a vertical series of elongated cells, interconnected by perforations in their walls in areas known as sieve plates. The perforations are present in smaller areas of each sieve plate. The sieve plates may occur in the end-walls or lateral walls of the sieve tube. The mature sieve plate is coated with a film of callus pad completely blocking the sieve plate. The sieve plates may occur in the end-walls or lateral walls of the sieve tube. The mature sieve plate is coated with a film of callus, which may increase in amount and form a callus pad completely blocking the sieve plate. The development of the callus pad may cause the sieve tube permanently functionless. In other cases the callus pad formed in the autumn is redissolved in the spring. The mature sieve tube lacks a nucleus, but while functional contains cytoplasm. Sieve tubes may be detected by recognition of the callus pads with some staining reagents. For example :

- *Alkaline solution of corallin* stains callose red.
- *Aniline blue* stains callose blue.
- *Chlor-zinc-iodine* stains callose a reddish-brown.
- *Solution of ammoniacal copper nitrate* does not dissolve callose.
- *Solution of potash* as even a cold 1% solution of potash dissolves callose, this should not be used as a clearing agent if it is afterwards desired to test the section for callose.

Due to their delicate structure and lack of lignification, sieve tubes are difficult to observe in commercial drugs. The sieve tubes are detected in Cascara bark when stained with corallin soda and in powdered Gentian.

The companion cells are associated with the sieve tubes both structurally and functionally. The sieve tube and the companion cells are derived from a common mother cell of the procambial strand in primary phloem or from a phloem mother cell derived from the cambium in secondary phloem. The phloem mother cell undergoes longitudinal division into two daughter cells of unequal size, the smaller of which becomes the companion cell. The companion cell is characterized by its dense proto-plast and well-developed nucleus, and by possessing a thin cellulose wall.

The cells of the phloem parenchyma are usually axially elongated, although they may remain isodiametric and be arranged in linear series. They remain typically thin-walled.

The phloem often contains secretory cells (e.g., ginger, cinnamon, cassia and jalap). Laticiferous tissue may also occur in the phloem (e.g. lobelia and taraxacum).

(ii) Xylem

The structural elements of xylem are tracheids, vessels or tracheae, xylem fibres, xylem parenchyma and rays.

Protoxylem and metaxylum are the parts of the primary xylem. Secondary growth in thickness of the stem and root forms secondary xylem.

Tracheids are elongated tubes pointed at both ends. Their cell walls are lignified and pitted. Vessels or tracheae constitute of elongated tubes but without any oblique perforated walls. The vessels of the protoxylem show annular or spiral thickenings. The later-formed xylem contains sclariform and reticulate thickenings. The secondary wall thickening is composed of lignocellulose.

The tracheid is an elongated water-conducting cell, with a lignified and variously thickened and pitted cell wall. At maturity it is a dead element. The pits are bordered and may appear simple. In gymnosperms the pits are present in the radial walls.

The secondary wall thickening may be annular, spiral, scalariform and reticulate tracheids. Transition forms between these types are not uncommon. Annular and spiral tracheids occur most frequently in protoxylem; scalariform and reticulate tracheids are pesent in metaxylem and secondary xylem. True vessels are absent in gymnosperms, in which the secondary xylem consists of a homo-geneous tracheidal system broken by narrow medullary rays and a slight development of xylem parenchyma. Cellulose wadding is made from high grade sulphite pulp usually prepared from coniferous wood with bordered pits and a small amount of wood parenchyma. The tissues are completely delignified in the preparation of the pulp. Tracheids

occur in the secondary xylem of some angiosperms (e.g., Ipecacuanha).

Vessels or *tracheae* are the fundamental con-ducting elements of the xylem of the angiosperms. The vessel is composed from a vertical series of cells, in which increase in diameter and dissolution of the end-walls forms a continuous tube. They have some of the scalariform pits of the adjacent end-walls which are broken down to give slit-like openings. The vessels of the protoxylem show annular or spiral thickening. The secondary wall thickening is composed of lignocellulose. Larger vessels may have a complete secondary wall perforated only by pits. These pits vary in size, form and crowding and sometimes bands of tertiary thickening are laid down within the secondary wall.

Spiral and annular vessels are typical of protoxylem, and present in the protoxylem of stems and roots, in small vascular bundles and in the veins of leaves, e.g., Gentian, Clove, Squill and most leaves (e.g., Senna, Belladonna, Hyoscyamus and Stramonium). Spiral and scalariform vessels occur in Lobelia stem. Reticulate vessels occur in Gentian, Ginger and Rhubarb. Vessels showing numerous bordered pits occur in Quassia, Jalap, Sandalwood, Hydrastis and the stems of Belladonna and Aconite.

The secondary xylem is made up of *rays* and *xylem parenchyma* which permeate the dead mass of mature vessels, tracheids and wood fibres. The xylem parenchyma cells are often axially elongated, often showing thickening and lignification. The walls are traversed by simple pits or, by half-bordered pits. Xylem parenchyma may function as a storage tissue, the cells becoming blocked with starch (as in Ipecacuanha). The xylem parenchyma cells may grow into the vessel cavities and form tyloses which block up the vessel and render it non-functional, as in the development of heartwood. The distribution of xylem parenchyma may be diffuse, vasicentric when it forms sheaths around the large vessels, or terminal when a zone of xylem parenchyma is formed towards the end of the year's growth. The formation of concentric zones of xylem parenchyma may give rise to 'false annual rings', as in Quassia.

A secondary xylem is composed of rays and xylem parenchyma. The xylem parenchyma cells

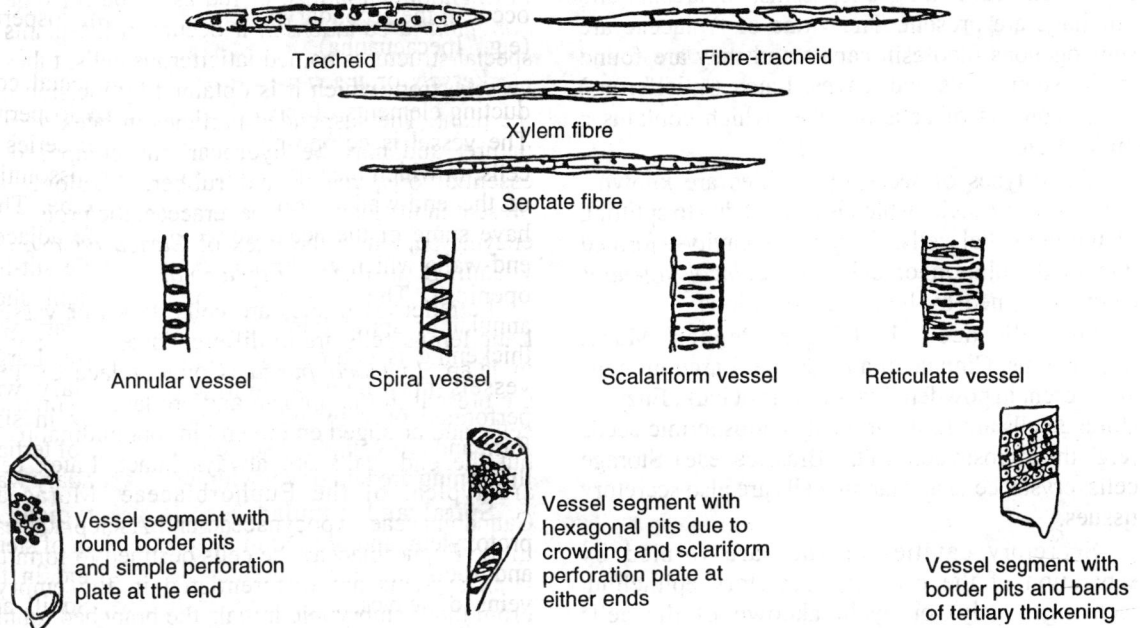

Fig. 5.7. Xylem components.

are often axially elongated, usually thick and lignified. The formation of concentric zones of xylem parenchyma may give rise to 'false annular rings'.

According to the mode of presence of the xylem and phloem the vascular bundles may be collateral, bicollateral, concentric, and radial.

(a) *Collateral* : This is the most common type of vascular bundle found in stems and leaves. In this system the xylem and phloem remain side by side arranged on the same radius, phloem on the outer side and xylem on the inner side. Collateral bundles may be open when cambium is present in between phloem and xylem or closed when cambium is absent.

(b) *Bicollateral* : When another patch of phloem is present on the inner side of the external phloem, then the vascular bundle is called as bicollateral.

(c) *Concentric* : In this system one kind of vascular tissue surrounds the other.

(d) *Radial* : Here the xylem and phloem occur in separate patches on alternate radii on the axis. Radial vascular bundles are characteristic of roots.

In dicot stems the vascular bundles are arranged in the form of a ring and in monocot, the bundles are scattered.

Cambium

Cambium is a meristematic tissue present between the phloem and xylem in dicot stems. It is absent in young roots, but appears on maturing the plant between the radially placed phloem and xylem. Then it forms a zigzag ring giving out secondary xylem on the inner side and secondary phloem on the outer side. The delicate primary structures are either crushed or poorly represented in developed plant parts.

Medullary rays are composed of parenchymatous cells, run diagonally and extend from pith (medulla) to the cortex through the secondary xylem and secondary phloem.

Secretory tissues

Secretory cells, secretory cavities or sacs, secretory ducts or canals and latex tissue are the secretory tissues. Cells containing oils, resins, oleoresins and mucilage are present. The vittae of Apiaceae are schizogenous oleoresin canals and they are found in the stem, roots and leaves. Latex (laticiferous) tissue consists of cells or tubes which contains a milky fluid.

Three types of secretory cavities are known : *Schizogenous* cavity which is formed due to splitting of the epithelial cells; *Lysigenous* cavity—formed due to dissolution of cells and *Schizolysigenous* cavity - formed by both the operations.

Oil cells occur in Ginger, Pepper, Mace, Cardamoms, Cinnamon and Cassia. Large oil cells are present in powdered sassafras root bark. Enzyme storage cells are found in many endospermic seeds (e.g., the myrosin cells of the Brassicaceae). Storage cells, crystal cells and tannin cells are also secretory tissues.

Secretory cavities or *sacs* are formed by separation of the cells and secretory epithelium (schizogenously) or by breakdown of the cells forming a cavity not bounded by a definite epithelium (lysigenously). Schizogenous oil cavities occur in Eucalyptus, lysigenous oil cavities in *Gossypium* species. Secretory products may appear in cells before break down of epithelium to give a lysigenous cavity. Schizolysigenous oil cavities are present in the Rutaceae and the Burseraceae. The oil cavity develops from a mother cell, which is divided to give daughter cells which separate, leaving a schizogenous central cavity. The walls of the cells surrounding this central cavity then break down, forming an oily secretion. Then the cavity increases in size lysigenously.

The vittae of the Apiaceae are schizogenous oleoresin canals and they are present in the stem, roots, fruits and leaves. The oleoresin ducts of *Pinus* species are also of schizogenous origin. Schizogenous oleoresin ducts which enlarge lysigenously are found in some plants of the Leguminosae (e.g., *Capaifera*).

Latex is an emulsion or a suspension, the continuous phase of which is an aqueous solution of mineral salts, proteins, sugars, tannins, alkaloids, etc., and the suspended particles are oil-droplets, resin, gum, proteins, starch, caoutchoue, etc. This turbid fluid is often white in colour, as in the Opium poppy, *Papaver somniferum*, but may be yellow, as in *Chelidonium majus*, or red as in the rhizome of *Sanguinaria canadensis*; it occurs in the plants in special structures named laticiferous cells, tubes or vessels, from which it is obtained by incision into the plant. The suspended particles in latex vary in nature, and may be hydrocarbons composed of essential oils, resins and rubber. Alkaloids are present in the latex of Papaveraceae, the proteolytic enzyme papain in the latex of *Carica papaya* and vitamin B_1 in that of *Euphorbia*.

Laticiferous tissues are cells, tubes or vessels. Laticiferous cells are of different sizes and shapes; in jalap, *Ipomoea purga* (Convolvulaceae), they are present in the phloem and are large cylindrical cells, and arranged end to end in longitudinal rows, but the end walls are always intact. Latex cells are typical of the Euphorbiaceae, Moraceae, Cannabinaceae, Apocynaceae and Asclepiadaceae. In the Euphorbiaceae the cells destined to form the latex systems are differentiated in the embryo. From these embryonic initials the branched tubular latex cells of the mature plant are developed. The latex cells have thickened walls and numerous nuclei, and contain latex in which characteristic dumb-bell-shaped starch grains may be present. Laticiferous tubes are of two types, branches and unbranched. Unbranched long tubes are found in the phloem of *Cannabis sativa*, where the cells arise in the growing-point and continually elongate as the plant grows in height, but transverse walls are not formed though the nucleus divides repeatedly, thus producing a coenocytic structure. Branched tubes occur in *Alstonia scholaris* (Apocynaceae). Each tube is developed from a single cell, which grows in length as the plant grows. Laticiferous vessels result from the fusion of numerous cells of the phloem parenchyma. Typical laticiferous vessels are present in Lobelia, *Lobelia inflata*, (Lobeliaceae) and in the Opium poppy *Papaver somniferum*. Cells of the parenchyma become filled with latex and the walls of contiguous cells break down thus forming irregular branching structures, which are easily distinguished from "tubes" because of irregularities in the walls and the occurrence of short projections at numerous places.

The walls of all these laticiferous structures are very resistant and consequently the structures can be isolated from the surrounding tissues by maceration on a water-bath in 5 per cent aqueous caustic potash or soda.

Laticifers are also formed by the fusion of a longitudinal series of cells. They are present in Convolvulaceae, Campanulaceae and the suborder Liguliflorae of the Asteraceae. The Papaveraceae possess latex elements intermediate in structure between latex cells and vessels. The laticifers of Ipomoea and Sanguinaria consist of longutudinal rows of cells which retain their transverse walls. In Chelidonium the marginal parts of the transverse walls persist; in *Papaver* and *Argemone* there is only slight evidence of the original transverse walls. The laticifers in the Liguliflorae form a continuous nonseptate series of passages usually occurring in the primary and secondary phloem. *Taraxacum officinale* shows concentric zones of anastomosing latex vessels in the phloem of both rhizome and root.

It is difficult to determine the mode of origin of the laticifers. A laticifer may arises from their association in some plants with idioblasts containing tannins and mucilage. Latex material may also occur in schizogenous canals.

ERGASTIC CELL CONTENTS

These cell contents are identified by microscopical examination or by physical and chemical tests. They include carbohydrates, proteins, fixed oil, fats, alkaloids, volatile oils, resins, gums, calcium oxalate and silica. As they are non-living, they are known as *ergastic*.

Starch

Starch occurs as granules most abundantly in roots, rhizomes, fruits and seeds. Starch of various sources differs in shape and size. It usually occurs in larger grains in storage organs than are to be found in the chlorophyll-containing tissues of the same plant. The small granules formed in chloroplast by the condensation of sugars are afterwards hydrolysed into small sugars so that they may pass in solution to storage organs where, under the influence of leucoplasts, large grains of reserve starch are formed.

Proteins

Protein is found in the form of aleurone grains. The ground mass of protein encloses one or more rounded bodies and an angular body known as the crystolloid. The simplest aleurone grain consists of a mass of protein surrounded by a thin membrane. Aleurone grains are best observed after defatting and removal of starch. Sections being examined for aleurone should be treated with the following reagents :

1. Millon's reagent stains the protein red on warming.
2. Ninhydrin yields pink or violet colour with proteins.
3. Picric acid stains the ground substance and crystalloid yellow.

The endosperm cells of Nutmeg each possess one large and several smaller aleurone grains. The large aleurone grains are 12-20 μm in diameter, and contain a large well-defined crystalloid. Aleurone grains, containing globoids, are present in the endosperm and cotyledons of Linseed. Some of the aleurone grains of the endosperm of Fennel contain a minute cluster crystals of calcium oxalate.

Aleurone grains vary much in size, shape and complexity. They are characteristic of particular seeds. They give information about the systematic position of the plant in which they occur. Many aleurone grains are small in size, very simple in structure, consist of an amorphous mass of protein enveloped by a more dense protein membrane. This type of grain is found in many Leguminous seeds (peas and beans), and in cereals. Other aleurone grains have inclusions embedded in an amorphous ground mass of protein surrounded by a denser protein envelope. Three kinds of inclusions are present : (1) well-formed crystals of protein, named *crystalloids*; (2) sphere crystals, termed *globoids*, which consist of calcium and magnesium in combination with an organo-phosphoric acid; (3) calcium oxalate in rosette form in prisms or needles. A grain may enclose one or two crystalloids and these may be accompanied by one or more globoids, as in *Ricinus communis*, in the soy bean, *Glycine hispida*, and in Linseed, *Linum usitatissimum*. In other seeds globoids occur as the only inclusions as in quince, *Pyrus cydonia*, and ispaghula, *Plantago ovata*. Aleurone grains consisting of a ground substance enclosing one or two rosettes of calcium oxalate are the most common grains of umbelliferous seeds. In *Myristica surinamensis*, globoid, crystalloid and calcium oxalate rosette are all present together in the same grain. The size of aleurone grains is smaller than that of many starch grains; those of *Linum usitatissimum* are about 15 μ, of *Ricinus communis*, about 10 μ, of *Brassica alba* about 7.5 μ and of *Foeniculum vulgare* about 5 μ.

Protein and aleurone grains are insoluble in ether, alcohol and glycerin; they are stained yellow by solution of iodine. Water dissolves part of the ground substance and a 5 per cent solution of sodium chloride and saturated aqueous solution of disodium phosphate dissolve the whole ground substance, leaving the crystalloid intact; globoids also gradually dissolve in the disodium phosphate. Aqueous caustic alkali, about 0.3 to 0.5 per cent, will dissolve the crystalloids and leave the globoids unaffected. The globoids are soluble in acetic, tartaric and mineral acids; in ammoniacal solution of ammonium chloride and ammonium phosphate, from which characteristic crystals of magnesium ammonium phosphate, ultimately separate, indicating the presence of magnesium in the globoids. Eosin in aqueous solution stains aleurone red, especially the ground substance and alcoholic picric acid stains it yellow, especially the crystalloids. Millon's reagent gives a white precipitate with proteins and the colour gradually changes to brick-red on standing or changes rapidly on warming gently.

Fixed oils and fats

Fixed oils and fats are widely found in both vegetative and reproductive structures. They often occur in seeds, where they may replace the carbohydrates as a reserve food material, and are not associated with protein reserves. As lipids, fats form an essential component of biological membranes.

Reserve fats are present in solid, or crystalline masses which melt on warming. Feathery crystalline masses of fat occur in the endosperm of Nutmeg. Fixed oils occur as small drops. Oil globules, associated with aleurone grains, are present in the cotyledons of Linseed and Colocynth and in the endosperm of Nux vomica and Apiaceae fruits. Oils and fats are soluble in ether-alcohol. Castor oil is sparingly soluble in alcohol. They are coloured brown or black with a 1% solution of osmic acid, and red with a diluted tincture of alkanna. The latter

stains slowly and should be allowed to act for at least 30 min. A cold mixture of equal parts of a saturated solution of potash and strong solution of ammonia slowly saponifies fixed oils and fats to yield soap crystals.

Gums and mucilages

Gums, mucilages and pectins are polysaccharide complexes formed from sugar and uronic acid units. They are insoluble in alcohol but dissolve or swell in water. They are formed from the cell wall (e.g., Tragacanth) or deposited on it in successive layers. When such cells are mounted in alcohol and irrigated with water, the stratification may often be seen.

The solution of Ruthenium Red stains the mucilage of Senna and Buchu leaves, Althaea, Linseed, Mustard and Sterculia gum but has less action on Tragacanth. A lead acetate medium can be used to prevent undue swelling. Mucilage of Squill is stained with alkaline solution of corallin. Others are stained by chlorzinc-iodine or methylene blue dissolved in alcohol and glycerin.

Gums are amorphous, translucent solids, insoluble in alcohol and in most organic solvents; they are, however, soluble in water to yield viscous, adhesive solutions, or are swollen by the absorption of water into a jelly-like mass. They consist of calcium, potassium and magnesium salts of complex substances, known as polyuronides, and can be hydrolysed by prolonged boiling with dilute acids to yield mixtures of sugars and organic acids. The sugars so formed are monosaccharides, usually pentoses such as arabinose, xylose or galactose. The acids liberated by hydrolysis are uronic acids, *i.e.*, acids derived from monosaccharides by the oxidation of the primary alcoholic group which they contain, two of the simplest uronic acids being glucuronic acid and galacturonic acid. In certain gums, *e.g.*, Acacia gum, part of the polyuronide complex is composed of units of aldobiuronic (aldobionic) acids, which are glycosidal compounds of one molecule of a uronic acid and one molecule of a sugar. In most gums the polyuronides are of mixed composition, being formed by glycosidic linkages between several uronic acid molecules and various sugar molecules. Pectins and hemicelluloses also yield, on hydrolysis, uronic acids and sugars, thus showing a relationship with gums.

Gums are yielded by trees and shrubs belonging to a number of families, but especially Leguminosae, Rosaceae, Rutaceae, Anacardiaceae, Combretaceae and Sterculiaceae. They are produced by the conversion of the cell walls of the tissues into gum (gummosis), presumably by means of an enzyme of the origin of which nothing definite is known.

Gums are abnormal products, resulting from pathological conditions brought about either by injury or by unfavourable conditions of growth and are usually formed by changes in existing cell walls.

Mucilages are similar in constitution to gums, but are normal products of cell activity, being secreted in the cell and laid down like hemicelluloses, often in such quantity as to completely fill the cells. In the epidermal cells of Linseed and of Ispaghula and in the cells of the root of *Althea officinalis* starch grains are present and are used up during the process of the formation of the mucilage.

The artificial gum (dextrin) produced from starch differs essentially from the gums in being entirely converted into dextrose by dilute mineral acids; it is strongly dextrorotatory, natural gums being slightly laevorotatory.

Volatile oils and resins

Volatile oils occur as droplets in the cell. They are sparingly soluble in water but dissolve in alcohol and fixed oils. They resemble fixed oils in their behaviour towards osmic acid and tincture of alkanna, but they are not saponified when treated with ammoniacal potash.

Resins may be associated with volatile oil or gum, or may be found in irregular masses which are insoluble in water but soluble in alcohol. Resins, oleoresins and gum resins are usually secreted into secretory cavities or ducts. They stain slowly with diluted tincture of alkanna.

Tannins

Tannins are widely present in solution in the plant cell sap and in distinct vacuoles. Tannins are soluble in water and alcohol. Sections of galls are cut dry and mounted in clove oil, plates of tannin may be observed. Sections containing tannins acquire a bluish-black or greenish colour when mounted in a dilute solution of ferric chloride.

Alkaloids and glycosides

These secondary metabolites are rarely visible in plant cells as such the application of specific chemical tests is required to study their distribution in the plants.

Calcium oxalate

The crystals of calcium oxalate occur in five different forms in plants. Prisms of calcium oxalate may occur singly or in small groups. Sphaeraphides (Druses) are spherical aggregates of sharp pointed angular crystals. Raphides are needle shaped single or collection of bundles. Microsphenoidal crystals appear like an amorphous mass in a cell. These crystals shine brightly when seen in polarized light.

Oxalic acid rarely occurs in the free state in plants but is very common as its calcium salt in the form of crystals. It is dimorphous and is found either as the trihydrate of the tetragonal system of crystals, or as the monohydrate of the monoclinic system.

Crystals of the tetragonal system are produced due to supersaturation of the cell sap with calcium oxalate. They have all three axes at right angles to one another; two of the axes are equal in length and the third, or principal axis, may be either shorter or longer. The tiny sandy crystals or microcrystals are found in the Solanaceae. Some shape may appear from an excess of oxalic acid in the cell sap. They have three unequal axes with the two lateral axes at right angles to one another. These crystals shine more brightly in polarized light than the trihydrate crystals.

The most common forms present are prisms (Senna, Hyoscyamus, Quassia, Liquorice, Cascara, Quillaia, Rauwolfia); rosettes (Rhubarb, Stramonium, Cascara, Senna, Clove, Jalap); single acicular crystals (Ipecacuanha, Gentian, Cinnamon); bundles of acicular crystals (Squill); micro-sphenoidal or sandy crystals (Belladonna).

The types of calcium oxalate crystal, their size and distribution be recorded. Cascara shows cluster

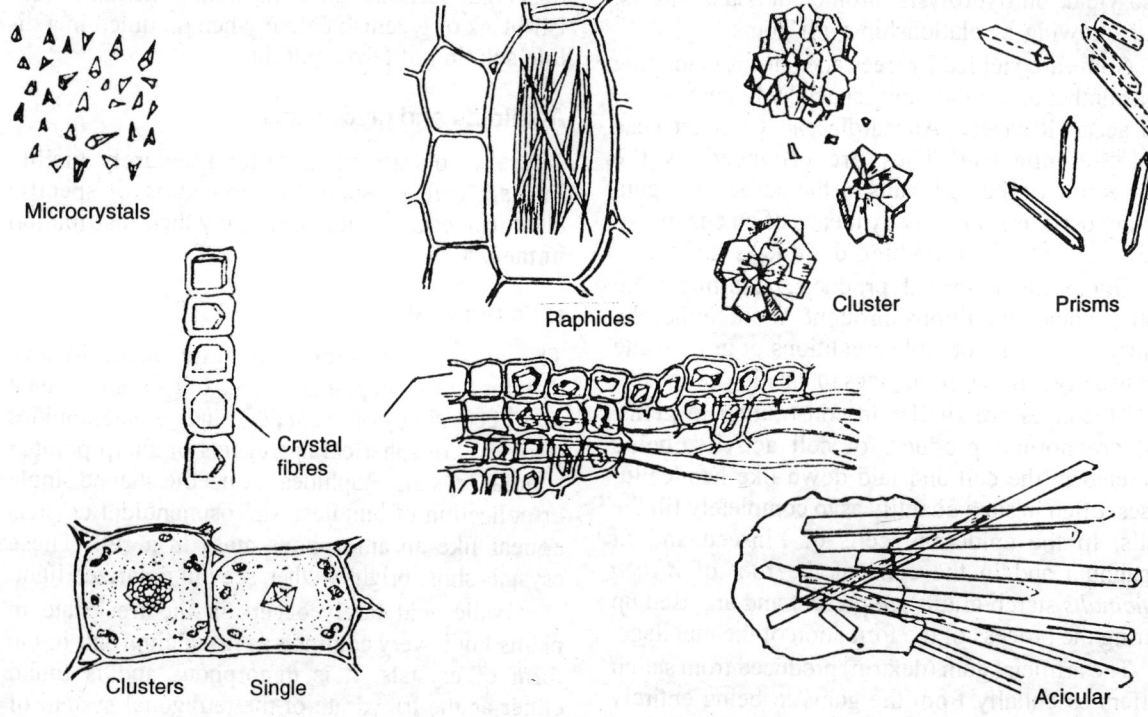

Fig. 5.8. Calcium oxalate crystals.

crystals in the ground mass of parenchyma and prisms are present in the rows of parenchymatous cells forming a sheath round the fibres. The prisms of calcium oxalate in calumba appear in the sclereids.

The cells containing calcium oxalate may differ from those surrounding them in size, form or contents, and are often called as idioblasts.

Calcium oxalate is usually present up to 1% in plants but in the rhizome of Rhubarb it may exceed 20% of the dry weight. The solanaceous leaves may be distinguished from one another, Belladonna by its sandy crystals, Stramonium by its cluster crystals and Henbane by its single and twin prisms. Phytolacca leaves and roots possess acicular crystals, Belladonna leaves and roots have sandy crystals.

Sections to be examined for calcium oxalate may be cleared with chloral hydrate or caustic alkali, as these reagents only very slowly dissolve the crystals. The polarizing microscope is useful in the detection of small crystals. Crystals of calcium oxalate are insoluble in acetic acid and caustic alkali, soluble in hydrochloric and sulphuric acids without effervescence and show, after solution in 50% sulphuric acid, a gradual separation of needle-like crystals of calcium sulphate at the site of the original crystals.

Calcium carbonate

This is embedded in or incrusted in the cell walls. Concretions of calcium carbonate formed on outgrowths of the cell wall are called cystoliths. They are present in the orders Urticaceae, Moraceae, Cannabianaceae and Acanthaceae, and in some of the Combretaceae and Boraginaceae. Well-formed cystoliths occur in the enlarged upper epidermal cells and in the clothing hairs of the lower epidermis of the leaf of *Cannabis sativa*. When the mineral substance of the cystolith is dissolved out in dilute acid, there remains a small, stratified, basis composed of cellulose. Calcium carbonate is soluble with effervescence in acetic, hydrochloric or sulphuric acid. If 50% sulphuric acid is used, needle-shaped crystals of calcium sulphate gradually separate.

Hesperidin and diosmin

These are present as feathery-like aggregates or sphaerocrystalline masses in the cells of the Rutaceae and in isolated plants of other families. Crystalline masses of diosmin are found in the upper epidermal cells of Buchu leaves. These crystals are insoluble in benzene, chloroform and alcohol but soluble in potassium hydroxide.

Silica

This substance forms the skeletons of diatoms (agar and kieselguhr). It is present as an incrustation on cell walls or as masses in the interior of cells (*e.g.*, in the cells of the sclerenchymatous layer of cardamom seeds). Silica is soluble only in hydrofluoric acid. It may be examined by igniting the material and treating the ash with hydrochloric acid, the silica remains unchanged.

6

Orders and Families of Herbal and Animal Drugs

The plant and animal kingdoms are each divided into a number of phyla, classes, orders, suborders and families.

ANGIOSPERMS : MONOCOTYLEDONS

Monocotyledons have an embryo with one cotyledon. Many members are herbs, usually with parallel-veined leaves. The stele has scattered, closed vascular bundles; the flowers are trimerous.

Table 6.1. The main orders and families of monocotyledons

Orders	Families
Bromeliales	Bromeliaceae
Cyperales	Cyperaceae
Graminales	Poaceae
Liliflorae	Liliaceae, Agavaceae, Alliaceae, Amaryllidaceae, Hypoxidaceae, Dioscoreaceae, Iridaceae
Microspermae	Orchidaceae
Principes	Palmae
Scitamineae	Musaceae, Zingiberaceae, Cannaceae, Marantaceae
Spathiflorae	Araceae, Lemnaceae

1. BROMELIALES : Bromeliaceae

The Bromeliaceae is the only family of the order. It contains about 44 genera and 1400 species; mainly tropical and subtropical, xerophytes and epiphytes. Fruit is a berry or capsule. Genera includes *Bromelia* and *Ananas*. *Ananas comosus* (syn. *A. sativus*) is the pineapple. Its juice contains bromelain, a protein-splitting enzyme. Many species contain gums, mucilages, tannins, phenolic acids and flavonoids.

2. CYPERALES : Cyperaceae

The Cyperaceae is the single family. It has about 90 genera and 4000 species; occurs as herbs. Genera includes *Cyperus*, *Scirpus* and *Carex*. Papyrus, used as paper, is derived from *Cyperus papyrus*. Some species of *Scirpus* and *Ampelodesma* serve as host plants for species of *Claviceps* to produce ergot-like sclerotia. Volatile oils, tannins, phenolic acids, flavonoids and sesqui-terpenoids are present in the plant of this family.

3. GRAMINALES : Poaceae (Gramineae)

The Poaceae contains about 620 genera and 10,000 species. These are mostly herbs with fibrous roots, annuals, biennials and perennials; universally distributed. Some important genera are *Bambusa*, *Arundinaria*, *Oryza*, *Arundo*, *Triticum*, *Agropyron*, *Hordeum*, *Secale*, *Avena*, *Sorghum*, *Zea*, *Saccharum*, *Andropogon*, *Cymbopogon*, *Phalaris* and *Vetiveria*. Products obtained are bamboos from species of *Bambusa* and *Arundinaria*, rice from *Oryza sativa*, wheat from *Triticum*, barley from *Hordeum*, rye from *Secale*, millet or guinea corn from *Sorghum vulgare*, maize or Indian corn from *Zea mays* and sugarcane from *Saccharum officinale*. *Andropogon*, *Cymbopogon* and *Vetiveria* are rich in volatile oils. These grass oils are relatively cheap and are used in perfumery, especially for scenting soap. They include citronella, lemongrass and palmarosa (geranium) oils from species of *Cymbopogon*; oil of vetiver from *Vetiveria zizanioides*. The roots of khus-khus are used both in perfumery and as a drug and are also woven into fragrant-smelling mats.

The Poaceae contains a very wide range of constituents, e.g., starches, sugar, volatile oils, alkaloids, phenolic acids, flavonoids, terpenoids, saponins and cyanogenetic substances.

4. LILIIFLORAE : Liliaceae, Agavaceae, Hypoxidaceae, Amaryllidaceae, Alliaceae, Dioscoreaceae, Iridaceae

The order contains five suborders and 17 families. The Liliaceae is further sub-divided into the Smilaceae and Ruscaceae.

The plants are perennial herbs having a bulb, corm or rhizome. The flowers are hermaphrodite, regular or zygomorphic. The perianth is usually petaloid; the ovary superior (e.g., Liliaceae) or inferior (e.g., Iridaceae). Fruit is a capsule or berry.

(i) Liliaceae

It is a widely distributed family with about 250 genera and 3700 species. The fruit is a loculicidal or septicidal capsule or a berry. The genera includes *Veratrum, Gloriosa, Colchicum*; *Herreria*; *Asphodelus, Bowiea, Funkia-Hosta, Kniphofia, Aloe*; *Gagea, Allium*; *Lilium, Fritillaria, Tulipa*; *Scilla, Urginea, Ornithogalum, Hyacinthus, Muscari*; *Asparagus, Polygonatum, Convallaria, Trillium, Paris*; *Ophiopogon*; *Aletris*; *Smilax*.

Some of these plants are cultivated for their flowers, vegetables including asparagus (*Asparagus officinalis*) and onion, garlic, shallot, leek and chives (species of *Allium*) and for drugs (Squill, Sarsaparilla, Veratrum, Colchicum seed and corm, Aloes and Cevadilla seed).

Many plants of the family contain alkaloids, which are of the steroidal, isoquinoline or purine types; sterols, cardenolides, bufadienolides and steroidal saponins. The amino acid azetidine-2-carboxylic acid occurs in many genera and is also found in the Agavaceae. Other constituents are quinones (benzoquinones, naphthoquinones, anthra-

quinones and anthrones); flavonoids (anthocyanins and flavonols); the γ-pyrone chelidonic acid; cyanogens; and fructosan-type carbohydrates. Some volatile oils of the family are antimicrobial in nature.

(ii) Agavaceae

It includes 20 genera and 670 species. The genera include *Yucca, Agave, Condyline, Dracaena, Sansevieria, Phormium, Nolina* and *Furcraea*. The drug Socotra dragon's blood is obtained from *Dracaena cinnabari*. Steroidal saponins are present in species of *Yucca, Agave* and *Furcraea*. *Sansevieria zeylanica* yields bow-string hemp and *Furcraea gigantea* Mauritius hemp. Alkaloids and cardeno-lides are absent in the family.

(iii) Amaryllidaceae

It includes 85 genera and about 1100 species. Many have bulbs or rhizomes. Fruit is a loculicidal capsule or berry. Genera include *Galanthus, Amaryllis, Leucojum, Nerine, Pancratium, Hymenocallis, Narcissus, Ungernia, Hippeastrum* and *Sternbergia*. An alkaloid, lycorine, from the family has antifungal activity.

(iv) Hypoxidaceae

This family has seven genera and 120 species. Herbs contain a tuberous rhizome or corm and used in traditional medicine as anti-inflammatory and anti-tumour drugs. A lipophilic extract is marketed in Germany, and the dried corm in South Africa, for treatment of prostate hypertrophy. The plants contain phenolic glycosides of the norlignan type.

(v) Dioscoriaceae

It is a family of five genera and about 750 species; occur in tropical or warm temperate as climbing herbs or shrubs. The plants have fleshy tubers (called yams) or rhizomes. The leaves are arrow-shaped; flowers dioecious; fruit a capsule or berry. The genera are *Dioscorea, Tamus, Rajana* and *Stenomeris*. *Tamus communis*, the black bryony, grown in Europe, has poisonous scarlet berries. Its rhizome contains a number of phenanthrone derivatives, dioscin and gracillin. The yams of *Dioscorea batatas* contain abundant starch and are used as foodstuffs in the tropics. Steroidal saponins are present in many species of *Dioscorea* and *Tamus*.

(vi) Iridaceae

This family includes more than 60 genera and 800 species as perennial herbs with corm (e.g., *Crocus*) or rhizome (e.g., *Iris*); flowers, hermaphrodite, regular or zygomorphic; fruit a loculicidal capsule with numerous seeds. The genera include *Crocus*, *Ramulea*, *Sisyrinchium*, *Tritonia*, *Freesia* and *Iris*. Saffron is present in *Crocus sativus*, orris root, and species of *Iris*. Constituents include quinones (naphthoquinones and anthraquinones), aromatic ketones (in *Iris*), carotenoid pigments (in Saffron), terpenoids and flavonoids.

5. MICROSPERMAE : Orchidaceae

The order contains a single family.

The Orchidaceae is one of the largest families of flowering plants, with some 735 genera, over 17000 species and many hybrids. These are perennial herbs, epiphytes (e.g., *Vanilla*). Genera include *Orchis*, *Cypripedium*, *Phalaenopsis*, *Dendrobium*, *Liparis*, *Malaxis*, *Vanda*, *Cryptostylis* and *Vanilla*. The economic products are orchids. Vanilla pods contain glycosides of vanilla, which produce vanillin and other aromatic substances by slow enzymic change. Alkaloids are of indolizidine, indole, pyrrolidine and pyrrolizidine. Other constituents include phenolic acids, tannin, flavonoids, coumarins and terpenoids.

6. PRINCIPES: Palmae

The order contains the single family Palmae.

It has 217 genera and about 2500 species. It is widely distributed in the tropics and subtropics as trees with an unbranched stem bearing a crown of large and branched leaves. Important genera are *Phoenix*, *Sabal*, *Copernicia*, *Metroxylon*, *Calamus*, *Areca*, *Elaeis*, *Cocos*, *Phytelephas* and *Daemonorops*. The economic plants are date palm, *Phoenix dactylifera*; sago from the stem of *Metroxylon rumpii* and *M. laeve*; rattan canes from species of *Calams*; areca or betel nuts from *Areca catechu*; palm oil and palm kernel oil from *Elaeis*

guineensis; coconut from *Cocos nucifera*; carnauba wax from *Copernicia cerifera*; and dragon's blood resin from the fruits of *Daemonorops* species. Seeds of *Phytelephas* spp. (*P. aequatorialis* in Equador) are used as the vegetable ivory. The family contains fixed oil, carbohydrates, leaf wax, saponins, tannins, catechins, flavonoids, terpenoids and ketones. Alkaloids occur in *Areca*. Steroidal substances occur (e.g., estrone) in the pollen of *Phoneix*.

7. SCITAMINEAE : Musaceae, Zingiberaceae, Cannaceae, Marantaceae

The order contains four families :

(i) Musaceae

It is a family of two genera and 42 species, namely *Musa* and *Enseta*. The plants are big herbs with 'false' aerial stems and sheathed leaves arising from a rhizome. The fruits of *Musa paradisiaca* (plantain) and *M. sapientum* (banana), are rich in starch. Manila hemp or abaca is derived from *Musa textilis*. Starch, fructosans, phenolic acids, anthocyanins, terpenoids and sterols are present in the plants.

(ii) Zingiberaceae

This family contains about 49 genera and 1300 species. The herbs are perennial, aromatic with fleshy rhizomes and tuberous roots; flowers in racemes, heads or cymes. Fruit a loculicidal capsule; seed with perisperm. Genera include *Curcuma*, *Alpinia*, *Zingiber*, *Amomum*, *Elettaria*, *Aframomum*; *Hedychium* and *Costus*. Products of the family include turmeric from the rhizomes of *Curcuma longa*; ginger, the rhizome of *Zingiber officinale*; cardamom fruits from *Elettaria cardamomum*; and grains of paradise, the seeds of *Aframomum melegueta*. Volatile oils and pungent principles are found in Ginger. Other constituents are the colouring matters (curcuminoids), tannins, phenolic acids, leucoanthocyanins, flavonoids, ketones and terpenoids.

(iii) Cannaceae

This family contains only the single genus *Canna* (55 spp.). The rhizome of *Canna edulis* yields starch.

(iv) Marantaceae

It is a family of 30 genera and 400 species of tropical herbaceous perennials. The genus *Maranta* contains *Muranta arundinacea*. Its rhizome yields arrowroot.

8. SPATHIFLORAE : Araceae

The order consists of two families, the Araceae and the Lemnaceae.

The Araceae has 115 genera and about 2,000 species; mainly herbs or climbing shrubs and over 90% tropical. Many plants contain poisonous latex, the poison being destroyed by heat. The genera include *Acorus, Arum, Monstera, Dracuncula, Amorphophallus* and *Cryptocoryne*. Calamus or sweet flag rhizome, from the perennial herb *Acorus calamus*, is widely distributed in Europe and North America. The species of *Arum* are poisonous; these plants contain amines and cyanogenetic compounds. The rhizome of *Cryptocoryne spiralis* is known as 'Indian ipecacuanha'. *Amorphophallus campanulatus* is the elephant-foot yam. Many members of the family are cyanogenetic. Pyridine or indole type of alkaloids are present in a few genera. Other constituents include saponins, tannins, phenolic acids, amines and terpenoids.

ANGIOSPERMS : DICOTYLEDONS

The angiosperms or flowering plants (2,50,000 species) are herbs, shrubs and trees. The phylum is divided into monocotyledons and dicotyledons.

The dicotyledons are herbs, shrubs or trees. Their seeds have two cotyledons. The leaves are reticulately veined and the stem contains a ring of open vascular bundles. Dicotyledonous flowers are usually pentamerous or tetramerous; unisexual (e.g., Salicaceae), but usually bisexual. The perianth may or may not be differentiated into sepals and petals.

The dicotyledons are divided into two groups:
  (i) Archichlamydeae, further subdivided into 37 orders and about 226 families; and
  (ii) Sympetalae contains 11 orders and about 63 families.

In Archichlamydeae, the flowers have either no perianth or a perianth that is differentiated into sepals and petals, the latter being free.

Table 6.2. Orders and families of Dicotyledons

Order	Family
A. Subclass Archichlamydeae	
1. Aristolochiales	Aristolochiaceae
2. Cactales	Cactaceae
3. Celastrales	Aquifoliaceae, Celastraceae, Buxaceae
4. Centrospermae	Phytolaccaceae, Caryophyllaceae, Chenopodiaceae
5. Cucurbitales	Cucurbitaceae
6. Fagales	Betulaceae, Fagaceae
7. Geraniales	Geraniaceae, Zygophyllaceae, Linaceae, Erythroxylaceae, Euphorbiaceae
8. Guttiferales	Paeoniaceae, Dipterocarpaceae, Theaceae, Guttiferae (Clusiaceae)
9. Juglandales	Myricaceae, Juglandaceae
10. Magnoliales	Magnoliaceae, Winteraceae, Annonaceae, Eupomatiaceae, Myristicaceae, Canellaceae, Schisandraceae, Illiciaceae, Monimiaceae, Calycanthaceae, Lauraceae, Hernandiaceae
11. Malvales	Elaeocarpaceae, Tiliaceae, Malvaceae, Bombacaceae, Sterculiaceae
12. Myrtiflorae	Lythraceae, Myrtaceae, Punicaceae, Rhizophoraceae, Combretaceae, Onagraceae
13. Papaverales	Papaveraceae, Fumariaceae, Capparaceae, Brassicaceae
14. Piperales	Piperaceae
15. Polygonales	Polygonaceae
16. Proteales	Proteaceae
17. Ranunculales	Ranunculaceae, Berberidaceae, Menispermaceae, Nymphaeaceae
18. Rhamnales	Rhamnaceae, Vitaceae
19. Rosales	Hamamelidaceae, Crassulaceae, Saxifragaceae, Rosaceae, Papilionaceae, Krameriaceae
20. Rutales	Rutaceae, Simaroubaceae, Burseraceae, Meliaceae, Malpighiaceae, Polygalaceae
21. Salicales	Salicaceae
22. Santalales	Olacaceae, Santalaceae, Loranthaceae
23. Sapindales	Anacardiaceae, Aceraceae, Sapindaceae, Hippocastanaceae
24. Sarraceniales	Serraceniaceae, Nepenthaceae, Droseraceae

(Contd.)

Order	Family
25. Thymelaeales	Thymelaeaceae, Elaeagnaceae
26. Umbelliflorae	Alangiaceae, Cornaceae, Garryaceae, Araliaceae, Apiaceae
27. Urticales	Ulmaceae, Moraceae, Cannabinaceae and Urticaceae
28. Violales	Flacourtiaceae, Violaceae, Turneraceae, Passifloraceae, Cistaceae, Bixaceae, Tamaricaceae, Caricaceae

B. Subclass Sympetalae

1. Campanulales	Campanulaceae (including Lobeliaceae), Asteraceae
2. Dipsacales	Caprifoliaceae, Valerianaceae, Dipsacaceae
3. Ebenales	Sapotaceae, Ebenaceae, Styracaceae
4. Ericales	Ericaceae
5. Gentianales	Loganiaceae, Gentianaceae, Men-yanthaceae, Apocynaceae, Asclepiadaceae, Rubiaceae
6. Oleales	Oleaceae
7. Plantaginales	Plantaginaceae
8. Plumbaginales	Plumbaginaceae
9. Primulales	Myrsinaceae, Primulaceae
10. Tubiflorae	Polemoniaceae, Convolvulaceae, Boraginaceae, Verbenaceae, Lamiaceae, Bignoniaceae, Solanaceae, Scrophulariaceae, Acanthaceae, Pedaliaceae, Gesneriaceae, Myoporaceae

A. SUBCLASS ARCHICHLAMYDEAE

1. ARISTOLOCHIALES : Aristolochiaceae

The order comprises three families.

The Aristolochiaceae has seven genera and about 500 species. Members occur in the tropics and warm temperate zones. Most are herbs or climbing shrubs. Oil-secreting cells occur throughout the family, often forming transparent dots on the leaves. The principal genera are *Aristolochia* and *Asarum*. Constituents of the family include alkaloids (aporphine and protoberberine), aristolochic acid, phenolic esters and ethers, volatile oils and flavonoids. Some species show tumour-inhibiting properties.

2. CACTALES : Cactaceae

The Cactaceae, the only family of the order, contains up to 150 genera and about 2,000 species. The plants are xerophytes and are all found in the Americas. They may thrive in deserts where there is a reasonable rainfall. Some cacti occur in rain forests as epiphytes (e.g., *Epiphyllum*). They are succulent and store water in their stems. The plant body is usually globular or cylindrical with wool, spines and flowers. In *Epiphyllum* the stems are flattened and consist of jointed segments, which are often mistaken for leaves. Among the genera are *Epiphyllum*, *Opuntia*, *Cephalocereus*, *Cereus* and *Echinocereus*. The leaves of *Opuntia* and *Nopolea* provide food for cochineal insects. Dried cactus flowers (*Opuntia* spp.) are used as an astringent herbal remedy. The Indian drug, *Opuntia dillenii*, useful in gonorrhoea and coughs, belongs to Cactaceae. *Lophophora williamsii* is the plant producing peyote. This contains the hallucinogenic alkaloid, mescaline. Several genera contain simple isoquinoline alkaloids; most species yield abundant mucilage.

3. CELASTRALES : Aquifoliaceae, Celastraceae, Buxaceae

It is an order of 13 families; trees and shrubs with simple leaves.

(i) *Aquifoliaceae* : It consists of two genera and about 400 species, all but one of which belong to the genus *Ilex*. Members are trees and shrubs found in the temperate and tropical regions. Mate or Paraguay tea is obtained from *Ilex paraguensis* and other species. Constituents reported in the family include caffeine, theobromine, cyclitols (shikimic acid and inositol), triterpenes and triterpenoid saponins.

(ii) *Celastraceae* : It is a family of 55 genera and 850 species; tropical and temperate trees and shrubs. The genera include *Euonymus*, *Celastrus*, *Cassine*, *Maytenus*, *Prionstemma*, *Catha*, *Tripterigum* and *Peripterygia*. *Catha edulis* leaves, known as Abyssinian tea, contain an alkaloid cathine (norpseudoephedrine). The root bark of *Euonymus atropurpureus* contains cardioactive glycosides. The family possess alkaloidal amines, alkaloids of the pyridine and purine types, sugar alcohols (dulcitol), saponins, cardenolides, terpenoids and substances having antitumour activity.

(iii) *Buxaceae* : This family possesses five genera and 100 species of tropical and temperate, usually evergreen, shrubs. The genera are *Buxus*, *Notobuxus*, *Sarcocolla*, *Pachysandra* and *Simmondsia*. The family contains alkaloids, phenolic acids and waxes.

4. CENTROSPERMAE : Phytolaccaceae, Caryophyllaceae, Chenopodiaceae

The order contains 13 families with the monochlamydeous type of flower (e.g., Phytolaccaceae and Chenopodiaceae) and the dichlamydeous type of flower (e.g., Caryophyllaceae). Most families of the order produce characteristic betacyanin and betaxanthin pigments.

The Phytolaceaceae is a family of 12 genera and 100 species, herbs, shrubs and trees, found in tropical America and South Africa. *Phytolacca* includes *Phytolacca americana* (Poke root), the leaves and roots of which are used as an adulterant of belladonna: its berries contain a dyestuff. The roots are used to cure rheumatic diseases. They contain antihepatotoxic neo-lignans.

The Caryophyllaceae has 70 genera and about 1,750 species, mostly herbs. The genera include *Saponaria*, *Stellaria*, *Arenaria*, *Spergularia*, *Herniaria*, *Silene*, *Lychnis*, *Gypsophila* and *Dianthus*. Many of these plants are rich in saponins. The root of *Saponaria officinalis* contains about 5% of saponins and is widely used as a domestic detergent.

The Chenopodiaceae contains 102 genera and 1,400 species; most grow naturally in soils containing much salt (halophytes). The genera include *Beta*, *Chenopodium*, *Salicornia*, *Atriplex* and *Anabasis*. *Chenopodium anthelminticum* yields the anthelmintic Mexican tea or 'wormseed' and its oil of chenopodium. The family Chenopodiaceae include the Indian drugs *Chenopodium album* (anthelmintic, laxatives), *C. ambrosioides* (anthelmintic) and *Spinacia oleracea* (used for urinary calculi, respiratory diseases, liver problems). The plants contain sterols, flavonoids and saponins.

5. CUCURBITALES : Cucurbitaceae

This order contains the single family Cucurbitaceae.

A family of about 110 genera and 640 species; tropical; mostly herbs climbing by tendrils. The fruit is fleshy. Most members have bicollateral vascular bundles. The genera include *Cucurbita*, *Cucumis*, *Ecballium*, *Citrullus*, *Luffa*, *Bryonia* and *Momordica*. *Cucurbita pepa* is a vegetable marrow. *C. maxima*, great pumpkin; *Cucumis melo*, the melon; *C. sativus*, the cucumber. *Echallum elaterum*, the squirting cucumber, yields the purgative elaterium; *Citrullus colocynthis* yields colocynth; *C. lanatus*, the water melon. The vascular network of the pericarp of *Luffa* is used as a bath sponge. The fruits and seeds of *L. acutangula* contain saponins and are used in Ayurvedic medicine. Bryony root, from *Bryonia dioica*, is used as a purgative and for the treatment of gout. It contains saponins. *Bryonia alba* contains antitumour substances. The enzyme elaterase hydrolyses the bitter glucosides to cucurbitacins and glucose. The cucurbitacins are triterpenoid bitter principles named A to Q, cucurbitacin-E (α-elaterin).

6. FAGALES : Betulaceae and Fagaceae

These families consist of monoecious trees and shrubs.

The Betulaceae has two genera, *Alnus* and *Betula*. Phenolic substances such as myricetin, delphinidin, ellagic acid and terpenoids such as lupeol and betulin are present in the species. The wood of *Betula alba* is used for charcoal.

The Indian plant *Betula utilis* (Betulaceae) is found throughout the Himalayan range. Its bark is used as antiseptic, carminative and to treat hysteria.

The Fagaceae has eight genera and about 900 species. *Fagus* includes the beech, *F. sylvatica* nuts yield oil; *Castanea* includes the sweet chestnut, *C. sativa*, which yields timber and a bark used for tanning. *Quercus* provides valuable timber, shikimic acid (a cyclitol), methyl salicylate and terpenoids. The capsules and unripe acorns of *Q. aegelops* (valonia) are used in tanning. *Q. ilex* and *Q. robur* yield tanning barks and *Q. tinctoria*, a yellow dye. *Q. suber* affords the commonly used cork. An extract of *Q. stenophylla* is used to eliminate renal and urethral calculi. Turkish galls, an important source of tannic acid, are obtained from *Q. infectoria*.

Quercus infectoria is found in Himalayas and belongs to the family Papilionaceae.

7. GERANIALES : Geraniaceae, Zygophyllaceae, Linaceae, Erythroxylaceae, Euphorbiaceae

The order Geraniales consists of nine families.

(i) The Geraniaceae consists of five genera and 750 species; mostly herbs. Members of the two large genera, *Geranium* and *Pelargonium* are popularly called 'geraniums'. The rose geranium oil is obtained from a *Pelargonium* species. The family contains volatile oils which are widely used in perfumery.

(ii) The Zygophyllaceae is a family of 25 genera and 240 species; mostly woody perennials, tropical and subtropical. Genera include *Zygophyllum, Tribulus, Guaiacum, Peganum* and *Balanites. Peganum harmala* and *Tribulus terrestris* are used in Indian medicine. Some members contain alkaloids, steroidal saponins or lignans.

(iii) The Linaceae is a family of 19 genera and about 290 species; mostly herbs or shrubs. About 230 of the species belong to *Linum*. Cyanogenetic glycosides, fixed oils, mucilages, diterpenes and triterpenes are present in the family. Flax and linseed and its oil are obtained from *Linum usitatissimum*.

(iv) The Erythroxylaceae comprises three to four genera with genera *Erythroxylum* and *Nectaropetalum. Erythroxylum* spp. are distributed widely in S. America and Madagascar. Alkaloids found in most species are principally esters of the tropane type together with related bases such as hygrine, hygroline and cuscohygrine, Cocaine and cinnamoylcocaine are present in the cultivated species *E. coca* and *E. novogranatense*. Phenolic constituents such as caffeic and chlorogenic acids, and flavonoids may have chemosystematic importance.

(v) The Euphorbiaceae is a large family of about 3000 genera and 6000 species. Most members are trees or shrubs, a few herbs. Some genera (e.g. *Euphorbia*) are xerophytic. The genera include *Euphorbia, Phyllanthus, Mallotus, Ricinus, Croton, Hevea, Jatropha, Manihot, Sapium, Poranthera, Securinega, Aleurites* and *Hippomane*. The products include castor seeds, castor oil, dye, taenicide kamala (from *Mallotus philippinensis*); rubber, from species of *Hevea, Manihot* and *Sapium*; manihot or cassava starch, from *Manihot esculentus (utilis)*; Chinese tallow, a fat, from *Sapium sebiferum*; a drying oil, from *Aleurites moluccana*, Amla from *Phyllanthus emblica*, croton oil from *Croton tiglium*, and cascarilla bark from *C. cascarilla* and *C. eleuteria*. In some cases the latex is poisonous or irritant. *Manihot esculentus* occurs in sweet and bitter varieties, only the latter yields prussic acid. Some members contain anthraquinones, triterpenoids, fatty acids, epoxides, unsaturated fatty acids and antitumour agents. Alkaloids are of the aporphine, pyridine, indole, quinoline or tropane types.

8. GUTTIFERALES : Paeoniaceae, Dipterocarpaceae, Theaceae, Guttiferae

Of the 16 families in the order, only the four above are important.

(i) The Paeoniaceae contains the single genus *Paeonia* with 33 species which are perennial rhizomatous herbs. Peony root is important in Chinese medicine obtained from *P. lactiflora*. It is a constituent of a herbal tea used for the treatment of children's eczema. The active anti-inflammatory ingredient is paeonol, 2'-hydroxy-4'-methoxy acetophenone, other constituents of the rhizome are monoterpenoid glycosides one of which, paeoniflorin, is used as a basis for the quality control of the drug.

(ii) The Dipterocarpaceae has 15 genera and about 580 species. Many are large trees yielding useful timbers. Oleoresins are present in the family. The genera include *Dipterocarpus, Shorea, Dryobalanops* and *Hopea*. Products include: gurjun balsam from *Dipterocarpus turbinatus*; varnish resins from species of *Shorea, Hopea* and *Balanocarpus*; an edible fat, used in chocolate manufacture, from the nuts of *Shorea macrophylla*; and Borneo camphor, from *Dryobalanops aromatica*.

(iii) The Theaceae or Ternstoremiaceae consists of 16 genera and about 500 species of tropical and subtropical trees and shrubs. The genera include *Camellia* and *Ternstroemia*. They contain purine bases in *Camellia*, saponins, tannins and fixed oils. *Camellia sinensis* yields tea and caffeine. The 'tea seed oil' is an edible oil which is a possible adulterant of olive oil and is obtained from *Camellia sasanqa*.

(iv) The Guttiferae (Clusiaceae) contains about 40 genera and 1,000 species. They are trees, shrubs or lianes. The main genera are *Hypericum*, *Kielmeyera*, *Clusea*, *Garcinia* and *Calophyllum*. Constituents of the family include resins, volatile oils, alkaloids, xanthones and seed oils. Products include resin from *Calophyllum* and gamboge from *Garcinia*. The edible fruit mangosteen is obtained from *Garcinia mangostana*.

9. JUGLANDALES : Myricaceae and Juglandaceae

The Myricaceae has about four genera of trees and shrubs with unisexual flowers. Some members contain volatile oil (e.g., *Myrica gale*). *Myrica esculenta* is an Indian drug belonging to the family Myricaceae. Its bark is used in fever, asthma and cough.

The Juglandaceae has eight genera. The walnut, *Juglans regia*, produces timber and edible nuts. *Juglans* contains the naphthoquinone juglone, the sugars raffinose and stachyose, flavonoids and phenolic acids.

10. MAGNOLIALES : Magnoliaceae, Winteraceae, Annonaceae, Myristicaceae, Canellaceae, Schisandraceae, Illiciaceae, Monimiaceae, Lauraceae and Hernandiaceae

This order contains 22 families.

(i) The Magnoliaceae contains 12 genera and about 230 species, which occur in both temperate and tropical regions. They are trees or shrubs with oil cells in the parenchyma. The genera include *Magnolia*, *Michelia* and *Liriodendron*. Tulip tree. *L. tulipifera* contains alkaloids (e.g., dihydroglaucine) and sesquiterpenes.

(ii) The Winteraceae comprises 7 genera and 120 species. *Drimys winteri* (Winter's bark) contains volatile oil used as a stimulant and tonic.

(iii) The Annonaceae contains 120 genera and about 2,100 species. The genera include *Uvaria*, *Xylopia*, *Monodora* and *Annona*. The seeds of *Monodora myristica* are used like nutmegs. The family contains mainly isoquinoline type alkaloids. *Annona reticulata*, *A. squamosa* and *Polyalthia longifolia* are Indian drugs of the family Annonaceae.

(iv) The Myristicaceae contains 18 genera and 300 species, mainly found in tropical Asia. The genera include *Myristica*, *Virola*, *Horsfieldia* and *Knema*. The flowers are dioecious and consist of three-lobed perianth with 3-18 monadelphous stamens or a solitary carpel containing a basal anatropous ovule. The fruit is a fleshy drupe. The single seed is completely enveloped in a lobed aril. Some species ('Nutmeg' and 'Mace') contain volatile oil and hallucinogenic substances.

(v) The Canellaceae contains five genera and 16 species; trees with gland-dotted leaves. Fruit is a berry. The genera include *Canella*, *Cinnamodendron* and *Warburgia*. Canella bark, a spice, is obtained from *Canella alba*, grown in the Bahamas and Florida.

(vi) The Schisandraceae comprises two genera and 47 species of climbing shrubs. *Schisandra* has 25 species; lignans are common constituents.

(vii) The Illiciaceae has the single genus *Illicium*, found in Asia. Atlantic North America and the West Indies. Star-anise belongs to this family.

(viii) The Monimiaceae includes 20 genera and 150 species of trees and shrubs, which contain volatile oil and resin. The genera include *Hedycarya* and *Peumus*. *Peumus boldo* bark yields a dye and its leaves contain the alkaloid boldine.

(ix) The Lauraceae has 32 genera and about 2,500 species. These are tropical or subtropical trees and shrubs with leathery, evergreen leaves; the fruit is a berry. The genera include *Persea*, *Ocotea*, *Cinnamomum*, *Aniba*, *Litsea*, *Neolitsea*, *Lindera*, *Laurus* and *Cryptocarya*. The bark of *Cryptocarya massoia* yields an essential oil with a coconut-like aroma and is used in shampoos. The bay laurel, *Laurus nobilis*, yields essential oil, the principal one being 1,8-cineole. The drugs are 'Cinnamon bark', 'Cassia bark' and 'Camphor'. The fruit is a berry or drupe. Alkaloids, volatile oils and fixed oils occur in many species. The Indian drugs of Lauraceae family are *Cassytha filiformis*, *Cinnamomum camphora*, *C. tamala*, *C. zeylanicum*, *Litsea glutinosa* and *L. monopetala*. The drugs contain volatile oils, sterols, flavonoids and phenolics.

(x) The Hernandiaceae has three genera and 54 species; occurs as tropical trees, shrubs or lianes with oil cells. Species of *Hernandia* contain tumour-inhibiting alkaloids and lignans including podophyllotoxin.

11. MALVALES : Elaeocarpaceae, Tiliaceae, Malvaceae, Bombacaceae, Sterculiaceae

It is an order of seven families.

Herbs, shrubs or trees; tropical and temperate. Many species contain mucilage.

(i) *Elaeocarpaceae* : A family of 12 genera and 350 species of tropical and subtropical trees and shrubs. Chief genera are *Elaeocarpus* and *Sloanea*. Indolizidine alkaloids are present in *Elaeocarpus*.

(ii) *Tiliaceae* : A family of 50 genera and some 450 species; usually trees or shrubs. The genera include *Corchorus* and *Tilia*. Jute fibre is obtained from *Corchorus capsularis* and *C. olitorius*. Lime tree flower, the dried inflorescences of *Tilia plantyphyllos* or *T. cordata*, is used in respiratory tract infections and as a nervine and tonic; constituents include volatile oil, flavonoids and phenolic acids. Cardiac glycosides are reported from *Corchorus*; alkaloids are absent.

(iii) *Malvaceae* : The family contains 75 genera and about 1,000 species of herbs, shrubs and trees;

tropical and temperate. The genera include *Malva*, *Gossypium*, *Hibiscus*, *Althaea*, *Pavonia* and *Thespesia*. The cottons, species of *Gossypium*, are used as seed hairs and seed oil. Marshmallow root, from *Althaea officinalis*, is used as a demulcent and, is rich in mucilage. Saponins, tannins, leucoanthocyanins and phenolic acids are present. The Indian drugs belonging to Malvaceae family are *Hibiscus esculenta*, *H. rosasinensis*, *Abutilon indicum*, *Sida cordifolia*, *Sida alba*, *Sida cordata* and *Urena lobata*.

(iv) *Bombacaceae* : A small family of about 20 genera and 180 species of tropical trees. The genera include *Bombax*, *Ceiba* and *Adansonia*. Kapok, the lignified, silky hairs from the fruits of *Bombax* and *Ceiba*, has been used for lifebelts and as a stuffing material.

(v) *Sterculiaceae* : A family of 60 genera and 700 species; mainly tropical. The genera include *Sterculia*, *Theobroma*, *Cola* and *Brachychiton*. Cocoa, oil of theobroma and chocolate are prepared from *Theobroma cacao*; kola or cola nuts are obtained from *Cola vera* and *C. acuminata*; and Sterculia or Karaya gum comes from *Sterculia urens*. Mucilage is common; purine bases are present in *Theobroma* and *Cola*.

12. MYRTIFLORAE : Lythraceae, Myrtaceae, Punicaceae, Rhizophoraceae, Combretaceae, Onagraceae

This order contains 17 families.

(i) *Lythraceae* : A family of 25 genera and 550 species; herbs, shrubs and trees. The genera include *Rotala*, *Lythrum*, *Decodon*, *Lagerstroemia*, *Heimia* and *Lawsonia*. The naphthoquinone lawsone occurs in leaves of *Lawsonia inermis*. Some species contain alkaloids. Indian drugs belonging to Lythraceae are *Ammania baccifera*, *Lagerstroemia indica*, *Lawsonia inermis* and *Woodfordia fruticosa*.

(ii) *Myrtaceae* : A family of about 100 genera and 3000 species of evergreen shrubs and trees; found in Australia, East Indies and tropical America. The family is divided into two subfamilies, the Myrtoideae (fruit a berry or drupe) and the Leptospermoideae (fruit a loculicidal capsule). The genera of the Myrtoideae include *Myrtus*, *Psidium*, *Pimenta*, *Eugenia*, *Pseudocaryophyllus* and *Syzygium* (*Jambosa*). To the Leptospermoideae belong *Eucalyptus*, *Leptospermum* and *Melaleuca*. The genera contains volatile oils, *e.g.*, cloves oil, eucalyptus oil, cajuput oil and pimento. *Psidium guajava* gives the edible fruit guava. Constituents of the family other than volatile oils are leucoanthocyanins, cyclitols, tannins, phenolic acids and esters.

(iii) *Punicaceae* : *Punica* is the single genus with two species. The fruit rind of *Punica granata*, the pomegranate, contains tannin; its stem and root bark yield tannin and the liquid alkaloids pelletierine and isopelleterine.

(iv) *Rhizophoraceae* : A family of 16 genera and 120 species; often trees. *Rhizophora* yields the tanning material mangrove cutch.

(v) *Combretaceae* : A family of 20 genera and 600 species; tropical and subtropical trees and shrubs; rich in tannin. The genera include *Terminalia*, *Combretum*, *Quisqualis* and *Anogeissus*. Myrobalans, the fruits of *Terminalia chebula*, are rich in tannin. *Combretum butyrosum* yields a butter-like substance, and *Anogeissus latifolia* yields the gum known as ghatti gum. Combretaceae includes *Terminalia indica*, *T. arjuna*, *T. bellerica*, *T. catappa*, *T. chebula*, *Anogeissus latifolia* and *Quisqualis indica* as important Indian drugs.

(vi) *Onagraceae* : A family of 21 genera and 640 species; mostly perennial herbs. The genera include *Fuchsia*, *Oenothera*, *Clarkia* and *Epilobium*. Many are cultivated for their flowers. Tannins and cyanogenetic compounds are recorded.

13. PAPAVERALES : Papaveraceae, Fumariaceae, Capparaceae, Brassicaceae

It is an order of seven families.

The Papaveraceae belongs to the suborder Papaverineae. The alkaloids of the Papaveraceae are related to those of the Ranunculaceae, and that thiogluconates are absent from the Papaveraceae but present in the other two families.

(i) The Papaveraceae is a family of 26 genera and about 300 species. The plants are usually herbs with solitary, showy flowers. The fruit is a capsule, with numerous seeds, each containing a small embryo in an oily endosperm. The genera include *Platystemon*, *Romneya*, *Eschscholtzia*, *Sanguinaria*, *Chelidonium*, *Bocconia*, *Glaucium*, *Meconopsis*, *Argemone* and *Papaver*. All members contain latex tissue. The family is rich in alkaloids. *Eschscholtzia californica*, used by the Californian Indians is a sedative. The important Indian plants belonging to Papaveraceae are *Argemone mexicana* and *Papaver somniferum*.

(ii) *Fumariaceae* : It contains 16 genera and about 55 species; they possess a watery juice. Isoquinoline alkaloids are a feature of the family. Fumitory is used for liver disorders.

(iii) *Capparaceae* : A family of 30 genera and 650 species; trees or shrubs, xerophytic. The genus *Capparis* includes *Capparis spinosa*, the buds of which are used in flavouring. The family has myrosin cells and mustard-oil glycosides such as glucocapparin.

(iv) *Brassicaceae* : A family of 375 genera and about 3,200 species; herbs and a few under shrubs. The fruit is called a siliqua. The testas of the seeds often contain mucilage. The genera include *Brassica*, *Sinapis*, *Nasturtium*, *Lepidium*, *Hesperis*, *Cheiranthus*, *Isatis*, *Erysimum*, *Crambe* and *Lunaria*. Cultivated *Brassica* species include: *B. nigra* (black mustard); *B. oleracea* (cabbage, cauliflower, broccoli, etc.); *B. campestris*, turnip; *B. napus* (rape or colza oil), *Sinapis alba* (white mustard); *Nasturtium officinale* (water cress); *Lepidium sativum* (garden cress); *Isatis tinctoria* (the dyestuff wood) and *Crambe maritima* (the sea kale). Cardiac glycosides occur in some genera and the seeds usually contain mucilage and fixed oil.

14. PIPERALES : Piperaceae

This order contains four families.

The Piperaceae includes four genera and about 2,000 species. The plants are tropical, mostly climbing shrubs or lianes, with swollen nodes and fleshy spikes of flowers. The leaves contain oil cells. The one-celled ovary has a single basal ovule and develops into a berry. The four genera are *Piper*, *Trianaeopiper*, *Ottonia* and *Pothomorphe*. The Piperaceae contains phenolic esters and ethers; pyrrolidine alkaloids; volatile oils and lignans. The peppers are widely used as condiments. In the South Pacific islands an aqueous extract of the roots of *P. methysticum* (kava-kava) is consumed as a stimulant; large doses cause intoxication. In herbal medicine the root is used as a diuretic, stimulant and tonic. The active principles are pyrone derivatives (kava lactones). The Indian medicinal plants belonging to Piperaceae are *Piper betle* (antiseptics, used in respiratory troubles), *P. cubeba* (carminative, stimulant, expectorant), *P. longum* (used in respiratory diseases, dysentery, skin problems), *P. nigrum* (aromatic, stimulant, stomachic) and *P. retrofractum* (useful in colic, dyspepsia and gastralgia). The drugs contain essential oils, sterols, piperine-type alkaloids and free organic acids.

15. POLYGONALES : Polygonaceae

It has about 40 genera and 800 species, mostly herbs. The genera include *Rheum*, *Rumex*, *Fagopyrum*, *Coccoloba* and *Polygonum*. The fruit is one-seeded, usually three-winged nut (e.g., dock and buckwheat). Anthocyanin pigments are common; also flavones and flavonols. Buckwheat, *Fagopyrum esculentum*, is a commercial source of rutin. Quinones (anthraquinones, phenanthraquinones anthrones and dianthrones) are found in many species of *Rheum, Rumex* and *Polygonum*. Garden rhubarb is obtained from *Rheum rhaponticum*. The Indian drugs belonging to Polygonaceae are *Polygonum recumbens* (haemostasis), *Rheum emodi* (astringent, bitter, stomachic), *Rumex maritimus* (demulcent) and *R. vesicarius* (laxative, diuretic). The important chemical constituents are flavonoid glycosides and anthraquinones.

16. PROTEALES : Proteaceae

The Proteaceae, contains 62 genera and 1,050 species. They occur as shrubs and trees in Australia, New Zealand and South Africa. The chemical constituents reported include cyanogenetic compounds, alkaloids, tannins, leucoanthocyanins, arbutin and the sugar alcohol polygalitol. The genera include *Protea, Grevillea, Persoonia, Hakea* and *Knightia*.

17. RANUNCULALES : Ranunculaceae, Berberidaceae, Menispermaceae and Nymphaeaceae

Among seven families, the above four are of medicinal interest. The families show a considerable variety of plant constituents and alkaloids are very common. The alkaloids are based on benzylisoquinoline, bisbenzylisoquinoline or aporphine.

(i) The Ranunculaceae comprises 59 genera and about 1,900 species. The plants are mostly perennial herbs with a rhizome or rootstock. Many members are poisonous. The fruit is an etaerio of achenes or follicles, or a berry. The genera include *Helleborus, Aconitum, Thalictrum, Clematis, Actaea, Ranunculus, Anemone, Delphinium, Adonis* and *Hepatica*. The chromosomes, based on size and shape, fall into two distinct groups, the *Ranunculus* type (R-type) and the *Thalictrum* type. The glycoside ranunculin has been found only in plants of the R-type. This glycoside hydrolyses to protoanemonin, which is vesicant. Isoquinoline-derived alkaloids occur in *Thalictrum, Aquilegia* and *Hydrastis*; diterpene-derived alkaloids in *Delphinium* and *Aconitum*. Saponins are present in *Ranunculus, Trollius, Clematis, Anemone* and *Thalictrum*; cyanogenetic glycosides in *Ranunculus* and *Clematis*; cardenolides in *Adonis*, bufodienolides in *Helleborus*. Black hellebore rhizome, from *Helleborus niger*, contains very powerful cardiac glycosides. Various aconite roots contain highly toxic alkaloids. Black Cohosh, rhizome of *Cimicifuga racemosa*; contains triterpenoid glycosides cycloartenol and isoflavones (formononetin). The drug is used in herbal medicine to treat menopausal and other female disorders, and also various rheumatic conditions.

(ii) The Berberidaceae has 14 genera and about 575 species, they are perennial shrubs usually with spiny leaves. The fruit is a berry with one to numerous seeds. The genera include *Berberis, Mohonia, Epimedium, Vancouveria* and *Leontice*.

The Berberidaceae contains alkaloids of the benzylisoquinoline, bisbenzylisoquinoline and aporphine types. Lignans such as dehydropodophyllotoxin occur; also triterpenoid saponins. The root tubers of *Leontice leontopetalum* contain saponin and alkaloids and are used for the treatment of epilepsy.

(iii) The Menispermaceae is a family of 65 genera and 350 species; mainly tropical twining shrubs, herbs or trees. The plants have palmately lobed leaves and dioecious flowers. The fruit is a drupe, the dorsal side of which develops more rapidly than the ventral. These contain the highly toxic substance picrotoxin.

The genera include *Chondodendron, Tiliacora, Triclisia, Anamirta, Coscinium, Tinospora, Jateorhiza, Abuta, Cocculus, Menispermum, Stephania, Cassampelos* and *Cyclea*. The family contains the same types of alkaloid as are found in the Ranunculaceae and Berberidaceae. Diterpene and triterpene alkaloids also occur (e.g., columbin in *Jateorhiza*). Saponins are present in many species. *Coscinium fenestratum* ('false calumba', 'tree turmeric') stems are widely used in SE Asia and India for the treatment of a variety of ailments. The principal alkaloid constituents are berberine and jatrorrhizine. *Stephania pierrii (S. erecta)* contains bisbenzylisoquinoline alkaloids and is used in Thai folk medicine as a muscle relaxant.

(iv) The Nymphaeaceae is a small family of about six genera and 70 species. Species of *Nymphaea* (water-lilies) are widely cultivated. The genera include *Nymphaea, Nuphar, Nelumbo* and *Ondinea*. *Nuphar variegatum* rhizomes contain antibacterial tannins.

18. RHAMNALES : Rhamnaceae, Vitaceae

The order contains three families.

(i) *Rhamnaceae* : This family contains 59 genera and about 900 species; cosmopolitan, trees or shrubs. The genera include *Rhamnus, Zizyphus, Scutia, Discaria, Columbrina, Maesopsis* and *Hovenia*. *R. purshiana* produces Cascara bark. The edible fruits of *Ziziphus jujuba* are used as a mild sedative. The constituents of the family include purgative quinones (anthraquinones, anthranols and their glycosides). Alkaloidal peptides occur in some genera; also terpenoids and triterpenoid saponins. Rhamnaceae includes *Ventilago denticulata, Zyzyphus jujuba* and *Z. oenoplia* as the Indian medicinal plants.

(ii) *Vitaceae* : *Vitis vitifera* produces grapes, wine, raisins and currants. Vitaceae includes *Cayratia pedata, C. trifolia, Cissus quadrangula, Leea indica* and *Vitis vinifera* as the Indian medicinal plants.

19. ROSALES : Hamamelidaceae, Crassulaceae, Saxifragaceae, Rosaceae, Leguminosae, Krameriaceae

The order Rosales consists of 19 families divided into four suborders: Hamamelidineae (Hamamelidaceae); Saxifragineae (Crassulaceae, Saxifragaceae and Pittosporaceae); Rosineae (Rosaceae); Leguminosineae (Leguminosae and Krameriaceae). The flowers are usually hermaphrodite (rarely bisexual), hypogynous, perigynous or epigynous.

(i) *Hamamelidaceae* : A family of 26 genera and 106 species of trees and shrubs, subtropical. Genera include Hamamelis leaves (*Hamamelis virginiana*), Levant storax (*Liquidambar orientalis*) and American storax or sweet gum (*L. styraciflua*). The family contains tannins, balsamic resins, phenolic acids and cyclitols; alkaloids are absent.

(ii) *Crassulaceae* : A family of 35 genera and 1,500 species; many perennial xerophytes. The genera include *Sedum, Sempervivum* and *Crassula*. The family contains isocitric acid. The carbohydrate sedoheptulose occurs in both the Crassulaceae and the Saxifragaceae. Cyanogenetic glycosides and cardiac glycosides occur in some species; tannins are common but alkaloids rare.

(iii) The Saxifragaceae is a family of 30 genera and about 580 species. The genera include *Saxifrage, Astilbe* and *Ribes*. The latter, includes fruits as the blackcurrent, red current and gooseberry. These are rich in citric and malic acids and in ascorbic acid. Black Current Syrup is used medicinally.

(iv) *Rosaceae* : It includes about 100 genera and 2000 species of herbs, shrubs and trees. The leaves are simple (e.g., *Prunus*) or compound (e.g., *Rosa*). The genera includes *Spiraea, Quillaia, Pyrus, Malus, Sorbus, Kerria, Rubus, Potentilla, Geum, Alchemilla, Agrimonia, Poterium, Rosa, Prunus, Laurocerasus* and *Crataegus*. Constituents of the Rosaceae include cyanogenetic glycosides, saponins, tannins, seed fats, sugar alcohols, cyclitols, terpenoids and mucilage. Important products are oil of rose (*Rosa damascena*), rose hips (*R. canina*), wild cherry bark (*Prunus serotina*), almond oil (*Prunus amygdalus*), quillaia bark (*Quillaia saponaria*), hawthorn (*Crataegus oxycanthoides*), cherry laurel leaves (*Prunus domestica*), raspberry fruits and leaves (*Rubus idaeus*) and morello cherries (*Prunus cerasus*). Rosaceae also includes Indian medicinal plants *Cydonia oblonga, Prunus domestica, P. puddum* and *Rosa damascena*.

(v) *Leguminosae* : This is the second-largest family of flowering plants and contains 600 genera and about 12,000 species. It includes more important drugs than any other family. It is divided into three subfamilies—the Papilionaceae, the Mimosoideae and the Caesalpinoideae, containing, respectively, about 377, 40 and 133 genera.

    a) *Papilionaceae* : Herbs, shrubs or trees; leaves simple or compound; flowers zygomorphic and papilionaceous (e.g., in broom); stamens 10, fruit a legume. The genera include *Myroxylon* (12), *Sophora, Crotalaria, Lupinus, Cytisus, Ononis, Medicago, Melilotus, Trifolium, Psoralea, Indigofera, Astragalus, Vicia, Lens, Lathyrus, Pisum, Abrus, Glycine, Erythrina, Mucuna, Phaseolus, Arachis, Trigonella, Butea, Derris, Lonchocarpus, Copaifera* and *Erythrophleum*. Drugs from this subfamily are Fenugreek seeds, Calabar bean, Tonco seed, Derris, Lonchocarpus, Tolu balsam, Peru balsam Arachis oil and Tragacanth gum. Economic products are hemp (*Crotalaria juncea*), lentas (*Lens esculents*), peas (*Pisum sativum*), soya bean (*Oscine hispida*), scarlet runner, betas (*Phaseolus* spp.), groundnut (*Arachis hypogaea*) and copaiba oleoresin and copals (*Copaifera* spp.). Species of *Indigofera* (*I. tinctoria*) are a source of indigo.

    b) *Mimosoideae* : Most members of this subfamily are trees or shrubs; leaves usually bipinnate; flowers regulate calyx usually gamosepalous; stamens equal in numbers, fruit a legume. Important genera are *Mimosa* and *Acacia*. Products include Acacia gum from *Acacia* spp. and wattle barks used in tanning from *Acacia* spp. and volatile oils such as oil of cassie (*A. farnesiana*), which are used in perfumery.

    c) *Caesalpinoideae* : Members are trees or shrubs; leaves pinnate or bipinnate; flowers zygomorphic. Drugs derived from this subfamily are Senna leaves and pods, Cassia pods and Tamarinds.

    Tannin sacs are common, particularly in the Mimosoideae and Caesalpinoideae. The constituents of the Leguminosae and Rosaceae contain cyanogenetic glycosides, saponins, tannins, mucilage and anthocyanins. Alkaloids are common in the Leguminosae but rare in the Rosaceae. The important Indian medicinal plants of Caesalpinioideae are *Bauhinia purpurea, Caesalpinia bonduc, Cassia senna, C. fistula, C. tora, Saraca indica* and *Tamarindus indica*.

    d) *Krameriaceae* : It is a family of one genus, *Krameria*, and 20 species. They are shrubs or herbs found from the southern USA to the Argentine. The flowers resemble the Caesalpinoideae, but two of the petals are modified into glands and there are only three stamens. They contain phlobatannins.

20. RUTALES : Rutaceae, Simaroubaceae, Burseraceae, Meliaceae, Malpighiaceae, Polygalaceae

The Rutales plants are mainly shrubs or trees. The flowers have a disc between the androecium and the gynaecium. Oil glands are present. The order contains 21 families and is divided into three suborders. The families Rutaceae, Simaroubaceae, Burseraceae and Meliaceae all belong to the same suborder, the Rutineae.

(i) *Rutaceae* : The family consists of about 150 genera and 900 species; mainly shrubs and trees; abundant in South Africa and Australia. Oil glands are present in the leaves and other parts. The fruits are of various types and include orange and lemon, lime (*Citrus limetta* and *C. medica* var. *acida*), citron, bergamot, shaddock and grapefruit. Other genera include *Zanthoxylum, Fagara, Choisya, Ruta, Dictamnus, Diosma, Galipea, Cusparia* (*Angostura*), *Ptelea, Toddalia, Skimmia, Limonia, Aegle, Moniera, Haplophyllum, Teclea, Esenbeckia* and *Murraya*. Buchu leaves (*Barosma* spp.); jaborandi leaves and their alkaloid, pilocarpine (*Pilocarpus* spp.); Japan pepper (*Zanthoxylum piperitum*); elephant-apple (*Limonia acidissima*); Brazilian angostura (*Esenbeckia febrifuga*); and angostura or cusparia (*Galipea officinalis*). Species of *Haplophyllum, Evodia, Clausena, Phellodendron*, and *Zanthoxylum* have all been used in traditional medicine. Bael fruit (*Aegle marmelos*), an important Ayurvedic medicine, contains coumarins and flavonoids (rutin and marmesin). Prickly Ash bark is derived from *Zanthoxylum clavaherculis*; it contain alkaloids, e.g., chelerythrine and nitidine, a lignanasarinin and an *n*-isobutyl polyeneamide. It is used as an antirheumatic. The bis-indole alkaloid yeuhchukene from *Murraya paniculata* has anti-implantation, contraceptive activity. Constituents of the Rutaceae are variety of alkaloids, volatile oils, rhamnoglucosides, coumarins and terpenoids. Alkaloids include alkaloidal amines, imidazole, indole, isoquinoline, pyridine, pyrrolidine, quinazoline and quinoline types. Many of the fruits are rich in citric and other acids and in vitamin C. The Indian drugs belonging to Rutaceae are *Aegle marmelos, Atalantia malabarica, Citrus aurantifolia, C. limon, C. medica, Glycosmis arborea, Murraya koenigii, Peganum harmala* and *Zanthoxylum alatum*.

(ii) *Simaroubaceae* : A family of 20 genera and about 120 species; tropical and subtropical shrubs and trees; without oil glands. Bitter principles are a characteristic of the family. The genera include *Quassia* (*Simarouba*), *Picrasma* (*Aeschrion*), *Brucea, Soulamea, Ailanthus* and *Perriera. Atlanthus glandulosa*, Tree of Heaven, is used to adulterate belladonna and mint.

(iii) *Burseraceae* : A family of about 16 genera and 500 species; tropical shrubs and trees. The leaves are gland-dotted. Oleoresin canals are found in the phloem and pith. The genera include *Commiphora, Boswellia, Bursera* and *Canarium*. The products of the family are Myrrh, Frankincense (*Boswellia* spp.), American elemi (*Bursera gummifer*), Manila elemi and Java almond from *Canarium luzonicum*.

(iv) *Meliaceae* : A family of 50 genera and about 1400 species; trees or shrubs. They yield timber (e.g., mahogany from *Swietenta maha-goni*); and seed oils. The genera include *Cedrela, Swietenia, Khaya, Carapa, Melia* and *Azadirachta. A. indica* (Neem) is an important Indian medicinal plant; bark, leaves and seeds are used. The chemical constituents of the family are triterpenoids and limonoids.

(v) *Malpighiaceae* : A family of 60 genera and 800 species, shrubs or small trees. The genera include *Malpighia* and *Banisteriopsis*. Some members have stinging hairs. *Banisteriopsis* contains indole alkaloids, and plants may be hallucinogenic.

(vii) *Polygalaceae* : A family of 12 genera and about 800 species, 600 species belong to *Polygala*; e.g., the milkwort, *Polygala vulgaris*. Other genera are *Monnina, Securidaca* and *Carpolobia*. Senega root is obtained from the North American *Polygala senega*. Important constituents are triterpenoid saponins and, in *Polygala*, the sugar alcohol polygalitol. Methyl salicylate is present in some plants.

21. SALICALES : Salicaceae

It contains only two genera, *Salix* and *Populus*. The dioecious flowers are in catkins.

Both genera contain phenolic glycosides such as fragilin, salicin and populin. Osiers (*Salix purpurea* and *S. viminalis*) are used for basket-making, and *S. alba* var. *caerulea* is used for cricket-bats. Species of *Populus* contain raffinose and stachyose. The dried winter buds of various species of poplar constitute Balm of Gilead Bud. The hive product propolis is derived from poplar bud exudates.

22. SANTALALES : Olacaceae, Santalaceae Loranthaceae

The order contains seven families.

The Olacaceae has about 27 genera and 250 species. Acetylenic acids occur in *Olax stricta*.

The Santalaceae contains about 30 genera and 400 species. Of the genera, *Santalum* contains 25 species and *Thesium* about 325 species. Monoterpenes and sesquiterpenes occur in several genera. The plants are hemiparasitic herbs, shrubs and small trees. *Santalum album* yields sandalwood and sandalwood oil and is rich in sesquiterpene alcohols. Australian sandalwood and its oil are obtained from another member of the family, *Eucarya spicata*.

The Loranthaceae is a large family of 36 genera and 1,300 species. The genus *Viscum* consists of about 60 species of parasitic evergreen shrubs, which contain cyclitols. The dried aerial parts of *Viscum album*, which grows on apple and other trees, are used for various circulatory conditions. It contains glycoproteins (the mistletoe lectins), polypeptides (viscotoxins) and lignans.

23. SAPINDALES : Anacardiaceae, Aceraceae, Sapindaceae, Hippocastanaceae

The Sapindales consist of 10 families.

(i) *Anacardiaceae* : A family of 60 genera and some 600 species; mainly tropical trees and shrubs. The genera include *Mangifera*, *Anacardium*, *Rhus*, *Pistacia*, *Toxicodendron*, *Lannea*, *Cotinus* and *Schinus*. Products include the mango, *Mangifera indica*; cashew nut, *Anacardium occidentale*; sumac leaves, used in dyeing and tanning, *Rhus coriaria*; the Japanese wax tree, *Thus succedanea*; mastic resin, *Pistacia lentiscus*; and pistachio nuts, *Pistacia vera*. The family contains dyeing and tanning materials and phenolic compounds some of which cause dermatitis (e.g., the vesicant constituents of the poison ivy, *Rhus toxicodendron*, other species of *Rhus* yield Japanese lacquer and Japan wax. Mastic resin contains triterpenoid acids and alcohols. The Indian drugs *Anacardium occidentale*, *Buchanania lanzan*, *Mangifera indica*, *Pistacia integerrima*, *Rhus succedanea*, *Semecarpus anacardium* and *Spondias pinnata* belong to Anacardiaceae.

(ii) *Aceraceae* : A family of trees and shrubs. The genus *Acer saccharum* yields maple sugar.

(iii) *Sapindaceae* : A family of about 150 genera and 2000 species; tropical and subtropical. The genera include *Paullinia*, *Sapindus*, *Cardiospermum*, *Eriocoelum*, *Blighia* and *Radlkofera*. The seeds of *Paullinia cupana* are made into a paste and dried to form guarana; this contains caffeine and is used as a beverage. *Sapindus saponaria* has been used in Brazil and India as a soap and for the treatment of several diseases; it contains saponins with hederagenin as an aglycone. Constituents of the family include saponins, cyanogenetic glycosides, cyclitols (e.g., shikimic acid); the seed fats contain a high proportion of oleic acid. Some species contain alkaloids, e.g., caffeine and theobromine in *Paullinia*. Sapindaceae includes *Euphoria longun*, *Litchi chinensis*, *Sapindus trifoliatus* and *S. mukorossi* as the Indian medicinal plants.

(iv) *Hippocastanaceae* : A small family of only two genera and 15 species; tropical trees and shrubs of southern Africa. *Aesculus* contains the horse chestnut, *A. hippocastanum*. Its seed fat contains a high proportion of oleic acid (70%).

24. SARRACENIALES : Sarraceniaceae, Nepenthaceae, Droseraceae

This order contains three small families of insectivorous plants which are of minor pharmaceutical interest.

The Sarraceniaceae consists of three genera and 17 species of pitcher-plants. The Nepenthaceae has two genera and 68 species, of which 67 belong to *Nepenthes*. In these plants the leaves are modified into pitchers, which attract insects by their colour and honey-like secretion. The Droseraceae has four genera and 105 species. In these common bog-plants the leaves are covered with glandular hairs which trap and digest insects. The constituents of plants of this order are tannins and phenolic compounds. The European sundew, *Drosera rotundifolia*, is an ingredient of a liqueur. It contains the naphthoquinone plumbagone, which has antimicrobial activity.

25. THYMELAEALES : Thymelaeaceae, Elaeagnaceae

It is an order of five families.

(i) *Thymelaeaceae* : This family contains 90 genera and 500 species; mostly temperate and tropical shrubs. The genera include *Gnidia, Daphne* and *Pimelea*. Some species of *Daphne* are poisonous and contain vesicant resins. Mucilage and coumarins are present in the family.

(ii) *Elaeagnaceae* : A family of three genera and about 50 species, including *Hippophae, Elaeagnus* and *Shepherdia*. Indole alkaloids and cyclitols are found in the family.

26. UMBELLIFLORAE : Alangiaceae, Apiaceae, Cornaceae, Garryaceae, Araliaceae

This is an order of seven families. Acetylenic compounds are present throughout the order.

(i) *Alangiaceae* : A family of 2 genera and 20 species, tropical trees and shrubs. Alkaloids and triterpenoid saponins occur. *Alangium lamarkii* is an Indian medicinal plant.

(ii) *Cornaceae* : A family of 12 genera and 100 species; trees and shrubs. The genera include *Cornus* and *Acuba*.

(iii) *Garryaceae* : It has only *Garrya*; shrubs containing alkaloids.

(iv) *Araliaceae* : A family of 55 genera and 700 species; mainly tropical trees and shrubs, some climbing (e.g., ivy). The genera include *Panax, Tetrapanax, Aralia, Hedera, Cussonia, Pseudopanax, Fatsia* and *Sciadodendron*. The drug is Ginseng, from *Panax schinseng* (*P. ginseng*). *Tetrapanax papyriferum* is the ricepaper tree, and *Hedera helix*, the common ivy. Resin passages are present in the family. Constituents include saponins, a few alkaloids, acetylenic compounds, diterpenoids and triterpenoids.

(v) *Apiaceae* (*Umbelliferae*) : The family contains about 275 genera and 2,850 species. The three subfamilies and main genera are as follows :

a) Hydrocotyloideae includes *Hydrocotyle*;

b) Saniculoideae includes *Eryngium, Astrantia* and *Sanicula*;

c) Apioideae includes *Chaerophyllum, Coriandrum, Smyrnium, Conium, Conium, Bupleurum, Apium, Petroselinum, Carum, Pimpinella, Seseli, Foeniculum, Oenanthe, Ligusticum, Angelica, Ferula, Peucedanum, Pastinaca, Laserpitium, Thapsia, Daucus, Ammi, Heracleum, Prangos* and *Anethum*.

The main umbelliferous fruits and their volatile oils used in pharmacy are Fennel, *Foeniculum vulgare* : Caraway, *Carum carvi;* Dill, *Anethum graveolens;* Coriander, *Coriandrum sativum*; Anise, *Pimpinella anisum*; and Cumin, *Cumminum cymium*. *Bupleurum falcatum* roots contain oleanene saponins and are an important antihepatotoxic drug. Visnaga, from *Ammi visnaga*, yields khellin, a dimethoxyfuranochromone. Among poisonous plants of the family are *Conium maculatum*, the spotted hemlock, which contains the alkaloid coniine; and *Oenanthe crocata*, the hemlock waterdropwort, which contains oenanthotoxin. Other popular plants of the family are celery, *Apium graveolens*; parsley, *Petroselinum crispum*; parsnip, *Pastinaca sativa*; and carrot, *Daucus carota*. Constituents of the family are volatile oils, resins, coumarins (e.g., umbelliferone), furocoumarins, chromonocoumarins, terpenes and sesquiterpenes, triterpenoid saponins and acetylenic compounds.

27. URTICALES : Ulmaceae, Moraceae, Cannabinaceae, Urticaceae

(i) The Ulmaceae contains 15 genera and 200 species of tropical or temperate shrubs and trees. The genera include *Ulmus, Celtis* and *Trema*. Members contain no latex (distinction from Moraceae). Mucilage is present in the barks of *Ulmus rubra* and *U. campestris*; raffinose and stachyose occur in *Ulmus*, an indole alkaloid is present in *Celtis*.

(ii) The Moraceae has about 53 genera and 1,400 species. They occur as shrubs or trees containing latex. The fruit is often multiple, as in *Ficus*, the fig. The large genus *Ficus* include *F. benghalensis* (banyan), *F. elastica* (Indian rubber tree) and *F. carica* (common fig). The latex is often anthelmintic, owing to the proteolytic enzyme ficin. Another genus *Castilloa elastica* yields Panama rubber or caoutchouc. The family also contains cardenolides and pyridine alkaloids. Species of *Morus* are used in oriental medicine. The Indian drugs *Artocarpus heterophyllus, A. lakoocha, Ficus benga-lensis, F. cunia, F. glomerata, F. heterophylla, F. hispida, F. infectoria, F. religiosa* and *F. rumphii* belongs to the family Moraceae. Triterpenes, sterols and flavonoids are common chemical constituents of the family.

(iii) The Cannabinaceae (Cannabidaceae) consists of the two genera *Cannabis* and *Humulus* and the three species *Cannabis sativa* (hemp), *Humulus lupulus* (common hop) and *H. japonica* (Japanese hop). *Cannabis* produces the best hemp and active constituents when grown in a temperate climate.

(iv) The Urticaceae has 45 genera and 550 species; tropical or temperate herbs or undershrubs without latex. Some genera have stinging hairs (e.g., *Urtica*), others lack such hairs (e.g., *Pilea, Boehmeria* and *Parietaria*).

28. VIOLALES : Flacourtiaceae, Violaceae, Turneraceae, Passifloraceae, Cistaceae, Bixaceae, Tamaricaceae, Caricaceae

This is an order of 20 families; includes herbs, shrubs and trees; tropical and temperate. Cyanogenetic glycosides occur in Flacourtiaceae, Turneraceae and Passifloraceae.

(i) *Flacourtiaceae* : A family of 93 genera and over 1,000 species. Genera include *Erythrospermum, Hydnocarpus, Flacourtia* and *Homalium. Hydnocarpus* seeds contain cyclic, unsaturated acids which are bactericidal towards the micrococcus of leprosy. Other constituents of the family are cyanogenetic glycosides, tannins and phenolic acids. Flacourtiaceae includes the Indian drugs *Casearia tomentosa, Flacourtia indica, F. sepiaria, Hydnocarpus kurzii* and *H. laurifolia.*

(ii) *Violaceae* : A family of 22 genera and about 900 species; cosmopolitan, herbs and shrubs. The genera include *Viola, Hybanthus* and *Hymenanthera*. The pansy (*Viola tricolor*), sweet violet (*V. odorata*) and dog violet (*V. canina*) are used medicinally and contain volatile oil, anthocyanin, flavonoid (rutin) and carotenoid pigments. *Hybanthus ipecacuanha* is found as an adulterant of genuine Ipecacuanha.

(iii) *Turneraceae* : A family of seven genera and 120 species of trees, shrubs and herbs. *Turnera diffusa* is the source of damiana leaves.

(iv) *Passifloraceae* : A family of 12 genera and 600 species; tropical and warm temperate; shrubs and trees, often climbers. The main genera are *Passiflora, Adenia* and *Tetrapathaea*. Some of the fruits are edible Passion fruits from *Passiflora edulis* are edibles. The dried aerial parts of *P. incarnata* are a sedative; they contain flavonoids, cyanogenetic glycosides, volatile oil and harmane-type alkaloids.

(v) *Cistaceae* : A family of eight genera and 200 species. Members are herbs and shrubs. The genera include *Helianthemum, Cistus* and *Halimium*. Species of *Cistus* yield the oleo-gum resin ladanum, used in perfumery and for embalming.

(vi) *Bixaceae* : It is a single genus *Bixa* with four species. *Bixa orellana* seeds under the name of 'annatto', are used as an edible colourant.

(vii) *Tamaricaceae* : A family of four genera and 120 species; herbs and shrubs. *Tamarix mannifera* yields the manna of the Bedouins.

(viii) *Caricaceae* : A family of four genera and 55 species; small trees found in tropical America and Africa. *Carica papaya* (papaw) is cultivated for the milky juice which is the source of the proteolytic enzyme papain.

B. SUBCLASS SYMPETALAE

In Sympetalae the petals are fused. The subclass consists of 11 orders and 63 families.

1. CAMPANULALES : Campanulaceae, Asteraceae

An order of eight families; mainly herbs with latex vessels or oils passages.

(i) *Campanulaceae* : A family of 70 genera and 2000 species. The subfamily Campanuloideae contains *Campanula*. The subfamily Lobelioideae contains *Lobelia.* Indian tobacco, *Lobelia inflata*, and Indian lobelia, from *L. nicotaniaefolia*, contains lobeline. Members of the family contain phenolic compounds, tannins and triterpenoid glycosides.

(ii) *Asteraceae* (*Compositae*) : The Asteraceae is the largest family of flowering plants and contains about 900 genera and some 13,000 species. The two subfamilies and their main genera are as follows:

a) *Tubuflerae* : In this subfamily latex vessels are absent, but schizogenous oil ducts are common. The genera include *Senecio, Xanthum, Ambrosia, Zinnia, Helianthus, Dahlia, Helenium, Tagetes, Solidago, Bellis, Aster, Erigeron, Achillea, Anthemis, Chrysanthemum, Matricaria, Tanacetum, Artemisia, Blumea, Inula, Doronicum, Calendula, Eupatorium, Arnica, Vernonia, Echinops, Carlina, Arctium, Carduus, Centaurea, Carthamus* and *Gerbera*; chamomile or Roman chamomile flowers, from *Anthemis nobilis*; German chamomile, *Matricaria chamomilla*; insect flowers, *Chrysanthemum cinerariaefolium*; wormseed or santonica, *Artemisa cina*; arnica flowers and rhizome, *Arnica montana*; calendula flowers, *Calendula officinalis*; yarrow hérb, *Achillea millefolium*; grindelia herb, *Grindelia camporum*; blessed thistle leaves, *Cnicus benedictus*; coltsfoot leaves, *Tussilago farfara*; wormwood herb, *Artemisia absinthium*; pellitory or pyrethrum root, *Anacyclas pyrethrum*; elecampane root, *Inula helenium*; Ngai camphor, from *Blumea balsamifera*. The florets of the safflower, *Carthamus tinctorius*, are used as dye and as a substitute for saffron.

b) *Liguliflorae* : In this subfamily latex vessels are present but volatile oil is rare. Genera include *Cichorium, Crepis, Hieracium, Taraxacum, Lactuca, Scorzonera* and *Sanchus*. Vegetables include lettuce, scorzonera root, chicory and endive. Medicinal plants are dandelion root, *Taraxacum officinale*; lactucarium or lettuce-opium, *Lactuca virosa*; mouse-ear hawkweed, *Hieracium pilosella*—which has antibiotic activity and has been used for the treatment of Malta fever. Chicory root and dandelion root have been used as an adulterants of or substitutes for coffee. A Turkestan dandelion, *Taraxacum koksaghiz*, is cultivated in Russia as a source of rubber latex.

Some of the volatile oils found in the Tubuliflorae contain acetylenic compound. Sesquiterpenes known as azulenes give the blue colour to freshly distilled oil of chamomile. Many sesquiterpene lactones include eudesmanolides (e.g., santonin), germacranolides, guaianolides and pseudoguaianolides; some of these have cytotoxic activity. The Senerio alkaloids cause liver damage and are, therefore, dangerous to livestock. Other alkaloids of pyridine, quinoline and diterpenoid types also occur in the family. Other constituents include the insecticidal esters of pyrethrum triterpenoid saponins of grindelia, cyclitols, coumarins and flavonols. *Stevia rebaudiana*, a herb indigenous to North eastern Paraguay, is the source of stevioside, an ent-kaurene glycoside used as a sweetener for soft drinks.

2. DIPSACALES : Caprifoliaceae, Valerianaceae, Dipsacaceae

It is an order of four families.

(i) *Caprifoliaceae* : A family of 12 genera and about 450 species; herbs and small trees. Important genera are *Viburnum, Lonicera* and *Sambucus*. Constituents reported in the family are valerianic acid, aucubin glycosides, saponins, coumarins and cyanogenetic glycosides.

(ii) *Valerianaceae* : A family of 13 genera and 360 species; mostly herbs. The genera include *Valeriana*, *Valerianella*, *Centranthus* and *Patrina*. The valerian roots of commerce are derived from *Voleriana officinalis* and the Indian valerian, *V. wallichii*. The family contains esters yielding isovalerianic acid, alkaloids, iridoids and valepotriates.

(iii) *Dipsacaceae* : A family of eight genera and about 150 species. The genera include *Scabiosa*, *Knautia* and *Dipsacus*. The constituents include a C-glycoside alkaloids and tannins.

3. EBENALES : Sapotaceae, Ebenaceae, Styracaceae

It is an order of seven families.

(i) *Sapotaceae* : A family of about 75 genera and about 800 species; most are tropical trees. The genera include *Mimusops*, *Mandhuca* (*Bassia*), *Achras*, *Pierreodendron*, *Palaquium* and *Butyrospermum*. Gutta-percha is the coagulated latex from species of *Palaquium* and *Payena*. Constituents present are latex, seed fats, cyanogenetic glycosides, saponins, tannins, leucoanthocyanins, pyrrolizidine alkaloids and the cyclitol D-quercitol.

(ii) *Ebenaceae* : A family of three genera and about 500 species; tropical trees and shrubs. The genera *Diospyros* and *Euclea* are important. Varieties of ebony are obtained from *Diospyros ebenum* and *Euclea pseudoebenus*. The fresh unripe fruits of *D. mollis* are used as an anthelmintic (hookworms and tapeworms). Naphthoquinones are present in the family.

(iii) *Styracaceae* : A family of 12 genera and 180 species of trees and shrubs. The genera include *Styrax* and *Halensia*. Benzoins are obtained from species of *Styrax*. Balsamic resins, phenolic acids, tannins and the benzofuran egonol are present in the family.

4. ERICALES : Ericaceae

An order of five families, including the Pyrolaceae, Epacridaceae and Ericaceae.

Ericaceae : A family of about 80 genera and 2,000 species. Members are shrubs or small trees.

The genera include *Rhododendron*, *Ledum*, *Erica*, *Calluna*, *Vaccinium*, *Gaylussacia*, *Gaultheria*, *Pieris*, *Lyonia*, *Arbutus* and *Arctostaphylos*. The family includes the wintergreen, *Gaultheria procumbens*, which yields natural oil of wintergreen and bearberry leaves from *Arctostaphylos uva-ursi*, which contain the phenolic glycoside arbutin. The family produces phenolic acids, phenolic glycosides (e.g., arbutin), aucubin glycosides, diterpenoids (grayanotoxin), triterpenoids (ursolic acid), cyclitols and leucoanthocyanins. A few species are cyanogenetic.

5. GENTIANALES : Loganiaceae, Gentianaceae, Menyanthaceae, Apocynaceae, Asclepiaceae, Rubiac

It is an order of seven family.

(i) *Loganiaceae* : A family of 18 genera and 500 species; trees, shrubs and herbs. The genera include *Strychnos*, *Logania*, *Gelsemium*, *Geniostoma*, *Anthocleista* and *Gardneria*. The seeds of *Strychnos nux-vomica* contains strychnine and brucine. The aucubin glycoside loganin, iridoids and alkaloids are present in the family.

(ii) *Gentianaceae* : A family of 80 genera and about 1,000 species; herbs and shrubs. The genera include *Gentiana*, *Exacum*, *Sebaca*, *Erythraea* (*Centaurium*), *Chironia*, *Swertia*, *Halenia* and *Enicostema*. Gentian root, from *Gentiana lutea* and *Swertia chirata* (Chiretta) are used to stimulate the appetite in anorexia. Some members are used in liqueurs. The family contains alkaloids; iridoid glycosides; flavones, xanthones and their glycosides; phenolic acids; tannins; and the trisaccharide gentianose. Gentianaceae includes the Indian drugs *Canscora decussata*, *Swertia chirata* and *Nymphoides hydrophyllum*.

(iii) *Menyanthaceae* : A family of five genera and 33 species. It consists of aquatic or marsh herbs. It contains bitter principles.

(iv) *Apocynaceae* : A family of about 250 genera and 2,000 species; woody climbers; tropics and subtropics. The fruits are follicles, a berry or capsules. Important genera are :

(a) *Plumieroideae*:   *Arduina-Carissa*,

Allamanda, Landolphia, Carpodinus, Hancornia, Pleiocarpa, Plumeria, Alstonia, Aspidosperma, Rhazya, Amsonia, Lochnera-Catharanthus, Vinca, Tabernaemontana, Voacanga, Alyxia, Rauwolfia, Ochrosia and *Cerbera,*

(b) *Apocynoideae* : *Echites, Dipladenia, Odontadenia, Mandevilla, Baissea, Funtumia, Apocyanum, Nerium, Strophanthus, Wrightia, Parsonia, Lyonsia* and *Malouetia.* Drugs include the *Cantharanthus roseus,* Strophanthus seeds; Rauwolfia roots; Kurchi or holarrhena bark; Alstonia barks; and Aspidosperma barks. Many species of *Landolphia, Carpondinus* and *Hancornia* yield rubber latex. The Indian medicinal plants belonging to Apocynaceae are *Alstonia scholaris, Holarrhena antidysenterica, Nerium indicum, Plumeria rubra, Rauwolfia serpentina, R. tetraphylla, Thevetia peruviana, Wrightia tinctoria* and *W. tonentora.*

Constituents of the Plumieroideae include indoline alkaloids. Steroidal alkaloids occur in *Holarrhena* and harman-type alkaloids in *Amsonia* and *Aspidosperma.* Cardioactive glycosides are present in *Acokanther, Carissa* and *Melodinus* and in *Apocyanum, Nerium* and *Strophanthus.* Other constituents of the family are cyanogenetic glycosides, leucoanthocyanins, saponins, tannins, coumarins, phenolic acids, cyclitols and triterpenoids.

(v) *Asclepiadaceae* : A family of 130 genera and 2000 species; tropical and subtropical shrubs, twining or perennial herbs. The genera include *Asclepias, Tylophora, Xysmalobium, Cryptostegia, Cynanchum, Marsdenia, Pergularia* and *Hemidesmus.* The family contains latex, alkaloids of the indole, phenanthroindo-lizidine and pyridine groups; cardenolides; cyanogenetic glycosides; saponins, tannins, and cyclitols.

(vi) *Rubiaceae* : A family of about 500 genera and 6,000 species; tropical trees and shrubs. The first subfamily Cinchonoideae includes *Oldenlandia, Condaminea, Cinchona,*

Uncaria, Nauclea, Gardenia and *Mitragyna.* The second subfamily, Rubioideae includes the genera *Coffea, Ixora, Pavetta, Psychotria, Cephaelis-Uragoga, Mitchella, Asperula, Godium* and *Rubia.* Products include Cinchona barks and their alkaloids (quinine), Ipecacuanha root, Catechu, from *Uncaria gambier,* and Coffee from *Coffea arabica.* Alkaloids are of the indole, oxindole, quinoline and purine types; anthraquinones occur in *Morinda, Rubia* and *Galium.* Anthocyanins are present in *Cinchona*; aucubin glycosides (e.g., asperulin), cyclitols (e.g., quinic acid), coumarins, depsides in *Coffea*; phlobatannins, catechins (e.g., in *Uncaria*); diterpenoids and triterpenoids and iridoid glycosides in *Genipa.*

6. OLEALES : Oleaceae

Oleaceae, the only family of the order, contains 29 genera and about 600 species. The genera include *Olea, Forsythia, Fraxinus, Syringa, Osmanthus, Jasminum* and *Ligustrum.*The manna is obtained by making incisions in the stem of *Fraxinus ornus.* The family contains olive oil, sugar alcohols (mannitol), saponins, tannins, coumarins and iridoid glycosides.

7. PLANTAGINALES : Plantaginaceae

Plantaginaceae consists of three genera and about 270 species; annual or perennial herbs. Four species belong to the genus *Plantago* (plantains). The seeds of several species are used in medicine.

8. PLUMBAGINALES : Plumbaginaceae

The Plumbaginaceae contains 19 genera and about 775 species; herbs or shrubs. The genera include *Plumbago* and *Ceratostigma.* Roots of *Plumbago* spp. are used in Indian medicine as immunosuppressive and antitumour agents. Phenolic acids, tannins, anthocyanin pigments and naphthoquinones (e.g., plumbagin) are present in the family.

9. PRIMULALES : Myrsinaceae, Primulaceae

It is an order of three families.

The Primulaceae consists of 20 genera and about 1,000 species; perennials herbs, with rhizomes or tubers. The genera include *Primula, Cyclamen,*

Anagallis and *Dionysia*. The flowers are rich in flavonoids. Anthocyanin pigments are common.

10. TUBIFLORAE : Polemoniaceae, Convolvulaceae, Boraginaceae, Verbenaceae, Lamiaceae, Solanaceae, Scrophulariaceae, Bignoniaceae, Acanthaceae, Pedaliaceae, Gesneriaceae, Myoporaceae

It is an order of six suborders and 26 families. The families are divided into the following suborders :

(a) *Convolvulineae* : Polemoniaceae and Convolvulaceae.

(b) *Boraginineae* : Boraginaceae.

(c) *Verbenineae* : Verbenacae and Lamiaceae.

(d) *Solanineae* : Solanaceae, Scrophulanaceae, Bignoniaceae, Acanthaceae, Pedaliaceae and Gesteriaceae.

(e) *Myopineae* : Myoporaceae.

(i) *Polemoniaceae* : A family of 15 genera and 300 species; herbs. Genera include *Phlox* and *Polemonium*. The family contains saponins and tannins.

(ii) *Convolvulaceae* : A family of about 55 genera and 1650 species. Annual or perennial herbs with twining stems; shrubs and trees. The genera include *Convolvulus*, *Ipomoea*, *Pharbitis-Ipomoea*, *Argyreia* and *Cuscuta*. An alcoholic extract of *Cuscuta reflexa* has hypotensive and bradycardiac effects. Convolvulaceae includes the Indian drugs *Convolvulus nervosus*, *Cuscuta reflexa*, *Evolvulus alsinoides*, *Ipomoea alba*, *I. batalas*, *I. paniculata*, *I. nil*, *I. quamoclit* and *I. turpethum*.

Brazilian arrowroot is the starch obtained from the tubers of the sweet potato, *Ipomoea batatas*. Many species contain hallucinogens such as ololiuqui, from *Rivea corymbosa*, and morning glory seeds, from species of *Ipomoea*. The family contains indole, isoquinoline, pyrrolidine and tropane alkaloids, purgative resins, phenolic acids and triterpenoid saponins.

(iii) *Boraginaceae* : A family of about 100 genera and 2,000 species; mostly perennial herbs. The genera include *Heliotropium*, *Cynoglossum*, *Symphytum*, *Borago*, *Anchusa*, *Alkanna*, *Pulmonaria* and *Lithospermum*. Products include species of *Lithospermum*, which have hormone activity; alkanna or anchusa root, from *Alkana tinctoria*, which contains red colouring matters. Naphthoquinones, the ureide allantoin, pyrrolizidine alkaloids, cyclitols, phenolic acids and tannins, occur in the family. Allantoin is present in the root of comfrey, *Symphytum officinale*. The Indian plants *Cordia dichotoma*, *C. wallichii*, *Heliotropium indicum*, *Trichodesma indicum* and *T. zeylanicum* belong to Boraginaceae.

(iv) *Verbenaceae* : A family of about 100 genera and 3,000 species; herbs, shrubs and trees. The genera include *Tectona*, *Lippia*, *Verbena*, *Callicarpa*, *Vitex*, *Nyctanthes*, *Duranta* and *Stilbe*. Teak is obtained from *Tectona grandis*; verbena oil from *Lippia citriodora*; and vervain, from *Verbena officinalis*. *Vitex agnus castus* has been used as a herbal preparation for the treatment of female conditions relating to the premenstrual syndrome and the menopause. Volatile oils, saponins, tannins, quinones, iridoids and piscicidal substances are present in the family. Verbenaceae includes the Indian drugs *Avicennia alba*, *Callicarpa nudiflora*, *Clerodendrum inerme*, *Gmelina arborea*, *Lantana camara*, *Prema corymbosa* and *Vitex trifolia*.

(v) *Lamiaceae (Labiatae)* : A family of about 200 genera and 3300 species; aromatic, annual or perennial herbs or undershrubs. The genera include *Ajuga*, *Teucrium*, *Rosmarinus*, *Scutellaria*, *Lavandula*, *Marrubium*, *Nepeta*, *Lamium*, *Ballota*, *Stachys*, *Salvia*, *Monanda*, *Satureja*, *Origanum*, *Thymus*, *Mentha*, *Pogostemon*, *Ocimum*, *Leonurus* and *Leonotis*. Many members of the family are used as culinary or medicinal herbs, as sources of volatile oils and constituents of the volatile oils such as menthol and thymol. The important plants are rosemary, lavender, peppermint and spearmint, note pennyroyal (*Mentha pulegium*), sweet majoram (*Origanum marjorama*), patchouli (*Pogostemon patchouli*), melissa (*Melissa officinalis*), germander (*Teucrium chamaedrys*), wood sage (*T. scorodonia*), wood betony (*Stachys officinalis*), sage (*Salvia officinalis*), sweet basil (*Ocimum basilicum*), savory (*Satureja* spp.), horehound (*Marrubium* spp.), hyssop (*Hyssopus officinalis*), thyme (*Thymus vulgaris*) and *Monarda punctata*. The other constituents of the family are diterpenoids and triterpenoids, saponins, a few pyridine and pyrrolidine alkaloids, insect-moulting hormones, polyphenols and tannins, iridoids and their glycosides, quinones, furanoids, cyclitols, coumarin, and the sugars raffinose and stachyose.

(vi) *Solanaceae* : A family of about 90 genera and over 2,000 species; tropical and temperate; herbs, shrubs or small trees. The genera include *Nicandra, Lycium, Atropa, Hyoscyamus, Physalis, Capsicum, Solanum, Lycopersicon, Mandragora, Datura, Solandra, Cestrum, Nicotiana, Petunia, Salpiglossis, Schizanthus, Scopolia, Withania, Duboisia, Acnistus* and *Fabiana*. The Indian drugs belonging to Solanaceae are *Atropa acuminata, Datura metal, Hyoscyamus muticus, Capsicum annuum, Nicotiana tobacum, Solanum indicum, S. nigrum, S. xanthocarpum, S. tuberosum* and *Withania somniferum*.

Products of the Solanaceae include Stramonium leaves; henhane leaves; belladonna herb and root; capsicum; potato starch from *Solanum tuberosum*, mandrake from *Mandragora officinarum*; duboisia, from Australia species of *Duboisia* which are used for the manufacture of tropane alkaloids; scopolia leaves and roots, sources of tropane alkaloids; tobacco, from *Nicotiana tabacum*. The family contains tropane, alkaloidal amine, indole, isoquinoline, purine, pyrazole, pyridine, pyrrolidine, quinazolizidine, steroid alkaloids, glycoalkaloids, steroidal saponins, withanolides, coumarins, cyclitols, pungent principles (e.g., in *Capsicum*), flavones, carotenoids and anthraquinones in *Fabiana*.

(vii) *Buddlejaceae* : A family of 6-10 genera and 150 spp.; principal genera are *Buddleja* and *Nuxia*. The genus produces flavonoids,

iridoids and iridoid glycosides, sesquiterpenoids, phenylethanoids, lignans and saponins (saikosaponins).

(viii) *Scrophulariaceae* : A family of 220 genera and about 3000 species; annual or perennial herbs or undershrubs, few are trees. Genera are *Verbascum, Calceolaria, Linaria, Anitirrhinum, Scrophularia, Penstemon, Mimulus, Gratiola, Veronica, Digitalis, Isoplexis, Melampyrum, Euphrasia, Bartsia, Pedicularis, Rhinanthus, Odontitis, Chaenorrhinum, Bacopa* and *Gratiola*. Important drugs are the leaves of *Digitalis purpurea* and *D. lanata* and their cardiac glycosides. Picrorhiza rhizome or 'Indian gentian' from *Picrorhiza kurroa* contains bitter iridoid glycosides; and is used to treat liver ailments. *Verbasum thapsus* (mullein), an adulterant of digitalis, is used as a herbal medicine for bronchial conditions. The family contains cardenolides, steroidal and triterpenoid saponins; cyanogenetic glycosides, aucubin glycosides; naphthoquinones and anthraquinones; aurones and iridoids.

(ix) *Bignoniaceae* : A family of about 120 genera and 650 species; mainly tropical trees and shrubs. The genera include *Jacaranda, Catalpa, Tecoma, Mussatia, Amphicome, Kigelia* and *Tecomella*. *Kigelia pinnata* bark contains napthoquinoids and iridoids. *Tecoma stans*, contains monoterpene alkaloids. In South America the leaves of *Mussatia hyacinthina* and other species are chewed alone or mixed with coca leaves for their sweetening, euphoric or medicinal effects. The constituents of the family include iridoids and iridoid glycosides, saponins, phenylpropanoids, tannins and quinones.

(x) *Acanthaceae* : A family of 250 genera and 2,500 species; shrubs and herbs. Genera include *Acanthus, Andrographis, Blepharis, Adhatoda* and *Barleria*. The leaves of *Adhatoda vasica*, used in India, contain the alkaloid vascine (peganine). *Andrographis paniculata* is also an important Indian drug plant. In addition to alkaloids, the family contains tannins, diterpenoids, cyanogenetic compounds and saponins.

(xi) *Pedaliaceae* : A family of 12 genera and 50 species; tropical herbs. The genera include *Harpagophytum*, *Pedalium* and *Sesamum*. *Sesamum indicum* yields the fixed oil sesame or gingili oil. *Harpagophytum procumbens* (Devil's Claw), found especially in the Kalahari desert and Namibian steppes, is used in Europe as an anti-inflammatory and anti-rheumatic herbal remedy; constituents include iridoid glycosides, flavonoids, phenolic acids and phenolics.

(xii) *Gesneriaceae* : A family of 120 genera and 2,000 species; mainly herbs. The genus *Streptocarpus* has 132 species. Tannins, naphthoquinones, chalcones and anthraquinones are present.

(xiii) *Myoporaceae* : A family of three genera and 240 species. The genus *Eremkophila* is Australian. *Myoporum* occurs in the South-West Pacific area and the monotypic *Bontia* is found only in the West Indies. The family contains terpenoids, tannins, cyanogenetic glycosides and furans.

THALLOPHYTES

Thallophyte are those plants which are not differentiated into root, stem and leaves. They include bacteria, algae, fungi and lichens.

BACTERIA AND ALGAE

1. BACTERIOPHYTA

The bacteria are unicellular organisms having size from 0.75 to 8 μm. They reproduce by binary fission. Most species of bacteria do not contain chlorophyll. In *Escherichia coli* the cell wall consists of a four-layer structure, the inner one being rigid, the three outer ones nonrigid. A protoplast membrane encloses the cytoplasm. The protoplast membrane acts as a permeability barrier and contains enzymes concerned with respiration and the active transport of metabolites.

Bacteria have the following characteristic shapes:

(i) Rod-shaped or bacillary forms (e.g., *Clostridium welchii*, *Escherichia coli* and *Bacillus subtilis*).

(ii) Spherical or coccal forms, found in aggregates, i.e., in chains (streptococci), in

Table 6.3. Order and families of Bacteria and Algae

Phyla	Orders	Families
1. Bacteriophyta	Eubacteriales	Rhizobiaceae, Micrococcaceae
2. Chrysophyta (Diatomeae)	Discales Pennatales	Actinodiscaceae Fragilariaceae, Naviculariaceae
3. Phaeophyta (Brown Algae)	Laminariales Fucales	Laminariaceae Fucaceae, Sargassaceae
4. Rhodophyta (Red Algae)	Gelidiales Gigartinales	Gelidiaceae Gracilariaceae, Gigartinaceae

groups of two (diplococci), four (tetracocci) or eight (sarcinae). Aggregates of irregular pattern are said to be of staphylococcal form.

(iii) Twisted or spirillar forms.

(iv) Branched forms (in *Mycobacterium*).

Bacteria possess flagella, thread-like processes. They form capsules consisting of polysaccharide material. They possess endospores, which are highly refractive bodies. Many bacteria are capable of elaborating complex colouring matters.

Bacteria carry out various chemical reactions, some of which are used for identification and differentiation. Bacterial action is used in the production of vinegar, acetone, butyl alcohol, lactic acid and L-sorbose. Bacteria are able to ferment carbohydrates with the formation of acidic and gaseous products. They digest protein and product of hydrogen sulphide from organic sulphur compounds.

Bacteria are most important as disease-producing organisms (about 10% of bacteria are probably pathogenic); for producing antibiotics; for effecting biochemical conversions; as agents in the deterioration of crude drugs and medicaments; in genetic engineering involving recombinant DNA (e.g., the production of human insulin). In the nitrogen cycle atmospheric nitrogen is fixed by *Azotobacter* or, by various species of *Rhizobium*, *Nitrosomonas* is able to oxidize ammonia to nitrite, while *Nitrobacter* can oxidize nitrite to nitrate. Bacteria are important in sewage purification, in the retting of fibres such as jute and flax, and in the ripening of cheese.

2(a). CHRYSOPHYTA : Discales : Actinodiscaceae

The Chrysophyta has three classes :
 (i) Bacillariophyceae (Diatomeae), contains about 10,000 species of diatom. They are unicellular algae, have a silica skeleton, and show different shape and in the cell wall;
 (ii) Centricae (in which Discales is one of the orders); and
 (iii) Pennatae (which includes the order Pennatales). The Centricae are centric or discoid in shape and generally marine, while the Pennatae are pennate or naviculoid and occur in fresh water.

Arachnoidiscus is an example of the family Actinodiscaceae found in Japanese agar and other genera are found in diatomite or kieselguhr.

2(b). CHRYSOPHYTA : Pennatales : Fragilariaceae and Naviculariaceae

Species of these two families occur in diatomite.

3(a). PHAEOPHYTA : Laminariales : Laminariaceae

The brown algae are mainly marine. They vary from microscopic branched filaments to leathery frond-like forms up to 60 cm in length. Their brown colour is due to the carotenoid pigment fucoxanthin, which masks the other pigments.

About 30 species of *Laminaria* are used for manufacture of alginic acid, mannitol and iodine.

3(b). PHAEOPHYTA : Fucales : Fucaceae and Sargassaceae

Examples of the Fucaceae are *Fucus* and *Pelvetia*; and of the Sargassaceae, *Sargassum*. These are collected for the production of alginic acid and its derivatives. *F. vesiculosus* gives water-soluble extracts that inhibit the activity of the HIV reverse-transcriptase enzyme.

4(a). RHODOPHYTA : Gelidiales : Gelidiaceae

The red algae are divided into 11 orders. The species are marine and are found in the tropics and subtropics. Their plastids contain chlorophyll, the red pigment phycoerythrin which mask the other pigments, sometimes the blue pigment phycocyanin.

Important genera of the Gelidiaceae are *Gelidium* and *Pterocladia* which are used in the preparation of agars.

4(b). RHODOPHYTA : Gigartinales : Gracilariaceae and Gigartinaceae

Gracilaria, a source of agar. *G. lichenoides,* is found in the Indian Ocean. In the Gigartinaceae *Chondrus crispus* yields carageenin or Irish moss, *Gigartina stellata* is a source of British agar.

FUNGI

The fungi, devoid of chlorophyll, are saprophytic or parasitic members of the Thallophyta. The plant body is made up of filaments or hyphae, which together constitute the mycelium. The hyphae may be aseptate and coenocytic but are often separate. The segments are uni-, bi- or multinucleate. In the formation of fruiting bodies the hyphae may become woven into dense masses of pseudoparenchyma (e.g., the sclerotium of ergot).

The protoplast of fungal cells consists of granular or reticulate cytoplasm. In older cells it is vacuolated. The nucleus may show a delicate reticulum and nucleoli. Its contents may be condensed into a chromatin body. The cell wall in many Archimycetes and some Phycomycetes (Oomycetes) and in the yeasts consists mainly of cellulose. In other fungi cellulose is replaced by the nitrogenous substance chitin.

Both sexual and asexual reproduction occur. The spores of the sporophyte generation are known as oospores (produced endogenously) or basidiospores (produced exogenously). The fungi also produce spores. They are borne on the gametophyte (Phycomycetes and Ascomycetes) or on the sporophyte (rusts and some Autobasi-diomycetes). These accessory spores often take the form of conidia, non-motile spores, borne externally on conidiophores.

In Archimycetes, the simplest fungi, the mycelium is absent or rudimentary. A member of this group produces wart disease in potatoes. The following groups and families are of pharmaceutical interest.

Table 6.4. Classification of fungi

Class	Order	Families
1. Ascomycetes	Protoascales	Saccharomycetaceae
	Plectascales	Aspergillaceae
	Sphaeriales	Hypocreaceae
	Clavicipitales	Clavicipitaceae
2. Basidiomycetes	Polyporinales	Polyporaceae
	Agaricales	Tricholometaceae
		Amanitaceae
		Agaricaceae
	Phallinales	Phallinaceae
3. Fungi Imperfecti	Moniliales	Dematiaceae
4. Phycomycetes	Mucorales	Mucoraceae

1(a). ASCOMYCETES : Protoascales : Saccharomycetaceae

This group includes the yeasts. Dried yeast is prepared from a strain of *Saccharomyces cerevisiae*. Cryptococcaceae includes *Candida utilis*, which produces torula yeast, a rich source of proteins and vitamins.

1(b). PLECTASCALES : Aspergillaceae

In this order the conidial stage is more pronounced than the ascal stage. *Penicillium* yields important antibiotics such as penicillin and griseofulvin. *P. islandicum* forms emodin. *Aspergillus oryzae* is used in the manufacture of soya sauce; *A. fumigatus* produces the antibiotic fumagillin; and *A. flavus* yields aflatoxin in poorly stored feeding materials.

1(c). SPHAERIALES : Hypocreaceae

Gibberella produces the plant growth regulators known as gibberellins, first reported from *G. fugikuroi*.

1(d). CLAVICIPITALES : Clavicipitaceae

The ascospores are produced in a sac or ascus. Genera of the Clavicipitaceae include *Claviceps* and *Cordyceps*.

2(a). BASIDIOMYCETES : Polyporinales : Polyporaceae

The Basidiomycetes produce basidiospores, borne externally on the spore mothercell or basidium. They have septate mycelia which form elaborate fruiting bodies (e.g., mushrooms). Some species are edible, others poisonous.

The Polyporaceae includes *Polyporus, Polystichus, Fomes, Ganoderma* and *Boletus*. *Polyporus officinalis* (white agaric) and *P. fomentarius* are used in medicine, *Ganoderma lucida* is used in Chinese medicine and it contains biologically active triterpenoids. *Boletus edulis* is edible.

2(b). AGARICALES : Tricholometaceae

The Tricholometaceae contains *Clitocybe* producing muscarine. Other families of the order contain *Stropharia, Psilocybe* and *Conocybe*, which yield hallucinogenic substances such as psilosin and psilocybin.

2(c). AGARICALES : Amanitaceae

The family includes *Amanita* and *Pluteus; Amanita muscaria* (fly agaric) and *A. pantherina* contain muscarine.

2(d). AGARICALES : Agaricaceae

The genus *Agaricus* (*Psalliota*) contains about 30 species. The common mushroom belongs to *A. campestris*.

2(e). PHALLINALES : Phallinaceae

Phallus impudicus is the stinkhorn, belonging to the family Phallinaceae.

3. FUNGI IMPERFECTI : Moniliales : Dematiaceae

The Fungi Imperfecti is devoid of sexual spores. Some members may be Ascomycetes which have completely lost the ascus stage.

The family Dematiaceae contains *Helminthosporium*. *H. graminium*, produces helminthosporin. The Tuberculariaceae, contains *Fusarium*. *Fusarium lini* will transform digitoxigenin into digoxigenin. Fungal spores are a common source of allergens.

4. PHYCOMYCETES : Mucorales : Mucoraceae

These fungi have an aseptate mycelium; e.g.,

Phytophthora infestans, which causes potato blight. In the Mucoraceae *Mucor* and *Rhizopus* are the moulds associated with badly stored food products. Some *Rhizopus* species are used industrially for the saccharification of starchy material and for producing D-lactic acid from glucose. They are important in the microbiological conversions of steroids.

LICHENS

A lichen is an association of an alga and a fungal partner. Some lichens of arctic regions are used as food. The deserts species *Lecanora esculenta* produces the biblical manna. The 'oak moss', used as a fixative in perfumery, is the lichen *Evernia prunastri*. Many lichens contain derivatives of orcinol, orcellic acid and lecanoric acid. These compounds are phenolic acids formed by the interaction of the carboxyl group of one molecule with the hydroxyl group of another. Depsidones (e.g., norstictic and psoromic acids) complex with metals and are probably responsible for the ability of lichens to flourish on mineral-rich soils including mine tailings and to accumulate large quantities of metals, such as copper, zinc, etc.

Lichen dyes are used in the textile industry. Litmus, produced from certain lichens (e.g., *Lecanora, Roccella* spp.) by fermentation, is used as an indicator.

Iceland moss, *Cetraria islandica*, is used for disguising the taste of nauseous medicines and with other species (e.g., *Cladonia* spp.) for the treatment of cough. It contains the very bitter depsidone, cetraric acid. Many lichens have antibiotic properties.

BRYOPHYTES AND PTERIDOPHYTES

These two phyla have some phytochemical interest.

BRYOPHYTA

The phylum is divided into two classes, Hepaticae (liverworts) and Musci (mosses). The gametophyte generation is a leaf-like thallus in the liverworts and a leafy plant with a stem in the mosses.

Peat, used as a domestic fuel, consists of partly decayed mosses and other plants. In Ireland deposits of bog moss (*Sphagnum* species) are many feet thick. Sphagnum moss, a mixture of various species of *Sphagnum*, is found in Britain and used as an absorbent dressing or compressed into sheets to prepare absorbent mattresses.

Table 6.5. Bryophyte orders, families and genera

Class	Order	Genera
1. Hepaticae	Jungerma-niinales	*Bazzania, Solenostoma, Gymnomitrion, Diplophyllum*
	Jubulineales	*Lunularia*
2. Musci	Sphagnales	*Sphagnum*
	Dicranales	*Dicranum*
	Funariales	*Funaria*

PTERIDOPHYTA

The Pteridophyta includes the Filices (ferns), Articulatae (horsetails) and Lycopsida (club mosses).

GYMNOSPERMS

Gymnospermae contains many fossil members.

The gymnosperms are the seed-bearing plants or spermaphyta. They have ovules which are not enclosed in an ovary. A perianth is absent except in the Gnetales. The seeds usually contain one mature embryo having two to 15 cotyledons. The wood is composed largely of tracheids.

Table 6.6. Classes, orders and families of Pteridophyta

Class	Order	Family	Genera
1. Articulatae	Equise-tales	Equiseta-ceae	*Equisetum*
2. Filices	Filicales	Polypodi-aceae	*Polypodium, Dryopteris, Pteris Pteridium, Onychium, Dennstaedtia, Adiantum, Athyrium, Asplenium*
3. Lycopsida	Lycopo-diales	Lycopo-diaceae	*Lycopodium*

Table 6.7. Orders and families of Gymnosperms

Orders	Families
1. Cycadales	Cycadaceae
2. Coniferae	Pinaceae, Taxodiaceae, Cupressaceae, Araucariaceae, Podocarpaceae, Cephalotaxaceae
3. Ginkgoales	Giakgoaceae
4. Gnetales	Ephedraceae
5. Taxales	Taxaceae

1. CYCADALES : Cycadaceae

The order contains only 10 genera and about 100 species. The family Cycadaceae contains the single genus *Cycas*. A sago is obtained from the pith of *Cycas circinalis* and *C. revolula*.

2(a). CONIFERAE (OR CONIFERALES) : Pinaceae

All members of the order are evergreen trees or shrubs; mostly with needle-like leaves; monoecious or dioecious. Sporophylls are usually in cones. Resin ducts occur in all parts.

The Pinaceae are trees. Important genera are : *Abies, Pseudotsuga, Tsuga, Picea, Larix, Cedrus,* and *Pinus*. Many species (e.g., *Pinus*) yield oleoresin ('Colophony resin and Turpentine'). Other species are *Abies balsamea*, yielding Canada balsam; *Pseudotsuga taxifolia* (Douglas fir); *Picea abies* (Norway Spruce); and *Larix europaeus* (larch). The barks of larch and hemlock spruce are tanning materials. *Pinus pinea* (the umbrella pine) produces large edible seeds (pignons). The Indian medicinal plants belonging to Pinaceae are *Abies spectabilis* (antipyretic), *Cedrus deodara* (used in fever, diarrhoea, dysentery and urinary diseases) and *Pinus roxburghii* (carminative, rubefacient).

2(b). CONIFERAE : Taxodiaceae

A small family of 10 genera, *Sequoia, Taxodium, Cryptomeria, Tetraclinis, Taiwania* and *Cunninghamia*; 16 species. The resin sandarac is obtained from *Tetraclinis articulata*.

2(c). CONIFERAE : CUPRESSACEAE

A family of 19 genera and 130 species of trees and shrubs.

The genera include *Callitris, Thuja, Cupressus, Chamaecyparis* and *Juniperus*. *J. communis* yields juniper berries and volatile oil; *J. virginiana*, the red cedar wood is used for pencils; and *J. sabina*, volatile oil of savin, *J. oxycedrus* yields oil of cade. This tar-like oil contains cadinene and phenols.

2(d). CONIFERAE : Araucariaceae

Two genera and 38 species of trees.

Araucaria provides useful timbers; and *Agathis*, the resins known as copals or amines, are used for varnish. Manila copal is obtained from the Malaysian *Agathis alba*; and kauri copal from *A. australis*, the kauri pine, occurs in Australia and New Zealand.

2(e). CONIFERAE : Podocarpaceae

Six genera and 125 species of trees and shrubs. The largest genus, *Podocarpus*, yields valuable timbers. They contain norditerpene and bisnorditerpene dilactones.

2(f). CONIFERAE : Cephalotaxaceae

A family of one genus (*Cephalotaxus*) and seven species of trees and shrubs (plum yews) is found from the eastern Himalayas to Japan. They contain antitumour constituents and the alkaloids (harringtonine and homoharringtonine) *C. harringtonia*.

3. GINKGOALES : Ginkgoaceae

Except *Ginkgo biloba*, the plants of this order are found only as fossils. They are used to cure diseases associated with the ageing process.

4. GNETALES : Ephedraceae

The order consists of three families (Gnetaceae, Ephedraceae and Welwitchiaceae).

The Ephedraceae contains the single genus *Ephedra*. Various species yield the drug Ephedra and the alkaloid ephedrine.

5. TAXALES : Taxaceae

It includes the genera *Taxus, Pseudotaxus, Torreya, Austrotaxus* and *Amentotaxus*.

The common yew, *Taxus baccata*, produces valuable wood. All parts of the plant are very poisonous. Cattle and horses can die very rapidly after eating the leaves and stems. Alkaloids, a cyanogenetic glycoside and antitumour agent have been reported in the genus.

Taxus brevifolia (Pacific yew), the bark of this species yields the promising anticancer drug taxol, a nitrogenous diterpene.

ANIMAL PRODUCTS

Animals are classified into Phyla, Classes, Orders, Families, Genera and Species. The number of crude drugs derived from animal sources is limited.

PROTOZOA

These are unicellular microorganisms including parasites causing malaria (*Plasmodium*), sleeping sickness (*Trypanosoma*) and dysentery (*Entamoeba*). Some dinoflagellates (*Prorocentrum, Dinophysis*) produce polyether toxins responsible for some shell-fish poisoning.

PORIFERA (Sponges)

From sponges the metabolites include bromophenols (antibacterial properties), cyclic peroxides and peroxyketals (antimicrobial, ichthyotoxic, cytotoxic activities) and modified sesquiterpenes (antimalarial, antifungal, antibacterial, anticancer activities). Siliceous sponge spicules are present in samples of kieselguhr and agar.

COELENTERATA (Jellyfish, sea anemones, corals)

The soft coral *Plexaura homomalla* yields a high amount of prostaglandin A_2. *Sacrophyton glaucum* contains diterpenoids (sarcophytols A and B) which inhibit tumour promotion.

PLATYHELMINTHES (Flatworms)

The Trematodes (the parasitic flukes, *e.g.*, liver fluke and *Schistosoma*) and the Cestoda (tapeworms) are included in this phylum.

NEMATODA (Roundworms)

Some are parasitic in man and animals.

MOLLUSCA

Class *Gastropoda* contains the snails, slugs and limpets. Some snails are vectors of parasites such as *Schistosoma*.

Class *Lamellibranchia* includes scallops, mussels, oysters and clams.

Class *Cephalopoda* includes the squids, cuttlefish and octopuses. Cuttlefish bone (from *Sepia officinalis*) is used in dentifrices and as an antacid.

ANNELIDA (Segmented worms)

The phyllum includes earthworms, lugworms and leeches. The potent neurotoxic agent nereistoxin is obtained from the Japanese species *Lumbriconereis heteropoda*.

ARTHROPODA

A very large phylum of jointed animals including the crustaceans, insects and arachnids.

Class Crustacea includes the shrimps, crabs, lobsters, centipedes and millipedes.

Class insecta

The following orders of this taxon have medicinal interest :

1. *Order Anoplura (Lice)* : Commonly found in birds and mammals. The human parasite is *Pediculus humanus* encountered as the body louse (*corporis*) and the head louse (*capitis*); it is carrier of typhus fever and an indirect transmitter of relapsing fever.

2. *Order Hemiptera (Bugs)* : The cochineal beetle is an important colourant. Shellac is a resinous substance prepared from a secretion of a scale insect *Laccifer lacca*.

3. *Order Coleoptera (Beetles)* : The blistering beetles of the genera *Cantharis* and *Mylabris*, possess vesicant properties and preparations of *C. vesicatoria* are used in the form of plasters and collodions as rubefacients and vesicants.

4. *Order Lepidoptera (Butterflies and moths)* : Some moths infest stored drugs. Silk is used in pharmacy in the form of oiled silk.

5. *Order Hymenoptera (Ants, bees, wasps)*: Hive products derived from *Apis mellifica* include honey, beeswax, royal jelly and propolis.

Class arachnida

Arthropods include spiders, scorpions and mites.

Order Acarina (mites) the common housemite is a cause of allergy in humans.

CHORDATA

The most important subphylum of the Chordata is the Vertebrata (Craniata) composed of all those animals with backbones, *e.g.*, the Pisces (aquatic vertebrates) and the Tetrapoda (terrestrial vertebrates). They are divided into the following four classes having medicinal significance :

1. Class *Osteichthyes (Bony fish)* : Cod and halibut are important for their liver oils which contain vitamins A and D and eicosapentaenoic acid (dietary supplement).
2. Class *Amphibia (frogs and toads)* : Dried and powdered toadskins contain cardioactive principles and used for the treatment of dropsy.
3. Class *Reptilia (Crocodiles, snakes and lizards)*: Snake venoms are important products.
4. Class *Mammalia (Warm-blooded animals which suckle their young)* : Subclass *Eutheria* embraces the placental mammals, *e.g.*, bats, rodents, carnivores, whales, ungulates and primates. The products include lard, suet, wool fat, wool, gelatin, musk, catgut, insulin, hormones, blood and liver products, vaccines, sera and spermaceti.

DESCRIPTION OF IMPORTANT FAMILIES

FAMILY : ACANTHACEAE

Vegetative characters

Habit and habitat : Majority are herbs, a few are shrubs (*Beloperone, Acanthus, ilicifolius*) and some are climbers (*Thunbergia* sp.). Many species of *Acanthus* grow in marshy places and under mangrove trees. *Cardentha difformis* and *Asteracantha longifolia* are aquatics, the latter has axillary spines. *Barleria, Blepharis* and *Aechmanthera* are xerophytic. Herbs may be annual or perennial, wild or cultivated as ornamentals or as medicinal plants.

Root : Much branched tap root. Adventitious stilt roots have been recorded in *Acanthus ilicifolius*.

Stem : Aerial; underground tubers in *Ruellia tuberosa*, mostly erect; sometimes climbing or twinning (*Thunbergia*); cylindrical or angular; usually branched; hollow or solid; woody or herbaceous; luspid and hairy in many species; spinous in *Acanthus ilicifolius* and *Asteracantha longifolia*; glabrous in many species.

Leaf : Cauline and ramal; exstipulate; petiolate; or sessile; opposite; simple; pinnately lobed in *Acanthus mollis*; mostly entire; hairy or glabrous; reticulate-unicostate. In some cases leaves bear conspicuous spots or markings (*Sanchezia nobilis, Aphelandra aurantiaca*).

Floral characters

Inflorescence

Usually a spike (*Acanthus, Adhatoda*); in terminal or axillary racemes (*Thunbergia laurifolia*); sometimes solitary axillary (*Bontia*) : in cymose clusters in *Peristrophe*.

Flower : *Bracteate* pedicellate or sessile; bracts and bracteoles are spinous in some genera (*Barleria*); complete; zygomorphic, bisexual, hypogynous, tetracyclic; variously coloured; usually small. Many have large and showy bracts (*Beloperons, Aphelandra*).

Calyx : In *Acanthus* there are 4 sepals, two large with one often spinous and two interior ones small and often scale like, 5-lobed in *Crossandra, Adhatoda*; mostly gamosepalous and bilabiate; very short and 10 to 15 toothed in *Thunbergia*; deeply cleft and segmented in *Strobilanthus* : 4-parted in *Barleria*; imbricate or convolute; hairy or glabrous inferior.

Corolla : Usually five; gamopetalous; bilabiate; imbricate or convoluted; irregular; variously coloured, inferior.

Androecium : Usually 4 (*Acanthus, Ruellia, Strobilanthus, Thunbergia*) and all fertile; in some cases two stamens are fertile and two are staminodes and sterile (*Adhatoda, Justicia, Beloperone*); epipetalous; attached to base of corolla tube (*Pachystachys, Adhatoda*), or at the middle (*Jacobinia*) or near the throat (*Peristrophe*); mostly didynamous; in *Beloperone* the connectives are elongated so that the anther lobes are separated; usually bithecous; monothecous in *Aphelandra;* dehiscence by slits, introrse. In *Penstemon*, there are five fertile stamens. The exine of pollen grains is variously sculptured and may be fissured, reticulate, spinous, echinulate, pored granulate and furrowed.

Gynaecium : Bicarpellary; syncarpous; superior; bilocular; ovules two or many in each loculus; axile placentation; ovary seated on a distinct nectariferous disc; style single, filiform; stigmas bifid or simple.

Fruit : A capsule with two chambers, dehiscing elastically by two valves; dehiscence loculicidal to the very base.

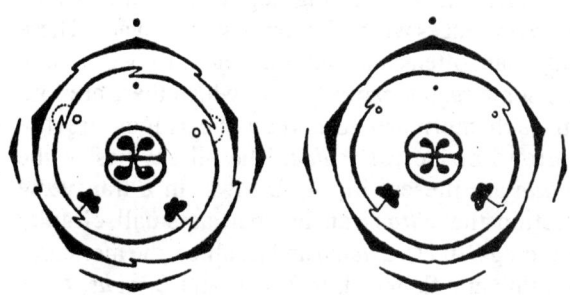

Fig. 6.1. Floral diagrams (two types) of *Acanthaceae*.

Seed : Non-endospermic; characteristic outgrowths called *retinaculae* or *jaculators* arise from the stalks of seeds. Jaculators are hooked in *Strobilanthus, Barleria, Ruellia, Acanthus* and *Crossanda*; minute, conical and scale like in *Cardanthera*; hard and stiff in *Asteracantha*. In *Ruellia, Blepharis* and *Crossandra* the seeds are covered with hygroscopic hair or scales that become mucilaginous when wet and help in the descent of seeds at the time of germination.

Pollination : By means of insects.

Floral formula : $\oplus \; \female \; K_{(4-5)} \; C_{(5)} \; A_{2-4 \; or \; 5} \; G_{(2)}.$

FAMILY : APIACEAE (UMBELLIFERAE OR CARROT FAMILY)

Vegetative characters

Habit and habitat : Mostly annual (*Foeniculum, Coriandrum, Carum carvi, Hydrocotyle*), perennial (*Caraway*) or biennial (*Pteroselinum crispum*) herbs; a few shrubs (*Ferula communis, Eryngiun giganteum*); the two East African species of *Pseudocarum* are climbers, with sensitive tendrils. All species of *Azorella* distributed over the

Antarctic islands and the Andes have very peculiar shape. The plants are evergreen and look very delicate, but are strong. They look like huge cushions and may be more than 100 years old. These are topped by new branches with new flowers during the next period of vegetation and so on. The plants are mostly aromatic due to the occurrence of oil ducts in all parts. The stem is usually hollow.

Root : A branched tap root; sometimes becoming tuberous due to storage of food as in Carrot (*Daucus carota, Apium graveolens*, etc.). Adventitious roots are found in *Cicuta virosa* (Cow-bane).

Stem : Aerial; climbing in *Pseudocarum*; reduced and discoid in young plants of *Daucus carota*; solid when young, becoming hollow at maturity due to shrinking of pith in the internodal region; branched; cylindrical (*Hecacleum, Coriandrum* etc.) or distinctly ribbed (*Foeniculum*) green; hairy (*Anthriscus sylvestris, Trachymene caerulea*), smooth glaucous or glabrous; in *Cicuta virosa* the stem is tuberous and bears adventitious roots.

Leaf : Cauline and ramal, radical in young plants of *Daucus carota*; usually, exstipulate; stipulate in *Hydrocotyle*; petiolate; alternate; opposite in some species of *Apiastrum*; simple; entire reniform and undivided in *Hydrocotyl*. In *Eryngium agavifolium*, the leaves are broadly linear and taper to a point and are parallel veined like the monocots (*E. aloifolium, E. yuccifolium* and *E. bromelifolium*); palmately lobed; finely dissected in *Foeniculum*; pinnately lobed and decompound in *Coriandrum* and *Daucus carota*; unipinnate-compound in *Pimpinella major*; the pinnate compound leaves in *Crithmum maritimum* are fleshy and succulent; venation reticulate unicostate (*Eryngium alpinum, Hydrocotyle*), reticulate multicostate (*Astrantia major, Eryngium planum*), parallel in *Eryngium agavifolium*. In *Acorella*, the leaves are reduced. In *Aegopodium podagraria*, the leaves are bipinnate and the leaflets have distinct petioles.

Floral characters

Inflorescence : It is an umbel; simple umbel in *Hydrocotyle*, mostly compound umbels (*Foeniculum, Coriandrum, Daucus*); in a compound umbel there is usually an involucre of bracts at a place from where the stalks of first order arise, there is again an other whorl of bracts at a place where the floral stalks arise from the top of the branches of first order. The former whorl of bracts is called *involucre* whereas the latter is called *involucel*. Involucre and involucel are absent in *Foeniculum, Heracleum* and *Anethum*, present in *Daucus carota*. In *Banicula*, the umbels are arranged in cymose grouping. In *Eryngium*, the flowers are sessile so that the umbel look like a head resembling a *Capitulum*. In *Eryngium giganteum*, the heads are large and surrounded by prickly bracts with ivory coloured veins. In *E. elpinum*, the bracts are long, blue and thorny. In some species of *Azorella* and *Xanthosia*, the inflorescence is reduced to a single flower. Each such flower is surrounded by an involucre of bracts which shows that it is a reduced umbel.

Flower : Bracteate (*Hydrocotyle*) or ebracteate (*Foeniculum*); pedicellate (*Coriandrum, Foeniculum, Daucus*) or sessile (*Eryngium*); actinomorphic (*Foeniculum, Hydrocolyle*) or zygomorphic (*Coriandrum*); usually bisexual; unisexual and monoecious in *Echinophora*, unisexual and dioecious in *Arctopus*. In *Astrantia*, the umbel has a few long pedicelled male flowers among a large number of short-pedicelled bisexual flowers (polygamomonoecium); epigynous; cyclic; usually pentamerous; small and often coloured white or yellow.

Calyx : Five; gamosepalous (*Coriandrum, Hydrocotyle*); reduced in *Foeniculum* and many other genera; valvate; green; rarely petaloid; superior.

Corolla : Five; choripetalous; regular (*Foeniculum, Heracleum*); or irregular (*Coriandrum*) with two small and three large petals; apex obtuse, rounded or acute, sometimes bifid (*Coriandrum*); truncate (*Orlaya grandiflora*); petals reflexed in *Anethum graveolens*; valvate (*Foeniculum*); imbricate (*Coriandrum*); white; yellow or blue; superior.

Androecium : Five; free; alternipetalous; filaments equal in length; longer or shorter than the corolla; anthers bithecous; basifixed and dorsifixed, rarely versatile; dehiscence longitudinal, introse.

Gynaecium : Bicarpellary; syncarpous; inferior; bilocular; placentation marginal parietal; one pendulous ovule in each loculus; styles two each terminating in a capitate or linear stigma. In many genera, the stigmas (*Saniculoideae*) are surrounded by a bilobed honey secreting disc called the *stylopodium*. In the *Apioideae*, the style penetrates through the *stylopodium*; the ovary is placed anteroposteriorly; ovules anatropous with ventral raphe.

Fruits : A cremocarp, which splits down a septum between the two carpels into two one-seeded mericarps. The two mericarps are, at first held together by a thin stalk, called the *carophore*, running up between them. The *carophore* generally gets forked at the apex. The pericarp is each one-seeded mericarp has 5 projecting ridges, two cut of which are at the edges where the splitting takes place. These ridges are often called *lateral ridges*. Between these are some *secondary ridges*, of which there are four in each mericarp. Between the ridges are the furrows or the *valleculae*. The oil cavities or the *vittae* are present in the furrows. In a transverse section the *vittae* can be seen as small circular openings. In *Herasleum* and its allies, the mericarps are thin and flattened. In *Torilis* and *Daucus*, fruits have hooked spines.

Seed : Endospermic, with small embryo. The seed is often united to a pericarp.

Floral formula : $\oplus$ or + or σ or $\female$ $K_{(5) \text{ or } 5}$ C_5 A_5 $G_{(2)}$.

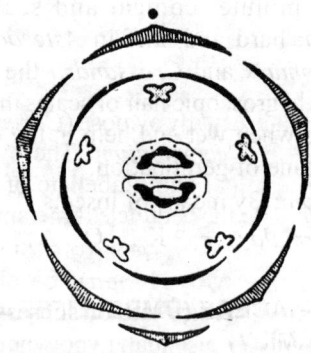

Fig. 6.2. Floral diagram of Apiaceae.

Pollination : By means of insects. The main visitors are flies; beetles and *Hymenoptera* are also frequent. Flowers are extremely *protandrous*, the male stage being most commonly over before the female begins. The massing of flowers in distinct-umbels makes them conspicuous and this is further aided by zygomorphism prevalent in some genera. Honey is secreted by stylopodium which is easily approach-able to the insects. In *Eryngium*, the flowers have their nectar tucked away in a tube several millimetres deep, and formed by the stiffy erect sepals. In this case beetles and short-tongued insects cannot effect pollination, only bees, bumblebees and butterflies pollinate the flowers.

FAMILY : APOCYNACEAE

Vegetative characters

Habit and habitat : Mostly trees and shrubs; or climbers; rarely perennial herb (*Vinca rosea*).

Root : A much branched tap root. In *Pachypodium bispinosum*, the root is turnip shaped (up to 45 cm diameter) and stores water.

Stem : Aerial; erect or climbing; cylindrical or angular; branched; unbranched in *Pachypodium*; herbaceous (*Vinca*); woody; usually solid; thorny (*Carissa*); glabrous (*Rauwolfia*). The stem is tuber-ous in *Adenium multiflorum*.

Leaf : Cauline (*Vinca rosea*) and ramal; exstipu-late; rarely interpetiolar or intrapetiolar gland like stipules are present (*Tubermaemontana, Vallaris*), petiolate or subsessile; alternate in *Thevetia, Rhazya* and *Ochrosia*; opposite in *Holarrhena, Strophan-thus*; whorled in *Nerium, Rauwolfia*; simple; shape of lamina varies with species.

Floral characters

Inflorescence : It is usually cymose (*Carissa, Vinca, Nerium*), spike in *Pachypodium*. The cymes may be axillary or terminal and umbellate or corymbi-form. In *Landolphia* the peduncle is metamorphosed into a tendril.

Flower : Bracteate (*Vinca*), or ebracteate (*Nerium, Carissa*), pedicellate or subsessile; com-plete; actinomorphic; bisexual; hypogynous; cyclic; pentamerous (except gynaecium); in some species large and beautifully coloured.

Calyx : Five; gamosepalous; mostly 5-lobed; sometimes deeply 5 lobed; lanceolate and ciliate in *Carissa*; 5-fid in *Rauwolfia*; calyx segments recurved in *Cerbera odollam*; imbricate (*Nerium*) or valvate (*Vinca minor*); sepals free in *Vinca*; usually green; inferior. In some species there are four sepals.

Corolla : Five; gamopetalous; funnel-shaped (*Thevetia*), salver form (*Vinca*), funnel-shaped with 5 broad or lacinate lobes in *Nerium*, tubular in *Amsonia*; rotate in *Vallaris*; usually twisted, some-times imbricate, rarely valvate. In *Strophanthus sarmentosus*, the corolla lobes are produced into long hair like processes; tomentose externally in *Epigynum*; glabrous in *Anodendron*; the throat of the corolla tube is often hairy or closed with a corona of scales; usually gaudily coloured; inferior.

Androecium : Five; epipetalous; alternipe-talous; the filaments are commonly free; the anthers are usually bithecous, sagittate and acute, free (*Vinca, Carissa*) or conivant round the stigma and fused with it (*Nerium, Leaumontia*). In *Nerium* the anthers have long hairy appendages at apex; filaments short (*Nerium*); or very long and dilated above in *Beaumontia*; anthers obtuse (*Plumeria, Garissa*); dehiscence longitudinal and introrse; pollen granu-lar; usually a hypogynous disc is present; disc absent in *Plumeria*.

Gynaecium : Mostly bicarpellary; syncarpous (*Arduina, Allemanda*), or apocarpous (*Pleio-carpa*), in *Alyxia, Cerbera, Vinca, Nerium indicum* the two ovaries are free and the styles are fused, superior (*Vinca, Nerium*), or semi-inferior (*Plumeria*); bilocular (*Thevetia*), or semi-inferior (*Plumeria*); bilocular (*Thevetia*) or unilocular (*Allemanda*); plasentation parietal (*Allemanda*); marginal (*Vinca, Nerium*), ovules one in each loculus in *Acokanthera*, two in each loculus in *Thevetia*, many in *Tabernaemoniana, Nerium* and *Vinca*; ovules anat-ropous, pendulous; style usually simple, rarely split above (*Pleiocarpa*), with a thickened head and a ring of hairs below it; stigma capitate (*Nerium*), and annular (*Vinca*), or bifid (*Plumeria, Carissa, Thevetia*). In *Vinca*, the stigma is densely covered with hair at its apex.

Fruit : A berry (*Acokanthera, Carissa*), a drupe in *Thevetia, Ochrosia*; two follicles in *Plumeria, Amsonia, Nerium*; and a capsule in *Allemanda*.

Seed : Endospermic, the seeds usually have a tuft of hair or are winged (*Plumeria*).

Pollination : Entomophilous.

Floral formula : $\oplus \ \male\female \ K_{(5)} \ C_5 \ A_5 \ G_{(2) \text{ or } 2 \text{ or } (2)}.$

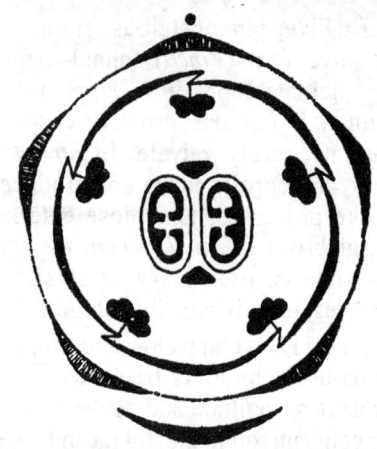

Fig. 6.3. Floral diagram of Apocynaceae.

FAMILY : ASCLEPIADACEAE

Vegetative characters

Habit and habitat : The family includes perennial herbs (*Calotropis*); shrubs and twinners and climbers. Some are epiphytes and few are succulent.

Root : Usually a branched tap root that grows very deep in soil in many species; adventitious roots are found in *Dischidia.*

Stem : Aerial; erect (*Calotropis*); weak and climbing; thick and succulent; in all 350 species have succulent stem. The stem is a sucker in *Dischidia rafflesiana* that occurs in Assam; cylindrical (*Calotropis*) or angular (*Leptadenia*); solid; branched; covered with waxy bloom (*Calotropis, Hoya*); spinous in *Hoodia*; milky latex present in most of the genera (*Calotropis, Cryptoslegia*); woody or woody below and herbaceous above. The stem is tuberous in some species of *Ceropigia*. Underground tuberous stems occur in *Brachystelma.*

Leaf : Cauline and ramal; exstipulate; petiolate; sometimes subsessile or sessile; usually opposite and decussate (*Calotropis*), rarely whorled (*Asclepias syriaca*), alternate in *Ulteria* (one species endemic in south India); simple; greatly reduced in succulent genera; fleshy and modified into pitchers in *Dischidia*; reduced to spines in *Stapelia*; succulent in *Hoya*; absent in *Hoodia* and some species of *Periploca.*

Floral characters

Inflorescence : Umbellate cymes in *Leptadenia, Heterostemma*; dichasial cymes in *Cryptoslegia; Cryptolepis* and *Toxocarpus*; large and solitary in *Stapelia grandiflora* and *Hoodia gordoni.*

Flower : Bracteate (*Calotropis, Cryptoslegia*), or ebracteate (*Hoodia, Stapelia*); pedicellate or subsessile; complete; actinomorphic; slightly zygomorphic in *Ceropegia*; bisexual; hypogynous; pentamerous (excluding gynaecium); cyclic; coronate; very large (30 cms in diameter) in *Stapelia gigantea* and *Hoodia*; waxy in *Hoya*; covered with hair in *Hoodia* and *Stapelia.*

Calyx : Five; free; sometimes fused (gamosepalous) as in *Leptadenia* and *Heterostemma*; imbricate; usually hairy; inferior.

Corolla : Five; gamopetalous; campanulate (*Calotropis, Raphistamma*); tubular (*Daemia*); funnel shaped (*Cryptostegia*); salver-shaped (*Toxocarpus*); vulvate (*Calotropis*) or twisted (*Cryptostegia*); corolla lobes ciliate in *Periploca calophylla*; waxy in *Hoya*; large and hairy in *Stapelia* and *Hoodia*. In *Ceropegia*, the five lobes of the corolla are separate at the bottom and fused at the tips so that the flowers appear to have 5-windows; strongly scented in *Stephonotis floribunda*, emits a foul smell in *Stapelia* and *Hoodia*; inferior.

Corona : The Asclepiadaceous flower is characterised by the presence of corona. The corona may be scaly or a hairy outgrowth from the petals or the staminal tube. In the former case it is called *Corolline corona*, whereas in the latter case it is called *staminal corona*. The corolline corona is present in *Cryptoslegia, Cryptolepis, Gymnema* and *Brachylepis*. Staminal corona is of wide occurrence (*Calotropis, Asclepias, Tylophora, Periploca, Hoya*). In *Calotropis* the corona lobes arise near the bast of the filaments and are free with coiled basal spurs. In *Hoya*, the 5 coronal lobes are convex, conical and star-shaped. In *Dischidia*, the staminal coronal lobes number 5 and are fused near base, each lobe is double hooked. In *Marsdenia*, the corona is in three whorls, the outer whorl is *corolline* whereas the inner two *staminal*. Coronal lobes are absent in a number of species.

Androecium : Five; uaually epipetalous and inserted at the base of the petals and alternating with

them. In *Cryptoslegia* and *Periploca* the free filaments bear anthers that are connate around the
stigma, in the former the anthers are strongly
appendaged, whereas in the latter the anthers bear
hair on their back. In all the cases stamens are fused
with the stigmatic disc to form a common structure
called the *gynostegium*. In case the filaments are
free (*Cryptoslegia, Periploca*) each filament is
closely appressed to the stigmatic head; in case the
filaments are fused to form a tube (*Calotropis, Hoya,
Cerropegia*) the apex of the tube is fused with the
stigma to form a 5-angled disc or the *gynostegium*.
The anthers are bithecous and commonly winged
and adherent to the stigmatic disc; the stigmatic surface of the lower side of stigma is exposed between
each pair of anthers. The edges of the adjacent anthers are so closely parallel that they form clefts
which leaf to the angles of the *gynostegium* where
there is lodged the *corpusculum* of the *translators*.
Below these clefts are spaces of varying size and
shape according to the form of stamens and the
stigma head. These spaces are called the
interstaminal chambers, in which the pollinia turn
from the insects legs become deposited. In
Calotropis the pollen grains of each cell of anther
become agglutinated to form a waxy mass called
pollinium. Each anther has two such *pollinia* (one
in each lobe). During floral development a material
is secreted from the surface of the stigma-head at
five points between the stamens. This material dries
to form ten stalk like structures. These 10 stalks fuse
at a point to form *translators*. Each such translator
has three parts : (i) a basal adhesive disc called the
corpusculum; (ii) two stalks called the *caudicles*;
and (iii) a spoon like apical portion called the *shovel.*
These translators are so arranged that the
corpusculum lies at each of the 5 angles of the stigmatic disc; the caudicles with their shovels receive
pollinia from the anther cells of two adjacent anthers. In some *Asclepiadaceae* the translators have
only one caudible and one pollinium mass attached
to the shovel. In this case the pollinia are not waxy
but are granular. In *Calotropis, Asclepias* and
Cryptostagia, each anther cell has only one pollinium mass so that the 5 anthers have pollinia. In
Secamone, Toxocarpum and *Gentianthas*, each cell
in the anther has two pollinia so that there are 20
pollinia in all the 5 anthers. In such cases translator
carries 4 pollen masses or *pollinia*.

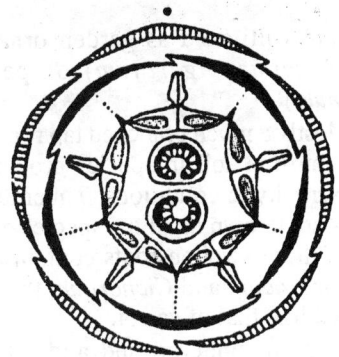

Fig. 6.4. Floral diagram of Asclepiadaceae (*Calotropis*).

Gynaecium : Bicarpellary; apocarpous; the
ovaries and the styles are separate except for the
stigmas that are fused to form a 5-angled disc with
an anther adnate to each side. In *Calotropis,
Asclepias* and many other genera the staminal tube
(formed by the fusion of filaments) completely
surrounds the gynaecium; each carpel is unilocular
with many ovules on marginal placenta; styles two,
separate, hairy in some cases; stigmas fused to forms
a 5-angled disc to which are fused the anthers. The
stigmatic disc with coherent anthers is called the
gynostegium.

Fruit : Etaerio of two follicles. In some cases
one of the follicles is reduced or abortive. The
follicles are usually greatly divergent (*Daemia
extensa, Calotropis*). In *Sarcolobus*, the follicles are
solitary.

Seed : Endospermic; compressed; usually
winged and surmounted by a dense tuft of hygroscopic hairs (*coma*). In *Sarcolobus*, the seeds are
devoid of hairs. The embryo is large with flat cotyledons and short radicle.

Floral formula : $\oplus \; \Male\Female \; K_{5 \text{ or } (5)} \; C_{(5)} \; A_{(5)} \; G_2$.

FAMILY : ASTERACEAE (COMPOSITAE)

Vegetative characters

Habit and habitat : Predominantly herbs, some
shrubs or undershrubs, few are woody climbers or
herbaceous climbers; rarely middle sized trees. The
genus *Senecio* with 1500 species in the world includes species that are annual or perennial herbs,
shrubs, or even middle sized trees. A few species of
this genus are succulents. In *S. brassica*, the 8 inches
long leaves overlap as cabbage (Band Gobhi) leaves

do. Many are cultivated as garden ornamentals; annuals (*Sonchus, Ageratum*) or perennials (*Senecio, Inula*).

Root : Mostly a much branched tap root that may grow deep into the soil in species growing under extremely xerophytic conditions. Tuberous adventitious roots are known in all the species of *Dahlia*. The cells of these swollen roots contain abundant inulin. In *Taraxacum* and *Cichorium*, the tap roots are thickened like that of carrot.

Stem : Aerial; underground and tuberous in *Helianthus tuberosus* (the tubers store inulin); erect (*Helianthus*) or weak and climbing (*Mikania scandens*); cylindrical or angular; solid or fistular; branched or unbranched; woody in arboreal forms, herbaceous in majority of the species; reduced in the young plants (*Sonchus, Geebera, Gaillardia*). In *Senecio kleinia*, the branches get transformed into succulent water storage organs. In *Zazania latifolia*, the underwater parts of the stem are pink in colour and sweetish to taste; in many species the stem contains latex (*Sonchus, Launea, Taraxacum, Parthenium*), mostly hairy; spinous in *Carthamus*; aromatic in *Artemisia*. The stem is winged in *Onopordum acanthium*.

Leaf : Radical cauline and ramal; exstipulate; petiolate (*Helanthus*) or sessile (*Inula, Zinnia*); alternate (*Vernonia*), opposite (*Zinnia, Dahlia*). In *Arnica montana* the leaves are arranged in opposite whorls. In *Odontospermum pygmaeum* the leaves are reduced to scales and in *Hoplophyllum* the leaves are metamorphosed into spines; simple; entire (*Gnapthatium, Calendula*) dentate (*Helianthus*); pinnately lobed, finely dissected in *Artemisia*; variously shaped; hairy (*Helianthus, Ageratum*), spinous (*Carthamus*), woolly or tomentose (*Gerbera*). In *Senecio radicans* the leaves are succulent and store water and about ½" thick, each leaf has a small aperture through which the light enters the vitreous interior and helps in photosynthesis. The leaves of *Artemisia* and *Launea* contain oil ducts and latex. In *Silybum marianum*, the leaves are variegated and studded with yellow spines.

Floral characters

Inflorescence : It is a capitulum, surrounded by an involucre of one or more series of free or connate bracts. The peduncle or the inflorescence axis be-

comes flattened (*Helianthus, Ageratum*), conical, or elongated and cylindrical (*Ratibida columnifera*) and is called *receptacle*. The receptacles become cup like and concave in *Epaltes*. It bears sessile flowers called the *florets*. The individual florets may be bracteate (*Helianthus*) or ebracteate (*Sonchus*). In many genera the florets are of two kinds : (i) *Ray florets* are arranged along the rim of the receptacle and have distinct strap-shaped and ligulate corollas; (ii) *Disc florets* are clustered in the central disc like part of the receptacle, the younger ones are near the centre and older ones toward the periphery of the disc, the disc florets are usually bisexual and actinomorphic. Such capitula are called *heterogamous*. In many other genera there is no distinction into ray florets and disc florets and all the florets are bisexual and actinomorphic. Such capitula are called *heterogamous*. *Xanthium* is characteristic in possessing unisexual capitula, the female heads consist of only two flowers, whereas the male heads are about the size of peas and are bundled closely together. *Xanthium* is wind pollinated. *Artemisia* is also wind pollinated and has small and inconspicuous capitula. In *Matricaria matricarioides*, the receptacle is hollow. In *Centauraea*, the marginal florets are transformed into large and sterile display organs. In *Mikania*, the capitual are small and made of only 4 flowers. In *Echinops*, the heads or capitula are one flowered and are arranged together in big compound capitula. Each Capitulum has one bisexual and actinomorphic flower surrounded by its own sheath and *involucral-bracts*. In *Carlina acaulis*, the ray florets are replaced by brilliant white bracts. In *Helichrysum, Helianthus* and *Gaillardia*, the heads are solitary terminal. In *Cicerbita alpina* the heads are arranged in erect racemes. In *Achillea*, the heads are arranged in compact umbels. In *Ageratum*, the capitula are arranged in a corymbose manner.

Flower : Bracteate, or ebracteae; sessile; ebracteolate; complete, or imperfect (ray florets of *Helianthus*, marginal florets of *Centaurea*); actinomorphic (disc florets of *Helianthus. Dahlia*, all the florets in *Ageratum*), zygomorphic (ray florets of *Helianthus, Dahlia* and all the florets in *Sonchus*); bisexual (*Ageratum, Sonchus*, disc florets of *Helianthus* and *Dahlia*), unisexual (*Xanthium*, ray florets of *Helianthus* and *Dahlia* are female; outer florets of *Centaurea* are sterile); epigynous; cyclic; inconspicuous; protan-drous.

Calyx : Represented by 2-3 scale like outgrowths in *Helianthus*, by 5 unequal scale like outgrowth in *Ageratum*, by numerous hair like outgrowths in *Sonchus* and *Dandelion* (*Taraxacum officinale*), by numerous stiff bristles in *Carthamus* and *Bidens*; it is extremely reduced or even absent in many cases (*Ambrosia*); free (*Helianthus*), or united (*Ageratum*); persistent in *Sonchus*, *Dandelion*, *Carthamus*, *Bidens* and helps in fruit dispersal; superior.

Corolla : Five; gamopetalous; tubular (*Ageratum, Centaurea*, disc florets of *Helianthus*, *Dahlia*); in *Helianthus* the corolla tube is swollen into a bulb like structure near its base; ligulate and strap-shaped (ray florets of *Helianthus* and *Dahlia*); valvate initiate in *Mutisia*; colour varies with species, superior.

Androecium : Five; filaments mostly free, slightly connate in *Silybum* epipetalous; synanthrous; anthers usually long and fused to form a tube around the style; in some cases (*Dahlia, Helianthus*), the connective is produced beyond the anther lobes into a sort of long sterile appendage; sometimes hair-like or scaly processes arise from the bases of the anther lobes and many remain free or united and thus conceal the low lying nectar secreting disc; anthers bithecous; dehiscence longitudinal and introrse, sometimes porous; superior.

Gynaecium : Bicarpellary syncarpous; inferior; unilocular, placentation basal; ovule one; anatropous; style single that passes through the synanthrous staminal tube and bifurcates into two stigmas. There is often a brush of hair on the style below the stigmas. Only inner surfaces of the stigmas are as a rule receptive to pollen.

Fruit : It is a *cypsela* (achenial fruit). In some species, the persistent calyx forms a hairy pappus. The hairs are hygroscopic and spread out in dry air and help the fruit, to float in air. Like this the fruits are carried to greater distances and are properly disseminated. During rainy season or in humid places the hair absorb moisture and become heavy thus helping the fruit to alight on the ground and germinate. In *Adenostemma*, the pappus is sticky and is carried by animals from place to place. In *Bidens* the pappus is made of barbed bristles that stick to animal bodies. In *Xanthium* the receptacle is provided with hooks, in *Arctium*, the involucral bracts become hooked at the tips and cling to animals.

Seed : The seed is non-endospermic or has scanty endosperm. The embryo is straight. In *Xanthium* the fruit has two seeds, the upper is permeable to O_2 and germinates under normal conditions. The lower seed is not permeable to O_2 and germinates only when placed under high O_2 conditions or its testa is punctured.

Pollination : It is effected by insects (entomophilous). The small and inconspicuous flowers are massed together in compact heads or *capitula* which enable a single insect to pollinate many flowers at the same time. This massing together of the numerous small flowers is of great advantage, as it enables large number of flowers to be pollinated in one insect visit. It saves time as the insect has not to fly from flower to flower pollinate them individually. It has saved unnecessary development of corolla and other beautifying devices of the flower and it affords a consolidated and a pleasing and attractive look, besides making the mechanism of pollination simple and effective. The honey is secreted by a ring-shaped nectary around the base of the style and is protected from rain and short tongued insects by the calyx tube. When the flower opens, the style with its stigmas tightly closed against each other is comparatively short. It grows and projects into the anther tube (formed by the synanthrous androecium). The flowers are *protaadrous* and anthers are mature and shed their pollen which is carried out slowly as the style with pressed stigmas grows up. The outer surface of the stigmas is sterile and not receptive so that self-pollination cannot take place. The device helps in bringing the pollen grains to the surface of the anther tube so that they come into contact with the visiting insects.

In *Artemisia vulgaris*, the capitulum is pendent, the anther tube projects beyond the corolla so that the dry and powdery pollen is exposed to wind. On the tips of the anthers are long bristles which together form a pollen-holder. Afterwards the style emerges and the large hairy stigmas spread out.

Floral formulae : The floral formulae are variable with the type of floral head. A few examples are given below :

Helianthus annuus

Ray floret : +♀ or neuter $K_{2 \text{ or } 3}$ $C_{(5)}$. A_{zero} $G_{(2)}$ or absent

Disc floret : ⊕ ♀ $K_{2 \text{ or } 3}$ $C_{(5)}A_{(5)}$ $G_{(2)}$

Sonchus : + ♀ $K_{(*)}C_{(5)}A_{(5)}$ $G_{(2)}$

Ageratum : $KC_{(5)}A_{(5)}G_{(2)}$

Xanthium

Male flowers : + ♂ K_{zero} $C_{(5)}A_{(5)}$ G_{zero}

Female flowers : + ♀ K_{zero} $C_{(5)}$ A_{zero} $G_{(2)}$

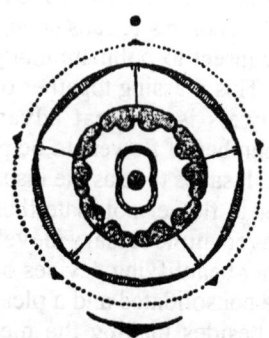

Fig. 6.5. Floral diagram of Asteraceae (Compositae) (disc floret).

FAMILY : CAESALPINOIDEAE (Caesalpiniaceae)

Vegetative characters

Habit and habitat : Majority are trees and shrubs, some are woody climbers.

Root : A branched tap root.

Stem : Aerial; erect, or climbing by means of hooked prickles and stem tendrils; woody; solid; branched; glabrous or sub-glabrous; sometimes tomentose (*Acrocarpus*); covered with prickles and spines, herbaceous in some annual species of *Cassia*.

Leaf : Ramal; leaf base pulvinate in some; stipulate or exstipulate; stipules reduced; petiolate; alternate; compound; unipinnate (*Cassia, Saraca, Tamarindus*), bipinnate (*Delonix, Caesalpinia, Peltophorum*).

Floral characters

Inflorescence : Simple or compound recemes; spike in *Dimorphandra*.

Flower : Bracteate; pedicellate; bracteolate in *Amherstia*; complete; zygomorphic; bisexual; perigymous; pentamerous; cyclic; large and beautifully coloured in some genera.

Calyx : Five, 4 in *Amherstia*; free (*Cassia, Caesalpinia, Delonix*), or united (*Bauhinia, Wagatea, Acrocarpus*); campanulate in *Wagatea* and *Acrocarpus*; imbricate; green or petaloid (*Amherstia*); odd sepal anterior.

Corolla : Five, in *Cassia, Delonix, Bauhinia* etc.; three to five in *Humboldtia*, 3 in *Amherstia* and *Tamarindus*; one in *Afzelia* and *Pahuda*; absent in *Hardwickia, Saraca* and *Dialium*; free; imbricate; the posterior petal is innermost; gaudily coloured. There are three large and two small petals in *Amborstia*.

Androecium : Ten; three in *Tamarindus*; seven in *Pahuda*; five in *Acrocarpus*; free; in *Cassia* three smaller stamens are sterile, 4 are medium sized, and three large and sickle-shaped; in *Saraca* 2-8 stamens are fertile.

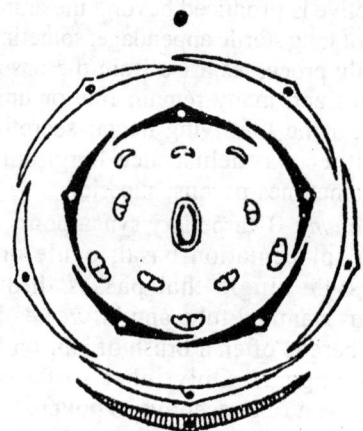

Fig. 6.6. Floral diagram of Caesalpiniaceae.

Gynaecium : Monocarpellary; superior; unilocular; ovules many; placentation marginal; ovary straight or curved or sickle-shaped; hairy or tomentose; style short or long, stigma simple, linear or capitate.

Fruit : A leguminous pod; dehiscent, or indehiscent and lomentaceous; cylindrical (*Cassia*) or flattened (*Delonix*).

Seed : Mostly non-endospermic.

Pollination : Entomophilous.

Floral formula : $+ \diamond$ $K_{5 \text{ or } (5)}$ $C_{5 \text{ or } 3 \text{ or } 1 \text{ or zero}}$ $A_{10 \text{ or } 7 \text{ or } (3)}$ G_1.

FAMILY : CONVOLVULACEAE (Sweet Potato Family)

Vegetative characters

Habit and habitat : Herbs (*Ipomoea muricata, I. alba, Evolvulus*), shrubs (*Ipomoea carnea, Blinkworthia*), herbaceous climbers, *Ipomoea digitata, Cuscuta* and *Convolvulus*), shrubby climbers (*Ipomoea leari, I. cairica* and *Porana*), large woody climbers (*Lettsomia aggregata*); annual or perennial; *Ipomoea aquatica* is an aquatic herb.

Root : Usually a much branched tap root. In *Convolvulus arvensis*, the plants send out extensive branched adventitious roots that act as soil binders. Adventitious roots also arise in *Ipomoea carnea*. In *Cuscuta*, the leafless stem bears adventitious parasitic roots called the haustoria. They penetrate into the host tissue and establish contact with the vascular bundles and absorb water and ready made food. The seeds of *Cuscuta* germinate to give a leafless and thread like stem which, in the absence of a host nearby, grows by creeping along the ground for some distance. Later the rear portion dies, while tip continues to grow for some time. If it happens to come across a host, it will twine around it and send haustoria into the stem. In case host is not available the plant dies. In *Ipomoea batatas* (Sweet potato, Shakar kandi), the adventitious roots, which develop

by the side of the leaf, store food and become swollen and tuberous and attain various sizes and shapes. The roots store sugar as well as starch and are edible.

Stem : Aerial : erect (*Ipomoea carnea*) or prostrate (*Evolvulus alsipoides*) or climbing; herbaceous or woody; cylindrical or flattened in *I. harbitis I. hederacea*; solid; branched; hairy (*Evolvulus alsinoides* and *I. cymosa*) pale green; shining and leaflets in *Cuscuta*; tubercled in *Neuropeltis racemosa*. In *Convolvulus scam-monia*, the stem is an underground rhizome and produces a purgative juice called Scammony.

Leaf : Cauline and ramal; exstipulate; petiolate; alternate; absent or scaly in *Cuscuta*; simple; entire or palmately lobed in *Quamoclit pannata* the leaves are regularly pinnately divided into nearly thread like lobes, reticulate-unicostate or reticulate-multicostate. Extra floral nectaries present in special flask-shaped cavities have been recorded in species of *Calonyction* and *Ipomoea*.

Floral characters

Inflorescence : Flower may be solitary axillary (*Quamoclit pennata*, some species of *Ipomoea, Evolvulus alsinoides*), in terminal cymose clusters (*Erycibe paniculata, Convolvulus cneorum*) or in axillary cymose clusters (*Convolvulus arvensis* and many species of *Ipomoea* and other genera). In *Ipomoea pes-tigridis*, the inflorescence is a dichasial cyme that later changes into a monochasial cyme.

Flower : Bracteate (*Cuscuta*) on ebracteate usually pedicellate; bracteolate in *Cuscuta*; complete; actinomorphic; bisexual; unisexual in *Hildenbrandtia*; hypogynous; cyclic; large sweetly scented and beautifully coloured in many genera (*Calystegia sepium, Ipomoea tricolor* and *I. carnea*).

Calyx : Five; free; sometimes gamosepalous; imbricate, persistent; usually green; inferior. In *Quamoclit sloteri*, the sepals have awn-like tips.

Corolla : Five; gamopetalous; campanulate; funnel-shaped, tubular, salverform; imbricate or valvate; variously coloured and scented. In *Convolvulus tricolor*, the corolla is blue with yellow centre and white edge; white with silvery hair in *Convolvulus cneorum*; inferior.

Androecium : Five; polyandrous; epipetalous;

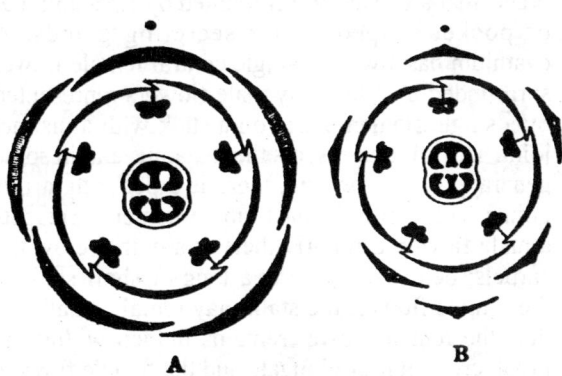

Fig. 6.7. Floral diagrams of Convolvulaceae. A. *Ipomoea*; B. dodder (*Cuscuta*).

alternate with the petals; inserted deep in the corolla tube; usually of unequal length; basifixed or dorsifixed; anthers bithecous; dehiscence longitudinal; introrse.

Gynaecium : Bicarpellary; syncarpous; superior, bilocular, tricarpellary and trilocular in *Ipomoea leari*; placentation axile; two ovules in each loculus; in some species of *Porana* there is a single ovule in each loculus, and the ovary has two ovules. The ovary is tetralocular in *Argyreia*. Style simple (*Ipomoea, Convolvulus* and *Evolvulus*) or two free from base (*Neuropeltis*) or united half their length (*Breweria*); in *Erycibe* the style is absent; stigma capitate (*Ipomoea leari*) or bifid (*Convolvulus, Ipomoea palmata*), sessile and lobed in *Erycibe,* bifid and linear in *Rivea*. The ovules are usually anatropous or semi-anatropous. A nectar secreting disc is usually present below the ovary (*Cuscuta*).

Fruit : Mostly capsular (*Convolvulus, Ipomoea,* etc.), sometimes baccate (*Erycibe, Argyreia*).

Seed : Endospermic; endosperm mucilaginous or cartilaginous; embryo with plicate cotyledons.

Pollination : Entomophilous.

Floral formula : $\oplus \ \varphi \ K_5 \ C_{(5)} \ A_5 \ G_{(2-3)}$.

FAMILY : EUPHORBIACEAE

Vegetative characters

Habit and habitat : The family includes large number of annual or perennial herbs (*Euphorbia dracunculoides, E. prostrata, E. pilulifera, E. hyporcifolia, Phyllanthus fraternus,* etc.) that may be unarmed or armed; shrubs and trees. Some genera (*Euphorbia* sp.) have milky latex.

Root : A much branched tap root.

Stem : Aerial; erect; prostrate (*Euphorbia prostrata*); armed (*Euphorbia splendens*) or unarmed (*Phyllanthus, Ricinus*); hairy (*Euphorbia hispida*), or glabrous, pubescent (*Putranjira*); cylindrical or angular; branched; hollow or solid; usually contain milky latex; in the genus *Euphorbia* the stem exhibits curious modifications as a consequence of adaptations to xerix environments, the leaves are reduced, scale like or absent and the stems become thick and succulent and store water. In some cases the stems become green and assimilatory and give a cactus like look, the leaves

and stipules often become modified into spines (*E. trigona, E. royleana*).

Leaf : Cauline and ramal; stipulate or exstipulate; petiolate or sessile; reduced and scale like in *Euphorbia trigona* and *E. royleana*, modified into spines in some species; caducous (*E. tirucalli, E. royleana*) or evergreen (*Buxus, Ricinus,* etc.); alternate (*Ricinus, Bridelia, Putranjiva, Phyllanthus, Euphorbia* sp.) or opposite (*Buxus, Trewla* and *Excoecaria*) or whorled (*Mischodon*); mostly simple; trifoliate compound in *Bischofia* and *Hevea*; simple leaves may be undivided (*Euphorbia, Barrus, Bridelia* and *Phyllanthus*), or divided (*Dalechampia*) or palmate (*Ricinus*). Undivided leaves may be entire (*Trewia, Phyllanthus fraternus*) or dentate or serrate; variously shaped; hairy or glabrous; reticulate unicostate or multicostate (*Ricinus*). In species of *Croton*, the leaves are variegated and densely clothed with minute orbicular and shining scales made up of radially arranged cells. Extra floral nectaries and diverse types of glands occur on the leaves (*Ricinus*). Stipules are modified into spines in *Euphorbia splendens*.

Floral characters

Inflorescence : In the genus *Euphorbia, Antho-stema* and *Pedilanthus*, the characteristic inflorescence is a *Cyathium*. The Cyathia may be solitary or variously arranged in cymose groups or dichasial cymes or in heads. A *cyathium* is a collection of unisexual flowers (both male and female) arranged in a cymose manner on an abbreviated axis and enclosed within a cup-shaped involucre of coloured or green bracts that are usually surmounted by 1.5 semilunar or pocket shaped nectar secreting glands. A cyathium has always a single central female flower surrounded by 2 to many male flowers represented by a single stamen borne on a stalk with a distinct joint. The joint represents the thalamus and in some genera *e.g., Anthostema*, there is a perianth at this points. This confirms that a single stamen represents a male flower. Similarly there is a point below the carpels; below the joint is a long or short stalk of the female flower, the stalk may remain small and thus the female flower remains hidden within the involucre or it may elongate and the female flowers come out of the involucre. The male flowers are arranged opposite the involucral lobes in a centrifugal manner. The female flowers ripen first. Branched hair are also visible amidst the male flowers. In *Euphorbia pulcherrima*, the leaves around the clusters of *Cyathia* become beautifully coloured. In *E. splenlens*, each cyathium has two red bracts that surround the involucre. These are additional measures to attract insects. In *Ricinus communis* the male and female flowers are arranged in panicles of racemes, the female flowers are at the top and male flowers below. In *Phyllanthus fraternus*, the male and female flowers arise singly or in clusters of 2 or 3 in the axis of simple leaves of a branch, the male flowers arise in axils of lower leaves whereas female flowers arise in the axila of upper or younger leaves of a branch. Simple racemes and spikes occur in *Acalypha, Tragia, Mallotus*, etc.

Flower : Bracteate; pedicellate or subsessile or sessile; unisexual; monoecious or dioecious; actinomorphic, hypogymous; usually 5-merous; cyclic; small and conspicuous.

Perianth : In *Phyllanthus*, there are 6 perianth lobes arranged in two whorls of three each. In *Croton*, the male flowers have two whorls of perianth whereas in female flowers there is usually one whorl of 5 lobes; free (*Phyllanthus fraternus*), or fused (*Ricinus*). In *Euphorbia*, the perianth lobes are usually wanting; usually there are 5 perianth lobes arranged in a single series; imbricate (*Actephila, Jatropha, Andrachne*), or valvate (*Ricinus*). A lobed or annular and 5 lobed disc is often present (*Phyllanthus*). In *Andrachae*, the disc bears 5 bifid nectar secreting glands; disc absent in many species (*Breynia, Sauropus*). Such a disc is present on the thalamus or as glands at the bases of perianth lobes.

Male flower : In *Euphorbia* and *Pedilanthus*, the male flowers are naked and represented by a single stamen borne on a short or a long stalk with a distinct joint representing the thalamus. In *Phyllanthus, Octodes, Givotia, Platystigma, Blachia* and *Croton*, the male flowers have free and biseriate perianth. In *Ricinus*, the perianth of 5 lobes is uniseriate and gamophyllous. In *Actephila* and *Andrachne*, the perianth is biseriate, the inner series is scale like. The perianth may be free (*Croton, Phyllanthus*) or united (*Ricinus*); imbricate or valvate. The perianth is distinguished into calyx and corolla in *Wielandia*.

Androecium : In *Euphorbia* and *Pedilanthus*, the

male flower has a single stamen. The male flowers in *Euphorbia splendens* and *E. pulcherrima* occur in 5 antipetalous groups of 5 flowers each. These flowers are arranged centrifugally, *i.e.*, older towards the centre and younger away from the centre. In *Manihot* there are free stamens. In *Buxus*, there are 4 stamens with bithecous anthers adnate to a thick connected. In *Bridelia* and *Bischofia*, there are five free stamens. In *Phyllanthus*, there are three stamens whose filaments fuse to form a central column with anthers borne at the tip. The anthers are usually bithecous; dehiscence may be longitudinal transverse, or by means of apical pores; anthers basifixed, forsifixed, or versatile.

Pistillode : Present or absent (*Hernonia, Ricinus* etc.).

Female flower : Perianth is as in male.

Gynaecium : Usually tricarpellary; syncarpous; superior; trilocular; placentation axile; ovule one or two in each loculus; there are three distinct styles, each style forks into two stigmas so that there are 6 stigmas; ovary usually trigonous. In *Bridelia*, the ovary is bilocular and has two bifid styles. In *B. minutiflora* there is only one style with a bifid stigma. In *Bischofia* the three styles are linear and ovary may be 3 to 4 locular. In *Glochidion* the carpels are connate into a 3-15 locular ovary with 2 ovules in each lobulus, the styles in this case are connate into a globose or cylindrical or clavate column that is lobed or notched at tip. In *Antidesma* the tricarpellary ovary is unilocular due to suppression of other two carpels and has only two ovules.

Staminodes : May be present or absent.

Fruit : The fruit is most commonly a schizocarpic capsule; rarely a drupe (*Bridelia, Drypetes, Antidesma, Givotia, Cometia*). It is a regma dehiscing into the three cocci in *Ricinus communis*.

Seed : Endospermic; embryo may have flat board cotyledons (*Phyllanthus, Euphorbia, Croton*) or narrow cotyledons (*Poranthera, Ricinocarpus*). Seeds are arillate in some genera (*Gelonium*).

Floral formula : *Male flower* : $\oplus \, \male \, P_{(3-5) \text{ or } 3+3 \text{ or zero}} \, A_{1-\alpha} \, G_{\text{zero or } (3-\alpha)}$.

Floral formula : *Female flower* : $\oplus \, \female \, P_{(3-5) \text{ or } 3+3 \text{ or } (5)} \, A_{\text{zero}} \, G_{(3)}$.

Pollination : In many genera with coloured flowers or bracts (*Jatropha, Manihot, Euphorbia splendens, E. pulcherrima*), the pollination is entomophilous. Unisexuality favours cross-pollination which is a rule in the family. In *Ricinus, Croton* and *Phyllanthus*, the pollination is effected by wind.

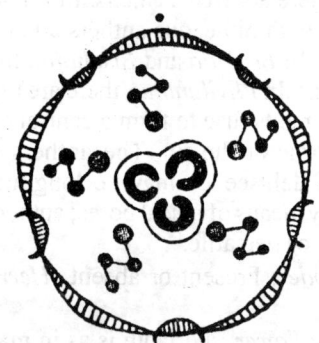

Fig. 6.8. Floral diagram of Euphorbiaceae (*Euphorbia*).

GNETALES

Gnetaceae

Gnetum

The genus Gnetum, with more than 30 spp. is confined to the humid and moist regions of the world.

Morphology : *Gnetum* plants are shrubs, trees or climbers with twinning stems, and in general habit resemble a dicotyledonous plant. The main stem bears two types of branches; a short shoot of limited growth (internodes present), and a long shoot of unlimited growth (internodes absent). The difference between the types of shoots is not very pronounced. In the climber *G. ala*, the short shoots bear leaves higher up near the branches of the supporting tree. The leaves lie crowded in one plane, in decussate pairs so that the branch looks like a pinnate leaf. The lamina is large, oval, entire with reticulate venation and gives a typically dicotyledonous appearance.

Several *Gnetum* spp. have articulated stems. The joints consist of two parts—one immediately above and the other immediately below the node, the two being separated by an annular groove. The internodes are shed at the joint, and lie in large numbers below the plant, resembling bones.

Reproduction : *Gnetum* is dioecious. The male and female strobili consist of a stout axis which bears a basal pair of opposite and connate bracts, and usually six to eight superposed cupules or collars. The cupules arise as annular protuberances in acropetal succession, and an annular rim is formed at the axillary position of each cupule. The cupules are tightly packed in a young strobilus, and the latter do not elongate appreciably during initiation of the annular rims. Later, the internode elongates so that the annular rims separate from the next upper cupule and the axillary position becomes pronounced. The annular rim develops as a hump from a few cells lying below each collar. Then this annular meristem comes to lie between the collar which bears it and the one below it, and gives the impression of axillary origin.

Male Strobilus : Three to six rings of male flowers develop basipetally above each collar. A single ring of abortive ovules may occur above the flowers. The flowers in different rings are arranged alternately.

A male flower consists of a stalk bearing two unilocular anthers enclosed in a perianth. On maturity, the stalk elongates and pushes the anthers (through an opening in the perianth) beyond the collars of the cone.

Male gametophyte : The mature pollen grain is shed at the three-celled stage. The division of the microscope nucleus results in a small lenticular and a large cell. The lenticular cell rounds up, does not divide further nor take part in the development of the pollen tube, and degenerates. The nucleus of the larger cell divides again and, of the two nuclei, one hyaline with a large nucleolus and is the first to enter the pollen tube. The second nucleus is rich in chromatin, has a cytoplasmic sheath of its own, and divides in the pollen tube to give rise to two male gametes.

These three nuclei have been variously interpreted. They represent the prothallial, tube and generative nuclei. They represent the tube nucleus, and stalk and body cells.

There is a new type of gametophyte development in *Gnetum ula*. The microscope divides and forms a small generative (body) cell on one side, and a large cell. The generative cell (which has its own sheath of cytoplasm) eventually lies free in the cytoplasm of the large cell, and then moves into the pollen tube and divides to form two male gametes.

The nucleus of the larger cell divides to become a binucleate cell.

Female strobilus : A female strobilus usually has six to eight collars and a single ring of ovules above each collar. Two to eight (usually five or six) ovular primordia differentiate from the annular rim. The latter becomes conspicuous before initiation of the ovules. Gradually, the ovules become visible on the upper edge of each collar. Generally, the upper few collars have no ovules.

Ovule : The cells in the epidermal and sub-epidermal layers of the ovular primordium divide actively. The dermal cells undergo both periclinal and anticlinal divisions. Simultaneously, each primordium can be distinguished into an upper region, which bears the ovule, and a lower, cushion-like area. Hairs differentiate from the surface of this cushion and from sterile cells between the ovules.

Three envelopes arise acropetally on ovular primordia and enclose the nucellus. The outer envelope (*oe*) is the first to differentiate. It arises laterally to the ovular primordium by peri- and anticlinical divisions in the dermal and subdermal cells and is of dual origin. At pollination, the *oe* increases in thickness. About 30 vascular strands are present at the level just above the junction between the inner envelope (*ie*) and the nucellus, and a few of them extend almost to the apex. Laticifer canals (do not form lateral connections) are scattered throughout the envelope, and numerous stomata occur in the outer layer.

After the *oe* is initiated, the apex of the ovule shows a clear uniseriate dermal layer. The middle envelope (*me*) and inner envelope (*ie*) have a subdermal origin.

The *me* arises next. Around pollination, it grows in thickness, only in the subapical part of the envelope, by periclinal divisions of the sub-dermal cells which elongate radially.

In *Gnetum*, the archegonia are absent. In *G. ula*, when a pollen tube enters the free-nuclear micropylar region of the gametophyte, one or more group/s of adjoining cells becomes densely cytoplasmic. Only one cell from each group function as the egg. The lower end of gametophyte becomes partly cellular. The egg in *G. ula* is a uninucleate or coenocytic cell. The functional female nuclei are large, and in prophase. In *G. africanum* also certain large and densely cytoplasmic cells in the micropylar region are potential egg cells.

In *G. gnemon*, one or more nuclei in the vicinity of the pollen tube become conspicuous by their larger size. They show striated cytoplasm around them, which later becomes delimited from the rest of the cytoplasm.

In the male cones, the female gametophyte (in the ovules) does not develop beyond the megaspore mother cell, or when the first meiotic division is completed (*G. ula*) or has 64 nuclei (*G. gnemon*). Rarely, only some of the ovules are functional, develop normally and ripen into seeds (*G. gnemon, G. africanum*).

Pollination : In *G. ula* and *G. gnemon*, a drop of surgery fluid exudes from the tip of the micropylar tube and catches pollen grains. The slimy pollination drop has appreciable quantities of reducing sugars in *G. gnemon*. Surface evaporation causes the contraction of the column of fluid, which brings about the withdrawal of pollen grains down to the nucellus.

Anemophily is probably concerned in the transfer of pollen to the female cone, through entomophily may also be involved. The male inflorescences emit a sweetish odour in the morning. The anthers open between 0.700 and 11.00 h. At about the same time, or earlier, nectar drops are present on fertile and sterile (in the male inflorescences) female flowers. All these characters are suggestive of insect pollination.

A dioecious (shrub species), *G. gnemon* var. *tenerum*, flowers in the evening. Both male and female strobili emit a putrid odour, that from male strobilus being longer than that from the female. Pollination droplets are secreted in the evening from ovules on female strobili and from sterile ovules on male strobili.

The bulk of the endosperm develops after fertilization, though cell formation may commence before fertilization. In *G. gnemon*, the female gametophyte is free-nuclear at the time of differentiation of the eggs. The lower part becomes cellular when the zygotes appear in the micropylar part. Wall formation is initiated either simultaneously with fertilization, or about that time. In *G. ula*, polyploid cells are produced at the chalazal end of the gametophyte before fertilization, but only uninucleate cells are produced after fertilization. With further growth, the endosperm broadens at the expense of adjoining nucellar cells which are consumed laterally as well as at the base. In *G. gnemon* and *G. africanum* the meristematic activity in the gametophyte is limited to the axial region and a few outer layers, especially at the two poles. Thus, the main mass of endosperm is formed and starch appears first in the outer cells at the lower end, later at the micropylar end, lastly in the inner cells. In older seeds, the cells become gorged with starch grains and may mask the nuclei. Oil droplets have also been detected; in later stages the cell walls show many simple pits.

Seed : In most species the mature seed is oval and green to red. The endosperm forms the bulk of the seed, and is surrounded by three envelopes. The nucellus is consumed except for a thin strip at the apex.

During the development of seed, the level of insertion of the inner envelope shifts distally. This is due to the development of an ovular tissue between the inner and middle envelopes, accompanied by an intercalary growth in the entire developing seed. The middle and outer envelopes show no such shift in their levels of insertion. A special term, endochalazal, was introduced for such an ovular structure.

The seed coat consists of three layers; (a) outer sarcotesta, (b) middle sclerotesta and (c) inner endotesta. The sarcotesta is free from the base up to apex, and is green and succulent. It is composed of a heavily cutinized epidermis and homogeneous parenchymatous cells. Diverse types of sclereids with lignified walls, and numerous branched fibers and laticifers also occur. In *G. ula*, *G. montanum* and *G. neglectum*, small astrosclereids or brachy-sclerids occur just below the outer epidermis. Additional astrosclereids are scattered in the deeper tissue. Haplochelic stomata, as in the leaves, occasionally develop on the outer epidermis.

The sclerotesta forms the protective layer of the seed. It has numerous sclereids of varying shape and may sometimes extend as a basal plate. Depending on the species, at maturity the middle layer may be nearly free from the outer layer, or may be partially or completely fused with it.

FAMILY : LAMIACEAE (LABIATAE)

Vegetative characters

Habit and habitat : Predominantly herbs (*Ocimum, Salvia, Mentha*), many shrubs (*Teucrium, Rosmarinus, Lavandula dentata*); annual or perennial; wild or cultivated (*Salvia, Ocimum*); rarely climbers or twinners (some species of *Scutellaria*). Majority are aromatic and yield ethereal oils. *Mentha aquatica* grows in water in ditches or wet places.

Root : Branched tap roots; but adventitious roots are found in some stoloniferous species and in *Mentha*, which propagate by suckers.

Stem : Aerial; erect; or sub-erect prostrate (*Glechoma hederacea*) or stoloniferous; underground sucker in *Mentha*; woody or herbaceous; hairy; squarish; branched; solid or hollow. In *Hedeoma*, the stems are green and assimilatory because the leaves are reduced.

Leaf : Cauline and ramal; radical in *Horminum*; exstipulate; petiolate or sessile; opposite and decussate; simple; entire; serrate or pinnatifid (*Perovskia*), kidney shaped in *Glechoma hederacea* (ground ivy); hairy; or glabrous; reticulate unicostate; green or variegated (*Coleus*); highly aromatic. In *Rosmarinus*, the leaf margins are revolute and the leaves are persistent. The leaves are reduced in some species of *Hedeoma*.

Floral characters

Inflorescence : It is very characteristic and mixed. The main axis of peduncle continues to grow and does not end in a flower. The primary form of inflorescence is, therefore, racemose. The unit of inflorescence which occurs in the axils of each opposite leaf or the bract is a few flowered dichasial cyme becoming monochasial in its later branching. The flowers of the two cymes at each node, being sessile or shortly stalked, overlap the bract axils and often look like a whorl. This apparent whorl of flowers at the node is called a *verticillaster*. In reality, it is a combination of two condensed dichasial cymes one on each side of the stem. The verticillasters are arranged in a racemose manner on the peduncle. In

Coleus, Physostegia and *Teucrium*, the inflorescence is a spike; simple racemes in *Scutellaria indica*; in dense head like clusters in *Monorda*.

Flower : Bracteate (*Coleus*), or ebracteate (*Salvia, Ocimum*); bracteolate in *Prunella*; pedicellate or sessile (*Coleus, Salvia, Physostegia*); complete; zygomorphic; bisexual; actinomorphic in *Mentha*; hypogynous; tetracyclic, beautifully coloured and scented; usually bilabiate. In *Iboza*, the flowers are unisexual and the plants are *dioecious*.

Calyx : Five; gamosepalous; tubular (*Lavandula, Nepeta, Marrubium*) or campanulate (*Teucrium*); bilabiate (*Salvia, Ocimum*). In *Salvia* the upper lip is entire or 3-toothed whereas the lower lip is 2 cleft. In *Ocimum basilicum* the upper lip is of one saucer shaped sepal, the lower is made up of 4 sepals that project beneath the upper lip like so many teeth. In *Hoslundia* the calyx is fleshy; usually green. In *Salvia farinosa*, the calyx is white to purplish with dense tomentum. In *S. azurea*, the calyx is greyish-green and finely puberulent, petaloid in many cultivated varieties of *Salvia*; persistent in *Salvia, Ocimum* and many other genera; inferior. In *Scutellaria*, the calyx has two entire lips and has a scale that grows over the back of upper lip.

Corolla : Five; gamopetalous; irregular; looks to be regular in *Mentha* due to the reduction of the upper lip to a small round lobe which is almost indistinguishable from the 3 lobes of the lower lip. In *Ajuga, Rosmarinus* and *Teucrium*, the corolla lacks upper lip; and all the five petals, constitute the 5-lobed lower lip. In *Pogostemon cablin*, the corolla is 4-lobed; in *Ocimum* and *Hyptis* the upper lip is composed of 4 petals and lower of one petal (4/1). In *Salvia* and *Lamium*, the upper lip is two lobed and the lower 3-lobed; variously coloured and scented; inferior.

Androecium : Usually 4 (*Ocimum, Mentha, Leucas*); sometimes two (*Salvia, Cunila, Monarda*), the posterior stamen is completely suppressed or reduced to a staminode. In *Salvia* and *Lycopus*, staminodes are lacking; filaments free; monoadelphous in *Coleus*; epipetalous. In *Salvia*, the anther lobes of the two fertile stamens are widely separated on a long slender connective articulated with the filament; the upper end of the connective bearing a fertile anther lobes, the lower end usually with

an imperfect one or none. In some cases the stamens are didynamous (*Lamium*). In *Scutellaria*, the anthers are hairy. In *Prunella*, the filaments are glabrous and 2-toothed at apex, lower tooth bearing the anther lobes; anther lobes divaricate in *Dracocephalum*; inferior.

Gynaecium : Bicarpellary; syncarpous; superior; bilocular; becoming tetralocular by the formation of a false septum, so that there is one ovule in each loculus; placentation axile; the carpel sometimes becomes deeply four lobed; ovary seated on a hypogynous nectariferous disc that may be well developed, thick, entire or lobed; style simple, *gynobasic*, (except in *Ajuga* and *Teucrium*); stigmas two, distinct. Ovules are anatropous.

Fruit : Mostly carcerulus (Schizocarpic), rarely a drupe (*Stenogyne*).

Seed : Non-endospermic with embryo having flat or plano-convex cotyledons and radical pointing downwards. Endospermic seeds are found in *Prostanthera*.

Floral formula : $\oplus \ \updownarrow$ rarely $K_{(5)} \ C_{(5)} \ A_{2-4 \ or \ (4)}$ $G_{(2)}$.

Pollination : It is effected by insects. The bilabiate corolla ensures that a visiting insect shall take a definite position in regard to the anthers and the stigma while searching for the nectariferous disc at the base of the ovary. The lower lip acts as a flag to attract the insects and also serves as a landing place, whereas the upper lip encloses the essential organs, which are so placed so as to touch the insect's back. The length of the corolla tube varies with species and determines the kind of insect visitor. Most of

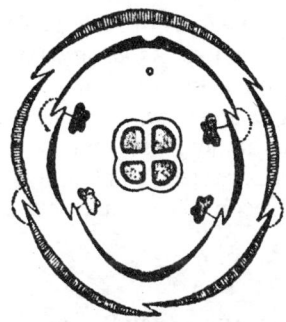

Fig. 6.9. Floral diagram of Lamiaceae.

the flowers are visited by bees; the long tubed flowers, e.g., those of *Monarda* are visited by butterflies. A few species of *Salvia* are visited by humming birds. In *Lamium* the flowers are homogenous.

FAMILY : LILIACEAE
Vegetative characters

Habit and habitat : Mostly herbs perennating by means of bulbs (*Tulipa, Hyacinthus, Lilium, Fritillaria, Asphodelus, Allium, Colchicum, Erythronium, Gagea, Urginea, Scilla*) or rhizomes (*Convallaria, Polygonatum, Mainathemum, Aloe*). *Aloe aristata* is the smallest species with plants only 15 cm in height, whereas *A. bainesii* and *A. dichotoma* grow up to 35 to 50 feet tall and possess thick aerial stems. In *Ruscus* and *Asparagus*, the stems are aerial and branched and the leaves are scale like bearing needle like or flattened leaf like cladodes in their axils. Both are herbs or sub-shrubs. *Smilax* is a climbing shrub, it climbs by means of stipular tendrils, which are regarded by some as coiled outgrowths of the leaf sheaths. In *Gloriosa* and *Sandersonia*, the leaf tips become tendrillar. Both are climbing herbs. *Protolirion* is a root parasite from Malayam Peninsula. Many are xerophytes and grow in dry and arid zones (*Aloe, Yucca*).

Root : Mostly fibrous adventitious roots. In *Asparagus* the roots become swollen and tuberous.

Stem : An underground bulb rhizome, the rhizome may be extensively branched (*Polygonatum*). In *Smilax, Asparagus, Yucca, Cordyline* and *Gloriosa*, the stems are aerial and branched and may be herbaceous or woody; solid or fistular; branched. In *Ruscus* and *Asparagus*, the aerial stems bear modified leaf-like branches called the *cladodes*. These arise in the axils of scale leaves and may be linear and needle like (*Asparagus*) or flattened and leaflike (*Ruscus*). In *Cordyline, Dracaena, Aloe. Yucca, Kingia* and *Xanthorrhoea*, the thick and woody stems undergo secondary growth by the activity of an extra stelar cambial ring that produces *leptocentric* secondary vascular bundles. The bulb in *Allium* is discoid.

Leaf

Radical (*Aloe, Allium, Lilium, Asphodelus,* etc.) or cauline and ramal (*Smilax, Gloriosa; Dracaena*);

exstipulate; petiolate or sessile; leaf base sheathing; leaves scale like in *Asparagus* and *Ruscus;* in *Aloe,* the leaves are thick and succulent and store water in the mucilage containing cells of the storage tissue. The leaves of *Phormium tenax* are 10 cm broad and up to 3 m long. Leaves are mostly alternate; opposite in *Scolyopus,* whorled in *Trillium;* simple; stems leafless in *Bowiea*. In *Aloe* and *Hamonthia,* the leaves have spinous apex and prickly margins. In *Gloriose,* and *Sandersonia* the leaf tips are tendrillar. In *Smilax* the stipules are modified into tendrils. Venation is usually parallel, reticulate in *Smilax* and *Trillium*. In *Chlorophytum comosum* var. *rariegatum,* the leaves are variegated. Leaves cylindrical or concentric in *Allium* and *Asphodelus;* leaf bases in *Allium* become thick and store food. Leaves only two in *Erythronium*.

Floral characters

Inflorescence : Solitary in *Clintonia uniflora, Tulipa, Uvularia,* some species of *Lilium* and *Erythromium*. In *Asphodelus,* the flowers are borne in racemes on a branched and leafless scape; simple racemes in some species of *Aloe;* in panicles of racemes in *Yucca* and *Dracaena*. In *Allium cepa,* the inflorescence is *scapigerous*, the flowers are borne in heads enclosed by one or more membranous bracts or spathes, the flower head is composed of many uniparous cymes disposed in an umbellate manner. Solitary or fascicled in *Ruscus*. In *Aspidistra* the flowers are borne singly at surface of ground beneath the foliage and are not often observed.

Flower : Bracteate (*Asparagus*) or ebracteate (*Helonias, Chamaelirium*); pedicellate; complete; or incomplete; actinomorphic; in *Haworthia* and *Haemerocallis* the flowers are zygomorphic; bisexual; unisexual in *Smilax (dioecious),* Ruscus and *Lomandra*; hypogynous; semi-inferior in *Ophiopogon* and *Aletris*; trimerous; cyclic. In *Colchicum autumnale,* the flowers appear in autumn and have their anthers and stigmas protruding above the ground whereas ovary, style and filaments of stamens remain below the ground where they are protected from cold. The fruit is raised above the ground in spring by the elongation of floral stalk. Flowers are protogynous in *Asphodelus* and protandrous in *Allium*.

Perianth : 6, in two whorls of three each, free (*Clintonia, Streptopus, Lilium, Erythronium*, or fused (*Asparagus, Aloe, Haworthia, Polygonatum, Allium*); perianth tube cylindrical or campanulate in *Polygonatum, Hyacinthus, aloe*; tube basally enlarged and curved above in *Gasteria*; funnel-shaped or bell-shaped (*Kniphofia, Chinodoxa*); cup-shaped (*Aspidistra*); rotate in *Anthericum*; urn-shaped in *Muscari*; distinguished into sepals and petals in *Trichium*. In *Mainanthemum*, there are 4 perianth lobes in two series of two each and gamophyllous, usually petaloid or sepaloid; inferior; superior in *Ophiopogon*. Perianth with basal glands in *Zigadenus*.

Androecium : Six; in two whorls of three each; four in *Maianthemum*; three in male flowers of *Ruscus*; in *Tofieldia* there are 9 to 12 stamens; free; opposite the perianth lobes; epiphyllous; in *Ophiopogon* the filaments are very short; in *Allium, Asparagus* and *Scilla*, the filaments are filiform; in *Asphodelus* and *Ornithogalum* the filaments are flattened and membranous; included or excerted; anthers bithecous; basifixed (*Tulipa, Erythronium Allium*, dorsifixed (*Ornithocalum, Scilla*), or versatile (*Asparagus, Lilium*), introrse (*Ophiopogon, Asphodelus, Allium, Aparagus*), or extrorse (*Xerophyllum*). In *Lilium martagon* the large orange anthers are attached by special joints to the long filaments. In *Ruscus* the three filaments are connate forming a short tube with anthers at its top.

Gynaecium : Tricarpellary, syncarpous; superior; semi-inferior in *Ophiopogon* and *Aletris*; trilocular; placentation axile with many ovules in each loculus; ovules anatropous. In *Maianthemum*, the grnaecium is bicarpellary, syncarpous and bilo-cular; in female flowers of *Ruscus*, the ovary is unilocular with two ovules. In *Asparagus* and *Asphodelus*, the trilocular ovary has two ovules in each loculus. Style simple (*Asparagus, Asphodelus, Allium*) or 3-parted (*Gloriosa*). In *Tricyrtis*, there are three styles, each with a bifid stigma. In *Asparagus*, the simple style bears a trifid stigma. In *Veratrum*, the three separate styles are persistent. In *Veratrum*, the three carpels are incompletely fused, their distal tips are free and divergent, the carpel margins are merely appressed and not histo-

logically fused. In *Tofieldia glutinosa*, there are 3 to 5 carpels that are almost free up to base. In *Aphyllanthes*, the unilocular ovary has only one ovule in marginal medium position.

Fruit : A loculicidal (*Aloe*) or a septicidal (*Tricyrtis, Stenanthium, Veratrum*) capsule. In *Smilax, Asparagus, Clintonia, Polygonahum* etc., the fruit is a berry.

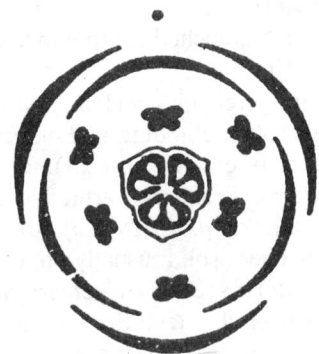

Fig. 6.10. Floral diagram of Liliaceae.

Seed : Endospermis, endosperm cartilaginous or horny, Endosperm is nuclear and helobial. It is a helobial in all the species of *Asphodelus*, in *Aloe lateritia* and *Halmarocalis fulva*. It is nuclear in *Colchicum autumnale, Gloriosa, Lilium* and *Hyacinthus*.

Floral formula : ⊕ ☿ rarely $P_{(3+3) \text{ or } 3+3}$ $A_{3+3 \text{ or } 2+2}$ $G_{(3) \text{ rarely } (3)}$.

Pollination : Flowers usually pollinated by the agency of insects; sometimes self-pollination is also effected. The flower emits its perfume especially at night and is then visited by the moths. The female moth effects pollination. It has a long ovipositor with which she can penetrate the tissue of the ovary of the flower. She begins collecting pollen a little before dark. The pollen is shaped into a pellet about three times as large as her head. She then flies to the next flower and deposits a few eggs in the ovary after piercing the ovary wall. Having done this, she climbs to the top and presses the pellet of pollen grains into the stigma. The ovules are thus fertilised and are so numerous that they are plenty for the larvae to feed upon and also to reproduce the plant.

FAMILY : MIMOSOIDEAE

Vegetative characters

Habit and habitat : Trees (*Acacia, Albizzia*), shrubs (*Mimosa rubicaulis*), herbs (*Mimosa pudica*) or climbers (*Entada*). *Neptunia* with its two Indian species is hydrophytic. Majority grow under xerophytic conditions. Many (*Acacia*) are armed and covered with spines or prickles, a few are unarmed (*Albizzia, Entada*).

Root : A much branched tap root that penetrates deep into the soil.

Stem : Aerial; erect or scandent, and straggling (*Mimosa rubicaulis*), climbing in *Entada*; woody; angular and twisted in (*Entada*); cylindrical (*Acacia, Albizzia, Prosopis*); armed with spines (*Acacia, Piptadaenia, Prosopis*), or unarmed (*Albizzia*); branched; solid; usually covered with a rough bark; various species of *Acacia* yield gums of many types from the stem. Stem spines occur in *Dichrostachys, Prosopis* and *Piptadaenia*.

Leaf: Cauline and ramal; stipulate stipules modified into spines in *Acacia*; in *A. sphaerocephala* the spiny stipules are hollow and provide shelter to insects; petiolate; in *Entada* the common petioles of a bipinnate leaf end in long and woody bifid tendrils, in some species of *Acacia*, the petiole becomes flattened into a phyllode and the leaflets fall down; alternate; once pinnate (*Inga*) or twice pinnate; leaflets opposite or alternate, sessile or subsessile or petiolate; the leaves of *Mimosa* and *Neptunia* are sensitive to touch and show sleep movements when touched. In *A. sphacrocephala* each pinnule terminates in small globule of parenchyma called Belts corpuscles that are eaten by ants.

Floral characters

Inflorescence : Cymose heads in *Parkia, Mimosa, Albizzia,* and *Acacia*; in some species of *Albizzia* the cymose heads are arranged in terminal panicles; spike in *Prosopis*, racemes in *Adenanthera.*

Flower : Bracteate; sessile (*Prosopis, Entada*); sub-sessile (*Albizzia, Acacia*) or pedicellate (*Adenanthera*); ebracteolate; complete; regular; antino-morphic; bisexual; perigynous; tetramerous in *Mimosa*; cyclic; small.

Calyx : Five; gamosepalous; cup-shaped in

Piptadaenia; shortly tubular and 5-toothed in *Entada* and *Xylia*; campanulate in *Acacia* and *Albizzia*; there are 4 fused sepals in *Acacia suma* and *Mimosa*; valvate; imbricate in *Parika*; odd sepal anterior; odd sepal posterior in *Parkia ofricana*; green or petaloid (*Acacia arabica*). In *Parkia africana*, the five sepals are free and unequal.

Corolla : Usually five; four free and valvate in *Mimosa* and *Acacia suma*; choripetalous or gamopetalous (*Acacia, Albizzia, Xylia*). In *Xylia*, the petals are linear and fused only at the base. In *Acacia* and *Albizzia*, the corolla is tubular and 5-toothed; valvate; inferior. In *Albizzia lebbeck*, the teeth of corolla tube are hairy.

Androecium : Four free in *Mimosa pudica*; 10 free in *Prosopis, Entada, Adenanthera* and *Xylia*; 10 and monoadelphous in *Parkia*; indefinite and free in *Acacia*; indefinite and monoadelphous in *Albizzia, Colliandra* and *Puhecolobium*; filaments longer than petals and filiform in *Acacia, Albizzia* and *Piptadaenia*; usually bitheous and introse.

Gynaecium : Monocarpellary; superior; unilocular; placentation marginal; ovules more than one or numerous in a carpel; style long and filiform; simple; stigma simple, linear or knobbed.

Fruit : A legume (*Albizzia*) or a lomentaceous pod (*Acacia*). In *Entada scandens* the pod is woody 2-4 feet long and 3-4 inches broad, consisting of 10-30 one-seeded flat or square or orbicular joints.

Seed : Nonendospermic.

Floral formula : $\oplus \ \male\female \ K_{(5) \text{ or } (4)} \ C_{4 \text{ or } 5 \text{ or } (5)} \ A_{4 \text{ or } 10 \text{ or } (10) \text{ or } \alpha \text{ or } (\alpha)} \ G_1.$

FAMILY : NYCTAGINACEAE

Vegetative characters

Habit and habitat : Mostly herbs (*Boerhavia, Mirabilis, Abronia*); few shrubs (*Pisonia aculeata*); climbers (*Bougainville*) or tres (*Pisonia alba*).

Root : A much branched tap root; thick and tuberous in *Mirabilis*; fusiform in *Boerhavia*.

Stem : Aerial; erect or climber or prostrate (*Boerhavia*); angled, branched; solid, hairy; woody in arboneal forms, otherwise herbaceous.

Leaf: Cauline and ramal; exstipulate; petiolate; opposite; equal or unequal (*Abronia*); simple; reticulate-unicostate.

Floral characters

Inflorescence : Usually cymose clusters, dichasial in the beginning but becoming monochasial later.

Flower : Bracteate, bracts reduced and mainly in *Boerhavia*, large and coloured in *Bougainvillea* (3), green and sepal like in *Mirabilis* where each flower has an involucre of five fused bracts; pedicellate; complete; actinomorphic; bisexual; unisexual in *Pisonia*; hypogynous; cyclic; variously coloured.

Perianth : Five, gamophyllous; campanulate (*Borrhavia*) or tubular (*Mirabilis, Bougainvillea, Abronia*), usually coloured like petals; persistent; the upper part of the persistent perianth usually falls down and the lower part surrounds the fruit and is variously modified to help in dispersal, this lower persistent part is called *anthocarp*; inferior.

Androecium : 3-5 in *Mirabilis* and *Abronia*, 5-10 in *Bougainvillea*, 1-5 in *Boerhavia*, sometimes the number rises to 15 or 20 or even 30 by branching; included (*Bougainvillea*) or exserted (*Mirabilis*); filaments equal or unequal; alternipetalous, anthers bithecous; basifixed or dorsifixed; dehiscence longitudinal, by lateral slits; Epiphyllous in *Boerhavia*.

Gynaecium : Monocarpellary; unilocular; superior; placentation basal; ovule one, anatropous or campylotropous; style long and filiform, simple; stigma simple. A nectariferous disc is present in *Mirabilis*.

Fruit : An indehiscent achene enclosed within persistent perianth that may become winged, ribbed or grooved or even hairy and mucilagenous.

Seed : Non-endospermic but with a distinct perisperm and a curved embryo with unequal cotyledons.

Floral formula : $\oplus$ $\male$ or $\female$ $P_{(5)}$ $A_{3\text{-}5 \text{ or } 5\text{-}10 \text{ or } 20\text{-}30}$ G_1

Pollination : The presence of brightly coloured bracts and large and coloured flowers suggest and entomophilous pollination.

FAMILY : PAPAVERACEAE

Vegetative characters

Habit and habitat : Predominantly herbaceous, a few shrubs and trees. Annuals or perennial. Most of the species are cultivated for their ornamentral and economical values, other grow wild. The stems and leaves contain a milky or coloured latex except in *Eschscholtzia* and *Hunnemannia* where the latex is colourless and watery.

Root : Mostly tap root, which is extensively branched and is usually a surface feeder.

Stem : Erect; branched; herbaceous or woody; may be smooth or hairy; rugose in trees and shrubby forms; hollow or solid (*Papaver orientale*); glaucous (*Argemone*) or glabrous.

Leaf : Radical in young plants; cauline and ramal in older plants; exstipulate; alternate; in some cases upper leaves are sub-opposite, rarely whorled; petiolate or sessile (*Argemone*); simple; entire or pinnately or plamately incised; hairy, sometimes spinous (*Argemone*); unicostate-reticulate or multicostate-reticulate.

Floral characters

Inflorescence : Solitary terminal or solitary axillary sometimes in racemes or in compound racemes; dichasial cymes with cincinnal tendency are also met with in some genera (*Chelidonium majus*).

Flower : Ebracteate; pedicellate; complete; regular; actinomorphic, bisexual; hypogynous; perigynous in *Eschscholtzia*, in this case the receptacle has a lower or basal vase-like portion and an upper flattened platform that spreads at right angles to the axis of the stem.

Calyx : 2 to 3; chorisepalous (free); sometimes fused (*Eschscholtzia*) to form a cap like or calpytrate structure covering the floral bud; usually caducous; hairy; green; imbricate or twisted; inferior.

Corolla : Four (*Papaver*) to six (*Argemone*) or eight or twelve; free (Choripetalous); usually biseriate (arranged in two whorls); sometimes uniseriate; rarely triseriate; crumpled (*Papaver*) in bud condition; large and variously coloured. The petals are absent in *Macleaya* and *Bocconia*; imbricate and usually fall down in mature flowers; inferior.

Androecium : Usually numerous, rarely four (*Pteridophyllum, Hypecoum*); free; in many whorls that alternate with each other, when few cyclic; filaments distinct; slender; coloured like the petal; sometimes flattened and alate; anthers dithecous; basifixed dehiscene longitudinal, introse; inferior.

Gynaecium : Polycarpellary (2-many); syncarpous; in *Platystemon* the numerous carpels are lightly united before fruit formation and separate at fruiting time; superior; unilocular or becoming multilocular by the formation of false septa; placentation parietal; ovules many; in *Bocconia* there is only one basal ovule; in *Papaver* the placenatae intrude towards the centre and result in a superficial placentation; ovules anatropous or campylotropous; style short, single or many as in *Platystemon*, sometimes indistinct; stigmas equal in number to the carpels; in *Papaver* the stigma is sessile and rayed forming a stigmatic disc, each lobe of which is opposite to the placenta.

Fruit : A capsule; dehiscence porous (*Papaver*) or septicidal (*Argemone*). Fruit is a follicle in *Platystemon*, rarely an indehiscent nut.

Seed : Endospermic, endosperm oily; embryo small.

Pollination : The flowers are mostly large and conspicuous and insect pollinated. Many contain no honey and are visited by pollen seeking insects; often protandrous.

Floral formula : $\oplus \; \male \female \; K_{2 \text{ or } 3 \text{ or } (2)} \; C_{2+2 \text{ or } 3+2} \; A_{\alpha \text{ or } 4}$ $G_{(2-\alpha)}$.

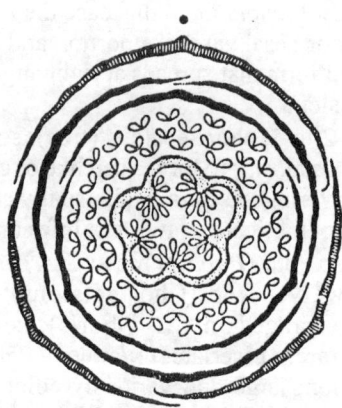

Fig. 6.11. Floral diagram of Papaveraceae (Argemone).

FAMILY : PAPILIONACEAE (PEA FAMILY)

Vegetative characters

Habit and habitat : The sub-family includes herbs; shrubs; woody climbers; herbaceous climbers. Some are twinners. They grow a in variety of habitats and may be xerophytic, hydrophytic, halophytic and mesophytic.

Root : A much branched tap root that usually bears modulated outgrowths which hoard millions of nitrogen fixing bacteria. *Dolichos falcatus* has tuberous roots.

Stem : Aerial; erect in trees, shrubs and many herbs, weak in twinners (*Dolichos, Atylosia*) and tendrillar climbers (*Pisum, Lathyrus*); woody or herbaceous (*Pisum*); branched; angular or cylindrical; glabrous tomentose and hairy in many species; solid of fistular.

Leaf : Cauline ramal; stipulate; leaf-base pulvinate in many plants; alternate; simple, trifoliate in many genera; pinnate with many leaflets in *Tephrosia, Cicer, Dalbergia* (leaflets alternate). In *Astragalus* the rachis of the compound leaf ends in a spine; modified into tendril in *Lathyrus aphaca* where the stipules become large and leafy to perform photosynthetic functions in *Pisum, Lathyrus* and some other plants the leaflets become tendrillar and help in climbing. In *Desmodium* the two lateral leaflets of a leaf perform autonomous movements.

Floral characters

Inflorescence : Racemose.

Flower : Bracteate; pedicellate or sub-sessile; bracteolate (*Arachis*) or ebracteolate; irregular; complete; zygomorphic; bisexual; perigynous; cyclic; pentamerous; small and large; showy (*Sophora*).

Calyx : Usually five; gamosepalous; campanulate; dentate teeth subequal; tubular in some species of *Astragalus* and *Cyamopsis*, inferior; odd sepal anterior; green; mostly hairy, persistent in *Tephrozia*.

Corolla : Five; choripetalous; papilionaceous (butter fly appearance); the posterior petal is large and conspicuous and encloses two posterolateral petals or the *wings* or *alae*, which in turn enclose the antero-lateral petals that fuse to form a boat-shaped structure called the *keel* or *carina*. The *keel* encloses the essential organs (stamens and carpels). In *Phaseolus*, the *keel* is prolonged into a long beak and is spirally twisted. In *Dumasia*, the wings and the keel are adherent and have long claws. In *Tephrozia*, the petals are green in young flowers and become violet in mature flowers.

Androecium : Mostly ten; nine in *Abrus* and *Dalbergia*; diadelphous (1 + 9) in *Pisum*, diadelphous (5 + 5) in *Smithia*. In genera with diadelphous stamens 1 + (9), the posterior stamen is free and the filaments of the rest nine are fused to form a tube like structure surrounding the ovary stamens of five each. The anthers are usually bithecous (4-celled) but in *Arachis hypogea* (groundnut), there are two posterior sterile anthers, two globose monothecous anthers, three oblong monothecous and three bithecous anthers. Pollen grains smooth walled in *Tephrosia*, triaperturate in *Tephrosia*.

Gynaecium : Monocarpellary; superior; unilocular; placentation marginal; ovules many; ovules anatropous or campylotropous; in *Butea, Flemingia* and *Heylandia* there are only two ovules in a carpel, in *Cylista* there is only one ovule in an ovary; ovary minute and sessile in *Rothia* and *Heylandia*, linear in *Crotolaria* and many other plants, flattened in *Lathyrus, Pisum* and *Tephrosia*, cylindrical and oblong in others (*Indigofera*); ovary sessile, subsessile, or stalked, hairy; style minute (*Rothia*), short (*Medicago*) or long and filiform (*Arachis hypogea*), hairy or without hair (*Mucuna*); stigma simple, spathulate or capitate (*Mucuna*), papillate in *Lathyrus, Pisum* and *Tephrosia*.

Fruit : The fruit is typically a legume opening by both sutures, but sometimes by one suture, or quite indehiscent (*Melilotus*). The fruit may be dry or fleshy; straight; curved (*Trigonella*) or spirally coiled (*Medicago*).

Seed : The seed is nonendospermic, the food is stored in the thick cotyledons. The seeds of many papilionate have hard seed coats and an external waxy coating. Seeds of *Trifolium resupinatum* are hard when they ripen during hot dry weather and soft when they ripen during rainy season.

Pollination : The flowers are insect pollinated. The stamens and the carpel are enclosed by the keel, the honey is secreted by the inner sides of stamens near their base and collects in the staminal tube around the base of the ovary. On either side of the base of the tenth free stamen, there are two openings that lead to the honey. The honey is thus concealed and is at some depth, so that only a clever insect with a tongue of moderate length is required to effect pollination. Bees are the suitable insects and *Papilionatae* are pollinated by bees. The bees alight on the wings and depress them by their weight, whilst they probe for honey under the *standard*. The wings are usually joined to the keel by a protuberance which fits into suitable hollow at the bases of the *keel*. This results in the depressing of the keel along with the wings or the alae. As the keel is depressed the stamens and the carpel emerge out of it, the stigma usually comes out first, so that there is a fair chance of cross-pollination.

Floral formula : $+ \ \male \female \ K_{(5)} C_{1+2+(2)} A_{(9)+1 \, \text{or} \, (9) \, \text{or} \, 10 \, \text{or} \, (5)+(5)} G_1.$

PINACEAE

Pinaceae is the largest and the most recent of the modern conifer families. The exact time of origin is not clear, but the family is evident by the early Cretaceous. Seed cones of this Cretaceous assemblage show considerable diversity but have more features characteristic of *Pinus* than of any other modern taxa. Anatomically also, the cones are distinctly *Pinus*-centred (which occurs only in the early Cretaceous).

The characteristic features of the family are : spirally arranged parts; two pollen sacs in a microsporophyll, pollen mostly bisaccate; ovuliferous scale free or slightly fused at the base of the bract scale, two ovules per scale and seed generally winged. There are over 200 spp. included in ten taxa; *Abies, Cathaya, Cedrus, Keteleeria, Larix, Picea, Pinus, Pseudolarix, Pseudotsuga* and *Tsuga*. All are trees, and the family is economically very important.

Pinus : The genus has about 80 valid species. They are divided into two natural subgenera with distinct characters:

(a) *Haploxylon* or soft pines—the scaly shoot at the base of the short shoot is deciduous, ray tracheids in secondary wood of stem and root have smooth wall; the needle (leaf) has a single vascular bundle.

(b) *Diploxylon* or hard pines—the scaly shoot present at the base of the short shoot is persistent; the ray tracheids have a corrugated wall, and the needle has two vascular bundles.

Morphology

Young pine trees are pyramidal with horizontal branches at regular intervals. This symmetry is lost as the tree matures and the crown becomes round, flat or spreading.

There is a primary tap root with a large number of laterals called long roots. The primary root soon becomes arrested while the long roots continue to grow and bear clusters of dwarf roots. Some of these roots branch dichotomously, form coralloid masses, have an ectotrophic mycorrhiza and are termed mycorrhizal roots.

At any level of phosphorus, could result from differences in diversion of carbohydrates from the host to the fungal structure.

Two types of branches are present: *long shoot* with unlimited growth; *dwarf shoot* with limited growth. The long shoots occur on the main stem as lateral buds in the axils of scale leaves, and terminate in an apical bud. The latter is enclosed by a number of bud scales closely surrounded by a thick mat of hairs. The lateral buds grow, nearly horizontally, to a certain length termed *nodal* growth. In *uninodal* pines a single internode, while in *multinodal* pines two or more internodes are formed in a year.

The dwarf shoot or foliar spur develops on a long shoot in the axil of a scale leaf and lacks a terminal bud. Each dwarf shoot initially has two opposite scales—prophylls followed by 5-13 cataphylls. Finally, needle-like foliage leaves develop on the spur shoot, in fascicles of one (*P. monophylla*), two (*P. sylvestris, P. merkusi*), three (*P. insularis, P. roxburghii, P. gerardiana*), four (*P. quadrifolia*) and five (*P. griffithii, P. wallichiana, P. armandi*). The number of needles present is constant for a species and is used for identification of different pines.

The plants are monoecious. The male and female cones are borne on different branches of the same tree. The male cones are modified dwarf shoots and appear in clusters on the lower branches of the tree. The number of cones is a cluster varies from 15 (*P. griffithii*) to 140 (*P. roxburghii*). Each cone arises in the axial of a scale leaf, replaces a dwarf shoot and is surrounded by several bracts. The female cones replace the terminal buds of the long shoot and are a modified long shoot. In the beginning, the female cones are protected by an involucre of bracts.

The cone has an average length of 1.5-2 cm and a diameter of 0.8-1 cm. The cone axis elongates (at the time of pollination) and the cone protrudes beyond the envelop the scales and is open to receive pollen grains. After pollination the cone closes. Originally, the cones are pale green but about the time of pollination the colour changes to reddish purple, and finally to glaucous green or purplish (*P. wallichiana*). The seeds are shed nearly 27 months from the time of initiation of the cone. The cones (at this time) are 20-24 cm in length and 5.5-6 cm in diameter. In most species the hard and woody mature female cone opens to release the seeds (*P. roxburghii, P. wallichiana*), in others the seeds are released only after the cones fall to the ground and rot.

Male cone : A male cone consists of a number of spirally arranged microsporophylls with upturned scaly apices. Two microsporangia are borne on the abaxial side and dehisce by a longitudinal slit.

Male gametophyte : The uninucleate microspore/pollen grain is the first cell of the male gametophyte. In all its divisions inside the microscope, the nucleus divides equally, but the cytoplasm becomes unequally distributed.

As the intine is being laid down, the divisions of microspore nucleus lead to the formation of two prothallial cells. Both the prothallial cells are ephemeral, and their remnants become embedded in the intine. After the formation of prothallial cells, the antheridial initial divides, giving rise to a small antheridial cell, which remains attached to the intine at the site of prothallial cells and a large vacuolate tube cell with a conspicuous nucleus. The electron density and organelle distribution of the antheridial and tube cells are similar, but there is a cytochemical difference in the amount of DNA, RNA and proteins.

From the end of April in northern Himalaya, India, 2000-3000 m, to the beginning of June. *P. wallichiana* pollen grains are shed at the four-celled stage, *i.e.*, two prothallials, antheridial and tube cell. The pollen germination is arrested and further development takes place on the nucellar apex.

Female cone: A young cone is small, elongated to spherical, and green in *P. roxburghii* and maroon in *P. wallichiana*. Each cone consists of 80-90 ovuliferous scales in the axial of bract scale, two together are termed seed-scale complex. They are arranged spirally on the cone axis. Independent vascular traces supply the ovuliferous and bract scale, in the former it is inversely oriented. The number of seed-scale complex varies with the species. Those present at the base and apex of the cone are sterile. An ovuliferous scale arises in the axial of a bract scale, which enclosed it till the time of pollination. It bears two ovules on its dorsal surface, their micropyles face the cone axis. Later, the ovuliferous scale outgrows the bract scale.

Ovule : The ovule is unitegmic. The integument is free from the nucellus except at the chalazal end, and forms a symmetrical tube well beyond the level of the nucellus. Adaxially, the edges of the integument extend into two long arms, which curve inwards before pollination, outwards during the curve back after pollination and finally dry up. There is no vascular supply to the ovule.

Megasporogenesis : The archesporial cell becomes distinguishable while the female cone is still covered by the scale leaves. It differentiates at the broad apical end of the nucellus and divides transversely to give rise to primary parietal and primary sporogenous cell. The former undergoes both vertical and transverse divisions, so that the sporogenous cell is pushed deep into the nucellus, and later functions as the megaspore mother cell. Starch grains accumulate at the chalazal end of the megaspore mother cell (*P. sylvestris*). The latter undergoes miosis-I and produces a dyad. Only a triad is formed if the upper dyad cell does not undergo meiosis II, or a tetrad if both the dyads undergo meiosis II. In a triad and linear tetrad, the upper dyad cell and the adjoining megaspores or the upper three megaspores in a tetrad usually degenerate. The chalazal megaspore functions so that the development of the gametophyte is monosporic.

Three to five layers of cells round the functional megaspore become densely cytoplasmic with prominent nuclei. This is the spongy or nutritive tissue. In the ovules, if the megaspore mother cell, or functional megaspore, fails to develop, the adjoining cells of the spongy tissue enlarge simulating a cellular gametophyte. The spongy tissue comprises a definite zone of physiologically active cells which are concerned in the nutrition of the young gametophyte, especially at the resting stage. The cells of this zone contain abundant starch.

Female gametophyte (first period of growth): The functional megaspore enlarges and shows a large vacuole even before the nuclear divisions commence. It forms a few free nuclei and apparently remains inactive for 8-9 months (first period of rest).

Pollination : Each tree produces an enormous number of pollen grains dispersed by wind. The surrounding area becomes clouded by the yellow powder (also known as sulphur shower). However, only a few pollen grains reach the pollen chamber and develop further.

A pollination drop is secreted (possibly from the nucellus), at the flared-out tip of the integument. The fluid contains sucrose, glucose and fructose. The secretion starts a few days after the female cones emerge out of the scale leaves and the ovuliferous scales separate sufficiently to permit the free entry of pollen. Under high humidity and cell turgor, the secretion begins around midnight, and by early morning the micropyle dries up. The arrival of the wind-borne pollen at the micropyle is purely a chance phenomenon. The pollen is caught in the pollination drop, grains stick to the two-pronged "stigmatic" micropylar canal and "migrate" to the nucellar tip.

The pollen grain has a germinal furrow which closes in dry weather, but remain wide open in high humidity, or when in contact with the pollination drop. The pollen tube emerges through this furrow.

Seed : The seed ripens within few weeks without much change in the size of the embryo.

In the young ovule the integument is three-layered. It becomes six- or seven layered at the time of pollination.

FAMILY : RANUNCULACEAE (BUTTER CUP FAMILY)

Vegetative characters

Habit and habitat : Herbs, vines (*Clematis, Naravelia*) or shrubs (*Xanthorhiza*), rarely trees (*Paeonia*); annual or perennial; cultivated as well as wild.

Root : Tap root and adventitious roots are found. In some cases, *e.g.*, *Ranunculus* sp. and *Aconitum*, the adventitious roots store food and swell to form a tuber-like structure that help the species to perennate.

Stem : Aerial and underground (*Helleborous*), thick rhizome or a row of tubers one formed each year. Sympodial rhizome is found in *Anemone*. The stem is climbing in *Naravelia* and *Clematis*; woody (*Paeonia*, *Clematis*) herbaceous (*Ranunculus*); annual or perennial; branched, branching racemose; solid as well as hollow; hairy or smooth.

Leaf : Radical, ramal and cauline; exstipulate, in some species of *Ranunculus*. The margins of the leaf base become expanded and appear like stipules; petiolate; leaf base sheathing; simple (*Ranunculus, Caltha, Coptis*) or palmately (*Clematis, Naravelia*) and pinnately compound (*Actaea, Xanthorrhiza*); simple leaves may be entire, (*Caltha, Coptis*), cordate (*Ranunculus ficaria*), palmately divided (*Ranunculus muricatus*), sometimes finely disected into fine segments (*Ranunculus aquatilis, Delphinium ajacis*).

Floral characters

Inflorescence : Solitary terminal, there is an involucre of green leaves below the flowers, the involucral leaves usually alternate with the outermost perianth leaves. In some species of *Nigella* and in *Aconitum* after the appearance of a terminal flower, the buds below develop in ascending order so that a raceme with an end flower is formed. In *Delphinium*, the inflorescence is a typical *raceme*. In *Ranunculus*, cymose clusters are formed.

Flower : Bracteate (*Nigella, Clematis*), ebracteate (*Anemone, Eranthis*); pedicellate; ebracteolate (*Ranunculus*) or bracteolate (*Delphinium*), complete or incomplete; regular or irregular (*Aquilegia, Delphinium*); bisexual or unisexual (*Thallictrum*, may be monoecious or dioecious); hypogynous; spiral or cyclic or spirocyclic (*Ranunculus, Delphinium*); variously coloured; large or small. Flowers usually protandrous but protogynous in *Helleborous*. In zygomorphic flowers, the calyx and corolla are produced into a spur. In *Delphinium*, there is a single spur whereas in *Aquilegia*, the flower has many spurs. The flowers are bracteolate in *Delphinium ajacis*.

Perianth

In *Helleborous*, the perianth is uniseriate and consists of variable (4-6) number of tepals that are coloured. In *Helleborous niger*, there is a differentiation between sepals and petals before fertilisation. After fertilisation the petals turn green. In *Delphinium* (Larkspur) the perianth is biseriate. The posterior lobes of perianth in the outer and inner whorl are produced into a spur which has a nectary at its base. The outer whorl of perianth has five sepals whereas the inner one has only four gamotepalous sepals, the anterior one being absent. Between the perianth lobes and stamens are present nectaries that are considered to be modified petals or by some to be modified stamens.

In some species sepals and petals are distinct (*Ranunculus*).

Calyx : Usually 5 (*Ranunculus*), 4 in *Clematis*, sometimes 3 to 6 (*Eranthis hyemalis*); chorisepalous (free); petaloid when petals are absent; valvate or imbricate; inferior. In *Nigella*, the petaloid calyx has 5 to 8 pocket-shaped nectaries internal to the sepals. The nectaries are protected by lid-like structures that prevent the insects from reaching the nectar. In some species of *Ranunculus* the sepals become reflexed.

Corolla : Usually Five but the number varies between three to twenty-three, some-times absent (*Clematis*); choripetalous (free); in *Helleborous* (10-20) and *Eranthis* there are small tubular petals that secrete honey. In *Eranthis* there are 6 sepals and many petals. In *Nigella* the petals are caducous and fall down very early, the sepals in this case become petaloid. The corolla is usually imbricate inferior.

Androecium : Numerous; polyandrous; spirally arranged; filaments short or long; anthers dithecous; dehiscence longitudinal, extrose; basifixed.

Gynaecium : Usually polycarpellary; apocarpous and spirally arranged (*Ranunculus, Ancmonr, Climatis*); sometimes bicarpellary syncarpous or 5-carpellary to polycarpellary syncarpous (*Nigella*); in *Aconitum* it is bi- to pentacarpellary syncarpous; the number of free carpels varies from 5-300; superior, unilocular; placentation basal (*Ranunculus*), marginal in *Delphinium*, parietal in *Aconitum*; ovaries 1-many, anatropous.

Fruit : Achens is *Ranunculus*; capsule in *Nigella* and baccate (berry) in *Actaea*; follicles in *Aconitum*, simple follicle in *Larkspur*.

Seed : Endospermic, endosperm abundant; embryo small and straight. In *Helleborous* the seeds bear small oil glands on their raphe. The oil attracts the ants which disseminate the seeds. In *Ranunculus ficaria* the embryo has a single cotyledon.

Pollination : Usually entomophilous, rarely by wind (*Thallictrum*).

Floral formula : $\oplus \ \male\female$ or $\oplus$ or $\male\female$ or $P_{4-6} \ A_6 \ G_{1-\alpha}$ or $_{(2-12)}$ or $\oplus \male\female \ K_{5 \ or \ 3-6} \ C_{5 \ or \ 5-23 \ or \ 0} \ A_\alpha \ G_\alpha$ or $\oplus\male\female \ P_{5+(4)} \ A_\alpha \ G_1$.

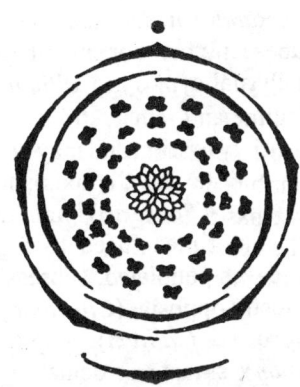

Fig. 6.12. Floral diagram of Ranunculaceae.

FAMILY : RUTACEAE

Vegetative characters

Habit and habitat : Cultivated or wild growing trees or shrubs (sometimes climbing), rarely herbs, abundantly in pellucid glands filled with essential oil.

Root : A branched tap root.

Stem : Aerial; etect; branched; armed with spines (*Aegle, Citrus, Zanthoxylum*) or unarmed. The stem is usually cylindrical and solid but angular or ribbed young shoots are also found in many plants. The stem surface may be glaucous, glabrous; spinous; gland-dotted; usually aromatic; younger parts pubescent or tomentose.

Leaves : Ramal and cauline; exstipulate; petiolate or subsessile; alternate (*Citrus, Aegle*) or opposite, simple (in *Evodia*) or compound (*Murraya, Zanthoxylum, Aegle*); compound leaves usually pinnate (mostly imparipinnate) multifoliate (*Murraya, Zanthoxylum*), trifoliate (*Aegle*), unifoliate (*Citrus, Skimmia*); the leaflets may be opposite (*Zanthoxylum*) or alternate (*Murraya*), dotted with translucent glands; aromatic (*Citrus, Skimmia*) or pungent (*Toddalia*). The leaflets are of various shapes and may be glabrous; glaucous, tomentose; venation is reticulate-unicostate.

Floral characters

Inflorescence : Usually axillary (*Citrus, Murraya*) or terminal cymes (*Clausena, Skimmia*). In *Atlantia racemosa*, the flowers occur in racemes. Rarely solitary, axillary in *Triphasia trifoliata* and *Paramignya*.

Flower : Ebracteate; pedicellate or subsessile; ebracteolate; complete or incomplete (*Zanthoxylum*), regular or irregular as in *Dictamnus*; actinomorphic; rarely zygomorphic; bisexual; unisexual in *Zanthoxylum alatum* (dioecious), hypogynous; usually pentamerous; in *Toddalia* the flowers may be bi-, tri-, tetra- or pentamerous. A distinct nectariferous disc is present below the ovary. The flowers are mostly cyclic with sepals and petals gland dotted and aromatic or fragrant or even pungent. In *Ruta*, the terminal flowers of the inflorescence are pentamerous whereas the lateral ones are tetramerous.

Calyx : Five or four; united or free; valvate or imbricate; inferior; odd sepal posterior; green; gland dotted.

Corolla : 5 (*Citrus, Murraya*), 4 (*Clausena, Zanthoxylum*) or even 3 (*Triphasia*); usually free but united in *Galipea, Correa* and *Ticorea*; valvate or imbricate; inferior; gland-dotted and sweet-smelling or aromatic and pungent; variously coloured, white (*Citrus Murraya*), greenish white in *Aegle marmelos*, bright yellow in *Zanthoxylum alatum*.

Androecium : Five, 8 or 10 (*Paramignya, Glycosmis, Murraya*), many (*Citrus*); free (*Aegle, Skimmia, Murraya*); monoadelphous in *Atlantia monophylla*; polyadelphous in *Citrus*; diplostemonous in *Murraya exotica*; anthers bithecous; dehiscence longitudinal and introse; inferior.

Gynaecium : 1-5 carpellary in *Zanthoxylum*; tricarpellary in *Triphasia;* tetracarpellary (*Limonia* with one ovule in each carpel, two ovules in each carpel in *Atlantia missionis*); pentacarpellary to polycarpellary in *Citrus*; syncarpous; in *Zanthoxy-*

lum, the ovaries are free whereas the styles are fused at the top; bilocular to multilocular; unilocular in *Feronia*; placentation axile; in *Feronia*, placentation in parietal. In *Zanthoxylum* there is a small gynophore. Ovules 1, many in each carpel; usually collateral or superposed; anatropous; styles as many as the carpels or united into one style; short; thick and fleshy; persistent in *Glycosmis*; united apically and free below in *Zanthoxylum*; stigma one, capitate or lobed (4 lobed in *Evodia*).

Fruit : Commonly berry (hesperidium in *Citrus*); in *Glycosmis pentaphylla*, the berry is irregularly globose; one to two seeded berry in *Murraya* and *Micromelum*. In *Aegle marmelos* the berry is large globoae, yellow and with a hard epicarp. The fruit may also be capsular, schizocarpic or a drupe (*Spathelia*).

Seed : Endospermic with a large, straight or bent embryo; non-endospermic in *Clausena*. Polyembryony is very common in this family.

Pollination : The flowers are markedly *protandrous* and are well adapted to insect pollination. The strong or sweet smell and gaudy colours attract insects. In *Ruta*, the flowers are visited by small files. In this case the flower is protandrous, the stamens lie in pairs in the boat-shaped petals. The stamens bend upwards one by one, dehisce and fall back; stigma ripens late. In case cross-pollination fails to occur, the stamens again move up, touch the stigma and effect self-pollination.

Floral formula : $\oplus$ or $\male$ or $\female$ $K_{(5) \text{ or } 3-5}$ $C_{3-5 \text{ or } (5)}$ $A_{5-\alpha \text{ or } (5-\alpha)}$ $G_{(2-\alpha) \text{ or } 1}$

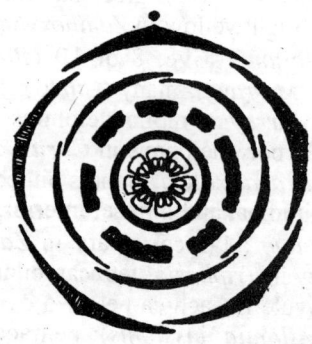

Fig. 6.13. Floral diagram of Rutaceae.

FAMILY : RUBIACEAE

The family includes 500 genera and 6,000 species. In India, the family is represented by 551 species belonging to more than 50 genera.

Vegetative characters

Habit and habitat : Trees, shrubs, and herbs; some are twinners (*Paederia*) and climbers (*Uncaria* climbs with hooked peduncles). Majority are perennials, few annuals; cultivated and wild. *Hymenopogon parasiticus* is an epiphyte.

Root : A branched tap root.

Stem : Aerial; erect or weak; cylindrical or angular, herbaceous (*Gallium*) or woody; armed with spines (*Ixora, Randia dumetorum*); mostly unarmed, glabrous; pubescent; hairy or smooth (*Stephegyne*); branched; dichasial cymes in *Gallium*.

Leaf : Cauline and ramal; stipulate, stipules exhibit a great variety of form and may be interpetiolar (between the petiole and the axis); leafy (*Rubia, Gallium*), divided (*Borreria*), hair-like (*Pentas, Houstonia*); sometimes fused to form a sheath (*Gardenia*); leaves petiolated, subsessile or sessile (*Gallium*); mostly opposite (*Cinchona*), sometimes whorled (*Saprosma, Gallium*), simple; entire (*Cinchona, Gallium*); sinuate or dentate (*Silvianthus*); glabrous or glaucous; reticulate-unicostate.

Floral characters

Inflorescence : Mostly a much branched cymose panicle (*Cinchona*); cymose heads (*Sarcocephalus, Nauclea, Uncaria, Coffea*) dehiscent cymes (*Gallium*); compound cymes in *Hedyotis* and *Mussaenda*; corymbs of cymes in *Webera*; solitary in *Gardenia, Condamenia* and *Saprosma ceylanica*.

Flower : Bracteate (*Randia uliginosa, Gardenia*), or ebracteate (*Sarcocephalus, Cinchona*); pedicellate; subsessile (*Gardenic*) or sessile (*Greenia; Randia*); bracteolate or ebracteolate; complete; imperfect sterile flowers known in *Gardenia turgida*; actinomorphic; zygomorphic in rare cases (*Posoqueria, Rondeletia*); mostly bisexual (*Coprosma* and *Anithospermum*); epigynous rarely perigynous; tetramerous or pentamerous; cyclic; variously coloured.

Calyx : Four, five; gamosepalous; tubular, campanulate; cup-shaped in *Urophyllum*, funneliform (*Mitchella*); in *Mussaenda* one of the five sepals is much larger and leaf-like and is brightly coloured to attract insects. Calyx lobes are inserted at the rim of the receptacle; superior; green or petaloid. Calyx is a very much reduced or obsolete in *Gallium*. Persistent in *Anthocephalus cadamba*.

Corolla : Four (*Gallium, Mitchella*) or five (*Coffea, Rubia*). 5-11 in *Gardenia*; gamopetalous; campanulate (*Coprosoma*), rotate in *Rubia* and *Gallium*, funnel-shaped in *Asperula* and *Rucharlia*, tubular (*Ixora*), salverform (*Coffea*); valvate (*Canthium, Cinchona*) or imbricate (*Guettarda*), twisted in *Octotropis*; throat of corolla tube usually glabrous in *Gardenia* and hairy in *Genipa*; inserted on the epigynous thalamus; superior; colours variable. The corolla is two lipped in *Roundeletia* and *Henriquezia*.

Androecium : Two (*Silvianthus*), 4 (*Gallium*), 5 (*Rubia, Cinchona*), 5-11 (*Gardenia*); epipetalous, alternipetalous; inserted near the mouth of corolla tube (*Coffea arabica*) or near base (*Nertera*), or middle (*Cinchona*); filaments very short or absent in *Ixora* and *Coffea*; anthers dorsifixed (*Coffea*) or basifixed (*Cinchona*); dehiscence longitudinal; introse.

Gynaecium : Bicarpellary in most of the genera; pentacarpellary in *Leptodermis*, 4-9 carpellary in various species of *Lasianthus*; syncarpous; inferior; superior in *Pagamea* and *Gaertnera*, half inferior in *Synaplanthera*, unilocular in *Gardenia*, mostly bilocular, 4-9 locular in *Lasianthus*, 5-locular in *Vangueria*, bilocular in lower part and tetralocular in upper part in *Anthocephalus cadamba*, ovules one (*Canthium*) to many in each loculus; placentation mostly axile, basal in *Hamiltonia, Paederia, Rudegea* and *Myrinecodia*, parietal in *Gardenia*; ovules anatropous; style single, long or short; styles bifid (*Hymenopogon*), multifid in *Leptodermis*; stigmas bifid or 3 to 9 (*Lasianthus*), simple and spindle-shaped in *Webera*, fusiform in *Sarcocephalus*. Usually a fleshy disc is present at the summit of the ovary.

Fruit : A berry (*Ixora, Coffea, Mussaenda*); drupe (*Webera, Gardenia*); capsular (*Anthocephalus cadamba, Uncaria, Cinchona*). In *Anthocephalus* the capsules are embedded in a fleshy receptacle.

Seed : Usually endospermic; nonendospermic in *Bobea, Malanea* and *Guelardia*. In *Cinchoma*, the seeds have broad wings with irregularly lacerated edge.

Floral formula : $\oplus$ or $+ \, \male K_{(4-5)} \, C_{(4-5)} A_{4-5} \, G_{(2-5)}$.

Pollination : Entomophilous; flowers with long and tubular corollas are pollinate by bees and lepidopteran insects; in *Rubia* the corolla is rotate and the honey is exposed or only slightly concealed and is visited by flies; heterostyly is quite common; honey is usually secreted by a distinct annular nectariferous disc present around the base of the style.

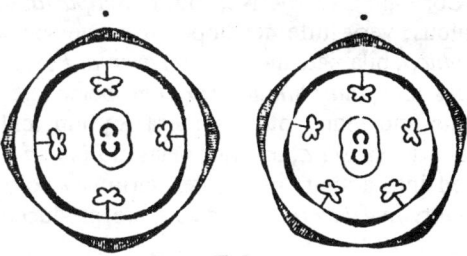

Fig. 6.14. Floral diagrams of Rubiaceae.

FAMILY : SCROPHULARIACEAE

Vegetative characters

Habit and habitat : Mostly herbs, a few are shrubs (*Brandsia discolor*) and trees (*Wrightia gigantea, Paulownia*), *Antirrhinum cirrhosum* climbs by means of sensitive leaf petioles. *Striga lutea* and *S. generioides* are root parasites. The African genera *Harveya* and *Hyobanche* are total parasites.

Root : A branched tap root.

Stem : Aerial; erect; climbing in *Antirrhinum cirrhosum* and a few other genera; cylindrical or angular; hollow or solid; branched; green or without chlorophyll (*Harveya*); herbaceous or woody (*Wrightia, Paulownia*); hairy or glabrous.

Leaf : Cauline and ramal; radical in *Mazua japonicus*; stipulate; petiolate or sessile; alternate (*Linaria* sp., *Antirrhinum crontium*), opposite (*Scoparia*), whorled (*Russelia*); glabrous, usually reticulate-unicostate.

Floral characters

Inflorescence : Racemose in *Linaria ramosissima*; a spike in *Verbascum thapsus*; solitary axillary in *Antirrhinum crontium*; axillary cymose clusters in *Scoparia dulcis*.

Flower : Bracteate or ebracteate; pedicellate or sessile (*Antirrhinum crontium*); usually zygomorphic rarely actinomorphic (*Verbascum thapsus*); bisexual; hypogynous; tetracyclic; small (*Linaria*), or large and beautiful (*Antirrhinum majus*).

Calyx : Mostly 5; rarely 4 (*Scoparia dulcis*); fused; imbricate; or valvate; persistent; in *Calecolaria, Synthyris* and some species of *Veronica* the odd sepal is abortive and the calyx is 4-parted; campanulate or shortly tubular; hairy in some species (*Antirrhinum crontium*); green; inferior.

Corolla : Usually five; four in *Scoparia*; gamopetalous; very little developed in some species of *Veronica*; bilabiate in *Linaria, Torenia, Penstemon, Mazus* and *Antirrhinum crontium*; personate in *A. mazus* and many other genera; cylindrical and tubular in *Russelia*; anterior petal in *Linaria* is produced into a spur; imbricate; variously coloured; inferior. In *Diascia*, two petals are produced into spurs.

Andorecium : Usually four (*Digitalis, Scoparia, Mazus, Antirrhinum*), all the five fertile in *Verbascum*; two in *Veronica, Veronicastrum*; epipetalous; polyandrous. In *Verbascum*, the three posterior or all the stamens are bearded. In *Penstemon*, 4 stamens are fertile, the fifth sterile stamen is as long as others; filaments woolly in *Chelone*. In *Torenia*, the four stamens are in two pairs of unequal length; basifixed or dorsifixed; bithecous, rarely monothecous; dehiscence is usually longitudinal, introrse.

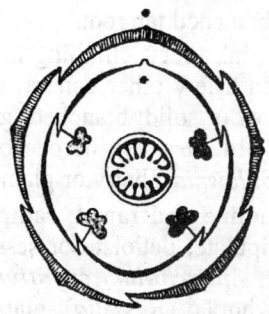

Fig. 6.15. Floral diagram of Scrophulariaceae.

Gynaecium : Bicarpellary; syncarpous; superior, bilocular placentation axile; ovules usually many in each loculus; ovules anatropous or amphitropous; style simple and undivided, short or long; stigma bilobed or capitate. A nectariferous disc is usually present below the ovary. It may be annular or unilateral. Ovary may become trilocular (*Antirrhinum erontium*) due to false septum.

Fruit : A capsule that usually dehisces by two valves, sometimes by 4 valves.

Seed : Endospermic; embryo slightly curved or straight.

Pollination : By means of insects.

Floral formula : $+$ or rarely $\oplus$ ⚥ $K_{(5)\ or\ (4)}$ $C_{(5)\ or\ (4)}$ $A_{4\ or\ 5\ or\ 2}$ $G_{(2)}$.

FAMILY : SOLANACEAE

Vegetative characters

Habit and habitat : Mostly herbs (*Petunia, Schizanthus*), a few shrubs and trees (*Solanum grandiflorum, S. macranthum*); *Solanum jasminoides* is an attractive woody climber. A few are armed with spines (*Solanum xanthocarpum*).

Root : A branched tap root. In *Mandragora officinarum* the roots are thick and forked and vaguely resemble a human being in miniature.

Stem : Aerial; erect; climbing (*Solanum jasminoides*), spinous in *Solanum xanthocarpum*; herbraceous or woody; cylindrical; branched; solid or hollow; hairy (*Petunia, Nicotiana, Withania*), or glabrous; Tuberous in *Solanum tuberosum* (Potato).

Leaf : Cauline and ramal; exstipulate; petiolate or sessile, usually alternate; sometimes opposite (*Atropa*), simple; entire (*Petunia*); pinnatisect (*Lycopersicon, Solanum tuberosum*); finely divided in some species of *Schizanthus*; reticulate unicostate.

Floral characters

Inflorescence : Solitary axillary (*Datura, Solandra*); extra axillary and leaf opposed cymes (called *Rhipidium*) in *Solanum nigrum*; helicoid cymes in *Solanum tuberosum*; in axillary umbellate cymes in *Withania*; solitary terminal or solitary in *Petunia*; in racemes or scorpioid cymes in various species of *Cyphomandra*.

Flower : Bracteate (*Petunia, Datura*) or ebracteate (*Solanum nigrum*); pedicellate or subsessile; ebracteolate; complete; actinomorphic; zygomorphic in *Schizanthus*; bisexual; hypogynous; cyclic; pentamerous; variously coloured; large and showy in many species.

Calyx : Five; fused (gamosepalous); imbricate (*Petunia*) or valvate; tubular (*Datura*); campanulate (*Solanum nigrum, Petunia*), unceolate when mature in *Withania*; persistent in some genera (*Withania, Physalis*, etc.); green; orange coloured or petaloid in *Juanulloa aurantiaca*; sometimes hairy (*Petunia, Datura*); inferior.

Corolla : Five; fused; rotate (*Solanum nigrum*); tubular (*Petunia, Datura*); funnel-shaped in *Scopolia*; urn-shaped in *Salpichroa*; in *Schizanthus* the corolla tube may be short or long and spreads into a bilabiate limb with deeply cut lobes (irregular); imbricate (*Petunia*) or valvate; hairy on the outside in *Petunia*; in some cases a woolly ring of scale like outgrowths arise from the throat of corolla tube (*Salpichroa, Browallia*); variously coloured; inferior. In *S. xanthocarpum*, the petals are covered with stellate hair on the outer side and are green when young and become violet later.

Androecium : Five; four in *Browallia*; epipetalous; filaments inserted in the middle or deep down the corolla tube; usually unequal; didynamous in *Browallia*; in some cases anther are large and conical and are connivant to form around the style and stigma (*Solanum xanthocarpum, S. nigrum*); but are not organically, fused; included or exserted; bithecous; in *Browallia* the shorter pair of stamens have anthers with one lobe undeveloped (a fifth staminode is also recognisable on the posterior petal); usually basifixed or dorsi-fixed; dehiscence longitudinal; introrse; by means of apical pores in *Solanum nigrum*. In *Schizanthus* there are two fertile stamens and three staminodes.

Gynaecium : Bicarpellary; syncarpous; superior; bilocular; becoming tetralocular by the formation of a false septa in *Datura*; unilocular in *Henoonia*; placentation axile; placenta swollen; ovules many in each loculus. In *Cestrum*, there are up to two ovules in each loculus; ovule one in *Henoonia*; ovary *obliquely placed*; in some cases a nectariferous disc is present below the ovary (*Petunia*); style usually simple and undivided; stigma bifid or capitate. In *Solanum xanthocarpum*, the style is covered with stellate hair.

Fruit : A berry (*Lycopersicon esculentum, Atropa, Capsicum*); a capsule in majority of genera (*Datura, Petunia*).

Seed : Endospermic; cotyledons plain (not plicate). Endosperm may be *Cellular* or *nuclear*. In *Hyoscymus niger*, the endosperm is peculiar and is regarded by some as helobial and by others as a modification of helobial type.

Pollination : Entomophilous; *Cestrum nocturnum* and *Nicotiana* are pollinated at night or after sunset by moths; butterflies are also common insect visitors of solanaceous flowers.

Floral formula : $\oplus + $ or $\cancel{Q}\, K_{(5)}\, C_{(5)}\, A_{5\ or\ 4}\, G_{(2)}.$

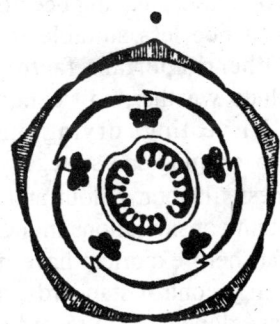

Fig. 6.16. Floral diagram of Solanaceae.

Production of Herbal Drugs

The crude drug, which reaches the pharmaceutical manufacturers, passes through different stages, all of which influence the nature and amount of active constituents present.

The quality of herbs is dependent on several variables; plant variety, growing conditions, cultural practices, drying and processing methods, storage and packaging. The genetic characteristics of a particular plant variety is a factor affecting quality, but problems for producers have arisen from mis-labelling, misunderstanding and ignorance, and also from seeds or cuttings having been of the incorrect variety and hence less suitable for the required markets. Other important factors influencing quality include weather, soil conditions, cultural practices, harvesting, drying and processing techniques, packaging and storage.

Cleanliness, flavour, colour and aroma are the most important considerations in the purchasing of herbs. So far, herb exporters have not established national quality control standards, although some countries have done so with regard to spices. Both buyers and sellers are recognising the need for specific quality standards together with accepted means of testing. Major herb and spice importing countries have developed specifications, which include definitions regarding botanical species, details relating to the correct part(s) of the plant to be used, colour and permitted levels of extraneous matter. Standards can vary and this can create problems, particularly for exporters. However, attempts are being made to standardise quality regulations.

Mentha piperita contains high proportion of pulegone in young plants; replaced by menthone and menthol as leaves mature. *M spicata* contains carvone as the major product in young plants and dihydrocarvone in older ones. *Cloves* yield 14-21% of oil; mother 'blown' cloves contain very little oil. *Coriandrum sativum* shows marked changes in oil composition at the beginning of flowering and fruiting. In *Achillea millefolium*, during flowering produces monoterpenes (principally 1,8-cineole) in oils from leaves and flowers. Oil obtained during the vegetative period contains mainly sesquiterpenes (92%) with germacrane-D as the major component. In *Cinnamomum camphora*, camphor is deposited in heartwood as tree ages; ready for collection at 40 years. *Taxus baccata* needles contain up to 0.1% 10-deacetyl-baccatin in summer and large amounts of 2,4-dimethoxyphenol in winter. In *Cannabis sativa*, young seedlings contain principally cannabichromeme; Δ^9-tetrahydro cannabinol is the major cannabinoid of adult plants. In *Digitalis purpurea*, glycoside content varies with age. Purpurea-glycoside A is formed in the last and reaches a constant maximum of 50% of the total glycoside. In *D. lanata*, the highest levels of total glycosides (lanatoside C) are observed in first-year leaves, and attain in the highest levels in second-year plants. In *Dioscorea tokoro*, changes in sapogenin content in first season's growth are observed.

In *Papaver somniferum*, morphine content of capsule is highest 3 weeks after flowering; the secondary alkaloids (codeine, thebaine, narcotine and papaverine) reach their maximum earlier. In *Datura stramonium*, the hyoscine/hyoscyamine ratio falls from 80% in young seedlings to 30% in mature fruiting plants. In *Duboisia myoporoides,* the hyoscine/hyoscyamine ratio depends both on the developmental stage of the plant and on the position of the leaves on the stem. In *Ipomoea violacea* seeds, lysergic acid amide/chanoclavine ratio increases as the seed matures. In *Solanum dulcamara* fruits, solasodine content fluctuates during maturation of the fruit; tomatidenol and soladulcidine predominate in the end. In Citrus glycosides and limonoids, limonin and naringin levels in grapefruit fall as fruit matures. In *Ammi visnaga*, unripe fruits are richest in both khellin and visnagin. In *Liquidambar formosona*, there is a seasonable variation of hydrolysable leaf tannins, most rapid changes occur in the spring. In *Vanilla planifolia*, the highest rate of vanillin biosynthesis occurs 8 months after flower pollination.

ENVIRONMENTAL CONDITIONS

Plant growth and the nature and quantity of secondary metabolites are affected by temperature, rainfall, length of day (including the quality of light) and altitude. Such effects have been studied by growing particular plants in different climatic areas and observing variations.

The seeds of Cannabis, grown in England, are rich in CBD and devoid of THC. The seeds when are cultivated in Sudan, start to produce THC in the first generation and in the second generation contained up to 3.3% THC with a further decrease of CBD. It is impossible to control all the variables in such experiments. A particular factor may lead to the development of a small plant. On a percentage dry weight basis, it indicates a high proportion of metabolite, even though the overall yield per plant could be quite low. Similarly, certain nutrients may produce large plants with low concentration of constituents on a percentage dry weight basis, but yield per plant may exceed that of the control.

Temperature

Temperature is a major factor for controlling the development and metabolism of plants. Each species adapts to its own natural environment. Plants are able to exist in a considerable range of temperature. Many tropical and subtropical plants will grow in temperate regions during summer months, but lack frost resistance to withstand the winter. The highest temperatures are observed near the Equator, but the temperature falls about 1°C for every 200 m of elevation. India has a tropical climate on the coast and a temperate one in the mountains. The annual variations in temperature are as important as the temperature of the hottest month. At Singapore the annual range of temperature is 1.5°C, whereas Moscow, with its hot summers and cold winters, has a range of 29.3°C. Night and day temperature must also be considered. In general, the formation of volatile oils appears to be enhanced at higher temperatures, although very hot days may lead to an excess physical loss of oil. The mean optimum temperature is 20°C for nicotine production in *Nicotiana rustica* (lower at 11°C and at 30°C).

Fixed oils produced at low temperatures contain fatty acids with a higher content of double bonds than those formed at higher temperatures.

A certain temperature is essential for all the vital functions of the plant. It markedly affects germination, growth, reproduction and movements. Temperature requirement is, however, different for plants growing in different climatic regions of the earth. Under certain conditions some organs of the plant are thermotropic; for instance, the opening and closing of flowers and of stomata and the drooping of leaves at night, are caused partly by heat. In many cases temperature helps the dehiscence of fruits and thus the dissemination of seeds. Plants normally prefer a temperature varying from 20°C to 40°C. Active tissues filled with water have much less ability than dry seeds and spores to withstand extremes of temperature. Most flowering plants are killed at a temperature below 0°C and above 45°C; while seeds remain uninjured at a temperature far beyond these limits. Freezing temperature or frost kills plants, but at high altitudes where frosts frequently occur plants become unusually resistant. Temperature has an important effect on plant geography. We find a considerable difference between the flora of tropical, sub-tropical, temperate, arctic and alpine regions.

Rainfall

Water is the most important factor. It is responsible for various structural modifications of plants. Water is indispensable for all the vital functions of the plant. Protoplasm is saturated with water. Over 90% of the total weight of active tissues is water. The source of water for terrestrial plants is rain. Rainfall has a marked effect on the geographical distribution of plants. Thus depending on the amount of precipitation of vegetation may broadly be of the following types: evergreen forest (with abundant rainfall), deciduous forest (with moderate or low rainfall), grassland (with low rainfall) and thorn scrub (with scanty rainfall). Availability of rain-water depends on the water-retaining capacity of the soil, and on plants themselves. The soil may be physically dry or sometimes physiologically dry due to the cold state of the ground on the preponderance of salts in it. Topographical factors are also very important in this respect. Cherrapunji in the Khasi Hills, the rainiest spot in the world with an annual rainfall of over 12,700 mm, has a very luxuriant vegetation; while Rajasthan with very little or no rain is extremely arid. Abundance or scarcity of available water determines the life-cycle of the plant, the duration of plant growth and the time of reproduction in addition to certain well-marked features of the plant. Two extremes are hydrophytes and xerophytes.

The production of volatile oil varies with the annual rainfall, its distribution throughout the year, its effect on humidity, its effect coupled with the water-holding properties of the soil and the development of glandular hairs. Continuous rain can lead to a loss of water-soluble substances from leaves and roots by leaching as in case of some alkaloids (particularly Solanaceae), glycosides and volatile oils. This could account for low yields of some active constituents in wet seasons from plants.

Sunlight and radiations

The amount and intensity of the light affect the growth of plants. In the wild state, the plant will be found where its shade requirements are met, and under cultivation similar shade must be provided. In some cases light is a factor which helps to determine the amount of glycosides or alkaloids produced. With Belladonna, Stramonium and *Cinchona ledgeriana* full sunshine gives a higher content of alkaloids than in shade. *Datura stramonium* var. *tatula* on long exposure to intense light yields hyoscine in high content at the time of flowering. Irradiation of intact plants with near ultraviolet light in the range 290-380 nm (peak 370 nm) stimulates the synthesis of dimeric alkaloids in catharanthus probably by inducing catharanthine oxidation as a trigger reaction. Under long-day conditions peppermint leaves contain menthone, menthol and traces of menthofuran; plants grown under short-day conditions contain menthofuran as a major component of the volatile oil. A long photo-period for young leaves activates the reduction of pathway with conversion of menthone to menthol. In flowers of *Nicotiana sylvestris* and other species a marked increase (about tenfold) in aromatic compounds including benzyl alcohol was detected at night, whereas no increase in the volatiles (e.g., linalool, caryophyllene) originating from the mevalonic acid pathway was noted.

The daily variation in the proportion of secondary metabolites is probably light-controlled. Many plants initiate flowers only in certain day-lengths.

The presence or absence of light, together with wavelength range, have a marked effect on the secondary metabolite production of some plants in tissue culture.

Physiologically light is a very important factor. It is responsible for the formation of chlorophyll and for carbon assimilation; it accelerates transpiration. Although strong light checks growth, it has a tonic effect on plants. Light induces certain kinds of movements like photonasty and phototropism. Relative length of day and night has a marked effect on the development of flowers and maturation of fruits. Of all parts of the plant the leaves undergo by far the greatest modifications under the action of light. Plants growing in shady places are called *sciophytes*, and they usually have large leaves which are thin in texture and sparsely distributed on the stem; the stem is thin with long inter-nodes; both the stem and the leaves are glabrous; palisade tissue is poorly developed; the leaf consists largely or entirely of spongy tissues; epidermis often contains chlorophyll and the cuticle is thin; stomata may be present on both sides. Common examples are *Begonia*, aroids, woodsorrel, ferns, mosses and liverworts. Plants which can only grow well in the light are called *heliophytes*, and they have small leaves which are thicker and crowded together on the stem; the stem is stouter with short internodes; the stem and sometimes the leaves are very hairy; palisade tissue is well developed; epidermis is provided with a thick cuticle, but no chlorophyll; stomata are present on the lower side, often sunken or occluded. Aqueous tissue is often present. Most thick-leaved plants are heliophytes.

Altitude

The coconut palm requires a maritime climate and the sugarcane is a lowland plant. Tea (1000-2000 m), cocoa (100-200 m), Saffron (1,700 m), Banafshah (2,000 m), Digitalis (2,000 m), Coffee (800-1800 m), medicinal Rhubarb, Tragacanth and Cinchona require elevation. In the case of *Cinchona succirubra*, the plants grow well at low levels but produce practically no alkaloids. The bitter constituents of *Gentiana lutea* increase with altitude, whereas the alkaloids of *Aconitum napellus* and *Lobelia inflata* and the oil content of Thyme and Peppermint decrease. Other oil-producing plants may reach a maximum at certain altitudes. Pyrethrum gives the best yields of flower-heads and pyrethrins at high altitudes on, or near, the Equator and, therefore, is grown in East Africa and northwest South America. However, vegetative growth is more pronounced under irrigated conditions at lower altitude.

Atmospheric composition

Digitalis lanata grown in greenhouses with a carbon dioxide-enriched atmosphere (1000 p.p.m. CO_2 during the whole of the growth period from April to November) produced 3.5 times the amount of digoxin ha^{-1} than did the field cultivated plants.

Wind

Wind has usually a destructive action on vegetation. It enhances transpiration; very strong and dry wind is often fatal to plants, particularly to young seedlings. In forests, some plants can resist the action of wind far better than others. On the seashore, coconut-palm is exposed to strong gusts of wind. The plant can withstand them well because its leaves are cut into narrow segments with stout mid-rib; the cuticle also is very thick. Wind is useful in disseminating seeds and fruits, particularly those provided with some kind of appendages. In deserts, there are certain species which, when the air is dry, roll up into balls and are driven by wind from one place to another. They strike roots and grow when the conditions are favourable.

EDAPHIC FACTORS : SOIL

Since most plants are fixed to the ground and draw their supply of essential food elements from the soil, with the exception of carbon dioxide and a little nitrogen in some cases, which are obtained from the air, it is evident that there is an intimate relationship between plants and soils. Thus the distribution of plants over different regions of the earth, and their structural peculiarities, are largely determined by edaphic factors. This being so, a study of soils in different aspects is as important as the study of plants themselves from ecological points of view.

Medicinal species vary enormously in their soil and nutritive requirements. Three important basic characteristics of soils are their physical, chemical and microbiological properties.

Variations in particular size produce clay, via sand, to gravel. Particle size is an important factor influencing water-holding capacity, and some plants (e.g., *Althaea officinalis*) which produce mucilage as a water-retaining material contain less mucilage when grown on soil with a high moisture content. In moist regions, as in Kashmir and Darjeeling, clay soils absorb excess water. Their high moisture content makes them cold and they are difficult to work on account of their stiffness. In drier regions, such as the Mediterranean, such soils are much esteemed for their power of absorbing and retaining moisture. The basic soil type is modified by the presence of humus, organic fertilizers, chalk and lime. Fine soils rich in humus and having a permeable substratum possess a degree of humidity which is generally favourable for plants. Sandy soils poor in humus and having a gravel subsoil are generally suitable for xerophilous plants. On calcareous soils, which are poor in humus, vegetation is markedly xerophilous. If humus is present, the moisture-absorbing power is much increased. Soils containing much humus and little lime are inclined to become acid, while those with abundant lime are alkaline. Although particular species have their own soil pH tolerances (*Datura stramonium* 6.0-8.2, *Majorana hortensis* 5.6-6.4), no marked influence of pH value within the tolerance range has been demonstrated for essential oils (*Mentha piperita*) and alkaloids (*D. stramonium*). All plants require calcium for their normal nutrition but plants known as caliphobous plants (*e.g., Pinus pinaster* and *Digitalis purpurea*) cannot be grown on chalky soils, probably owing to the alkalinity. In some cases different varieties of the same species may grow on different soils. *Valeriana officinalis* var. *sambucifolia* is common on the coal measures, but avoids the limestone, where it is replaced by *Valeriana officinalis* var. *mikanii*. Nitrogen fertilizers increase the size of the plants and the amounts of alkaloids produced. The effects of nitrogen on glycoside and essential oil contents appear variable. Nitrogen fertilization increases the silymarin content of the fruits of *Silybum marianum* grown on reclaimed ground. The effect of potassium on alkaloid production shows no consistent trend. The increase in putrescine production takes place in barley grown on a potassium-deficient medium, where the organic base has been formed to act as a substitute for potassium ions.

Trace amounts of manganese are necessary for the successful production of *Digitalis purpurea*. A regimen of manganese and molybdenum feeding over the two years of development of *D. grandiflora* gives significant increases in glycoside yield. Soil bacteria of the genus *Agrobacterium* are finding application in the production of 'hairy root' cultures.

Biotic factor

The term 'biotic factor' includes all influences exerted by living organisms to bring about any change in the vegetation of a locality. The most important in this respect are the human beings and the grazing animals. Man acts as a powerful agent, influencing profoundly the original vegetation of a locality in a number of ways: cultivation, terrace cultivation in the hills, reclamation of land, cutting down trees for wood and fuel, deforestation and afforestation. Grazing by domesticated animals destroys many herbaceous plants in pastures and places round about villages of agriculturists. Grazing constantly interferes with the normal development of the vegetation of particular areas. The relation of a species to other living organisms is apparent in many cases. There is the competition with its neighbours for food, water and sunlight. It may be attacked and sometimes wholly destroyed by parasitic plants or animals, or it may be fed upon by animals; in some cases plants are of mutual help to each other, *e.g.*, symbionts. Symbiosis between bacteria and leguminous plants may be recalled to mind in this connection. Soil bacteria, protozoa, earth-worms and rats are useful agents in altering the soil. They also damage vegetation. This leads us to see how closely interwoven are the lives of plants and animals.

Topographic factor

This has an important bearing on vegetation, particularly in mountainous regions such as the Himalayas. Altitude is the dominant factor in this respect, determining zonal distribution of vegetation, *e.g.*, tropical, sub-tropical, temperate, subtemperate and alpine. Within the zone rainfall plays an important part. Slope is another important factor, either retaining water in the soil after rainfall or draining it down. It influences the type of vegetation. Besides, exposure to sun, monsoon rain and wind also affect vegetation. Thus the southern slope of the Himalayas develops luxuriant deciduous and evergreen forests, whereas the northern side develops only dry forests.

PLANT DRUGS

At present some drugs are obtained from cultivated plant, e.g., Cardamoms, Indian Hemp, Ginger, Peppermint, Spearmint for oil production, Ceylon cinnamon, Linseed, Fennel, Cinchona, Flux, Opium poppy and Coca. In other cases both wild and cultivated plants are used. Some plants are now grown because supplies of the wild plants are insufficient to meet the demand or due to limited distribution or inaccessibility, collection is difficult. Cultivation is required for drugs such as Indian hemp and Opium, which are subject to government control and to improve quality of the drug. The improvement may be due to the power to confine collections to species, varieties or hybrids which have the desired characters (e.g., Aconite, Cinnamon, Fennel, Cinchona and Valerian).

It may be for better development of the plants owing to improved conditions of the soil, pruning, and the control of insect pests and fungi or for better facilities for treatment after collection. For example, drying at a correct temperature in the cases of Digitalis, Colchicum, Belladonna and Valerian, and the peeling of Cinnamon and Ginger.

The conditions under which the plant flourishes in the wild state are reproduced or improved. Small changes in ecology can affect plant products; thus, satisfactory rubber trees grow wild in the Amazon basin but cleared areas converted to rubber plantations have been a failure.

Propagation from seeds

For better crop the seeds must be collected when perfectly ripe. They should normally be stored in a cool and dry place and must not be kiln-dried. The seeds of cinnamon, coca and nutmegs rapidly lose their power of germination if allowed to dry or if stored for quite short periods. Long storage of all seeds usually decreases the percentage which germinate. Seeds are naturally sown at the season when they ripen.

In some cases, immediate sowing of the fresh seed is available. If the seeds of *Colchicum autumnale* are air-dried even for a few days, only about 5% germinate in 1 year and some may not germinate for 5 years. If these seeds are sown as soon as the capsules dehisce, 30% will germinate in the first year. With *Erythroxylum coca* and *E. novogranatense*, the seeds stored at 4°C for 24 days gave, respectively, 29% and 0% germination.

Seeds may, if slow germinating, be soaked in water or a 0.2% solution of gibberellic acid for 48 h before sowing. Some drastic methods, such as soaking in sulphuric acid in the case of henbane

seeds, or partial removal of the testa by means of a file or grindstone, have also been recommended.

Time of seed-sowing may affect the active constituents. *Chamomilla recutita* gave a significantly higher yield of oil if the seeds were spring-sown rather than autumn-sown and the oil composition also varied.

Vegetative propagation

The vegetative propagation is carried out by the following means :

1. By the development of bulbs (*e.g.*, Squill); corms (*e.g.*, Colchicum); tubers (*e.g.*, Jalap and Aconite); or rhizomes (*e.g.*, Ginger).
2. By division in a plant which has a number of aerial stems or buds, *e.g.*, Althaea, Rhubarb, Gentian and Male fern.
3. By runners or offsets (*e.g.*, Chamomile and the mints).
4. By suckers or stolons (*e.g.*, Liquorice and valerian).
5. By cuttings or portions of the plant capable of developing roots, *e.g.*, the propagation of mints, lavender, rosemary, duboisias, tree daturas, coca and vanilla.
6. By layers : A layer is a branch or shoot which is induced to develop roots before it is completely severed from the parent plant. This is done by partly interrupting the food supply by means of a cut or ligature and embedding the part. The slit portion of the branch is enclosed in moist peat, surrounded by moss, and the whole enclosed in polythene, *e.g.*, the propagation of Cascara.
7. By grafting and budding : Grafting is an operation in which two cut surfaces of different and closely related plants are placed so as to unite and grow together. The rooted plant is called the *stock* and the portion cut off the *scion* or *graft*. *Cinchoma ledgeriana* scions are grafted on *Cinchona succirubra* root-stocks, eventually giving a tree which produces bark rich in the alkaloid quinidine. Grafting of female scions of *Myristica fragrans* on male stocks may be used to increase the proportion of fruit-bearing trees in the plantation. Budding consists of the introduction of a piece

of bark bearing a bud into a suitable cavity or T-shaped slit made in the bark of the stock. Budding is largely used for *Citrus* species. Selected strains of sweet orange are budded on sour stocks.

8. By fermentation : This process is applied for the production of moulds and bacteria, used in the manufacture of antibiotics, lysergic acid derivatives and some vitamins.

10. By cell culture followed by differentiation.

Production of drug

Drug are obtained from both wild and cultivated plants. There is still some controversy as to which types are best, some arguing that herbs collected wild in their natural habitat have more flavour than those cultivated commercially, whereas others believe the opposite. Many culinary herbs are now cultivated with success, but some which are collected wild (*e.g.,* rosemary) have so far proved uneconomic when cultivated. In most cases the demand for culinary herbs is such that collection from the wild would be totally insufficient to satisfy market requirements. In addition, it is often inefficient and unprofitable for the picker. The industrial and tourist developments in the main drug producing countries, combined with the employment opportunities provided by neigh-bouring countries, have made labour more expensive and reduced the quantity of herbs which are collected from the wild or hand-picked. This trend is not only found in the traditional herb producing countries of the Mediterranean, but also in eastern Europe countries, such as East Germany, Hungary and Bulgaria. The expected increase in demand for drugs can only be satisfied by the wider cultivation of herbs in short supply. Cultivation of drugs offers a number of advantages. Drugs grown under cultivation can give a high yield, and allow the production of plants with more consistent properties than plants growing wild. Cultivation assists crop husbandry by facilitating weeding, the control of insects and disease, and permits mechanisation, speedy and planned harvesting, quick transportation to the drying sheds and correct preparation, drying and storage of the herb, all of which help to maintain the aroma and flavour as far as possible. These advantages will become more important and should be quality specifications for herbs.

Drug production can be undertaken using either labour-intensive techniques, as for example in North Africa, or capital-intensive harvesting and processing methods, as in the USA. In the past few years drugs have been increasingly grown on a large scale, employing methods similar to those used for other field crops, including mechanical harvesting with machines specially adapted for the purpose. Production is mainly undertaken in temperate and Mediterranean countries, but if developing countries with temperate or subtropical climates have adequate labour resources, satisfactory cultural conditions and practices, and can produce acceptable quality drugs at competitive prices, they should be able to supply a growing proportion of the rising demand for drugs. For example, Egypt has become an important supplier of several drugs, including mint and marjoram. Moreover, many drugs are only harvested once a year and, therefore, the seasons crop only reaches the various users in the autumn. Consequently, dried drugs brought before May or June in any year are almost certainly from the previous years harvest. Therefore, a new producer capable of supplying the market at a different period of the year would have certain marketing advantages.

However, one should not minimise the difficulties that a new drug producer would have to face in order to satisfy the increasingly stringent quality requirements. A prospective producer will need to ensure that the cuttings or seeds obtained are of the correct type and strain. There have been several instances of seeds, bought under a certain name, proving on germination to be a different plant and unsuitable for the market. Another complicating factor is that sometimes a given plant is sold under several different names. Some crops require two or more years of care before a crop can be harvested for sale, and a particular areas climate and soil can greatly influence the aroma and flavour of a herb. A new producer must be aware of the diverse diseases and pests that can affect herbs, and the correct methods of eradication. In several markets buyers are worried about fertiliser and pesticide residues, and considerable care must be taken in the choice of them.

Whether grown wild or cultivated, only certain parts of the plant are collected for commercial use; in some cases the underground parts (*e.g.,* root, rhizome, tuber or bulb) are collected, whilst in others it is the aerial parts, such as the leaf, herbage, flower, fruit or seed.

Harvesting

An important factor influencing the quality of the drug is the time at which it is harvested, since the essential oil content, therefore, the aromatic and flavouring qualities, vary during the life cycle of a plant. Leaves are gathered throughout the whole growing period, although young leaves tend to be the most suitable. They are either picked singly, or else the entire stem is cut off and the leaves afterwards stripped. The leaves should be healthy, free from disease and insect pests, clean and dry, without any trace of moisture from dew or rain. The aerial or top parts of the plant (herbage) are collected with the flower-bearing stem just before, or at the beginning of the flowering stage. Usually they are cut off several centimetres above the ground. For cultivated crops specially adapted harvesting machines are used. In older plants, where the bottom section of the stems have become woody, only the non-woody parts are collected. Fruit and seeds are collected when mature. In cultivated crops, which are harvested by machine, this is done just before they are fully ripe so as to avoid crumbling of the fruit or loss of the seeds. It is vitally important in harvesting herbs that they are delivered to the drying shed as quickly as possible. Care should be taken that they are not packed too tightly, and that they do not sweat during transportation.

Collection

Drugs may be collected from wild or cultivated plants, by casual, unskilled labour (*e.g.,* Ipecacuanha) or by skilled workers in a highly scientific manner (*e.g.,* Digitalis, Belladonna and Cinchona). The amount, and the nature of the active constituents is not constant throughout the year as in cases of Podophyllum, Ephedra, Rhubarb, Wild Cherry and Aconite. Rhubarb contains no anthraquinone derivatives in winter but anthranols which in summer are converted by oxidation into anthraquinones. The contents of C-glycosides, O-glyco-sides and free anthraquinones in the developing shoots and leaves of *Rhamnus purshiana* fluctuate markedly throughout the year.

The age of the plant governs the total quantity of active constituents produced and the relative proportions of the components of the active mixture. Some ontogenetic variation of constituents must exist for all plants. The composition of a number of secondary plant metabolites varies appreciably throughout the day and night.

Daily variations of the alkaloids of the poppy, hemlock, lupin, broom, the solanaceous plants, ergot, the steroidal alkaloids of 'industrial shoots' of *Solanum laciniatum*, the cardiac glycosides of *Digitalis purpurea* and *D. lanata*, the simple phenolic glycosides of *Salix* and the volatile oil content of *Pinus and Salvia*, have been reported. Leaves are collected as the flowers are beginning to open, flowers just before they are fully expanded, and underground organs as the aerial parts die down. Leaves, flowers and fruits should not be collected when covered with dew or rain. Any which are discoloured or attacked by insects or slugs should be rejected. Even with hand-picking, it is difficult, certainly expensive, to get leaves, flowers or fruits entirely free from other parts of the plant.

In Senna leaf and Digitalis the official monographs allow a certain percentage of stalks to be present or a limited amount of foreign matter. Similarly, with roots and rhizomes a certain amount of aerial stem is often collected and is permitted in the cost of Senega root. The harvesting of umbelliferous fruits resembles that of corn. Reaping machines are used, and the plants, after drying in stocks, are threshed to separate the fruits. Special machines are used to harvest ergot and lavender flowers. Barks are usually collected after a period of damp weather, as they then separate most readily from the wood. For the collection of gums and gum resins, dry weather is selected and care should be taken to exclude vegetable debris as far as possible.

Underground organs must be freed from soil. Shaking the drug before, during and after drying, or brushing it, may be sufficient to separate a sandy soil. In the case of a celay or other heavy soil, washing is necessary. Valerian is washed in the streams on the banks of which it usually grows. Before drying, any wormy or diseased rhizomes or roots should be rejected. Those of small size are often replanted. In certain cases the rootlets are cut off. Rhubarb, Ginger and Marshmallow are usually peeled. All large organs, such as calumba root and inula rhizome, should be sliced to facilitate drying. Before Gentian root is dried, it is made into heaps and allowed to ferment. Seeds of Nux vomica and Cocoa, which are obtained from mucilaginous fruits, are washed to free from pulp before drying.

Drying

Slow drying at a moderate temperature is necessary for Orris rhizome, Vanilla pods, Cocoa seeds and Gentian root. Drying should take place as soon as possible after collection, if enzymic action is not desired. Drugs containing volatile oils lose their aroma if not dried or if the oil is not distilled from them immediately. All moist drugs are liable to develop mould. For these reasons, drying apparatus and stills should be situated as near to the growing plants as possible.

The duration of the drying process varies from a few hours to many weeks. In open-air drying depends very largely on the weather. In suitable climates open-air drying is used for Clove, Colocynth, Cardamom and Cinnamon. In warm and dry climates arrangements have to be made for getting the drug under the cover of sheds or tarpaulins at night or during wet weather. For drying in sheds the drugs may be suspended in bundles from the roof, threaded on strings. Chinese rhubarb is placed on trays made of sacking of tinned wire-netting. Papers spread on a wooden framework are also used for fruits from which the seeds are collected.

Drying by artificial heat is more rapid than open-air drying. It is necessary in tropical countries *e.g.*, West Africa, where the humidity is very high, and Honduras for drying Cardamom fruits. In Europe, continuous belt driers are used for large crops such as Digitalis. Alternatively, heat may be applied by means of open fires (*e.g.,* Nutmegs), stoves or hot-water pipes. There must be a space of at least 15 cm between superimposed trays, and air must circulate freely.

Rapid drying helps flowers and leaves to retain their colour and aromatic drugs their aroma. The temperature used must be controlled according to the constituents and the physical nature of the drug.

The leaves, herbs and flowers may be dried between 20 and 40°C, and barks and roots between 30 and 65°C. For rural tropical areas, solar dryers have some distinct advantage over conventional artificial heat dryers. If leaves and other delicate structures are overdried, they become very brittle and tend to break in transit. Drugs such as Aloes and Opium may require further drying after importation.

With some natural products, such as vanilla, processes of fermentation or sweating are necessary to bring about changes in the constituents. Such drugs require special drying processes, usually called "curing."

Correct and proper drying is vital for the production of a satisfactory herb which is to be traded internationally. Drying involves reducing the moisture in the harvested herb to a maximum of 5-10 per cent, thus minimising spoilage. If properly dried, a herb will retain much of its original colour, and this is an important criterion used by purchasers to judge quality. The method of drying will depend on the species of the plant and the parts of it to be dried. A considerable quantity of herbs is dried naturally in the shade, but artificial drying is increasingly being used since it produces, according to some sources, a superior product, retaining much more of the original flavour and avoiding a hay-like taste. Modern methods now make it possible to dry some herbs which formerly could not be satisfactorily dried by natural methods. In all cases the drying area should be spotlessly clean, free of dust, and protected from animals and other sources of contamination. The drying room should also be well ventilated, and drying should take place on rust-free steel-meshed or firm fabric-meshed frames. Handling of the herbs should be limited to the absolute minimum to avoid crumbling. In most cases the herbs should be spread in thin layers to speed drying and to prevent spoilage by moisture condensation and overheating. However, some herbs can be dried by tying the aerial parts in bunches and hanging them up to dry. Tender leaf herbs, such as basil or mint, should be dried rapidly to avoid discoloration and mould.

The duration of drying varies according to the particular plant, its level of moisture content, and the drying temperature. Flowers and leaves tend to dry more quickly than stems. The drying temperature has a vital influence on quality. If herbs are dried naturally, it is done in the shade with good air circulation. Artificial drying in special rooms, where space is limited, required higher temperature. The temperature should not exceed 40ºC for culinary herbs because the essential oils, and hence the flavour, are often lost at higher temperatures. The moisture level of herbs varies, and the drying ratio expresses the weight relationship between the fresh herb and the dried herb.

Nearly all herbs entering international trade are in the dried form and have not been further processed. There are several reasons for this. Firstly, it is difficult to check the level of contamination of ground herbs, compared with crude herbs. Secondly, ground herbs lose their essential oil constituents and characteristic aroma much more rapidly, and thus cannot be stored for as long as crude or unground herbs. Thirdly, grinders argue that it is much easier to maintain quality control standards by keeping stocks of unground herbs of varying quality, and blending these to purchasers' specifications. Food manufacturers do not usually import or process herbs, but purchase them from grinders and processors to suit their own specifications.

Garbling

Garbling is the final step in the preparation of a crude drug. Garbling consists of the removal of extraneous matter, such as other parts of the plant, dirt and added adulterants. This step is done to some extent during collection, but should be carried out after the drug is dried and before it is baled or packaged. Garbling may be done by mechanical means in some cases.

Storage

The large-scale storage of drug is very important. Except in a few cases, e.g., Cascara bark, long storage is not to be recommended. Drugs such as Indian hemp and Sarsaparilla deteriorate even when carefully stored. Drugs stored in the usual containers, e.g., sacks, bales, wooden cases, cardboard boxes and paper bags, reabsorb about 10-12% or more of moisture.

Plastic sacks will effectively seal the contents. The permissible moisture contents of Starch, Acacia gum and other drugs are mentioned in some pharmacopoeias.

The combined effects of moisture and temperature on humidity and the then water-condensation when the temperature falls, must be considered in drug storage. Drugs such as Digitalis and Indian hemp should never be allowed to become air-dry since they lose a part of their activity. They may be kept in sealed containers with a dehydrating agent. For large quantities, the bottom of a case may be filled with quicklime and separated from the drug by a perforated grid or sacking. If the lime becomes moist, it should be replaced. Volatile oils and fixed oils, especially cod-liver oil, should be stored in sealed, well-filled containers in a cool, dark place. In case of cod-liver oil, the air in the containers is sometimes replaced by an inert gas. Air-dried drugs are always susceptible to the attack of insects and other pests. Therefore, they should be examined frequently during storage and any showing mould or worms should be either rejected or treated with a suitable method. Sterilization of some plant materials before storage is necessary to reduce undesirable microbial contamination and to prevent the development of other living organisms.

Ethylene oxide or methyl chloride may be used, and drugs so treated should comply with an acceptable limit for toxic residues, *e.g.,* for Senna pods, 50 ppm of ethylene oxide.

Different types of storage can influence the quality of a herb considerably. Although herbs can retain their aroma and flavour for a long period if kept under correct conditions, they tend to lose their flavour a little faster than spices such as Pepper, Ginger and Cloves. Dried herbs store best in the whole (or leaf) form, and consequently most buyers choose this form of storage. A further important consideration in storage is to limit contamination. Most authorities recommend storage in airtight containers in a dry, dark place at a temperature not exceeding 18ºC. Heat loses herbs of their flavour whilst dampness causes ground herbs to cake and deteriorate. Satisfactory packaging materials include laminated paper bags, cardboard containers, tins or hessian (jute) sacks, as well as various containers made of other natural or artificial fibres. The herbs for the retail market should be available in small quantities, preferably in jars or packets not exceeding about 30 g, to ensure periodic replacement.

Packaging and preservation

The packaging of drugs depends on their final utilization. In commerce, if transportation, storage, and ultimate use are considered, it is important to choose the type of packaging that provides protection to the drug and occupies economy of space. Leaf and herb material is powdered, made into a solid compact mass and then sewn into a cover. Bales that are shipped overseas weigh from 50 kg to 100 kg. Senna leaves from India come in bales of 200 kg; Stramonium from Argentina in bales of 350 kg. Drugs that are likely to deteriorate from absorbed moisture (Digitalis, Ergot) are packed in moisture-proof cans. Gums, resins, and extracts are shipped in barrels, boxes or casks.

Packaging is typical for certain drugs. The standard package for Balsam of Peru, Balsam of Tolu, Colophony and all grades of Aloe is a 55-gallon steel drum. Matting-covered packages of cinnamon from the far East, (bales covered with cowhide) (seroons) containing Sarsaparilla from South America, lead flasks with oil of rose from Bulgaria, and many other odd forms of packaging are used in the drug trade.

Proper storage and preservation are required for maintaining a high degree of quality of the drug. Hard-packed bales, barks and resinous drugs usually reabsorb some moisture. But leaf, herb and root drugs that are not well packed tend to absorb 10, 15 or even 30% moisture of the weight of the drug. Excessive moisture increases the weight of the drug, reduces the percentage of active constituents, favors enzymatic activity and facilitates fungal growth.

Light causes highly coloured drugs unattractive and undesirable changes in constituents. The oxygen in the air increases oxidation of the constituents of drugs, especially when oxidases are present. Therefore, the warehouse should be cool, dark and well ventilated with dry air.

The drugs are protected against attacks by insects. The insects that infest vegetable drugs belong mainly to the orders Lepidoptera, Coleoptera, and Diptera.

For prevention of insects attacks, a number of methods have been used. The simplest method is to expose the drug to a temperature of 65°C for preventing insect attacks and many other forms of deterioration. For the fumigation of large lots of crude drugs in warehouses and manufacturing plants, methyl bromide is used.

Small lots of drugs may be stored in tight, light-resistant containers, e.g., tin cans, covered metal bins or amber glass containers. Drugs should not be stored in wooden boxes or in drawers and never in paper bags where deterioration is hastened, odours are communicated from one drug to another, attacks by insects are facilitated, and destruction by mice and rats may occur. If drugs in small quantities stored in tight containers, insect attack can be controlled by adding to the container a few drops of chloroform or carbon tetrachloride from time to time. A suitable cartridge containing a nonliquefying, inert, dehydrating substance may be introduced into the tight container in case of Digitalis and Ergot, whose moisture content must be maintained every time.

High temperatures accelerate all chemical reactions and then deterioration, drugs must always be stored at as a low temperature as possible. The ideal temperature is just above freezing. Certain drugs, such as the biologics, must be stored at a temperature between 2° and 8°C.

ANIMAL DRUGS

Animal drugs are produced from wild (whale, musk deer) or domesticated animals. Their collection parallels the collection of vegetable drugs. Many animal drugs are obtained from domesticated animals. When drugs consist of insects, the drugs are either collected from wild insects (cantharides) or from cultivated forms, e.g., honey bees. Drugs such as lanolin, milk products, endocrine products, hormones and some enzymes are obtained from domesticated hogs, sheep or cattle. Glandular products and enzymes are obtained from a slaughter-house.

Drug Adulteration

An adulterated drug means one which does not conform to the official requirements. Adulteration involves incorporation of impurities, spoilage, deterioration, admixture, sophistication and substitution. The genuine drugs are substituted with spurious, inferior, defective or harmful substances. The spoiled or deteriorated drugs represent the greatest percentage of drug adulteration. In some cases the dealers substitute the drugs with cheap materials in case of scarcity or when the price of a drug is high. The adulteration may be due to faulty collection, imperfect preparation and incorrect storage as described hereunder :

FAULTY COLLECTION

In some cases the proportion of medicinally-active constituent reaches a maximum at a particular season, stage of development, or age. But collection of correct part of genuine plant without regard to time factors causes adulteration. The following are some examples :

(i) *Season* :

Table 8.1. Adulteration due to season

Drug	Season of maximum activity
Solanaceous leaves	Flowering stage of the drug (summer)
Wild Cherry bark	Autumn
Colchicum corm	Early summer
Male fern	Late autumn

(ii) *Stage of development and age* :

Table 8.2. Adulteration due to plant age

Drug	Stage and age of maximum activity
Linseed	When fully ripe
Coriander	When fully grown and ripe
Wild Cherry bark	Bark of young stems
Belladonna root	Root of 3-4 years old

(iii) *Collection of less valuable part* : Sometimes adulteration is done by collection of other less valuable part of a genuine plant. For example:

Table 8.3. Adulteration due to different parts

Drug	Official part	Less valuable parts
Buchu	Leaves	Stems
Clove	Flower-buds	Flower-stalks
Senega	Root	Stems
Serpentary	Rhizome and roots	Sub-aerial stem

(iv) *Collection of drugs from other species* : Ignorance or neglect on the part of collectors may lead to unintentional collection of drugs from the allied or foreign species. Such plants may bear a superficial resemblance to the genuine plant. In place of the genuine drugs, substituted products are available in the market. These substituents are identical in appearance. Some example are as :

Table 8.4. Adulteration due to allied drugs

Drug	Official source	Source of adulteration
Aconite	Aconitum napellus	Aconitum deinorrhizum and other species of Aconitum
Buchu	Barosma betulina	Barosma crenulata, Barosma serratifolia
Cascara sagrada	Rhamnus purshiana	Rhamnus californica
Myrrh	Commiphora molmol	Commiphora erythaea var. brescens
Belladonna leaf	Atropa belladonna	Scopolia carniolica, Phytolacca decandra, Ailanthus glandulosa
Indian belladonna	Atropa acuminata	Roots of Althaea officinalis, leaves of Phytolacca acinosa, Solanum nigrum and other species of Solanum and Datura
Pale Catechu	Uncaria gambier	Acacia catechu
Chamomile	Anthemis nobilis	Chrysanthemum parthenium
Digitalis	Digitalis purpurea	Verbascum thapsus; Symphytum officinale; Primula vulgaria; Digitalis thapsi
Tragacanth	Astragalus gummifer	Sterculia urens and other species of Sterculia
Chirata	Swertia chirata	Swertia angustifolia, S. alata, Rubia cordifolia and Andrographis paniculata
Cinnamon	Cinnamomum zeylanicum	Cinnamomum cassia
Balsam of Tolu	Myroxylon balsamum	Mixture of vanillin, Rosin, cinnamic and benzoic acids
Kalmegh	Andrographis paniculata	Chirata (Swertia chirata)
Ispaghula	Plantago psyllium	Salvia aegyptiaca, P. arenaria, P. lanceolata, P. major
Linseed oil	Linum usitatissimum	Vegetable oils of rapeseed, cottonseed, soyabean, sunflower and safflower and rosin, mineral and fish oils
Ipecac	Cephaelis ipecacuanha	Richardia scabra, Cryptocoryne spiralis, Psychotria emetica, Manettia ignita, Hybanthus ipecacuanha, Asclepias curassavica, Anodendron paniculatum, Calotropis gigantea
Galanga	Alpina officinarum	Acorus calamus
Saffron	Crocus sativus	Flower and floral parts of some Asteraceae family, e.g., Calendula species, Carthamus tinctorius; corn silk
Saussurea oil	Saussurea lappa	Elecampane oil
Punarnava	Boerhaavia diffusa	Trianthema portulacastrum
Rauwolfia	Rauwolfia serpentina	Rauwolfia beddomei, R. densiflora, R. micrantha, R. perakensis, R. nitida, R. tetraphylla; Ophiorrhiza mungos and Clerodendrum species
Nux-vomica	Strychnos nux-vomica	S. potatorum and S. nux-blanda
Pyrethrum	Chrysanthemum cinerariaefolium	C. leucanthemum
Datura	Datura stramonium	Xanthium strumarium, Carthamus helenioides, Chenopodium hybridum
Cardamom	Elettaria cardamomum	Orange seeds, unroasted coffee grains
Calamus	Acorus calamus	Alpinia galanga; Aconitum species
Areca nut	Areca catechu	Sogo palm nuts (Metroxylon sps.), tapioca (Manihot esculenta), potato (Ipomoea batatas), nuts of Caryota urens
Liquorice	Glycyrrhiza glabra	Abrus precatorius
Ashoka bark	Saraca indica	Trema orientalis bark
Kurchi bark	Holarrhena antidysenterica	Wrightia tinctoria bark
Devadru bark	Polyalthia longifolia	Saraca indica bark
Hindi-sana leaves	Cassia angustifolia	Cassia auriculata leaves

IMPERFECT PREPARATION

Collection of other and less valuable parts of the genuine plant may cause adulteration. For example, stems are collected with leaves. The adulteration done by non-removal of inert or undesirable parts of the drugs is illustrated by the following examples:

Table 8.5. Adulteration due to imperfect preparation

Drug	Official composition	Inert and undesirable part
Ginger	Rhizome freed from cork	Cork
Male fern	Rhizome and leaf bases	Roots and dead portions
Orange and lemon peels	Outer part of the pericarp	Inner white spongy part of pericarp
Ipecac	Roots or rhizomes	Aerial stem
Fennel	Fruit	Undeveloped or mould attack fruits
Saffron	Stigma and style-tops	Parts of corolla
Quillaia	Inner part of the bark	Rhytidome
Tamarind	Fruits freed from the brittle outer part	Outer part of pericarp
Pyrethrum	Flower heads	Stem and leaf

Neglect of proper conditions for drying leads adulteration in the following drugs :

Table 8.6. Adulteration due to drying conditions

Drug	Faulty treatment
Colchicum corm	Drying at a temperature above 65°C which accelerates the rate of hydrolysis of colchicine
Digitalis	Leaving in a wilted condition for long period, thereby, providing suitable conditions for the decomposition of the glycosides by enzymes, or drying above 60°C, thereby, promoting hydrolysis of the glycosides
Gentian	Allowing excessive fermentation before drying in which sugars are converted to alcohol and carbon dioxide and the proportion of water-soluble extract is reduced below the official minimum.
Cod-liver oil	Excessive heat used in separating the oil from the livers affects the proportion of vitamins, odour and colour

INCORRECT STORAGE

Incorrect storage spoils many drugs. The quality, value or usefulness of the drug has been impaired or destroyed by the action of moisture, light, temperature and microorganisms (fungi and bacterial) and the article becomes unfit for human consumption. Many examples of spoilage are found in food industry. All drugs which are unfit for human or animal consumption are legally considered as adulterated. The impairment of the quality or value of an article by the abstraction or destruction of valuable constituents by distillation, extraction, ageing, moisture, heat, fungi, insects or other means deteriorate the drugs considerably. Few examples are :

Table 8.7. Adulteration due to incorrect storage

Drug	Storage condition
Cascara sagrada	To be collected at least one year before being used
Male fern	To be used after the internal green colour is lost
Digitalis, Belladonna leaf, Hyoscyamus and Stramonium	To be preserved in a dry place or a container which prevents excess of moisture to stop enzymatic hydrolysis
Cod-liver oil	Protected from light, which would decompose vitamin A
Volatile oil	Protected from light, and stored in well-closed containers in a cool place
Lard	Protected from moisture
Squill	Powdered squill hardens by absorption of moisture
Coffee	Caffeine is lost by over-heating
Ergot	Protected from molds

DELIBERATE ADULTERATION

Substitution of exhausted drugs : Many drugs are extracted on a large scale for the isolation of an active constituent or volatile oil, or for the preparation of an extract. The exhausted material may be used entirely or in part as a substitute for the genuine drug. This extraction procedure does not bring any change in the morphology of the drug. Some example are :

Table 8.8. Adulteration due to exhausted drugs

Drug	Constituent removed
Clove	Volatile oil
Umbelliferous fruits	Volatile oil
Indian hemp	Resin
Glycyrrhiza	Glycyrrhizin and other water-soluble matter
Jalap	Resin
Balsam of Tolu	Balsamic acid
Ginger	Gingerol, volatile oil and resin
Tea	Caffeine
Cardamom	Volatile oil
Saffron	Volatile oil
Cardamom powder	Hulls powder

Sometimes foreign matters are added which are cheap in comparison with the drug and are usually

Table 8.9. Adulteration due to foreign materials

Drug	Foreign or fictitious matters
Cochineal	Barium sulphate, barium carbonate, lead carbonate and animal charcoal
Myrrh	Quartz and other mineral matter
Resins and Copaiba	Colophony
Black pepper	Seeds of papaya
Saffron	Materials coloured with coal-tar dye, oil and glycerine
Papain	Arrowroot starch, dried milk of cactus, gutta-parcha, rice flour and pepsins
Nux-vomica powder	Olive stone powder
Pyrethrum powder	Lead chromate, turmeric and fustic
Coca leaves	Novacaine, boric acid, sodium carbonate and bicarbonate, lime chalk, starch, lactose and quinine
Honey	Cane sugar, corn syrup and artificial invert sugar
Asafoetida	Gum arabic, gum-resins, rosin, gypsum, red clay, chalk, barley or wheat flour, slices of potato, etc.
Clove	Clay material
Caraway	Clay material
Lemon oil	An admixture of citral and other terpenes
Balsam of Peru	An admixture of synthetic benzyl benzoate, Storax, Benzoin and Balsam of Tolu
Nutmeg	Broken kernels moulded with clay; shaped pieces of wood

dense and inconspicuous upon cursory examination. Replacement wholly or in part by a fictitious mixture of similar composition is occasionally a cause of adulteration. Admixture with non-plant substances resembling to a particular drug is commonly practised. For example :

DETERIORATION BY MOULDS, BACTERIA AND INSECTS

The factors causing deterioration of drugs are moisture content, temperature, light and the presence of oxygen. When these conditions are suitable, living organisms (bacteria, moulds, mites and insects) will rapidly multiply, using the drug as a source of nutrient.

Primary factors

Air-dried drugs contain about 10-12% of moisture and in some cases (*e.g.*, Digitalis) this may be sufficient to activate enzymes present in the leaves and bring about decomposition of the glycosides. Powdered Squill, which contain mucilage, rapidly absorb moisture and become a sticky mass. The shipment of drugs can lead to spoilage due to excessive condensation of moisture on the inner metal walls. It is a particular problem with cargoes in transit from humid moist climates to temperate regions. An increase in temperature and moisture, may accelerate enzyme activity. A high temperature rise leads to a loss of volatile constituents (e.g., essential oils from dried plant material). In absorbent cotton-wool, a reorientation of the small amount of fatty material present causes non-absorbency or lower absorbency. Direct sunlight can cause decomposition of certain constituents (e.g., vitamins in cod-liver oil) and produces a bleaching of leaves and flowers. Oxygen causes the resinification of volatile oils and the rancidification of fixed oils.

Mould and bacterial attack

The moulds like *Rhizopus, Mucor, Penicillium* and *Eurotium* species found in deteriorating drugs are usually the same as those present in poorly stored food products. Their presence is indicated by a mass of hyphae which bind the particles of drug and by a characteristic smell. Bacterial attack of crude drugs is less common unless chromogenic species are involved or effects produced such as dustiness in cotton-wool by attack on the fibres. Certain pathogenic bacteria such as Salmonellae and *Escherichia coli* are tested in some crude drugs taken internally (Digitalis, Sterculia, Tragacanth, Gelatin).

Coleoptera or beetles

Beetles are insects and belong to animal kingdom, comprising about 250,000 species. About 600 species are associated with stored food products or drugs. They may be found in the wood of packing-cases. Beetles have a body which is divided into head, thorax and abdomen. To the lower side of the thorax are attached three pairs of legs, while the upper surface usually bears two membranous hind-wings which are folded beneath horny elytra (fore-wings). They complete life cycle through egg, larval, pupal and adult stages, and cause damage both as adults and as larvae. They have well-developed biting mouth-parts and a head which is darker in colour than the rest of the body.

Carpophilus spp., e.g. *C. hemipterus* (dried fruit beetle) Family Nitidulidae (sap-feeding beetles), is obovate or oblong about 4 mm long; 11-segmented antennae with a compact club. Elyta shortened exposing two-three apical abdominal segments.

Oryzaephilus mercator (merchant grain beetle) and *O. surinamensis* (saw-toothed grain beetle) Family Silvanidae, are dark brown, narrow, distinctly flattened beetles, about 3 mm long. Clubbed antennae. Attack nuts and dried fruits.

Calandra granaria (granary weevil) Family Curcu-lionidae (weevils), is dark brown to black insects, about 3-4 mm long. Hind-wings absent, with characteristic snout and antennae. Bore into seeds and fruits and lay eggs in the cavity by means of the ovipositor. Larvae develop and pupae within the seeds.

Calandra granaria (granary weevil) (Curculionidae) is similar, hind-wings present, 2-5 mm long.

Siegobium paniceum (*Sitodrepa panicea, Anobium paniceum*) (drugroom beetle) Family Anoblidae ('furniture beetles'), are pale reddish-brown in colour; greyish hairs, 2-3 mm long. Antennae 11-segmented, with three terminal segments forming a loose club. Common in many stored vegetable drugs, formerly frequent in ships biscuits.

Anobium punctatum (common furniture beetle) (Anoblidae) is similar to *Stegobium paniceum*, 3-5 mm long. The prothorax exhibits a distinct hump. Does not attack drugs but may occur in wood of packing-cases, floors, etc.

Lasioderma serricorne (tobacco, cigar or cigarette beetle) (Anoblidae) is reddish colour, about 2 mm long. Found in many stored products, ginger and liquorice.

Pitnus fur (white-marked spider beetle); *P. tectus* (Australian spider beetle); *P. hirtellus* (brown spider beetle); *Trigonogenius globulus*; *Niptus hololeucus* (goldenspider beetle, cloth bug); and *Gibbium psylloides* Family Ptinidae ('spider beetles'), all are similar, somewhat resembling spiders, with long legs and antennae, stout bodies and hairy covering 2-4 mm long. Some species (e.g., *Niptus hololeucus*) are densely covered with hairs others (e.g., *Gibbium* spp.) are glabrous with a shining cuticle. They occur widely in stored products, e.g., —food, spices, cocoa, cereals, almonds, capsicum, ginger and nutmegs, etc.

Tribolium confusum (confused flour beetle); and *T. castaneum* (rust red flour beetle) Family Tenebrionidae, are reddish-brown beetles, 2-4 mm long. Found in many foodstuffs including flour and nuts. Infested flour has lingering pungent odour. They are more common in crude drugs, e.g. rhubarb.

Lepidoptera

The Lepidoptera include the moths and butterflies. A small number of moths cause injury to drugs. The damage is caused by the larva and not by the mature insect; but since moths are very mobile and lay eggs, infestation tends to spread rapidly.

Ephestia kuehniella, the Mediterranean flour moth; *E. cautella*, the fig moth; *F. elutella*, the cocoa moth, and *Plodia interpunctella*, the Indian meal moth all belong to the family, the Phycitidae. Various members of the family Tineidae, which cause damage to clothes and carpets are also found in drugs.

Ephestia kuehniella is about 25 mm long. It has dark brownish-grey scaly forewings and dirty-white hindwings. The larvae are whitish except for the brownish anterior and the dark hairs on each segment. They remain in the food material, where they form pupae. The grubs of *E. elutella* migrate away from the food and leave the food containers completely 'webbed' with their silky threads. They enter cracks in walls, where they spun cocoons and remain until they pupate in the spring.

Ephestia kuehniella is found in almond, capsicum, cocoa, cotton seed and ground-nut.

E. cautella is present in Tonco bean and cocoa.

E. elutella attacks cocoa, tobacco, rose petals and pomegranate root bark.

Plodia interpunctella destroys Cinnamon bark and yeast cake.

Tinea pellionella occur in Aconite root, almonds, capsicums, mustard seed, ginger, linseed, orris, saffron and tobacco.

Arachnida (Mites)

The mature forms have eight legs but possess no antennae. The members of the Tyroglyphidae, (*e.g.*, *Tyroglyphus dimidiatus*, the cheese-mite) are much smaller than the insects, and individuals can only be seen with a lens. If the suspected 'dust' is scraped into a pile, it will be seen to move.

Tyroglyphus farinae (*Acarus siro*), the flour or meal mite is common in cereal products, oil-seed cakes and many other commodities.

The Tyroglyphidae may themselves be attacked by other mites such as *Cheyletus eruditus*.

Different mites attack cantharides, causing considerable damage. Ergot, quince and linseed are very liable to attack.

Mites *Dermatophagoides pteronyssinus, D. culinar, Glycyphagus domesticus* (the house mite) and *Tyroglyphus farinae* (the flour mite), commonly exist in ordinary house dust as found under carpets and in mattresses. These mites are the allergens responsible for house dust sensitivity for many people. It is now possible to diagnose this condition by prick tests which utilize an extract prepared from *Dermatophagoides culinae.* This mite does not show the marked division of the body into two parts exhibited by the *Tyroglyphus* spp.

Control of infestation

The detection, prevention and eradication of mite and insect infestation are important hygienic and economic steps. Effective preventive measures involve good hygiene in the warehouse, *e.g.*, removal of spillages, old debris and packaging materials; elimination of sources of infestations such as floor cracks and crevices. Regular inspection, rotation of stock, early recognition of infestation for effective stock control, optimum storage conditions by maintenance of cool, dry environment and good packaging in woven sacks and bags, multiply paper sacks stitched at the seams, paper, polythene film, filmy cardboard are all penetrable by insects and mites.

If material becomes infested it is advisable to discard a small consignment before contamination of other materials. After a contaminated drug has been removed, pallets, shelves, walls and floors should be thoroughly cleaned and sprayed with a contact insecticide such as chlorpyriphos-methyl or pirimiphos-methyl. Weekly air-spraying with pyrethrins or synthetic pyrethroids, and the use of slow-release dichlorvos strips, control air-borne insects. Various dust formulations may be used in cracks.

Fumigation is used for killing insects and mites in bulk consignments. Methyl bromide and ethylene oxide are commonly used under gas-proof sheets or in other suitable gas-tight enclosures or chambers. Before drugs are used, the fumigants must be completely removed as, if they are consumed, they may constitute a health hazard.

Low-temperature storage reduces insect attack and if a sufficiently low temperature be used, gradually destroy insects, larvae and eggs. The eggs of *Ephestia elutella* and *E. kuehniella* are rapidly destroyed at -15°C and more slowly at higher temperatures.

The eggs of the flour mite can withstand exposure to -10°C for up to 12 days or 0°C for several months.

Ionizing radiations (e.g., from a ^{60}Co source) on cereal pests small doses inhibit reproductive ability and large ones destroy both mites and their eggs.

The quantitative determination of insect infestation in powdered vegetable drugs is based on the acetolysis of the weighed sample for the quantitative isolation of the insect fragments present. These fragments are suspended in a suitable medium with a weighed quantity of lycopodium spores. The number of strial punctures per elytron is characteristic for a particular beetle. By counting the strial punctures evident on the fragments of elytra present under the microscope, the number of beetles present may be determined. The use of lycopodium spores (94000 spores mg^{-1}) eliminates the necessity for counting all the strial punctures present in a particular volume (or weight) of the suspension.

Spoilage by rodents

Rodent faeces usually contain the animal's hairs. The drug samples, which on microscopical examination show the presence of these hairs, should be rejected.

CONFUSION OF COMMON VERNACULAR NOMENCLATURE

Common vernacular names of some plants in different regions of India cause this type of adulteration. In different regions the same plant is known by different names. Sometimes many drugs are known by the same name. For example, the drugs *Trianthema portulacastrum* and *Boerhavia diffusa* are known by the common name "Punarnava". In most of the states "Brahmi" is obtained from the plant *Hydrocotyle asiatica* while in eastern parts of India the plant '*Herpestis monniera* is used as "Brahmi". The plants *Evolvulus alsinoides, Convolvulus microphyllus* and *Clitoria ternatea* are sold by the name "Shankhpushpi". Similarly for "Boch" the rhizomes and roots of *Acorus calamus, Alpinia officinarum* and *Anacyclus pyrethrum* are available. Rasna is also a controversial drug and three different plants - *Pluchea lanceolata* (in north India), *Vanda roxburghii* (in Bihar and Bengal) and *Alpinia officinarum* (in south India) are sold as Rasna. Other examples are :

- **Agnimath :** It is an ingredient of *Dashmool*. Under this name the drug of family Verbenaceae used are *Clerodendrum indicum, C. phlomidis, C. infortunatum, Premna latifolia, P. obtusifolia* and *P. barhata*. Another plant, *Solanum torvum* (Solanaceae) is used as Agnimath.
- **Amahaldi :** *Curcuma amada, C. aromatica* (Zingiberaceae).
- **Arlu :** *Ailanthus excelsa* (Simaronbaceae), *Oroxylum indicum* (Bignoniaceae), *Orchis latifolia* (Orchidaceae).
- **Ashoka :** *Saraca indica* (Caesalpiniaceae), *Polyalthia longifolia* (Annonaceae).
- **Bharangi :** *Elaeodendron glaucum* (Celastraceae), *Gardenia latifolia* (Rubiaceae), *G. turgida, Picrasma quassioides* (Simarubiaceae).
- **Bijasar :** *Bridelia montana* (Euphorbiaceae), *Pterocarpus marsupium* (Papilionaceae), *Terminalia tomentosa* (Combretaceae).
- **Danti :** *Baliospermum montanum, Croton oblongifolius, C. tigilium, Jatropha curcas* and *Ricinus communis*. All these plants belong to the family Euphorbiaceae.

- **Gajpippali :** *Borossus flabellifer* (Arecaceae), *Piper chaba* (Piperaceae), *Scindapsus officinalis* (Araceae).
- **Gaojban :** *Anisomelis indica* (Lamiaceae), *Arnebia indica* (Lamiaceae); *Heliotropium ophioglossum, Onosma bracteatum, Trichodesma indicum, T. zeylanicum* (Boragi-naceae).
- **Indrayana :** *Citrullus colocynthis, Cucumis trigonus* (Cucurbitaceae).
- **Jivanti :** *Dregea vulubilis, Gymnema sylvestre, Holostemma annulare, Leptadenia reticulata, Sarcostemma acidum* (all belong to Asclepiadaceae), *Cimicifuga foetida* (Ranunculaceae), *Pholidota articulata* (Orchidaceae).
- **Laxamana :** *Atropa mandragora* (Solanaceae), *Biophytum sensitivum* (Geraniaceae), *Ipomoea sepiaria* (Convolvulaceae), *Mandragora autumnalis* (Solanaceae), *Smithia geminiflora* (Papilionaceae).
- **Nagkeshar :** *Calophyllum enophyllum, Mesna ferrea* and *Ochrocarpus longifolius* (all belong to Guttiferae).
- **Parpat :** *Fumaria parviflora* (Funariaceae), *Mollugo oppositifolia* (Ficoidaceae), *Oldenlondia aspera* (Rubiaceae), *Polycarpea corymbosa* (Caryophyllaceae), *Rungia repens* (Acanthaceae).
- **Pashanbhed :** *Bergenia ligulata* (Saxifraginaceae), *Coleus aromaticus* (Lamiaceae), *Didymocarpus pedicellata* (Gesneriaceae).
- **Priyangu :** *Aglaia elaeagnoidea* (Meliaceae), *Prunus mahaleb* (Rosaceae).
- **Punarnava :** *Boerhavia diffusa* (Nyctaginaceae), *Trianthena portulacastrum* (Ficoidaceae).
- **Rasna :** *Alpinia galanga* (Scitaminaceae), *Aristolochia indica* (Aristolochiaceae), *Enicostemma littorale* (Gentianaceae), *Inula racemosa* (Asteraceae), *Catharanthus roseus* (Apocynaceae), *Pluchea lanceolata* (Asteraceae), *Rauwolfia serpentina* (Apocynaceae), *Viscum album* (Loranthaceae), *Vanda roxburghii* (Orchidaceae), *Withania coagulens* (Solanaceae).
- **Ratanjot :** *Arnebia nobilis, A. benthamii, A. euchroma, A. hispidissima, Onosma hispidum,*

O. hookeri, Alkanna tinctoria (all belong to family Boraginaceae), *Clausena pentaphylla* (Rutaceae), *Geranium wallichianum, G. nepalense* (Geraniaceae), *Potentilla nepalensis* (Rosaceae), *Anemone obtusiloba* (Ranunculaceae), *Jatropa curcus* (Euphorbiaceae), *Vinca rosea* (Apocynaceae), *Anchusa tinctora* (Papilianaceae) and *Maharanga emodi.*

- **Rudanti** : *Astragalus candolleanus* (Papilianaceae), *Capparis monii* (Capparidaceae), *Cressa cretica* (Convolvulaceae).

- **Savira** : *Cryptoletis buchanani, Decalepis hamiltonii, Hemidesmus indicus* (all belong to family Asclepiadaceae), *Ichnocarpus frutescens* (Apocynaceae), *Vallaris solanacea* (Apocynaceae).

- **Shankhpushpi** : *Evolvulus alsinoides* (Convolvulaceae), *Convolvulus pluricaulis* (Convolvulaceae), *Canscora diffusa* (Gentianaceae), *Clitoria ternatea* (Papilionaceae), *Lavendula bipinnata* (Lamiaceae).

- **Somalata** - *Ephedra gerardiana* (Ephedraceae), *Sarccostemma brevistigma* (Asclepiadaceae).

- **Talispatra** : *Abies webbiana* (Pinaceae), *Rhododandron anthopogon* (Ericaceae), *R. campanulatum* (Ericaceae), *Taxus baccata* (Taxaceae).

- **Agaru** : *Aquilaria agallocha; Commiphora roxburghii, Exocoecaria agallocha.*

- **Akasbel** : *Cassytha filiformis, Cuscuta reflexa.*

- **Al** : *Morinda umbellata, Morinda citrifolia.*

- **Babuna** : *Matricaria chamomilla; Cotula anthemoides; Corchorus depressus.*

- **Banda** : *Viscum album; Dendrophthoe falcata; Hedera helix.*

- **Bhangra** : *Indigofera linifolia; Eclipta alba; Wedelia calendulacea; Sonchus arvensis.*

- **Chitra** : *Plumbago indica; Berberis asiatica; Drosera lunata.*

- **Hing** : *Ferula narthex; Anchusa strigosa; Ferula narthex; F. foetida.*

- **Kasni** : *Cichorium endivia; C. intybus.*

- **Luban** : *Boswellia serrata; Styrax benzoin.*

Evaluation of Drugs

We have not achieved benefit of even 2% of the total flora provided by nature. The major pitfalls in the plant-drug research include lack of standardization, confusion in nomenclature, controversial botanical identification, danger of extinction of some plants being extensively over exploited, lack of proper dosage formulations, or frustrating experiences of searching for single active principle. Therefore, future of plant drugs depends upon the maintenance of quality control/standardization, therepeutic credibility, proper research finding and sincere commitment to research on plant drugs. We shall contribute better if we mingle our folklore and modern science for the future development of safe and efficacious drugs.

Evaluation of drugs deals with the correct identification of the plant and determination of quality and purity of the crude drugs. Actual collection of the drug is done from the identified plant or animal. For this purpose research gardens have been maintained. The characters of an unknown sample are compared with the authentic monographs written in the pharmacopoeias. The high quality of the drug is maintained by collection of the drug from the correct natural source at proper time; preparation of samples of the collected drugs by proper cleaning to free from dirt, drying and proper preservation of the cleaned, dried and pure drug.

The evaluation of a drug is done by studying its organoleptic, microscopic, chemical, physical and biological properties.

ORGANOLEPTIC EVALUATION

Organoleptic evaluation means study of a drug with the help of organs of sense which includes its external morphology, colour, odour, taste and sound of its fracture.

Morphological characters : To study morphology of a drug, its shape and size, colour and external markings, fracture and internal colour, odour and taste and examined. The organized drugs are classified into :

1. *Barks* : Which are tissues in a woody stem outside the inner fascicular cambium, *e.g.*, Cinnamon, Cinchona, Quillaia, Ashoka and Kurchi.

2. *Underground structures* : Which may be rhizomes, roots, bulbs, corms and tubers; they are often swollen due to storage of carbohydrates and other chemicals, *e.g.*, roots (Podophyllum, Liquorice, Jatamansi, Rauwolfia), rhizomes and stolons which are underground stems and have buds, scale leaves and scars, (Ginger, Turmeric, Dioscorea).

3. *Leaves* : These are photosynthetic organs arising from a node on a stem. The shape, margin, base, apex and venation of the leaves help in the identification of the drugs. Senna, Tulsi, Vasaka and Digitalis leaves can easily be identified.

4. *Flowers* : These are reproductive organs of a plant and possess different shapes, size and colour, *e.g.*, Saffron, Banafsha and Pyrethrum.

5. *Fruits* : Fruits arise from the ovary and contain seeds, *e.g.*, Cardamom, Colocynth, Almond, Vidang, Bahera, Amla and Bael.
6. *Seeds* : Seeds are developed from the ovules in carpels of the flowers and characterized by the hilum, micropyle and sometimes raphe. The seed drugs are Ispaghula, Linseed, Nux-vomica and Psoralia.
7. *Herbs* : The whole aerial part is sometimes used as a drug, *e.g.*, Brahmi, Chirata, Kalmegh, Pudina and Shankhpushpi.

The shape of a drug may be cylindrical (Sarsaparilla), sub-cylindrical (Podophyllum), conical (Aconite); fusiform, ovoid or pyriform (Jalap), and terete or disk-shaped (Nux-vomica). The drug may be simple, branched, curved or twisted. The length, breadth and diameter are measured in millimeters or centimeters. In case of conical drugs the size of both parts is mentioned.

External markings are mentioned as furrows, ridges, wrinkles, annulations, fissures, nodules, projections, scars of leaf, stem-base, root, bud and bud-scale.

The fractures may be complete, incomplete, short, fibrous, splintery (breaking irregularly), brittle (easily broken), tough and weak.

Sensory characters : Colour, texture, odour and taste are useful in the evaluation of drugs. This method is especially applicable to drugs containing volatile oils or pungent principles (*e.g.*, Capsicum), and to the detection of the effects of inadequate drying or damp storage. The external colour varies from white to yellowish grey, brown, orange or brownish black. The colour of some drugs changes if they are dried in sunlight in place of shade.

The odour of a drug may be either distinct (characteristic) or indistinct. The terms used to define odours are aromatic, balsamic, spicy, allia-ceous (garlic-like), camphoraceous (camphor-like), terebinthinate (turpentine-like) and others. Leaves of different species of *Mentha* can be distinguished by smell. Clove and exhausted clove are differentiated by odour. Deteriorated Cantharides have ammonical smell while spoiled Ergot has rancid and ammonical smell.

Taste is a particular sensation production by certain substances when these come into contact with taste buds present in epithelial layer of the mouth. The taste may be sour (acidic), salty (saline), sweet (saccharine), bitter, alkaline and metallic. Substances possessing no taste are mentioned as tasteless. The tastes due to a characteristic odour are grouped as aromatic, balsamic, spicy, alliaceous, camphoraceous and terebinthinate. The taste produced by distinct sensations to the tongue are classified as mucilaginous, oily, astringent (producing a contraction of the tissue of the mouth), pungent (warm biting sensation), acrid (unpleasant, irritating sensation) and nauseous (causing vomiting).

The drugs like Ginger and Capsicum have pungent taste; Gentian, Chirata and Kalmegh have bitter taste; Glycyrrhiza and Honey are sweet in taste. Linseed and Isphagula are mucilaginous; fixed oils have bland taste; calcium oxide is astringent; Podophyllum, Kaladana, Jalap and Ipomoea are acrid; while Ipecac, Acorus and *Tylophora indica* contain nauseous taste.

Glycyrrhiza has hard and fibrous fracture due to the presence of fibrous and woody tissues. Aconite has a horny fracture due to gelatinization of starch.

Colour of drugs are standardized and determined by the Inter-Society Colour Council - National Bureau of Standard method. For example, reserpine is described as a "white or pale buff to slightly yellowish, odourless crystalline powder".

MICROSCOPIC OR ANATOMICAL EVALUATION

Schleiden (1847) used microscope for the examination of drugs. Microscopic examination of section and powder drugs, aided by stains, help in distinction of anatomy in adulterants. Further, microscopical examination of epidermal trichomes and calcium oxalate crystals is extremely valuable, especially in powdered drugs. In the powdered drugs the cells are mostly broken, except lignified cells. The cell contents such as starch, calcium oxalate crystals and aleurone are scattered in the powder. Some fragments are specific for each powder which may consist of parts of cells or groups of cells.

Plant parts are made up of specific arranged tissues, spores (Lycopodium) or hairs (Lupulin). Histological characters are studied from very thin transverse, or longitudinal sections properly mounted in suitable stains, reagents or mounting media.

The size, shape and relative positions of the different cells and tissues, chemical nature of the cell walls and of the cell contents are determined. The basic arrangement of tissues in each drug is fairly constant. Fibres, sclereids, tracheids, vessels and cork are least affected by drying. Starch, calcium oxalate, epidermal trichomes and lignin are examined carefully.

Microscope is also used for quantitative evaluation of drugs and adulterated powders. This is done by counting a specific histological feature such as stomatal index, vein-islets and vein termination numbers and palisade ratio. These features are compared with the standard samples.

Leaf measurements : Leaves are measured to distinguish between some closely related species not easily identified by general microscopy.

Palisade ratio : The average number of palisade cells beneath each epidermal cell is called as palisade ratio. It is determined from powdered drugs with the help of camera lucida.

Method : Pieces of a leaf (2 mm square) are cleared by boiling with chloral hydrate solution, mounted and examined with a 4 mm objective. A camera lucida is arranged to trace the epidermal cells and the palisade cells lying below them. First a number of groups each of four epidermal cells are traced and their outlines inked in to make them more conspicuous. The palisade cells lying beneath each group are then focused, traced and counted in each

Table 9.1. Palisade ratio

Species	Palisade ratio
Agathosma betulina	10 to 26
Agathosma ovata	5 to 14
Ailanthus glandulosa	7 to 13
Atropa belladonna	6 to 10
Datura stramonium	4 to 7
Digitalis purpurea	3.7 to 4.2
Xanthium strumarium	3 to 4
Solanum nigrum	2 to 4

group; those being included in the count which are more than half-covered by the epidermal cells. The figure obtained divided by 4 gives the palisade ratio of that group. The range of a number of groups from different particles should be recorded.

Stomatal number : The average number of stomata per square millimeter of the epidermis is known as stomatal number. The range and average value for each surface are recorded.

Method : Fragments of leaf from the middle of the lamina are cleared with chloral hydrate solution. The number of stomata in 12-30 fields are counted and from a knowledge of the area of the field the stomatal number is calculated. The camera lucida method described for vein-islet numbers may also be used, the position of each stomata being indicated on the paper by a small cross.

Replicas of fresh leaf surface are satisfactory for the determination of stomatal number and stomatal index. Gelatin and water gel are liquefied on a water-bath and smeared on a hot slide. The fresh leaf is added, the slide is inverted and cooled under a tap and after about 15-30 min the specimen is stripped off. The imprint on the gelatin shows a clear outline of epidermal cells, stomata and trichomes.

Examples : Stomatal numbers are useless for distinguishing between closely allied species. In some cases the ratio between the number of stomata on the two surfaces may be of diagnostic importance. *Datura innoxia* can be distinguished from other species of *Datura* by this means.

Stomatal index : The percentage proportion of the number of stomata form to the total number of epidermal cells of a leaf is termed as the stomatal index :

S.I. = $S/E+S \times 100$; where S = number of stomata per unit area, E = number of ordinary epidermal cells in the same unit area.

Stomatal number varies considerably with the age of the leaf but the stomatal index is highly constant for a given species.

Method : Pieces of leaf except extreme margin or midrib are suitably cleared and mounted. The lower surface is examined by a microscope with a 4 mm objective and an eyepiece containing a 5 mm square micrometer disc. The numbers of epidermal cells and of stomata are counted within the square grif. The two guard cells and ostiole being considered as one unit. A cell is counted if at least half of its area lies within the grid. Successive adjacent fields are examined until about 400 cells have been counted and the stomatal index value calculated from these figures. The stomatal index may be determined for both leaf surfaces.

Stomatal index values may be used to distinguish between leaves of cogeneric species.

Table 9.2. Stomatal index values

Species	Stomatal index	
	Upper surface	Lower surface
Atropa acuminata	1.7 to 12.1	16.1 to 18.3
Atropa belladonna	2.3 to 10.4	20.2 to 29.9
Cassia senna	11.3 to 13.3	10.8 to 12.5
Cassia angustifolia	17.1 to 20.8	17.1 to 19.2
Datura inermis	18.2 to 18.7	24.5 to 25.2
Datura metel	12.7 to 19.3	21.1 to 24.0
Datura stramonium	16.5 to 20.5	24.1 to 26.2
Datura tatula	15.4 to 22.2	28.3 to 31.1
Digitalis lanata	14.0 to 14.6	15.0 to 17.7
Digitalis lutea	2.5 to 8.6	21.6 to 25.1
Digitalis purpurea	1.6 to 4.1	18.1 to 19.6
Digitalis thapsi	6.0 to 7.9	12.0 to 13.5
Erythroxylum coca	—	12.2 to 14.2
Erythroxylum truxillense	—	9.1 to 10.7
Phytolacca acinosa	—	15.2
Phytolaca americana	3.0 to 5.7	13.1 to 13.4

Vein-islet number : The word 'Vein-islet' is used for the minute area of photosynthetic tissue encircled by the ultimate divisions of the conducting strands. *Vein-islet number* is defined as the number of vein-islets per square mm calculated from four contiguous square mm in the central part of the lamina, midway, between the midrib and the margin.

Method : The leaves are cleared by boiling in chloral hydrate solution in a test-tube placed in a boiling water bath. Alternately, the leaves, after soaking in water, be treated with sodium hypochlorite to bleach, 10% hydrochloric acid to remove calcium oxalate, and finally chloral hydrate.

A camera lucida is set up and the paper is divided into squares of 1 mm^2 using a 16 mm objective with the help of stage micrometer. The micrometer is then replaced by the cleared preparation and the veins are traced in four contiguous squares, either in a square 2 mm × 2 mm or a rectangle 1 mm × 4 mm. When counting, each vein-islet is numbered on the tracing. Each numbered area must be completely enclosed by veins, and those which are incomplete are excluded from the count if cut by the top and left-hand sides of the square or rectangle but included if cut by the other two sides.

Table 9.3. Vein-islet numbers

	Species	Range of vein-islet numbers
1. Senna	*Cassia senna*	14.9-29.4
	Cassia angustifolia	19.5-22.7
2. Digitalis	*Digitalis purpurea*	2-5.6
	Digitalis lanata	2-2.4
		3-7.9
	Digitalis lutea	1-1.6
	Digitalis thapsi	8.5-16.1
3. Coca	*Erythroxylum coca*	7.9-12
	Erythroxylum truxillense	15-26.1

The vein-islet number helps to distinguish closely related plants. In the case of Buchu, some species which cannot be distinguished from *Barosma betulina* by their palisade ratios, are differentiated by their vein-islet numbers.

Veinlet termination number : It is defined as the number of veinlet termination per mm^2 of leaf

Table 9.4. Veinlet termination number

Atropa acuminata	1.5-3.6
Atropa belladonna	6.4-10.2
Cassia angustifolia	25.8-32.9
Cassia senna	32.8-40.1
Datura stramonium	12.7-20.2
Digitalis purpurea	2.6-4.3
Erythroxylum coca	16.9-21.2
Ervthroxylum truxillense	23.2-32.2
Hyoscyamus niger	12.5-19.1

surface. A vein termination is the ultimate free termination of a veinlet or branch of a veinlet. By this character different Coca leaves and Senna leaflets are differentiated.

LYCOPODIUM SPORE METHOD

Lycopodium (syn. Club-moss spores, Lycopodium seeds; vegetable sulphur) consists of the spores of the clubmoss, *Lycopodium clavatum* Linn. (Fam. Lycopodiaceae, Phyllum Pteriodophyta); grows in the North America, Russia, Poland, India and Pakistan. The sporangial spikes are cut, dried and the spores are separated by shaking. Lycopodium is a light yellow, extremely mobile and flammable powder without odour or taste. It contains about 50% fixed oil, which consists mainly of glycosides of lycopodiumoleic acid; sugars (3%), phytosterin and alkaloids of the annotine type.

Lycopodium spores are exceptionally uniform in size (about 25 μm) and 1 mg of lycopodium contains an average of 94,000 spores. The number of spores per milligram is determined by direct counting and by calculation based on specific gravity and dimensions of the spores. It is possible to evaluate many powdered drugs if well-defined particles may be counted as in case of pollen grains or starch grains; or if single layered tissues or cells of the area of which may be traced at a definite magnification and the actual area calculated; or if characteristic particles of a uniform thickness, the length of which can be measured at a definite magnification and the actual length calculated. Mounts containing a definite proportion of the powder and lycopodium are used and the lycopodium spores counted in each of the fields in which the number of area of the particles in the powder is determined.

Counting of particles : In this method the material is powdered and moisture content of the powdered material is determined. A mixture of weighed quantity of the powder and lycopodium spores is suspended in a suitable viscous liquid. A drop of this suspension is mounted and examined with a 4 mm objective. The number of lycopodium spores and the number of characteristic particles are counted in 25 various fields. The same experiment is repeated with a second similar suspension. From the mean of these results and a knowledge of the weights of lycopodium and powder in the mixture, the number of characteristic particles in 1 mg of the powder may be determined.

By employing lycopodium spore method the number of pollen grains in pyrethrum powder (1000-2000/mg), starch granules in wheat powder (400 granules/mg) and starch grains in Ginger (261400 grains/mg) have been determined. The percentage of ginger present when admixed with other drugs can, therefore, be determined. The estimation of insects in powdered drugs may be performed by using the count of elytral strial punctures.

Measurement of area : Lycopodium spore method is also used to determine size of a particular type of particle in powders such as epidermal fragments of leaves, single layer of scalerenchyma, or isolated fibres. The procedure is almost the same as used for counting of particles. Weighed quantities of the powder and lycopodium spores are mixed as before and may be cleared with chloral hydrate or stained with phloroglucinol and hydrochloric acid to assist identification of the characteristic particles. A camera lucida and drawing-board are fitted up and by means of a stage micrometer the magnification produced with a 4 mm objective is determined. A magnification of about 400 is suitable. The cleared or stained suspension is mounted and a suitable area is examined. If the particles to be traced are fairly numerous, 25 fields at this magnification will be sufficient, but if the number of particles is small, an area of about 40 mm^2 should be examined. In each field the spores are counted and the characteristic particles are traced. The particle size is traced with the help of camera lucida and the spores are counted. The tracings are cut out and weighed and their area calculated by weighing a sheet of known area of the paper used. This area divided by the magnification used (420)^2 gives the actual area of the particles in a certain weight of the powdered drug, which is calculated from the number of spores counted and the weight of spores and powder in the suspension. By this method epidermal area of Indian Senna stalk (100 cm^2), sclerenchyma layer in Linseed, fibres in the Cinnamon bark and number of beaker cells in testa of Cinnamon seed have been measured.

The epidermal area per gram of dried Indian Senna and Ailanthus leaves are 270 cm^2 and 318 cm^2, respectively. As the particles of Ailanthus are easily distinguished from those of Senna, it is possible to determine the percentage of each in a mixture. A mixture containing 2% Ailanthus was used and duplicate determinations gave 1.73% and 2.15% of Ailanthus; an area of 42.6 mm^2 was examined.

The epidermal area per gram of Indian Senna stalk is 100 cm^2 and the percentage of stalk in a sample of powdered Indian Senna may thus be determined.

Powdered Linseed contains a well-marked layer of sclerenchyma one cell in thickness. The area per gram of this tissue is to average 34.3 cm^2 in material dried at 100°C and 49.7 cm^2 in defatted and dried material.

For barks containing fibres, the area of fibres per gram of the powdered bark is a constant and can be used to determine the amount of Cassia in Cinnamon and vice versa, and also to assess the quality of Cinnamon powders. The average value for genuine Cinnamon powder is 92.5 cm^2 per gram and for cassia is 13.1.

The number of beaker cells per square millimetre of the testa of Cardamom seed is a constant for each variety. The area of this layer of cells per milligram of powdered seed is also a constant and may be used to determine the percentage of powdered Cardamoms in a mixture.

Measurement of length : For the determination of Nux vomica powder, the length of lignified ribs of the trichomes per milligram of air-dry seed was 184 cm. The ribs were stained by treating with 1% safranin in 50% alcohol, followed by decolorization of non-lignified tissue by addition of a definite amount of 10% hydrochloric acid; 24 fields, at a magnification of ×350 (4 mm objective) on two mounts are examined. The method was used to determine the Nux vomica content of two veterinary medicines.

CHEMICAL EVALUATION

Chemical evaluation involves the determination of active constituents by a chemical process. Chemical tests are used to identify crude drugs to determine purity. Chemical tests for alkaloids, carbohydrates, steroids, phenolic compounds, saponins, proteins, amino acids, fixed oils and volatile oils are performed. Titrimetric assay, iodine value, saponification value, acid value, acetyl value, ester value, peroxide value, hydroxyl value and ash value are determined. Tropane alkaloids in Datura, Belladonna and Stramonium are determined by Vitali-Morin reaction. Potassium chlorate and hydrochloric acid are used to estimate emetine in Ipecac. Strychnine in Nux-vomica is detected with ammonium vanadate and sulphuric acid. Borntrager's test is useful for detecting anthraquinone glycosides present in Senna, Rhubarb, Cascara and Aloe. Alkaloid contents can be evaluated by determining total alkaloidal contents by acid-base titration.

Preparation of an extract by an appropriate solvent is sometimes applied to determine the quality of drugs. The solvent may extract a single constituent, e.g., fixed oil from crushed Linseed. Further examples, the use of extractive tests are useful in cases of Gentian, Colocynth seeds, Indian hemp, Ginger, Calumba, Rhubarb, Glycyrrhiza and Myrrh.

Drugs containing volatile oils are examined for authenticity and quality by determining the percentage of volatile oil yielded by steam distillation in a suitable apparatus. Standards for content of volatile oil in drugs usually allow a somewhat smaller percentage from powdered drugs as compared with the whole drug due to inevitable loss on grinding, volatilization and decomposition.

On ignition of crude drugs a residue of mineral substances or ash remains is derived from the cell wall and cell contents. The ash value is useful in determining authenticity and purity of drugs. For a number of official drugs, a limit is placed on the yield of acid-insoluble ash, i.e., the ash remaining after extraction of the total ash with dilute acid. This residue consists chiefly of silica, partly derived from the constituents of the cells and their walls and partly from foreign mineral matters, mainly soil. Acid-insoluble ash limits are imposed especially in cases where foreign silica may be present or when the calcium oxalate contents of the drug is high. Pharmacopoeial limits for acid insoluble ash vary from 0.5 (Agar) to 12 per cent (Hyoscyamus). Glandular trichomes present in Hyoscyamus have a capacity of retaining clay and thus the acid insoluble ash value is higher in such cases. In case of Glycyrrhiza, the total ash figure is of importance which indicates the care taken in the preparation of the drug. For the determination of total ash values the carbon must be removed below 450°C, since alkali chlorides would be lost due to volatile at high temperature. The total ash usually consists of carbonates, phosphates, silicates and silica. In case of Ginger, a minimum percentage of water-soluble ash is determined to detect the presence of exhausted ginger.

PHYSICAL EVALUATION

Physical constants such as elasticity in fibres, viscosity of drugs containing gums, swelling factor of mucilage containing materials, froth number of saponin drugs, congealing point of volatile and fixed oils, melting and boiling points and water contents (loss on drying at 110°C) are some important parameters used in the evaluation of drugs. Ultraviolet light is also used for determining the fluorescence of extracts of some drugs (Gambir, Senna) and colours of alkaloids as : Aconite (light blue), berberine (yellow), emetine (orange) and quinine (dense fluorescence in dilute sulphuric acid). The florescence of Belladonna leaf and root, Wild Cherry bark and Jalap is due to the presence of a coumarin, β-methyl asculetin. Pale Catechu shows fluorescence in alkaline solution due to gambir-fluorescin. Aloe exhibits a green fluorescence in a solution containing borax. Many other drugs show a marked intensity of colours or a characteristic colour under UV light. Rhubarb is differentiated from Rhapontic, Chinese or Indian Rhubarb by its marked fluorescence in UV light.

Physical constants are extensively applied to the active principles of drugs, such as alkaloids, volatile oils and fixed oils. Solubility expresses number of ml of solvent require to dissolve one gram of the drug. For example, 1 g of codeine sulphate is soluble in 30 ml of water, and in 1300 ml of alcohol. Alkaloids and other nitrogenous compounds are soluble in dilute hydrochloric acid. Melting points are recorded for solid fixed oils (fats) and alkaloids.

According to WHO guidelines, the approximate solubility of medicinal plant materials should be determined at 20°C. Solubility is expressed in terms of "parts", representing the number of millilitres (ml) of the solvent, in which 1 g of the solid is soluble. Descriptive terms are sometimes used to indicate the solubility of a substance, with the following meanings :

Table 9.5. Solubility and terms and their meanings

Terms	Meaning
Very soluble	Less than 1 part
Freely soluble	1-10 parts
Soluble	10-30 parts
Sparingly soluble	30-100 parts
Slightly soluble	100-1000 parts
Very slightly soluble	1000-1000 parts
Practically insoluble	More than 10000 parts

Most of the monoterpenes have asymmetric carbons. Therefore, they are optical active. For example, Peppermint oil has optical rotation as –18° to –32°. Specific gravity is important with nutgalls. The galls that will not sink in water are considered to be inferior quality. In Jalap, the specific gravity should be higher than water. This constant is also important for volatile oils and fixed oils. It is in between 1.45-1.46 for Peppermint oil at 20 degree.

Spectrocopic analysis (UV, IR, NMR, Mass), and radioimmuno assays are applied more frequently to the active individual drugs components. Chromatographic techniques such as paper, column, thin-layer, gas-liquid (GLC) and high performance liquid chromatography (HPLC) provide information about the chemical constituents present in the drug.

The foreign organic (animal, animal excreta, insects, fungi, bacteria or mould) and inorganic matters should be in pharmacoepeal limits. They are determined by sedimentation or floatation method. If the drug is not prepared properly, the total ash value will be more.

BIOLOGICAL EVALUATION

The drugs, which cannot be assayed satisfactorily by chemical or physical means, are evaluated by biological methods. Tests are carried out on intact animals, animal preparations, isolated living tissues or micro-organisms. Since living organisms are used, the assays are called 'biological assays'. Biological standardization procedures are generally less precise, more time consuming and more expensive to conduct than chemical assays. Therefore, they are generally used if the chemical identity of the active principle has not been fully elucidated; if, no adequate chemical assay has been derived for the active principle as in case of insulin; if the drug is composed of complex mixture and activity, *e.g.*, Digitalis; if the purification of crude drug is not possible, *e.g.*, separation of vitamin D from irridiated oils; and if the chemical assay is not a valid indication of biological activity.

A biological assay measures the actual biological activity of a given sample. In any one test the animals of only one strain are used. For some assays a specific sex must be used. The male rat has faster growth rate than the female. Therefore, use of both male and female in a growth test should be avoided. Bioassays are conducted by determining the amount of a solution of unknown potency required to produce a definite effect on suitable test animals or organs under standard conditions. To minimize the source of errors resulting from animal variation, standard reference preparations are used in certain bioassay procedures.

Bacteria such as a *Salmonella typhi* and *Staphylococcus aureus* are used to determine antiseptic value of certain drugs. In another microbiological methods the living bacteria, yeast and molds are used for assaying vitamins and to determine the activity of antibiotic drugs. Mice are used to test Rabies vaccine, Diphtheria toxoid and other biologics. The 'rat line test' is utilized for the assay of vitamin D preparation. Guinea pigs are employed to test the toxicity and antigenicity of diagnostic Diphtheria toxin and tetanus toxoid. Oxytocic activity of vasopressin injection is also tested on guinea pigs. Oxytocic injection is assayed on young domestic chickens by injecting into an exposed crural or brachial vein and observing changes in blood pressure. Digitalis glycosides are assayed on pigeons by transfusing the drug through the alar vein into the blood stream and noting the lethal effects. Cats are utilized in tests for drugs with depressor activity and glucagon injection. Mydriatic drugs such as atropine are evaluated on cat's eye. Curare alkaloids, *e.g.*, tubocurarine chloride, and pyrogens in antibiotic solutions are assayed on rabbits. Ophthalmic preparations are tested on rabbit eyes. Dogs are the test animals to determine pressor activity in drugs and to assay Veratrum viride preparations. Anthelmintic drugs (Male fern) are evaluated on earthworms. Evaluation of Ergot is carried out on cock's comb or rabbit intestine or its uterus. Human beings are also used to note the activity of drugs in clinical trial.

There are some disadvantages of bioassays. Quantitative accuracy is usually less than observed with most chemical analyses. Techniques and interpretations involved vary with different oporators. The effect measured in the test animals is different from that observed in treating patients.

A simple bioassay utilizing brine shrimp (*Artemia salina*) is available for determining new biological activities in plant extracts. The eggs of this creature, which serve as food for tropical fish, are allowed to hatch in a brine solution. The shrimp are exposed to different concentrations of the test material and an IL_{50} (median lethan concentration) value in $\mu g/ml$ is calculated. A broad range of compound show toxic effect to the shrimp. The procedure is rapid, reliable and cheap. Another procedure, called potato-disc assay, involved observation of the inhibition of crown gall tumors induced on potato discs by *Agrobacterium tumefaciens* by plant extracts or isolated compounds. This method is used for detecting in preliminarily fashion anticancer activity.

CHAPTER 10

Quality Control and Standardization

World Health Organization currently encourages, recommends and promotes traditional herbal remedies in National Health Care Programmes because such drugs are easily available at low cost, are comparatively safe and the people have faith in such remedies. Plant materials and herbal remedies derived from them represent a substantial proportion of the global drug market and in this respect internationally recognized guidelines for their quality assessment are necessary. The WHO emphasizes the need to ensure quality control of medicinal plant products by using modern techniques and applying suitable standards.

For pharmaceutical purposes, the quality of medicinal plant material must be as high as that of other medicinal preparations. However, it is impossible to assay for a specific chemical entity when the bioactive ingredient is not known. In practice, assay procedures are not carried out even for those medicinal plant materials where there are known active ingredients. For example, Ginseng or Valerian is bought and sold on the basis of its sensory characters. For medicinal purposes Ginseng should be assayed for its ginsenoside content and Valerian for its valepotriates. Further problem is posed by those preparation which contain complex heterogenous mixtures.

Standardization problem arises from the complex composition of drugs which are used in the form of whole plant, parts of the plant(s) and of plant extracts. Standardization of the presumed active compounds of drug in general does not reflect reality. Only in few cases drug activity depends upon a single component. Generally, it is the result of combined activity of several active compounds and of inert accompanying substances. Though these inert component do not directly affect pathological mechanism, might influence bioavailability and excretions of the active component. Further, inert plant components may increase drug activity and the rate of side effects be minimized. If there are different active compounds present in a plant drug, they might have additive or potentiating effect.

As the material to be examined has complex and inconsistent composition, the analytical limits cannot be so precise as for the pure chemical compound. Vegetable drugs are inevitably "inconsistent" because their composition and, hence, their standardization, may be influenced by several factors such as age and origin, harvesting period, method of drying, storage conditions and so on. To eliminate some of the causes of inconsistency, one should use cultivated rather than wild plants which are often heterogenous in respect of the above factors and consequently in their content of active principles.

The purpose of standardizing traditional remedies is to ensure therapeutic efficacy. The Indian Council of Medical Research (ICMR) has adopted a disease oriented strategy for validating the claims of efficacy of traditional herbal remedies, and have initiated clinical trials of such drugs in the areas of anal fistula, bronchial asthma, viral hepatitis, urolithiasis, diabetes and filariasis.

A standardization centre should prepare protocols for the correct identification, botanical authentication right from the source of collection of the plant material, its drying, powdering, extraction, in-process quality control, preparation of formulation, standardization of the finished product, stability studies, packing and labelling for the preparation of standardized drugs for clinical trials at various hospitals in different parts of the country.

Due to availability of modern methods of analysis the quality control of plant drugs used in the allopathic system of medicine has become very well established. The standards relating to authenticity, general quality and purity, and the assay of active constituents are included in all the principal pharmacopoeias, e.g. *British Pharmacopoeia (BP)* and Addenda, the *European Pharmacopoeia (EP)*, the *United States Pharmacopoeia—The National Formulary (USP* XXII/NF XV; *India Pharmacopoea* and other official national publications.

However, the quality of many herbal drugs used by manufacturers or sold directly to the public is not so well established. At present the European legislation ensures that product licences are not efficacy and safety, there is the question of safeguarding the quality of the product. To meet this requirement, official reference monographs for individual drugs are required. These will give macroscopical and microscopical descriptions; tests for identity, chromatographic behaviour, foreign and exhausted material, microbial contamination, pesticide residues and radioactivity; an assay method for the active constituents is also desirable with stated acceptable limits for the drug. For those plant materials with long-established commercial use the compilation of such monographs is necessary. But it requires cooperation between the various bodies involves together with financial backing and dedicated scientists.

Germany, the largest user of herbal medicines in Europe, has produced about 200 monographs on herbal drugs and the *Chinese Pharmacopoeia* (1980) has monographs covering 509 drugs.

In India, two government organizations, e.g., Central Council for Research in Unani Medicine (CCRUM) and Central Council for Research in Ayurvedic Medicine (CCRAM) are working for quality control of plant drugs.

In herbal medicines, the maximum effectiveness of the drug derives from the whole drug or its crude extract rather than from isolated components. When an assay is lacking, it is important that the crude drug is properly authenticated, its general quality verified and all formulations of it are prepared in accordance with good manufacturing practice. Attention should also be paid to the shelf-life of the crude drug and its preparations. Official standards are necessary to control the quality of drugs.

There is a considerable variation that occurs between different batches of a natural product. It is necessary to set relatively low standards which allow the use of commercial material available in any season. This has resulted in the tendency for manufacturers to reduce all of their material to the lowest requirement. For example, in a good year the alkaloid-rich leaves of Belladonna herb may be used for the manufacture of galenicals and the residue of the herb, containing much stem, used to give the powdered drug. Similarly, high-quality volatile oils may be mixed with lower grades and still remain within official limits.

STANDARDIZATION OF CRUDE DRUGS

A number of standards can be applied to the quality control of crude drugs.

Authentication

The plant material collected from an appropriate region of the country at an appropriate stage of its growth is well authenticated by detailed taxonomical study and the correct botanical identity is established.

For bulky drugs a different method of sampling is required from that involving broken or powdered drugs.

According to WHO guidelines, medicinal plant materials are categorized according to sensory, macroscopic and microscopic characteristics. An examination to determine these characteristics is the first step towards establishing the identity and the degree of purity of such materials, and should be carried out before any further tests are undertaken.

Visual inspection provides the simplest and quickest means by which to establish identity, purity and, possibly, quality. If a sample is found to be significantly different, in terms of colour, consistency odour or taste, from the specifications, it is considered as not fulfilling the requirements.

Macroscopic identity of medicinal plant materials is based on shape, size, colour, surface characteristics, texture, fracture characteristics and appearance of the cut surface. It is often necessary to substantiate the findings by microscopy and/or physiochemical analysis.

Microscopic inspection of medicinal plant materials is indispensable for the identification of broken or powdered materials; the specimen may have to be treated with chemical reagents.

Comparison with a reference material will often reveal characteristics not described in the requirements which might otherwise have been attributed to foreign matter, rather than normal constituents.

Any additional useful information for preparation or analysis should also be included in the test procedures for individual plant materials, for example, the determination of vein-islets and the palisade ratio.

Wrinkled and contracted leaves, herbs or flowers should be softened and stretched flat. Certain fruits and seeds may also require softening before dissection and observation of internal characteristics.

A graduated ruler in millimetres is adequate for the measurement of the length, width and thickness of crude materials. Small seeds and fruits may be measured by aligning 10 of them on a sheet of calibrated paper, with 1 mm spacing between lines, and dividing the result by 10.

For determination of colour, examine the untreated sample under diffuse daylight. If necessary, an artificial light source with wavelengths similar to those of daylight may be used. The colour of the sample should be compared with that of a reference sample.

For surface characteristics, texture and fracture characteristics, examine the untreated sample. If necessary, a magnifying lens (6x to 10x) may be used. Wetting with water or reagents, as required, may be necessary to observe the characteristics of a cut surface. Touch the material to determine if it is soft or hard; bend and rupture it to obtain information on brittleness and the appearance of the fracture plane—whether it is fibrous, smooth, rough and granular.

Foreign matter

According to WHO guidelines, a foreign matter is material consisting of any or all of the following :

- parts of the medicinal plant material or materials other than those named with the limits specified for the plant material concerned;
- any organism, part or product of an organism, other than that named in the specification and description of the plant material concerned;
- mineral admixtures not adhering to the medicinal plant materials, such as soil, stones, sand, and dust.

Medicinal plant material should be entirely free from soil, stones, dust, insects and other animal contamination including animal excreta.

It is difficult to obtain vegetable drugs in an entirely pure condition. The pharmacopoeias contain statements as to the percentage of other parts of the plant or of other organic matter which may be permitted. Drugs containing appreciable quantities of potent foreign matter, animal excreta, insects or mould should be rejected even though the percentage of such substances be insufficient to cause the rejection of the drug on the percentage of foreign matter.

A weighed quantity (100-500 g), of a drugs sample is spread in a thin layer on paper. It is examined as ×6 magnification and the foreign matter is picked out, weighed and the percentage recorded.

During storage, products should be kept in a clean and hygienic place, so that no contamination occurs. Special care should be taken to avoid formation of moulds, since they may produce aflatoxins.

Macroscopic examination can conveniently be employed for determining the presence of foreign matter in whole or cut plant materials.

ORGANOLEPTIC EVALUATION

Organoleptic examination refers to evaluation by means of organs of sense and includes the macroscopic appearance of the drug, its odour and tastes, occasionally the sound or "snap" of its fracture and the feel of the drug to the touch.

The macroscopical and sensory characters are used to identify a drug. The general appearance of the sample indicates whether it is likely to comply with such standards as percentage of seed in Colocynth, of ash in Valerian or of matter insoluble in alcohol in Asafoetida. Drugs may comply with the descriptions given in the pharmacopoeias. It is difficult to describe deterioration of drugs owing to faulty harvesting, shipment or storage or deterioration due to age. In such cases the trained worker will be able to identify the sample from its appearance. The following examples will serve to indicate the type of evidence to look for.

For determining odour, an innocuous material is placed in the palm of the hand or a beaker of suitable size, and slowly and repeatedly inhaled the air over the material. If no distinct odour is perceptible, crush the sample between the thumb and index finger or between the palms of the hands using gentle pressure. If the material is known to be dangerous, crush by mechanical means and then pour a small quantity of boiling water onto the crushed sample in a beaker. First, determine the strength of the odour (none, weak, distinct, strong) and then the odour sensation (aromatic, fruity, musty, mouldy, rancid, etc.). A direct comparison of the colour with a defined substance is advisable (e.g., peppermint should have an odour similar to menthol, cloves an odour similar to eugenol).

If leaves are packed before being properly dried, much discoloured material may be found in the middle of the packet. Overdrying makes leaves very brittle and causes them to break in transit. If starch-containing drugs break with a horny fracture, it may be inferred that the temperature of drying has been very high and that the starch has been gelatinized. A pale colour of chamomiles indicates that the drug has been collected in dry weather and carefully dried. The colour of the fractured surface of gentian shows that it has been correctly fermented. Some drugs are deteriorated during shipment or storage,

and become damp (*e.g.*, Cascara). Under moist conditions moulds are readily attacked themselves on drugs having a high mucilage content (*e.g.*, Psyllium, Linseed, Squill and Cydonia).

The price of some drugs depends on factors as size and colour, which are not necessarily related to therapeutic value, e.g., Senna leaflets, Senna pods, Chamomile flowers, Ginger, Nutmegs, Rhubarb and Capsicum.

MICROSCOPICAL EXAMINATION

Microscopical examination of the plant drugs is essential to the study of adulterants and for the correct identification. Different sections of the drug, *e.g.*, T.S. and L.S., vein termination number, stomatal index, vein islet number, pallisade ratio and characters of powdered samples are studied under microscope and compared with the literature values.

According to WHO guidelines, the coarseness or fineness of a powder is classed according to the nominal aperture size expressed in μm of the mesh of the sieve through which the powder will pass, and is indicated as follows :

Table 10.1. Powder size and particle character

Powder	Particle character
In coarse (2000/355)	All the particles will pass through a No. 2000 sieve, and not more than 40% through a No. 355 sieve
In moderately coarse (710/250)	All the particles will pass through a No. 710 sieve, and not more than 40% through a No. 250 sieve
In moderately fine (355/180)	All the particles will pass through a No. 355 sieve, and not more than 40% through a No. 180 sieve
In fine powders (180)	All the particles will pass through a No. 180 sieve
In very fine powders (125)	All the particles will pass through a No. 125 sieve

Powdered drugs or adulterants which contain a constant number, area or length of characteristic particles/mg (*e.g.*, starch grains, epidermis and trichome ribs) can be determined quantitatively by microscopy using lycopodium spores as an indicator diluent.

Crude fibre

The preparation of a crude fibre is required for resistant cellular material of drugs for microscopical examination. It is useful for rhizomes such as Ginger which contain large amounts of oleoresin and starch. The technique involves defatting the powder (2 g) and then boiling with a standard 0.12 M of sulphuric acid and 0.313 M sodium hydroxide solution and with suitable washing of the insoluble residue obtained at the different stages. The crude fibre so obtained can also be used quantitatively to assay the fibre content of foods and animal feedstuffs and also to detect excess of certain materials in powdered drugs, *e.g.*, clove stalk in Clove.

An apparatus (Fibertec M) for a less laborious determination of crude fibre involves integral extraction and filtration with no sample transfer, thus eliminating loss of sample as in the older filtration methods. Up to six samples can be processed simultaneously.

VOLATILE MATTER

Volatile oils are characterized by their odour, oil-like appearance and ability to volatilize at room temperature. Chemically, they are usually composed of mixture of monoterpenes, sesquiterpenes and their oxygenated derivatives. Aromatic compounds predominate in certain volatile oils.

They are considered to be the "essence" of the plant material, and biologically active, they are also known as "essential oils".

In order to determine the volume of oil, the plant material is distilled with water and the distillate is collected in a graduated tube. The aqueous portion separates automatically and is returned to the distillation flask. If the volatile oils possess a mass density higher than or near to that of water, or are difficult to separate from the aqueous phase owing to the formation of emulsions, a solvent with a low mass density and a suitable boiling-point may be added to the measuring tube. The dissolved volatile oils will then float on top of the aqueous phase.

Minimum standards for the percentage of volatile oil present in a number of drugs are mentioned in many pharmacopoeias. The weighed drug is placed in a distillation flask with water or a mixture of water and glycerin and connected Clavenger apparatus. On distillation, the oil and water condense and the volatile oil which collects in the graduated receiver as a layer on top of the water is measured. For oils with relative densities around or greater than 1.0, separation from the water is assisted by placing a known volume of xylene in the receiver and reading off the combined oil and xylene. Alternatively, for oils with relative densities greater than water (*e.g.*, Clove oil, 1.05), a receiver similar for the determination of water in crude drugs can be used without addition of xylene.

The time taken to complete the distillation of the oil varies with the nature of the drug and its state of comminution but about 4 h is usually sufficient. Solution of the volatile oil in a fixed oil (e.g. in powdered fruits of the Apiaceae may retard distillation. The pharmacopoeial standards for volatile oil contents of powdered drugs are lower than those for the corresponding whole drugs.

SWELLING INDEX

Many medicinal plant materials are of specific therapeutic or pharmaceutical utility because of their swelling properties, especially gums and those containing an appreciable amount of mucilage, pectin or hemicellulose.

This is defined as the volume in millilitres occupied by 1 g of a drug, including any adhering mucilage, after it has swollen in an aqueous liquid for 4 h. The drug is treated with 1.0 ml ethanol (96%) and 25 ml water in a graduated cylinder, shaken every 10 min for 1 h and allowed to stand as specified. The standard is applicable to those drugs containing mucilage and is official for Agar ($\geq$10), Linseed ($\geq$4) and Plantago ($\geq$10).

ASH VALUE

The presence of ash in medicinal plant materials is determined as total ash, acid insoluble ash and sulphated ash. When vegetable drugs are incinerated, they leave an inorganic ash which in the case of many drugs varies within fairly wide limits and these values are of significance for the purpose of plant drug evaluation. This includes both "physiological ash", which is derived from the plant tissue itself, and "non-physiological" ash, which is the residue of the extraneous matter (*e.g.* sand and soil) adhering to the plant surface.

Acid-insoluble ash is the residue obtained after boiling the total ash with dilute hydrochloric acid, and igniting the remaining insoluble matter. This measures the amount of silica present, especially as sand and siliceous earth.

Water-soluble ash is the difference in weight between the total ash and the residue after treatment of the total ash with water.

In some drugs (e.g., Rhubarb) it varies within wide limits and is, therefore, of little value for purposes of evaluation. In other cases (e.g., Liquorice), the *total ash* figure is of importance. In the determination of total ash values the carbon must be removed at low temperature (450°C). Alkali chlorides, which may be volatile at high temperatures, would be lost. If carbon is still present after heating at a moderate temperature, the water-soluble ash may be separated and the residue again ignited or the ash may be broken up, with the addition of alcohol, and again ignited. The total ash usually consists mainly of carbonates, phosphates, silicates and silica. To produce a more consistent ash a *sulphated ash* is produced by treatment of the drug with dilute sulphuric acid before ignition. In this all oxides and carbonates are converted to sulphates and the ignition is carried out at a higher temperature (600°C).

If the total ash be treated with dilute hydrochloric acid, the percentage of *acid-insoluble ash* may be determined. This consists mainly of silica, and a high acid-insoluble ash in drugs such as Senna, Cloves, Liquorice, Valerian and Tragacanth indicates contamination with earthy material. Senna leaf has a low acid-insoluble ash (2.5%); hyoscyamus has a higher value (12%). For Ginger a minimum percentage of *water-soluble ash* is demanded for detecting the presence of exhausted ginger.

Determination of total ash

Place about 2-4 g of the ground air-dried material, accurately weighed, in a previously ignited and tared crucible (usually of platinum or silica). Spread the material in an even layer and ignite it by gradually increasing the heat to 500-600°C until it is white, indicating the absence of carbon. Cool in a desiccator and weigh. If carbon-free ash cannot be obtained in this manner, cool the crucible and moisten the residue with about 2 ml of water or a saturated solution of ammonium nitrate. Dry on a water-bath, then on a hot-plate and ignite to constant weight. Allow the residue to cool in a suitable desiccator for 30 minutes, then weigh without delay. Calculate the content of total ash in mg per g of air-dried material.

Acid-insoluble ash

To the crucible containing the total ash, add 25 ml of hydrochloride (~70 g/l), cover with a watch-glass and boil gently for 5 minutes. Rinse the watch-glass with 5 ml of hot water and add this liquid to the crucible. Collect the insoluble matter on an ashless filter-paper and wash with hot water until the filtrate is neutral. Transfer the filter-paper containing the insoluble matter to the original crucible, dry on a hot-plate and ignite to a constant weight. Allow the residue to cool in a suitable desiccator for 30 minutes, then weigh without delay. Calculate the content of acid-insoluble ash in mg per g of air-dried material.

Water-soluble ash

To the crucible containing the total ash, add 25 ml of water and boil for 5 minutes. Collect the insoluble matter in a sintered-glass crucible or on an ashless filter-paper. Wash with hot and ignite in a crucible for 15 minutes at a temperature not exceeding 450°C. Subtract the weight of this residue in mg from the weight of total ash. Calculate the content of water-soluble ash in mg per g of air-dried material.

MOISTURE CONTENT

Some drugs (e.g., aloes, gelatin, gums) contain excess water. At suitable temperature, moisture activates enzymes and produces suitable conditions to the development of living organisms. As most vegetable drugs contain all the essential food requirements for moulds, insects and mites, deterioration can be very rapid.

Limits for water content should, therefore, be set for every given plant material. This is especially important for material that absorb moisture easily or deteriorate quickly in the presence of water.

The *azeotropic method* gives a direct measurement of the water present in the material being examined. When the sample is distilled together with an immiscible solvent, such as toluene or xylene, the water present in the sample is absorbed by the solvent. The water and the solvent are distilled together and separated in the receiving tube on cooling. If the solvent is anhydrous, water may remain absorbed in it leading to false results. It is therefore, advisable to saturate the solvent with water before use.

Loss of drying

The loss in weight in the samples is mainly due to water and small amounts of other volatile materials. For materials (digitalis, starch, aloes, fibres), which contain some volatile material, direct drying (105°C) to constant weight can be used. The moisture balance combines both the drying process and weight recordings. It is suitable where large number of samples are handled and where a continuous record of loss in weight with time is required. For materials such as balsams which contain a large proportion of volatile material, the drying may be done by spreading thin layers of the weighed drug over glass plates and placing in a desiccator over phosphorus pentoxide. Vacuum drying over an absorbent at a specified, temperature may be carried out.

Preparation of material

Prepare a suitable quantity of the sample by cutting, granulating or shredding the unground or unpowdered material, so that the thickness of the parts does not exceed 3 mm. Seeds of fruits smaller than 3 mm should be cracked. Avoid the use of high-speed mills in preparing the sample, and take care that no appreciable amount of moisture is lost during preparation. It is important that the portion is large enough to be a representative sample.

Azeotropic method (Toluene distillation)

The apparatus consists of a glass flask connected by a tube to a cylindrical tube fitted with a graduated receiving tube and a reflux condenser. The receiving tube is graduated in 0.1 ml divisions so that the error of readings does not exceed 0.05 ml. The preferred source of heat is an electric heater with a rheostat control, or an oil-bath. The upper portion of the flask and the connecting tube may be insulated.

Thoroughly clean the receiving tube and the condenser of the apparatus, rinse with water and dry. Introduce 200 ml of toluene and about 2 ml of water into a dry flask. Heat the flask to distil the liquid over a period of 2 hours, allow to cool for about 30 minutes and read off the volume of water to an accuracy of 0.05 ml (first distillation).

Weigh accurately a quantity of the material expected to give about 2-3 ml of water and transfer to the flask. Add a few pieces of porous porcelain and heat the flask gently for 15 minutes. When boiling begins, distil at a rate of 2 drops per second until most of the water has distilled over, then increase the rate of distillation to about 4 drops per second. As soon as the water has been completely distilled, rinse the inside of the condenser tube with toluene. Continue the distillation for 5 more minutes, remove the heat, allow the receiving tube to cool to room temperature and dislodge any droplets of water adhering to the walls of the receiving tube by tapping the tube. Allow the water and toluene layers to separate and read off the volume of water (second distillation). Calculate the content of water as a percentage using the formula :

$$\frac{100(n_1 - n)}{w}$$

where w = the weight in g of the material being examined.

n = the number of ml of water obtained in the first distillation

n_1 = the total number of ml of water obtained in both distillations

Loss on drying (Gravimetric determination)

Place about 2-5 g of the prepared air-dried material, or the quantity specified in the test procedure for the plant material concerned, accurately weighed, in a previously dried and tared flat weighing bottle. Dry the sample by one of the following techniques :

– in an oven at 100-105°C;

– in a desiccator over phosphorus pentoxide under atmospheric pressure or reduced pressure and at room temperature.

Dry until two consecutive weightings do not differ by more than 5 mg, unless otherwise specified in the test procedure. Calculate the loss of weight in mg per g of air-dried material.

Separation and measurement of moisture

The determination of water is carried out by separating and evaluating the water obtained from a sample. This can be achieved by passing a dry inert gas through the heated sample and using an absorption material (specific for water) to collect the water carried forward. Such methods can be extremely accurate, as applied for the determination of hydrogen in organic compounds by combustion analysis.

Methods based on distillation are used for moisture determination. The sample to be analysed is placed in a flask together with a suitable water-saturated immiscible solvent (toluene, xylene, carbon tetrachloride) and pieces of porous pot and is distilled. The water in the sample has a sufficient partial pressure and co-distils with the solvent, condensing in the distillate as an immiscible layer. A simple apparatus devised by Dean and Stark permits the direct measurement of the water obtained and the less dense solvent (toluene, xylene) is continuously returned to the distillation flask.

To determine the loss of water due to solubility in the solvent a preliminary distillation of the solvent with added water (about 2 ml) is carried out; the exact volume of water separating as a layer is measured and then the drug added to the flask and distillation resumed. Water separated from the drug is calculated from the combined final volume. The method is applicable to crude drugs and food materials. It has the disadvantage that relatively large quantities of the sample (5-10 g) may be required.

Gas-chromatographic methods are widely used for moisture determination due to their specificity and efficiency. The water in the weighed, powdered sample can be extracted with dry methanol and the extract is submitted to chromatography on a column on either 10% carbowax on Fluoropak 80 or Porapak, a commercial polymer suitable for GLC. The water separated by this means is determined from the resulting chromatogram. Teflon-6 coated with 10% polyethylene glycol 1500, with n-propanol

as an internal standard is also used for the determination of moisture in crude drugs.

Chemical method for measurement of moisture

Karl Fischer method is a chemical method used for water determination in the pharmaceutical, food, chemical and petrochemical industries. It is applicable for expensive drugs and chemicals containing small quantities of moisture. Dry extracts of alkaloid-containing drugs, alginic acid, alginates and fixed oils for parenteral use may be evaluated. For crude drugs such as Digitalis and Ipecacuanha the powdered material can first be exhausted of water with a suitable anhydrous solvent (dioxan) and the extract is taken for titration.

The reagent consists of a solution of iodine, sulphur dioxide and pyridine in dry methanol. This is titrated against a sample containing water, which causes a loss of the dark brown colour when no water is available at the end-point. The basic reaction is a reduction of iodine by sulphur dioxide in the presence of water. The reaction is completed by the removal of sulphur trioxide as pyridine sulphur trioxide, which in turns reacts with the methanol to form the pyridine salt of methyl sulphate.

$$H_2O + I_2 + SO_2 \rightleftharpoons 2HI + SO_3$$

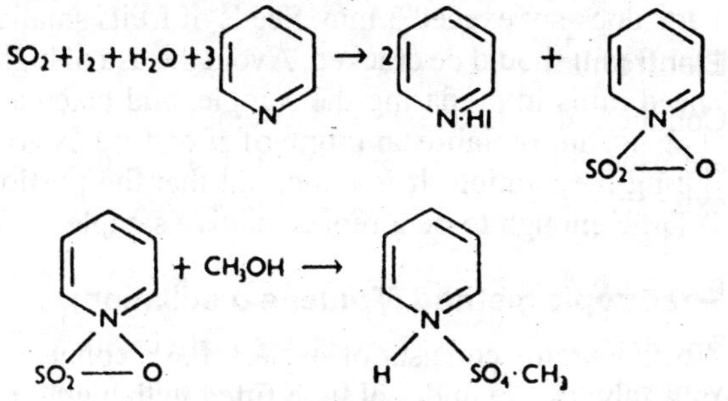

Fig. 10.1. Karl Fischer reaction.

In the absence of methanol, the pyridine sulphur trioxide reacts with another molecule of water. The reagent should be standardized immediately before use and this can be done by using of a standard solution of water in methanol or by use of a hydrated salt, *e.g.*, sodium tartrate ($Na_2C_4H_4O_62H_2O$). The titration is carried out under an atmosphere of dry nitrogen to eliminate interference from atmospheric moisture. The end-point is recorded amperometrically. Equipment is now available for a completely automated determination in which sample handling and weighing, introduction to the Karl Fischer cell, titration and data completion are done automatically.

The instability of the the reagent and the possibility of substances in the sample, other than water, which may react with the reagent, are the main drawbacks of the Karl Fischer method.

Other chemical methods for water determination include treating the sample with various carbides, nitrides and hydrides and measuring the gas evolved. The liberated gas is analyzed by gas chromatography.

Spectroscopic method

Water absorbs energy at various wavelengths throughout the electromagnetic spectrum and on this basis it can be determined quantitatively. Measurements can be made in both the infrared and ultraviolet regions suitable for very small quantities of water in drugs and gases. Nuclear magnetic resonance (NMR) spectroscopy is used for the determination of moisture in starch, cotton and other plant products.

Electrometric method

Conductivity, dielectric and coulometric methods are used for estimation of water but are not used extensively for pharmaceutical products.

EXTRACTIVE VALUES

The determination of extractable matter with a solvent refers to the amount of constituents in a given amount of medicinal plant material. Such extractive values proved an indication of the extent of polar, medium polar and non-polar components present in the drug.

As suitable assays become available (e.g., with

the anthraquinone-containing drugs), the extractive tests are no longer required as pharmacopoeial standards. In some cases extraction of the drug is by maceration by a continuous extraction process. The Soxhlet extractor is useful to prepare extractives. In this apparatus extraction is by boiling solvent followed by percolation; finally, evaporation yields the extract and the recovered solvent ready for the next sample.

Method 1 : Hot extraction

Place about 4.0 g of coarsely powdered air-dried material, accurately weighed, in a glass-stoppered conical flask. Add 100 ml of water and weigh to obtain the total weight including the flask. Shake well and allow to stand for 1 hour. Attach a reflux condenser to the flask and boil gently for 1 hour; cool and weigh. Readjust to the original total weight with the solvent specified in the test procedure for the plant material concerned. Shake well and filter rapidly through a dry filter. Transfer 25 ml of the filtrate to a tared flat-bottomed dish and evaporate to dryness on a water-bath. Dry at 105°C for 6 hours, cool in a desiccator for 30 minutes, then weigh without delay. Calculate the content of extractable matter in mg per g of air-dried material.

Method 2 : Cold maceration

Place about 4.0 g of coarsely powdered air-dried material, accurately weighed, in a glass-stoppered conical flask. Macerate with 100 ml of the solvent specified for the plant material concerned for 6 hours, shaking frequently, then allow to stand for 18 hours. Filter rapidly taking care not to lose any solvent, transfer 25 ml of the filtrate to a tared flat-bottomed dish and evaporate to dryness on a water-bath. Dry at 105°C for 6 hours, cool in a desiccator for 30 minutes and weigh without delay. Calculate the content of extractable matter in mg per g of air-dried material.

For ethanol-soluble extractable matter, use the concentration of solvent specified in the test procedure for the plant material concerned; for water-soluble extractable matter, use water as the solvent. Use other solvents as specified in the test procedure.

Table 10.2. Extractives used for drug evaluation

Drug	Method of evaluation
Benzoin, Catechu and Tolu balsam	Limits of ethanol-insoluble matter
Colocynth	Limit of light petroleum extractive
Gentian and Glycyrrhiza	Percentage of water-soluble extractive
Ginger, Ipomoea and Jalap	Percentage of ethanol (90%) extractive
Linseed powder	Percentage of ether-soluble extractive
Quillaia	Percentage of ethanol (45%) extractive
Valerian	Percentage of ethanol (60%) extractive

Chromatographic profile and marker component

Thin layer chromatography (TLC) is widely adopted for the rapid and positive analysis of plant drugs. TLC provides semi-quantitative information about the chief constituents of the plant drug and, thus, enables an assessment of drug quality. Furthermore, TLC provides drug finger print. It is suitable for monitoring the identity and purity of drugs, and for detection of adulteration and substitution. TLC-densitometer scanner is used for obtaining finger print profile of extracts of many drugs. High Performance Liquid Chromatography (HPLC) is used to plant drugs like *Andrographis paniculata* where hepatoprotective bioactive compound andrographolide is known and the same has been quantitatively estimated. A reverse phase HPLC method of estimating vasicine, the major bioactive alkaloid of *Adhatoda vasica*, has been employed to standardize two polyherbal formulations used for the treatment of bronchial asthma in Ayurvedic system of medicine.

Pharmacopoeias are using thin-layer chromatography as a means for assessing quality and purity of herbal drugs.

The R_F value (rate of flow, *i.e.*, distance moved by solute divided by distance moved by solvent front) of a compound, determined under specific conditions, is characteristic and can be used as an aid to identity. $R_F (R_F \times 100)$ values are in the range 0-100. Quantitative extracts of crude drugs are prepared and compared chromatographically with standard reference solutions of the known constituents. Intensities of the visualized chromatographic spots can be visually compared and the method can be used to eliminate inferior or adulterated drugs. In this way semiquantitative tests for the principles of drugs (Peppermint, Saffron, German Chamomile, Digitalis) are rapidly evaluated.

Gas chromatographic retention times and peak areas can be used for the examination of volatile oils and other mixtures.

MICROBIAL CONTAMINATION

Medicinal plant materials normally carry a great number of bacteria and moulds, often of soil origin. With natural bacteria and fungi of herbs, aerobic spore forming bacteria frequently predominate. Current practice of harvesting, handling and production often causes additional contamination and microbial growth. The determination of *E. coli* and mould may indicate good production and harvesting practices. In addition, the presence of aflatoxin in plant material can cause health hazards if absorbed even in very small amounts. Therefore, they should be determined after using a suitable clean-up procedure.

A number of drugs (e.g., Acacia, Agar, powdered Digitalis, etc.) should be free of *Escherichia coli* in the quantity of material stated; others (e.g., Alginic acid, Cochineal, Tragacanth) are also tested for the absence of *Salmonella*. There is a limit for total viable aerobic count, *e.g.*, for Acacia 10^4 micro-organisms g^{-1}. Generally, manufacturers will ensure that, for crude drugs to be taken internally, the limits for bacterial and mould contamination as applied to foodstuffs are adhered to. The drugs are sterilized in special equipment by treatment with ethylene oxide.

About 24% crude drug samples are contaminated at the level of 10,000 organisms g^{-1}, which is above the FIP requirements for non-sterile pharmaceutical preparations. From 50 crude drugs, 74 *Aspergillus* and 28 *Penicillium* strains are isolated; other common genera are *Mucor*, *Rhizopus* and *Thamnidium*.

Moulds may produce strongly toxic substances in the crude drug and herbal preparations. They may be the embryotoxic, teratogenic, mutagenic and carcinogenic substances as produced by some species in peanuts, corn, wheat and rice. The roots (e.g., *Acorus calamus, Picrorrhiza kurroa*) and seeds (Neem and *Datura*) stored under traditional storage conditions in India develop unacceptable levels of mycotoxins, principally aflatoxin B. By the use of mass spectrometry, mycotoxins in food products such as cereals, oil seeds and milk are regularly determined at levels of one part per billion and below.

Test for specific microorganism

The conditions of the test for microbial contamination are designed to minimize accidental contamination of the material being examined; the precautions taken must not adversely affect any microorganisms that could be revealed.

Procedure

Pretreatment of the material being examined

Depending on the nature of the crude medicinal plant material, grind, dissolve, dilute, suspend or emulsify the material being examined using a suitable method and eliminate any antimicrobial properties by dilution, neutralization or filtration.

Water-soluble materials

Dissolve or dilute 10 g or 10 ml of plant material, unless otherwise specified in the test procedure for the material concerned, in lactose broth or another suitable medium proven to have no antimicrobial activity under the conditions of the test, adjust the volume to 100 ml with the same medium. (Some materials may require the use of a large volume). If necessary, adjust the pH of the suspension to about 7.

Non-fatty materials insoluble in water

Suspend 10 g or 10 ml of material, unless otherwise specified in the test procedure for the material concerned, in lactose broth or another suitable medium proven to have no microbial activity under the conditions of the test; dilute to 100 ml with same me-

dium. (Some materials may require the use of a larger volume). If necessary, divide the material being examined and homogenize the suspension mechanically. A suitable surfactant, such as a solution of polysorbate 80 containing 1 mg per ml may be added. If necessary, adjust the pH of the suspension to about 7.

Fatty materials

Homogenize 10 g or 10 ml of material, unless otherwise specified in the test procedure for the material concerned, with 5 g of polysorbare 20R or polysorbate 80R. If necessary, heat to not more than 40°C. (Occasionally, it may be necessary to heat to a temperature of up to 45°C, for the shortest possible time). Mix carefully while maintaining the temperature in a water-bath or oven. Add 85 ml of lactose broth or another suitable medium proven to have no antimicrobial activity in the conditions of the test, heated to not more than 40°C, if necessary. Maintain this temperature for the shortest time necessary until an emulsion is formed and, in any case, for not more than 30 minutes. If necessary, adjust the pH of the emulsion to about 7.

Enterobacteriaceae and certain other Gram-negative bacteria

Detection of bacteria

Homogenize the pretreated material appropriately and incubate at 30-37°C for a length of time sufficient for revivification of the bacteria but not sufficient for multiplication of the organisms (usually 2-5 hours). Shake the container, transfer 1 g or 1 ml of the homogenized material to 100 ml of enterobacteriaceae enrichment broth-Mossel and incubate at 35-37°C for 18-48 hours. Prepare a subculture on a plate with violet-red bile agar with glucose and lactose. Incubate at 35-37°C for 18-48 hours. The material passes the test if no growth of colonies of Gram-negative bacteria is detected on the plate.

Quantitative evaluation

Inoculate a suitable amount of Enterobacteriaceae enrichment broth-Mossel with quantities of homogenized material prepared, appropriately diluted as necessary, containing 1.0 g, 0.1 g and 10 µg, or 1.0

ml, 0.1 ml and 10 µl, of the material being examined. Incubate at 35-37°C for 24-48 hours. Prepare a subculture of each of the cultures on a plate with violet-red bile agar with glucose and lactose in order to obtain selective isolation. Incubate at 35-37°C for 18-24 hours. The growth of well-developed colonies, generally red or reddish in colour, of Gram-negative bacteria constitutes a positive result. Note the smallest quantity of material that gives a positive result. Determine the probable number of bacteria.

Escherichia coli

Transfer a quantity of the homogenized material in lactose broth, prepared and incubated and containing 1 g or 1 ml of the material being examined, to 100 ml of Mac-Conkey broth and incubate at 43-45°C for 18-24 hours.

Prepare a subculture on a plate with Mac-Conkey agar and incubate at 43-45°C for 18-24 hours. Growth of red, generally non-mucoid colonies of Gram-negative rods, sometimes surrounded by a reddish zone of precipitation, indicates the possible presence of *E. coli*. This may be confirmed by the formation of indole at 43.5-44.5°C or by other biochemical reactions. The material passes the test if no such colonies are detected or if the confirmatory biochemical reactions are negative.

Salmonella species

Incubate the solution, suspension or emulsion of the pretreated material prepared at 35-37°C for 5-24 hours, as appropriate for enrichment.

Primary test

Transfer 10 ml of the enrichment culture to 100 ml of tetrathionate bile brilliant green broth and incubate at 42-43°C for 18-24 hours. Prepare subcultures on at least two of the following three agar media: deoxycholate citrate agar; xylose, lysine, deoxycholate agar; and brilliant green agar. Incubate at 35-37°C for 24-48 hours. Carry out the secondary test, if any, colonies are produced that conform to the description.

Secondary test

Prepare a subculture of any colonies showing the characteristics of triple sugar agar using the deep inoculation technique. This can be achieved by first inoculation the inclined surface of the culture medium followed by a stab culture with the same inoculating needle and incubating at 35-37°C for 18-24 hours. The test is positive for the presence of *Salmonella* spp. if a change of colour from red to yellow is observed in the deep culture (but not in the surface culture), usually with the formation of gas with or without production of hydrogen sulfide in the agar. Confirmation is obtained by appropriate biochemical and serological tests.

The material being examined passes the test if cultures of the type do not appear in the primary test, or if the confirmatory biochemical and serological tests in the secondary test are negative.

Pseudomonas aeruginosa

Pretreat the material being examined using buffered sodium chloride-peptone solution, pH 7.0, or another suitable medium shown not to have antimicrobial activity under the conditions of the test, in place of lactose broth. Inoculate 100 ml of soybean-casein digest medium with a quantity of the solution, suspension or emulsion thus obtained containing 1 g or 1 ml of the material being examined. Mix and incubate at 35-37°C for 24-48 hours. Prepare a subculture on a plate of cetrimide agar and incubate at 35-37°C for 24-48 hours. If no growth of microorganisms is detected, the material passes the test. If growth of colonies of Gram-negative rods occurs, usually with a greenish fluorescence, apply an oxidase test and test the growth or soybean-casein digest medium at 42°C. The following method may be used. Place 2 or 3 drops of a freshly prepared 0.01 g/ml solution of N, N, N', N'-tetramethyl-*p*-phenylenediamine dihydrochloride R on filter-paper and apply a smear of the suspected colony; the test is positive if a purple colour is produced within 5-10 seconds. The material passes the test if cultures of the type described do not appear or if the confirmatory biochemical test is negative.

Staphylococcus aureus

Prepare an enrichment culture as described for *Pseudomonas aeruginosa*. Prepare a subculture on a suitable medium such as Baird-Parker agar. Incubate at 35-37°C for 24-48 hours. The material passes the test if no growth of microorganisms is detected. Blank colonies of Gram-positive cocci often surrounded by clear zones may indicate the presence of *Staphylococcus aureus*. For catalase-positive cocci, confirmation may be obtained, for example, by coagulase and deoxyribonuclease tests. The material passes the test if cultures of the type described do not appear or if the confirmatory biochemical test is negative.

Validation of tests for specific microorganisms

If necessary, grow separately the test strains listed on the culture media indicated at 30-35°C for 18-24 hours. Dilute portions of each of the cultures using buffered sodium chloride-peptone solution pH 7.0 so that the test suspensions contains about 10^3 microorganisms per ml. Mix equal volumes of each suspension and use 0.4 ml (approximately 10^2 microorganisms of each strain) as an inoculum in tests for *Escherichia coli*, *Salmonella* species, *Pseudomonas aeruginosa* and *Staphylococcus aureus*, in the presence and absence of the material being examined, if necessary. The test method should give a positive result for the respective strain of microorganism.

Total viable aerobic count

The total viable aerobic count of the material being examined is determined, as specified in the test procedure, for the plant material concerned using one of the following methods: membrane-filtration, plate count or serial dilution.

Pretreatment of the material being examined

Pretreat the material as described in the "Test for specific microorganisms", but in place of lactose broth use buffered sodium chloride-peptone solution pH 7.0, or another suitable medium shown not to have antimicrobial activity under the conditions of the test.

Membrane filtration

Use membrane filters with a nominal pore size of not greater than 0.45 μm, the effectiveness of which in retaining bacteria has been established. For example, cellulose nitrate filters are used for aqueous, oily and weakly alcoholic solutions, and cellulose acetate filters for strongly alcoholic solutions. The technique described uses filter discs of about 50 mm in diameter. For filters of a different diameter, adjust the volumes of the dilutions and washings accordingly. Sterilize the filtration apparatus and the membrane by appropriate means. They are designed to permit the solution being examined to be introduced and filtered under aseptic conditions, and the membrane to be transferred to the culture medium.

Transfer 10 ml or a solution containing 1 g of the material to each of two membrane filters and filter immediately. If necessary, dilute the pretreated material to obtain an expected colony count of 10-100. Wash each membrane, filtering three or more successive quantities of approximately 100 ml of a suitable liquid such as buffered sodium chloride-peptone solution, pH 7.0. For fatty materials, a suitable surfactant may be added, such as polysorbate 20R or polysorbate 80R. Transfer one of the membrane filters, intended primarily for the enumeration of bacteria, to the surface of a plate with casein-soybean digest agar and the other, intended primarily for the enumeration of fungi, to the surface of a plate with Sabouraud glucose agar with antibiotics. Incubate the plates for 5 days, unless a more reliable count can be obtained otherwise, at 30-35°C for the detection of bacteria and at 20-25°C for the detection of fungi. Count the number of colonies formed. Calculate the number of microorganisms per g or per ml of the material tested, if necessary, counting bacteria and fungi separately.

Plate count

For bacteria : Use Petri dishes 9-10 cm in diameter. To one dish add a mixture of 1 ml of the pretreated material and about 15 ml of liquefied casein–soybean digest agar at a temperature not exceeding 45°C. Alternatively, spread the pretreated material on the surface of the solidified medium in a Petri dish. If necessary, dilute the pretreated material as described above to obtain an expected colony count of not more than 300. Prepare at least two dishes using the same dilution and incubate them at 30-35°C for 5 days, unless a more reliable count is obtained in a shorter period of time. Count the number of colonies formed and calculate the results using the plate with the largest number of colonies, up to a maximum of 300.

For fungi : Use Petri dishes 9-10 cm in diameter. To one dish add a mixture of 1 ml of the pretreated material and about 15 ml of liquefied Sabouraud glucose agar with antibiotics at a temperature not exceeding 45°C. Alternatively, spread the pretreated material on the surface of the solidified medium in a Petri dish. If necessary, dilute the pretreated material as described above to obtain an expected colony count of not more than 100. Prepare at least two dishes using the same dilution and incubate them at 20-25°C for 5 days, unless a more reliable count is obtained in a shorter period of time. Count the number of colonies formed and calculate the results using the dish with not more than 100 colonies.

Serial dilution

Prepare a series of 12 tubes each containing 9-10 ml of soybean-casein digest medium. To each of the first three tubes add 1 ml of the 1 : 10 dilution of dissolved, homogenized material prepared. To the next three tubes add 1 ml of a 1 : 100 dilution of the material and to the next three tubes add 1 ml of a 1: 1000 dilution of the material. To the last three tubes add 1 ml of the diluent. Incubate the tubes at 30-35°C for at least 5 days. No microbial growth should appear in the last three tubes. If the reading of the results is difficult or uncertain owing to the nature of the material being examined, prepare a subculture in a liquid or a solid medium, and evaluate the results after a further period of incubation. Determine the most probable number of microorganisms per g or ml of the material.

If, for the first column, the number of tubes showing microbial growth is two or less, the most probable number of microorganisms per g or per ml is less than 100.

Effectiveness of the culture medium and validity of the counting method

The following strains are normally used :

Staphylococcus aureus : NCIMB 8625 (ATCC 6538-P, CIP 53.156) or NCIMB 9518 (ATCC 6538, CIP 4.83).

Bacillus subtilis : NCIMB 8054 (ATCC 6633, CIP 52.62).

Escherichia coli : NCIMB 8545 (ATCC 8739, CIP 53.126).

Candida albicans : ATCC 2091 (CIP 1180.79) or ATCC 10231 (NCPF 3179, CIP 48.72).

Allow the test strains to grow separately in tubes containing soybean-casein digest medium at 30-35°C for 18-24 hours, except for *Candida albicans* which needs a temperature of 20-25°C for 48 hours.

Dilute portions of each of the cultures using buffered sodium chloride–peptone solution pH 7.0 to obtain test suspensions containing about 100 viable microorganisms per ml. Use the suspension of each microorganism separately as a control of the counting methods, in the presence and absence of the material being examined, if necessary.

To validate the method, a count for the test organism should be obtained differing by not more than a factor of 10 from the calculated value for the inoculum. To test the sterility of the medium and the diluent, as well as aseptic performance, carry out the total viable aerobic count using sterile buffered sodium chloride–peptone solution pH 7.0 as the test preparation. There should be no growth of microorganisms.

Test for aflatoxins

This test is designed to detect the possible presence of aflatoxins B_1, B_2, G_1 and G_2, which are highly dangerous contaminants in any material of plant origin.

Procedure

Preparation of samples

Grind or reduce not less than 100 g of crude medicinal plant material to a moderately fine powder (sieve no. 355/180). The larger the sample size, i.e., 500 g–1 kg or more, the greater the possibility of detecting pockets of contamination.

Weigh 50 g of the powdered material, transfer to a conical glass-stoppered flask, and add 170 ml of methanol R and 30 ml of water. Using a mechanical device, shake vigorously for not less than 30 minutes. Filter through a medium-porosity filter-paper. If a special clean-up procedure is required, collect 100 ml of filtrate (A) from the start of flow; otherwise discard the first 50 ml and collect 40 ml of filtrate (B).

In order to eliminate interfering plant pigments use a special clean-up procedure; transfer 100 ml of filtrate A to a 250 ml beaker and add 20 ml of zinc acetate/aluminium chloride TS and 80 ml of water. Stir, allow to stand for 5 minutes, add 5 g of a filter aid, such as diatomaceous earth, mix and filter through a medium-porosity filter-paper. Discard the first 50 ml and collect 80 ml of filtrate (C).

Transfer either filtrate B or C to a separating funnel. Add 40 ml of sodium chloride (100 g/l) TS and 25 ml of light petroleum R, and shake for 1 minute. Allow the layers to separate and transfer the lower layer to a second separating funnel. Extract twice with 25 ml of dichloromethane R and shake for 1 minute. Allow the layers to separate and combine each of the lower layers in a 125 ml conical flask. Add several boiling chips and evaporate almost to dryness on a water-bath. Cool the residue, cover the flask and keep it for the determination by thin-layer chromatography or for a further clean-up procedure by column chromatography.

If necessary, remove further interfering compounds using a column 300 mm long with an internal diameter of 10 mm, a stopper and either a medium-pore sintered disc or a glass-wool plug. Prepare a slurry by mixing 2 g of silica gel with 10 ml of a mixture of 3 volumes of ether and 1 volume of light petroleum, pour into the column and wash with 5 ml of the same solvent mixture. Allow the adsorbent to settle and add to the top of the column a layer of 1.5 g anhydrous sodium sulfate. Dissolve the residue from above in 3 ml of dichloromethane and transfer it to the column. Rinse the flask twice with 1 ml portions of dichloromethane and add them to the column, eluting at a rare not faster than 1 ml/min. Then add successively to the column 3 ml of light petroleum, 3 ml of ether and 3 ml of dichloromethane, and elute at a rate not faster than 3 ml/min. Discard the eluates. Add to the column 6 ml of a mixture of 9 volumes of dichloromethane and 1 volume of acetone and elute as a rate not faster than 1 m/min, preferably without using vacuum. Collect this eluate in a small vial, add a few boiling chips and evaporate just to dryness on a water-bath.

Method

To either of the residues obtained above, add 0.2 ml of a mixture of 98 volumes of chloroform and 2 volumes of acetonitrile, close the vial and shake vigorously until the residues are dissolved, preferably using a vortex mixer.

Carry out the test by thin-layer chromatography, using silica gel G as the coating substance and a mixture of 85 volumes of chloroform, 10 volumes of acetone R and 5 volumes of 2-propanol as the mobile phase. Apply separately to the plate 2.5 µl, 5 µl, 7.5 µl and 10 µl of aflatoxin mixture TS, then apply three volumes, each of 10 µl, of the sample residues. Further superimpose on one of these spots 5 µl of aflatoxin mixture TS. Place the plate in an unsaturated chamber and develop. After removing the plate from the chromatographic chamber, allow it to try in air and examine the chromatogram in a dark room under ultraviolet light (365 nm).

Four clearly separated blue fluorescent spots are obtained from the aflatoxin mixture. Observe any spot obtained from the solutions of the residues that coincides in hue and position with those of the aflatoxin mixture. Any spot obtained from the solutions of the residues with the superimposed aflatoxin mixture should be more intense than the corresponding spot for the test solution, and should show no sign of separation or trailing, which would be a sign of dissimilar compounds.

Interpretation of results

No spots corresponding to aflatoxin should be obtained from any of the sample residues. If any such spot is obtained, compare its position with the spots obtained from the aflatoxin mixture to identify the type of aflatoxin present. An approximate estimation of the concentration of aflatoxin in the sample may be obtained by comparing the intensity of the spots with those of the aflatoxin mixtures.

PESTICIDE RESIDUES

The use of biocidal agricultural chemicals, known as pesticides, has greatly reduced the presence of insects, fungi and moulds in foods. Medicinal plants are liable to be affected by pesticide residues which accumulate from agricultural practices of spraying, treating soils during cultivation and through the administration of fumigants during storage. Since many medicinal plant preparations are taken over long periods of time, limits for pesticide residues should be established following the recommendations of the Food and Agriculture Organization (FAO) and the WHO. These recommended guidelines include analytical methodology of pesticide residues. Pesticides of persistent nature containing Hg, DDT, HCH (BHC), aldrin, dieldrin, melipax and toxaphene are not allowed for medicinal plants.

In some countries regulations exist to cover limits of these residues in foods, cosmetics, drugs and spices. Most spices exported from India contain pesticide residues. Chamomile (principally DDT) and Valerian root (DDT) contain the residues within acceptable levels. Thin-layer chromatography (TLC) and gas chromatographic methods are available for the determination of organochlorine and urea derivatives, enzymatic methods for organophosphorus compounds, colorimetric methods for urea derivatives, and spectroscopic techniques for paraquat, triazines and heavy metals.

Toxic residues may be reduced or eliminated by the use of infusions of the dried plant material and by the extraction of the useful plant constituents. Storage of Senna pods at 30°C reduces the ethylene oxide residues to tolerable levels.

Only the chlorinated hydrocarbons and related pesticides (e.g., aldrin, chlordane, DDT, dieldrin, HCH) and a few organophosphorus pesticides (e.g. carbophenothion) have a long residual action. Most other pesticides have very short residual actions. Therefore, it is suggested that, where the length of exposure to pesticides is unknown, the medicinal plant material should be tested for the presence of organically bound chloride and phosphorus, or the content of these two substances should be determined.

Determination of pesticide residues

Chromatography (mostly column and gas) is recommended as the principal method for the determination of pesticide residues. Samples are extracted by a standard procedure, impurities are removed by partition and/or adsorption, and the presence of a moderately broad spectrum of pesticides is measured in a single determination. Some pesticides are satisfactorily carried through the extraction and clean-up procedures, others are recovered with a poor yield, and some are lost entirely. In chromatography, the separations may not always be complete, pesticides may decompose or metabolize, and many of the metabolic products are still unknown. It is not yet possible to apply an integrated set of methods that will be satisfactory in all situations.

It is, therefore, desirable to test plant materials of unknown history for broad groups of compounds rather than for individual pesticides. Chlorinated hydrocarbons and other pesticides containing chlorine in the molecule can be detected by the measurement of total organic chlorine; insecticides containing phosphate can be measured by analysis for total organic phosphorus, while pesticides containing arsenic and lead can be detected by measurement of total arsenic or total lead, respectively. Similarly, the measurement of total bound carbon disulfide in a sample will provide information on whether residues of the dithiocarbamate family of fungicides are present.

If the pesticide to which the plant material has been exposed is known or can be identified by suitable means, an established method for the determination of that particular pesticide residue should be used.

General aspects of analytical methodology

The sample should be tested as quickly as possible after collection, before any physical or chemical changes occur. If prolonged storage is envisaged, the samples should preferably be stored in air-tight containers under refrigeration.

Light can cause degradation of many pesticides, and it is, therefore, advisable to protect the samples and any extracts or solutions from undue exposure.

The type of container or wrapping material used should not interfere with the sample or affect the analytical results.

Solvents and reagents used in the analytical method should be free from substances that may interfere with the reaction, alter the results or provide degradation of pesticide residue in the sample. It is usually necessary to use specially purified solvents or to distil them freshly in all-glass apparatus. Blank determinations with the solvents should be carried out, concentrating and testing them as specified in the test procedure for the plant material concerned.

The simplest and quickest procedure should be used to separate unwanted material from the sample (clean-up procedure) in order to save time when many samples have to be tested.

The process of concentrating solutions should be undertaken with great care, especially during the evaporation of the last traces of solvent, in order to avoid losses of pesticides residues. For this reason, it is often not advisable to remove the last traces of solvent. Agents, such as mineral oil or other oils of low volatility, that may help to preserve the solution could be added to retard the loss of relatively volatile pesticides, especially when the last traces of solvent are being evaporated. However, these agents, while satisfactory in colorimetric procedures, are usually not desirable in gas chromatographic methods. It may be necessary to evaporate heat-labile compounds using a rotary vacuum apparatus.

Maximum limit of pesticides for medicinal plant material

The toxicological evaluation of pesticide residues in medicinal plant materials should be based on the likely intake of the material by patients. In general, the intake of residues from medicinal plant materials should account for no more than 1% of total intake from all sources, including food and drinking-water. Certain plant materials may contain extremely high levels of pesticide residues, but the levels remaining after extraction are usually much lower, because of the low solubility in water or ethanol. It is, therefore, important to determine the actual quantity of residues consumed in the final dosage form.

Where the nature of the pesticide to which the plant material has been exposed is unknown, it is sufficient to determine the content of total chlorine and to base the calculation on the acceptable residual level (ARL) of the most toxic chlorine-containing pesticide (e.g., aldrin or dieldrin).

An ARL (in mg of pesticide per kg of plant material) can be calculated on the basis of maximum acceptable daily intake of the pesticide for humans (ADI), as recommended by FAO and WHO, and the mean daily intake (MDI) of the medicinal plant material.

Some countries have established national requirements for residue limits in plant materials. Where such requirements do not exist, the following formula may be used :

$$ARL = \frac{ADI \times E \times 60}{MDI \times 100}$$

where ADI = maximum acceptable daily intake of pesticide (mg/kg of body weight);

E = extraction factor, which determines the transition rate of the pesticide from the plant material into the dosage form;

MDI = mean daily intake of medicinal plant product.

The 60 in the numerator represents mean adult body weight, while the denominator incorporates a consumption factor of 100 reflecting the fact that no more than 1% of the total pesticide residue consumed should be derived from medicinal plant material.

This formula is based on the acceptable daily intake (ADI) determined by FAO and WHO.

Determination of total chlorine and phosphorus

Most pesticides contain organically bound chlorine or phosphorus.

Procedure

Preparation of samples

The plant powder is extracted with a mixture of water and acetonitrile. Most pesticides are soluble in this mixture, while most cellular constituents (e.g., cellulose, proteins, amino acids, starch, fats and related compounds) are sparingly soluble and are thus removed. A number of polar and moderately polar compounds may also be dissolved; it is, therefore, necessary to transfer the pesticides to light petroleum. For pesticides containing chlorine, further purification is seldom required, but for those containing phosphorus, further purification by column chromatography may be necessary, eluting with mixtures of light petroleum and ether.

Preparation of the column

Use Florisil grade 60/100 PR (or equivalent), activated at 650°C, as the support. If this material is obtained in bulk, transfer it immediately after opening to a 500 ml glass jar or bottle with a glass stopper or foil-lined, screw-top lid. Store in the dark. Before use, heat at not less than 130°C, cool in a desiccator to room temperature and heat once again to 130°C after 2 days.

Prepare a Florisil column (external diameter, 22 mm) which contains, after settling, 10 cm of activated Florisil topped with about 1 cm of anhydrous sodium sulfate. Pre-wet the column with 40-50 ml of light petroleum. Place a graduated flask under the column to receive the eluate.

Method

Plant material powder (20-50 g) is kept into a blender, add 350 ml of acetonitrile with a water content of 35% (to 350 ml of water add sufficient acetonitrile to produce 1000 ml). Blend for 5 minutes at a high speed. Filter under vacuum through an appropriate funnel, diameter 12 cm, fitted with filter-paper, into a 500 ml suction flask.

Transfer the filtrate to a 250 ml measuring cylinder and record the volume. Transfer the measured filtrate to a 1 litre separating funnel and carefully add 100 ml of light petroleum. Shake vigorously for 1-2 minutes, add 100 ml of sodium chloride (400 g/l) and 600 ml of water. Hold the separating funnel in a horizontal position and mix vigorously for 30-45 seconds. Allow to separate, discard the aqueous layer and gently wash the solvent layer with two 100 ml portions of water. Discard the washings, transfer the solvent laer to a 100 ml glass-stoppered cylinder, and record the volume. Add about 15 g of anhydrous sodium sulfate and shake vigorously. The extract must not remain in contact with this reagent for longer than 1 hour. Transfer the extract directly to a Florisil column; if necessary, reduce the volume first to 5-10 ml. Allow it to pass through the column at a rate of not more than 5 ml per minute. Carefully rinse the cylinder with two portions, each of 5 ml, of light petroleum, transfer them to the column, rinse with further small portions of light petroleum if necessary, and then elute at the same rate with 200 ml of

ether/light petroleum. Change the receiver and elute with 200 ml of ether/light petroleum. Again change the receiver and elute with 200 ml of ether/light petroleum. Evaporate each eluate to a suitable volume, as required, for further testing.

- The first eluate contains chlorinated pesticides (aldrin, DDE, TDE (DDD), o,p'- and p,p'-DDT, HCH, heptachlor epoxide, lindane, methoxychlor), polychlorinated biphenyls (PCB), and phosphated pesticides (carbophenothion, ethion and fenchlorphos).
- The second eluate contains chlorinated pesticides (dieldrin and endrin) and phosphated pesticides (methyl parathion and parathion).
- The third eluate contains phosphated pesticide (malathion).

Combustion of the organic matter

Combustion of the organic matter in oxygen is the preparatory step for the determination of chlorine and phosphorus. The pesticide is extracted from the sample and purified, if necessary. The extract is concentrated, evaporated to dryness, transferred to a sample holder, and burner in a suitable conical flask flushed with oxygen. The gases produced during combustion are then absorbed in a suitable solution. The absorbed choline is determined as chloride and the absorbed phosphorus as orthophosphate, both colorimetrically.

Determination of chlorides

The determination is made with a spectrophotometer capable of measuring absorbance at 460 nm using absorption cells with path-lengths of 2 cm and 10 cm.

Determination of phosphates

The phosphomolybdate method is based on the reaction of phosphate ions with ammonium molybdate to form a molybdophosphate complex, which is subsequently reduced to form a strongly blue-coloured molybdenum complex. The intensity of the blue colour is measured spectrophotometrically. This method is applicable for the determination of any phosphates that have undergone a prior separation procedure.

Naturally occurring phosphates are present in most samples, and are often not removed during the clean-up procedure. In order to obtain background values, therefore, it is necessary to proceed with the determination of all samples, even those with no phosphate-containing pesticides. These background values should be subtracted from the results obtained on testing pesticide residues. Extracts of most uncontaminated materials contain about 0.05-0.1 mg/kg of phosphorus. Therefore, no contamination with organophosphate pesticides can be assumed for results in this range.

Apparatus

The determination is made with a spectrophotometer capable of measuring absorbance at 820 nm using an absorption cell with a path-length of 1 cm.

Determination of arsenic and heavy metals

Contamination of medicinal plant materials with arsenic and heavy metals can be attributed to many causes including environmental pollution and traces of pesticides.

Limit test for arsenic

The amount of arsenic in the medicinal plant material is estimated by matching the depth of colour with that of a standard strain.

STANDARDS APPLICABLE TO VOLATILE AND FIXED OILS

Some standards are mainly appropriate to volatile oils and fixed oils.

Refractive index

The refractive index of a substance is the ratio between the velocity of light in air and the velocity in the substance under test. For light of a given wavelength, (the D line of sodium, has a double of lines at 589.0 nm and 589.6 nm), the refractive index of a material is given by the sine of the angle of incidence divided by the sine of the angle of refraction. The refractive index varies with the temperature.

Refractive index is measured by Abbe refractometer in which the angle measured is the 'critical angle' for total reflection between glass of high refractive index and the substance to be examined.

By this means, and by selecting a particular wavelength of light at which to make the measurements, it is possible to calibrate the instrument directly in terms of refractive index. The emergent beam is viewed in the instrument, and the critical angle is indicated by the edge of the dark part of the field of view. In this instrument the monochromatic light source is a dispersion 'compensator' placed at the base of the telescope tube of the refractometer. This consists of two direct-vision prisms made accurately direct for the D sodium line; the prisms can be made to rotate in opposite directions. The system of variable dispersion which these prisms form can be made to counterbalance the resultant dispersion of the refractometer prism and the material being examined. The temperature of the sample is adjusted by a water jacket.

Automatic refractometers, e.g., the Leica Auto Abbe refractometer, measure refractive index with precision to the fifth decimal place, as decimal places for the visual refractometer. A reflected light principle is used and light is not transmitted through the sample and hence problems with dark or coloured samples are avoided. The shadow-line location is determined by the instrument software, eliminating variations in readings caused by individual subjective interpretations.

Measurements of refractive index are important for purity assessments of volatile and fixed oils. Oils of Cassia, Cinnamon and Cinnamon leaf have refractive indices of about 1.61, 1.573-1.600 and about 1.53, respectively. The refractive index of lemon oil is 1.474-1.476, for English lavender oil 1.460-1.474.

Optical rotation

The optical rotation of a liquid is the angle through which the plane of polarization of light is rotated either clockwise or anticlockwise when the polarized light is passed through a sample of the liquid. The observed rotation is dependent on the thickness of the layer examined, its temperature and the nature of the light employed. Sodium light, layer 1 dm thick and a temperature of 20°C are generally used.

Most volatile oils contain optically active components and the direction of the rotation, and its magnitude, is a useful criterion of purity, *e.g.*, caraway oil, +74° to +80°; lemon oil, +57° to +70°; terpeneless lemon oil, –5° to +2°, cinnamon oil, 0° to –2°; citronella oil, Java, –5° to +2°; citronella oil, Ceylon, –9° to –18°; peppermint oil, –10° to –30°; spearmint oil, –45° to –60°, oils from East Indies (+10° to +25°), the West Indies (+25° to 45°).

Many natural materials are optically active and the rotation of their solutions in water, ethanol or chloroform are measures in a similar way,

$$\text{Specific rotation} = \frac{\text{Angular rotation per dm of solution}}{\text{Grams of optically active substance per ml of solution}}$$

$$[\alpha]_D^t = \frac{100\alpha}{lc} = \frac{100\alpha}{ldp}$$

where α is the observed rotation in degrees, l is the length of the observed layer in dm, c is the number of grams of substance contained in 100 ml solution, d is the density and p is the number of grams of substance contained in 100 g of solution. The specific rotation of a compound should include the solvent used, its concentration, the type of light employed (sodium D line of 589.3 nm or mercury green line of 546.1 nm) and temperature.

Quantitative chemical tests

Some qualitative chemical tests, *e.g.*, acid value, iodine value, saponification value, ester value, unsaponifiable matter, acetyl value and volatile acidity, are applicable to the fixed oils.

Some tests are also useful in the evaluation of resins (acid value, sulphated ash), balsams (acid value, ester value, saponification value), volatile oils (acid value, acetyl value, ester value) and gums (methoxyl determination, volatile acidity). Gas chromatography is useful to determine the individual methyl esters of the acids produced by the hydrolysis of fixed oils to ascertain the source of the oil and to detect the presence of foreign oils.

QUALITY CONTROL OF INDIAN ESSENTIAL OILS

The more important essential oils currently produced in India are Citronella, Lemongrass, Sandalwood, Palmarosa, Eucalyptus, Himalayan cedarwood and Vetiver. Small quantities of 'Khus', ajowan, gingergrass, rose and geranium oils are also produced. Of this only sandalwood is produced on a cottage/small scale industry basis.

India exports essential oils of lemongrass, citronella, sandalwood and palmarosa in adequate volume. A substantial quantity of essential oils namely cardamom, kokam, ginger and eucalyptus oil are being exported. India also imports considerable quantities of essential oils of peppermint, patchouli, clove, geranium, lavender and resinoids.

Standardization of essential oils

Soon after the establishment of ISI in 1947, the Essential Oils and Allied Products Sectional Committee, CDC 11 was set up for formulation of National Standards on essential oils. This Committee with the growth in diversity of work is now designated as Natural and Synthetic Perfumery Materials Sectional Committee, PCDC 18 under the Petroleum, Coal and Related Products Department (PCDC) of ISI.

ISI has been able to formulate 18 standards on essential oils, 36 on aromatic chemicals and one on resinoids. The pattern of testing of physico-chemical requirements and olfactory assessment has been standardized. Standards of essential oils had been prepared and used in various countries earlier than India, such as EOA (Essential Oil Association), USA, Givaudan Index, New York, and also the leading manufacturers of aroma and flavour had created their own standards for maintaining quality control in production and sale.

Development of an Indian standard

For preparation of national standards, ISI functions through a network of technical committees. The conflicting viewpoints of different interests are resolved and the latest developments in technology incorporated. Besides the technical committee critically examines the subject, the documents prepared by it are distributed widely to obtain comments of the individuals and organisations which are not represented on the Committee. The documents are also circulated abroad so as to keep abreast with the trends in other countries. This process of extensive circulation of draft standards no doubt cause some delay in their formulation, but ensures, that they are acceptable to the concerned interests, and implemented.

Standard methods of test for essential oils

Methods of Sampling and Test for Natural and Synthetic Perfumery Materials: Any consumer when buying a product is definitely interested in knowing whether he is getting his money's worth and also that the product is fit for the purpose intended. Standard methods of testing, therefore, form the most important basis for use of standard specifications. It is insufficient to specify that a material shall possess certain physico-chemical requirements without reference to specified test methods which should be used to determine them. Different methods of test are bound to yield results at variance. Additional parts to include latest techniques like gas chro-matography.

Methods for Olfactory Assessment of Natural and Synthetic Perfumery Materials : Olfactory assessment of essential oils is of paramount importance. The method is based on subjective olfactory response wherein conditions, environment, reagents and procedure all have been standardized as far as possible. Separately under the Sensory Evaluation Sectional Committee, standards on sensory evaluation for *intense* flavour, ghee, food and beverages have been developed.

In Indian Standards on essential oils and synthetic chemicals, the non-perfumery use of the material for food and flavour industry has also been mentioned. An essential oil or synthetic chemical conforming to the requirements as stipulated in the printed ISS may have to specify certain additional requirements in order to be acceptable to the food and flavour industry.

Material specifications for essential oils

Oil of Lemongrass : It ranks second in India's export of essential oils. Indian lemongrass oil, also known as East Indian Lemongrass oil, is produced mainly in Northern and Central Kerala by distillation of the grass known as *Cymbopogon flexuosus* Stapf., Fam : Poaceae, the Indian oil has found acceptance in the world market for its uniformly high citral content and its solubility in 70 per cent alcohol. The oil produced in other countries, most notably West Indies, is insoluble in 70 per cent alcohol. The specification has stressed the need to evaluate the oil on the basis of its citral content as the oil is essentially used for the preparation of citral. The oil is consequently preferred over the oil produced in other countries which does not conform to these requirements of the chemical industry.

HEAVY METALS

Contamination of medicinal plant materials with arsenic and heavy metals (like cadmium and lead) may cause environmental pollution and traces of pesticides. The limits (parts per million) of such heavy metals in medicinal plants should remain within specifications.

Arsenic or red sulphide of mercury is included as part of the formula, while other herbal preparations may contain large quantities of lead. The plating on a metal spoon used for herbal medicine may contain about 65% lead and 10% antimony. This could result in the ingestion of dangerous quantities of lead by young children. Many other herbal compounds contain unacceptably high levels of metals (*e.g.*, Khamira gaozaban, which includes 130 p.p.m. of zinc). A clay material, chewed by pregnant women known as sikor organi, contains very high levels of lead (50 p.p.m. or more).

ASSAYS FOR QUALITY CONTROL

A crude drug may be assayed for a particular group of constituents, *e.g.*, the total alkaloids in Belladonna, the total glycosides of Digitalis and the reserpine content of *Rauwolfia* species. Biological assays are used for the assays of those potent drugs (e.g., Digitalis) for which no other satisfactory assays is available. In pharmacopoeias, now these have been replaced by chemical and physical assays for routine standardization. However, the biological assays are important for screening plant materials and their fractionated extracts in the search for new drugs. Simple biological assays (*e.g.*, brine shrimp toxicity) can be carried out by a phytochemist without any special procedures used by pharmacologists.

Spectroscopic analysis

The electromagnetic vibrations used in spectroscopic analysis are divided into the ultraviolet (185-380 nm), the visible (380-780 nm), the near-infrared (780-3000 nm) and the infrared (3-40 μm) regions. In spectroscopic analysis, the capacity of certain molecules to absorb vibrations at specific wavelengths is utilized. Thus, the butenolide side-chain of cardiac glycosides is responsible for a strong absorption at 215-220 nm; the conjugated double bonds of lycopene (a carotene of tomatoes) absorb light at a wavelength of 470 nm, giving a red colour; and the carbonyl group of ketones, carboxylic acids and esters has a strong absorption in the infrared at about 1850-1670 cm^{-1}. The absorption spectrum of a molecule in the infrared region is complex, since the energies involved are too small to bring about electronic transitions but large enough to produce numerous vibrational and associated rotational energy changes.

The ultraviolet absorption characteristics as standards for benzylpencillin, lanatoside C and a number of alkaloids—for example, emetine, morphine, reserpine, cocaine, colchicine and tubocuraine chloride, are mentioned in pharmacopoeias (Table 10.4).

If the light of a particular wavelength is passed through a solution of a substance, the transmission $T = I / I_0$, where I_0 is the light reaching the detector (a photoelectric cell) when solvent alone is used in the light-path and I is the light reaching the detector when a solution of the substance under investigation is examined. The most useful value is $\log_{10}(I_0/I)$, decimal optical density or simply the optical density (E). The optical density is proportional to the number of absorbing units in the light-path (Beer's law).

For the *quantitative evaluation* of a substance, a standard curve is first prepared by measuring the optical densities of standard solutions of the pure compound by use of light of a suitable wavelength. The solutions must be sufficiently dilute to obey Beer's law. The optical density of the solution to be evaluated is then determined and its composition ascertained from the standard curve. Individual components of a mixture having different absorption maxima can be determined by ultraviolet absorp-

Table 10.3. Type of assays for crude drugs

Types of assay	Examples
Separation and weighing of active constituents	Colchicine is Colchicum corn and seed. Resins of Podophyllum, crude filicin in male fern, total balsamic esters of peru balsam
Chemical	'Total alkaloids' of many drugs, Strychnine in Nux vomica, morphine in Opium, cinnamic aldehyde in oil of Cinnamon, free alcohols in Peppermint oil. carvone in oil of Caraway
Physical	Cineole in eucalyptus oil
UV spectrometry	Compounds having conjugations
IR spectrometry	Compounds having functional groups
Biological	Cardioactive drugs, antibiotics, vitamins, taenicides, anthraquinone derivatives, mydriatic drugs, saponins, antitumour drugs, anti-amoebic drugs, ginkgolides (anti-PAF activity)
Enzyme-immunoassay	Quassin, neoquassin, 18-hydroxy-quassin (*Quassia* and *Picrasma* spp.), podophyllotoxin, tropane alkaloids, artemisinin in *Artemisia annua*, pyrrolizidine alkaloids, ergot alkaloids
Radioimmunoassay (RIA)	Hesperidin, limonin and niringin (*Citrus*), cardenolides sennosides (*Cassia augustifolia*), tropane alkaloids, morphine and related alkaloids, lysergic acid derivatives (Ergot), quinine ajmaline (*Rauwolfia* spp.), vincristine and related alkaloids (*Catharanthus roseus*), solasodine (*Solanum* spp.)

tion. The reported E values at the wavelength (l) indicated are 312 at 262 nm for strychnine and 216 at 300 nm for brucine. When pure solutions are not available for analysis, colorimetric analysis is often preferable, if the reaction used to produce the colour is highly specific for the compound under consideration.

Colorimetric analyses can be carried out with a suitable spectro-photometry, *e.g.*, simpler colorimeters in which suitable filters are used to select the correct wavelengths of light. In these instruments a simple light-source is used and, between the lamp and the solution to be analysed, a filter is placed which transmits that range of wavelengths absorbed by the compound under test. The transmitted light is recorded by a photoelectric cell and the composition of the solution determined by reference to a standard curve.

Fluorescence analysis

Many substances, *e.g.*, quinine in dilute sulphuric acid solution, emit light of a different wavelength or colour from that which falls on them when the exciting light is removed.

In fluorescence, the fluorescent light is always of greater wavelength than the exciting light. Light rich in short wavelengths is very active in producing fluorescence. For this reason strong ultraviolet light produces fluorescence in many substances which does not visibly fluoresce in daylight. Fluorescence lamps are usually fitted with a suitable filter which eliminates visible radiation from the lamp and transmits ultraviolet radiation of the desired wavelength. The eyes are properly protected in the presence of ultraviolet radiation.

For examination, solids may be placed directly under the lamp, whereas liquids may be examined in non-fluorescent dishes or test tubes or after spotting on to filter paper. Many alkaloids in the solid state show distinct colours, *e.g.*, aconitine (light blue), berberine (yellow) and emetine (orange). Pieces of cinchona bark when placed under the lamp show a number of luminous yellow patches and a few light blue ones. If the inner surface of the bark is touched with dilute sulphuric acid, the spot immediately turns blue. Ipecacuanha root has a brightly luminous appearance. The wood of hydrastis rhizome shines golden yellow. Areca nuts when cut show a light blue endosperm. Calumba pieces appear intensely yellow, with the cambium and phloem distinguished by their dark-green colour. Precipitated and prepared chalks may be differentiated from one another.

Most oils, fats and waxes show some fluorescence under filtered ultraviolet light. Fixed oils and fats fluoresce least, waxes more strongly, and mineral oils (paraffins) most of all.

Powdered drugs detected in UV light are ergot in flour, of cocoa shells in powdered cocoa, and of rumex in powdered gentian. Different varieties of rhubarb may be distinguished from one another. *Rheum officinale, R. tanguticum* and *R. emodi* have a brown fluorescence, and *R. compactum, R. undulatum, R. ribes* and *R. rhaponticum* show a violet colour. Ultraviolet is mainly used for the location of separated compounds on paper and thin-layer chromatograms.

Plant extract chromatograms are examined in ultraviolet light even if the constituents that one is investigating are not themselves fluorescent. In this way the presence of fluorescent impurities may be detected.

Sometimes fluorescence-quenching is used to locate non-fluorescent substances on thin-layer chromatograms. For this, an ultraviolet fluorescent background is prepared by the incorporation of a small amount of inorganic fluorescent material into the thin layer. The separated substances cause a local quenching of the background fluorescence and they appear as dark spots on a coloured background.

The fluorescence produced by a compound in ultraviolet light is also used for quantitative evaluation. The instrument used is a fluorimeter and consists of a suitable ultraviolet source and a photoelectric cell to measure the intensity of the emitted fluorescent light. The intensity of the fluorescence for a given material is related to its concentration. A narrow range of wavelengths is selected for measurement by inserting a filter between the fluorescing solution. With plant extracts it is important to ascertain that the substance being determined is the only one in the solution producing a fluorescence at the measured wavelength and there are no substances in the solution which absorb light at the wavelength of the fluorescence.

Quinine is assayed by the measurement of the blue fluorescence (366 mm) produced by irradiation of the alkaloid in a dilute sulphuric acid solution at about 450 nm. Alexandrian senna is assayed by measuring the fluorescence produced in the Borntrager reaction under specified conditions. Hydrastine in Hydrastis root is determined by oxidizing an extract of the drug with nitric acid and measuring the fluorescence of the hydrastinine produced. By this method berberine and canadine, other alkaloids of Hydrastis, are excluded from the assay. Emetine and papaverine are determined fluorimetrically after oxidation with acid permanganate and noscapine after oxidation with persulphate. The individual constituents of a mixture of cardiac glycosides may be separated by paper chromatography and the fluorescence of the separated glycosides is measured after treatment with a suitable spray and irridiation with ultraviolet light. The individual glycosides may be eluted from the paper with a suitable solvent and the fluorescence of the solutions can be measured. For the estimation of reserpine in *Rauwolfia* species, the green fluorescence is produced when reserpine in acetic acid is oxidized with hydrogen peroxide. Fluorimetric methods are used for the estimation of the ergot alkaloids, umbelliferone and aflatoxin.

NMR spectroscopy

This technique is associated with structure-determinations of organic compounds. The ^{1}H-NMR spectroscopy is used for the assay of atropine and hyoscine in extracts of Belladonna, Hyoscyamus and Stramonium.

Immunoassays

These assays are highly sensitive and specific. They are used for the quantitative determination of many compounds in biological fluids.

Radioimmunoassays (RIA)

The assays depends on the highly specific reaction of antibodies to certain antigens. The saturation method has been developed for phytoanalysis. Small molecules (below MW 1000) constituting the secondary plant metabolites are not involved in such immuno responses, but when bound covalently to protein carriers, as haptens, they do become immunogenic. Haptens combine with antibodies but do not stimulate their production unless linked to a carrier molecule. A hapten of known specific activity is prepared in the labelled condition (e.g., ^{3}H- or ^{125}I-labelled), mixed with an unknown amount of unlabelled hapten and added to an antibody in the form of a serum, then there will be competition between the labelled and unlabelled antigen for the restricted number of binding sites available. This results in some bound and some unbound hapten; these can be separated and a determination of the radioactivity in either fraction, with reference calculated. The antiserum is raised in rabbits.

Table 10.4. Ultraviolet spectrometric analysis of drug constituents

Constituents	Wavelength for measurement of optical density
Alkaloids :	
Lobeline	249 nm
Reserpine	268 nm
Vinblastine	267 nm
Vincristine	297 nm
Tubocurarine chloride	280 nm
Morphine	286 nm
Colchicine	350 nm
Cardioactive glycosides with butenolide side-chain	217 nm
Quassinoids	254 nm
Cassia oil—aldehyde content	286 nm
Bergamot oil—bergapten content	313 nm
Flavaspidic acid from male fern	290 nm
Capsaicin	248 and 296 nm
Vanillin	301 nm
Vitamin A (cod-liver oil)	328 nm
Withanolides	222 nm
Flavones	250-280, 310-350 nm
Isoflavones	245-275, 310-330 nm

RIA has the advantage that only small amounts of plant material are required; it is usually specific for a single, or small range of metabolites. It is an efficient tool for the screening of large numbers of plants, 200-800 specimens may be assayed in 1 day.

The assays can be performed on quantities of sample ranging from 0.5 mg to a few milligrams. Structures as small as anther filaments can be studied.

A considerable specialized expertise is requi-red to set up the assays. There is a possibility of cross-reactions with components of the plant extract other than those under investigation.

The RIA for hyoscine is highly specific but norhyoscine reacts strongly, the cross-reaction with 6-hydroxyhyoscyamine is less, and with hyoscyamine, very much less. In the assay for solasodine, tomatidine, will cross-react.

Table 10.5. Visible spectrometric analysis of drug constituents

Alkaloids

Ergot (total alkaloids)	550 nm with p-dimethyl-amino-benzaldehyde reagent; 532 nm with vanillin in concentrated hydrhchloric acid
Morphine	442 nm by the nitroso reaction
Reserpine	390 nm by the treatment of alkaloid with sodium nitrite in dilute acid
Tropic acid esters of hydroxytropanes	555 nm by treatment of alkaloid with fuming nitric acid followed by dryness and addition of methanolic potassium hydroxide solution to an acetone solution of the nitrated residue (Vitali–Morin reaction)
Anthraquinones	500 nm after treatment with alkali, 530 nm for the cochineal colour value
Capsaicin in Capsicum	730 nm after reaction with phosophomolybdic acid and sodium hydroxide solution; 505 nm after treatment with diazobenzene-sulphonic acid in 10% sodium carbonate solution
Cardioactive glycosides:	
based on digitoxose-moiety	590 nm by Keller-Kiliani reaction
based on lactone ring	620 nm by reaction with m-dinitrobenzene
Cyanogenetic glycosides : (cyanide determination)	630 nm by the pyridine-parazolone colour reaction
Tannins :	
Rhatany	750 nm using phosphomolybdic acid and sodium carbonate solution
Volatile oils :	
Menthol from peppermint oil	500-579 nm (green filter) by use of p-dimethylamino-benzaldehyde reagent

Table 10.6. Infrared spectrometric analysis of drug constituents

Alkaloids :	
Quinine and strychnine mixtures	$1645\text{-}1790 \text{ cm}^{-1}$
Steroidal sapogenins	$920\text{-}1080 \text{ cm}^{-1}$
Volatile oils :	
o-Methoxycinnamaldehyde in cassia oil	$1450 \text{ and } 1490 \text{ cm}^{-1}$

Enzyme-linked immunosorbent assays (ELISA)

In this method, there is a competition for an immobilized antibody with a modified form of the compound under analysis that has an enzyme bound to it. The compound-enzyme complex is released from the binding site. The determination of the enzyme activity enables the original solution to be quantified.

The method is very sensitive. The pyrrolizidine alkaloid retronecine can be measured in the parts per billion range and one sclerotium of ergot is detectable in 20 kg of wheat.

Tandem mass spectroscopy (MS-MS)

Mass spectroscopy is usually associated with the structure elucidation of compounds. However, by the simultaneous use of two mass spectrometers in series it is possible to determine quantitatively the amount of a particular targeted compound in complex mixtures, plant extracts or in dried plant material.

It is an important analytical tool for analytical problems. The method has been used for the analysis of cocaine in plant materials, pyrrolizidine in *Senecio* and other genera, taxanes in needles of *Taxus cuspidata*, aflatoxin B_1 in peanut butter, xanthones, steroids and antibiotics. It is the best method for determination of taxol, cephaloman-nine and baccatin in *T. brevifolia* bark and needle extracts. The chemotaxonomy of the Cactaceae has been investigated by this method.

QUALITY EVALUATION OF SPICES

The term 'flavour' is used generally to mean aroma, but sometimes to denote taste also. It is the sum total of all perceptions in the mouth when a food is eaten; it thus includes the responses of the receptors in the gustatory and nasopharyngeal regions to the various stimuli in the foods. The well recognized basic tastes are saltiness, sweetness, sourness, bitterness, pungency and astringency.

Aroma evaluation

Aroma is generally the major component of flavour. Unlike the stimuli for taste, aroma stimuli are found in large numbers and types but in trace amounts in bulk food. In spices they are in larger amounts as volatile oils. These are analyzed by techniques for separation and analysis of components at micro levels. Several hundreds of components have been identified in volatiles of individual foods by GC-MS.

Flavour of spices has qualitative, quantitative and hedonic (preference/rejection) components and the ultimate decisions on quality could only be by human perception. Flavour is a sensorily perceived quality and can at best be described with words. Unlike colour and texture or shape, which can be measured, flavour requires human sensory instrument for its meaningful analysis. Sensory analysis of flavour quality has been considered highly variable, due to psycho-physical bias of the instrument used. Studies during the last two or three decades have shown that considerable objectivity can be built into sensory test procedures to minimize this bias. It is necessary to carefully choose and train the human measuring instrument to obtain the required accuracy and reliability, the same as one would do while selecting instruments or conditions for physical or chemical measurements. Additionally, in sensory tests, statistical design and analysis are used to much greater measure to obtain the most valid and meaningful results that show the significance of the differences between samples. The sensory panel analysis is better than reliance on one or few experts, who inspite of their highly developed perception capabilities are restricted by the samples they have earlier experienced and the consequent fixation of concepts. For example, a 'tea taster' from Cochin may respond differently for a 'tea taster' in Darjeeling and unlikely to be useful as a 'wine taster'.

In the study of ginger, for selecting the descriptors for the profile, 'TLC-aromagram' technique was adopted. Here, the extracts from authentic samples were first fractionated by the versatile preparative thin-layer chromatography using suitable solvents. A co-chromatographed area only was sprayed with a chromogenic reagent (5% vanillin-H_2SO_4). Based on the position of the coloured spots, corresponding areas on the silica layer were scraped and extracted in sugar solution and tasted for describing the component aroma. The panel is able to perceive the component aromas of the total extract, now fractionated. This technique has many advantages over column fractionation: (i) visualizing separation of components which provides a basis for collecting the fractions, (ii) multiple developments or use of different developing solvents, (iii) recombination of different separated areas to determine relative significance to total aroma. A typical set of TLC-aromagram of a sample of good ginger oil.

The main differences between fresh and dry ginger aroma as analyzed by GC and flavour profile lie in the higher levels of fresh green, lemony and camphory, pungent green and flowery notes in green ginger. In dry ginger there is a dominance of pungent dry, woody/rooty notes while the other notes are lower. In the sequence of evaluation a decision initially whether the sample is 'dry' or 'green' type is made and next the component profiles are analyzed for their intensity and finally a scoring of overall quality is made as green or dry ginger.

Pungency evaluation

Pungency is the other valued attribute of spices making generally insipid yet highly nutritious meal acceptable for eating. Pungency is 'stinging', 'irritating', 'hot' or 'piquant'. The importance of the usage of the term pungency to the gustatory response when the food with the spice is eaten. At concentrations slightly above their thresholds, the different, pure stimuli are indistinguishable from one another even by trained panelists. The differences recorded could be explained by intrinsic intensity, concentration and solubility of the stimuli along with aroma interactions.

The chemistry of pungency stimuli from major spices have been well studied over the years. Those responsible for pungency in chillies (*Capsicum* spp.) are the capsaicinoids, a group of 5 related compounds, vanillylamides of monocarboxylic acids, varying in length (C_8-C_{11}), and have been estimated by GC after silylation reversed phase TLC and by HPLC. Capsaicin and dihydro-capsaicin (80 to 90% of total capsaicinoids) are found to be the major pungent components while the other three homologs nordihydrocapsaicin, homodihydrocapsaicin and homocapsaicin (10 to 20% of total capsaicinoids) are either half or less as pungent as capsaicin or dihydrocapsaicin. The method involves frontal elution of the capsaicinoids using buffered methanol (pH 9.6), when the capsaicinoids are clearly separated from fat and the colour components which remain absorbed on the paper at the origin. Separated capsaicinoids are reacted with the sensitive Gibbs reagent (2,6-dichloro-p-benzoquinone-4-chlori-mine) and per cent capsaicinoids in sample is calculated from the average $E^{1\%}/1$ cm value for the reaction with pure capsaicin.

In pepper, the pungency has been shown to be due to piperine, 5-(3,4-dioxymethylene phenyl)-2-*trans*, 4-*trans*; pentadienoic acid piperi-dide. The homologs, piperittine (trienoic), piperanine (mono-enoic) and the pyrrolidine analog, pyrroperine are present in very small percentage as also to have low or no pungency. The UV absorption at 342 nm, characteristic of compounds with conjugated diene system attached to an aromatic ring, is used for estimation of piperine and related compounds. The percent piperine in extracts are calculated from a standard curve made with crystallized piperine.

Ginger is valued for pungency besides the dominant aroma has been examined for pungent compo-nents. A mixture of o-methoxy phenyl alkyl ketones, gingerols and their dehydration products shogaols were considered to be the pungent components. A part of the area representing the homologous gingerols and shogaols are pungent; using temperature programmed gas chromatography combined with thin layer chromatographic separation, the identity of the (6)-(8)- and (10)-homologs and that the pungency is essentially due to (6)-gingerol and (6)-shogaol has been confirmed. The active shogaol is more pungent than gingerol. The estimation of the (6)-homolog of these components has been achieved by separation by the wedged-tip TLC technique with a selected solvent, (hexane: ether, 1.5:1, v/v), and colorimetry determining with Folin-Ciocalteau reagent and vanillin as standard. These values have also been shown to be significantly correla-table to estimates of pungency.

Pungency is estimated by determining the highest dilution at which it is recognized, the reciprocal of which is expressed as Scoville Heat Units.

A reproducible and reliable estimates of pungency in Scoville value can be obtained when tested

Table 10.7. Structure and pungency of natural stimulants in spices

Formula	Name	Source	Pungency SU 10^5
	Capsaicin	Capsicum	160
	Piperine	Pepper	1.0
	(6)-Gingerol	Ginger	0.8
	(6)-Shogaol	Ginger	1.5

under standardized conditions, adopted and described in the Indian Standard.

Determination of bitterness value

Medicinal plant materials that have a strong bitter taste ("bitters") are employed therapeutically, mostly as appetizing agents. Their bitterness stimulates secretions in the gastrointestinal tract, especially of gastric juice.

Bitter substances can be determined chemically. However, since they are mostly composed of two or more constituents with various degrees of bitterness, it is first necessary to measure total bitterness by taste.

The bitter properties of plant material are determined by comparing the threshold bitter concentration of an extract of the materials with that of a dilute solution of quinine hydrochloride. The bitterness value is expressed in units equivalent to the bitterness of a solution containing 1 g of quinine hydrochloride in 200 ml.

Safe drinking water should be used as a vehicle for the extraction of plant materials and for the mouth-wash after each tasting. Tasting buds dull quickly if distilled water is used. The hardness of water rarely has any significant influence on bitterness.

Sensitivity to bitterness varies from person to person, and even for the same person it may be different at different times (because of fatigue, smoking, or after eating strongly flavoured food). Therefore, the same person should taste both the time. The bitter sensation is not felt by the whole surface of the tongue, but is limited to the middle section of the upper surface of the tongue. A certain amount of training is rerquired to perform this test. A person who does not appreciate a bitter sensation when tasting a solution of 0.058 mg of quinine hydrochloride R in 10 ml of water is not suitable to undertake this determination.

The preparation of the stock solution of each individual plant material (S_T) should be specified in the test procedure. In each test series, unless otherwise indicated, the determination should start with the lowest concentration in order to retain sufficient sensitivity of the taste buds.

Procedure

Caution : This test should not be carried out until the identity of the plant material has been confirmed.

Preparation of solutions

Stock and diluted quinine hydrochloride solution

Dissolve 0.100 g of quinine hydrochloride in sufficient safe drinking-water to produce 100 ml. Further dilute 5 ml of this solution to 500 ml with safe drinking water. This stock solution of quinine hydrochloride (S_q) contains 0.01 mg/ml. Use nine test-tubes for the serial dilution for the initial test.

Stock and diluted solutions of the plant material

Prepare the solution as specified in the test procedure for the given plant material (S_T). Use 10 test tubes for the serial dilution for the test.

Method

After rinsing the mouth with safe drinking water, taste 10 ml of the most dilute solution swirling it in the mouth mainly near the base of the tongue for 30 seconds. If the bitter sensation is no longer felt in the mouth after 30 seconds, spit out the solution and wait for 1 minute to ascertain whether this is due to delayed sensitivity. Then rinse with safe drinking water. The next highest concentration should not be tasted until at least 10 minutes have passed. The threshold bitter concentration is the lowest concentration at which a material continues to provoke a bitter sensation after 30 seconds. After the first series of tests, rinse the mouth thoroughly with safe drinking water until no bitter sensation remains. Wait for at least 10 minutes before carrying out the second test.

DETERMINATION OF HAEMOLYTIC ACTIVITY

Many medicinal plant materials of the families Caryophyllaceae, Araliaceae, Sapindaceae, Primulaceae, and Dioscoreaceae contain saponins. The most characteristic property of saponins is their ability to cause haemolysis: when added to a suspension of blood, saponins produce changes in erythrocyte membranes, causing haemoglobin to diffuse into the surrounding medium.

The haemolytic activity of plant materials, or a preparation containing saponins, is determined by comparison with that of a reference material, saponin, which has a haemolytic activity of 1000 units per g. A suspension of erythrocytes is mixed with equal volumes of a serial dilution of the plant material extract. The lowest concentration to effect complete haemolysis is determined after allowing the mixtures to stand for a given period of time. A similar test is carried out simultaneously with the saponin.

Procedures proposed for the determination of the haemolytic activity of saponaceous medicinal plant material are all based on the same principle although the details may vary, e.g., the source of erythrocytes, methods for the preparation of the erythrocyte suspension and the plant material extract, the defined haemolytic activity of the reference material of saponin, and the experimental method. In order to obtain reliable results, it is essential to standardize the experimental conditions, and especially to determine the haemolytic activity by comparison with that of saponin.

Procedure

To prepare the erythrocyte suspension fill a glass-stoppered flask to one-tenth of its volume with sodium citrate (36.5 g/l) swirling to ensure that the inside of the flask is thoroughly moistened. Introduce a sufficient volume of blood freshly collected from a healthy ox and shake immediately. Citrated blood prepared in this way can be stored for about 8 days at 2-4°C. Place 1 ml of citrated blood in a 50 ml volumetric flask with phosphate buffer pH 7.4 and carefully dilute to volume. This diluted blood suspension (2% solution) can be used as long as the supernatant fluid remains clear and colourless. It must be stored at a cool temperature.

To prepare the reference solution, transfer about 10 mg of saponin, accurately weighed, to a volumetric flask and add sufficient phosphate buffer pH 7.4 to make 100 ml. This solution should be freshly prepared.

The extract of plant material and dilutions should be prepared as specified in the test procedure for the plant material concerned, using phosphate buffer pH 7.4.

Preliminary test

Prepare a serial solution of the plant material extract with phosphate buffer pH 7.4 and blood suspension (2%) using four test tubes.

As soon as the tubes have been prepared, gently invert them to mix, avoiding the formation of foam. Shake again after a 30 minute interval and allow to stand for 6 hours at room temperature. Examine the tubes and record the dilution at which total haemolysis has occurred, indicated by a clear, red solution without any deposit of erythrocytes. Proceed as follows :

- If total haemolysis is observed only in tube no. 4, use the original plant material extract directly for the main test.
- If total haemolysis is observed in tubes 3 and 4, prepare a two-fold dilution of the original plant material extract with phosphate buffer pH 7.4.
- If total haemolysis is observed in tubes 2, 3 and 4, prepare a five-fold dilution of the original plant material extract with phosphate buffer pH 7.4.
- If, after 6 hours, all four tubes contain a clear, red solution, prepare a ten-fold dilution of the original plant material extract with phosphate buffer pH 7.4 and carry out the preliminary test again as described above.
- If total haemolysis is not observed in any of the tubes, repeat the preliminary test using a more concentrated plant material extract.

Main test

Prepare a serial dilution of the plant material extract, undiluted or diluted as determined by the preliminary test, with phosphate pH 7.4 and blood suspension (2%) using 13 test tubes.

Carry out the dilutions and evaluations as in the preliminary test but observe the results after 24 hours. Calculate the amount of medicinal plant material in g, or of the preparation in g or ml, that produces total haemolysis.

To eliminate the effect of individual variations in resistance of the erythrocyte suspension to saponin solutions, prepare a series of dilutions of saponin in the same manner as described above for the plant material extract. Calculate the quantity of the saponin in g that produces total haemolysis.

Calculate the haemolytic activity of the medicinal plant material using the following formula:

$$100 \times \frac{a}{b}$$

where 1000 = the defined haemolytic activity of saponin in relation to ox blood

a = quantity of saponin that produces total haemolysis (g),

b = quantity of plant material that produces total haemolysis (g).

DETERMINATION OF TANNINS

Tannins (or tanning substances) are substances capable of turning animal hides into leather by binding proteins to form water-insoluble substances that are resistant to proteolytic enzymes. This process, when applied to living tissue, is known as an "astringent" action and is the reason for the therapeutic application of tannins.

Chemically, tannins are complex substances; they usually occur as mixtures of polyphenols that are difficult to separate and crystallize. They are easily oxidized and polymerized in solution; if this happens they lose much of their stringent effect and are, therefore, of little therapeutic value.

Procedure

To prepare the plant material extract, introduce the quantity specified in the test procedure for the plant material concerned, previously powdered to a known fineness and weighed accurately, into a conical flask. Add 150 ml of water and heat over a boiling water-bath for 30 minutes. Cool, transfer the mixture to a 250 ml volumetric flask and dilute to volume with water. Allow the solid material to settle and filter the liquid through a filter-paper, diameter 12 cm, discarding the first 50 ml of the filtrate.

To determine the total amount of material that is extractable into water, evaporate 50.0 ml of the plant material extract to dryness, dry the residue in an oven at 105°C for 4 hours and weigh (T_1).

To determine the amount of plant material not bound to hide powder that is extractable into water, take 80.0 ml of the plant material extract, add 6.0 g of hide powder R and shake well for 60 minutes. Filter and evaporate 50.0 ml of the clear filtrate to dryness. Dry the residue in an oven at 105°C and weigh (T_2).

To determine the solubility of hide powder, 6.0 g of hide powder R, add 80.0 ml of water and shake well for 60 minutes. Filter and evaporate 50.0 ml of the clear filtrate to dryness. Dry the residue in an oven at 105°C and weigh (T_0).

Calculate the quantity of tannins as a percentage using the following formula :

$$\frac{[T_1 - (T_2 - T_0)] \times 500}{w}$$

where w = the weight of the plant material in grams.

DETERMINATION OF FOAMING INDEX

Many medicinal plant materials contain saponins that can cause a persistent foam when an aqueous decoction is shaken. The foaming ability of an aqueous decoction of plant materials and their extracts is measured in terms of a foaming index.

Procedure

The plant coarse powder (1 g) is weighed accurately and transferred to a 500 ml conical flask containing 100 ml of boiling water. Maintaining at moderate boiling for 30 minutes. Cool and filter into a 100 ml volumetric flask and add sufficient water through the filter to dilute to volume.

Pour the decoction into 10 stoppered test tubes (height 16 cm, diameter 16 mm) in successive portions of 1 ml, 2 ml, 3 ml, etc. up to 10 ml, and adjust the volume of the liquid in each tube with water to 10 ml. Stopper the tubes and shake them in a lengthwise motion for 15 seconds, two shakes per second. Allow to stand for 15 minutes and measure the height of the foam. The results are assessed as follows :

(i) If the height of the foam in every tube is less than 1 cm, the foaming index is less than 100.

(ii) If a height of foam of 1 cm is measured in any tube, the volume of the plant material decoction in this tube (a) is used to determine the index. If this tube is the first or second tube in a series, prepare an intermediate dilution in a similar manner to obtain a more precise result.

(iii) If the height of the foam is more than 1 cm in every tube, the foaming index is over 1000. In this case repeat the determination using a new series of dilutions of the decoction in order to obtain a result.

Calculate the foaming index using the following formula :

$$\frac{1000}{a}$$

where a = the volume in ml of the decoction used for preparing the dilution in the tube where foaming to a height of 1 cm is observed.

RADIOACTIVE CONTAMINATION

A certain amount of exposure to ionizing radiation cannot be avoided since there are many sources, including radionuclides occurring naturally in the ground and the atmosphere.

Dangerous contamination may be the consequence of a nuclear accident. The World Health Organization, in close collaboration with several other international organizations, has developed guidelines for use in the event of widespread contamination by radionuclides resulting from a major nuclear accident. The health risks from food accidentally contaminated by radionuclides depend not only on the specific radionuclide and the level of contamination but also on the quantity of food consumed.

The range of radionuclides that may be released into the environment as the result of a nuclear accident might include long-lived and short-lived fission products, actinides, and activation products. The nature and the intensity of radionuclides released may differ markedly and depend on the source (reactor, reprocessing plant, fuel fabrication plant, isotope production unit, etc.).

The amount of exposure to radiation depends on the intake of radionuclides and other variables such as age, metabolic kinetics, and weight of the individual (also known as the dose conversion factor).

Even at maximum observed levels of radioactive contamination with the more dangerous radionuclides, significant risk is associated only with consumption of quantities of over 20 kg of plant material per year so that a risk to health is most unlikely to be encountered given the amount of medicinal plant materials that would need to be ingested. Additionally, the level of contamination might be reduced during the manufacturing process. Therefore, no limits for radioactive contamination are proposed.

Method of measurement

Since radionuclides from accidental discharges vary with the type of facility involved, a generalized method of measurement is so far not available. Suspect samples can be analysed by a competent laboratory. Details of laboratory techniques are available from the International Atomic Energy Agency (IAEA).

11

Pharmacological Active Drugs

The drugs act on the nervous systems, heart and blood vessels, lungs, gastrointestinal tract, kidneys, liver, reproductive organs, skin and mucous membranes. The hormones, vitamins and chemotherapeutic drugs are used to treat infections and malignant diseases. Some plants (*e.g.*, *Papaver*, ipecacuanha and liquorice) contain a range of compounds with differing pharmacological properties.

A single plant is used to treat different diseases and it is difficult to co-related all the action of the drug with pharmacological activities.

DRUGS ACTING ON THE NERVOUS SYSTEM

In human body, the nervous system coordinates and regulates the various voluntary and involuntary activities of the body. The central nervous system (CNS) and the autonomic nervous system are interlinked and some drugs which affect the CNS may also produce reactions associated with the autonomic system.

Drugs involved with the CNS may have a general stimulatory or depressant action with anti-convulsant and psychopharmacological activities. Some useful natural drugs of the group are the narcotic (opioid) analgesics. Hallucinogenic drugs have important sociological implications.

Lysergic acid diethylamide (prepared from ergot alkaloids), mescaline (obtained from peyote cactus) and cannabis act as hallucinogenic agents. Purine bases (*e.g.*, caffeine, theophylline, theo-bromine) stimulate mental activity. Cocaine is one of the earliest drug used as a mental stimulant. Reserpine depresses mental activity and is useful in psychiatric treatment. Yohimbine (found in Apocynaceae species) has similar action to reserpine but its antiadrenaline reactions and effect on heart muscle render it of no clinical use. Valerian and Passiflora are sedative and hypnotic. Picrotoxin (obtained from *Anamirta cocculus* berries) is analeptic, previously used to treat barbiturate poisoning. Lobeline, an analeptic drug, is a respiratory stimulant. Strychnine is a weak analeptic, toxic doses produce spinal convulsions. Camphor is also a weak analeptic. Tropane alkaloids (atropine and hyoscine) are used to treat travel sickness and delirium tremens. Gelsemium root, though highly toxic, is used as antispasmodic and acts as central depressant of motor function. The analgesic drug morphine is effective for relief of severe pain. It has depressant action on the cough and respiratory centres. Codeine is less active than morphine. It is a much safer drug for the relief of mild pain and for use as a cough suppressant.

The autonomic nervous system supplies the smooth muscle tissues and glands of the body. Its has complex function. It is composed of two divisions, the sympathetic (thoracolumbar or adrenergic) division, which arises from the thoracic and lumber regions; and the parasympathetic division, originating in the brain and in the sacral region. An increase in activity of the sympathetic system stimulates the body for immediate action, whereas stimulation of the parasympathetic or vagal system produces effects more associated with those occurring during sleep and with energy conservation. Acetylcholine and noradrenaline and its derivatives are two important neurotransmitter substances of the autonomic nervous system.

Acetylcholine-like drugs are pilocarpine, arecoline, muscarine and physostigmine. Physostigmine is a cholinesterase inhibitor. The drugs acting as antagonists of acetylcholine are tropane ester alkaloids (*e.g.*, atropine and hyoscine), neuromuscular blocking agents (*e.g.*, tubocurarine) and ganglion blocking agents (*e.g.*, tubocurarine). Ephedrine is an adrenaline-like drug. Ergot alkaloids (*e.g.*, ergotamine) acts as antagonists of adrenaline. Reserpine has an antihypertensive effect resulting from dilation of heart and circulatory vessels and belongs to noradrenaline depletion category. Atropine, hyoscine, physostigmine and pilocarpine are used in ophthalmic preparations for the eye, being under the control of the autonomic nervous system.

THE HEART, CIRCULATION AND BLOOD

The coronary and circulatory diseases now are the principal cause of human mortality. With increased public awareness of the importance of the heart diseases, healthier living states on diet, supplementary food factors and exercise are very important.

Cardioactive glycosides

There is a group of drugs which affect the heart's performance. A number of plants scattered throughout the plant kingdom contain C_{23} or C_{24} steroidal glycosides which exert a states effect on the failing heart. The glycosides of various *Digitalis* species are extensively used. The pharmacological activity of these glycosides is dependent on both the aglycones and the sugar attachments.

Digitalis acts in competition with K ions for specific receptor enzyme (ATPase) sites in the cell membranes of cardiac muscle and is particularly successful during the depolarization phase of the muscle when there is an influx of Na^+ ions. The clinical effect of congestive heart failure is to increase the force of myocardial contraction (the positive inotropic effect) resulting in a complete emptying of the ventricles. Due to depression of conduction in the bundle, the atrioventricular conduction time is increased, showing an extended P-R interval on the electrocardiogram. Arising from their vagus effects, the digitalis glycosides are also used to control supraventricular (atrial) cardiac arrhythmias. The diuretic action of digitalis arises from the improved circulatory effect.

Digitalis, Strophanthus, Convallaria, Nerium, Thevetia and *Erysimum* species contain cardioactive glycosides.

Antiarrhythmic drugs

The cardiac glycosides can be used to control supraventricular (atrial) cardiac arrhythmias. The alkaloid quinidine (obtained from Cinchona barks) act on both supraventricular and ventricular arrhythmias. Its salts and quinidine itself find prophylactic use in recurrent paroxysmal dysrhythmias such as atrial fibrillation or flutter.

Antihypertensive drugs

Primary hypertension usually requires hospitalization. Rauwolfia and its principal alkaloid reserpine together with Veratrum extracts are used in allopathic medicine. Other plants regularly employed include misletoe, Crataegus, Yarrow, Tilia and Fagopyrum.

Platelet activating factor (PAF) antagonists

In the circulatory system thrombi may be caused on the arterial side as due to the adhesion of blood platelets to one another and to the walls of the vessels. This platelet aggregation is triggered by the platelet activating factor which is released from activated basophils. PAF from the rabbit was characterized as a 1-O-alkyl-2-acetyl-*n*-glyceryl-3-phosphorylcholine. Some prostaglandins and thromboxanes are also involved in the aggregation mechanism and thromboxane A_2, synthesized from arachidonic acid, is particularly potent. In undamaged vessels thromboxane A_2 is possibly balanced by a prostaglandin, *e.g.*, prostacyclin of the arterial intima which has deaggregation properties.

In the treatment of cerebrovascular or cardiovascular diseases, aspirin acetylates the platelet enzyme cyclo-oxygenase. The neolignan kadsurenone is obtained from *Piper futokadsura*, a plant long used in Chinese traditional medicine for allergy treatments. Other plants of traditional medicine reported to have anti-PAF activity include species of *Forsythia, Arctium, Centipeda, Tussi-lago, Pyrola, Populus* and *Peucedanum*. The active constituents include lignans, sesquiterpenes, coumarins, pyrocatechol and salicyl alcohol.

Extracts of the maidenhair tree, *Ginkgo biloba*, are used to treat various circulatory disorders. Certain fish oils (*e.g.*, cod-liver, halibut-liver) decrease the ability of platelets to aggregate by virtue of their high eicosapentaenoic acid content; this acid tends to favour the biosynthesis of thromboxane A_3, a weaker stimulator of platelet aggregation than thromboxane A_2.

DRUGS ACTING ON BLOOD VESSELS

These drugs are vasoconstrictor or vasodilator substances. Some of the drugs (*e.g.*, ergot) are useful in relation to specific systems. Ergotamine (tartrate) from *Claviceps purpurea* produces a correct constrictor effect in vascular smooth muscle; the reversal of the dilation of cranial vessels leads to its use at the onset of classical migraine attack. Ergotoxine is similar to ergotamine. Ephedrine prolongs action on blood pressure, 'Nervous System'.

Nicotine shows vasoconstrictor effects from its action on sympathetic ganglia, and by it promoting release of vasopressin and adrenaline.

Most of the drugs (*e.g.*, picrotoxin) stimulate the central nervous system and the vasomotor centre in the medulla, producing a rise in blood pressure.

Papaverine (an opium alkaloid) acts directly on the blood vessels by causing relaxation of smooth muscle. An intravenous injection is used for the treatment of pulmonary arterial embolism.

Xanthine derivatives (caffeine, theobromine and theophylline) act as papaverine; they also have a central vasoconstrictor action counteracting the peripheral effect. Ergotamine is an adrenaline antagonist. In resperpine therapy vasodilatation is produced by a peripheral and central action. Veratrum alkaloids (from *Veratrum* spp.) act as bradycardia and peripheral vasodilatation by sensitization of cardiac, aortic and carotid sinus baroreceptors.

DRUGS FOR DIGESTIVE DISORDERS

The upper and the lower portions of the gastrointestinal tract are most susceptible to disorder and are consequently associated with the greatest number of drugs for their treatment.

Bitters are used in liquid medicaments to stimulate appetite. The bitter constituents stimulate the gustatory nerves in the mouth and give rise to an increase in the psychic secretion of gastric juice. Extracts of Calumba, Cinchona (or quinine), Nux vomica (or strychnine) are used.

Anticholinergic drugs are hyoscine and hyoscyamine which help disturbances caused by gastric mobility and muscle spasm particularly with some ulcer patients.

Emetics are Ipecacuanha preparations which on oral administration have a delayed emetic action produced by irritation of the mucous membranes. Picrotoxin stimulates the vomiting centre through its general effect on the central nervous system.

Carminatives are aromatic substances which assist the eructation reflex; their mode of action is obscure. Dill oil is used for the relief of flatulence, especially in babies. Other plants or oils used as carminatives include Caraway, Fennel, Peppermint, Thyme, Nutmeg, Calamus, Pimento, Ginger, Clove, Cinnamon, Chamomile and Matricaria. Chalk is used as an antacid and charcoal as an adsorbent.

Ulcer therapy includes derivatives of glycyrrhetinic acid (a triterpenoid of Liquorice root) for the treatment of peptic ulcer. Deglycyrrhizinized liquorice has also been employed. Other antiulcer agents are alginic acid, marshmallow and comfrey.

Demulcents soothe and protect the alimentary tract and overlap with some materials used in ulcertherapy. Iceland moss, orris and elm bark are used as denulcent.

Laxatives and purgatives may be classed according to their mode of action :
  – Agar and Ispaghula are hydrophilic colloids which function as bulk-producing laxatives.
  – Bran is an indigestible vegetable fibre which absorbs water and provides bulk.

- Senna (leaves and fruit) contains anthraquinone derivatives which are hydrolysed in the bowel to stimulate Auerbach's plexus in the wall.
- Cascara, Rhubarb, Aloes and Castor oil act as Senna. They contain glycerides which on hydrolysis yield riconoleic acid, irritant to the small bowel.
- Podophyllum resin, Jalap resin and Colocynth are drastic purgatives. They are prescribed with belladonna to reduce gripping.

Rectal and colonic drugs are Arachis oil, Esculin, Hamamelis, Pilewort and balsam of Peru. They are used as suppositories. Antidiarrhoeal drugs are morphine and codeine which act by increasing the smooth muscle tone of the bowel and by reducing its mobility. They are prescribed with kaolin.

THE NASAL AND RESPIRATORY SYSTEMS

There are numerous proprietary preparations for the treatment of infections of the respiratory tract.

Aromatic inhalations include benzoin, cincole, eucalyptus oil, menthol, peppermint, pumilo pine oil, balsam of Tolu, thymol and turpentine.

Plant expectorants are Ipecacuanha, Senega root, Liquorice root, Squill bulb, Tolu balsam, pine oil, Lobelia, Grindelia, Angelica root and leaf, Storax, Cocillana, Coltsfoot, sweet violet and bloodroot. Codeine and atropine are antiexpectorants. Morphine, codeine, noscapine and Wild Cherry are used as cough depressant. Marshmallow, verbascum, plantago, Iceland moss and honey act as demulcent.

Bronchodilators and nasal decongestants are Ephedra, ephedrine and xanthines (theophylline).

HEPATOPROTECTIVE DRUGS

The liver is the principal organ of metabolism and excretion and is effected by a number of diseases such as liver cirrhosis (cell destruction and increase in fibrous tissue), hepatitis (inflammatory disease) and hepatitis (noninflammatory condition). The most common plant drug used for its antihepatotoxic properties is *Silybum marianum*. In India the plants used as hepatoprotective drugs are *Arnica montana, Cichorium intybus, Picrorhiza kurroa, Apium graveolens, Andrographis paniculata, Curcuma longa, Berberis vulgaris, Boerhavia diffusa, Phyllanthus fraternus, Swertia chirata* and *Vitex negunda.*

DRUGS FOR URINARY AND REPRODUCTIVE SYSTEM DISORDERS

Plant diuretics are xanthine derivatives as present in many beverages (tea, coffee, etc.) and promote dilation of the renal medullary blood vessels. Digitalis glycosides improve the failing heart thereby increasing renal perfusion and glomerular filtration.

Diuretics and urinary antiseptics include Buchu, Bearberry, Juniper and Copaiba. These include drugs used for the treatment of cystitis and urethritis.

Drugs acting on the uterus are the preparations of Ergot used in childbirth; now replaced by the isolated alkaloid ergometrine. Its salts has a direct stimulant action on the uterine muscle and reduces the incidence of postpartum haemorrhage. Ergotamine acts similarly with marked peripheral vasoconstrictor action and not used for obstetric purpose.

Black haw is a uterine tonic and sedative used for the prevention of miscarriage and for dysmenorrhoea after childbirth.

Hydrastis is used for menorrhagia and other menstrual disorders.

Male impotence is treated by papaverine.

Oral contraceptives for female are 'Steroids' and for male, gossypol.

DRUGS FOR SKIN AND MUCOUS MEMBRANE DISORDERS

Drugs affecting the skin may act as emollient, absorbents, astringents, irritants or antiseptics. A number of substances are easily absorbed through the skin and are useful to treat skin diseases.

Emollients and demulcents are used as ointments, creams and lotions which contain fixed oils (e.g., Olive, Arachis, Coconut, Theobroma), fats (Wool-fat, Lard), waxes of animal origin (Beeswax, Spermaceti), gums (Acacia, Tragacanth) and mucilages (Psyllium, Elmbark).

Starch, alginates and charcoal act as absorbents. Astringents are tannins (e.g., tannic acid), Krameria, Catechu, galls, *Aspidosperma*, Hamamelis, Pomegranate rind and kinos.

Counter-irritants are Camphor, turpentine, Capsicum, Aconite, methyl salicylate and mustard seed. Tars, eucalyptus oil, thyme oil, eugenol, thymol and cajuput are antiseptic drugs. Corticosteroids are used locally as anti-inflammatory agents.

Psoriasis and eczema are treated with comfrey, allantoin, cade oil, evening primrose oil, chrysarobin, *Lithospermum*, savin, myrrh and grindelia.

Wound covering (occlusive, nonocclusive, haemostatic) are in the healing process and these are alginates and cotton fibres.

STEROIDS AND ANTI-INFLAMMATORY DRUGS

Corticosteroidal hormone are the (1) glucocorticoids, which regulate carbohydrate and protein metabolism and possess a strong anti-inflammatory action, and the (2) mineralocorticoids, which influence the electrolyte and water balance of the body. The compounds are used in replacement therapy, Addison's disease, reduction of lymphatic tissues (leukaemias), suppression of lymphopoiesis and as anti-inflammatory agents for rheumatoid arthritis, cerebral oedema and raised intracranial pressure.

These hormones are produced naturally in the adrenal cortex. Many semi-synthetic drugs are also used. These are synthesized using plant steroids as intermediates; diosgenin, steroidal alkaloids of the Solanaceae and hecogenin being the principal sources. There is a large world demand for these compounds, for the synthesis or oral contraceptives.

NON-STEROIDAL ANTI-INFLAMMATORY DRUGS

Aspirin is one of the most widely-used mild analgesic and non-steroidal anti-inflammatory drugs (NSAID). It occurs as salicylates and glycosides in willow bark, long used for the treatment of rheumatic diseases, gout and painful conditions of all types.

Enzymes are used to detect anti-inflammatory activity of plants. Galangin, a flavonoid of *Alpinia officinarum* (Zingiberaceae; galangal rhizome) is a cyclo-oxygenase inhibitor. Lipoxygenase inhibitors are present in *Spilanthes oleracea* (Asteraceae) used

to cure rheumatic disorders and in *Echinacea purpurea* root, (Asteraceae), which contains isobutylamides.

Flavonoids possess anti-inflammatory activity. Gilead bud, cumicifuga rhizome, Equisetum, Jamaica Dogwood, Matricaria flowers, Meadow sweet, Red Clover flower and Willow Bark contain flavonoids. An infusion of Matricaria flowers (*Chamomilla recutita*) is used for its anti-inflammatory action in the treatment of acute gastritis. The flavonoids and not the volatile oils are responsible for activity. However, in *Calendula officinalis* the terpenoids are active constituents. With liquorice root (*Glycyrrhiza glabra*) both the triterpenoid saponin, glycyrrhizin, and the flavonoids have anti-inflammatory activity.

Colchicine, an alkaloid of *Colchicum autumnale*, is used to treat acute attack of gout. It may act by reducing the inflammatory response caused by deposits of urate crystals in the joint and by reduction of phagocytosis of the crystals. Its use has been replaced by allopurinol (inhibition of xanthine oxidase) and by phenylbutazone. Guaiacum resin is used to cure chronic rheumatic conditions and gout; it contains a mixture of lignans. The dried root of *Harpagophytum procumbens* (Devil's claw) (Pedaliaceae) is prescribed to treat painful rheumatic conditions; iridoid glycosides, *e.g.*, harpagoside, are the main constituents. Pineapple juice of *Ananas comosus* (Bromeliaceae) contains at least five proteolytic enzymes, called bromelin or bromelain. The enzyme has ability to dissolve fibrin in conditions of inflammatory oedema.

Ginkgolides (C_{20} terpenes from *Ginkgo biloba*) are potent antagonists of platelet activating factor.

ANTIDIABETIC DRUGS

Many plants are used orally to treat diabetes; *e.g.*, karela fruit (*Momordica charantia*), cumin fruit, ginseng, *Teucrium oliverianum*, neem (*Azadirachta indica*), onion, *Aloe* spp., Job's tears (*Coix lachrymajobi*), *Galega officinalis*, *Cyamopsis tetragonolobus*, *Gymnema sylvestris*, *Pterocarpus marsupium*, Jamun (*Syzygium cumini*) and *Swertia chirata*.

ANTISEPTIC DRUGS

Many higher plant constituents have anti-bacterial properties. Moulds and streptomyces are the principal sources. Quinine is the most effective agent for the treatment of malaria. Artemisinin (Qinghaosa), a sesquiterpene lactone, is the active constituent of Chinese drug, *Artemisia annua*. It is effective against chloroquine resistant strains of *Plasmodium vivax* and *P. falciparum* and against cerebral malaria.

Emetine as a salt, an alkaloid of ipecacuanha, is used to cure amoebic dysentery. Extract of male fern is used for tapeworm infections.

Santonin possesses a powerful action in paralysing round-worms; due to its high toxicity, it is replaced by piperazine. Oil of chenopodium acts like santonin; is widely used in hookworm disease.

Thymol is given in hookworm treatment.

ANTITUMOUR DRUGS

Catharanthus alkaloids, taxol and podophyllum are plant drugs used to treat some malignant diseases.

ANTI-ALLERGIC DRUGS

A large number of materials produce allergic conditions in sensitive individuals. Extracts containing specific allergies are available as diagnostic kits or for desensitization. Examples of plant allergens are grass, flower and tree pollens, dried plants and moulds.

ORAL ANTICOAGULANTS

These compounds inhibit the clotting mechanism of the blood and are useful in arterial thrombosis; they have no effect on platelet aggregation. 4-Hydroxycoumarins from plants act by antagonizing the effects of vitamin K. Warfarin sodium is one of the most widely used drugs. Plants used in herbal medicine which contain coumarin derivatives and possess anti-vitamin K activity include *Melilotus officinalis, Galium aparine* and *Lavandula officinalis*.

Other anticoagulants are heparin, hirudin, produced by the leech; hirudin, a polypeptide of 65 amino acids, can also be obtained from modified *Saccharomyces*.

HYPOLIPIDAEMIC DRUGS

Treatment of hyperlipidaemia is mainly dietary along with other natural therapy. Natural products include nicotinic acid and fish oils containing high quantities of ω-3-marine triglycerides. The latter involve eicosapentaenoic acid and docasahexaenoic acid which, possess the first double bond at C-3.

Gastric drugs lowers serum total cholesterol and improves the lipid profile. Low-density lipoprotein are reduced and high-density lipoprotein is increased giving a more favourable HDL-LDL ratio.

Drug Constituents

The medicinal value of a crude drug depends on the presence of one or more chemical constituents of physiological importance. They may be glycosides, alkaloids, organized resins and enzymes. A vegetable drug is composed of a number of tissues such as cells, fibres, vessels and other structures. The cell walls may consist of cellulose, lignins, tannins or cork cells. The cells of aromatic drugs like Cinnamon and Coriander contain volatile oils occurring in specialized cells or glands. The glycosides and alkaloids may occur in solution in the cell sap and deposit in the cells later on. The total contents of the cells are not used as physiological importance. For example, calcium oxalate occurs as a crystalline deposit and protein may be present as solid aleurone grains. Both these components are rejected in the preparation of a tincture or extract of the drug.

The unorganized drugs possess no cellular structure but consist of extracts, exudation, secretions and other products of the plants. The value of gums, gum-resins, oleo-resins, starch, fixed oils, catechu, and opium depends on the whole of the material present. The constituents of drugs of medicinal value generally belong to one of the following group: glycosides, enzymes, anthraquinone derivatives, alkaloids, tannins and other phenols, proteins, carbohydrates, gums, resins, fixed oils, fats, waxes and volatile oils.

HYDROCARBONS

The least polar organic natural products are the a liphatic hydrocarbons. They usually have an odd number of carbon atoms, due to decarboxylation of their fatty acid counterparts. Hydrocarbons may be either saturated or unsaturated. The unsaturated ones contain multiple bonds. Each double bond results in two less hydrogen atoms relative to the saturated counterpart, and is thus in a higher oxidation state. Those highly branched hydrocarbons derived from isoprene can exist as hydrocarbons.

Saturated hydrocarbons are the simplest and least polar organic natural products. Common hydrocarbons such as hexane, $CH_3(CH_2)_4CH_3$, are not generally found in plants, but are derived from fossilized plant and animal matter. Turpentine, commonly used as paint remover, consist of simple hydrocarbons, particularly n-heptane, as found in conifers. In living plants, saturated hydrocarbons are universally distributed as the waxy coatings on leaves, and as cuticle waxes on the surfaces of fruits. Several plants are rich in aliphatic hydrocarbons used in vegetable oils. For example, olive oil contains hydrocarbons ranging from C_{13} to C_{28}. Branched simple alkanes rarely occur in significant quantity in plants.

The simplest unsaturated hydrocarbon is ethylene, an important plant hormone. Larger unsaturated hydrocarbons are also common as plant waxes. High amounts of alkenes have been detected in rye pollen, rose petals, and sugar cane. As the chain length and degree of unsaturation increases, the hydrocarbons become waxy and then solid at room temperature.

Unsaturated natural products contain double and

Name	Formula
Methane	CH_4
Ethane	CH_3CH_3
Propane	$CH_3CH_2CH_3$
n-Butane	$CH_3(CH_2)_2CH_3$
n-Pentane	$CH_3(CH_2)_3CH_3$
n-Hexane	$CH_3(CH_2)_4CH_3$
n-Heptane	$CH_3(CH_2)_5CH_3$
n-Octane	$CH_3(CH_2)_6CH_3$
n-Nonane	$CH_3(CH_2)_7CH_3$
n-Decane	$CH_3(CH_2)_8CH_3$
n-Undecane	$CH_3(CH_2)_9CH_3$
n-Dodecane	$CH_3(CH_2)_{10}CH_3$
n-Tridecane	$CH_3(CH_2)_{11}CH_3$
n-Tetradecane	$CH_3(CH_2)_{12}CH_3$
n-Eicosane	$CH_3(CH_2)_{18}CH_3$
n-Heneicosane	$CH_3(CH_2)_{19}CH_3$
n-Docosane	$CH_3(CH_2)_{20}CH_3$
n-Tricosane	$CH_3(CH_2)_{21}CH_3$
n-Heptacosane	$CH_3(CH_2)_{25}CH_3$
n-Pentatriacontane	$CH_3(CH_2)_{33}CH_3$
n-Tetracontane	$CH_3(CH_2)_{38}CH_3$
n-Pentacontane	$CH_3(CH_2)_{48}CH_3$

Fig. 12.1. Hydrocarbon natural products

triple bonds. The polyacetylenes are naturally occurring hydrocarbon derivatives characterized by one or more acetylenic groups in their structures. The *sp* hybridization of the triple bond results in a linear shape for this region of the molecule. The domestic carrot contains four polyacetylenes, the major one being falcarinol, which is a mild neurotoxin found only to be present in 2 mg kg^{-1} (dry weight) of carrot roots. The water dropwort, *Oenanthe crocata*, found near streams in the Northern Hemisphere, contain several toxic poly-acetylenes.

Polyacetylenes are also found in the higher fungi, where their typical chain length is from C_8 to C_{14}, whereas the polyacetylenes from higher plants are typically from 14 to 18 carbons in length.

Biosynthetically, the polyacetylenes are likely to be derived by enzymatic dehydrogenation from the corresponding olefins. Both wyerone acid in the broad bean (*Vicia faba*) and safynol in safflower oil from *Carthamus tinctorius* have been shown to act as natural phytoalexins, helping to deter the micro-organisms which attack these plants. Simple functionalized hydrocarbons are pre-sent in small amounts in plants.

The marine plants are used as a source for hydrocarbons that contain both chlorine and bromine. Hundreds of different halogenated natural products have been isolated, particularly from the red algae and the animals that feed upon them. Various species of red algae from the genus *Laurencia* contain numerous halogenated natural products, including laurinterol, spirolaurenone, and laurencin.

ALCOHOLS

A large variety of volatile alcohols, *e.g.*, aldehydes, ketones, and esters, occur in small concentrations in plants. Due to their strong odours, they attract insect pollinators and animal seed disseminators. All of the straight-chain alcohols from C_1 (wood alcohol) to C_{10} have been found in plants in either free or esterified form. Ceryl alcohol, $CH_3(CH_2)_{24}CH_2OH$, is a constituent of cuticular waxes.

SULPHIDES

Hydrocarbon sulphides are found in some plants which possess obnoxious odors. Sulphides are common in the species of *Allium*, many of which are lachrymators and have pungent odours. Thiophenes are present in the Asteraceae family, in association with the polyacetylenes. The glucosinolates or mustard oil glucosides are also readily detected and help to create the flavors of the mustard, radish, onions and garlic. The most common sulphur containing natural products are the amino acids cysteine and methionine.

Simple aldehyde and ketone plant natural products are rarely found in plants. Hentriacontan-14, 16-dione ($C_{31}H_{60}O_2$) is a major wax constituent of cereals and other grasses.

ESTERS

Esters are the condensation products of alcohols and acids. They tend to have strong and pleasant odours. Strawberries contain ethyl butyrate, ethyl isovalerate, isoamyl acetate, ethyl caproate and 2-hexenyl acetate. Ethyl acetate, ethyl butyrate, ethyl valerate and propyl butyrate are pressnt in apple. Pineapples possess ethyl acetate, methyl isocaproate, methyl isovalerate, methyl caprylate and ethyl acrylate.

FATTY ACIDS

Fatty acids are the simplest lipids characterized by a polar hydrophilic head region connected to a long hydrophobic hydrocarbon tail. Some lipids, including the fats, are used for energy storage but most are used to form lipid constituents of membrane which surround cellular organelles and protoplasts (the plasma membrane).

The most common fatty acids in plants are oleic and palmitic acid. The hydrocarbon chain may be saturated, as in palmitic acid, or unsaturated, as in oleic acid. Fatty acids differ from each other primarily in chain length and the locations of multiple bonds. Thus, palmitic acid (16 carbons, saturated) is symbolized 16:0 and oleic acid, which has 18 carbons with one *cis* double bond at carbon 9 is symbolized $18:1^{\Delta 9}$. Double bonds are assumed to be *cis* unless otherwise indicated.

Fatty acids are utilized as building-block components of the saponifiable lipids, only traces occur in the free-acid form in cells and tissues. Normally these exist in various bound forms and may be present up to 7% of the weight of dried leaves. They include long chain esters (waxes), triacylglycerols (fats), glycerophospholipids and sphingolipids (membrane lipids). The common fatty acids are lauric, myristic, palmitic, stearic, arachidic, behenic, oleic, linoleic and arachidonic acids.

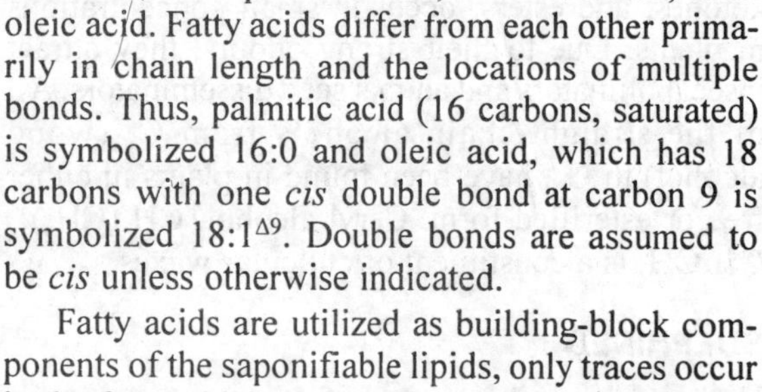

$$
\begin{array}{ll}
\underset{C-OCOR^1}{\overset{H_2}{|}} & \underset{C-OCOR^1}{\overset{H_2}{|}} \\
\underset{CH-OCOR^2}{|} & \underset{CH-OCOR^2}{|} \\
\underset{\underset{H_2}{C-OCOR^3}}{|} & \underset{\underset{H_2}{C-OPO_2H}}{|}
\end{array}
$$

$$CH_3(CH_2)_{12}CH=CHCH(OH)CH(NH_3^+)CH_2OH$$

Fig. 12.2. Sphingosine

Some common lipids are tristearin, lecithin and sphingosine.

The various fatty acids of higher plants have an even number of carbons ranging from C_{14} to C_{22}. Unsaturated fatty acids predominate in higher plants.

Waxes containing polymeric esters formed by the linking of several hydroxy-acids are prominent in the waxy coatings of conifer needles. The two common acids in such waxes are subinic [$HOCH_2(CH_2)_{10}CO_2H$] and juniperic acids [$HOCH_2(CH_2)_{14}CO_2H$]. The lipid constituents of cork and cuticle are known as suberin and cutin, respectively, and are composed of high molecular weight fatty acid esters.

CARBOHYDRATES

Sugars or carbohydrates are the primary products of photosynthesis and universal constituents of living organisms. They act as a source of energy to plants. They are stored as starch or fructans and polymerized to form cellulose. They combine to form glycosides of many fundamental groups of natural products including terpenes (to form saponins), phenols, and alkaloids. In plants, carbohydrates are found as support elements (celluose), as energy reserves (starch) which store solar energy captured by the photosynthetic process, as constituents of various metabolites (nucleic acid and coenzymes) and as required precursors for all other metabolites.

Sugars are optically active aliphatic polyhydroxylated compounds which are readily water soluble. This is due to the hydrophilic nature of the hydroxyl functionality and does not involve the salt formation. The sugars are classified into three groups depending on their size: monosaccharides, such as glucose; oligosaccharides, including sucrose; and polysaccharides, which include cellulose.

The most common monosaccharides are glucose and fructose. Less common are xylose, mannose, rhamnose and galactose. The individual sugars may be physically separated either enzymatically or by treatment with acid.

The oligosaccharides normally include from two to five saccharide (or sugar) units. These are joined by any of three possible ether linkages that can complicate structure elucidation. Common oligosaccharides include sucrose, trihalose, stachyose and raffinose.

Most of the carbohydrates found in plants occur as polysaccharides of high molecular weight. The polysaccharides (or glycans) have a wide variety of functions in plants. Cellulose serves as a structural material whereas in animal keratin and collagen act similar structural roles. Cellulose is the most abundant organic compound in plants and the most abundant single polymer in the biosphere. A simple straight-chain polymer without branching is formed using β-(1,4) ether linkages and forms the main structural polysaccharides of the cell wall. *Amylose*, which is used as a storage, contains α-(1,4) linkages. Amylopectin has α-(1,4) and α-(1,6) linkages. The linkages of cellulose form straight ribbons that line up side by side forming polymers of high mechanical strength and limited extensibility. Other structural polysaccharides include the poly-galacturonans (pectic polysaccharides), xylans, glucomannans, chitins, and the glycosaminoglycans.

The complex cell-wall polysaccharides act as *recognition signals*. The saccharide sequence of these heteropolysaccharides is informational. Poly-saccharides are not sweet in taste.

Gum, mucilage and pectin are derived carbo-hydrates which are composed of acid or ester forms. Gums are polyuronides formed due to combination of sugar and uronic acid units. Gums are used as emulsifier, suspending agents, tablet binders and thickeners.

Chemically, mucilages are similar to gums but differ in the nature of sugar and acid residue. They may contain sulphate groups or their salts. They form a clear colloidal solution and are used mainly as suspending agent. Mucilage is present in Agar, Plantago seeds and Linseed.

Mucilage soaks up water producing a sticky jelly-like mass. Mucilage lines the mucous mem-branes of the digestive tract and protect them against acidity, irritation and inflammation. This soothing and protective action is also seen in mucous mem-branes of the throat, lungs, kidneys and urinary tubules.

Pectins are consisted of methoxylated poly-galacturonic acids. They are present in the inner portion of the rind of Citrus fruits and in apples. They swell in water and form stiff jellies.

TERPENES

The *terpenes* are the most common natural pro-ducts. Terpenes are a unique group of hydrocarbon-based natural products biogenetically derived from isoprene.

Terpenes are classified by the number of 5-car-bon units they contain as hemiterpenes (C_5), mono-terpene (C_{10}), sesquiterpene (C_{15}), diterpene (C_{20}), sesterterpene (C_{25}, rare), triterpene (C_{30}) and tetra-terpenes (C_{40}).

The terpenes are of a similar biogenetic origin, in which isopentenyl pyrophosphate and dimethyl-allyl pyrophosphate combine to yield geranyl pyrophosphate and dimethylallyl pyrophosphate combine to yield geranyl pyrophosphate, leading to monoterpenes. Similarly, compounds derived from farnesyl pyrophosphate lead to sesquiterpenes, and triterpenes are formed from two equivalents of farnesyl pyrophosphate. These various combinations and oxidations give rise to a large variety of terpenes.

The terpenes have ecological and physiological actions. Many of them inhibit the growth of competing plants (allelopathy). Some are insecti-cidal; others attract insect pollinators. The plant hormone, abscissic acid, is one of the sesqui-terpenes. Gibberellic acid is one of the major plant hormones.

Hemiterpenes : C_5

Isoprene itself does not occur free in nature but several five-carbon compounds are known which contain the isopentane skeleton, including isoamyl alcohol, isovaleraldehyde, tiglic acid, angelic acid, β-furoic acid, isovaleric acid and senecioic acid.

Monoterpenes : C_{10}

The monoterpenes are derived from the C_{10} geranyl pyrophosphate and constitute important components of volatile oils.

A volatile steam-distillate fraction of an aromatic plant responsible for characteristic aroma is the principal source of monoterpenoids (*ca.* 90%). They are C-10 compounds whose carbon skeletons are made up by combination of two isoprene molecules united in a head-to-tail manner. The essential oil is usually present in the plants belonging to families Asteraceae, Lauraceae, Zingiberaceae, Lamiaceae, Myrtaceae, Pinaceae, Rosaceae, Rutaceae and Apiaceae. Sulphurous compounds are detected in the plants of Brassicaceae and Liliaceae families. In the angiosperms, the orders Asterales, Cornales, Lamiales and Rutales are the most important sources of mono-terpenoids. They are widely distributed in insects. Some monoterpenoids have been isolated from the fungi and marine algae. The alarming chemical constituents (pheramones) produced by some insects are composed of a mixture of mono-terpenes. Monoterpenes are usually hydrocarbons, alcohols, aldehydes and ketones and are more abundant in nature and are more easily synthesized. They have been utilized as flavours, perfumes, insecticides, herbicides, pharmaceuticals, food products, beverages, cosmetics and paints.

Most of the monoterpenes are present in common plants. Myrcene is found in the essential oil of bay leaves and hops. It is used as an intermediate in the manufacture of perfumes. Geraniol, which is isomeric with linalool, constitutes the major part of the oil of roses, citronella, lemon grass, and others. Menthol is found in the essential oil of peppermint and other members of the mint family. Carvone is one of the main odoriferous components of caraway seed (*Carum carvi*). Linalool is the principle constituents of coriander (*Coriandrum sativum*), a common spice. Safranal is responsible for the characteristic odor of saffron (*Crocus sativus*). Eucalyptol (cineole) is the main component of the essential oil of eucalyptus leaf (*Eucalyptus* spp.). Eucalyptol, along with camphor, form the major constituents of rosemary oil. Mullein, a common tomentose biennial, produces a number of iridoid glycosides, including aucubin.

Sesquiterpenes : C_{15}

The C_{15} sesquiterpenes, derived from three isoprene units, exist in a wide variety of forms, including linear, bicyclic and tricyclic frameworks. Like the monoterpenes, most of the sesquiterpenes are present in essential oils because they belong to the steam distillable fraction often containing the characteristic odoriferous components of the plant. Farnesol pyrophosphate serves as a key intermediate in terpenoid biosynthesis.

The cadinenes occur as essential oils from juniper and cedar trees and santonin is an antihelmintic that is isolated from wormwood (*Artemisia maritima*).

Acorine, a sesquiterpene dilactone, is present in the essential oil of sweet flag (*Acorus catamus*). Over 6000 sesquiterpene lactones are known. They are particularly present in the Asteraceae.

Many sesquiterpenes possess antitumour, antileukaemic, cytotoxic and antimicrobial activities. They can be responsible for skin allergies in humans and they also act as insect-feeding deterrents.

Chemically, the compounds can be classified according to their carbocyclic skeletons. From the germacranolides can be derived the guaianolides, pseudoguaianolides, eudesmanolides, eremophilanolides, xanthanolides, etc. A structural feature of all these compounds is the α,β-unsaturated γ-lactone.

Sesquiterpene lactones of the Apiaceae differ in their stereochemistry from the analogous compounds of the Asteraceae.

The conformation of the *trans, trans*-farnesyl diphosphate precursor is different in the two cases.

Iridoids

The iridoids are cyclopentan-[c]-pyran monoterpenoids. *Iridomyrmex*, a genus of ants produces these compounds as a defensive secretion.

There are many secoiridoids in which the pyran ring is open, and in a few the pyran ring oxygen is replaced by nitrogen.

They are present in Valerian, Gentian and Harpagophytum. Loganin is a precursor of the nonindole portion of some alkaloids.

Iridoids and *seco*-iridoids usually occur as glycosides and provide a structural link between terpenes and alkaloids. They are common in a variety of animals and dicotyledonous plants belonging to Scrophulariaceae, Rubiaceae, Verbenaceae, Bignoniaceae, Acanthaceae, Lamiaceae, Gentianaceae and some other families. They are natural cyclopentanoid monoterpenoids characterized by a cyclopenta [c] pyran skeleton. The nomenclature of iridoids has been denoted as iridane (*cis*-2-

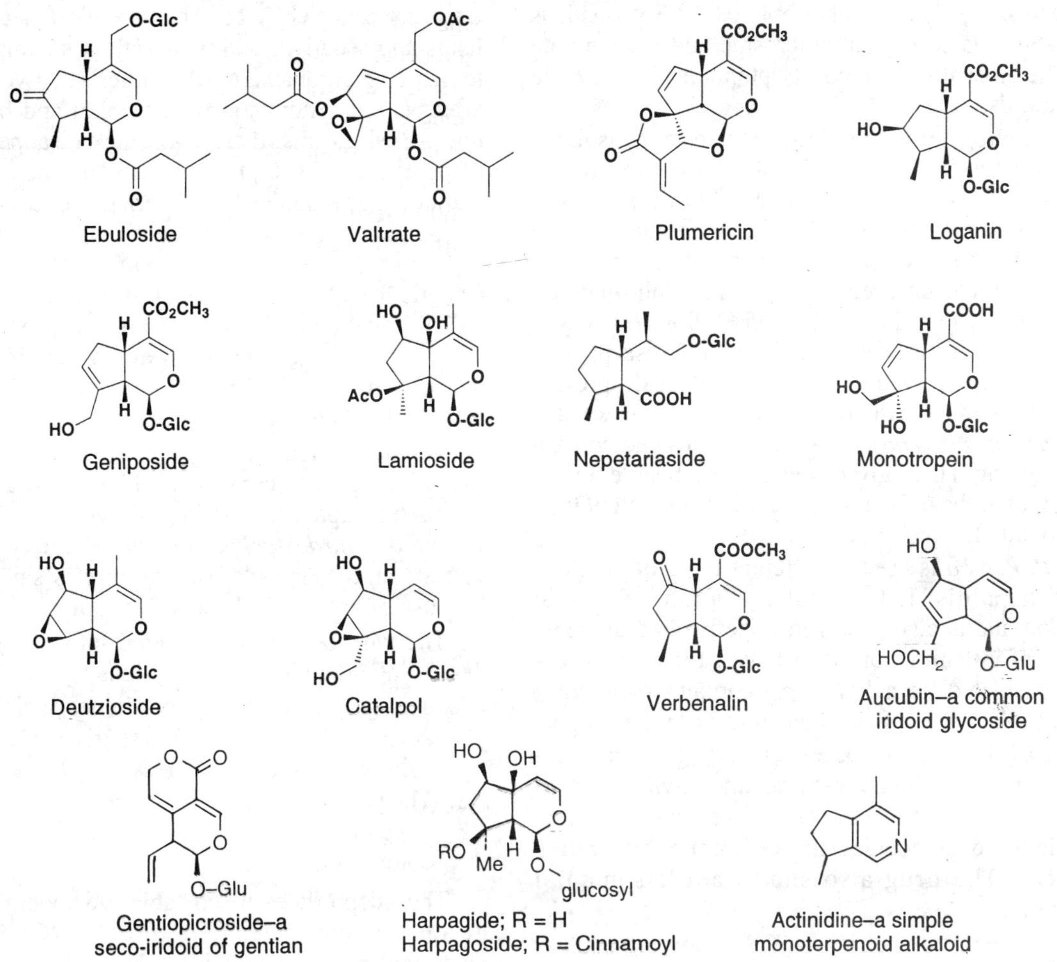

Fig. 12.3. Iridoids.

oxobicylo-[4.3.0]-nonane). Their carbon skeleton consists of eight to ninteen carbons but ten or nine carbons are the most frequent compounds containing thirteen (fulvopluminerin), fourteen (pulmericin) and ninteen carbons (oruwacin). *Seco*-iridoids are characterized by the structural feature of a 7, 8-*seco* ring. Glucose is the most common monosaccharide which occurs frequently at C-1. In addition, other sugars like apiose, 4-deoxyhexose, xylose, rhamnose, allose, gentiobiose and β-serotinose are found to attach to the iridane aglycone. Besides sugars, additional substituents like cinnamoyl, dihydrocaffeoyl, coumaroyl, caffeoyl, isovaleroyl, benzoyl, gentisoyl, vanilloyl, foliamenthoyl, menthiafoloyl,

nerol-8-oyl, etc. have been detected as substituents. If the sugar moiety is removed by enzymatic or acidic cleavage of glycosidic bonds, the resulting aglycone often decomposes.

Iridoids belonging to the sub-group of the chromogenic glycosides, which mostly give blue-shaded colour under acidic condition, were named as "pseudoindicanes" or "aucubin glycosides".

Iridoid glycosides of *Picrorhiza kurroa* are used as bitter tonics, stomachics, digestive and febrifuge. Gentiopicroside is found in many species of *Gentiana* and *Swertia*. Gentiopicroside is a bitter crystalline water soluble glucoside with a bitter value of 12000. Swertiamarin, found in *Swertia* species, is 5-hydroxy-gentiopicroside. Sweroside is closely related to gentiopicroside and participitate in the biosynthesis of non-tryptophan part of indole alkaloids.

Amarogentin is the bitterest substance isolated from natural products and tastes bitter even in 1 × $10^{5.8}$ or 5.8 lac dilution (5,80,00,000). It is present in Gentian roots and Chirata. Amarogentin is a phenolcarbonic ester of sweroside. It imparts bitter taste to the drug even if present in small quantity. Amaroswerin (bitter value : 5,80,000, 0001 and amaropanin (bitter value 2,00,00,000 also present in the drug. Picrosides I and II and kutkoside, present in the sub-terranean parts of Indian katuki (*Picrorhiza kurroa*), are C_9 glycosides and contain epoxy ring. These glycosides are responsible for the activity of the drug. Picroside II is more potent than picroside I.

P. kurroa is used in different types of jaundice and hepatitis. It has cholagogue and chloretic action and is also useful in infective and amoebic type of inflammation of the liver. Picroliv, an extract isolated from *P. kurroa*, contains picroside I and kutkoside as major constituents in the proportion of 1 : 5 and possesses very good hepatoprotective and immuno-stimulant activity. A standardized extract of *P. kurroa* consisting a mixture of irridoid glycosides shows immunorestorative effect. The drug also shows antileishmanial activity.

Valtrats, Valepotriats or Valtratums are another group of epoxy iridoid esters isolated from fresh or stabilized roots of Valerian. They are neither glycoside nor lactone and are said to be active primary components of the valerian. They are triesters of polyhydroxy cyclic pentanopyran, esterified with isovaleric, acetic, isocaproic and beta-acetoxy valeric acids. They are about 0.5% in European valerian (*Valeriana officinalis*) and 2% in Indian valerian (*Valeriana wallichii*). They are classified into conjugated dienes: Valtrat and Acevaltrat give blue colour with HCl and acetic acid, and monoenes : Didrovaltrat and isovaleroxy hydroxy-didrovaltrat (IVHD) give yellow brown colour with HCl. Together with these compounds, a water soluble iridoid ester glycoside valeriosidat without epoxy ring, is also found. Valtrats are highly unstable compounds getting decomposed easily during drying into

Baldrinal and free acids. They are used as tranquilizers and sedatives and their action is comparable to that of meprobamate. Like other sedatives, their effect is not synergistic with alcohol and barbiturates. Besides this, there is a quick disappearance of abstinaunce symptoms of alcohol and opium addicts. Large number of Valerian products, often in combination with other sedatives, are marketed, e.g., Valman, a well known formulation of Kali-Chemie from Hannover, contains valtrat, acevaltrat and didrovaltrat in the proportion of 15:5:80. Cytotoxic and anticancer activities are present in valtrat and didrovaltrat. Valtrat is more potent in these actions than didrovaltrat.

Valerian also contains other sedative and tranquilizing active constituents like valeric acid and valeranon. Japanese valerian (*V. angustifolia*) and Jatamansi (*Nardostachyas jatamansi*) are devoid of valtrats and their sedative property is said to be because of valeric acid and valeranon.

The valepotriates are divided into two groups depending on their colour reactions :

1. The group of conjugated dienes which with acids (HCl + CH_3COOH) give blue salts soluble in water.
2. The group of monoenes which react with non-oxygen acids and give a non-specific brown colouration.

The valepotriates are unstable and undergo rapid decomposition at temperature > 40°C and are destroyed by mineral acids (pH < 3) and alkalis (pH > 11).

The main valepotriates isolated from *Valeriana wallichii* are valtrate, isovaltrate, homovaltrate, acevaltrate, homoacevaltrate and IVHD-valtrate. All these compounds degrade to yield baldrinal, homobaldrinal and their corresponding acids depending on the nature of the compounds.

Evaluation of valepotriates

The contents of valepotriates vary depending upon the variety, origin, time of collection and the method of drying the herb. Many European varieties of *Valeriana* do not contain any valepotriates at all. The quantitative ratios of the three main valepotriates are also different in plants of different varieties. For example, valtrate clearly dominates in *Valeriana officinalis*, whereas the three compounds (valtrate, acevaltrate and didrovaltrate) are almost in equal quantities in *V. wallichii*. This enable to chemically differentiate the two varieties and identify the herb for study. The most important step in the evaluation of the drug is qualitative and quantitative determination of the valepotriates content. A number of methods are known in the literature for the quantitative determination of valepotriates in the drug and its preparations. The estimation is often made either by spectrophotometry or colorimetry. Colorimetric and titration methods can be used to evaluate the total esters present in the sample. UV method of analysis can measure only the dienes present in the sample but to determine quantitatively each component, HPLC is the method of choice.

(a) U.V. spectrophotometry

The derivatives that absorb in UV (valtrate and acevaltrate with conjugated diene system λ_{max}^{256}) are estimated by UV spectrometry after chromatographic separation and elution of the spots.

A known volume (0.03 ml) of extract is applied on TLC plates coated with silica gel GF 254. The chromatograms are developed for 15 minutes by using a mixture of hexane-methyl ethyl ketone (8:2), dried at a temperature of 20°C and observed in UV 254 nm light. The spots of fluorescence-suppressing substances (which appear as blue spot on green ground coat) are marked with a needle and the marked zones of adsorbent are transformed quantitatively to a small filtrate made of sintered glass G-4 and eluted with 3 portions of methanol and volume made up to 10 ml. Absorption of the solution is measured at 256 nm and the valtrate content is determined by using the coefficient $E_{1\%}^{1\,cm} = 379$. This method gives an accuracy of $\pm 8\%$.

(b) Colorimetry or densitometry

The technique is based on the highly exhibited coloration reaction. The reaction principle consists in the formation of a hydroxamic acid by hydroxylamine in highly alkaline medium by the rupture of ester function according to the following scheme:

$$RCOO\text{---}R' + NH_2OH \longrightarrow RCO\text{---}NHOH + R'OH$$

$$\longrightarrow \quad \underset{\underset{OH}{|}}{RC = NOH}$$

The hydroxamic derivatives formed, give in acid medium, a coloured ferric complex with $FeCl_3$ of the formula, $(R\text{---}CO\text{---}NHO)_3$ Fe whose intensity of colouration is proportional to the quantity of the hydroxamate formed and, therefore, to that of the ester.

The method consists in subjecting the dichloromethane extract of drug to TLC. The individual zones treated with standard solutions of alkaline NH_2OH followed by acidic $FeCl_3$ (in absolute ethanol or methanol) and resulting colour determined at 512 nm. Pure compounds are used as reference.

Densitometric method

The densitometric method enables us to estimate the isolated spot without the risk of interference. It is independent estimation of total esters in a sample. A modified method consists in dissolving a known weight (W) of the extract in a known volume (V_1) of methanol. An aliquot volume (V_2) of this solution is neutralized with 0.01N NaOH using phenophthalein as indicator. Subsequently 10 ml more of 0.01N NaOH are added and contents heated as 56-59°C for 3 min, diluted with 200 ml of water, cooled and titrated with 0.01N H_2SO_4. From this, the amount of alkali consumed for the hydrolysis of the esters is obtained and percentage of total valepotriates in terms of valtrate is obtained by the following relation:

$$\text{Percentage of total (V.P.)} = \frac{0.00106 \times V_1 \times V_3 \times 100}{W \times V_2}$$

V_1 = Total volume of the extract.
V_2 = Aliquot volume of the solution used.
V_3 = Volume of 0.01N NaOH consumed.
W = Weight of extract.

Diterpenes: C_{20}

The diterpenes are formed from four isoprene groups, most of which are of limited distribution in the plant kingdom. Because of their higher boiling points, they are not considered to be essential oils. They are present in resins, the material that remains after steam distillation of a plant extract. The diterpenes exist in various structural types.

The C_{20} compounds include resin acids as (+)- and (–)-pimaric acid and their isomers and abietic acids of pine resin. The gibberellins, first obtained from fungi of genus *Gibberella* and so found in higher plants, are diterpenoid acids which have a marked effect on growth of seedlings. Phytol, $C_{20}H_{39}OH$, an unsaturated alcohol, is a component of the chlorophyll molecule. Vitamin K_1, an anti-haemorrhagic compound is also a phytol derivative. Vitamin A, a diterpenoid, is a carotene. Furano-diterpenes constitute the bitter principles of calumba root. *Teucrium chamaedrys*, wall germander, and *T. scorodonia*, wood sage, (Lamiaceae) are both used in herbal medicine as diaphoretics and antirheumatics. Besides containing small amount of volatile oil, flavonoids and tannins, both herbs produce diterpenes of the neoclerodane type. The alkaloids of species of *Aconitum*, *Delphinium* and *Garrya* are diterpenes. Some diterpenes from *Kalmia latifolia* (Ericaceae) have antifeedant pro-perties with respect to the gypsy moth.

Forskolin (coleonol), a diterpene isolated from *Coleus forskohlii* (Lamiaceae) is a polyoxygenated diterpenes.

Preparations of *Coleus* species are used for the treatment of heart diseases and abdominal colic. Forskolin has hypotensive, spasmolytic, cardiotonic and platelet aggregation inhibitory activity; due to its unique adenylate cyclase stimulant activity it is a promising drug for the treatment of glaucoma, congestive cardiomyopathy and asthma.

Tiglianes, daphnanes and ingenanes are three related groups of diterpenoid compounds found in the Euphorbiaceae (e.g. *Croton tiglium*, *Euphorbia* spp.) and the Thymelaeaceae (e.g. *Daphne, Lasiosiphon, Pimelia* and *Gnidia* spp.). Biologically, they produce intense inflammation on appli-cation to the skin and have both tumour-promoting and antitumour activity. Phorbol (a tigliane derivative) is the 12,13-diester, 12-O-tetrade-canoylphorbol-13-acetate, which is extensively used in pharmacologi-cal investigation although *Croton tiglium* contains some 10 others. They substitute for diacyglycerol in the activation of the phosphorylating enzyme pro-tein kinase C; the shape of the molecules, with their long-chain ester groupings, seems to match the side-chains on the natural second messenger, diacyl-glycerol. The 12,13,20-triesters of phorbol are termed 'cryptic irritants' because they do not exhibit pro-inflammatory activity on mammalian skin unless the C-20 acyl group is removed by hydro-lysis.

The cyclic ether zoapatanol is used as an aborti-facient. A number of clerodanes have been isolated from the *Ajuga, Salvia*, and *Teucrium* species, and have been found to possess insecticidal activity. A variety of cytotoxic lactones have been isolated from *Podocarpus* species. These *podolactones* have plant regulatory properties and antileukemic activity. The gibberellins comprise an important group of plant hormones. Marrubin is a diterpene lactone from white horehound (*Marrubium vulgare*), which has been used as a bitter and choleretic in digestive and biliary complaints. Taxol, discovered by Wani et al. (1971), is a wholly unique antimitotic agent which binds to microtubules and stabilizes them as opposed to all other antimitotics of the tubulin-bind-ing type, such as vincristine, the podophyllotoxins, and colchicine.

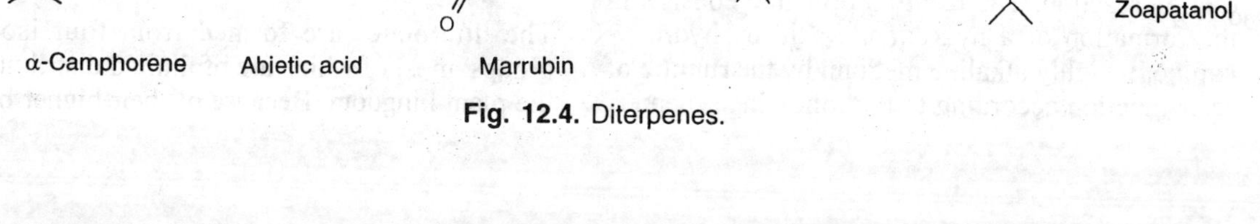

α-Camphorene   Abietic acid   Marrubin   Zoapatanol

Fig. 12.4. Diterpenes.

Triterpenes : C_{30}

The C_{30} terpenes are based on six isoprene units and are biosynthetically derived from squalene. They are often melting colourless solids and are distributed among plant resin, cork and cutin. There are several important groups of triterpenes, including common triterpenes, steroids, saponins, sterolins, and cardiac glycosides. Among these is azadirachtin, a powerful insect antifeedant from Neem oil. They may be aliphatic (e.g. the squalene in animals and oils of arachis and olive) tetracyclic (lanosterol) or pentacyclic (α- and β-amyrins). They may occur in free state, as esters or glycosides.

Tetracyclic triterpenes also include the limonoids, the sterols found in wool fat and yeast and the cardioactive glycosides. Only a few of the common triterpenes are actually widely distributed among plants. The amyrins and ursolic and oleanic acids are common on the waxy coatings on leaves and as a protective coating on some fruits. Other triterpenes include the limonins and the cucurbitacins.

Tetraterpenes: C_{40}

The most common tetraterpenoids are the carotenoids, a widely distributed group of C_{40} compounds. The carotenoids are generally derived from lycopene. Cyclization at one end gives γ-carotene and at both ends provides β-carotene. This pigment is the most common of all of these pigments and virtually universal in the leaves of higher plants. Numerous double-bond isomers are possible for these basic structures, all of which can provide brightly coloured pigments varying from yellow to red. In plants, carotenoids serve both as necessary pigments in photosynthesis and as colouring agents in flowers and fruits. They protect plants from over-oxidation catalyzed by other light absorbing pigments such as the chlorophylls.

In association with chlorophyll, carotenes participate in photosynthesis. They have vitamin A activity and are industrially important as food colourants. The colours of the red tomato and the orange are due to the carotenoids lycopene and citraurin, respectively. Some carotenoids are oxygenated derivatives.

Plant carotenoids are responsible for the red, orange and yellow pigments found in fruit and roots such as tomatos, red peppers, pumpkins, and carrots. They are present in the petals of many flowers and are the primary pigments responsible for the fall coloration of deciduous trees. Carotenoids are synthesized in the terpenoid pathway as

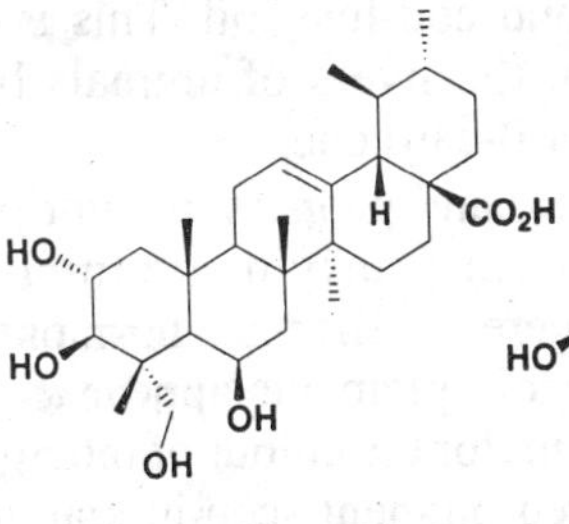

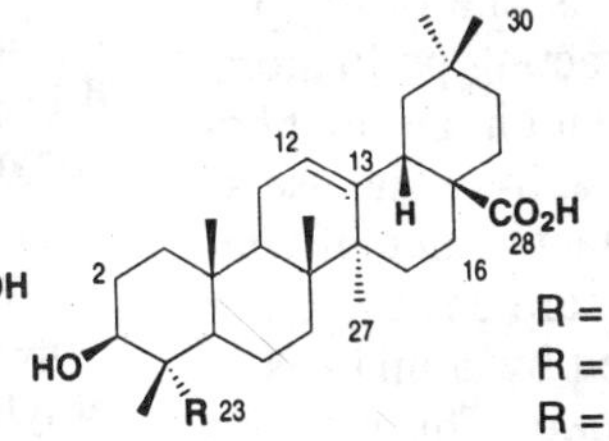

R = CH_3 : Oleanolic acid
R = CH_2OH : Hederagenin
R = CH_2OH, OH 2β, 16α : Polygalacic acid
R = CHO : Gypsogenin
R = COOH, OH 2β : Medicagenic acid
R = COOH, OH 2β, 27 : Presenegin

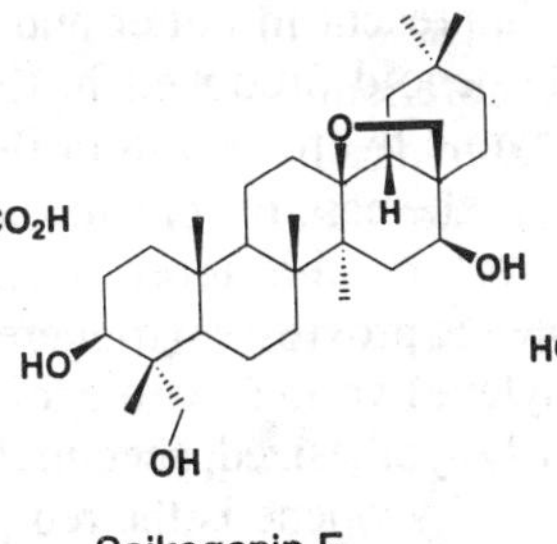

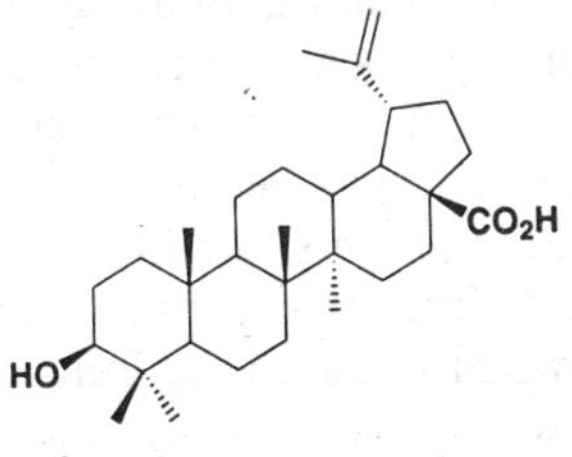

Madecassic acid   Saikogenin F

Betulinic acid 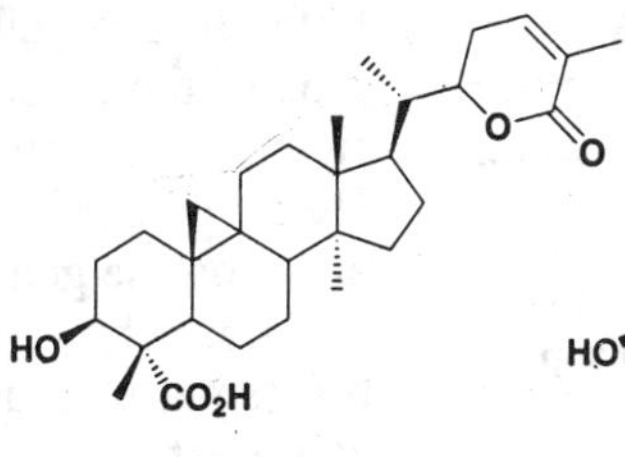   Abrusogenin

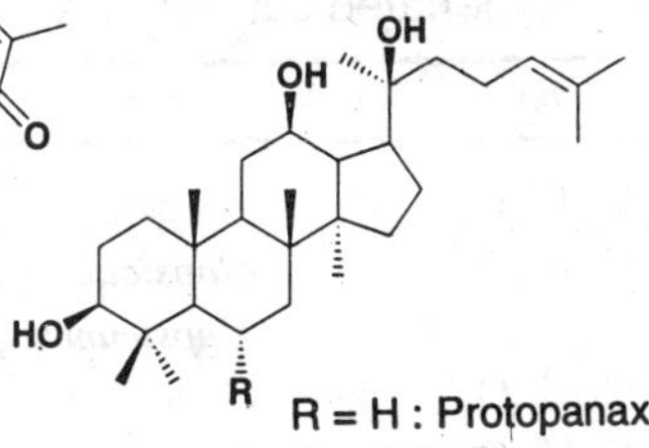

R = H : Protopanaxadiol
R = OH : Protopanaxatriol

Fig. 12.5. Triterpenes.

C_{40} tetraterpenes derived from the condensation of eight isoprene units starting with isopentenyl diphosphate. There are two basic types of carotenoids: (1) carotene which contains no oxygen atoms and (2) xanthophyll which does contain oxygen. At the center of each carotenoid molecule, the linkage order is reversed, resulting in a molecule which is symmetrical. A set of double bonds in the molecule is responsible for the absorption of light in the visible portion of the spectrum. This has an important impact on the absorption of a wider range of light wavelengths for use in photosynthesis. In photosynthetic organisms, carotenoids are an integral structural component of photosynthetic antenna and reaction center complexes, but they also protect against the harmful effects of photooxidation processes. Like chlorophyll, carotenoids are found in the thylakoids of green leaves and stems. In fruits and flowers they are also found in plastids, but these plastids have structural differences and are referred to as chromoplasts to indicate that they contain pigments other than chlorophyll.

β-Carotene is the orange pigment in carrot roots, pumpkin fruits, leaves of deciduous trees, and some flower petals. Zeaxanthin and violaxantin are bright yellow and found in autumn-coloured leaves and flower petals. Coloration of flowers is very important to the survival success of the plant producing them. The colour of the flowers is one of the primary factors involved in the attracting pollinators. For humans, β-carotene is important in our diet because of its purported anticancer activity, its use as a food coloring, and as an important source of vitamin A that is synthesized from β-carotene and other carotenoids. Vita-min A produced by animals is in turn converted to the pigment, *retinal*. This pigment is one of the essential components in the light receptors of the eye that allow us to see.

Table 12.1. Oxygenated carotenoids

Carotenoid	Formula	Source
Bixin	$C_{25}H_{30}O_4$	Annatto
Capsanthin	$C_{40}H_{58}O_3$	*Capsicum* spp.
Capsorubin	$C_{40}H_{60}O_4$	*Capsicum* spp.
Crocetin	$C_{20}H_{24}O_4$	Saffron
Crocin	$C_{44}H_{64}O_{24}$	Saffron
Fucoxanthin	$C_{40}H_{60}O_6$	Brown algae

Carotenoid pigments act in fruit and seed dispersal by attracting animals which in turn spread the seeds. Most fruits also produce odour compounds such as monoterpenes to help attract these organisms, and the sugars produced and stored in the fruits act as a positive reward. In ripening fruits, chlorophyll pigments gradually break down in chloroplast thylakoid membranes, revealing the carotenoid pigments that were masked by the chlorophyll pigments. During ripening there is also significant synthesis of new carotenoid pigments.

Test for carotenoids

Carotenoids on treatment with strong sulphuric acid, give dark blue, green or violet colours. This reaction serves for distinguishing them from other natural pigments such as the anthocyanins. The test is best carried out by reacting an ether or chloroform solution of the carotenoid with 85% sulphuric acid, when a blue colour is formed at the junction of the two layers. Most carotenoids give a blue colour with antimony trichloride in chloroform (Carr-Price test), or a dark-blue colour with concentrated hydrochloric acid containing a little phenol.

Important C_{40} compounds are yellow or orange-red carotenoid pigments of which about 180 have been reported. A fat-soluble growth factor, vitamin A, is present in butter and cod-liver oil. This is a diterpenoid produced in the livers of animals by enzymic hydrolysis from β-carotene.

In the case of tomatoes and peppers, the unripe fruits are characteristically bright green. As ripening progresses (triggered by the plant hormone, ethylene) various carotenoid pigments appear and, newly synthesized, account for the colour of the ripe fruits. Lycopene is the red pigment seen in mature tomato and red pepper fruits. Tomatoes can have both red and yellow fruits depending on the genotype of the parent. In some peppers, we encounter ripe fruits which are seen at maturity (bell peppers). Here ripe peppers may be yellow or red depending again on the genotype of the parents. Similar types of colour chan-ges occur in fruts of ripening cucurbits (squash, gourds, pumpkins) and in the fruits of egg plant.

Red maple (*Acer rubrum*) trees produce red-coloured flowers and leaves, yet they are wind polli-

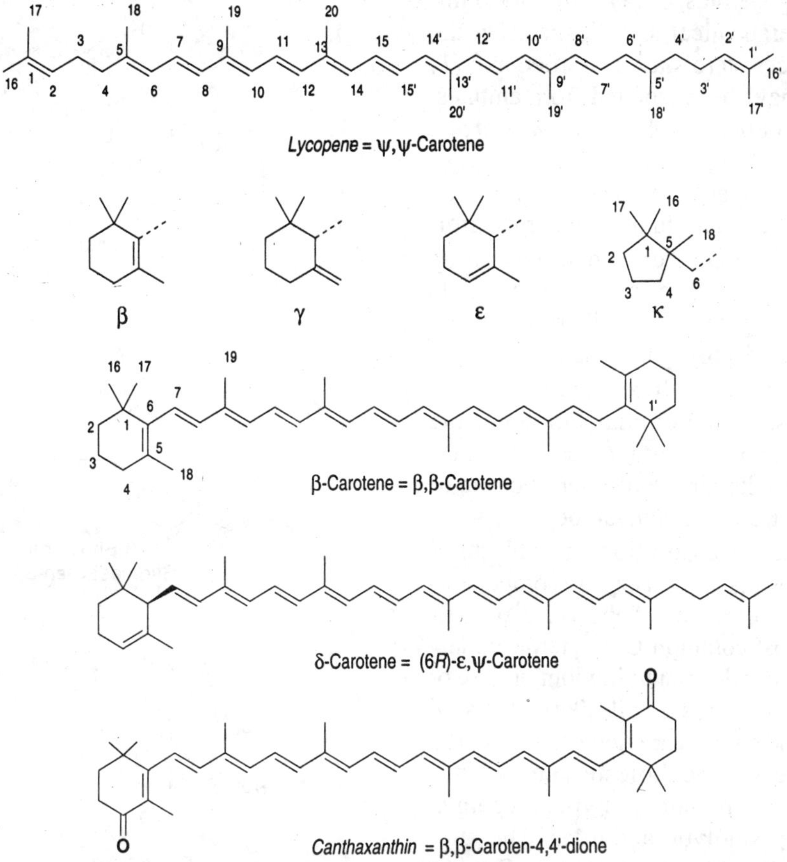

Lycopene = ψ,ψ-Carotene

β γ ε κ

β-Carotene = β,β-Carotene

δ-Carotene = (6R)-ε,ψ-Carotene

Canthaxanthin = β,β-Caroten-4,4'-dione

Fig. 12.6. Tetraterpenes.

nated. These plants do not have to attract pollinators. The pigments help to warm the flowers or leaves during early spring or late fall. This extra heat would greatly aid seed development and photosynthetic processes in early spring allowing the plant to get a head start on growth over other plants and provide a longer period to produce energy.

Polyterpenoids

Polyterpenes are composed of many isoprene units. These are macro-molecules of molecular weight over 100000, are found in india-rubber and gutta-percha. Chemically, pure rubber is *cis*-1,4-polyisoprene $(C_5H_8)_n$ present in *Hevea brasiliensis*. Gutta-percha is *trans*-1,4-polyisoprene, and chicle, obtained from *Manilkara sapota*, contains a mixture of low molecular weight *cis*- and *trans*-polyisoprenes.

STEROIDS

Steroids in general are tetracyclic compounds characterized by the presence of a perhydro-1, 2-cyclopentenophenanthrene ring system. The three cyclohexane rings are designated as A, B, C and the cyclopentane ring is the D ring. They are colourless crystalline compounds and widely distributed in animals and plants. All the steroids give among other products 'Diels' hydrocarbon on dehydration with selenium at 360°C. They possess an alcoholic group and may be saturated (plant sterols) or unsaturated (animal and many plant sterols). Mammalian endocrine glands are the source of several hundred naturally occurring steroids, many with biochemical, clinical or therapeutical significance. On the basis of their sources sterols are classified as : (1) *Zoosterol*, which have been isolated from animals, *e.g.*, cholesterol, coprostanol, (2) *Phytosterols*, which are obtained from plant sources, e.g., sitosterol, stigmasterol; and (3) *Mycosterols*, which are obtained from yeast and fungi, *e.g.*, ergosterol.

On the basis of the number of hydroxyl group the sterols may be mono-hydroxysterols (*e.g.*, cholesterol, stigmasterol), dihydroxysterol, tri-hydroxysterols and polyhydroxysterols.

All plant steroids are hydroxylated at C-3 and are in fact sterols. In the animal kingdom, the steroids have profound importance as hormones, coenzymes, and provitamins. However, the role of the phytosterols is less well understood.

Sterols prevent the absorption of cholesterol from the gastro-intestinal tract. They are components of the unsaponifiable matter of the fixed oils. β-sitosterol is the most common C-29 sterol, widely distributed throughout the plant kingdom, in free or in glycosidal form. Various seed oils like cotton seed oil, soyabean oil and corn oil are rich in β-sitosterol. Such drugs possess hypocholesteraemic, antithrombotic, anti-inflammatory, hypoglycaemic, antifertility and spasmolytic activities. The antiinflammatory activity of β-sitosterol from *Cyperus rotundus* is similar to hydrocortisone and oxyphenbutazone and the antipyretic activity is similar to aspirin. β-Sitosterol from *Cyperus rotundus* is similar to hydrocortisone and oxy-phenbutazone and the antipyretic activity is similar to aspirin. β-Sitosterol possesses a wide margin of safety with minimum ulcerogenic activity. In Germany, several formulations containing β-sitosterol are used to treat noninfective prostatitis and prostata adenosa.

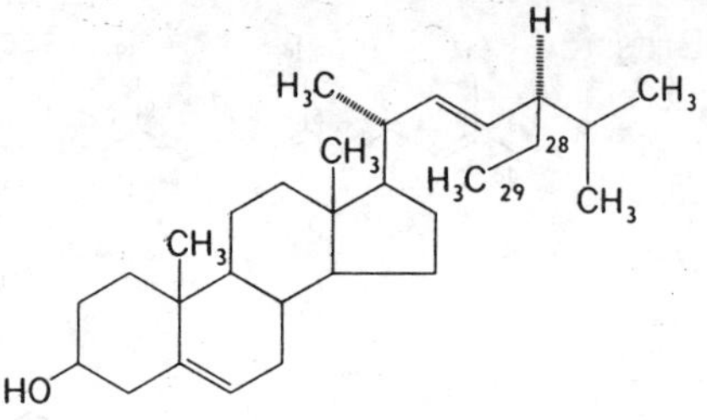

Utilization of natural steroids in pharmaceutical industry

There is a great demand for natural products which will serve as starting materials for their partial synthesis.

Cortisone and its derivatives are 11-oxosteroids. The sex hormones, including the oral contraceptives, and the diuretic steroids have no oxygen substi-

Stigmasterol
Stigmasta-5,22-dien-3β-ol

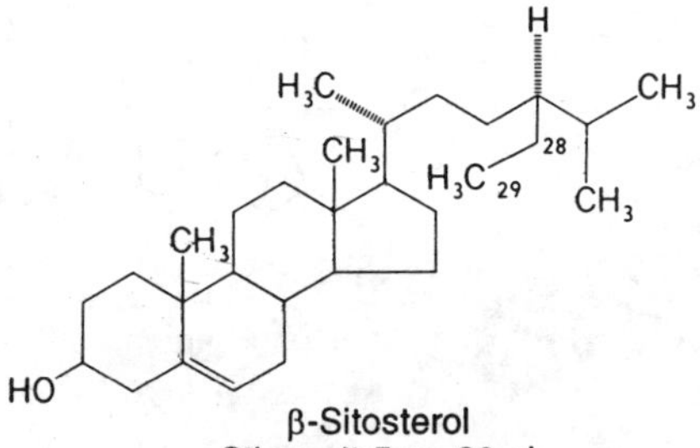

β-Sitosterol
Stigmast-5-en-3β-ol

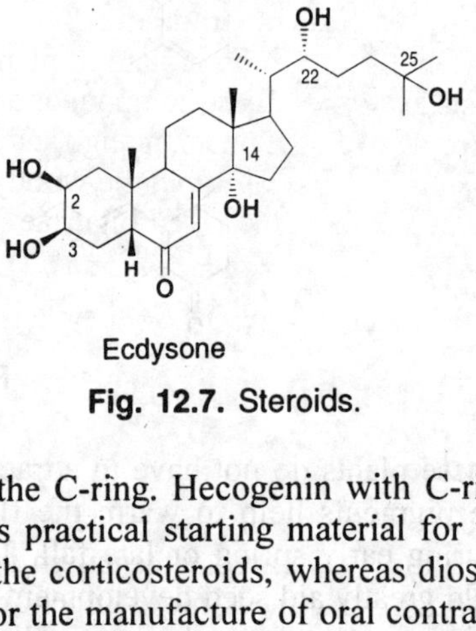

Ecdysone

Fig. 12.7. Steroids.

tution in the C-ring. Hecogenin with C-ring substitution is practical starting material for the synthesis of the corticosteroids, whereas diosgenin is suitable for the manufacture of oral contraceptives and the sex hormones. Diosgenin can also be used for corticosteroid synthesis, of a microbiological fermentation to introduce oxygen into the 11α-position of the pregnene nucleus.

In the plant, cholesterol is a precursor of insect-moulting hormones. They are formed together with bufadienolides and saponins.

Cucurbitacins

These tetracyclic triterpenoids possess cytotoxic and antitumour properties. They occur in the Cucurbitaceae and other families such as the Euphorbiaceae and Brassicaceae. They are hydrolysed by the enzyme elaterase.

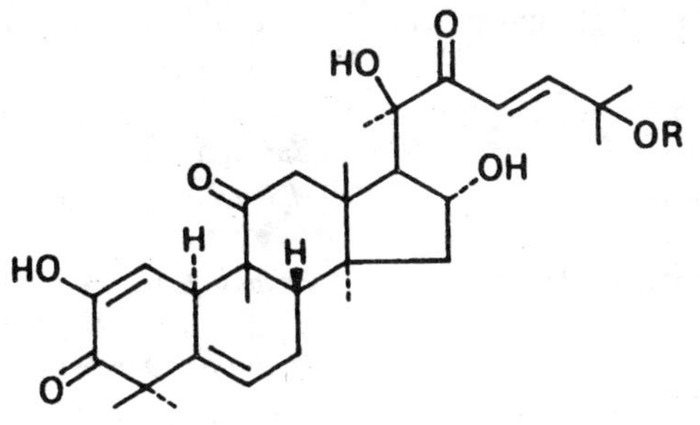

Cucurbitacin E (elaterin); R = CH₃CO
Cucurbitacin I (elaterin B); R = H

Fig. 12.8. Cucurbitacins.

Cycloartanes

The ring closure of squalene 2,3-oxide yields cycloartenol as an intermediate in plant sterol biosynthesis. However, these compounds are also found in the free state in the neem, mango and olive plants, *Euphorbia* spp., *Hypericum*, the woody nightshade and in members of the Cucurbitaceae.

The plant *Ajuga decumbens* (Lameaceae) contains the steroidal lactone ajugalactone; this compound has an α,β-unsaturated carbonyl group and inhibits insect metamorphosis.

Ecdysones

The ecdysis of insects is a state in which larvae undergo during their transformation into an adult. Ecdysones, or insect-moulting hormones, are

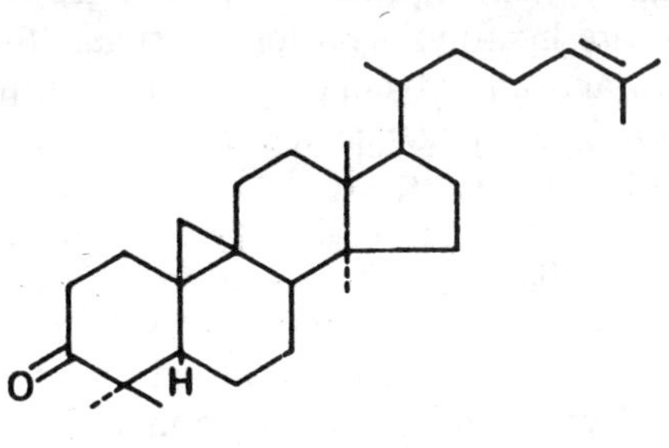

Cycloartenone

Fig. 12.9. Cycloartenone.

substances which stimulate changes, *e.g.*, ecdysone, isolated from silk-worm pupae. In plants they occur in abundance. Ecdysterone (20-hydroxy-ecdysone) is obtained from both plant and insect sources. Insects do not themselves biosynthesize steroids and rely on plant materials for suitable precursors.

SAPONINS

Saponins are high-molecular-weight triterpene glycosides containing a sugar group attached to either a sterol or other triterpene. They are widely distributed in the plant kingdom and composed of two parts: glycone (sugar) and aglycone or genin (triterpene). Typically, they have detergent properties, readily form foams in water, have a bitter taste, and are piscicidal (toxic to fish). Many of the plants that contain saponins have been used as soaps. These include soaproot (*Chlorogalum pomeridianum*), soapbark (*Quillaja saponaria*), soapberry (*Sapindus saponaria*) and soapnut (*Sapindus mukurossi*).

Saponins are constituents of many plant drugs and folk medicines, especially among Asian peoples.

The aglycones, or genins as they are sometimes called, may be of the triterpene, steroid, or steroid alkaloid class. Saponins may be mono- or polydesmodic, depending on the number of attached sugar moieties.

The saponins are comprised of six isoprene units and are derived from squalene. Commercially important preparations based on saponins include sarsaparilla root (*Sarsaparilla* spp.), licorice (*Glycyrrhiza* spp.), ivy leaves (*Hedera* spp.), primula root (*Primula* spp.), as well as Ginseng (*Panax* spp.).

The ammonium and calcium salts of glycyrrhizinc acid are referred to as the *glycyrrhizins*. At 50 to 100 times sweeter than sucrose, these are the active ingredients in locorice root (*Glycyrrhiza glabra*), with expectorant, bacteriostatic, and antiviral activity. The ginsenosides are one of many triterpene saponins from ginseng (*Panax ginseng*) believed to be responsible for its immunostimulant activity.

There are two types of saponins - triterpenoid and steroidal saponins. The steroidal saponins are similar to the human body's own naturally occur-

Table 12.2. Natural pentacyclic triterpenoid saponins

Saponin	Genin	Sugar components	Source
Aescin	Aescigenin	2 glucose, 1 glucuronic acid, 1 tihlic acid	*Aesculus hippocastanum*
Calendulasaponin A	Oleanolic acid	2 glucose, 1 galactose, 1 glucuronic acid	*Calendula officinalis*
Glycyrrhizic acid	Glycyrrhetinic acid	2 glucuronic acid	*Glycyrrhiza* spp.
Guaianin	Noroleanolic acid	1 rhamnose, 1 glucose, 1 arabinose, 1 fucose, 1 rhamnose	*Gypsophila* spp. and other Caryophyllaceae
Hederacoside A (hederin)	Hederagenin	1 glucose, 1 arabinose	*Hedera helix* (ivy)
Primula-saponin	Primulagenin	1 rhamnose, 1 glucose, 1 galactose, glucuronic acid	*Primula* spp.
Quillaia-saponin	Quillaiac acid (hydroxygypsogenin)	Glucuronic acid, 6 sugars and acyl moieties	*Quillaja saponaria*
Saikosaponin A	Saikogenin F	1 glucose, 1 fructose	*Bupleurum* spp.

ring steroid hormones. Many plants containing steroidal saponins have a marked hormonal activity, *e.g.*, *Dioscorea* species. Triterpenoid saponins, *i.e.*, *Glycyrrhiza glabra*, are often strong expectorant and may add in the absorption of nutrients.

Steroidal saponins are the plant glycosides which form colloidal soapy solutions in water. They can effect haemolysis of red blood cells at high dilution and act as fish poison. These plant products have the C_{27}-framework of cholesterol rather than that of the C_{29}-sitosterols. The sapon-genin side chain differs in having two oxidic bridges linked at C_{22} in a ketospiroacetal grouping, which is transformed into many other compounds.

The pentacyclic triterpenoid saponins are rare in monocotyledons. They are abundant in many dicotyledonous families, *e.g.*, the Caryophyllaceae, Sapindaceae, Polygalaceae Sapotaceae, Phytolaccaceae, Chenopodiaceae, Ranunculaceae, Berberidaceae, Papaveraceae, Linaceae, Zygophyllaceae, Rutaceae, Myrtaceae, Cucurbitaceae, Araliaceae, Apiaceae, Primulaceae, Oleaceae, Lobeliaceae, Campanulaceae, Rubiaceae and Asteraceae.

In these saponins the sapogenin is attached to a chain of sugar or uronic acid units, or both, often in the 3-position. Biosynthesis involves ring-closure of squalene similar to that of steroids.

Triterpenoid saponins may be classified into three groups represented by α-amyrin, β-amyrin and lupeol. The related triterpenoid acids are formed from these by replacement of a methyl group by a carboxyl group in positions 4, 17, 20, or 29.

Primula root contains these saponins about 5-10%; liquorice root about 2-12% of glycyrrhizic acid, quillaia bark up to about 10% of the mixture known as 'commercial saponins'; the seeds of the horse-chestnut up to 13% of aescin. Oleanolic acid occurs as a saponin in sugar beet, thyme, *Guaiacum* spp. and in the free state in olive leaves and clove buds.

Sugar residue may be linked via a single hydroxyl group (usually C–3–OH) of the aglycone monodesmoside saponins or more rarely via two hydroxyl groups or a single hydroxyl group and a carboxyl group (bis-desmoside saponins). Usually the sugars like D-glucose, D-galactose, D-xylose, L-rhamnose and L-arabinose occur in the glycosides.

The most important saponin-containing drugs are Quillaia and Senega. Most of the saponins are neutral and soluble in water. Like other glycosides, saponins are hydrolyzed to form a sugar (usually dextrose) and an aglycone, generally known as sapogenin. The sapogenins are insoluble in water, but soluble in weak alcohol. Their aqueous solutions form froths on shaking; produce stable emulsion on shaking with oils and fats; absorb and retain in solution a volume of gas (*e.g.*, CO_2) several times greater than absorbed by an equal volume of water; an aqueous solution added to red blood corpuscles causes haemolysis, *i.e.*, disintegration and solution of the corpuscles to form a clear red liquid.

Withanolides

This group of compounds, present only in some members of the Solanaceae, constitutes another class of steroidal lactone. *Withania somnifera* (Ashvagandha) is used as adaptogenic, aphrodisiac, tonic, sedative, antirheumatic and diuretic drugs; extracts of the plant also have a potent antimitotic activity. It contains withaferin A.

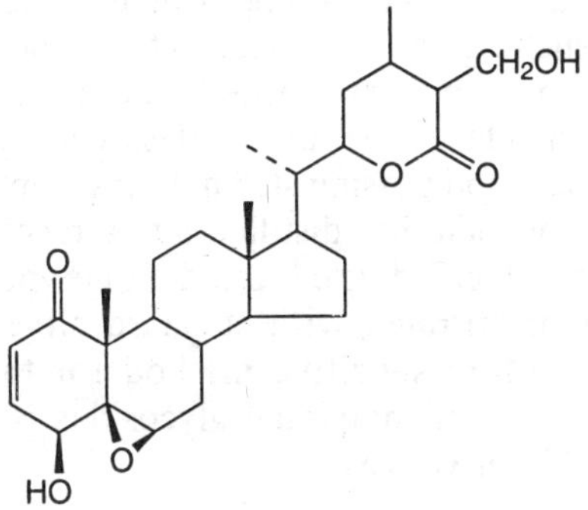

Withaferin A

Fig. 12.10. Withanolide.

AROMATICS

All plants contain different aromatic or phenolic natural products. The vivid colours that light up the plants are derived from the tetrapyrroles, principally chlorophyll; the terpene-based carotenes; and the aromatics, or the acetogenins. Several thousand aromatics are known and new structures are continuously being discovered. The polyphenolic lignins serve as structural components of the cell wall. Aromatic compounds are formed by several biosynthetic routes, including the polyketide and shikimate pathways, and from terpenoid origins. Due to the acidity of the phenol functionality (pK_a of 8 to 11), phenolic substances are water soluble and frequently form ether linkages with carbohydrate residues.

Non-phenolic aromatics

Several important natural products do not contain this functionality. These include the amino acids, tryptophan and phenylalanine, the indole alkaloids, and auxin (indole-3-acetic acid), an important plant hormone.

Tetrapyrroles

The chlorophylls are perhaps the most well-known plant constituents. As the primary catalysts of photosynthesis, they occur in several similar cyclic tetrapyrole forms and are located in the chloroplasts of all photosynthetic plant tissues.

Other porphyrin pigments occur in plants in much smaller amounts. The cytochromes, are critical components in the respiratory chain of both plants and animals. Finally, the linear tetrapyrroles, including phytochrome, phytoerythrin, and phytocyanin, are the critical components for plant morphogenesis, the process by which numerous important plant developmental processes are initiated.

GLYCOSIDES

Glycosides are compounds which upon hydrolysis give rise to one or more sugars (glycone) and a compound which is not a sugar (aglycone or genin). The aglycone is usually a compound containing one or more hydroxyl groups. The glycoside is formed by the elimination of a molecule of water between a hydroxyl group of the aglycone and a hydroxyl group of the sugar. The aglycone may be an alcohol (salicin), anthraquinone derivative, phenol, aldehyde, acid, ester, or other compound.

The other important glycosides are anthraquinone glycosides, cardiac glycosides, cyanophore glycosides and isothiocyanate glycosides.

Anthraquinone derivatives

The laxative action of certain drugs is attributed to derivatives of anthraquinones, $C_6H_4 (CO)_2 C_6H_4$. Various derivatives are obtained by replacing the hydrogen atoms by alkyl, hydroxyl and other groups. Many such derivatives occur in nature and often are combined with a sugar forming a glycoside. For example:

Chrysophanol : A dihydroxy methyl anthraquinone present in Rhubarb.

Emodin : A trihydroxy methyl derivative present in Cascara and Rhubarb.

Aloe-emodin : The primary alcohol derived from chrysophanol, present in Aloe, Rhubarb and Senna.

Rhein : The acid derived from aloe-emodin, present in Rhubarb and Senna.

The anthraquinone derivatives are often orange red coloured compounds. For their detection the filtrate is shaken with benzene or chloroform and set aside to form two layers. The organic layer is separated and shaken with an equal volume of solution of ammonia. A pink to red colour is developed.

Anthraquinones have an irritant laxative effect on the large intestine, causing constractions of the intestinal walls and stimulating a bowel movement. They also make the stool more liquid, facilitating bowel movements.

Cyanogenetic Glycosides

The cyanogenetic glycoside manihotoxin is present in *Manihot utilissima*. Amygdalin from bitter almonds, linamarin from linseed and phaseolunatin from a bean, *Phaseolus lunatus*, have been isolated. These yield prussic acid on hydrolysis and were the first discovered cyanogenetic or cyanophoric glycosides. Over 2000 plant species involving about 110 families are cyanogenetic. The presence or absence of HCN is of taxonomic importance and it is used as a character for separating the subfamilies of the Rosaceae. The presence or absence of prussic acid may denote varieties or different chemical races of the same species (e.g., *Prunus amygdalus* yields both bitter and sweet almonds).

Most of these glucosides are derived from the nitrile of mandelic acid and their structure is that of O- and not N-glycosides. The sugar portion of the molecule may be a monosaccharide or a disaccharide such as gentiobiose or vicianose. If a disaccharide, enzymes present in the plant may bring about hydrolysis in two stages, as in the case of amygdalin (amygdaloside).

Tests

The powdered material is placed in a small flask with sufficient water to moisten. In the neck of the flask a suitably impregnated strip of filter-paper is suspended by means of a cork. The paper may be treated in either with sodium picrate (yellow), which is converted to sodium isopurpurate (brick-red), or a freshly prepared solution of guaiacum resin in absolute alcohol which is allowed to dry on the paper and treated with very dilute copper sulphate solution. The guaiacum resin test-paper turns blue with prussic acid. If the enzymes present in the material have not been destroyed or inactivated, the hydrolysis takes place within an hour when the flask is kept in a warm place. More rapid hydrolysis will result if a small amount of sulphuric acid is added and the flask gently heated. The intensity of colour produced with sodium picrate paper can be used for semiquanti-tative evaluations.

For materials containing a high percentage of cyanogenetic glycosides (*e.g.*, bitter almonds), the amount may be determined quantitatively by placing the plant material in a flask with water and tartaric acid and passing steam through until all the hydrocyanic acid has distilled into a receiver. The distillate is then adjusted to a definite volume and aliquots are titrated with standard silver nitrate solution. More sensitive method for the direct determination of individual glycosides is GLC of their TMS derivatives.

Phenols and phenolic glycosides

Phenols are the largest group of plant secondary metabolites. Phenols are important constituents of some medicinal plants and in the food industry they are utilized as colouring agents, flavourings, aromatizers and antioxidants. The phenolic classes include simple phenolic compounds, tannins, coumarins and their glycosides, anthraquinones and their glycosides, naphthoquinones, flavones and related flavonoid glycosides, anthocyanidins and anthocyanins, lignans and lignin. The biosynthetic origin of some of these compounds involves the shikimic acid pathway. Phenols may also have aromatic rings derived by acetate condensation.

Most of the simple phenols are monomeric components of the polymeric polyphenols and acids which make up plant tissues, including lignin, melanin, flavolan, and tannins. These individual components are obtained by acid hydrolysis of plant tissues. The components include p-hydroxybenzoic acid, protocatechuic acid, vanillic, syringic, salicylic and gallic acids. Free phenols which do not require degradation of cell-wall polymers are relatively rare in plants. Hydroquinone, catechol, orcinol, and other simple phenols are found in relatively low concentrations.

Table 12.3. Some natural cyanogenetic glycosides

Glycoside	Source (Family)	Composition
Amygdalin	*Prunus amygdalus* (Rosaceae)	D(-)-Mandelonitrile-gentiobioside
Linamarin	*Linum usitatissimum* (Linaceae)	Acetone cyanohydrin-glucoside
Manihotoxin	*Manihot utilissima* (Euphorbiaceae)	Identical with linamarin
Dhurrin	*Sorghum vulgare* (Poaceae)	β-Glucoside of p-hydroxymandelonitrile
Prulaurasin	*Prunus laurocerasus* (Rosaceae)	DL-Mandelonitrile-D-glucoside
Phaseolunatin	*Phaseolus lunatus* (Papilionaceae)	Identical with linamarin
Prunasin	*Prunus serotina* (Rosaceae)	D(-)-Mandelonitrile-D-glucoside
Sambumgrin	*Sambucus nigra* (Caprifoliaceae)	L(+)-Mandelonitrite-D-glucoside
Vicianin	*Vicia angustifolia* (Papilionaceae)	Mandelonitrite-vicianoside

Thymol, which comprises 30 to 80% of the essential oil of Thyme (*Thymus vulgaris*), has been used as an expectorant.

Many of the phenols also exist as their methyl ethers. Khellin and visnagin are the active coumarin derivatives of the *Ammi visnaga* fruit trans-Anethole is mainly responsible for the taste and smell of Anise seeds (*Pimpinella anisum*). Apiol is a major constituent of the essential oil of parsley seed and is a powerful diuretic.

Catechol (*o*-dihydroxybenzene) is present free in Kola seeds and in the leaves of *Gaultheria* spp. and its derivatives are the urushiol phenols of the poison oak and poison ivy. Derivatives of resorcinol (*m*-dihydroxybenzene) constitute the narcotic principles of cannabis and the glucoside arbutin involves quinol (hydroquinone, *p*-dihydroxybenzene). The taenicidal constituents of Male fern are phloroglucinol derivatives.

The phenolic compounds often possess alcoholic, aldehydic and carboxylic acid groups; they include eugenol (a phenolic phenylpropane), vanillin (a phenolic aldehyde) and various phenolic acids, such as salicylic, ferulic and caffeic acids. Glycoside formation is common, and the glycoside coniferin and other derivatives of phenolic cinnamic alcohols are precursors of lignin.

A considerable number of plant substances are phenolic compounds, *e.g.*, the anthraquinone derivatives, morphine and the resinotannols. They form coloured compounds with ferric chloride. Certain plant pigments are also phenolic. For example:

1. *Hydroxy flavone glycosides* : They are derived from flavones or the related compound xanthones. These glycosides themselves are colourless, but form yellow salts. They occur in Clove, Hamamelis, Catechu, Buchu, Senega, Gentian, Digitalis and Stramonium. They yield a dull green or reddish-brown colour with ferric chloride. Thymol is a main phenol of Thyme (*Thymus vulgaris*).

2. *Anthocyanins* : They are phenolic plant pigments which may be red, blue, or purple. The exact colour depends upon the hydrogen ion concentration of the solution. For example, haematien is a reddish coloured anthocyanin of logwood which changes to blue upon addition of lime water.

Simple phenolic compounds are found in many plants and have different pharmaceutical uses. Vanillin is the aglycone of the glycosides of Vanilla pods and is used in confectionary and in perfumary. Similarly, eugenol (Clove), salicin, and arbutin are simple phenolic compounds. Salicylic acid, the main compound for aspirin preparation, is found in many plants. Phenols are antiseptic and reduce inflammation when taken internally. However, they have an irritant effect when applied to the skin.

GLUCOSINOLATE COMPOUNDS

Sinigrin and sinalbin are present in crystalline form in black and white mustards. Such glycosides are reported from many plants, particularly used as condiments (*e.g.*, norseradish) or in folk medicine. The general structure is as :

$$R-C \overset{\displaystyle N-O.SO_2.O.X}{\underset{\displaystyle S.C_6H_{11}O_5}{}}$$

where R represents $CH_2 = CHCH_2$ in sinigrin and p-$HOC_6H_4CH_2$ in sinalbin; in sinigrin the X is potassium but can take the form of a more complex cation, e.g., sinapine ($C_{16}H_{25}O_6N$), in sinalbin. The anion of the formula is designated a glucosinolate; thus, sinalbin becomes sinapine, 4-hydroxybenzyl-glucosinolate. Many such glycosides, with a variety of side-chains, including indolyl; all contain the β-D-1-gluco-pyranosyl residue and are found only in dicotyledonous plants mainly abundant in the families Brassicaceae, Capparidaceae, Resedaceae, Euphorbiaceae, Tovariaceae, Moringaceae, Tropaeolaceae and Caricaceae. The enzyme myrosinase is also widely distributed. The mustard oil glycosides significantly increase the non-specific resistance of the plants to microorganisms which disrupt plant-cells. They do not affect the resistance of these plants to club root infections. Many glucosinolates have an antithyroid and goitre-including effect in man.

LIPIDS-FIXED OILS, FATS AND WAXES

Lipids are water-insoluble biomolecules which are soluble in nonpolar solvents. They contain a large hydrocarbon chain in their structure. Biologically, lipids are the main structural components of membranes, act as fuel for storage and transport, and protective surface coatings. The lipid-based cell components also may be involved in cell recog-nition, species specificity and tissue immunity.

The term lipid is used for fixed oils, fats and waxes. Fixed oils are liquid at normal temperature while fats are solids or semi-solids at this temperature. Chemically, they are esters of glycerol with long chain fatty acids. These esters are termed as glycerides.

Fixed oils and fats are nonvolatile, insoluble in water and are lighter than it and form a permanent stain on a paper. They are sparingly soluble in cold alcohol (except Castor oil), but soluble in other organic solvents like petroleum ether, diethyl ether, chloroform, etc.

Waxes are esters of a higher alcohols (e.g. cetyl alcohol) with higher fatty acids. They are insoluble in water, soluble in many organic solvents and can be saponified by alcoholic alkali.

VOLATILE OILS

Volatile oils are flavouring constituents which evaporate on exposure at ordinary temperature. They are present in various plant parts such as flower petals (Saffron), fruits (Fennel), bark (Cinnamon), etc. They are secreted in particular secretory cells like glandular hairs, modified parenchyma cells, vittae or in lysigenous or schizogenous cavities.

Volatile oils are colourless liquids or crystalline or amorphous solids. They are slightly soluble in water, but highly soluble in ether, alcohol and other organic solvents. Like fixed oils they do not form permanent strains and cannot be saponified by alkalies.

Chemically, volatile oils are the mixture of monoterpenes and sesquiterpenes. They may be simple hydrocarbons, alcohols, ketones, aldehydes, phenols, ethers, oxides, esters, acids, aromatic or aliphatic compounds.

Phenolic volatile oils are present in drugs like Thyme, Clove, Creosote and Pine tar. They have antibacterial, antifungal and antiseptic properties.

RESINS, GUM-RESINS AND OLEO-RESINS

The resins are derived from living natural sources and most of them are plant products (except Shellac). The resinous exudation may consist almost entirely of resins (e.g., Benzoin), or it may be associated with volatile oil (e.g., Turpentine, Copaiba); or resin associated with gum (gum resin). If a considerable amount of volatile oil is present, the substance is called an oleo-gum-resin (e.g., Myrrh). The resins or oleo-resins, which contain benzoic or cinnamic acid either free or combined, are commonly called balsams (e.g., Benzoin, Balsam of Tolu, Balsam of Peru and Storax).

All resins are practically insoluble in water, soluble in organic solvents (*e.g.*, alcohol) and terpentine oil.

A solution of a resin in a volatile solvent, on painting on a smooth surface, is dried rapidly and completely to form a hard transparent film. This film should not be darken with age or become impaired upon exposure to light or moisture.

Resins are not single chemical compounds, but

are mixtures of various substances of complex chemical characters.

Resins are used as purgative, cathartic, hydragogue, sedative, counter-irritant, anthelmintic, expectorant and laxative. Externally they are used as mild antiseptic in the form of cerates, ointments and plasters.

Anthocyanidins and Glycosides

Anthocyanidins are flavonoids structurally related to the flavones. Their glycosides are known as anthocyanins. They are sap pigments and the actual colour of the plant organ is determined by the pH of the sap. For example, the blue colour of the cornflower and the red of roses is due to the same glycosides and both of these plants on hydrolysis with hydrochloric acid yield cyanidin hydrochloride.

The most common anthocyanidin, cyanidin, occurs in about 80% of permanently pigmented leaves, 69% of fruits and 50% of flowers. Cyanidin is followed in order of frequency by delphinidin and pelargonidin.

Anthocyanidins are precipitated from aqueous solutions as lead salts or as picrates. After hydrolysis with 20% hydrochloric acid, anthocyanidin hydrochlorides, being only slightly soluble, often crystallize out. Chromatographic methods are widely used for the separation and identification of both the aglycones and sugars.

The sugar components are usually attached in the 3- or 5-position. In flavone glycosides the attachment is usually in the 7-position. They may be monosaccharides (glucose, galactose, rhamnose or arabinose); disaccharides (*e.g.*, the rhamnoglucoside of *Antirrhinum* spp.); or trisaccharides (*e.g.*, the 5-glucoside-3-rutinoside of certain Solanaceae such as *Atropa* and *Solanum*). Diglucosides, in which separate glucose molecules are attached in both the 3- and 5-positions, are common (*e.g.*, *Campanula* and *Dahlia* spp.).

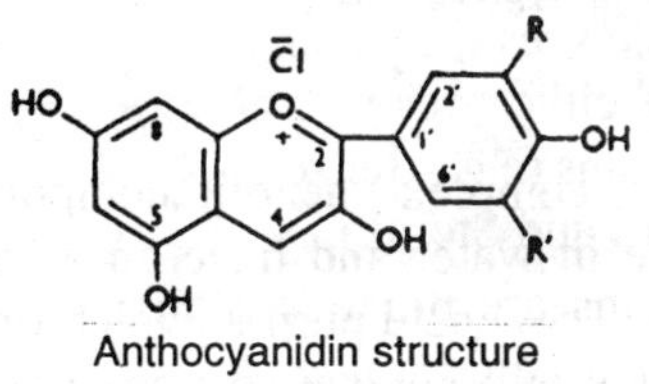

CHROMONES AND XANTHONES

These compounds are structural derivatives of benzo-γ-pyrone. Chromones are isomeric with the coumarins. A simple derivative is eugenin found in the clove plant, *Eugenia aromatica*. More complex are the furanochromones, the active constituents of the fruits of *Ammi visnaga*.

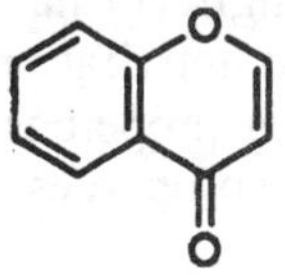

Benzo-γ-pyrone
(Chromone)

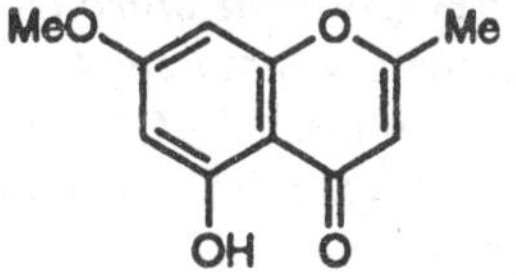

Eugenin

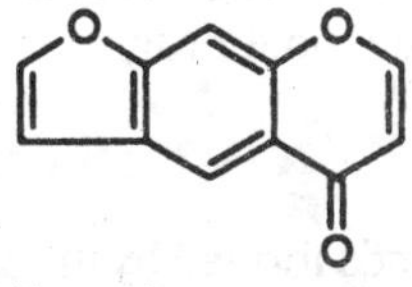

Furanobenzo-γ-pyrone
(Furanochromone)

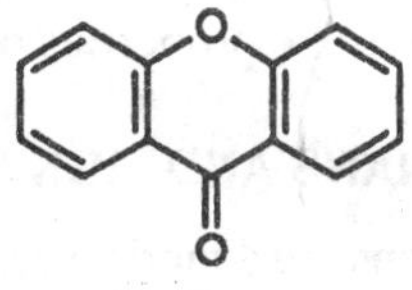

Xanthone

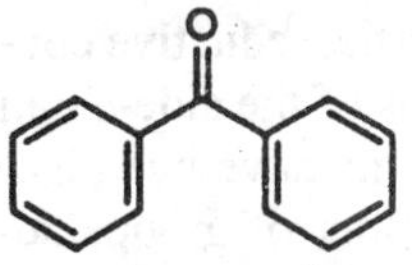

Benzophenone

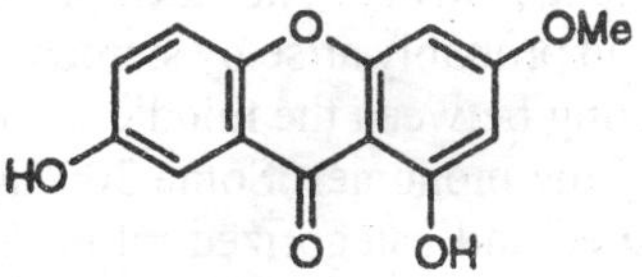

Gentisin

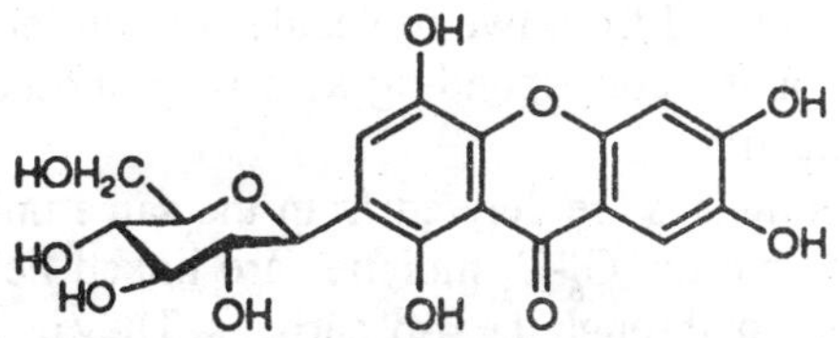

Mangiferin

Fig. 12.12. Chromones and xanthones.

Anthocyanidin structure

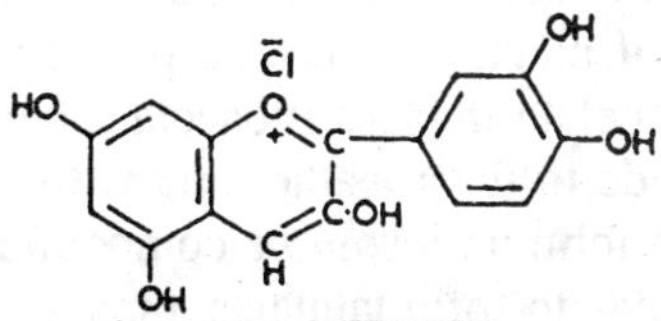

Cyanidin chloride

Fig. 12.11. Anthocyanidins.

Xanthones occur mainly in the Gentianaceae, Guttiferae, Moraceae and Polygalaceae. The characteristic oxygenation pattern of these compounds derived from the higher plants indicated that they were of mixed shikimate acetate origin. The xanthones derived from fungi show a characteristic acetate derivation. Their biosynthesis involves the oxidative coupling of hydroxylated benzophenones. Simple oxygenated derivatives, such as gentisin which contributes to the yellow colour of fermented Gentian Root, are found in both the Gentianaceae and Guttiferae. More highly oxygenated compounds and O-glycosylxanthones are distributed in the Gentianaceae whereas prenylated xanthones, several of which have antimicrobial properties, are isolated from Guttiferae. The C-glycosyl xanthone, mangiferin, is found in several species of *Hypericum* and in *Cratoxylem pruniflorum* and Chiretta (*Swertia chirata*). Mangiferin has anti-inflammatory, antiheptotoxic and antiviral properties. In contrast to its CNS-stimulant properties other xanthones exhibit CNS depressive properties in rats and mice.

The mycotoxin pigments of *Claviceps purpurea* (ergot), called secalonic acids, are complex xanthones. They contribute, with the ergot alkaloids, to the toxic properties of the whole drug.

LIGNANS AND LIGNIN

Lignans are dimeric compounds formed by the union of two molecules of a phenylpropene derivative. They are offshoots of the principal lignin biosynthetic pathway. They are optically active compounds and probably arise by stereospecific, reductive coupling between the middle carbons of the side-chain of the monomer. Some 300 lignans have been isolated and categorized into a number of groups according to structural features. Important pharmaceutical examples are the lignans of *Podophyllum* spp. which formed from two molecules of coniferyl alcohol or the corresponding acid with subsequent modification.

Neolignans are derived from the same units as lignans but the C_6-C_3 moieties are linked head to tail and not through the β-β' carbons. They occur in the heart-woods of trees of the Magnoliaceae, Lauraceae and Piperaceae.

Lignin is a polymeric substance, $(C_6$-$C_3)_n$, present in a matrix of cellulose microfibrils to strengthen certain cell walls. It is an essential component of most woody tissues and involves vessels, tracheids, fibres and sclereids. Lignins from different biological sources differ in composition, depending on the distinct monomeric units of which they are composed.

Variations in lignin constitution are due to random condensations of the appropriate alcohols with mesomeric free radicals formed from them by the action of a laccase-type (oxidase) enzyme. As there is no template for this non-enzymic condensation the structure of lignin molecules vary. Lignin is not isolated as a compound of defined composition.

a-Guaiaconic acid (*Guaiacum officinale, G. sanctum*). A furano-type lignan.

Macelignan (*Myristica fragrans*, Nutmeg). A dibenzylbutane-type lignan

(–)-Cubebin (*Piper cubeba*, Tailed pepper) A tetrahydrofuran-type lignan.

Podophyllotoxin (*Podophyllum* spp.) An aryltetralin-type lignan
Wuweizisu C (*Schisandra chinensis*) A dibenzocyclooctadiene-type lignan.
Eleutheroside E [(–)-syringaresinoldiglucoside] (*Silybum marianum*)
Urtica dioica (Stinging nettle)
Viscum album (Mistletoe)
Eleutherococcus senticosus
(*Acanthopanax senticosus*)
Tetrahydrofuran-type lignans

TANNINS

Tannins are complex phenolic compounds which are soluble in water and have an astringent and bitter taste. They yield purple, violet, or black precipitates with iron compounds; are precipitated by a number of metallic salts like potassium dichromate, lead acetate and lead subacetate; combine with skin and hide to form leather and with gelatin and isinglass to form an insoluble compound; combine with alkaloids to form tannates, most of which are insoluble in water, and they yield a bulky precipitate with phenazone.

The tannins are common to vascular plants existing primarily within woody tissues. Tannins consist of various phenolic compounds that react with proteins to form water-insoluble copolymers. This reaction with proteins has been used industrially for the conversion of animal skins into leather. Plant tissues with high tannin content have a strong bitter taste and are avoided by most feeders. The astringent taste of tannin containing bark and leaves makes them unpalatable to insects and grazing animals. Tannins contract the tissues of the body, hence, they are used to tan leather. They draw the tissues closer together and improves their resistance to infections. Tannins may be either *condensed* or *hydrolyzable*. Condensed tannins are formed biosynthetically by the condensation of *catechins* to five polymeric networks. Hydrolyzable tannins are derived from gallic acid.

The tannin containing drugs are Cinchona, Clove, Catechu, Cinnamon, Hamamelis and Krameria.

COUMARINS

Derivatives of benzo-α-pyrone such as coumarin (the lactone of O-hydroxycinnamic acid), aesculetin, umbelliferone and scopoletin are common in plants both in the free state and as glycosides. About 1000 natural coumarins have been isolated. Coumarin itself has been found in about 150 species belonging to over 30 different families; it is present in the undamaged plant as *trans-O*-glucosyloxycinnamic acid. Enzyme activity in the damaged tissue leads to a loss of a glucose and a *trans* → *cis* isomerization followed by ring closure. Coumarin gives a characteristic odour of new-mown hay and occurs in sweet clover, melitot, tonco beans and in woodruff, *Asperula odorata* (Rubiaceae).

In ammoniacal solution these compounds have a blue, blue-green or violet fluorescence, which is used as a qualitative test for certain umbelliferous resins such as asafoetida and galbanum. The fluorescence is more marked if examined in filtered ultra-violet light and is used for the chromatographic visualization of the compounds.

The furanocoumarins are similar to the coumarins and occur in the Rutaceae and Apiaceae. Celery fruits contain rutaretin and its dehydrated derivative apiumetin. Bergapten occurs in bergamot

oil and in the Chinese root-drug derived from *Peucedanum decursivum* (Apiaceae) which also contains pyranocoumarins. Marmesin derivatives and archangelicin have a reduced furanocoumarin structure consisting of coumarin and a C_5 sub-unit. Other prenylated compounds are the 3-isoprenylcoumarins, rutamarin of the genus *Ruta*. They show a wide range of biological activities. *Amni* species contain furano-methoxycoumarins but are more important for their content of furanobenzo-γ-pyrones.

Bicoumarins are formed from two coumarin moieties. Dicoumarol is formed at C3-C3' through a methylene group. It is found in fermenting hay and is formed by microbial action of coumarin. It is a powerful anticoagulant and haemorrhagic and can cause the death of animals consuming the spoiled folder.

Table 12.4. Natural hydroxy and methoxy coumarins

Compound	Source
Umbelliferone	Belladonna and Stramonium (Solanaceae): *Daphne mezereum* (Thymeliaceae); *Ferula* species yielding asafoetida and galbanum
Herniarin	*Lavandula spica* (Lamiaceae), *Ruta graveolens* (Apiaceae)
Aesculetin	Horse-chestnut (Hippocastanaceae), and *Fraxinus* (Oleaceae)
Scopoletin	Roots of Gelsemium, Oat, Jalap, Scammony, Scopolia and Belladonna; leaves of Tobacco, Stramonium, Chicory
Fraxin	*Fraxinus* spp. (Oleaceae)
Chicorin	*Cichorum intybus* herb

The phenylpropanoids contain a three-carbon side chain attached to a phenol. They include the hydroxycoumarins, phenyl propenes, the lignans and hydroxycinnamic acids, including the caffeic and coumaric acids. Coumarin is common to numerous plants and is the sweet-smelling volatile material which is released from newly mowed hay. The phenylpropenes are not phenols since they lack the hydroxyl functionality. They are not water soluble but are essential oils and include eugenol, the major principle of oil of cloves. Anethole and

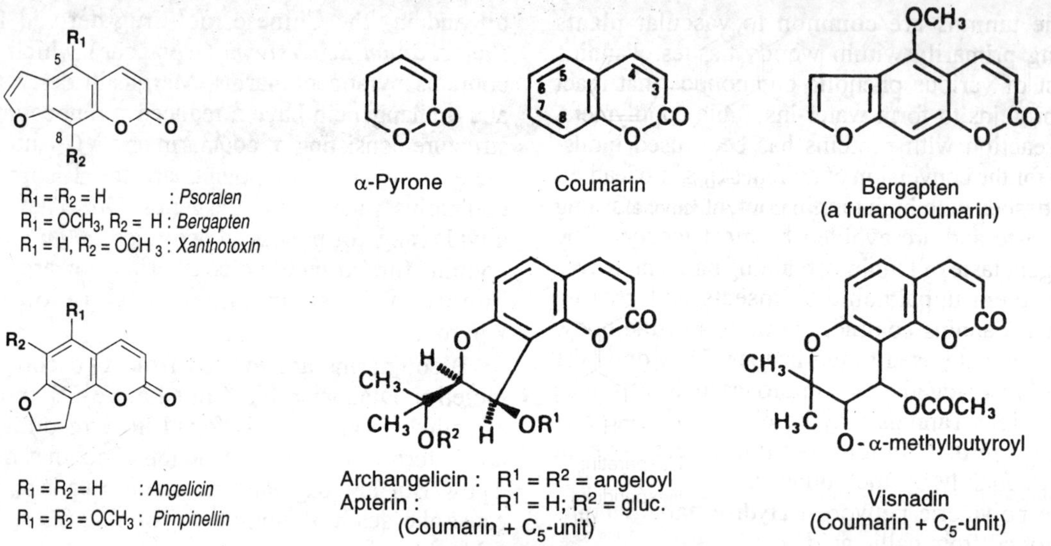

$R_1 = R_2 = H$: *Psoralen*
$R_1 = OCH_3, R_2 = H$: *Bergapten*
$R_1 = H, R_2 = OCH_3$: *Xanthotoxin*

α-Pyrone

Coumarin

Bergapten
(a furanocoumarin)

$R_1 = R_2 = H$: *Angelicin*
$R_1 = R_2 = OCH_3$: *Pimpinellin*

Archangelicin : $R^1 = R^2$ = angeloyl
Apterin : $R^1 = H; R^2$ = gluc.
(Coumarin + C_5-unit)

Visnadin
(Coumarin + C_5-unit)

O - α-methylbutyroyl

Fig. 12.13. Coumarins.

myristicin, the principles of nutmeg, are also phenylpropanoids.

Umbelliferone and scopoletin are coumarin phenylpropanoids that have been isolated from the roots of *Scopolia japonica*. The phenylpropene, eugenol, is used as a dental analgesic.

FLAVONE AND RELATED FLAVONOID GLYCOSIDES

The flavonoids occur both in the free state and as glycosides. They are the largest group of naturally occurring phenols. More than 2000 of these compounds are known, with nearly 500 occurring in the free state. They are formed from three acetate units and a phenylpropane unit with oxygenation of the C_3 unit, *i.e.*, C-2,3,4. They have a γ-pyrone moiety with the exception of the chalcones.

The flavones are often yellow (Latin *flavus*, yellow). They are more common in the higher plants and in young tissues, where they occur in the cell sap. They are used as chemotaxonomic markers and are abundant in the Polygonaceae, Rutaceae, Leguminosae, Apiaceae and Astera-ceae.

They occur both in the free state and as *O*-glycosides. Dimeric compounds with, a 5', 8-carbon-carbon linkage are also known (biflavonyls). The glycosides are generally soluble in water and alcohol, but insoluble in organic solvents; the genins

are sparingly soluble in water but are soluble in ether. Flavonoids dissolve in alkalis, giving yellow solutions which on the addition of acid become colourless.

The flavonoids exhibit anti-inflammatory, anti-allergic, antithrombitic and vasporotective properties, inhibition of tumour promotion and as a protective for the gastric mucosa. These effects are due to the influence of flavonoids on arachidonic acid metabolism. Many flavonoid-containing plants are diuretic (e.g., Buchu and Broom) or anti-spasmodic (e.g., Liquorice and Parsley). Some flavonoids have anti-tumour, antibacterial or anti-fungal actions. Fustic from the wood of *Morus tinctoria* and sumac (leaves of *Rhus* spp.) are colouring and tannin materials.

Pure flavone is colourless, present on the surface of some species of *Primula*. Many flavones are phenolic or methoxyl derivatives and form sap-soluble glycosides. The intensity of their yellow colour increases with the number of hydroxyl groups and with increase of pH. Isoflavones are found in the heartwood of *Prunus* and *Iris* species. Rotonenone present in the roots of *Derris* and *Lonchocarpus* species is an isoflavonoid.

About 2% of all carbon photosynthesized by plants is converted into flavonoids. Most of the tannins are derived from flavonoids.

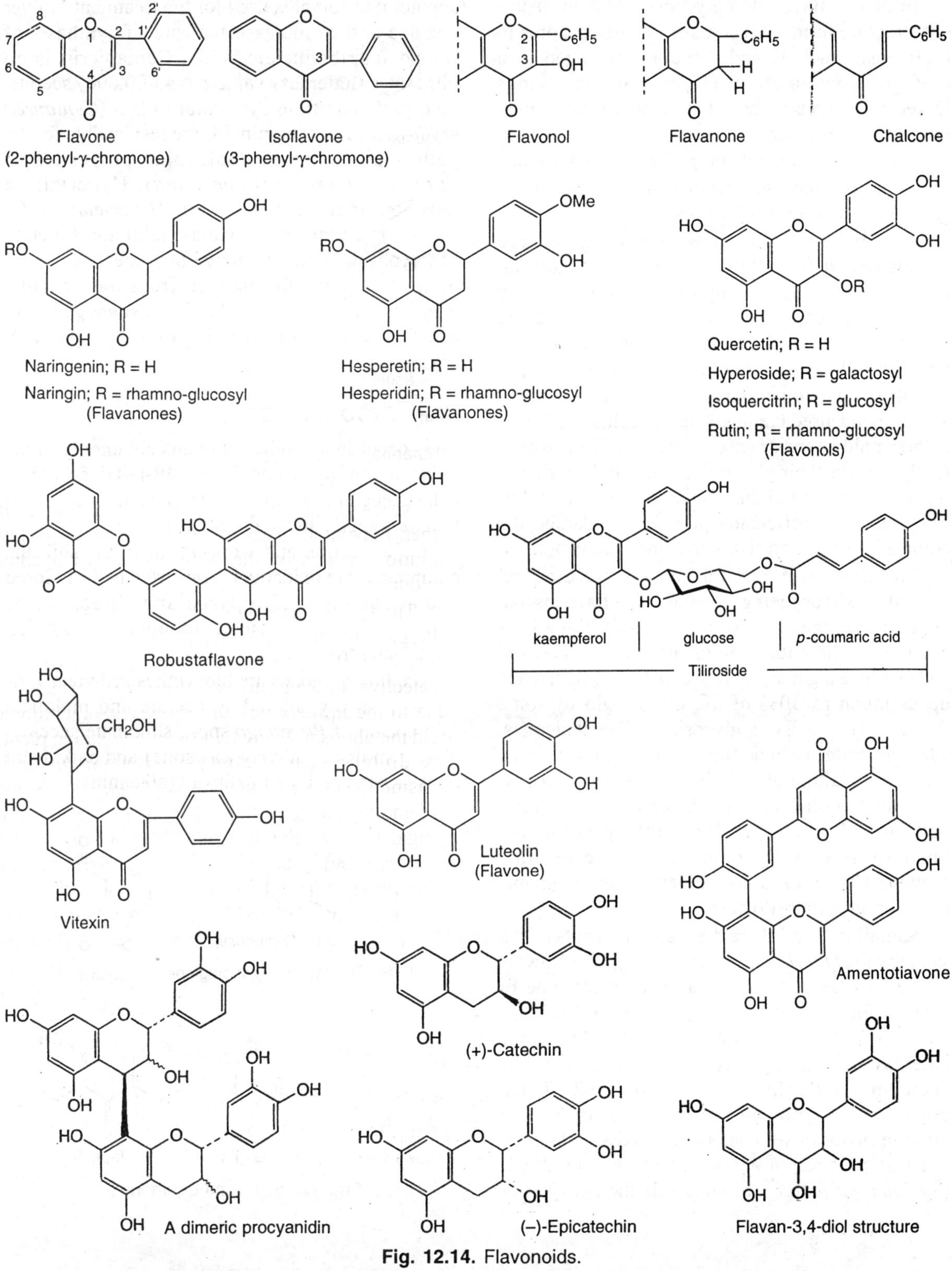

Flavone
(2-phenyl-γ-chromone)

Isoflavone
(3-phenyl-γ-chromone)

Flavonol

Flavanone

Chalcone

Naringenin; R = H
Naringin; R = rhamno-glucosyl
(Flavanones)

Hesperetin; R = H
Hesperidin; R = rhamno-glucosyl
(Flavanones)

Quercetin; R = H
Hyperoside; R = galactosyl
Isoquercitrin; R = glucosyl
Rutin; R = rhamno-glucosyl
(Flavonols)

Robustaflavone

kaempferol | glucose | p-coumaric acid
Tiliroside

Vitexin

Luteolin
(Flavone)

Amentotiavone

A dimeric procyanidin

(+)-Catechin

(–)-Epicatechin

Flavan-3,4-diol structure

Fig. 12.14. Flavonoids.

In plants, flavonoid aglycones occur in different structure forms. All contain 15 carbon atoms in their basis nucleus and these are arranged in a C_6-C_3-C_6 configuration; *i.e.*, two aromatic rings linked by a three carbon units which may or may not form a third ring.

A common biosynthetic pathway of flavonoids incorporates precursors from both the "Shikimic" and "Acetate-Malonate" pathways.

The different classes within the group are distinguished by additional oxygen-containing heterocyclic rings and hydroxyl groups. These include the catechins, leucoanthocyanidins, flavanones, flavanonols, flavones, anthocyanidins, flavonols, chalcones, aurones and isoflavones.

Other common groups include the xanthones and the condensed tannins. The catechins and leucoanthocyanidins are structurally very similar and only rarely exist as their glycosides. They polymerize to form condensed tannins which give tea its color. They also are sufficiently prevalent to darken the color of streams and rivers in some woody areas.

The flavanones and flavanonols are rare and normally exist as their glycosides. The flavones and flavonols are the most widely distributed of all the phenolics. The anthocyanins are the common red and rare blue pigments of flower petals and can make up as much as 30% of the dry weight of some flowers. They exist as glycosides. The chalcones, such as butein, lack the pyran ring found in flavonoids, although this is often subject to pH-controlled equilibria. The chalcone is more fully conjugated and normally brightly coloured. Phlorizin is a strong inhibitor of apple seedling growth. The *aurones* are golden yellow pigments common in certain flowers.

Santalins A and B are the major pigments of red sandalwood (*Pterocarpus santalinus*). The flowers of the hawthorne tree provide hyperoside, one of the principle flavonoids from this source (*Crataegus laevigata*). Neohesperidin is responsible for the bitter taste of orange peels (*Citrus aurantium*), while quercitin is the active ingredient of birch (*Betula pendula*). Silybin, one of the silymarins, is a mixture of various flavanone derivatives (flavonolignans) and present in the fruit of the milk thistle (*Silybum marianum*). Silymarin is the active anti-

hepatotoxic complex used for the treatment of liver damage and to increase the rate of synthesis of ribosomal ribonucleic acids. Centapicrin is an ultrabitter (bitterness value *ca*, 4,000,000) secoiridoid glycoside from the century plant (*Centaurea erythraea*). The cucuminoids are responsible for the yellow pigment and cholagogic properties of Turmeric (*Curcuma domestica*). Hypericin, a flavonoid from St. John's wort (*Hypericum perforatum*), is a monoamine oxidase inhibitor. Emetine and cephaeline are the active ingredients of syrup of Ipecac, powerful emetics from ipecacuanha (*Cephaelis ipecacuanha*). The isoflavones genistein and daidzein are found in high concentrations in soybeans (*Glycine max*).

NAPHTHOQUINONES

They occur in a number of plants commonly in the reduced and glycosidic forms. 4β-D-Glucoside of α-hydrojuglone is a constituent of walnut tree leaves (*Juglans regia*, Juglandaceae).

On extraction and work-up, or in the soil, the compounds are oxidatively converted to the colored naphthoquinone. *Diospyros* spp. (Ebenaceae) naphthoquinones occur as monomers, complex dimers and trimers.

Naphthoquinones are biosynthesized via a variety of pathways including acetate and malonate (plumbagin of *Plumbago* spp.), shikimate/succinyl CoA combined pathway (lawsone) and shikimate/mevalonate combined pathway (alkannin).

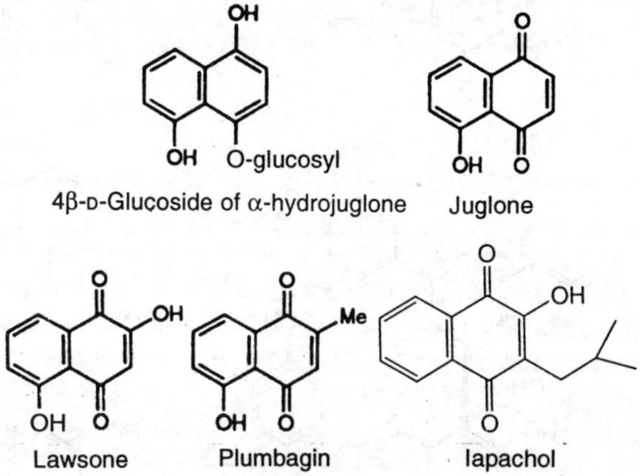

Fig. 12.15. Naphthoquinones.

Quinones

The *quinones* are strongly coloured pigments covering the entire visible spectrum. They are found in the internal region of the plant and thus do not impart a colour to the exterior of the plant. Generally, quinones are derived from benzoquinone, naphthoquinone, or anthroquinone structures.

A wide variety of quinones exist in plants many of which are of medicinal interest.

ALKALOIDS

Alkaloids are complex substances, occurring in plants or animals, are basic or alkali-like and possess physiological activity. The term is usually restricted to compounds having one or more heterocyclic rings containing nitrogen. They are the derivatives of pyridine, quinoline or isoquinoline and contain carbon, hydrogen, oxygen, and nitrogen but a few are without oxygen. Mostly alkaloids are solid colourless crystalline products but few alkaloids, which generally do not possess oxygen, *e.g.*, nicotine, coniine, spartein, are volatile colourless liquids. Some alkaloids are coloured, *e.g.*, berberine (yellow) and sanguinarine (red).

Many of the common drugs are alkaloid based, e.g., caffeine, quinine, nicotine, cocaine, morphine and strychnine. Biosynthetically, they may be derived from amino acids, terpenes, or aromatics depending on the specific alkaloid structure. They are often derived from the plant source rather than being produced synthetically. They may be grouped on the basis of the ring system present.

Whereas the phenols are weakly acidic, the alkaloids are distinguished by the amine functionality. This makes them basic in nature. Thus, the free amines are relatively polar lipophilic substances, whereas treatment with acid forms water soluble salts.

Nicotine may comprise up to 8% of the dry weight of Tobacco leaves (*Nicotiana tabacum*). Morphine, a powerful and addictive pain killer, may include up to 14% of the weight of high-grade Opium. Chelidonine is an alkaloid present in Celandine (*Chelidonium majus*). Quinine is a well-known alkaloid from Cinchona bark (*Cinchona pubescens*). Lycodopine is the principal alkaloid (with more than 100 other alkaloids) isolated from the stagshorn clubmoss (*Lycopodium clavatum*). Senicione, with its unique 12-membered ring, is one of several haemostyptic alkaloids from senecio (*Senecio nemorensis*). Intermedine is one of several pyrrolizidine alkaloids present in Comfrey root (*Commiphora abyssinica*). Caffeine, a popular stimulant, is present in tea, coffee, mate leaves, guarana paste and cola nuts. Hygrine is a simple pyrrolidine alkaloid. Scopolamine exists in various members of the nightshade family (Solanaceae) and can act as a powerful hallucinogen. Cocaine is a well-known controlled substance present in Coca leaves (*Erythroxolum coca*). The yellow alkaloid berberine, isolated from the barberry shrub (*Berberis* spp.), shows antimicrobial and cytotoxic activity. Papaverine, a smooth muscle relaxant and cerebral vasodilator, is also a constituent of Opium. Psilocybin occurs in the fruiting bodies of the Mexican hallucinogenic fungus, *Psilocybe mexicana*. Colchicine is a major alkaloid of *Colchicum autumnale*. *Strychnine* is present in the seeds of *Strychnos nux-vomica* and other Strychnos species.

Alkaloids combine with acids to give salts and are used in this form. A water-soluble alkaloidal salt or other compound is more useful than one insoluble in water. Alkaloids are fairly soluble in organic solvents, *e.g.*, chloroform, ether, alcohol and benzene.

In plants alkaloids are found in various parts as in seeds (strychnine), in fruits (Piper), in leaves (Belladonna, Datura), in roots (Rauwolfia), in rhizomes and roots (Ipecac), in corm (Colchicum) and in bark (Kurchi, Cinchona).

AMINO ACIDS AND AMINES

The common plant amines can be subdivided into aliphatic monoamines, aliphatic polyamines, and aromatic amines. Simple aliphatic amines exist as low-boiling liquids and include most of the primary amines from methy-lamine, CH_3NH_2, through hexylamine, $CH_3(CH_2)_5NH_2$. These molecules typically have strong, fish-like aromas. In cow parsley (*Heracleum sphondylium*), they act as insect attractants by stimulating the smell of carrion.

Common polyamines include putrescine, NH_2 $(CH_2)_4NH_2$; agmatine, $NH_2(CH_2)_4NHC(=NH)NH_2$; spermidine, $NH_2(CH_2)_3NH(CH_2)_4 NH_2$; and spermine. $NH_2(CH_2)_3NH(CH_2)_4NH (CH_2)_3NH_2$. Both putrescine and S-adenosylme-thionine are used for the formation of spermine and spermidine. These polyamines are thought to have many functions and are invariably found complexed with nucleic acids, including both DNA and RNA.

Many of the known aromatic amines are physiologically active. The most known member of this class is mescaline. It is the active principle of the peyote cactus, *Lophophora williamsii*, and is a potent hallucinogen. Similarly, three compounds critical to brain metabolism in animals are noradrenaline, histamine, and serotonin. All three occur in common plants.

Amino acids occur in plants both in the free state and as the basic units of proteins and other metabolites. They contain one or more amino groups and one or more carboxylic acid groups. They occur in nature as α-amino acids with an asymmetric carbon atom with the general formula $R-CH(NH_2)$ COOH. About 20 different ones have been isolated from proteins, all having an L-configuration. Other amino acids occur in the free state and some having the D-configuration are isolated from plants and microorganisms, where they may form antibiotic polypeptides.

Amino acids contain carbon, hydrogen, oxygen, nitrogen and other atoms (*e.g.*, sulphur in cystine and iodine in thyroxin). More than one amino group may be present (*e.g.*, lysine, diamino-caproic acid) and more than one carboxylic acid group (*e.g.*, aspartic or aminosuccinic acid). Some amino acids are aromatic such as phenylalanine, and tyrosine or heterocyclic such as proline (pyrrolidine nucleus), tryptophan (indole nucleus) and histidine (imidazole nucleus).

Amino acids are generally soluble in water but only slightly soluble in alcohol. With ninhydrin amino acids give a yellow, pink, blue or violet colour. Amino acids do not respond to the biuret test (compare polypeptides and proteins). Certain amino acids are detected by more specific tests (*e.g.*, histidine gives colour reactions with diazonium salts).

Protein bound amino acids

These include α-alanine, arginine, asparagine (amide of aspartic acid), abundant in many plants, aspartic acid; aminosuccinic acid, involved in the biosynthesis of purines; cysteine, which contains sulphur; cystine or dicysteine (in hair and insulin); 3,5-di-iodotyrosine (in thyroid); glutamic acid (a component of the folic acid vitamins); glutamine (free in animals and plants, *e.g.*, sugar beet); glycine (aminoacetic acid); histidine; δ-hydroxylysine (in gelatin); hydroxypyroline (in gelatin); leucine (α-aminocaproic acid); isoleucine; lysine; methionine (contains a sulphur atom); 3-monoiodo-tyrosine (in thyroid); phenylalanine; proline; serine (in phosphoproteins such as casein); threonine (in casein); thyroxin (the iodine-containing thyroid-hormone); 3,5,3'-triiodothyronine (in thyroid); tryptophan; tyrosine; and valine.

The protein amino acids are normally considered to be 20 in number for plants. The amino acids are high melting, water soluble, zwitterionic colourless solids. Since they have both basic (amine) and acidic (acid) functionalities, the amino acids have specific pK_a's unique to each amino acid.

Free amino acids

Compounds that contain nitrogen as part of a chain belong to this category of natural products. For the amino acids this results in molecules to form *zwitterionic* (a dipolar ion) depending on the pH of the environment.

Several hundred of these amino acids have been characterized and only a few (*e.g.*, γ-aminobutyric acid, α-aminoadipic acid, pipecolic acid and δ-acetylornithine) occur widely. Seeds and fleshy organs of plants are the principal sites for the accumulation of these compounds where they may serve as a nitrogen reserve. Other free amino acids are: β-alanine (β-aminopropionic acid); citrulline (an intermediate in the cycle of urea synthesis); creatine; ergothionine (a sulphur-containing constituent of some animal tissues and of ergot); and taurine (a component of bile acids). 3-N-Oxalyl-L-2, 3-diaminopropanoic acid is a neurotoxin of the seeds of *Lathyrus sativus*.

A nonprotein amino acid that is regularly found in plants is *d*-amino-butyric acid. Several hundred other amino acids are known.

PEPTIDES AND PROTEINS

The term 'peptide' includes compounds varying from low to very high molecular weights and showing marked differences in physical, chemical and pharmacological properties. The lowest members are derived from only two molecules of amino acid. The higher members have many amino acid units and form either peptides, simple proteins (albumins, globulins, prolamines, glutalins, etc.) or complex proteins, conjugated proteins, in which other groupings form part of the molecule, *e.g.*, carbohydrate in muco-proteins, the very complex chlorophyll molecule in the protein of chloroplasts, phosphorus-containing proteins such as casein, nucleoproteins, in which proteins are combined with nucleic acid, and the lipoproteins of the cytoplasm, in which protein is combined with lipids. Some proteins with low molecular weight are antibiotics which have a cyclic polypeptide structure (*e.g.*, gramicidin, bacitracin and polymyxin); peptide hormones such as oxytocin and vasopressin from the posterior pituitary gland; and glutathione found in nearly all living cells.

These complex compounds have two or more molecules of amino acid united by a peptide linkage which results from the elimination of water, a hydroxyl coming from one amino acid and a proton from the other. Thus, a dipeptide is formed:

A dipeptide of the Sapindaceous plant *Blighia sapida* has hypoglycaemic properties. Penicillin has a dipeptide structure. Tripeptides have three amino acid components and polypeptides from ten upwards. Peptides are usually defined as protein-like substances having molecular weights below 10000. In typical proteins the molecular weight is higher ranging from about 30000 to 50000 in the simple prolamines.

Proteins are high molecular weight polymers of amino acids. They are synthesized based on the triplet basic code of DNA in the nucleus of a cell. The individual amino acids makes proteins in plants and animals. The polypeptide has a nonrandom form which gives rise to a particular three-dimensional shape, flexibility and conformational lability.

The genetic information contained within each cell of plants and animals is expressed as proteins. Proteins are made up from large chains of amino acids and small oligomers comprise peptides. Proteins play a variety of roles. Some carry out the transport and storage of small molecules, while others make up a large part of the structural framework of cells and tissues. The most important class of proteins are the enzymes, the biological catalysts that promote the variety of reactions that channel metabolism into essential pathwafys. Individual types of cells may contain several thousand kinds of proteins.

Enzymes and other proteins

Enzymes are defined as organic catalysts produced by plants and animals with molecular weight from 13,000 to 8,40,000. At ordinary temperatures they bring about chemical changes, both synthetic and analytic. Most enzymes are insoluble in alcohol, ether and other organic solvents, but are soluble in water. In some cases the enzymes are combined with the protoplasm which must be killed by an organic solvent (*e.g.*, $CHCl_3$, toluene) or by mechanical means before extraction of the enzyme. Some enzymes do not pre-exist in the tissues, but are formed from substances termed *'zymogens'*. In nature, decomposition of the zymogen is carried out by a complex substance, known as *kinase,* to form the enzyme when needed.

The term *substrate* is used to a substance which reacts with the enzyme. In nature, enzyme and substrate are sometimes present in the same cell and the reaction may take place continuously. In other cases, enzymes and substrate are found in different cells. The reaction starts on diffusion of one of the substance; the reaction is controlled by the plant. Some enzymes are combined with the protoplasm, and this represents one method of preventing diffusion.

The rate of chemical change brought about by enzyme is affected by certain factors. For examples, some substances, like *paralysers,* inhibit the action of the enzymes. The substances, called *co-enzymes,* are required for the action. The substances known as *accelerators* or *activators,* greatly accelerate the rate of reaction.

Temperature is another important factor in enzyme action. For each enzyme there is a particular temperature, called the optimum temperature and lies between 35°-45°C, at which reaction proceeds most rapidly. Most of the enzymatic reactions are inhibited below 10°C, and destroyed by heating to 100°C.

Enzymes are usually soluble in water. They are accompanied with glycosides. Some drugs like Wild Cherry, Almonds, Mustard and Wintergreen, owe their value not to the glycoside present, but to its decomposition products by the enzymes.

Some important enzymes of medicinal importance are pancreatin of pancereas used to treat pancreatitis; trypsin of ox pancrease is prescribed to cure wounds, ulcers, abscesses and fistulas and as anti-inflammatory agent; chymotrypsin of pancreas of ox used identically as trypsin; fibrinolysin utili-zed to control venous thrombosis and pulmonary embolism; pepsin of the gastric juice employed to treat achylia gastrica; hyaluronidase found in microorganisms, leaches, snake venom and mammalian testes, and used to facilitate the administration of fluids by hydronermolysis.

Papain is the dried and purified latex of the fruit of *Carica payaya* and used as a digestant. Chymopapain is a nonpyrogenic proteolytic enzyme obtained from the latex of *Carica payaya* and employed in the treatment of herniated lumbar intervertebral discs. Bromelain is a mixture of protein-digesting and milk-clotting enzymes obtained from the juice of the pineapple, *Ananas comosus*. It is used as adjunctive therapy to reduce inflammation and oedema and to reduce tissue repair.

Gelatin is obtained from animal collagen and is a pharmaceutical aid. Other protein based drugs are Absorbable Gelatin sponge and film, microfibrillar collagen surgical sutures, penicillamine, heparin sodium, heparin calcium, protamine sulphate and levodopa.

Peptide Hormones

Hormones are secreted by endocrine glands of animals. Thyroxine, conjugated oestrogens, insulin, epinephrine, oxytocin, vesopressin and gonadotropins are important mammalian hormones released directly into the blood. Thyroxin hormone of thyroid gland is used to treat thyroid insufficiency. Menopausal symptoms in females and dysmenor-rhea are treated with conjugated oestrogens. Insulin, a polypeptide hormone secreted by the beta cells of the islets of Langerhans of pancrease gland, is prescribed to cure diabetes. Adrenal medulla of mammals secretes the hormone epinephrine (adrenaline) which is utilized as vasoconstrictor to cure acute asthma. Oxytocin, a polypeptide hormone secreted by posterior pituitary gland, causes contraction of uterine muscles, stimulates the ejection of milk in lactating mothers, induce labour in pregnant women and stop haemorrhage after child birth. Another peptide hormone of the posterior lobe of pituitary gland, vasopressin, is used in the treatment of intestinal paralysis and diabetes. Gonadotropins are secreted by the interior lobe of the pituitary gland which control the production of sex hormones. They are taken to cure infertility and in cryptoichidism.

BITTERS

Bitters are various type of chemical constituents. The bitterness itself stimulates secretions by the salivary glands and digestive organs. Such secretions dramatically improve the appetite and strengthen the overall function of the digestive system, the body is nourished and strengthened. *Swertia chirata* and *Andrographis paniculata* are the bitter containing herbs.

MICRO-ORGANISMS

Microorganisms (microbes) are the viruses, bacteria and rickettsiae which are sources of many biological substances of immunization importance. These drugs possess immunity against various infectious diseases. Immunity is acquired by administration of a vaccine, toxoid or antitoxin like diphtheria. Vaccines are suspended micro-organisms which may be obtained from viruses, bacteria and rickettsiae. On introduction into body, a vaccine stimulates the production of antibodies against pathogenic microbes. Viral vaccines are prophylactic agents used against polio, smallpox, rabies, influenza, measles and mumps. Rickettsial vaccine, prepared from Gram-negative microorganisms, is the typhus vaccine which produces active immunity against typhus fever. Bacterial vaccine is the suspension of pathogenic bacteria in sodium chloride or other solvent and includes Typhoid vaccine, Cholera vaccine, Plague vaccine, Pertussis vaccine (for whooping cough) and BCG vaccine (for tuberculosis).

The waste products of bacteria, called toxins, are dissolved in the surrounding culture medium after excretion. On treatment with formaldehyde their toxic properties are reduced but their antigenic property is not effected. These products are called fluid toxoids which are precipitated with alum, aluminium hydroxide or aluminium phosphate. The toxoids are used to induce artificial activity immunity in susceptible individual. For example, tetanus toxoid and diphtheria toxoid are the microbial products used to produce immunity in young children against diphtheria, tetanus and whooping cough.

NUCLEOSIDES, NUCLEOTIDES AND NUCLEIC ACIDS

Nucleic acids act as the repositories and transmitters of genetic information for every cell tissue and organism. These include DNA and RNA which are polymers comprised of five different monomers: adenine thymine (DNA only), uracil (RNA only), cytosine, and guanine. These individual monomers are composed of a sugar (ribose for RNA, deoxyribose for DNA), a base (purine or pyrimidine), and a phosphate linker. When the individual monomer contains all three components, it is referred to as a nucleotide, and when it lacks the phosphate, it is a nucleoside. These five bases can be isolated in trace amounts from plants. 5-Methylcytosine is found in the DNA of wheat germ. The pyrimidine glycosides, vicine and convicine, are present in certain legume seeds. The methylated purines, theobromine and caffeine, occur in plants and are valued for their stimulant effects. Substituted purines constitute the cytokinins, which act as plant growth regulators and initiators of cell division. The purines and pyrimidines are only slightly soluble in water.

There are two major nucleic acids : Deoxyribonucleic acid (DNA) and ribonucleic acid (RNA). These are chain-like macromolecules that store and transfer genetic information. They are major components of all cells, comprising up to 15% of their dry weight. The monomeric units of DNA are the deoxynucleotides and for RNA, the ribonucleotides. Each of these nucleotides consists of three main components: (1) a nitrogenous heterocyclic purine or pyrimidine base, (2) a pentose sugar, and (3) a molecule of phosphoric acid. DNA contains two pyrimidine bases (cytosine and thymine) and two purines (adenine and guanine). RNA has the same nitrogenous bases except that uracil replaces thymine. When the phosphate group of a nucleotide is absent, the remaining structure is called a nucleoside. Like the free purines and pyrimidines, free nucleosides occur only in trace amounts in most plant cells. The nucleotides can be present in significant amounts.

In addition to the common bases, many other purine and pyrimidine derivatives have been isolated. The function of many of these rare bases is not well understood. Transfer RNA may contain up to 10% of these minor components.

MARINE PRODUCTS

Marine products are used as thickening, emulsifying and suspending agents. Carrageenan from *Chondrus crispus* (Irish Moss) and alginates from species of *Laminaria. Ascophyllum, Ecklonia, Nereocystis* and *Macrocystis* are used in adhesive formulations and as stabilizers, ingredients of ointment bases, suspending agent and tablet disintegrating agents. Agar, obtained from species of *Gelidium* and *Gracilaria,* is used as laxative, emulsifier, suspending agent and in the preparation of vaginal capsules, suppositories and nutrient media in bacteriological culture. Spermaceti, a solid waxy substance obtained from the oil of the sperm whale, *Physeter macrocephalus,* is used as a pharmaceutical aid for creams, ointments, cerates, soaps and cosmetics. Shark liver oil, a fixed oil obtained from the liver of shark fish, *Hypoprion brevirostris,* is nutritive and used as a tonic and to treat xerophthalmia occurring due to deficiency of vitamin A. The marine fungus, *Cephalosporium acremonium,* produces the antibiotic cephalosporin C identical to penicillins. The strongly basic protein of low molecular weight, protamine, is obtained from the testes of the fish salmon. It is used as a heparin antagonist. Pralidoxine is produced from electric eel which acts as antidote for certain types of insecticide poisoning in humans. The Japanese drived red algae, *Digenea simplex*, contains the amino acid known as kainic acid from which an anthelmintic drug is prepared. Cod-liver oil is the source of vitamins A and D.

An anticoagulant agent has been isolated from the sea-anemone, *Rhodactis howesii.* Very potent anticancer agents, named dolastins 1-9, are present in Indian ocean sea-hare. The marine annelid, *Lumbriconereis heteropoda,* is toxic to some insects. The richest natural source of prostaglandin is the soft coral *Plexaura homomalla.* Many toxins occur throughout the complete range of marine life; they include irritants, CNS stimulants and depressants, haemolytic substances and protoplasmic poisons. Extracts of various marine algae contain vitamin C, folic acid, folinic acid, niacin and vitamin B.

VITAMINS

Vitmains are organic compounds which are not synthesized within the body. They are essential in small amounts for the maintenance of normal health. The lack of specific vitamins causes diseases such as beriberi, rickets, scurvy and xerophthalmia. Vitamin B_2 (niacin) and pantothenic acid act as coenzymes. Vitamin B_{12} and folic acid take part in the biosynthetic transfer of 1-carbon unit. In the biosynthesis of hydroxyproline, vitamin C is required. Vitamin B_1 and B_6 are involved in the metabolism of carbohydrates. Many vitamins take part in metabolic oxidation-reduction reactions.

Vitamin A is obtained from animal products and involved in vision, growth and tissue differentiation. Vitamin B is a complex mixture of compounds. Liver and yeast are the main sources of the B vitamins. Vitamin C (ascorbic acid) prevents scurvy and is used as antioxidant. Good dietary sources of vitamin C are citrus fruits, tomatoes, strawberries, fresh fruits and vegetables. Vitamin D is essential for the absorption and utilization of calcium. It is obtained from fish liver oils, milk, cereals and synthesized in the body in sunshine. Vitmain E, a mixture of tocopherols, is widely distributed in plant oils, vegetables, grains, eggs and meats. Its deficiency causes muscular dystrophy, coronary disease and sterility. Vitamin K is widely distributed in diary products and many fruits and vegetables. It is necessary for normal clotting of blood.

ANTIBIOTICS

Antibiotics are the chemical substances produced by microorganisms and they have the capacity, in low concentration, to inhibit microorganisms through an antimetabolic mechanism. Penicillin G, obtained from a strain of *Penicillium chryso-genum,* is an agent acting against many pathogenic Gram-positive bacteria and used to treat syphilis. Cloxacillin, dicloxacillin, methicillin, nafcillin and oxacillin are semisynthetic penicillins which are used for treatment of staphylococcal infections. Ampicillin has special clinical value for the treatment of infections caused by *Haemophilus influenza, Salmonella* species and *Shigella* species. Clavulanic acid is a fermentation product of *Streptomyces clavuligerus* and it controls many infectious diseases. Other antibiotics are cephalosporins (from *Cephalosporium acremonium),* chloramphenicol (from *Streptomyces venezuelae),* lincomycin (from *S. lincolnensis),* cycloserine (from *S. orchidaceus),* dactinomycin (from *S. parvullus),* vidarabine (from *S. antibioticus),* polymyxin B *(Bacillus polymyxa),* colistin *(B. poly-myxa),* tyrothricin *(B. brevis),* vancomycin *(S. orientalis),* bleamycin *(S. verticillus),* tetracyclines *(S. aureofaciens),* mitomycin *(S. caespitosus),* erythromycin *(S. erythreus),* amphotericin B *(S. nodosus),* navamycin *(S. natalensis),* griseofulvin *(Penicillium griseofulvum),* rifampin *(S. mediterranei),* nooobiocin (*S. niveus* and *S. spheroides),* streptomycin *(S. griseus)* neomycin and paromomycin *(Streptomyces fradiae* and *S. rimosus* var *paromomycinus),* kanamycin *(S. kanamyceticus),* gentamicin *(Micromonospora purpurea),* tobramycin or nebramysin factor 6 or nebrarius, amikacin (semisynthetic antibiotic derived from kanamycin A by acylation), netilmicin *(Micromonospora inyoensis)* and spectinomycin *(Streptomyces spectablis* and *S. flavopersicus).*

MISCELLANEOUS DRUGS

Ichthamol is a black tarry distillate obtained from bituminous schists containing fossil fish and possesses antiseptic and stimulant properties. Diatomaceous earth (siliceous earth, kieselguhr), made of shells of fossilized unicellular algae, is utilized in face powders, filtering aids, dentifrices and as chromatographic adsorbent.

Liver and stomach of healthy animals are converted into suitable preparations which are used as replacement therapy in pernicious anemia. Bile contains sodium salts of bile acid dehydrocholic, taurocholic and deoxycholic acids. Bile acids, obtained from ox bile, are used in deficiency of biliary secretion and parenterally as sodium salts to increase diuresis. Carmine, a colouring principle obtained from Cochineal insects, cantharidin, an irritant constituent of Cantharides insects, Heparin, Wool fat and Lanolin are the other animal products which are used in some formulations and in cosmetics.

13

Basic Metabolic Pathways and Secondary Metabolites

In nature, a plant is able to synthesize complex molecules from simple ones through highly specific reaction mechanisms. The reactions involved are either difficult or expensive to duplicate by classical chemical methods. In certain cases, it is, therefore, economical to allow part of the synthesis being carried out by the plant in nature and the subsequent steps by chemical methods. Some of the examples are synthesis of Vitamin A starting from citral present in lemongrass oil, the synthesis of corticosteroids including the whole range of cortisones, like prednisone, predinisolone and the sex hormones both androgens and estrogens starting from diosgenin present in certain species of Dioscorea tubers or solasodine present in solanum berries and leaves.

In the case of certain compounds present as active principles of plant, where different steric forms are possible, chemical synthesis yields a mixture of isomers which may be difficult to separate. The product obtained by synthesis may, therefore, be toxic or have different therapeutic effects than what is obtained in nature. In the plant these reactions take place at normal biological temperatures and pressures and the type and quantity of substance produced will be the one that it needs for its own metabolism and hence normally free from toxic ingredients.

Some basic metabolic pathways are identical in both plants and animals. The majority of vegetable drugs exhibit their therapeutic activity due to the presence of secondary plant metabolites, *i.e.*, those

not involved in the essential metabolism of the cell. The production of these secondary metabolites is dependent on the fundamental metabolic cycles of the living tissues.

The living plant cell possesses a highly organized structure with various organelles having distinct biochemical characteristics. The organelles allow the creation of different chemical environments within one cell by their structure which are all important in biological systems.

ENZYMES

Most of the reactions occurring in the cell are enzyme-dependent. They are organic catalysts produced by animal and vegetable cells. Their wide distribution and the delicacy of their operation has long been determined. The enzymes are proteins, coded by specific genes in the plant's DNA and are made via processes called transcription (conversion of DNA to RNA via the enzyme RNA polymerase) and translation (conversion of RNA to protein via enzymatic reactions associated with complex structures called ribosomes). When there is a series of enzymatically catalyzed reactions in a well-defined sequence of steps, we have a *metabolic pathway*. Some enzymes may be involved in metabolic pathways requiring just a few, as in the synthesis of starch from the sugar nucleotide, adenosine diphosphate (ADP)-glucose or many enzymatic steps, as in the synthesis of gibberellin hormones from mevalonic acid. Some enzymes may be involved in pathways that break down compounds (as in the hydrolysis of starch to sugars by α- and β-amylases). Still other enzymes may be involved in making storage forms of given compounds, such as glucosides, amides, or esters of the plant hormone indole-3-acetic acid (IAA). These different enzymatic pathways involved in the synthesis, breakdown, and creation of storage forms of a compound regulate the level of the given compound. The regulation of each pathway and each of its enzymes is, however, extremely complicated.

An enzyme usually acts on one substance or class of substances, since it is specific for a particular atomic group or linkage. Lipases are not highly specific, whereas fumarase acts only upon L-malate and fumarate, and D-malate is a competitive inhibitor of fumarase. Enzymes are also stereo- and regio-specific in their actions.

There is an enzyme potential for carrying out single-step transformations with complete stereochemical change, an aspect important in the synthesis of many drugs.

An enzyme will convert many thousand times its own weight and the gradual diminution in activity which takes place is probably due to secondary reactions which bring about formation of the enzyme.

The enzymology of the secondary metabolic pathways in plants has been investigated by studying cell cultures which are a better source for the isolation of enzymes than is the differentiated plant. In some cases, e.g., cell cultures of volatile oil-containing plants, little or no oil accumulates in the culture due to the absence of storage receptacles but the relevant enzymes for terpenoid synthesis are still manufactured and preparations of them can be made.

The enzyme strictosidine synthase governs the key reaction for the commencement of the biosynthesis of many monoterpenoid indole alkaloids, namely the condensation of tryptamine and secologanin to give 3α(S)-strictosidine.

By means of a new technology, enzymes can be immobilized on a suitable carrier either in whole plant cells or as the isolated enzyme. In this way these biocatalysts can be repeatedly used in analytical and clinical chemistry, or to effect specific chemical transformations.

Enzymes influence the rate of a reaction without changing the point of equilibrium. For example, lipase catalyses either the synthesis of glycerides from glycerol and fatty acids or the hydrolysis of glycerides, the final point of equilibrium being the same in either case. Similarly, β-glucosidase (prunase) has been used for both the synthesis and the hydrolysis of β-glucosides. In plants such reversible reactions may proceed in one direction or the other under different conditions, often resulting in variations in the accumulation of metabolites.

Enzymes are colloidal in nature. They may be partly purified, and in some cases isolated, by the methods of protein chemistry (*i.e.*, by fractional precipitation, dialysis and gel and affinity chromatography).

Most enzymes are soluble either in water or in dilute salt solutions and are precipitated by alcohol or acetone (acetone powders) and by high concentrations of salts. They are inactivated by heat, ultraviolet light and X-rays or by any treatment which brings about denaturation of proteins.

The activity of enzymes is markedly affected by the reaction of the medium and the presence of salts. Pepsin works only in an acid medium and trypsin in an alkaline one. Carbohydrases have pH optima of 3.8-7.5 and lipases optima of pH 5-8, while enzymes which act on bases all have optima more alkaline than pH 7.

The heat effects enzymes in the drying of drugs. At low temperatures enzymic changes are not usually marked. The proteolytic or protein-splitting enzymes in cod livers do bring about some hydrolysis at temperatures approaching zero. The optimum working temperatures of different enzymes vary, but they usually lie between 35 and 50°C. At temperatures of about 60°C destruction of the enzymes is rapid. When dry, enzymes show increased resistance to heat. Zymase, which in the presence of moisture is rapidly inactivated at 50°C, will, when dry, resist a temperature of 85°C.

Chemical nature

Urease and many other enzymes have been prepared in a crystalline form and their protein nature has been established. Their molecular weights vary from about 9000 (hydrogenase) to about 1,00,0000. In many cases the component amino acids are known.

During the isolation of an enzyme, the purified protein (apoenzyme) may be inactive but regains its activity in the presence of an essential coenzyme or activator, which may be organic or inorganic.

Coenzymes

Some enzymes contain smaller organic molecules which are called as coenzymes. They can participate in a large number of biochemical reactions. The coenzymes may consist of esters of phosphoric acid and various nucleosides. The adenosine and uridine phosphates contain one basic unit each (mononucleotides); they act to transport energy in the form of high-energy phosphate bonds. This energy is made available for biochemical reactions in the presence of the appropriate enzyme by hydrolysis of the bond. The terminal phosphate bond of the adenosine triphosphate (ATP) on hydrolysis to adenosine diphosphate (ADP) yields 50000 J mol^{-1}.

Uridine triphosphate (UTP) is involved in the synthesis of sucrose via diphosphate glucose and in the formation of uronic acids and cellulose.

Nicotinamide-adenine dinucleotide (NAD) and nicotinamide-adenine dinucleotide phosphate (NADP) contain two basic units each and are called dinucleotides. They function in oxidation-reduction systems with appropriate enzymes. The oxidized

Fig. 13.2. NAD and NADP.

forms are written NAD$^+$ and NADP$^+$ and the reduced forms NADH and NADPH, respectively.

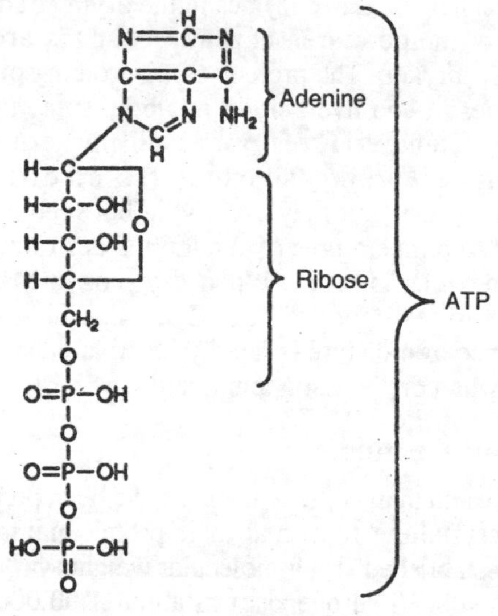

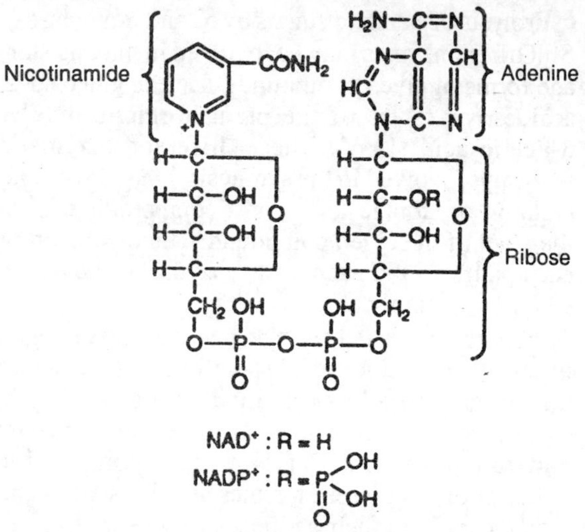

Coenzyme A (CoA) contains the units adenosine-3,5-diphosphate, pantothenic acid-4-phosphate and thioethanolamine. It participates in the transfer of acetyl and acyl groups, acetyl-CoA (active acetate) having a key role in plant and animal metabolism.

Riboflavine is made up of the two coenzymes flavin mononucleotide (FMN) and flavin adenine dinucleotide (FAD). They participate in the biological oxidation-reduction system, and FAD helps in

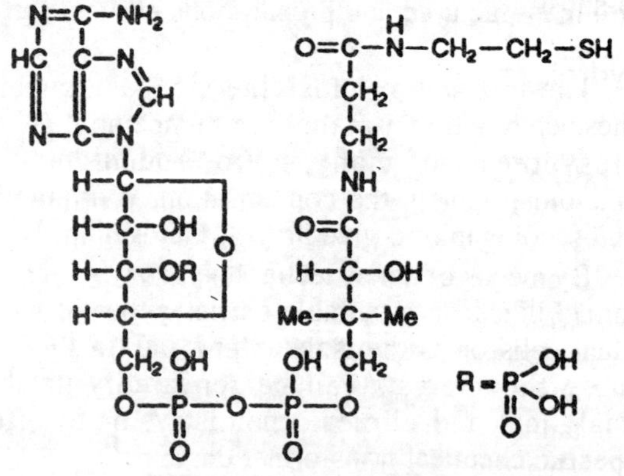

Fig. 13.1. ATP.

Fig. 13.3. Coenzyme A

the transfer of H^+ ions from NADH to the oxidized cytochrome system.

Other coenzymes are the decarboxylation coenzymes thiamine, biotin and pyridoxine. Folic acid derivatives participate in enzymatic reactions which involve one-carbon fragment transfers.

Some quinones, e.g., plastoquinone and ubiquinone are present in plants, animals and microorganisms and take part in biological electron transfer processes.

The enzymes are denoted by the name of the substrate and the termination '-ase'. The general term 'esterase' includes lipases, which hydrolyse fats and chlorophyllase hydrolyses chlorophyll.

Oxidoreductases

Oxidation and reduction involve simultaneously. The names 'oxidase' and 'reductase' may be applied to a single type of enzyme. Eleven different groups of oxidoreductases are known. Many oxidases (that is, enzymes which utilize molecular oxygen as acceptor) convert phenolic substances to quinones. They act on guaiacum resin to produce a blue colour which is used as a test for their detection. Oxidases include laccase present in lac, and ascorbate oxidase. Oxalate oxidase, a flavoprotein present in mosses and the leaves of higher plants, oxidizes oxalic acid into carbon dioxide and hydrogen peroxide. Peroxidases use hydrogen peroxide and not oxygen as the hydrogen acceptor. Catalase catalyses the decomposition of hydrogen peroxide. An oxidoreductase of the morphine biosynthetic pathway catalyses the stereoselective reduction of salutaridine to 7(S) salutaridinol using NADPH as co-substrate.

Hydrolases

These enzymes are :

1. *Hydrolysing esters* : These include lipases, which may be vegetable or animal origin and which hydrolyse glycerides. Mammalian lipases hydrolyse phenyl salicylate, acetylcholine and atropine. Other esterases are chlorophyllase, which hydrolyses chlorophyll, and tannase, which hydrolyses ester links in tannins.
2. *Hydrolysing sugars and glycosides* : Gycoside hydrolases are those enzymes which hydrolyse sugars, carbohydrates and glycosides. Those hydrolysing sugars include β-fructofuranosidase (sucrase or invertase), lactase, maltase, gentiobiase and trehalase. Polysaccharide enzymes are represented by α-amylase, β-amylase, cellulase, lichenase and inulase. Among the glycoside-hydrolysing enzymes are β-glucosidase or β-D-glucoside glucohydralase, which has a wide specificity for β-D-glucopyranosides. More specific glucoside-hydrolysing enzymes are those acting on salicin, amygdalin, sinigrin and cardiac glycosides.
3. *Hydrolysing the C-N linkage* : Many enzymes acting on peptide bonds are pepsin, rennin, trypsin, thrombin and plasmin, and the vegetable enzymes papain (from *Carica papaya*) and ficin (from species of fig). Other enzymes acting on linear amides are asparaginase (present in liquorice) and urease. Cyclic amides are hydrolyzed by penicillinase.

PHOTOSYNTHESIS

By photosynthesis the carbon dioxide of the atmosphere is converted into sugars by the green plant. It is one of the fundamental cycles on which life on Earth depends. The basic overall reaction is as :

$$CO_2 + H_2O \xrightarrow{\text{light}} (CH_2O) + O_2$$

Photosynthesis occurs in the chloroplasts: green, disc-shaped organelles of the cytoplasm which are bounded by a definite membrane, are autoreproductive and separated from the rest of the cell. The chloroplasts can carry out the complete process of photosynthesis. The cells of the red algae contain chlorophyll as the principal pigment and other tetrapyrrole derivatives—the phycobilins.

The chloroplasts have a highly organized structure in which the chlorophyll molecules are arranged within orderly structures (grana), each granum being connected with others by a network of fibres or membranes. The flat chlorophyll molecules themselves are orientated between layers of protein and lipid molecules so that the whole chloroplast acts as a battery containing several cells (the grana), each cell possessing layers of plates (the chlorophyll molecules).

Photosynthesis involves the production of adenosine triphosphate (ATP) from adenosine diphosphate (ADP) and phosphate and the light-energized decomposition of water.

$$H_2O \xrightarrow{\text{hv}} 2[H] + \tfrac{1}{2}O_2$$

ATP is a coenzyme and the high energy of the terminal phosphate bond is available to the organism for the supply of the energy necessary for endergonic reactions. The Hill reactions produces free oxygen and hydrogen ions which bring about the conversion of the electron carrier, NADP, to its reduced form NADPH.

In this complicated process, two systems, Photosystem I and Photosystem II (pigment system I and II) involve two chlorophyll complexes which absorb light at different wavelengths (above and below $\lambda = 685$ nm). Photosystem II produces ATP and Photosystem I supplies all the reduced NADP and some ATP. In these light reactions the chlorophyll molecule captures solar energy and electrons become excited and move to higher energy levels; on returning to the normal low-energy state, the electrons give up their excess energy, which is passed through a series of carriers like Photosystem II plastoquinone and several cytochromes to generate ATP. Photosystem I involves an electron acceptor and the subsequent reduction of ferredoxin in the production of NADPH. An alcoholic solution of chlorophyll possesses, in sunlight, a red fluorescence—no carriers are available to utilize the captured energy and it is re-emitted as light. The isolated chloroplasts, when exposed to light, are capable of producing oxygen, provided that a suitable hydrogen acceptor are present. The oxygen liberated during photosynthesis is derived from water and not from carbon dioxide.

Following the light reactions, a series of dark reactions then utilize NADPH in the reduction of carbon dioxide to carbohydrate. The terrestrial plants can be classified as C_3, C_4, intermediate C_3-C_4 and CAM plants in relation to photosynthesis.

C_3 plants

Calvin *et al.* determined the carbon reduction cycle by methods dependent on exposing living plants (*Chlorella*) to ^{14}C-labelled carbon dioxide for precise periods of time. The radioactive compounds produced were then isolated and identified. In this way a sequence for the formation of compounds was obtained. 3-Phosphoglyceric acid, a C_3 compound, was the compound first formed in a labelled condition but later on a number of 4-, 5-, 6- and 7-carbon systems has been isolated. Ribulose-1, 5-diphosphate reacts first with carbon dioxide first reacts go give two molecules of phosphoglyceric acid. An unstable intermediate in this reaction is 2-carboxy-3-ketopenitol.

C_4 plants

Some semi-arid plants growing in a high light intensity possess an additional carbon-fixation system which is more effective in its use of carbon dioxide, so lowering photorespiration and loss of water. Such plants are known as C_4 plants, because they synthesize, in the presence of light, oxaloacetic and other C_4 acids. Carbon assimilation is based on a modified leaf structure and biochemistry. In the mesophyll cells pyruvate is converted via oxaloacetate to malate, utilizing carbon dioxide, and the malate, or aspartate, is transported to the vascular bundle cells, where it is oxidatively decarboxylated to pyruvate again, carbon dioxide and NADPH, which are used in the Calvin cycle. Pyruvate presumably returns to the mesophyll cells. Plants possessing this facility exhibit two types of photosynthetic cells which differ in their chloroplast type. Intermediate C_3-C_4 pathways are also known.

CAM plants

Crassulacean acid metabolism (CAM) occurs in the Crassulaceae, Liliaceae, Cactaceae and Euphorbiaceae families in which the distinctive character of a build-up of malic acid during hours of darkness was first observed. Similar to C_4 plants, this is an adaptation of the photosynthetic cycle of plants which can exist under drought conditions. When water is not available, respiratory carbon dioxide is recycled, under conditions of darkness, with the formation of malic acid as an intermediate. Carbon dioxide and water loss to the atmosphere are eliminated, a condition which would be fatal for normal C_3 plants.

Fructose, produced in the Calvin cycle, is converted into glucose, sucrose and starch. Erythrose is a precursor in the synthesis of some aromatic compounds. Glucose-6-phosphate is formed by photosynthesis and it is an important intermediate in the oxidative pentose phosphate cycle and for conversion to glucose 1-phosphate in polysaccharide synthesis.

CARBOHYDRATE UTILIZATION

The starch of plant or the glycogen of animals is made available for energy production by conversion to pyruvate and then acetate. Acetyl-coenzyme A, then passes into the tricarboxylic acid cycle. As a result of this, the energy-rich carbohydrate is oxidized to carbon dioxide and water. During the process, the hydrogen atoms liberated are carried by coenzymes into the cytochrome system, in which energy is released in stages, with the possible formation of ATP from ADP and inorganic phosphate. In the end hydrogen combines with oxygen to form water.

One pathways for the initial metabolism of glucose involves compounds which are found in the photosynthetic cycle, and it appears as a reversal of this cycle but the mechanism is quite different. Another pathway is the Embden-Meyerhoff scheme of glycolysis molecules of pyruvate, each of which is converted to acetate, and one molecule of carbon dioxide. One turn of the TCA cycle represents the oxidation of one acetate to two molecules of carbon dioxide, giving rise to twelve molecules of ATP. The overall reaction for the metabolism of one molecule of glucose in terms of ADP and ATP is :

$$C_6H_{12}O_6 + 6CO_2 + 38ADP$$
$$+ 38P \text{ (inorganic)} \rightarrow 6H_2O + 6CO_2 + 38ATP$$

The above scheme are fundamental for the building up and breaking down of reserve foodstuffs for the biosynthesis of all other groups of compounds found in plants.

GLYCOSIDES

Glycosides are formed in nature by the interaction of the nucleotide glycosides, e.g., uridine diphosphate glucose (UDP-glucose) with the alco-holic or phenolic group of a second compound. Such glycosides, called O-glycosides, are the most abundant in nature. In other glycosides the linkage is through sulphur (S-glycosides), nitrogen (N-glycosides) or carbon (C-glycosides).

The formation and hydrolysis of an O-glycoside such as salicin may be represented are reversible reactions :

$$R. \ OH + H \ O.X \ \rightleftharpoons R.OX + H_2O$$
Sugar   Aglycone   Glycoside

or

$$C_6H_{11}O_5OH + HO.C_6H_4.CH_2OH \rightleftharpoons$$
Glucose   Salicyl alcohol
(saligenin)

$$C_6H_{11}O_5.O.C_6H_4.CH_2OH + H_2O$$
Salicin

In plants, glycosides are both synthesized and hydrolysed under the influence of specific enzymes. While glycosides do not themselves reduce Fehling's solution, the hydrolyzed products simple sugars produces cuprous oxide.

The sugars found in glycosides may be monosaccharides such as glucose, rhamnose and fucose or deoxysugars such as the cymarose found in cardiac glycosides. More than one molecule of such sugars may be attached to the aglycone either by separate linkages, or as a di-, tri- or tetrasaccharide. These complex glycosides are formed by the stepwise addition of sugars to the aglycone molecule.

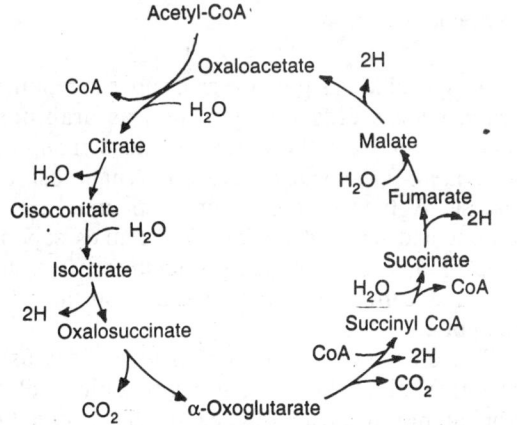

Fig. 13.4. Tricarboxylic acid cycle (TCA) or Krebs cycle.

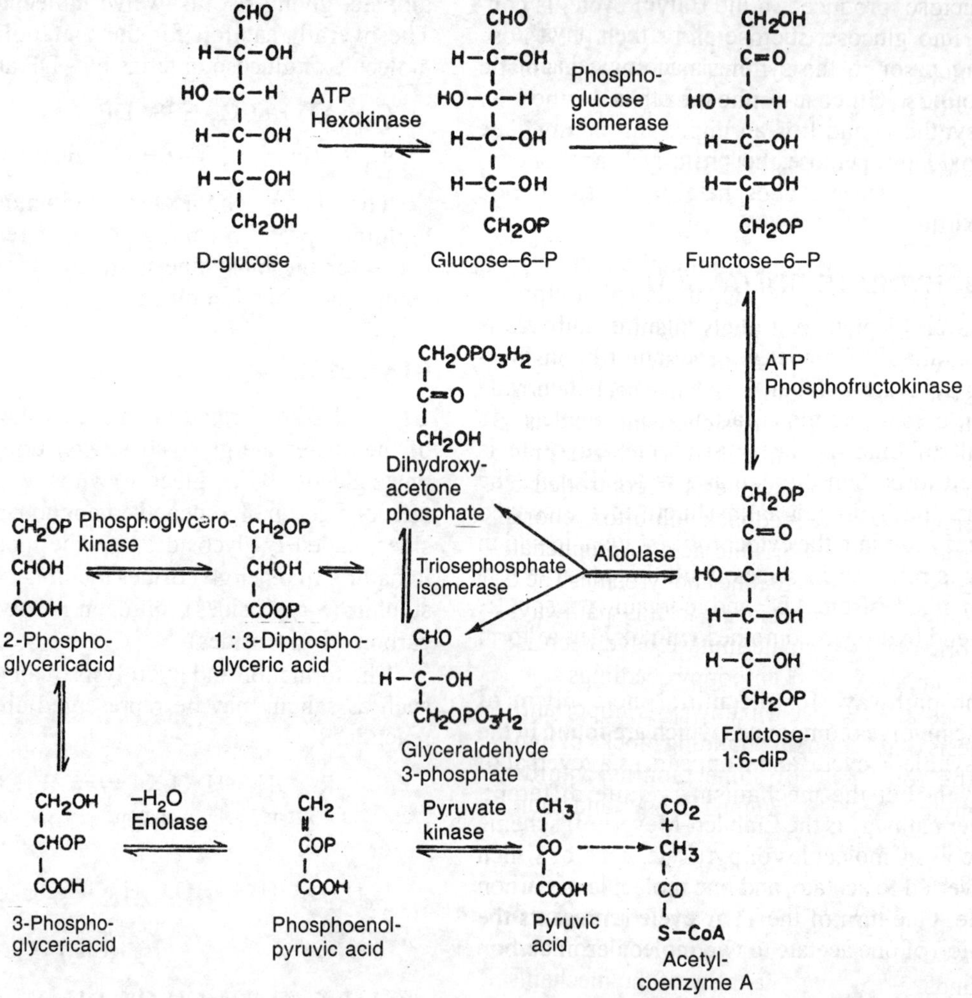

Fig. 13.5. Embden-Meyerhoff scheme of glycolysis.

The isomeric α- and β-forms of glycosides are theoretically possible. Practically all natural glycosides are of the β-type. The α-linkage is found in nature in sucrose, glycogen and starch. In *k*-strophanthoside, a glycoside of the aglycone strophanthidin with strophanthotriose (cymarose + glucose + glucose), the outer glucose molecule has the α-linkage and the inner glucose the β-linkage. Isomeric glycosides may be prepared synthetically from glucose and methyl alcohol by introducing methyl group into the OH groups to yield α- and β-methyl glucosides.

A glycoside has glucose as a sugar component; a *pentoside* yields a sugar such as arabinose; *rhamnosides* yield the methyl-pentose rhamnose; and *rhamnoglucosides* yield both rhamnose and glucose. Aglycones are generally phenol, anthraquinone and sterol glycosides. The names 'saponin' (soap-like), 'cyanogenetic' (producing hydrocyanic acid) and 'cardiac' (having an action on the heart) are applied to these substances.

The older system of naming glycosides using the termination '-in' (e.g., senegin, salicin, aloin, strophanthin) has been replaced by the termination '-oside' (e.g., sennoside).

In glycosides, the aglycones are of varied nature and complexity. Therefore, their physical and chemical properties and pharmacological action are very much different from each other.

AROMATIC BIOSYNTHESIS

Shikimic acid pathway

It is an important route from carbohydrate for the biosynthesis of the C_6-C_3 units (phenylpropane derivatives) as that of phenylalanine and tyrosine. The presence of the enzyme system responsible for the synthesis of shikimic acid has been determined. Anthranilate synthase uses chorismic acid as a substrate to give anthranilic acid which is a precursor of tryptophan. The synthesis is controlled by the latter acting as a feedback inhibitor; chorismate mutase converts chorismic acid to prephenate, the precursor of phenylalanine and tyrosine. The opium alkaloids are synthesized via this pathway. Two isoforms of chorismate mutase have been isolated and characterized from poppy seedlings.

The shikimic acid pathway is important in the genesis of the aromatic building blocks of lignin and in the formation of some tannins, vanillin and phenylpropane units of the flavones and coumarins.

Acetate hypothesis

It is possible to devise many routes for acetate condensation to give a variety of aromatic compounds. The general validity of the mechanism has been established by the use of labelled compounds. Thus, the incorporation of $[1^{-14}C]$ acetate into 6-methylsalicylic acid by *Penicillium griseofulvum* takes place.

The production of the mould anthraquinone

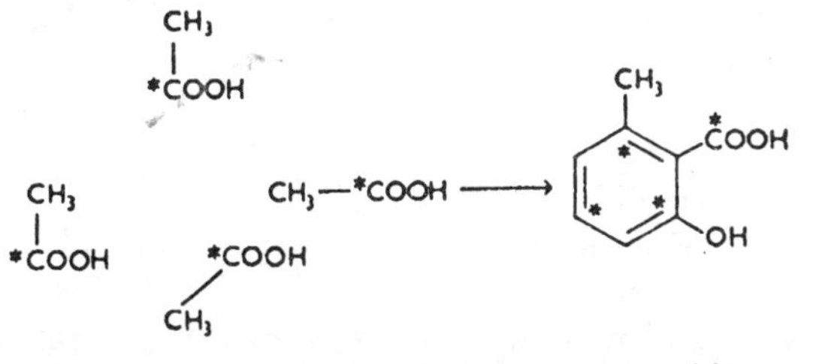

Fig. 13.6. Formation of an aromatic acid.

metabolite endocrocin takes place from eight C_2 units. Decarboxylation of endocrocin affords emodin. The original chain lengthening is the same as in fatty acid production but does not require the reduction of $=CO$ to $=CH_2$. In malonic acid pathway, the chain is built up from the combination of malonyl units with a terminal acetyl unit. Sometimes the starter unit is acetate, as involved in the formation of the tetracycline antibiotics from nine units; here malonamide-SCoA is the starter unit. Higher plants also utilize the polyacetate-malonate pathway for the biosynthesis of emodin-type anthraquinones.

The structures of anthraquinones such as alizarin, rubiadin, pseudo-purpurin and morindadiol, pigments of the Rubiaceae and other families, cannot be explained on the acetate hypothesis.

These compounds might be formed from naphthoquinones with the participation of mevalonic acid, a key precursor in the formation of isopentenyl units. The mevalonate is involved in this formation as shown by tracer experiments with *Rubia tinctorum*; ring C and carbon side-chain of pseudopurpurin and rubiadin are derived from mevalonate, and in the same plant shikimic acid has been shown to be incorporated into ring A of alizarin.

The aromatic rings of some compounds can be derived from both the shikimic acid and the acetic acid pathways. A phenylpropane formed by the former route may undergo chain lengthening by the addition of acetate units to give a polyketide and then, by ring closure, gives a flavonoid derivative.

Isoflavones and rotenoids are formed in the same manner, with a rearrangement of the aryl-B ring in relation to the three carbons.

Coumarins

Umbelliferone is the precursor of most furanocoumarins, and an enzyme has been isolated from *Ruta graveolens*, which catalyzes the reaction between this coumarin and dimethyl allyl pyrophosphate giving demethyl suberosin, the precursor of the linear furanocoumarins. Osthenol, the precursor of the angular furanocoumarins, is biosynthesized by a similar reaction. Ring closure of

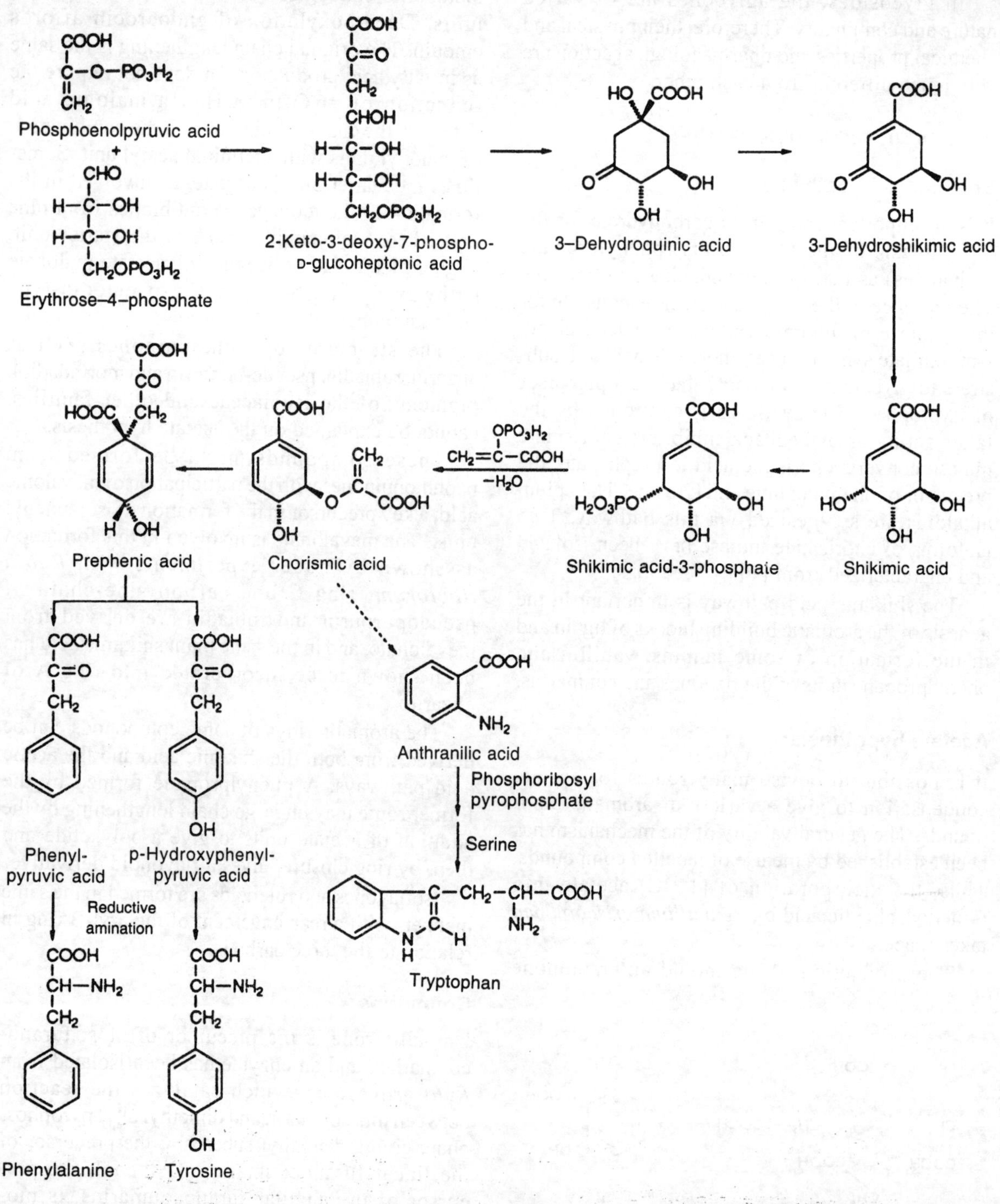

Fig. 13.7. Biosynthesis of aromatic compounds via the shikimic acid pathway.

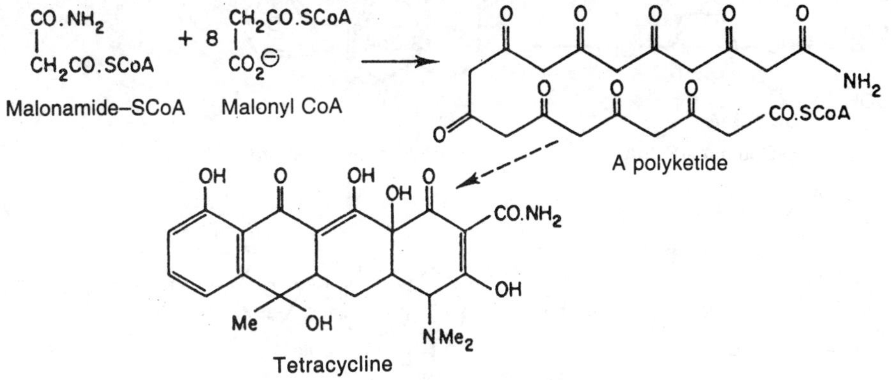

Fig. 13.8. Formation of tetracycline.

the dimethyl allyl derivatives gives marmesin and columbianetin, respectively, subsequent degradation of the side chain resulting psoralen from *Psoralea corylifolia* and angelicin from *Angelica archangelica*.

In the biosynthesis of coumarin, umbelli-ferone, glycosylation occurs at the 4-hydroxy-cinnamic acid (*p*-coumaric acid) stage, the glucoside, skimmin, is

formed before the free coumarin. Glucosylation of the 2-hydroxy group of trans-cinnamic acid derivatives is necessary to effect cyclization of lactone ring.

BIOSYNTHESIS OF FLAVONOIDS

The flavonoids and isoflavonoid ring structures are of mixed biosynthetic origin. Ring A is derived from

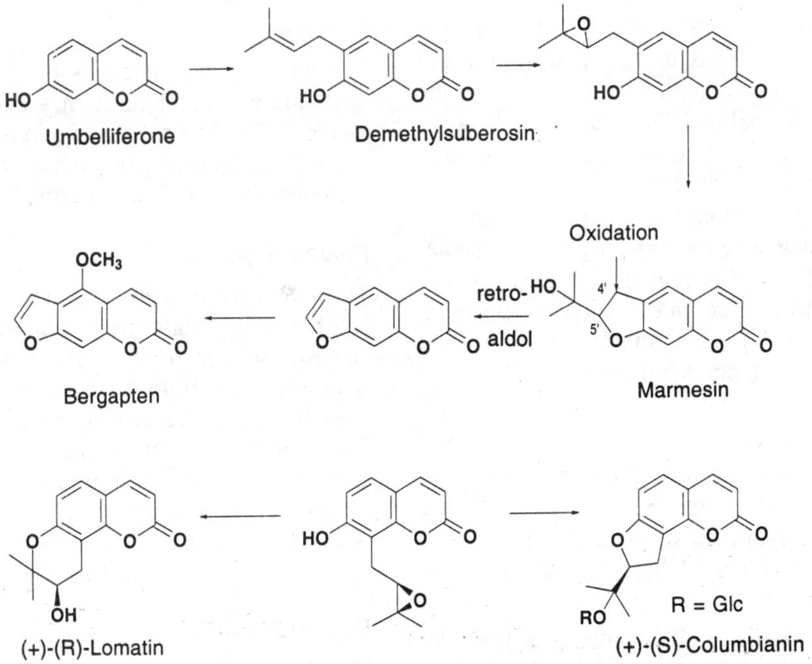

Fig. 13.9. Biosynthesis of furanocourarins.

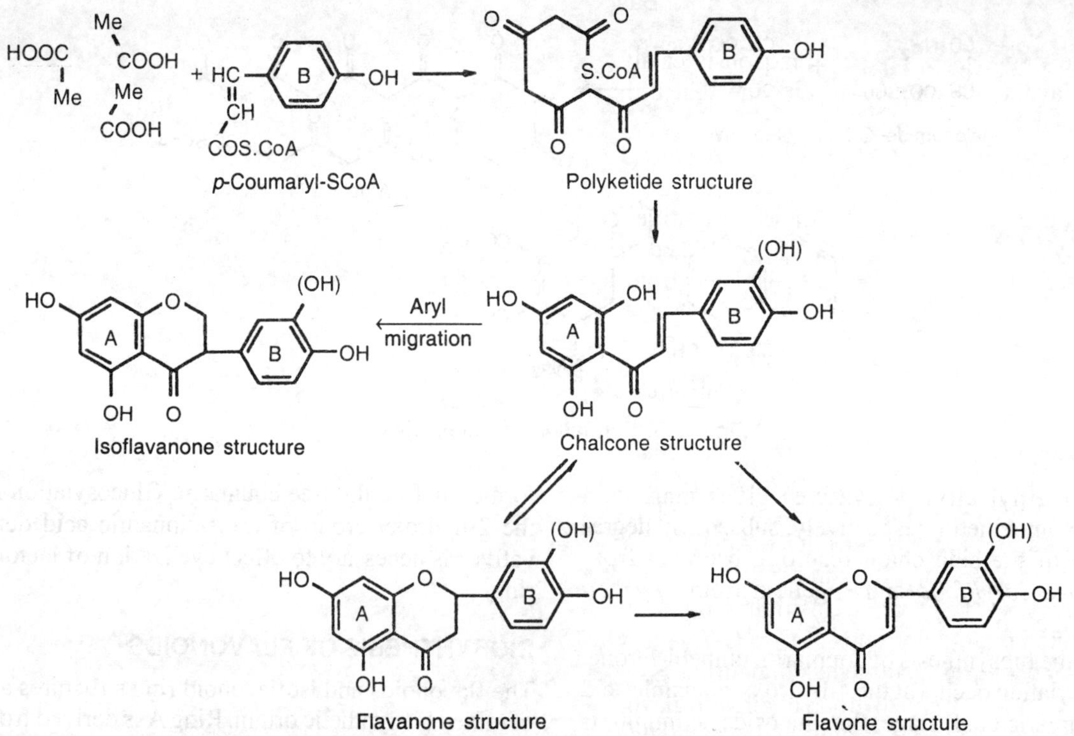

Fig. 13.10. Formation of flavanones, isoflavanones and flavones.

three acetate units condensed head to tail, while ring B and the three carbons of the central ring are derived from cinnamic acid. The acetate units are first converted to malonyl CoA, both the acetate-malonate and the shikimic acid pathways contribute to flavonoid biosynthesis.

The addition of malonyl Co-A units to cinnamic acid derivatives is catalyzed by the enzyme, flavanone synthase. This enzyme is highly specific and will only utilize p-coumaric acid as a substrate. Hydroxylation of the various flavonoids must occur after the flavanone synthase stage.

Chalcones

Chalcones are considered as the precursor of all other classes of flavonoid. Such compounds are biosynthesized from three malonyl units with p-coumaric acid or with 4-hydroxyphenylpyruvic acid.

Reduction of the α, β-unsaturated bond of chalcones gives the colourless dihydrochalcones.

Aurones

The aurone ring system is biosynthesized from a chalcone precursor through a coumaranone intermediate. Cell free extract of *Glycine max* (soybeans) converts 2', 4', 4-trihydroxychalcone to hispidol with the coumaranone as an intermediate.

Flavanones

The isomerization of chalcones to flavanones is catalyzed by chalcone-flavanone isomerase, an enzyme isolated from several plants. This enzyme is present in different isoenzymes which are specific for particular A ring hydroxylation patterns. The chalcone-flavone isomerase from parsley only catalyzes the isomerization of 2', 4', 6', 4-tetrahydroxychalcone. Chalcone-flavanone isomerase will only utilize free chalcones as substrates and has nc action on the glucosides.

Flavone

The 2,3-dehydrogenation of flavanones yields a

flavone ring system and the reaction is catalyzed by a flavanone oxidase, an enzyme that utilizes molecular oxygen.

Artocarpin from *Artocarpus heterophyllus* (Jack fruit) and mulberrin from *Morus alba* are probably biosynthesized from a chalcone derivative and dimethylallyl pyrophosphate. The postulated intermediate, artocarpesin, has been isolated from the Jack fruit.

Flavonols

A chalcone is the precursor of flavonols. Hydroxy group at C-3 is possibly introduced at the chalcone stage or even derived from phenylpyruvic acid through the formation of α-hydroxychalcones. Flavones are not converted into flavonols, despite the similarity of their structures.

Flavonols are present in higher plants with substituted hydroxyl groups at C-5, C-7, C-3', C-4' and C-5' or fully substituted as digicitrin.

Reduction of the keto group of dihydro-flavonols gives first the flavan- 3,4- diols and then the flavan-3-ols (catechins). These compounds exist as two series of stereoisomers - those compounds in which the 2,3-hydrogen atoms are *trans*, known as catechins. In *epi*-catechins, these hydrogen atoms are *cis*. The chiral C-2 and C-3 give rise to (+)– and (–)– optical isomers, those occurring naturally being (+)– catechin and (–)– *epi*-catechin.

Flavan –3,4– diols are also known as leucoanthocyanidins, as on treatment with acids, they give the corresponding anthocyanidin.

Proanthocyanidins

Condensation of catechin or *epi*-catechin with flavan-3,4-diols gives the dimers such as procyanidin B, with one linkage between the monomers, and those such as proanthocyanidin A_2, with two such linkages. Further polymerization eventually gives the condensed tannins which is non-enzymatic and similar to lignin formation.

Anthocyanins

These pigments are glycosides of the unstable anthocyanidins, compounds based on the flavylium ion. Glucose is the most common sugar to occur in anthocyanidin glycosides. Acylation of sugar with *p*-coumaric, caffeic, ferulic or sinapic acids also occur.

Anthocyanidins are biosynthesized from di-hydroflavonols. The biosynthesis is affected by light.

Anthocyanins are flavonoid-type compounds responsible for most of the red, pink, purple, and blue pigments found in roots, stems, leaves, seeds, and fruits. Examples include the red anthocyanins in red radish, red leaves of some Norway maple cultivars (e.g., *Acer saccharum* cv. '*Schwedleri*'), red fruits of some peppers, apples, and cherry (*Malpighia glabra*), and the red, pink, purple, and blue flowers of *Rhododendron, Hibiscus*, and *Fuchsia*. Anthocyanin pigments occur in the vacuoles of plant cells. They are synthesized from the aromatic amino acid, phenylalanine, in the phenylpropanoid pathway. This is the same pathway that is responsible for the synthesis of tannins, flavonones like maringenin, flavonols, flavonoids, isoflanonoids like genistein and daidzein, lignin, lignans, and coumarin.

The primary enzyme that commits the pathway to biosynthesis of the anthocyanin pigments is chalcone synthase (CHS). There is a whole gene family of CHS genes within most plants. Some of the genes are expressed in very specific tissues. CHS(A), for example, is only expressed in the petals and stamens of flowers that produce anthocyanins. In petunia, genetic loci controlling the synthesis of most of these enzymes have been located with the exception of 5GT (5-glucosyl transferase). The different coloured anthocyanins arise from precursors that include dihydrokaempferol (a precursor of the purplish red anthocyanin, pelargonidin), dihydroquercetin (a precursor of the purplish red anthocyanin, cyanindin), and dihydromyricetin (a precursor of the bluish purple anthocyanin, delphinidin). All of these antho-cyanidins are converted to their glucose such as pelargonidin-3-glucoside, cyanidin-3-glucoside, and delphinidin-3-glucoside which allows them better solubility in the aqueous solution of the vacuole.

The glucosyl moieties are typically glucose and rhamnose sugars. The colour of anthocyanins is affected by the number of hydroxyl and methoxyl groups in the B ring of the anthocyanidin, but apart

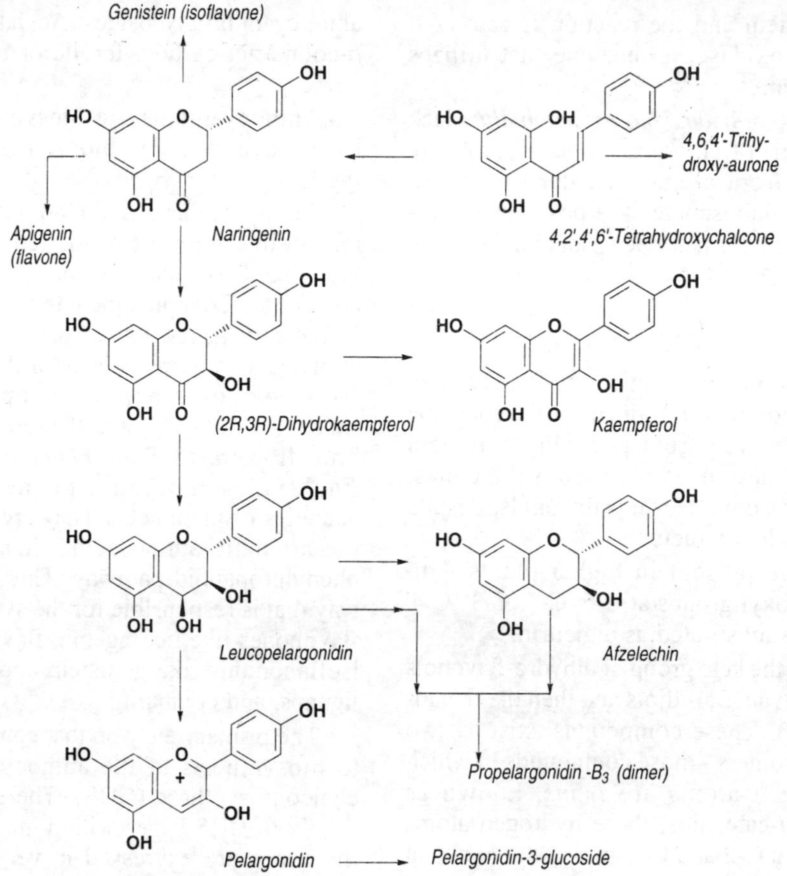

Fig. 13.11. Biosynthesis of pelargonidin.

from structure, colour is also affected by the presence of chelating metals such as iron and aluminium, the presence of flavone or flavonol co-pigments, and the vacuolar pH where these pigments are stored. In Hydrangea flowers, where the vacuolar pH is acidic, the flower petals appear blue; where it is alkaline, they appear pink. So the vast variety of colouration of many leaves, flowers, and fruits is often the result of several different pigments—chlorophylls, carotenoids, and anthocyanins.

Anthocyanins serve many diverse functions in plants, including attraction of insect and bird pollinators to flowers and dispersal of seeds and fruits by birds and mammals. In some cases, they are feeding deterrents and, like other flavonoids, can also protect the plant against damage from UV irradiation.

In roses, chrysanthemums and carnations, synthesis of the blue pigment, delphinidin-3-glucoside, does not normally occur because the 3,5 hydroxylase is not normally expressed.

Table 13.1. Factors controlling cyanin colour in flowers

Hydroxylation pattern of the anthocyanidins (*i.e.*, based on pelargonidin, cyanidin, or delphinidin)

Pigment concentration

Presence of flavone or flavonol co-pigment

Presence of chelating metal (blue effect)

Presence of aromatic acyl substituent (blue effect)

Presence of sugar on B-ring hydroxyl (red effect)

Methylation of anthocyanidins (red effect)

Presence of carotenoids (brown effect)

One interesting application in the use of naturally occurring anthocyanin pigments is developed from the red roots of radish, *Raphanus sativus*. This water-soluble pigment is extracted from these roots and is currently used to dye Maraschino cherries bright red instead of using a synthetic red dye as was done previously.

Isoflavonoids

The isoflavonoids are biosynthesized from chalcone precursors and ring migration has been postulated as an oxidation of a flavanone intermediate leading to an isoflavone.

In *Phaseolus aureus* (mung bean), the isoflavanone, dihydrodiadzein, is biosynthesized from 2', 4', 4- trihydroxychalcone, with the isoflavone, diadzein, as an intermediate.

Isoflavones are probably the precursors of the other classes of isoflavonoids. Coumestrol is derived from diadzein in the mung bean seedlings.

The rotenoid amorphogenin is biosynthesized from 2'-methoxyisoflavones.

BIOSYNTHESIS OF LIGNIN

Lignin is a complex polymer that exists as a 3-dimensional matrix around the polysaccharides of secondary cell walls found in plant fibers and in the tracheids and vessel elements of secondary xylem (wood). It is composed of varying amounts of the aromatic phenylpropanoid subunits (monolignols), *para*-coumaryl alcohol, coniferyl alcohol, and sinapyl alcohol made via the shikimic acid pathway. These monolignols are usually synthesized from the amino acid l-phenylalanine, although tyrosine can also be used. These monolignols are present in the ER and Golgi bodies, but the polymerization of lignin itself occurs outside the plasma membrane.

Lignin makes up between 15 and 35% of the dry weight of woody tissue, and it acts to provide additional rigidity and compressive strength to cell walls. Because lignin is hydrophobic, it also makes cell walls that become lignified impermeable to water. In plants, there is a simple tests involving the use of phloroglucinol/HCl or para-rosaniline HCl. The cell walls stain deep reddish brown in colour.

BIOSYNTHESIS OF AMINO ACIDS

As amino acids are the precursors of some secondary metabolites, they arise at various levels of the glycolytic and TCA systems. Nitrogen enters the metabolism of the organism by reductive amination of α-keto acids; pyruvic, oxalacetic and α-ketoglutaric acids give alanine, aspartic acid and glutamic acid, respectively. By transamination reactions with other appropriate acids, alanine, aspartic acid and glutamic acid act as α-amino donors in the formation of other amino acids.

$$R—CH(NH_2)—COOH \quad + R'—CO—COOH \rightleftharpoons$$
$$R—CO—COOH \quad\quad + R'—CH(NH_3)—COOH$$

Glutamic acid is a central product in amino acid metabolism and glutamic acid dehydrogenase. The enzyme acts in conjunction with NAD:

$$a\text{-ketoglutaric acid} + NH_3 + NADPH$$
$$\rightleftharpoons \text{glutamic acid} + NAD$$

The nitrogen of ammonia first appears in the dicarboxylic amino acids and is later transferred to other nitrogen compounds.

Proline, hydroxyproline, ornithine and arginine

These amino acids are involved in the secondary metabolism of some plants. They are precursors of a number of alkaloids. They are metabolically connected to glutamic acid and their formation in plant cells is complex. The enzymes involved in the formation of ornithine are the *N*-acetyl derivatives. Arginine is synthesized from ornithine in all organisms via the reactions of the urea cycle.

Serine and glycine

Together with cysteine and cystine, these amino acids are formed at the triose level of metabolism. Preparations from rat liver use the pathway for the formation of serine.

In animal tissues tetrahydrofolic acid (THFA) removes the hydroxymethyl group of serine to form hydroxymethyl-tetrafolic acid. This compound acts as a source of formate and methyl groups in many reactions, the β-carbon of serine may be their original source; this applies to the formation of methion-

$$CH_3-CO-COOH \xleftarrow{NH_3} CH_3-CH(NH_2)-COOH$$

Pyruvic acid   Alanine

$$HOOC-CH_2-CH_2-CO-COOH \qquad HOOC-CO-CH_2-COOH$$

α-Ketoglutaria acid   Oxalacetic acid

$$\big\updownarrow NH_3 \qquad\qquad\qquad \big\updownarrow NH_3$$

$$HOOC-CH_2-CH_2-CH(NH_2)-COOH \qquad HOOC-CH_2-CH(NH_2)-COOH$$

Glutamic acid   Aspartic acid

$$\big\updownarrow NH_3 \qquad\qquad\qquad \big\updownarrow NH_3$$

$$H_2N-OC-CH_2-CH_2-CH(NH_2)-COOH \qquad H_2N-OC-CH_2-CH(NH_2)-COOH$$

Glutamine   Asparagine

Fig 13.12. Reductive and trans-amination in the formation of amino acids.

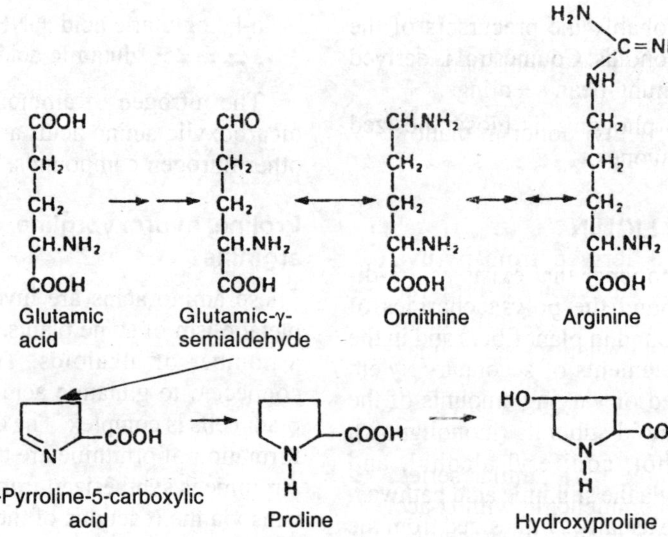

Glutamic acid → Glutamic-γ-semialdehyde ↔ Ornithine ↔ Arginine

Δ^1-Pyrroline-5-carboxylic acid → Proline → Hydroxyproline

Fig. 13.13. Origin of proline, hydroxyproline, ornithine and arginine.

$$COOH-CHOH-CH_2OPO_3H_2 \longrightarrow COOH-CO-CH_2OPO_3H_2$$

3-Phosphoglyceric acid   3-Phosphophydroxypyruvic acid

$$COOH-CH.NH_2-CH_2OH \longleftrightarrow COOH-CH.NH_2-CH_2OPO_3H_2$$

Serine   3-Phosphoserine

$$CH_2OH-CH.NH_2-COOH \rightarrow HCHO + CH_2.NH_2-COOH$$

Fig. 13.14. Formation of serine and glycine.

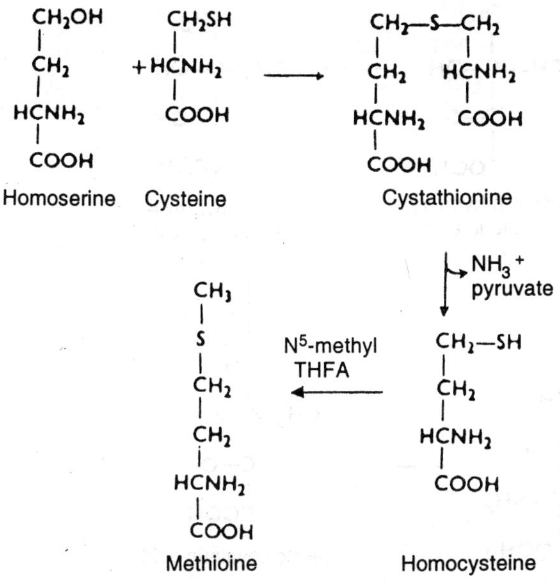

CH2OH   CH2SH

$$
\begin{array}{ccc}
CH_2OH & CH_2SH & CH_2\!-\!S\!-\!CH_2 \\
| & | & |\qquad| \\
CH_2 & +HCNH_2 & CH_2\quad HCNH_2 \\
| & | & \longrightarrow\qquad|\qquad| \\
HCNH_2 & COOH & HCNH_2\quad COOH \\
| & & | \\
COOH & & COOH \\
\text{Homoserine} & \text{Cysteine} & \text{Cystathionine}
\end{array}
$$

$$
\begin{array}{cc}
CH_3 & \raise2pt{\searrow NH_3{}^+}\;\text{pyruvate} \\
| \\
S & \\
| & CH_2\!-\!SH \\
CH_2 & | \\
| & CH_2 \\
CH_2 & | \\
| & HCNH_2 \\
HCNH_2 & | \\
| & COOH \\
COOH \\
\text{Methioine} & \text{Homocysteine}
\end{array}
$$

(arrow labelled N^5-methyl THFA)

Fig. 13.15. Biosynthesis of methionine.

ine, itself an important methyl donor in plant biochemistry.

Alanine, valine and leucine

These amino acids are derived from pyruvate. α-Ketoisovaleric acid is aminated to form valine and it also condenses with acetate to form an intermediate which on decarboxylation and amination affords leucine (Fig. 13.16).

Isoleucine

This amino acid is formed by a similar series of reactions to valine but commencing with α-aceto-α-hydroxypyropionic acid instead of α-acetolactic acid.

Lysine

Lysine, $H_2N\!-\!(CH_2)_4\!-\!CH(NH_2)\!-\!COOH$, is derived in plants from aspartate involving a pathway utilizing 2,3-dihydropicolinic acid and diaminopimelic acid. It is the precursor of some alkaloids of *Nicotiana*, *Lupinus* and *Punica*.

BIOSYNTHESIS OF PROTEINS

Protein synthesis takes place in association with the ribosomes, which are small bodies found in the cytoplasm and in the endoplasmic reticulum area. The amino acids are brought to the ribosomes associated with a transfer-RNA molecule and by the action of the ribosomes, using a sequence coded by a particular messenger-RNA molecule, are linked to form the peptide chains of the particular protein.

ISOPRENOID COMPOUNDS

Isoprene is a fundamental building block for rubber. 'Biogenetic isoprene rule' could be used to explain the formation of rubber monoterpenes, and many other natural products, including sterols and triterpenes with complex constitutions.

Acetic acid is involved in the synthesis of cholesterol, squalene, yeast sterols and rubber. The use of methyl and carboxyl-labelled acetic acid with animal tissues indicated that the methyl and carboxyl carbons alternated in the skeleton of cholesterol or squalene and that the lateral carbon atoms all come from acetyl-coenzyme A, the so-called 'active acetate'. Mevalonic acid (3,5-dihydroxy-3-methyl-valeric acid) is a C_6 acid and, as such, is not the 'active isoprene' unit which forms the basic building block of the isoprenoid compounds.

The C_5 compound is isopentenyl pyrophosphate; it is derived from mevalonic acid pyrophosphate by decarboxylation and dehydration. Isoprenoid synthesis then proceeds by the condensation of isopentenyl pyrophosphate with the isomeric dimethylallyl pyrophosphate to yield geranyl pyrophosphate. Further C_5 units are added by the addition of more isopentenyl pyrophosphate.

From geranyl and farnesyl pyrophosphates various structures can be built up. The use of stereospecifically ${}^3H-$ and ${}^{14}C$-labelled mevalonic acids have shown the stereochemical mechanism of the initial stages of isoprenoid formation. Only the (R)-form of mevalonic acid gives rise to the terpenoids, the (S)-form appearing to be metabolically inactive. In the formation of isopentenyl pyrophosphate, the elimination is *trans* and the removal of the proton in the isomerization to the dimethylallyl pyrophosphate is also stereospecific.

In the subsequent additions of the C_5 isopentenyl pyrophosphate units to form the terpenoids,

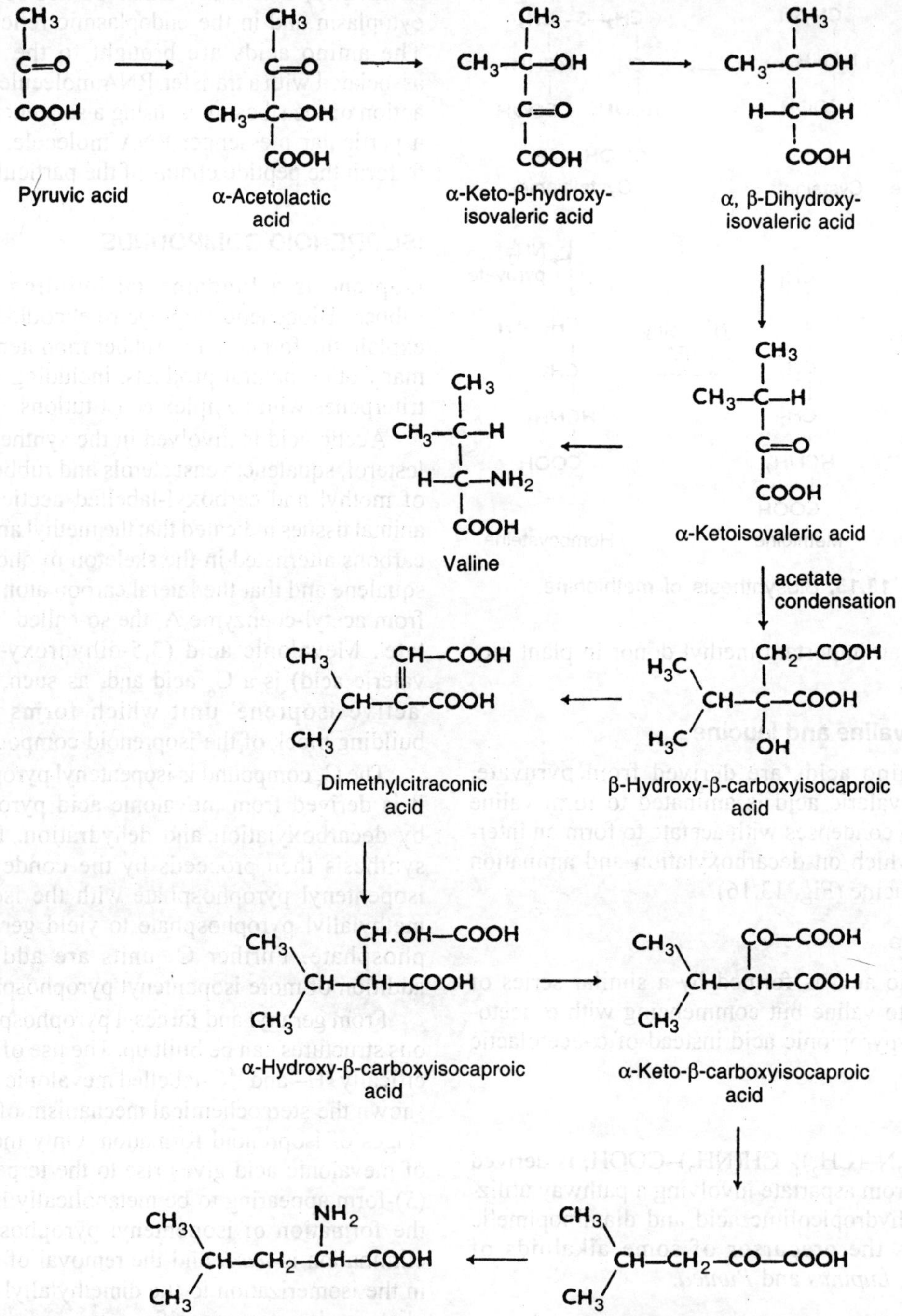

Fig. 13.16. Formation of valine and leucine.

R—CH(NH₂)COOH + R′—CH(NH₂)COOH ⟶

Amino acid   Amino acid

R—CH(NH₂)CO—NH—CH—R′ + H₂O
                        |
                      COOH
              Dipeptide

Fig. 13.17. Formation of dipeptide.

the elimination of hydrogen is *trans*. In the biogenesis of rubber, however, the hydrogen elimination produces a *cis* double bond.

A simple change in orientation of the isopentenyl pyrophosphate on the enzyme surface could produce this change without altering the reaction mechanism. In the enzymology of the isoprenoid pathway one key regulatory enzyme is hydroxymethylglutaryl-CoA reductase (mevalonate kinase). The situation is complicated by the existence of more than one species of enzyme and a plant may possess multiple forms each having a separate subcellular location associated with the biosynthesis of different classes of terpenoids. Some metabolites of mixed biogenetic origin involve the mevalonic acid pathway; prenylation is common, with C_5, C_{10} and C_{15} units associated with flavonoids, coumarins benzoquinones, cannabinoids and alkaloids.

Secondary metabolites

The basic metabolic pathways constitute the origins of secondary plant metabolism and give rise to different compounds; some of these are responsible for the characteristic odours, pungencies and colours of plants, culinary, medicinal or poisonous virtues and of obscure value to the plant.

The secondary metabolites are biosynthesized to aid the producer's survival. Various insects sequester specific alkaloids, iridoids, lactones and flavonoids serve as defensive agents or are converted to male pheromones.

Stereospecific reactions in terpenoid biogenesis involves the formation from mevalonic acid (MVA) of isopentenyl pyrophosphate (IPP) by *trans* elimination; isomerization to dimethylallyl pyrophosphate (DMAPP), association of the two 5-C units with *trans* elimination of hydrogen, and involving formation of *cis* double bends as found in rubber.

Biosynthesis of monoterpenes in leaves of peppermint

The leaves can synthesize a variety of monoterpenes from geranyl pyrophosphate (GPP). GPP production in the terpenoid pathway is the universal precursor of all monoterpenes. Monoterpenes, and some sesquiterpenes, serve as anti-herbivore agents that have significant insect toxicity while having negligible toxicity to mammals. Mixtures of these low molecular weight volatiles, called essential oils, give their characteristic odours, and many are commercially important in flavouring foods and in making perfumes.

In peppermint, the biosynthesis of *l*-menthol and *l*-menthyl acetate from *l*-menthone and the enzymes that lead to their biosynthesis occur in the glandular hairs that arise from leaf epidermal tissue. The products are stored in a modified extracellular space between the cuticle and the cell wall. Well known to repel insects, menthol at the very surface of the leaves (in hairs) seems to deter herbivores before

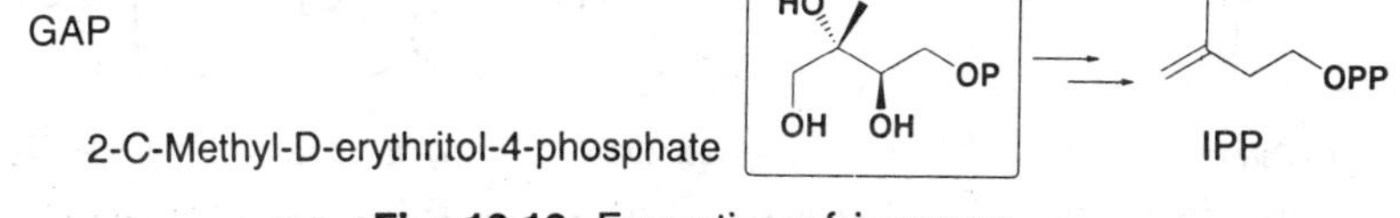

Fig. 13.18. Formation of isoprene

they even get a chance to take a trial bite. The synthesis of *d*-neomenthol and *d*-neomenthyl glucoside occurs not in the epidermal hairs, but, in the photosynthetic mesophyll tissue of the leaves that lies inside the epidermis. The ultimate product, *d*-neomenthyl glucoside, is then translocated from the leaf mesophyll tissue to the phloem in the leaf vascular bundles, and from there to the roots of the plant where it is stored.

The flowers of many plant species attract pollinators by producing different complex mixtures of volatile compounds within the various floral organs (i.e., stigma, style, ovary, filaments, petals, or sepals). It is the combinations of the constituents of this scent mixture that give each flowering plant species a unique fragrance. The insects can distinguish between these different floral scent mixtures which is the key to the reason that many specific plant species often have specific pollinator species. For example, plants that make flowers which produce linalool (a monoterpene) very often attract moth pollinators during the night, while species that may look very similar and live in the same area but do not produce linalool do not attract moths. They are pollinated by other insects, usually bees or butterflies during the daytime. Thus, the components of a floral scent have important implications for the pollination success of the plant that produce them.

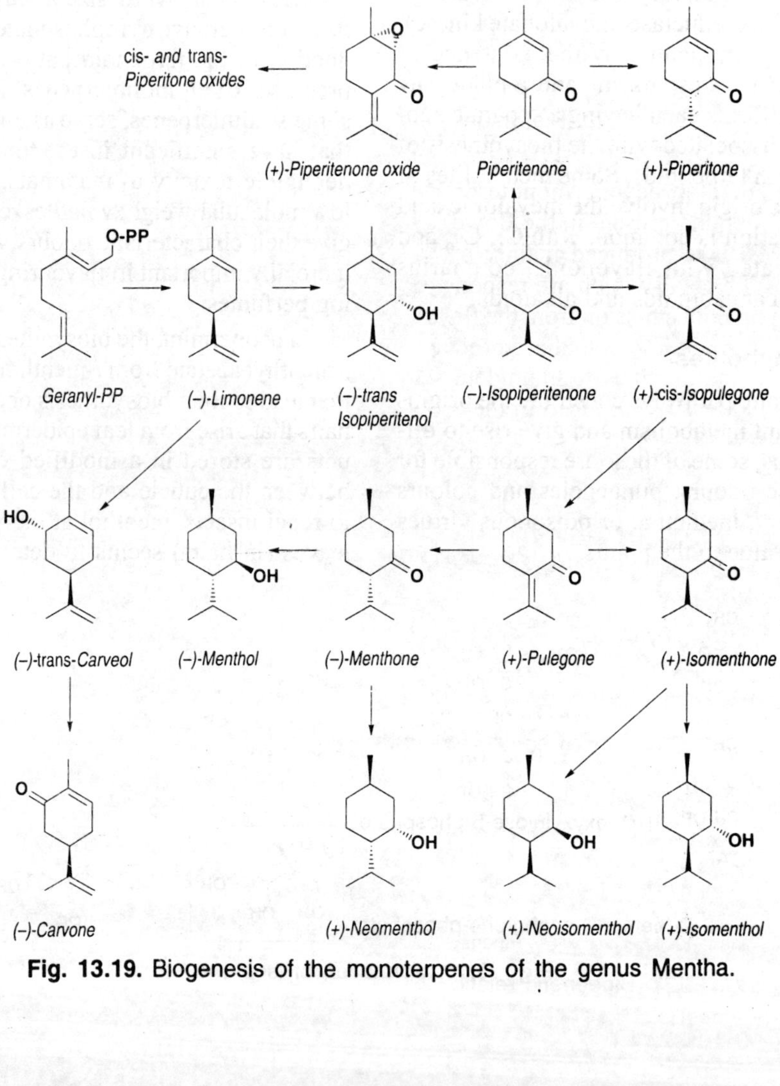

Fig. 13.19. Biogenesis of the monoterpenes of the genus Mentha.

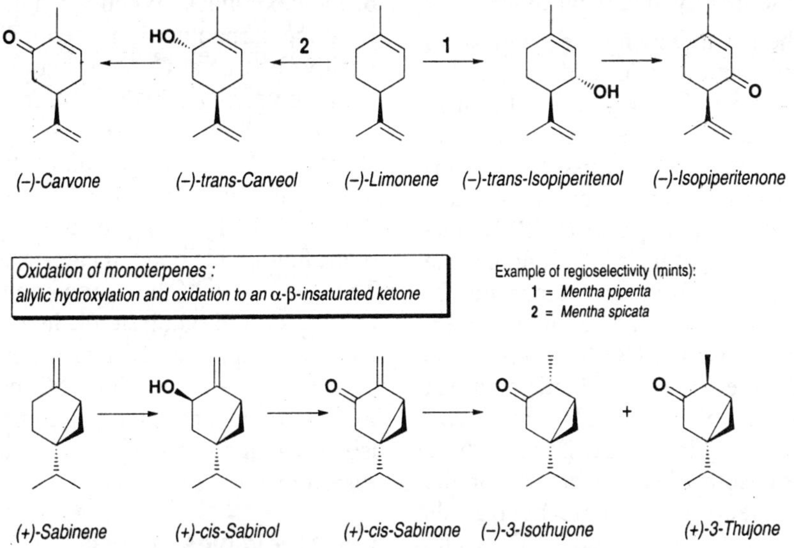

(−)-Carvone   (−)-trans-Carveol   (−)-Limonene   (−)-trans-Isopiperitenol   (−)-Isopiperitenone

Oxidation of monoterpenes :
allylic hydroxylation and oxidation to an α-β-insaturated ketone

Example of regioselectivity (mints):
1 = Mentha piperita
2 = Mentha spicata

(+)-Sabinene   (+)-cis-Sabinol   (+)-cis-Sabinone   (−)-3-Isothujone   (+)-3-Thujone

Fig 13.20. Biosynthesis of (−)-carvone and (+)-3-thujone.

Linalool is a common acyclic monoterpenoid floral aromatic compound present in the flowers of many plant species. It is produced mainly by the epidermal cells of the petals which are responsible for the majority of linalool emission from the flower. Linalool also has its oxide forms that are produced through an epoxide intermediate by an unidentified epoxidase. These oxides are produced in the trans- mitting tissue of the stigma and style of each flower where pollen tubes grow during pollination. The oxides, however, are a minor component of the floral scent mixture. Both linalool and its oxides are only produced when the flower is open. This timing has a distinct advantage for the plant since it avoids wasted energy by the production of compounds when they are not needed. Linalool is

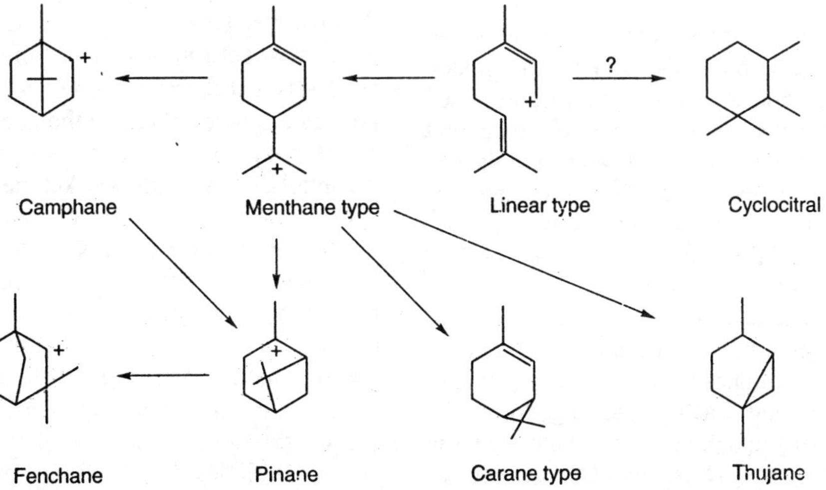

Camphane   Menthane type   Linear type   Cyclocitral

Fenchane   Pinane   Carane type   Thujane

Fig. 13.21. Biogenetic relationships between some monoterpene types.

toxic to some insects such as fleas. Linalool production is also toxic to young plant tissue.

In the biosynthetic pathway for the synthesis of monoterpene olefins and abietic acid the starting substrate in the pathway is acetyl-CoA. From it, oleoresin biosynthesis proceeds stepwise via mevalonate, isopentenyl pyrophosphate, dimethylallyl pyrophosphate, farnesyl pyrophosphate, and geranylgeranyl pyrophosphate (GGPP). The GPP leads directly to synthesis of monoterpene olefins such as α- and β-pinene, 3-carene, β-phellandrene, and limonene catalyzed by monoterpene cyclases. The substrate, GGPP, leads to the synthesis of the diterpenoid resin, abietic acid, via four enzymatic steps involving a single cyclase, two hydroxylases, and a dehydrogenase. Each of these enzymes has been isolated and assayed for the production of respective products by liquids scintillation spectrometry, using $[1(2)\text{-}^{14}C]$ acetic acid as the starting substrate.

BIOSYNTHESIS OF STEROIDS

Steroids are formed biosynthetically from isopentenyl pyrophosphate and involve the same sequence of reactions as does terpenoid biosynthesis. In fact, the triterpenoid squalene is an intermediate in steroid biosynthesis. The familiar acetate → → mevalonate → → isopentenyl pyrophosphate →, → squalene → → cholesterol pathway is proposed.

Squalene is transformed into sterols by its stereospecific conversion into S-squalene 2,3-epoxide by squalene epoxidase. The key enzyme involved in the cyclization of squalene 2,3-epoxide to the first cyclic sterol precursor in animals and fungi is 2,3-oxidosqualene : lanosterol cyclase. Lanosterol is replaced in photosynthetic organisms by its isomer cycloartenol, and the enzyme involved is 2,3-oxidosqualene : cycloartenol cyclase. Squalene is an acylic molecule with 6 double bonds, and the lanosterol molecule has 4 rings and 7 asymmetric centers. A proton initiates the cyclization by attacking the epoxide bond. Each of the rings form successively involving attack by a π bond on a specific carbon. The reactions are fast and stereochemistry is preserved as the rings form. Each π-bond attack

leaves behind a carbonium ion, which is the target of the next attack. When the rings are formed, the resulting carbonium ion intermediate, which has a positive charge at C-20, is stabilized by rearrangements involving 2 hydride shifts (17 → 20, 13 → 17) and 2 methyl shifts (14 → 13, 8 → 14). These shifts result in the migration of the positive charge to C-8 and, with the loss of a proton from C-9, either the 9,10,19-cyclopropane ring of cycloartenol or the 8,9-double bond of lanosterol may be formed. The conversion of the C_{30} compound, lanosterol, to the C_{27} steroid, cholesterol, involves the loss of 3 methyl groups, the shift of a double bond, and a reduction of a double bond. Consequently, numerous intermediates, including zymosterol, have been isolated that represent various stages in this transformation.

Carotenoid biosynthesis

Carotenoid biosynthesis involves the geranylgeranyl pyrophosphate (C_{20}) stage, two molecules of which join to give the straight-chain isoprenoid phytoene (nine double bonds). The newly formed central bond has the *cis* configuration compared with all the others, which are *trans*. Successive dehydrogenations produce phytofluene, ξ-carotene, neurosporene and lycopene (10, 11, 12, 13 double bonds, respectively). Terminal cyclizations from neurosporene, involving a common intermediate, form eventually the α- and β-ionone moieties of α- and β-carotene. Crocin (C_{20} structure), the yellow pigment of saffron is derived from a carotene.

The actual chemical properties of particular compounds are determined by the acquisition of functional groups. Thus, terpenes may occur as alcohols (menthol), ethers (cineole), ketones (carvone), etc., and as such have similar chemical properties to nonterpenoid compounds possessing the same group; aldehydes may be of aliphatic origin (citronellal), aromatic (cinnamic aldehyde), steroidal (some cardioactive glycosides); and resulting from the introduction of a heterocyclic system.

Some compounds may also involve different biogenetic entities. The complex indole alkaloids contain moieties derived from both the shikimate and isoprenoid pathways.

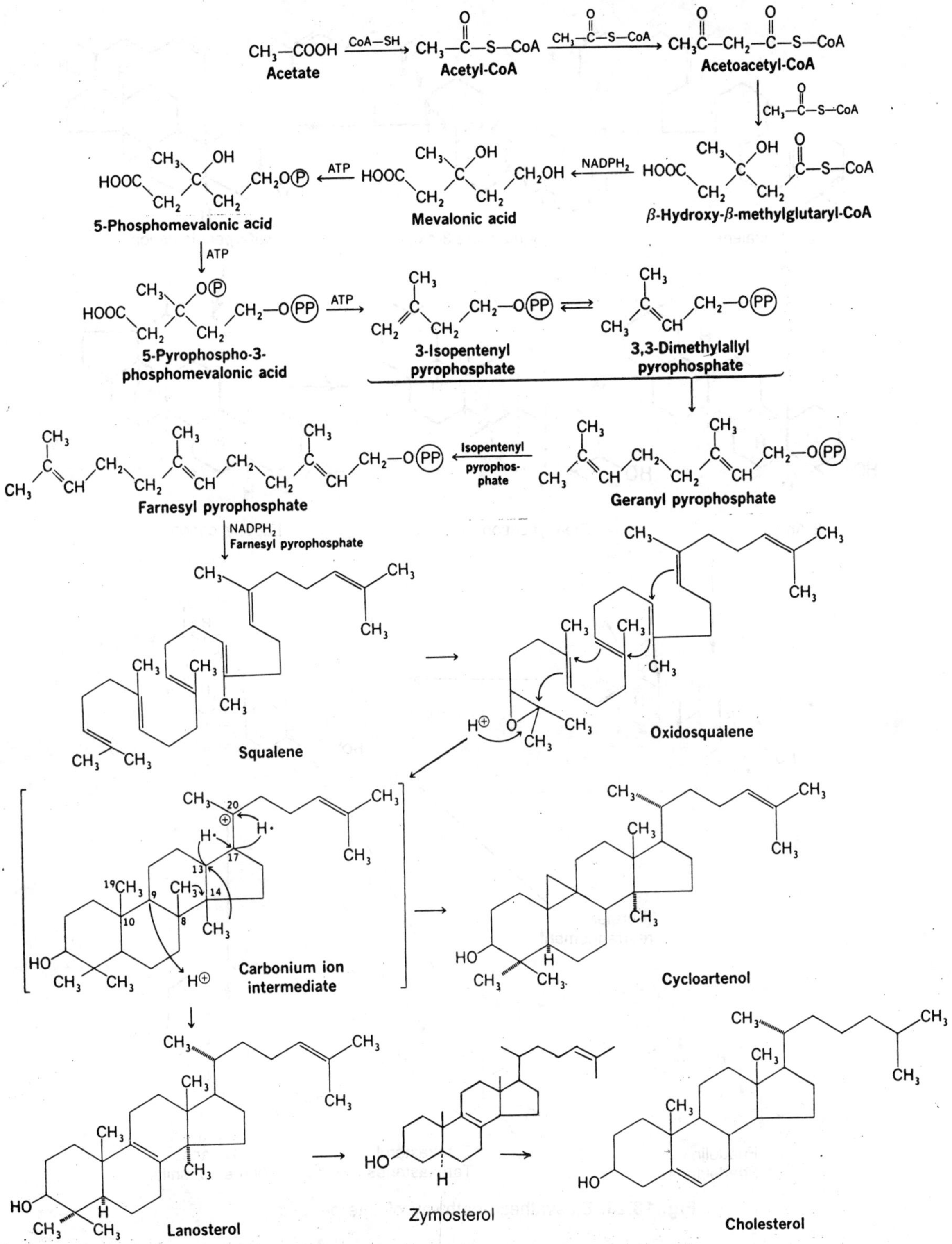

Fig 13.22. Biosynthesis of cholesterol.

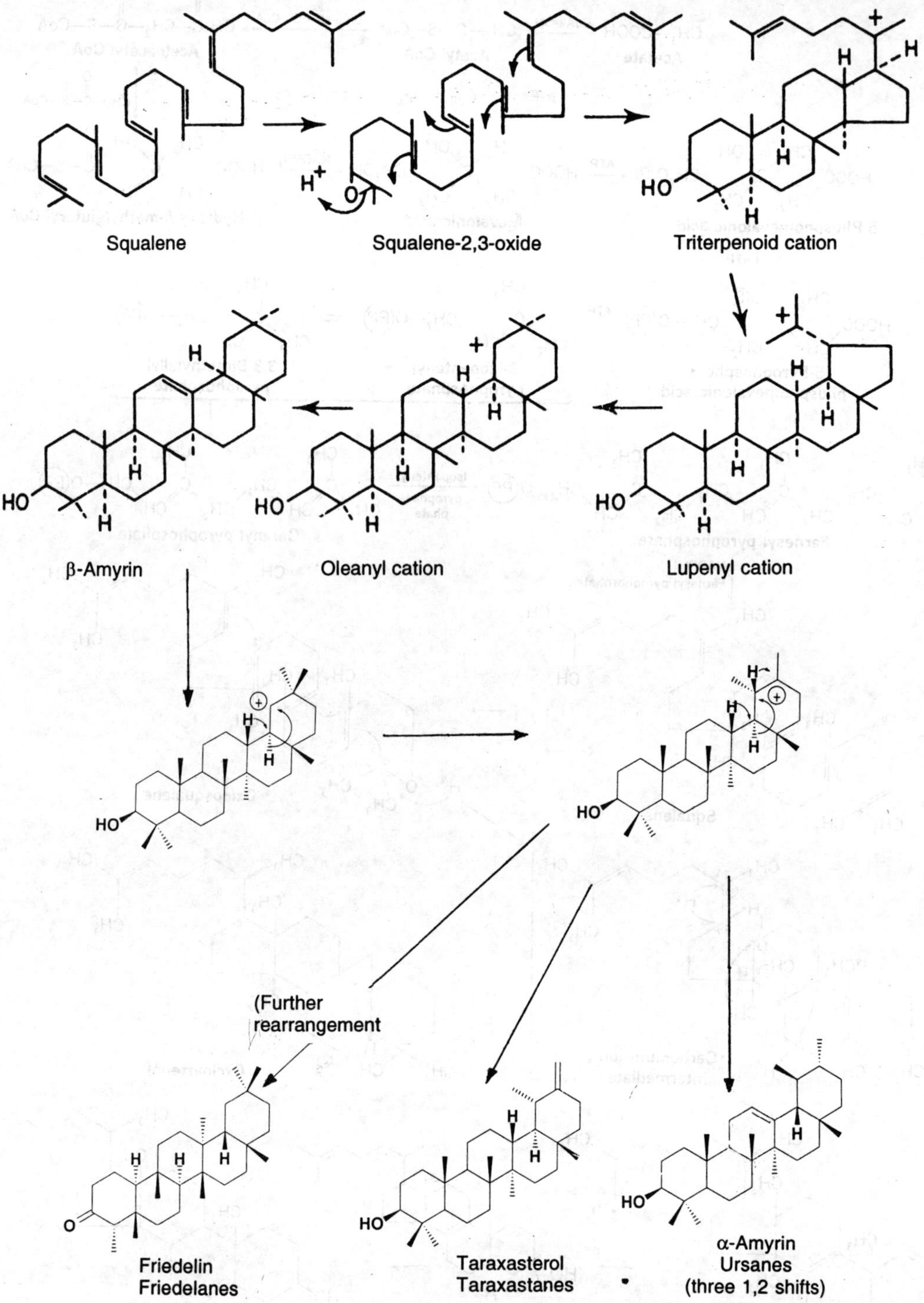

Fig. 13.23. Biosynthetic pathway of triterpenoids.

Squalene

Squalene-2,3-oxide

Triterpenoid cation

β-Amyrin

Oleanyl cation

Lupenyl cation

(Further rearrangement

Friedelin
Friedelanes

Taraxasterol
Taraxastanes

α-Amyrin
Ursanes
(three 1,2 shifts)

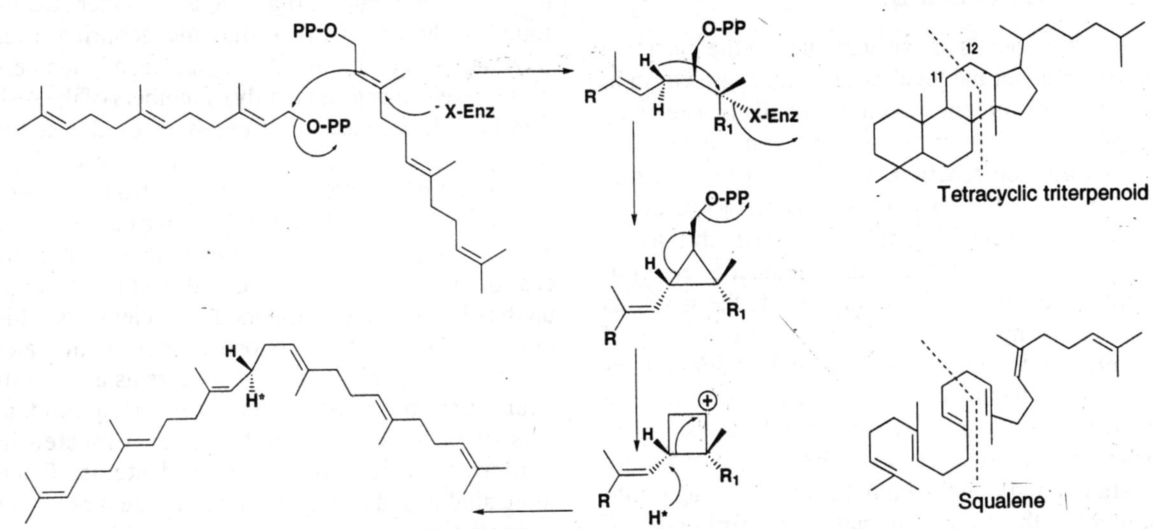

Fig. 13.24. Biosynthesis of terpenes : formation of squalene.

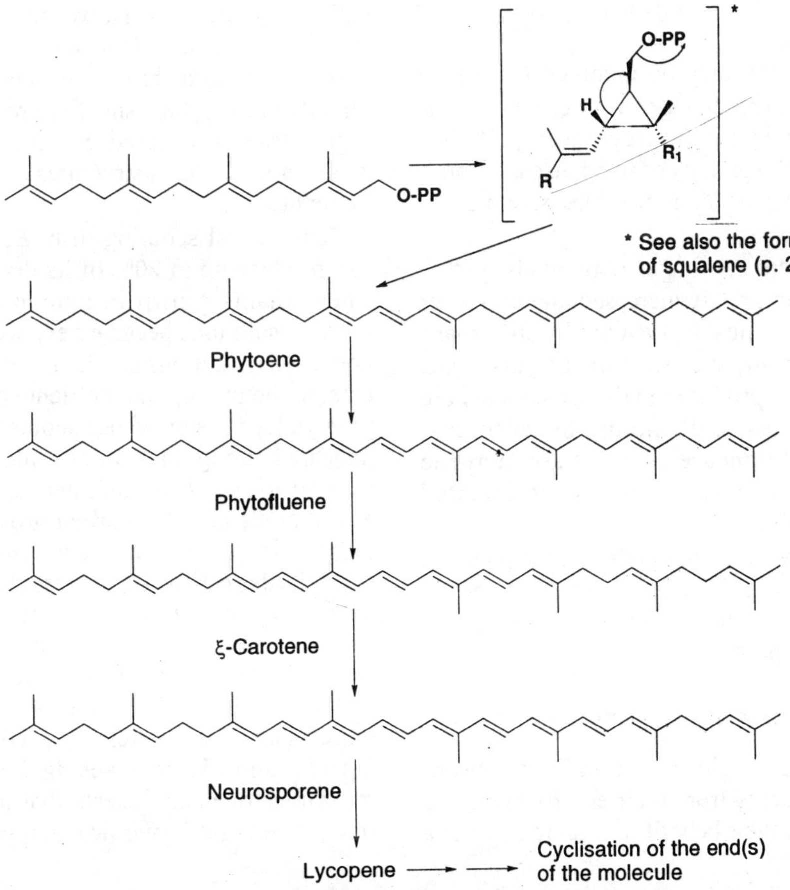

* See also the formation
of squalene (p. 271)

Phytoene

Phytofluene

ξ-Carotene

Neurosporene

Lycopene ⟶ ⟶ Cyclisation of the end(s)
of the molecule

Fig. 13.25. Carotenoid biosynthesis.

STRESS COMPOUNDS

These compounds are accumulated in the plant to a higher than normal level as a result of some form of injury, or disturbance to the metabolism. They may be products of either primary or secondary metabolism. Common reactions involved in their formation are the polymerization, oxidation or hydrolysis of naturally occurring substances; which may be secondary in their formation. A number of environmental and biological factors promote the synthesis of stress compound, *e.g.*, mechanical wounding of the plant, ultraviolet irradiation, dehydration, treatment with chemicals, and microbial infection. The production of such compounds has also been observed in cell cultures subjected to antibiotic treatment and in cells immobilized or brought into contact with calcium alginate, *e.g.*, formation of acridone alkaloid epoxides by *Ruta graveolens*, the increased production of echinatin and the novel formation of a prenylated compound by *Glycyrrhiza echinata* cultures.

Stress compound may be involved in various crude drugs formed pathologically (*e.g.*, some gums and oleoresins) and potential drugs (gossypol); they are implicated in the toxicity of some diseased foodstuffs and they play a role in the defensive mechanism of the plant.

Phytoalexins are antifungal compounds synthesized by a plant in greatly increased amounts after infection. The antifungal isoflavonoid pterocarpans are produced by many species of the Leguminosae. Other phytoalexins produced in the same family are hydroxyflavanones, stilbenoids, benzofurans, chromones and furanoacetylenes. Sesquiterpene phytoalexins have been isolated from infected *Gossypium* species.

Chemically, stress compounds include phenols, resins, carbohydrates, hydroxycinnamic acid derivatives, coumarins, bicyclic sesquiterpenes, triterpenes and steroidal compounds.

BIOGENIC SILICA AND SILICIFICATION

Some plants have developed the ability to absorb inorganic constituents from their environment and use them towards their benefit. Biogenic silica is a polymer of biological origin that is characteristically found in the cell walls of diatoms, scouringrustes (*Equisetum* spp.) or horsetails, grasses (all members of the Poaceae or grass family), members of the rush family (Juncaceae), and members of the sedge family (Cyperaceae). Silica found in these silica-accumulating plants has its origin from silicates found in soil minerals. It is taken up as monosilicic acid, $Si(OH)_4$ via the roots (or cell membrane in the case of the single-cell diatoms) from which it moves up the plant in the xylem-conducting elements. This upward movement of monosilicic acid with water and other mineral compounds occurs as a result of "transpirational pull" mediated by transpirational loss of water from stomatas (pores) located in epidermal tissues of leaves and stems. Once monosilicic acid arrives in stems and leaves where transpiration in occurring, it irreversibly polymerizes as amorphous silica gel, $SiO_2 . nH_2O$, mostly in cell walls which are hydrogen bonded to cellulose molecules. However, in grasses, within specialized silica cells located in the epidermis of leaves and floral bracts, it can also polymerize directly in the cytoplasm after breakdown of all cell organelles has occurred. Silica secretions can also result in specialized structures such as the needles on nettles.

The annual scouring rush, *Equisetum arvense*, can produce up to 20% of its dry weight as silica. These plants grown in silicon-free hydroponic nutrient solutions became very weak and appeared collapsed. Additions of silicon, as sodium metasilicate, to the hydroponic nutrient solution at only 80 ppm yielded plants whose shoots were upright and appeared strong and robust. Silica provides direct support of the shoot and, hence, is considered an essential element for normal growth and development in these types of plants. The primary role of silica in the cell wall is to provide support to the shoot in addition to that provided by cellulose and lignin. Amorphous silica gel is deposited in outer cell walls of epidermal tissue of leaves and stems and forms very hard and often very sharp structures which can deter attack by predacious animals, insects, and disease-causing fungi. In fact, the mandibles of many insects that attack rice plants (e.g., green and brown leaf hoppers that transmit tungro virus pathogens) get worn down and rendered ineffective in piercing the leaves of the rice plants. Likewise, the teeth of sheep get worn down significantly by eating high silica-containing pasture grasses. Fortunately, these animals can replace their worn-down teeth with new teeth.

Marine algae can absorb calcium in the form of calcium carbonate that they deposit on their surface as crusty support compounds, like biogenic silica, which seem to prevent the plants from getting damaged by crashing waves. Some plants can absorb toxic elements such as selenium (Se) or bromine which help ward off herbivores. *Astragalus* (loco weed) accumulates Se and incorporates it into certain amino acids and proteins. The plant itself can distinguish if a protein has Se, so there is no toxic effect to the plant. Se is toxic to most other plants also allows *Astragalus* to avoid competition in soils that certain Se. These soils often occur around uranium deposits, so *Astragalus* has been used as an indicator species in botanical prospecting. Other plants such as alpine penny-cress (*Thalspi caerulescens*) will take up elements such as zinc and cadmium making them very useful when planted in polluted areas needing bioremediation.

14

Carbohydrates

The carbohydrates include simple sugars and polysaccharides. They are carbonyl alcohols containing the elements carbon, hydrogen and oxygen. The last two elements are usually present in the same proportion as in water. Carbohydrates are the primary products of photosynthesis and from them the plant synthesizes various chemical constituents by subsequent organic reactions. They are most abundant components of both plants (cellulose, starch, sugars) and animals (glycogen). Sugars are united with many compounds to form glycosides.

Generally carbohydrates are divided into two groups :

1. Monosaccharides or simple sugars, and
2. Polysaccharides.

Monosaccharides

Monosaccharides are simple sugars which are a ketonic or aldehydic substitution product of a polyhydroxy alcohol. These sugars contain from three to nine carbon atoms. On the basis of number of carbon atoms in the molecule monosaccharides are classified as trioses (with three carbon atoms), tetroses (four carbon atoms), pentoses (five carbon atoms), and hexoses (six carbon atoms). The simplest sugars existing in nature are glyceraldehyde and dihydroxyacetone. The tetroses are not found in the free state. The pentoses and hexoses are accumulated in plants in greatest quantity. These are the products of hydrolysis of hemicellulose,

gums and mucilages. Hexoses are the first detectable sugars synthesized by plants and form the units from which most of the polysaccharides are produced. There are 16 possible aldohexoses and 8 ketohexoses; only levulose and dextrose occur in the free state. Hydrolysis of starch yields glucose, whereas inulin yields fructose. Monosaccharides like glucose possessing aldehydic group are called aldoses, ketone group containing sugars (fructose) are known as ketoses.

Glucose is an aldohexose whereas fructose is a ketohexose. The hexoses are 6-membered, open-chain compounds. Five of the carbon atoms have alcohol substituents, and the sixth carbon atom is an aldehyde or ketone group. Glucose and other hexoses often exist in cyclic forms and in straight chain structures. Glucose generally forms a 6-membered pyranose ring. Fructose can exist in two cyclic forms. Fructopyranose is the structure of the crystalline sugar and the furanose structure (5-membered ring) is present in oligosaccharides and polysaccharides. The furanose structure is relatively unstable but may be stabilized on glycoside formation. The fructose phosphate of furanose form is an intermediate in glycolysis. The anaerobic degradation of hexoses provides energy for metabolism. Naturally, fructose is always in furanose form. However, in crystalline form, it has a pyranose structure.

Formation of glucuronic acid from glucose and galacturonic acid from galactose by oxidation of the terminal groups to carboxylic (COOH) group gives uronic acids.

Biosynthesis of monosaccharides

Different monosaccharides are produced from the photosynthetic cycle. D-Fructose-6-phosphate and D-glucose-6-phosphate occur universally. Free sugars may accumulate due to hydrolysis of the phosphorylated sugars or the latter may be utilized in respiration, converted to sugar nucleotides (*e.g.*, uridine-diphosphoglucose—UDPG) or, by the action of various epimerases, give rise to other monosaccharides (e.g., galactose).

The reverse process, hydrolysis, is brought about by suitable enzymes or by boiling with dilute acid. The same sugars may be linked to one another in various ways.

Di-, tri- and tetrasaccharides

These sugars are derived from two, three or four monosaccharide molecules, respectively, with the elimination of one, two or three molecules of water. A plant sugar occurring in free state is sucrose (α-D-glucopyranosyl-β-D fructofuranoside). It is a non-reducing sugar and present in fruit juices, sugarcane, sugar beet and maples. On hydrolysis, sucrose is converted into invert sugar, which is made up of glucose and fructose in equimolecular amounts.

The disaccharides maltose, cellobiose, sopho-rose and trehalose are composed of two molecules of glucose joined by α-1,4-, β-1,4-, β-1,2- and α, α-1,1-(nonreducing) linkages, respectively.

Maltose (4-O-α-D-glucopyranosyl-D-gluco-pyranose) is also a disaccharide present in the cell sap. It is produced on large scale by the hydrolysis of starch during the germination process of barley and other grains. It is a reducing sugar. Hydrolysis of maltose yields 2 molecules of glucose.

Galactose is a constituent of lactose and raffi-nose. Trehalose is widely distributed in the fungi. Lactose is a reducing sugar containing an alde-hydic group and is present in milk.

Sugars are polyhydroxy-aldehydes or ketones and contain an unbroken chain of carbon atoms. Oligosaccharides are carbohydrates whose mole-cules consist of two to ten monosaccharide units

linked through oxygen. They are subdivided into disaccharides, trisaccharides, etc. They are hydrolyzed with water in the presence of catalysts or enzymes to produce monosaccharide molecules. Sugars are crystalline compounds, sweet in taste and soluble in water.

Table 14.1. Some di-, tri- and tetrasaccharides

Name	Monosaccharide units
Disaccharides	
Sucrose	Glucose, fructose
Maltose	Glucose, glucose
Lactose	Glucose, galactose
Cellobiose	Glucose, glucose
Trehalose	Glucose, glucose
Sophorose	Glucose, glucose
Trisaccharides	
Gentianose	Glucose, glucose, fructose
Melezitose	Glucose, fructose, glucose
Planteose	Glucose, fructose, galactose
Raffinose	Galactose, glucose, fructose
Manneotriose	Galactose, galactose, glucose
Rhamninose	Rhamnose, rhamnose, galactose
Scillatriose	Rhamnose, glucose, glucose
Tetrasacchariside	
Stachyose or manneotetrose	Galactose, galactose, glucose, fructose

Glucose, fructose, sucrose and maltose are the most common sugars in vegetable drugs. Certain other sugars, occur to a limited extent in nature, either in the free state or in glycosidal combination; *e.g.*, the monosaccharides : mannose (occurring in mannosans) and galactose (a constituent of lactose and raffinose), and the disaccharides : trehalose (in the fungi) and lactose (milk sugar). Lactose possesses a functional aldehyde group and is a reducing sugar. Trehalose is a non-reducing sugar.

Polysaccharides

Polysaccharides are derived from monosaccha-rides by condensation involving sugar phosphates and sugar nucleotides in an exactly similar manner to the formation of di-, tri- and tetra-saccharides. In polysaccharides the number of sugar units is much larger. The hydrolysis of polysaccharides, by enzymes or reagents, results in a succession of cleavages. The final products are hexoses or pentoses, their derivatives, sulphate esters, uronic acids or amino sugars.

Polysaccharides are substances of very high molecular weight consisting of large number of monosaccharide units linked through oxygen. The polysaccharide, yielding hexose are called hexosans; starch yielding glucose is known as glucosan and inulin producing fructose is termed as fructosan. The fundamental unit of plants is made of a polysaccharide, cellulose, which consists of glucose units joined by β-1, 4-linkages. The other plant constituents of high molecular weight are hemicelluloses which are more soluble and more easily hydrolyzed. Gums and mucilages are related to hemicelluloses. Gums consist largely of pentose and hexose moeties and hydrolysis yields galactose and arabinose. Hemicellulose on hydrolysis produces another type of sugars like glucose, mannose and xylose. Gums are formed by decomposition of the cellulose or by injuring the plant and some of them constitute an important group of drugs as emulsifying agents, suspending agents for insoluble powders in mixtures, as adhesive in pills and tablets, and for the preparation of hand lotions and other cosmetic items. Pectins are also related to cellulose in structural skeleton. Polysaccharides are neither sweet nor crystallizable, insoluble in water and do not form colloidal solutions.

Chemical tests

1. **Fehling's solution test :** The substance (0.5 g) is heated with dilute hydrochloric acid to hydrolyse a polysaccharides. The reaction mixture is neutralized by addition of sodium hydroxide solution and then Fehling's solutions 1 and 2 are added. Red precipitate of cuprous oxide is produced on heating in case of reducing sugars (all monosaccharides, and many disaccharides like lactose, maltose, cellobiose and gentiobiose). Non-reducing sugars include some disaccharides (sucrose and trihalose) and polysaccharides, which on boiling with acids are converted into reducing sugars.

2. **Molisch test :** A solution of carbohydrate in water is treated with alcoholic solution of α-naphthol. On addition of concentrated sulphuric acid along the side of test tube a purple ring is formed on the junction below aqueous layer. With insoluble carbohydrates (e.g., cellulose) the colour will produce on shaking the reaction mixture.

3. **Osazone formation :** A sugar on heating with phenylhydrazine hydrochloride, sodium acetate and acetic acid forms yellow crystals of osazone. Glucose and fructose form the same osazone (glucosazone, m.p. 205°C). The osazones are purified by recrystallization from alcohol. Sucrose does not form an osazone, but under the conditions of the above test sufficient hydrolysis takes place for the production of glucosazone.

4. **Resorcinol test for ketoses (Selivanoff's test):** A crystal of resorcinol is added to the solution and heated with an equal volume of concentrated hydrochloric acid. Pink colour is produced in case of ketoses (e.g., fructose, honey or hydrolyzed inulin).

5. **Test for pentoses :** A solution of the material is heated with equal volume of hydrochloric acid containing a little phloroglucinol. A red colour is formed in case of pentoses.

6. **Keller-Kiliani test for deoxysugars :** A deoxysugar (found in cardiac glycosides) is dissolved in acetic acid containing a trace of ferric chloride and transferred to the surface of concentrated H_2SO_4. A reddish-brown colour is formed at the junction which turns blue latter on.

7. **Furfural test :** A carbohydrate sample is heated in a test tube with a drop of syrupy phosphoric acid to convert it into furfural. A disk of filter paper moistened with a drop of 10% solution of aniline in 10% acetic acid is placed over the mouth of the test tube. The bottom of the test tube is heated for 30-60 seconds. A pink or red stain appears on the reagent paper.

8. **Enzyme reactions :** Some carbohydrate reactions are only brought about by certain specific enzymes, such enzymes may be used for identification.

9. **Chromatography :** Chromatography methods are used to drug extracts containing a number of carbohydrates in very small amounts and

may be used to study the products of hydrolysis of polysaccharide complexes such as gums and mucilages. Many pure sugars, uronic acids and other sugar derivatives are commercially available as standard samples. The carbohydrate spots obtained after separation are identified by their positions and by reagents. It may be useful to examine them in ultraviolet light. The reagents for reducing sugars are freshly prepared ammoniacal silver nitrate solution and aniline hydrogen phthalate (in water and phosphoric acid). These are applied to the chromatogram with a spray.

HONEY

Synonyms : Purified honey, Mel, Clarified honey, Strained honey, Madhu (Ayurveda).

Biological source : Honey is a sugary secretion deposited by the honeybees, *Apis mellifera* Linn. and other species of *Apis* in the honeycomb. It must be free from foreign substances such as parts of insects and leaves, but may contain pollen grains. (Family : Apidae).

Habitat : Honey is produced mainly in England, West Indies, California, Canada, Chile and in some parts of Africa, Australia and New Zealand.

Collection : Honeybees live in swarms which are gathered into hives. A hive contains :
1. a single queen bee,
2. the males or drones, and
3. the worker bees which are undeveloped females.

The worker bees possess a long, hollow tube to insert into the nectaries of the flowers. The tube is formed from the maxillae and labium. They take nectar from the flowers and pass it through the oesophagus into the honey-sac or crop. The nectar, which is an aqueous solution of sucrose (25%), is mixed with salivary secretion containing the enzyme invertase and then is hydrolyzed into the invert sugar. On returning at the hive, the worker bees deposit the contents of the honey sac in the previously prepared cell of the honeycomb. The filled cell is sealed by wax. For collecting the honey, the honeycomb is smoked to remove bees, the comb is cut and honey is collected either by drainage or by expression. The honey obtained by latter procedure is contaminated with the wax. For getting purified honey, it is heated at 80°C when the impurities float on the surface which are removed. The honey is diluted to a weight of 1.35-1.36 g per ml at 20°C.

The best honey is that derived from flowers such as clover and heather, obtained from hives that have never swarmed, and separated from the cut comb either by draining or by means of a centrifuge. Honey obtained by expression is liable to be contaminated with the wax.

Characters : Honey is thick, syrupy, translucent liquid when fresh. The colour is pale yellow or reddish-brown and it possesses pleasant odour and sweet taste which are dependent upon the floral source of the product. The honey obtained from *Eucalyptus* and *Banksia* species has somewhat unpleasant odour and taste and the honey collected from *Datura stramonium* is poisonous. On storage it becomes opaque and granular due to the crystallization of dextrose.

Chemical constituents : Honey consists chiefly of glucose (30-40%), fructose (40-50%) and small amounts of sucrose (0.1-10%), dextrin, formic acid, volatile oil and pollen grains. In addition to these, traces of enzymes, vitamins, proteins, maltose, melezitose, pentosans, gums, trace elements, amino acids and colouring matter are also present in honey.

Uses : Honey shows mild laxative, bactericidal, sedative, antiseptic and alkaline characters. It is used for cold, cough, fever, sore eye and throat, tongue and duodenal ulcers, liver disorders, constipation, diarrhoea, kidney and other urinary disorders, pulmonary tuberculosis, marasmus, rickets, scurvy and insomnia. It is applied as a remedy on open wounds after surgery. It prevents infection and promotes healing. Honey works quicker than many antibiotics because it is easily absorbed into the blood stream. It is also useful in healing of carbuncles, chaps, scalds, whitlows and skin inflammation; as vermicide; locally as an excipient, in the treatment of aphthae and other infection of the oral mucous membrane. It is recommended in the treatment of pre-operative cancer. Honey, mixed with onion juice, is a good remedy for arteriosclerosis in brain. Diet rich in honey is recommended for infants, convalescents, diabetic patients and invalids.

Honey is an important ingredient of certain lotions, cosmetics, soaps, creams, balms, toilet-waters and inhalants. It is used as a medium in preservation of cornea.

Adulterants : Honey is adulterated with cane sugar, corn syrup and artificial invert sugar which is obtained by acid hydrolysis of sucrose. The sugar contains furfural which gives red colour with resorcinol in the presence of hydrochloric acid. On prolonged heating or storage of the honey, furfural may be formed in the genuine honey.

Chemical tests : Adulteration in honey is determined by the following tests :

1. *Fiehe's test for artificial invert sugar* : Honey (10 ml) is shaken with petroleum or solvent ether (5 ml) for 5-10 minutes. The upper ethereal layer is separated and evaporated in a China dish. On addition of 1% solution of resorcinol in hydrochloric acid (1 ml) a transient red colour is formed in natural honey while in artificial honey the colour persists for sometime.

2. *Reduction of Fehling's solution* : To an aqueous solution of honey (2 ml) Fehling's solutions 1 and 2 are added and the reaction mixture is heated on a stream bath for 5-10 minutes. A brick red colour is produced due to the presence of reducing sugars.

3. *Limit tests* : The limit tests of chloride, sulphate and ash (0.5%) are compared with the pharmacopoeial specifications.

SUCROSE

Sucrose is a natural non-reducing sugar obtained from *Saccharum officinarum* Linn. (Fam. Poaceae), *Beta vulgaris* Linn. (Fam. Chenopodiaceae), and other sources. It is α-D-glucopyranosyl-(1-2)-β-D-fructofuranoside and the principal form of transport and temporary storage of energy in plants. It accumulates in certain fleshy roots.

Sucrose, known as *saccharum* or *sugar*, is widely distributed in plants. It is obtained commercially from sugarcane and sugar beets, but is also obtained from the sugar maple (*Acer saccharum*, Fam. Aceraceae). Cane sugar is produced in Cuba, Puerto Rico, Louisiana, the Philippines, Hawaii, Indonesia and India, while beet sugar is largely produced in Germany, Austria, Russia, France and the United States. Sugar beets are grown in places other than tropical and semitropical countries.

Production : The juice is obtained from sugarcane by crushing the stems between a series of heavy iron rollers. It is boiled with lime to neutralize the plant acids and to coagulate albumins. The juice is filtered, decolourized with SO_2, concentrated and crystallized. The residue, dark coloured syrup, is molasses.

Uses : Sucrose is used as a demulcent, nutrient, bacteriostatic, as preservative to prepare syrups, to mask disagreeable tastes in troches and tablets, as excipient for tablets and other forms for oral administration and to retard oxidation of some preparations. In pharmaceutical industry, sucrose is modified physically to render it directly compressible. A simple syrup is obtained by dissolving 650 g of sucrose in 1 L of hot purified water and by adding antimicrobial agents.

Biosynthesis of sucrose

Sucrose is an important metabolic product in higher plants. Sucrose is the first sugar formed in photosynthesis and the main transport material. Newly formed sucrose is probably the usual precursor for polysaccharide synthesis. However, a reaction between glucose 1-phosphate and fructose is responsible for sucrose production in certain microorganisms.

Fructose 6-phosphate, derived from the photosynthetic cycle, is converted to glucose 1-phosphate which, in turn, reacts with UTP to form UDP-glucose. UDP-glucose either reacts with fructose 6-phosphate to form first sucrose phosphate and ultimately sucrose, or with fructose to form sucrose directly. Once formed, the free sucrose may either remain in situ or be translocated via the sieve tubes to various parts of the plants. A number of reactions, *e.g.*, hydrolysis by invertase or reversal of the synthetic sequence, convert sucrose to monosaccharides from which other oligosaccharides or polysaccharides may be derived.

STARCH

Synonym : Amylum.

Biological source : Starch of pharmaceutical use consists of polysaccharide carbohydrate occurring as discrete granules in the mature grain of corn, *Zea mays* Linn. (Fam. Poaceae) or of wheat, *Triticum aestivum* Linn. (Poaceae), or tubers of potato, *Solanum tuberosum* Linn. (Solanaceae) or rice, *Oryza sativa* Linn. (Poaceae), or arrowroot, *Maranta arundinacea* Linn. (Marantaceae). Commercial starch is also obtained from tapioca or cassava starch, *Manihot utilissima* Pohl. (Family : Euphorbiaceae).

Geographical source : Commercially the starch is produced in USA, Argentina, India, China, Japan and other tropical and sub-tropical countries.

Starch is a main constituent of carbohydrate, the green plant and is found especially in seeds and underground organs. The green parts of plants exposed to sunlight contain small granules of transitional starch which are produced from photosynthesis. During the hours of darkness these are removed to the storage organs. Starch occurs in the form of granules. The shape and size of starch grains are characteristic of the species.

Preparation of starches

Commercial starches are not chemically pure and contain small amounts of nitrogenous and inorganic matter.

Cereal starches have to be freed from cell debris, oil, soluble protein matter and the abundant insoluble proteins (glutelins and prolamins) known as 'gluten'. Potato starch is associated with vegetable tissue, mineral salts and soluble proteins.

Preparation of maize corn starch

The clean grain is first softened by soaking at 50ºC for about 2 days in a 0.2% solution of sulphurous acid for disintegration, enabling the embryo or germ to be easily liberated intact and permitting the starch to be readily freed from fibre. During this time lactic acid bacteria are active and metabolize soluble sugars extracted from the maize. The grain, in water, is then disintegrated by attrition mills in which the liberated oil-containing embryos is not broken.

The germs are continuously separated from the suspension by liquid cyclones (hydroclones). The germs are used for the preparation of germ oils, which are an important source of vitamins. The remainder of the grain is ground wet and the starch and gluten separated from fibrous material in rotating, slightly inclined stainless steel reels covered with perforated metal sheets. The retained fibre is washed and the total mixture of starch and protein (mill starch) is fractionated into gluten and starch by the use of special starch purification centrifuges; as gluten is higher than starch, separation occurs. In another processes this separation was accomplished by repeated 'tabling', in which the suspension was allowed to flow very slowly through troughs about 40 m long and 0.7 m wide, when the heavier starch was deposited first. The starch suspension from the centrifuge is further purified in other centrifuges and hydroclones, which reduces the protein level. The starch is dried by flash dryers or a moving-belt dryer.

Zea mays oil contain β-sitosterol. The kernels possess di-O-(indole-3-acetyl)-myoinositol and tri-O-(indole-3-acetyl)-myoinositol. Three cinnamoyl citric acids, 2-O-*trans-p*-coumaroyl-, 2-O-*trans*-feruloyl- and 2-O-*trans*-caffeoyl-hydroxy-citric acids and cyanidin-β- and 2-O-*trans*-caffeoyl-hydroxycitric acids and cyanidin-β-glucoside are isolated from maize. 2-Heptanol and geosmin are the main constituent of the maize volatile oil. *Z. mays* also contain C-glycosyl-flavone maysin, 6C-glycosylated derivatives of chrysoeriol and apigenin, sorbitol, zeanin (in immature kernels), glycosides of kaempferol and quereetin (in pollens), and glucuronoxylo-oligosaccharides I-VI from corn hulls.

Preparation of rice starch

Rice is soaked in successive quantities of 0.4% caustic soda until the material can be easily disintegrated. The softened grain in a dilute suspension ground for separating the compound grains into their components which is repeatedly screened, and the starch separated by standing or by means of a centrifuge. The dump starch is next cut into blocks and dried at 50-60ºC for 2 days. The brown outer layer formed outside the blocks is then scraped and drying is continued at a lower temperature for about 14 days, during which time the blocks gradually crack into irregular masses. It is then powdered.

Preparation of potato starch

The potatoes are washed and a fine pulp is prepared in a rasping machine or in a disintegrator of the hammer-mill type. Much of the cell debris is removed from the pulp by rotary sieves and the milky liquid which passes through the sieve contains starch, soluble proteins, salts, and some cell debris. On standing, the starch separates more rapidly than the other insoluble matter. High speed centrifugal separators are used for separation of potato starch. At two or three points during the isolation, sulphur dioxide is added to prevent discoloration of the product by the action of oxidative enzymes. The washed starch is collected, dried to contain about 18% moisture and packaged. After corn, potato tubers are the second worldwide source of starch. One quintal of potatoes yields 15 to 23 kg of potato starch.

Preparation of wheat starch

To the wheat flour water is added to prepare dough and then kept for one hour to allow gluten to swell. The balls of dough are shaken with water on grooved rollers. Liquid containing starch falls below from which it is separated by centrifugation, washed and dried.

Characters

Starch occurs in irregular, angular powder or a white mass, insoluble in cold water and forms a colloidal solution on boiling with about 15 times its weight of water. In hot water, the granules first swell and then undergo gelatinization. On cooling the solution forms a translucent jelly. It produces deep blue colour with iodine solution. Starch granules undergo gelatinization on heating or by treating with sodium hydroxide solution of concentrated solution of calcium or zinc chlorides or chloral hydrate. Maize starch is almost neutral, rice starch is slightly alkaline and potato starch is slightly acidic.

Starches generally form colloidal sols in water. If a suspension of starch in cold water is added to boiling water while stirring, the opaque granules swell and finally

rupture to give a translucent sol. If this sol is concentrated, it sets to a firm jelly on cooling. Swelling and ultimate rupture of the starch granules to form pastes take place in cold, concentrated aqueous solutions of the caustic alkalies, chloral hydrate, ammonium thiocyanate, or hydrochloric acid.

Microscopic characters

Starches are mounted in water or Smith's starch reagent (equal parts of water, glycerin and 50% acetic acid). The size, shape and structure of the starch granules from any particular plant vary within definite limits. It is possible to distinguish between the starches derived from different species. Starch granules may be simple or compound. In some cases the compound granule is formed by the aggregation of a large number of simple granules (e.g., rice and cardamoms).

The starting point of formation of the granule in the amyloplast is marked by the hilum, which may be central or eccentric. Granules with an eccentric hilum are usually longer than broad. On drying, fissures are appeared in the granule originating from the hilum. The hilum takes the form of a rounded dot or of a simple, curved or multiple cleft.

The size of starch granule is increased by the deposition of successive layers around the hilum.

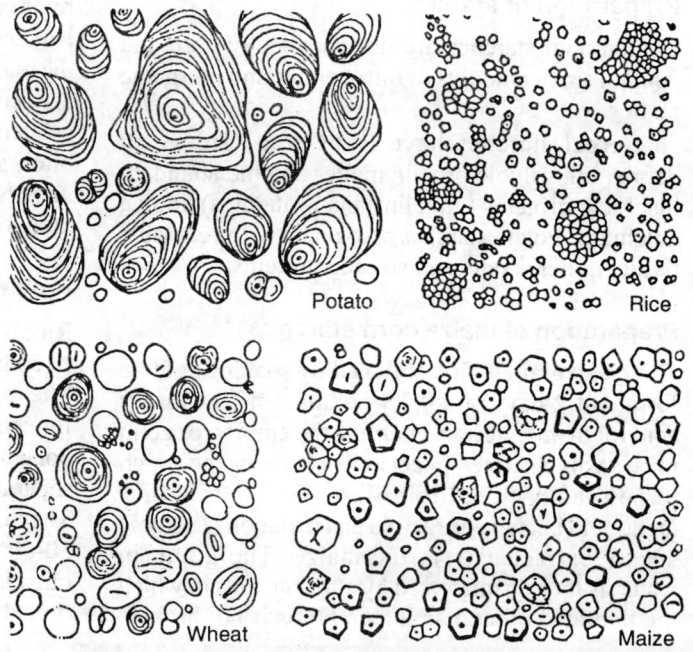

Fig. 14.1. Starch granules.

The concentric rings or striations are clearly visible in larger granules, *e.g.*, potato. The striations arise from the diurnal deposition of the starch giving variations in refractive index, density and crystallinity. The position and form of the hilum and the presence or absence of well-defined striations are used in the characterization of starches.

Starch granules show double refraction when placed between crossed Nicols. The starch behaves like a sphaerocrystal.

Microscopically, starch granules contain central or eccentric hilum, concentric rings or striations and differ in size and aggregation. In maize starch granules are 10-35 μm in size, angular, polyhedral, hilum is central, distinct and contain a cavity or from 2 to 5 rayed cleft. The striations are absent. Maize granules from the outer horny endosperm are muller-shaped. Granules from the inner mealy endosperm are polyhedral or sub-spherical. In commercial starch all the granules are simple. Hilum is central triangular or 2- to 5-stellate cleft. No striations are present.Tapioca starch contain mostly simple, subspherical, muller-shaped or round polyhedral granules. Hilum is punctate or cleft. Concentric striations are present. Rice starch is composed of 2-10 μm diameter compound and simple granules with an angular outline and aggregated from 2 to 150 components. The granules are polyhedral with sharp angles. Striations are absent and hilum is centric. Wheat starch contains larger granules lenticular, smaller ones globular, size is from 2 to 45 μm. Few compound granules are present. The hilum is central and unclaft. Concentratic and faint striations are observed. Potato starch contains most of simple granules, wedge or mussel-shaped. The diameter is from 2 to 110 μm. Hilum is in the form of a point, near the narrower point and eccentric. Concentric striations are well-marked. Few compound granules of 2 or 3 components are fused together.

Chemical constituents

Starches are generally mixtures of two types of polymers :

1. amylose, a linear (1-4)-α-D-glucan, and
2. amylopectin, a branched D-glucan with mostly α-D (1-4) and approximately 4% α-D (1-6) linkages.

Amylopectin or α-amylose is the main constituent of most starches (over 80%). The molecule has branched chains each consisting of 20-26 α-1,4-linked glucose residues. Several hundred of these chains are linked by α-1,6 glycosidic bonds to neighbouring chains giving a molecule containing some 50,000 glycosyl units. The branching pattern throughout the molecule is not uniform yielding amorphous (high degree of branching) and crystalline forms of starch.

Some starches contain up to 20% of amylose or β-amylose. It consists of linear chains of α-1,4-linked glucose residues. Several thousand glucose units constitute a chain. It has a very limited branching (α-1,6-linkages) to the extent of 2-8 branches per molecule.

Amylose is water-soluble and gives an unstable solution, which irreversibly precipitates. It is mainly responsible for the deep blue coloration ($\lambda_{max}c$, 660 nm) given by starch. Iodine as I_5 trapped as an inclusion complex in the amylose helix due to the strong affinity of amylose for iodine, it will take up to 19% of its weight of iodine and this figure can be used in the determination of amylose in starch. Dilute solutions in water or alkali have an appreciable viscosity and the molecule is extensively degraded by β-amylase to maltose. Hydrolysis is determined by treating with iodine and observing the colour changes (starch giving a blue; dextrins purple to reddish-brown; maltose, and glucose, if acid hydrolysis, no colour); by testing portions at intervals with Fehling's solution (the amount of reduction increases with the amounts of sugar formed); or by successive measurements of viscosity (viscosity decreases as hydrolysis proceeds). The solutions of amylopectin are stable, give purple colour with iodine (λ_{max} *c*. 540 nm), and the iodine-binding is low. Amylopectin is hydrolysed by β-amylase to the extent of 50-60% only by the enzyme; complete hydrolysis takes place with mineral acids and other enzymes.

Starch contains a very small amount of covalently bound phosphate and its exact location within the molecule is uncertain. The phosphorylation may be of some 1 in 300 glucose molecules. Cereal starches contain about 1% of lipid.

The starch in corn contains approximately 27%

amylose and 73% amylopectin. These two polymers are so associated in the crystal lattice that they are practically insoluble in water or alcohol. In amylose from 250 to 300 D-glucopyranose units are uniformly linked and the molecule acquires a helix-like shape. The amylopectin consists of 1000 or more glucose units. Due to these structural differences amylose is more soluble in water than amylopectin. Amylose reacts with iodine to form a deep-blue complex while amylopectin gives a blue-violet or purple colour. Due to these structural differences, amylose is more soluble in water than is amylopectin, and this characteristic may be used to separate the two components. More efficient separations are effected by complexing and precipitating the amylose with various alcohols or nitroparaffins. Amylose reacts with iodine to form a deep blue complex, amylopectin gives a blue-violet or purple colour. Amylopectin is responsible for the crystallinity of starch.

Most starches have a similar ratio of amylose to amylopectin, averaging about 25% of the former to 75% of the latter. Certain waxy or glutinous starches contain either no amylose or less than 6 per cent.

α-**Amylase** (α-1,4-glucan 4-glucano-hydrolase), an enzyme present in pancreatic juice and saliva, hydrolyzes starch by splitting of α-1,4-glucosidic linkages. Amylose thus yields a mixture of glucose, maltose, and amylopectin, a mixture of branched and unbranched oligosaccharides containing α-1,6 bonds.

β-**Amylase** (α-1,4-glucan maltohydrolase) removes maltose units from the non-reducing ends of polysaccharide molecules to produce pure maltose. The hydrolytic action of β-amylase on the α-1,4 linkages of amylopectin continues until a branch point is approached. The enzyme is unable to hydrolyze α-1,6 bonds, the reaction stops, leaving polysaccharide fragments known as dextrins as the product of incomplete hydrolysis.

During the course of hydrolysis iodine colour changes successively from blue-black to purple to red to no reaction.

Hydrolysis of starch with mineral acids, (HCl, H_2SO_4) produces glucose in quantitative yield. The reaction may be brought by an enzyme (α-amylase, β-amylase or amyloglucosidase) and yields more specific products. β-Amylase, for example, breaks off mostly into maltose units and amyloglucosidase yields mainly D-glucose.

Uses

Starch is used internally as mild astringent, nutritive, demulcent, protective and absorbent. It is given as an antidote in iodine poisoning. It is employed as pharmaceutical aid, as tablet disintegrant, filler, diluents, desintegrants, anticaking, and binder. Externally it is prescribed as an absorbent, emollient, in dusting powders and in ointments. Starch is the starting material for the preparation of glucose, dextrose, and dextrin. Some official preparations of starch are mucilage of starch B.P.C., Zinc Starch Dusting powder B.P.C., and Zinc oxide paste, I.P.

Starch is used in dusting powders due to its absorbent properties. In mucilage form it is used as a skin emollient, as a basis for some enemas and as an antidote in the treatment of iodine poisoning. Maize starch is converted to high-fructose corn syrup by a process involving hydrolysis (glucose producing) and subsequent isomerization. Starch products are used in the plastic industry, *e.g.*, biodegradable polyvinylchloride and polyethylene plastics. Starch is a starting material for the production of dextrins, cyclodextrins, polyalcohols, gluconates and bio-industrial products.

Sterilizable maize starch is used as a lubricant for surgeons gloves; it is maize starch subjected to physical and chemical treatments so that it does not gelatinize on exposure to moisture of steam sterilization. It is completely absorbed by body tissues.

Starch has many commercial uses, such as paper sizing, cloth sizing, and laundry starching. It is the starting material from which liquid glucose (corn syrup), dextrose, dextrins and high-fructose sweeteners are made.

Pregelatinized starch is starch that has been chemically or mechanically processed to rupture all or part of the granules in the presence of water. It is subsequently dried. The material is modified to enhance compressibility and flow characteristics. Pregelatinized starch is slightly soluble in cold water and is used as a tablet excipient.

Sodium starch glycolate, a semisynthetic material, is the sodium salt of a carboxymethyl ether of starch. It is used as a disintegrating agent in tablet formulations.

Hetastarch is a semisynthetic material. It is approximately 90% amylopectin, and 7 or 8 hydroxyethyl substituents are present for each 10 glucose units. A 6% solution of hetastarch is used as a plasma expander.

It is used in treatment of shock caused by hemorrhage, burns, surgery, sepsis, or other trauma. The duration of the improved hemodynamic status is 24 to 36 hours. The polymer is degraded, and molecules with molecular weights of less than 50,000 are eliminated rapidly by renal excretion.

Brazilian arrowroot

This is the starch obtained from the tubers of the sweet potato, *Ipomoea batatas* (Convolvulaceae). The granules are rounded, polyhedral or muller-shaped, the larger ones being 25-55 μm in diameter.

Portland arrowroot

The tuberous rootstock of the English hedgerow plant, *Arum maculatum* (Araceae), is rich in starch. It causes dermatitis among laundrymaids.

Soluble starch

Soluble starch is prepared by treating commercial potato starch with hydrochloric acid. After washing, it forms a limpid, almost clear solution in hot water. It has little reduction with Fehling's solution and gives a deep blue colour with iodine. On heating with 5% potassium hydroxide solution, it gives a canary-yellow colour; no colour is afforded by ordinary starch. Dextrins give a brown colour when similarly treated.

Commercial dextrins

High-grade dextrins are prepared by moistening starch with a small quantity of dilute nitric acid and then heating. It is dried at 110-115°C. The product is white dextrin. Inferior dextrins, which have a yellow or brown colour, are prepared by roasting starch at 150-250°C without the addition of acid.

White dextrins may contain up to 15% of soluble starch and 85% erythrodextrin. Yellow dextrins are

more completely hydrolysed and contain mainly maltose. It is detected and estimated with Fehling's solution.

Mutant varieties

Mutant varieties of maize and other crops produce abnormal starch grains. Thus 'waxy' maize starch contains mainly amylopectin producing a tapioca-like starch. It has shiny appearance due to the broken endosperm. Another mutant, 'amylose extender' is deficient in one of the enzymes responsible for producing the branching of the amylopectin molecule. About six specific enzyme deficiencies have been identified which are associated with abnormal maize starch mutants.

Tests for identification

1. Dissolve starch (1 g) in water (15 ml) by heating on a water bath. A viscous translucent jelly is formed on cooling.
2. Fehling's solution test is positive.
3. It shows Molisch's test for carbohydrates.
4. Solution of starch (1 ml) forms a deep blue colour on addition of iodine solution (1 drop). On warming the colour disappears and reappears on cooling.

Starch is the most common storage polysaccharide found in plants and serves as a primary food source for humans, domestic animals, birds, insects, and microbes. Starch is essentially made up of monomers of sugars linked end to end in long chains through α-1,4 linkages along the chain and with α-1,6 linkages as branch points. Amylose is unbranched and composed exclusively of α-1,4-linked glucan. In rice gains, there are varying amounts of amylose (straight-chain starch) and amylopectin (branched chain starch), depending on the cultivar. In sticky, short-grain rice (Japonica cultivars), amylopectin predominates. Such rice is better for soups and for eating with chopsticks.

A large amount of free sugar in a cell will cause the cytosol to become thick and syrupy. This causes a hypertonic osmotic condition in the cell which will result in excessive water uptake and potential damage. So, one of the primary benefits of producing starch is to make sugars osmotically inactive by making them insoluble within the cell. The starch produced by chloroplasts is the primary storage form that is mobilized for translocation to other plant parts during night periods. It often aggregates into starch grains which can be hydrolyzed to D-glucose, can be used for ATP synthesis via aerobic respiration to maintain turgor pressure in growing cells via its osmotic effects and for synthesis of cellulose and other polysaccharides in the cell wall. Translocated sugars and starch are also important in the development of storage organs such as the rice grains.

Large quantities of starch can be found in storage organs such as tubers and tuberous roots, taproots, stems located above ground and seeds. They allow the plant to survive on stored energy for long periods of winter or drought. In potatoes, under warm weather conditions starch gets hydrolyzed to sugar used for growth of new shoots. Starch also occurs in the root caps located at the tips of growing roots in the soil. It is stored in specialized colourless plastids in rootcap cells called *amyloplasts*. The starch-filled amyloplasts are dense, heavy bodies which fall downwards in the rootcap cells when a root is placed horizontally. These serve as gravisensors that trigger signal transduction events resulting in asymmetric growth of the root downward. If the rootcaps are removed from corn roots, the roots will not curve down when placed horizontally and thus will not grow into the soil where nutrients are located. When the rootcaps are replaced, gravisensitivity is restored. The starch grains in chloroplasts, as in amyloplasts of root caps, can serve as gravisensors in prostrated stems of plants.

Human eat starch in products such as potatoes, cereal grains, taro, and tapioca. It is also important in beer brewing as a "modified barley substrate" used in secondary fermentations. Starch in barley is hydrolyzed to maltose (a disaccharide) and eventually to D-glucose. This hexose is used as a substrate (food) for beer fermenting yeast which, under anaerobic conditions, convert the sugar to ethyl alcohol (*ca.* 3.5 to 4.5%) and carbon dioxide. Starch is easily visualized in storage organs, such as potatoes, or in swollen joints (pulvini) of cereal grass stems by the use of 1% solution of iodine-potassium (1:1).

Biosynthesis of starch

Synthesis of the amylose fraction of starch is initiated by enzymes known as transglycosylases. The reaction involves the elongation of chains of identical composition by the addition of single glucose residues. In certain microorganisms, glucose 1-phosphate is the glucose donor, and the enzyme that catalyzes the transfer is phosphorylase. Various sugar nucleotides, such as UDP-glucose and ADP-glucose, out as glycosyl donors in higher plants. Primer is essential to the reaction and must be a chain of at least 3 α-1,4-linked glucose units. UDP-glucose is the source of the glucose residues.

$$(\text{Glucose}) + \text{UDP-glucose} \longrightarrow (\text{Glucose})_{n+1} + \text{UDP}$$
$$(\text{Glucose})_{n+2} + \text{UDP-glucose} \rightarrow (\text{Glucose})_{n+2} + \text{UDP, etc.}$$

Amylopectin, the branched component of starch, is formed from amylose by the action of a transglycosylase Q-enzyme. This enzyme effects the splitting of a monosaccharide chain containing at least 40 glucose units into 2 fragments. The fragment that carries the newly exposed reducing end first forms an enzyme-substrate complex and is then transferred to an appropriate acceptor chain, establishing an α-1,6 branch.

The final stages of the synthesis of starch are associated with amyloplasts—double membrane organelles which develop, like chloroplasts, from protoplasts. Sucrose is the primary substrate which by the mediation of the reversible sucrose synthase and other enzymes is converted to fructose, glucose-1-phosphate and glucose-6-phosphate in the cytosol.

GUMS, MUCILAGES AND DIETARY FIBRES

Gums are natural plant hydrocolloids classified as anionic or non-ionic polysaccharides or salts of polysaccharides. They are translucent, amorphous substances produced in higher plants as a protective after injury. Useful hydrocolloids are present in some seed embryos or other plant parts (pectins), in various marine algae, and selected microorganisms. A number of semisynthetic cellulose derivatives are used for their hydrophilic properties.

Gums are heterogeneous in composition. Upon hydrolysis, arabinose, galactose, glucose, mannose, xylose, and various uronic acids are obtained. The uronic acids may form salts with calcium, magnesium, and other cations. The presence of methyl ether and sulfate ester substituents further modify the hydrophilic properties of some natural polysaccharides.

Gums are ingredients in dental and other adhesives and in bulk laxatives. These hydrophilic polymers are useful as tablet binders, emulsifiers, gelating agents, suspending agents, stabilizers and thickeners. In difficult utilization of hydrocolloids, some alteration in the hydration of the polymer is done; for example, gums are precipitated from solution by alcohol and by lead subacetate solution.

Gums and mucilages have similar constituents and on hydrolysis yield a mixture of sugars and uronic acids. Gums are pathological products formed upon injury of the plant or owing to unfavourable conditions, such as drought, by a breakdown of cell walls (extracellular formation; gummosis). Mucilages are generally normal products of metabolism formed within the cell (intracellular formation) and may represent storage material, a water-storage reservoir or a protection for germinating seeds. They are present in the epidermal cells of leaves, *e.g.*, senna, in seeds coats (linseed and psyllium), roots (marsh-mallow) and barks (slippery elm).

The gums are dissolved highly in water, whereas mucilages form slimy masses. Dilute solutions of the gums are precipitated by addition of ethanol. They are optically active. Mucilages are physiologic products and gums are pathologic products. The hydrocolloids may be linear or branched; may have acidic, basic, or neutral properties. Basic polymers have limited uses; acidic and neutral hydrocolloids are widely used.

Gums having linear polymer chains are less soluble than those with branched constituents. The linear hydrocolloids yield solutions with greater viscosity due to good alignment and intermolecular hydrogen bonding among linear molecules. The solutions of linear polysaccharides are less stable (tend to precipitate), at low temperature, than solutions of branched molecules. This property significantly influence the shelf life of product formulations. When linear polymers contain uronic acid residues, coulombic repulsion reduces inter-molecular associations and gives more stability to solutions. The hydrocolloids with acid groups also have the potential for anionic-cationic interaction to give precipitation or to alter the hydrophillic properties.

Branched hydrocolloids form gels and not viscous solutions at higher concentrations.

The sources of commercially useful gums of hydrocolloids are as follows :

> *Shrub or tree exudates*—Acacia, Karaya, Tragacanth.
> *Marine gums*—Agar, Algin, Carrageenan.
> *Seed gums*—Guar, Locust bean, Psyllium.
> *Plant extracts*—Pectins.
> *Starch and cellulose derivatives*—heta-starch, carboxy-methylcellulose, ethy-cellulose, hydroxypropyl methylcellulose, methyl-cellulose, oxidized cellulose.
> *Microbial gums*—dextrans, xanthan.

Mucilages pre-exist in specialized cells or canals commonly in Malvales and Fabales. They retain water and have an active role in germination. Their formation would involve the Golgi apparatus.

Gums and mucilage are highly branched heteropolysaccharides, very hydrophobic, insoluble within the plant cell, and often difficult for animals to digest. The animal spends its time eating yet gets nothing out of the process. For the plant, these polysaccharides can function as a storage reserve for carbohydrates, matrix that surrounds the walls of some cells. This matrix is called the *glycocalyx* and is mostly seen on the surfaces of roots where it may serve to protect the plant against microbial invasion. They are also found in bacteria and animals where they act in cell–cell recognition of symbionts or pathogens. In carnivorous plants like Sundew (*Drosera* spp.), mucin in produced to catch unwary insects in nutrient-poor environments. Gums are also useful in sealing wounds in leaves and stems. For example, when a cherry tree is injured, it will produce a thick substance called gum arabic that fills in the wound thus preventing infection. This also acts as a human cosmetic.

Cellulose, pectin, lignin, waxes, gums and mucilages are some of the many types of dietary fibre. Fibre is simply the insoluble polymers of plants and most come from cell walls. Fibre stimulates the gastrointestinal tract and acts as a laxative. Fibre containing pectins reduces blood cholesterol by adsorbing cholesterol molecules. Fibre inhibits many cancers, especially colon cancer, by binding the carcinogens and preventing them from entering the body while they pass through the system. One problem, however, is that fiber may also adsorb vitamins thus carrying them out of the body before they can be absorbed. So, a balance of fibers in the diet is essential. .

LOCUST BEAN GUM

Locust bean gum is the hydrocolloid-containing powdered endosperm of the seed of *Ceratonia siliqua* Linn. (Fam. Papilionaceae), a tree native to the Mediterranean region. The slow development of the tree, *i.e.*, about 15 years for initial seed production is the limited factor to meet expanding demands for hydrocolloids.

A powder of the flesh of the mature seed pods of the tree resembles chocolate and can be used in a variety of food products.

Locust bean gum is a galactomannan and is similar to guar gum. The locust bean gum has less frequency of galactose substituents on the linear mannose chain. Every fourth or fifth mannose residue is substituted. Locust bean gum is incompletely dispersed in cold water.

Locust bean gum is used as a thickener, stabilizer and a hydrocolloid is indicated.

XANTHAN GUM

Xanthan gum is a high-molecular weight microbial anionic polysaccharide prepared by the action of *Xanthomonas campestris* on suitable carbohydrates. The exocellular gum is recovered from the fermentation broth by precipitation with isopropyl alcohol. Xanthan gum is available as the sodium, potassium, or calcium salt.

The main component of xanthan gum is a branched, partially acetylated polysaccharide containing D-glucose, D-glucuronic acid and D-mannose. The polymer is consisted of repeating units of 16 sugar residues; 13 units form a linear chain, and 3 sugar residues are single-sugar side-chain substituents. The gum dissolves in hot and cold water to give high viscosity solutions, and it has good compatibility with a wide range of salts. The viscosity remains unchanged by temperature and pH changes. It tolerates alcohol concentrations up to 50 per cent. It does not form gels by itself, but forms thermally reversible gels in the presence of galactomannans of Papilionaceae family.

Xanthan gum is used as an emulsifying and suspending agent. The pseudoplastic properties of this gum enable toothpastes and ointments both to hold their shape and to spread readily. It is a common ingredient of sauses, soups, jellies, canned products and bakery products.

ACACIA GUM

Synonyms

Acacia, Gum Acacia, Gum Arabic, Acaciae gummi.

Biological source

Acacia gum is the dried gummy exudate obtained from the stem and branches of *Acacia senegal* Willd. and of some related species like *Acacia arabica* Linn. Family Mimosoideae (Mimosoceae).

Habitat

A. senegal is found in Sudan, Central Africa, West Africa and north-western India particularly Haryana, Gujarat and rocky hills of Rajasthan.

Collection

Acacia plant is a 6 m high thorny tree. The gum is produced by living and physiologically active cells of the phloem under certain pathological conditions by rod-shaped bacteria (*Bacterium acaciae*) found conspicuously in all the tissues. A transverse incision in the bark is made for peeling the loosened bark above and below the cuts. The cambium measuring 0.5-1.0 m in length and 5-7.5 cm in breath is exposed. Within a month new phloem cells are produced in the cambium. The tears of gum are formed on this exposed surface due to bacterial action or the action of a ferment which flow on its own and are collected in leather bags. The gum is garbled to free it from sand and vegetable debris and occasionally exposed to sunlight for 3-4 months to bleach it. During this bleaching process numerous minute cracks are formed on the outer surface of the tears due to which the surface becomes semiopaque. During drying process, the gum lost about 30% of its weight. The tears are graded finally on the basis of external appearance, packed and exported.

Trees growing in sandy plains and semi-rocky sites give higher gum-yield than those growing in rocky areas.

Three grades are usually exported namely hand-picked selected Kordofan, cleaned Kordofan and talka. Gum arabic is sold in one currency only ($US), and the currency changes affect the price. The Senegal Acacia gum is largely used for pharmaceutical purposes. This also occurs in three grades, namely 'gomme du bas du fleuve', gomme du haut du fleuve' and 'gomme friable'.

Spray-dried acacia, produced by the importers, is becoming of increasing importance. It has a low viable bacterial count.

Characters

Acacia gum occurs in rounded or ovoid, opaque, irregular or broken tears, 1-3 cm in diameter. Other surface contains numerous fine cracks. Colour is white or pale yellow. The gum is very brittle and the exposed surface is transparent and glassy. It is odourless and taste is bland and mucilaginous. The tears break rapidly with a glassy fracture, and much of the drug consists of small pieces. It is odourless and has a bland and mucilaginous taste.

Cleaned gum has fewer cracks which causes it to be more transparent, and in being more yellowish or pinkish in colour. The tears are less uniform in size, some being small, while others have a diameter of 4 cm or more. Some of the tears are vermiform in shape and the gum is more yellowish in colour. It is freely soluble in equal weight of water to form a viscous, adhesive laevorotatory and acidic solution. The gum is insoluble in alcohol and other organic solvents.

The aqueous solution is slightly acid and becomes more acidic on keeping, especially if hot water is used to make the solution. It is viscid, but not glairy, and when dilute form does not deposit on standing.

A 10% aqueous solution is laevorotatory, gives no precipitate with dilute solution of lead acetate (distinction from Tragacanth and Agar), gives no colour with solution of iodine (absence of starch and dextrin) and gives no reaction for tannin with ferric chloride. The mucilage gives a blue colour when treated with solution of benzidine and a few drops of hydrogen peroxide, which indicates the presence of a peroxidase distinction from (Tragacanth). Because benzidine has carcinogenetic properties, this test is no longer used.

Chemical constituents

Acacia gum contains chiefly arabin which is the mixture of calcium, magnesium and potassium salts of arabic acid. On hydrolysis, arabic acid yields L-rhamnopyranose, galactopyranose, L-arabofuranose and the aldobionic acid 6-β-D-glucuronosido-D-galactose. Further hydrolysis yields L-arabinose, D-galactose, D-glucuronic acid and rhamnose. The gum also possesses enzymes like oxidases, peroxidases and pectinases. It yields 2.7-4% of ash.

The composition of the gum is extremely complex and has not been fully elucidated. The major branched polysaccharide fraction of β-(1,3)-linked galactose units combines with side-chains of arabinose, rhamnose and uronic acids linked through the 1,6-positions. The gum also contains small amounts of protein, including arabino-galactan-proteins.

The degraded gum of *A. arabica* is composed of galactose (10 units) and glucuronic acid (4 units).

A. arabica bark contains 2-O-β-L-arabinofuranosyl-L-arabinose, 3-O-β-L-arabinopyranasyl-L-arabi-nose, gallic acid quercetin, (+)-catechin, (–)-epi-catechin, (+)-dicatechin, (+)-leucocyanidine; epigallocatechin, polyphenolic phlobaphenes, octacosanol, β-amyrin, β-sitosterol, betulin, catechin-5-gallate and naringenin.

Biosynthesis

The synthesis of amylose is a chain-lengthening process. The transfer of glucose from ADP-D-glucose to primer is catalyzed by starch (glucan) synthase. Primer glucan from parent cells is bound to the starch synthase of daughter cells. Soluble starch synthase exhibits absolute specificity towards ADP-D-glucose. However, an insoluble, granule-bound starch synthase can also utilize UDP-D-glucose, although the ADP-glucoside is the more efficient donor.

The formation of the α-(1 → 6) bonds of amylopectin are catalyzed by 1,4-α-glucan branching enzyme, also known as Q-enzyme. The branching is effected by transfer to short chains of α-(1 → 4) linked glucose units from a 1 → 4 linkage to a 1 → 6 linkage. Thus, the reaction is a transglucosylation involving the breaking of a 1 → 4 bond and the formation of a 1 → 6 bond. The enzyme(s) catalyzing the formation of 1 → 4 linkages of amylopectin may not be identical with the starch synthase of amylose.

Sucrose is incorporated into starch and this is effected through the formation of ADP-D-glucose and UDP-D-glucose catalyzed by sucrose synthase.

Uses

Acacia gum is demulcent, emollient and used as emulsifying and suspending agent for the administration of insoluble drugs. It is employed as an adhesive and binder in tablets especially in lozenges. Due to its demulcent properties, it is used in various formulations for cough, diarrhoea and throat problems. Internally, Acacia gum is used in inflammation of intestinal mucosa. It is also used to cover inflamed surfaces such as burns and sore nipples.

It is incompatible with readily oxidized materials such as phenols, and the vitamin A of cod-liver oil. It is used in the food, drinks and other industries.

Purity tests

An aqueous solution of the Acacia gum (5 g) is prepared by dissolving in water (15 ml) to perform the following tests for identity :

1. The aqueous solution is slightly acidic and becomes more acidic on keeping.
2. On standing it does not form viscous gelly-like mass. No sediment should be deposited on standing in case of pure gums.
3. To the aqueous solution (5 ml) few drops of dilute solution of lead acetate are added. No precipitate is formed due to absence of Tragacanth and Agar.

4. It does not form blue or brown colour with iodine solution due to absence of Tragacanth and Agar.
5. With ferric chloride solution it does not produce any violet or green colour due to absence of tannins.
6. To the solution of gum Acacia resorcinol (0.1 g) and hydrochloric acid (2 ml) are added and then heated on a water-bath. No yellow or pink colour is developed due to absence of sucrose or fructose.
7. Fine powder of the gum (5 g) is dissolved in distilled water (100 ml), dilute hydrochloric acid (10 ml) is added and the reaction mixture is boiled gently for 15 minutes. The hot solution is filtered by suction through a sintered glass crucible, washed thoroughly with hot water, dried at 105°C and weighed. The insoluble matter should not exceed 50 mg in case of pure gum.

Test for identification

1. To the aqueous solution (5 ml) borax (0.1 g) is added. A stiff translucent mass is obtained.
2. To the dilute aqueous solution few drops of lead sub-acetate are added. A white, bulky precipitate is produced.
3. To the aqueous solution (5 ml) few drops of 1% alcoholic solution of benzidine are added along with 10% hydrogen peroxide (0.5 ml). On shaking blue colour is produced due to enzyme oxidase.
4. Gum Acacia responds positively to Fehling's solution test of reducing sugars and Molisch's test of carbohydrates.
5. To the aqueous solution (5 ml), alcohol (10 ml) is added gradually by shaking. The cloudy liquid on addition of glacial acetic acid (0.5 ml) forms a white precipitate. It is filtered and to the clear filtrate ammonium oxalate solution (50 ml) is added. The filtrate becomes cloudy again.

Allied drugs

Gatti gum (Indian gum) is obtained in India and Sri Lanka from *Anogeissus latifolia* Wallich (Fam. Combretaceae). Its tears are of different colour and the outer surface is dull. Some of tears are vermi-form in shape and their surface shows fewer cracks than the natural acacia. Aqueous solution of this gum has the viscosity between those of Acacia and Sterculia gums. With lead subacetate solution, it forms very slight precipitates. The gum contains D-mannose, D-galactose, L-arabinose, D-xylose and D-glucuronic acid.

Starch, Tragacanth, Talka gum, Dextrin and cheaper gums from Acacia species are other adulterants of Acacia gum.

West African gum Combretum, obtained from *Combretum nigricans*, is not permitted as a food additive but is used as an adulterant of gum arabic. In gum Combretum, rhamnose and uronic acid units are located within the polysaccharide chain.

Talka gum is much broken and of very variable composition, some of the tears are almost colourless and others brown.

TRAGACANTH

Synonyms

Gum tragacanth, Anjira (Hindi).

Biological source

Tragacanth is the air-dried gummy exudation obtained by incision from the stems of *Astragalus gummifer* Labil. (White gavan) or other Asiatic species of *Astragalus* such as *A. kurdicus, A. adscendens* and *A. strobiliferus*. (Family : Mimosoceae)

Habitat

Tragacanth plant is most widely found in Iran, also in Asia Minor, Syria, Anatolia, Iraq, Turkey, Greece and Afghanistan.

Collection

The Tragacanth plants are 1 meter high thorny branching shrubs. The gum is produced physiologically in the plant cells. When a one or two years old plant is injured, the cell wall of the pith and then of the medullary rays are gradually converted into gum. The gum exudes immediately after injury whereas the gum is slowly produced after injury. A section of a tragacanth stem shows that the cell walls of the pith and medullary rays are gradually transformed into gum, the change being termed 'gummosis'. It is centripetal and the gum accumulates in the medulla and the medullary rays, the cell walls of which later collapse. The gum absorbs water and a considerable pressure is set up within the stem. The gum immediately exudes from the centre a stream of soft, solid tragacanth, pushing itself out like a worm, 2 cm long, within half an hour. In contact of the air it is hardened due to evaporation of water. The shape of the gum depends on the shape of the incision made. The gum is collected by the natives and packed.

Gum can be obtained from the plants in their first year but it is of poor quality and unfit for commercial use. The plants are tapped in the second year. The earth is taken away from the base to a depth of 5 cm and the exposed part is incised with a sharp knife. A wedge-shaped piece of wood is used to force open the incision so that the gum will exude more freely. The wedge is generally left in the cut for 12-24 h before being withdrawn. The

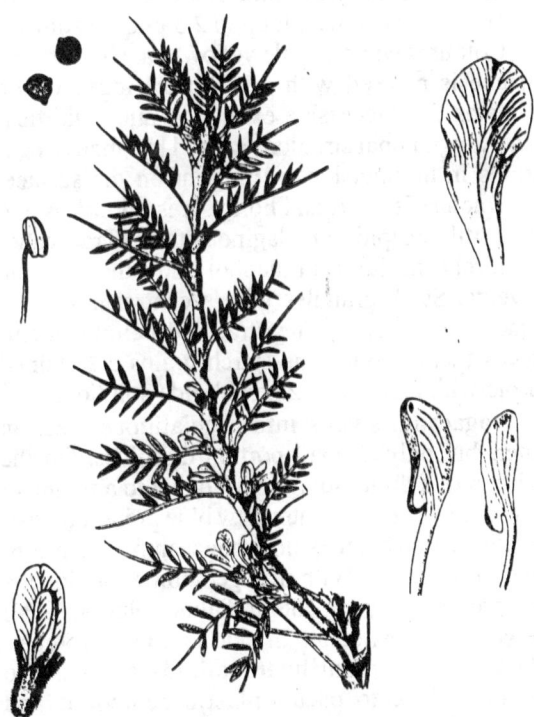

Fig. 14.2. Tragacanth twig.

gum exudes is collected 2 days after the incision. Some of the plants are burned at the top after having had the incision made. The plant then sickens and gives off a greater quantity of gum. Many plants are killed by the burning. The gum obtained after burning is of lower quality than that obtained by incision only, and is reddish and dirty looking. The crop becomes available in August-September.

Grades

Tragacanth is graded into several qualities; *e.g.*, Ribbon No. 1, 2,.., 5 and Flake No. 26, 27...., 55. The best grades are included as the official drugs, while the lower grades are used in the food, textiles and other industries.

Tragacanth is an expensive commodity due to limited supply and the extra treatment and tests required to meet the current microbial requirements have added to the cost.

Characters

Tragacanth occurs as thin, flattened, curved or ribbon-like flakes, length up to 2.5 cm, breadth 1.2 cm. Colour is white or pale yellow, translucent. The surface is marked with concentric ridges which indicates the successive exudation and solidification. Longitudinal striations caused by small irregularities in the incision are present on the surface. The fracture is short and horny. It is odourless and has a little insipid, mucilaginous taste. Tragacanth is entirely insoluble in alcohol and other organic solvents. Stach granules with a central hilum are present in the gum. The stratified cellular membranes that surround the starch grains are stained purple with iodine and zinc chloride solution.

Tragacanth swells into a gelatinous mass in water, but only a small portion dissolves. On the addition of a dilute solution of iodine to a fragment previously soaked in water, few blue points are visible (distinction from Symrna tragacanth, which contains more starch). With stronger iodine solution the gum produces a green colour. Dilute solutions (1%) are very viscous, stable in acid and heat, compatible with most plant hydrocolloids and easy to conserve. Due to pseudoplastic behaviour and anionic character of the solutions, Tragacant is a good stabilizer for suspensions.

Chemical constituents

Tragacanth consists of tragacanthin (water-soluble portion) and bassorin (water-insoluble portion). The insoluble portion swells to a gel and consists of 60-70% bassorin which is a complex of polymethoxylated acids. Tragacanthin is probably demethoxylated bassorin consisting of 30-40% of the gum. Tragacanthin is neutral and forms a colloidal solution with water. Bossorin is acidic and precipitates with ethanol. The gum is composed of sugar and uronic acid units. On hydrolysis of Tragacanth, galacturonic acid, D-galactopyranose, L-arabofuranose and D-xylopyranose are obtained. Starch and proteins are also present in Tragacanth.

Tragacanthin and bassorin have molecular weights of the order of 840,000. Both are insoluble in alcohol. Tragacanthin and bassorin may be separated by ordinary filtration of an extremely dilute mucilage. The tragacanthin may be estimated by the evaporation of an aliquot portion of the filtrate. The best grades of gum contain the least tragacanthin. If the tragacanthin content and moisture content are known, the amount of bassorin may be calculated.

In the tragacanthin fraction there are no methoxyl groups, but that the bassorin fraction contained about 5.38% methoxyl. The gums with high methoxyl contents and high bassoorin contents give the most viscous mucilages. Heating or fine powdering produces demethylation with loss of viscosity. The gum-exudates of the three species of Turkish gum-producers are proteinaceous polysaccharides and represent a protein content of about 3-4%, involving 18 amino acids. The relative amino acid proportions differed in the three gums.

For determination of minimum apparent viscosity of the powdered gum, a *flow time* for gum to be used in the preparation of emulsions, and a microbial limit test. Peroxidase enzymes are absent, but their presence has been detected in commercial samples of genuine drug. The presence of peroxidase enzymes is due to starch (3%) content; both disappear as gummosis occurs.

Uses

Tragacanth is used in pharmaceutical as com-pounding and dispensing agent, *e.g.*, to suspend heavy insoluble powders, as an excipient for tablets and to impart consistency to touches; also in making emulsions and emulsifying agents for oils and resin; as stabilizer, thickener and texturizer in food. As Tragacanth is resistant to acid hydrolysis, it is preferred for use in highly acidic conditions. It has demulcent and emollient properties and is used in various cosmetic formulations like hand lotions. It is also used in adhesives (mucilages, pastes); in textile sizing, textile printing and general printing inks, and in dyeing with insoluble colour lakes. Tragacanth is used for the treatment of constipation.

Allied drugs

Tragacanth of lower grades, known as *hog gum* or *hog tragacanth*, is used in textile industry and pickle manufacture. The pieces are of different shape, yellow to black in colour and contaminated with earth. Their ashes give a strong reaction for iron. The viscosity of mucilages prepared from these grades of tragacanth falls rapidly from the No. 1 to the No. 55, marked difference in price. It is adulterated with *Chitral gum* obtained from *Sterculia urens* and insoluble *Shiraz gum* of unknown origin imported from Iran. Good quality of *Shiraz gum* resembles Kordofan acacia. It contains no starch and gives a reaction for oxidase enzyme. Vermicelli tragacanth is obtained from *Astragalus cylleneus*, a species found in Greece.

Test for identity

1. Tragacanth contains about 30% of water soluble portion.
2. On boiling with sodium hydroxide solution a brown or yellow colour is formed.
3. It responds positively with Molisch's test and Fehling's solution test.
4. It swells and forms a smooth, nearly uniform stiff, opalescent mucilage free from cellular fragments.
5. Powdered material (0.5 g) is dissolved in water (1 ml) to form a homogenous mucilage. The mucilage is diluted with water (5 ml) and barium hydroxide solution added. A slightly flocculent precipitate is formed. On heating for ten minutes, it gives an intense yellow colour.
6. TLC analysis of the gum hydrolysate with H_2SO_4 and spraying with aminohippuric acid shows the presence of fucose, xylose, galactose and arabinose and absence of methylcellulose.
7. The foreign substances must not exceed 1% by weigh. The gum must pass a limit test for total viable aerobic count up to 10^4 micoorganisms/g and tests for *E. coli* and *Salmonella.*

STERCULIA GUM (KARAYA GUM)

Synonyms

Kadaya, Mucara, Kullo, Katilo, Kuteera, Indian Tragacanth, Bassora Tragacanth.

Biological source

Sterculia is the dried gummy exudate of the tree *Sterculia urens* Roxb., *S. villosa*, *S. tomentosa*, *S. tragacantha* (Family : Sterculiaceae) or from *Cochlospermum gossypium* Decand. (Family : Cochlospermaceae). It is the air-hardened product of the viscous exudate from the trunk and branches of the plant.

Habitat

The tree is found mainly in India (Gujarat, Maharashtra, Tamil Nadu, Rajasthan and M.P.), Pakistan and to some extent in Africa.

Collection

The gum exudes naturally or from incisions made to the heartwood and is collected twice a year, before and after the monsoon season (April-June and September). The gum of first collection has the highest viscosity. The dried irregular masses of several kilograms in weight are picked up, bark pieces are removed, packed and exported.

The first collection gives a gum with the highest viscosity. Blazes, up to one square foot in area, are made in the larger trees and the gum immediately starts to exude. The flow is greatest during the first 24 h and continues for several days. It is graded according to colour and presence of foreign organic matter. It is sold as a granulated, or finely powdered product.

Characters

A genuine gum occurs in irregular, colourless, translucent, striated masses weighing up to 25 g or more.

Medium grades have a marked pinkish tinge, while the lower grades are very dark and contain a considerable amount of bark. The gum has a marked odour of acetic acid, and when hydrolysed with 5% phosphoric acid, has a volatile acidity of not less than 14%. Sterculia has a methoxyl value of 0. When boiled with solution of potash, it becomes slightly brownish. It contains no starch and stains pink with solution of ruthenium red.

In water, sterculia gum has solubility but swells to many times its original volume. The coarser granulated grades give a discontinuous grainy dispersion, whereas the fine powder affords an apparently homogeneous dispersion.

Chemical constituents

Sterculia gum consists of an acetylated, branched heteropolysaccharide (glycanorhamno galacturonan) with a high composition of D-galacturonic acid and D-glucuronic acid moieties. Its basic unit is consisted of alternating α-D-galacturonic acid link through the C-4 position and α-L-rhamnose linked through the C-2 position. The chain is substituted on the galacturonic acid hydroxyl groups in C-2 or C-3 and on some of the rhamnose hydroxyl groups in C-4 by D-galactose and D-glucuronic acid.

Hydrolysis of the gum affords D-galactose, L-rhamnose, D-galacturonic acid, aldobiouronic acid, acetic acid and an acid trisaccharide. Uronic acid residues are present in 40% amount in the gum and the degree of acetylation is about 8%.

Tests for identification

It releases acetic acid upon heating, stains pink with ruthenium red, gives uronic acid (detected by dihydroxynaphthalene) and galactose and rhamnose (indicated by amino-hippuric acid) after sulphuric acid hydrolysis and has swelling index not less than 13 in a 37% v/v ethanol solution. A 1% aqueous solution of the gum has pH 5.5. The foreign matter insoluble in hot acidified (HCl) water should be less than 5%.

Uses

Sterculia gum is used as a bulk laxative, emulsifying and suspending agent and a dental adhesive. The powdered gum is used in lozenges, pastes and denture fixative powder. It is also employed in wave set solution, skin lotions, textile and printing industries, in the preparation of compositae building materials and as an adhesive for stoma appliances. It is indicated in symptomatic treatment of constipation and used as an adjunct in weight loss diets and for its zero-calorie bulk to provide a feeling of satiation. Due to its adhesive properties, the gum is used for colostomy apparati and to affix dental prostheses.

KATIRA GUM

Synonyms : Kumbi, galgal.

It is obtained from *Cochlospermum religiosum* (Linn.) Alston, syn. *C. gossypium* DC (Family Cochlospermaceae).

The plant is a small or medium sized, deciduous, soft wooded tree, 3-6 m high, with palmately 5-lobed leaves and large bright yellow flowers in terminal panicles.

The tree is found throughout India from Garhwal to Bengal, Orissa, central and southern India. It is particularly common in hot, dry and stony regions. It is often cultivated in gardens and near temples for its beautiful yellow flowers.

The gum exudes from the fibrous, deeply furrowed bark. It is similar to Sterculia gum and is also known as Hog gum. The gum is pale, semitransparent, transversely striated with a tendency to split into flat scales. On exposure to moist air, it gives off acetic acid slowly. It is insoluble in water, but swells into a pasty transparent mass in contact with water.

The gum contains about 50% pentosans and galactans. Hydrolysis of the gum yields acetic acid (14%), gondic acid ($C_{23}H_{26}O_{21}$), α-cochlospermic acid, xylose and galactose. It is exported from India to use in cigar paste and icecream industry. The gum is used as a substitute for Tragacanth in calico printing, marbling paper and leather dressing. The gum has sweetish, cooling, sedative properties and useful in coughs.

AGAR

Synonym

Agar-agar, Gelose; Japan agar, Bengal isinglass; Ceylon isinglass, Chinese isinglass, Japanese isinglass; Vegetable Gelatin, Kanten.

Biological source

Agar is the dried, hydrophilic, colloidal, polysaccharide complex extracted from the agarocytes of algae known as *Gelidium amansii, Gelidium cartilagineum* (L.) Gaillon (Family Gelidiaceae), *Gracilaria confervoides* (L.) Grev. (Family Sphaerococcaceae) and some other species of *Acanthopeltis, Ceramium,* and *Pterocladia.* (Family : Rhodophyceae). *Gelidium* provides about 35% of the total agar source.

About 18 important species of marine red algae occur in Indian coasts. The seven species, viz., *Gracilaria corticata, G. crassa, G. edulis, G. foliifora, G. verrucosa, Gelidiella acerosa* and *Pterocladia capillacea* are used to prepare Agar.

Habitat

Agar is prepared in Japan, Korea, South Africa, Mexico, Atlantic and Pacific coasts of USA, Spain and New Zealand. About 6500 tonnes are produced annually, of which about one-third originates from Japan. The genus *Gelidium* provides about 35% of the total source material.

Collection and preparation

Algae are cultivated on the coast. The development of algae takes place on poles which are withdrawn from time to time to strip off the algae. The seawood is washed for 24 hours in running water, beaten and shaken to remove sand and shells, extracted in steam heated digesters with dilute acids and then with water for 30 hours. The hot mucilaginous decoction is filtered through linen. On cooling a jelly is formed which is cut into bars. The bars are converted into strips by passing through wire netting. Water is removed by successively freezing, thawing and drying at about 35°C. The agar ice block weighing about 150 kg is crushed, melted, and filtered through a rotary vacuum pump. The moist agar flakes so obtained are dried by currents of dry air in tall cylinders.

Characters

Agar occurs in the form of a transparent or translucent, agglutinated, yellowish-white slender, lustrous, flattened strips or as fine or granulated powder. It is tough in damp, brittle in dried form,

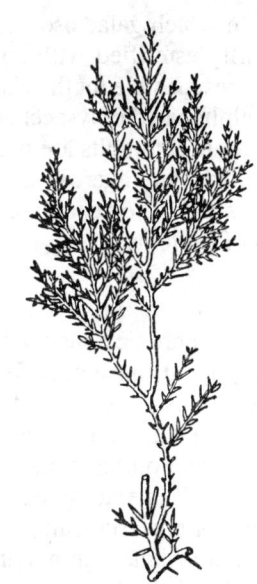

Fig. 14.3. *Gelidium amansii.*

odourless or with a slight odour and taste is mucilaginous. Agar is insoluble in cold water and alcohol, slowly soluble in hot water to form a viscid solution and its 1% solution forms a stiff firm jelly on cooling. Agar occur in two forms : (1) bundles of agglutinated, translucent, yellowish-white strips, these being about the thickness of leaf gelatin, 4 mm wide and about 60 cm long; (2) coarse powder or flakes. Agar swells in cold water but only a small fraction dissolves. A 1% solution is prepared by boiling and a stiff jelly separates from this on cooling.

Chemical constituents

Agar is composed of the calcium salt of acidic polysaccharides. It can be separated into a natural gelling fraction, *agarose*, and a sulphated non-gelling fraction, *agaropectin*. The structure is believed to be a complex range of polysaccharide chains having alternating α-(1 → 3) and β-(1 → 4) linkages. On hydrolysis Agar yields galactose and sulphate ions. It is a heterogeneous polysaccharide. Agarose, responsible for the gel strength, consists of alternate residue of 3,6-anhydro-L-galactose and D-galactose. The viscosity of agar solutions is due to the presence of agaropectin which is a sulphated polysaccharide in which galactose and uronic acid moieties are partly esterified with sulphuric acid. The agaropectin, responsible for the viscosity of agar solutions, is a sulphonated polysaccharide in which galactose and uronic acid units are partly esterified with sulphuric acid. Pure agarose is commercially available and its gels are recommended for the electrophoresis of proteins.

Uses

Agar is used to treat chronic constipation, as a laxative, suspending agent, an emulsifier, a gelating agent for suppositories, as surgical lubricant, as a tablet excipient, disintegrant, in production medicinal encapsulations and ointment and as dental impression mold base. It is extensively used as a gel in nutrient media for bacterial cultures, as a substitute for gelatin and insiglass, in making emulsions including photographic, gel in cosmetics, as thickening agent in food especially confectionaries and dairy products, in meat canning; sizing for silk and paper; in dyeing and printing of fabrics and textiles; and in adhesive. Agarose forms double helical three-dimensional network able to retain water molecules. It cannot be assimilated and is non-toxic. It increases the bulk and hydration of feels and acts as a mechanical laxative and as a gastrointestinal protective agent.

Chemical tests

1. Agar responds positively to Fehling's solution test.
2. Agar gives positive test with Molisch's reagent.
3. Aqueous solution of Agar (1%) is hydrolyzed with concentrated hydrochloric acid by heating for 5-10 minutes. On addition of barium chloride solution to the reaction mixture, a white precipitate of barium sulphate is formed due to the presence of sulphate ions. This test is absent in case of Starch, Acacia gum and Tragacanth.
4. To agar powder a solution of ruthenium red is added. Red colour is formed indicating mucilage.
5. Agar is warmed in a solution of potassium hydroxide. A canary yellow colour is formed.
6. An aqueous solution of agar (1%) is prepared in boiling water. On cooling it sets into a jelly.
7. To agar solution an N/20 solution of iodine is added. A deep crimson to brown colour is obtained (distinction from Acacia gum and Tragacanth).
8. To a 0.2% solution of Agar an aqueous solution of tannic acid is added. No precipitate is formed indicating absence of Geltain.
9. It does not gives any precipitate with Millon's reagent due to absence of Gelatin.
10. On heating Agar with soda lime no ammonia is evolved due to absence of Geltain.
11. If agar is ashed and the residue, after treatment with dilute hydrochloric acid, examined microscopically, the silica skeletons of diatoms and sponge spicules are detected. More perfect diatoms are isolated by centrifuging a 0.5% solution. The large discoid diatom *Arachnoidiscus*, which is about 0.1-0.3 mm in diameter, species of *Grammato-phora* and *Cocconeis*, and sponge spicules are detected in the ash of Japanese agar.

Agar is required to comply with tests for the absence of *Escherichia coli* and *Salmonella*, and general microbial contamination should not exceed a level of 10^3 microorganisms per g^{-1}, as determined by a plate count. It has a swelling index of not less than 10.

ISPAGHULA (PLANTAGO)

Synonyms

Psyllium seed; Flea seed; Plantain seed; Isabgol; Ishabgul; Spogel seed.

Biological source

Ispaghula consists of cleaned, dried, ripe seed of *Plantago psyllium* Linn., or of *Plantago indica* Linn. (*P. arenaria* Wald.), known as Spanish or French Psyllium seed, or of *Plantago ovata* Forsk, known as Blonde Psyllium or Indian Plantago. (Family : Plantaginaceae).

Habitat

P. psyllium is indigenous to the Mediterranean region and west Asia, presently cultivated in France,

Spain and Cuba. *P. ovata* is found in Punjab hills and other parts of north-west India, Sind and Baluchistan and is cultivated in Bengal, Karnataka, Gujarat and Maharashtra.

Cultivation and collection

The plant is a stemless or subcaulescent soft, hairy annual herb. It is cultivated by spreading seeds in November in well drained loamy soil. To the fields ammonium sulphate fertilizer is added and they are irrigated at an interval of 8-10 days for about 8 times. The crop is harvested in four months in March/April. The plants are cut just above the ground, dried and seeds are separated by thrashing.

Characters

The seeds of *P. ovata* are 2.0-3.3 mm in length, 1-16 mm in breadth; dull, pinkish grey-brown; long to elliptical in outline, boat shaped; the dorsal surface is convex with a small elliptical or elongated shining reddish brown spot while the ventral surface is concave with a deep furrow, not perfectly reaching to either end of the seeds. At the furrow a hilum is present which is covered by a thin membrane and appears as a red spot in the centre. The outer surface is smooth, hard and translucent. The seeds are odourless and taste is bland but mucilaginous.

Chemical constituents

The seeds contain hydrocolloidal polysaccharide (mucilage) in the outer seed coat (20-30%), fixed oils, tannin, aucubin glycoside (iridoid), sugars, sterols and protein. The mucilage of Ispaghula is colloidal in nature and its composition varies with the conditions of preparation. It is mainly com-posed of xylose, arabinose and galacturonic acid; rhamnose and galactose have also been reported. Two polysaccharide fractions have been separated from the muscilage. One fraction is soluble in cold water and on hydrolysis yields xylose (46%), an aldobiouronic acid (40%), arabinose (7%) and insoluble residue. The other fraction in soluble in hot water forming a highly viscous solution which sets as a gel on cooling and yields on hydrolysis xylose (80%), arabinose (14%), aldobiouronic acid (0.3%) and trace of galactose. The fatty oil is composed of linolenic, linoleic, oleic, palmitic, stearic and lignoceric acids. *P. ovata* is a good source of linoleic acid. The amino acids reported in the seeds are valine, alanine, glycine, glutamic acid, cystine, lysine, leucine and tyrosine.

P. lanceolata and *P. major* seeds contain aucuboside and catalpol. Palmitic, myristic, stearic, oleic and linoleic acids are present in the seeds, leaves and flowers of *P. psyllium*. Hydrolysis of mucilage of *P. lanceolata* yields galactose, arabinose, glucose, rhamnose, mannose, xylose and fucose. A phenyl propanoid glycoside, plantamajoside, is present in *P. asiatica*. 9-Oxo-octadec-*cis*-12-eonic acid and 9-hydroxyoctadec-*cis*-12-eonic acid are present in the seeds of *P. ovata*. Aucubin, catalpol, globularin and desacetylasperulosidic acid methyl ester are present in *P. lanceolata*. The seeds of *P. asiatica* yield oleanolic acid, acetoside, luteolin, its 7-0-glucoside, β-sitosterol, campesterol, stigmasterol, iridoids plantarenaloside, ixoroside, asperuloside, melampyroside and aucubin. Plantamajoside showed antibacterial activity against *Escherichia coli* and *Staphylococcus aureus*.

Uses

Seeds are demulcent, cooling, diuretic and used in inflammatory conditions of mucus membrane of gastrointestinal and genitourinary tracts. They are used to cure chronic dysentery, diarrhoea, duodenal ulcer, gonorrhoea, constipation and piles. Isabgol preparations are given after colostomy to assist the production of smooth solid faecal mass. The mucilage is not digested by enzymes and intestinal bacteria in the gut and comes out unchanged. Jelly-like mucilage absorbs irritating products and toxins of the gut and they are expelled from the body. The seeds are used in febrile conditions and the affections of kidneys, bladder and urethra. A decoction of seeds is prescribed in cough and cold, and the crushed seeds made into poultice are applied to rheumatic and glandular swellings. Recently anticancer, antitoxic, anti-atherosclerosis, hypocholesteremic, hypoglycemic, hypotensive, cardiac depressant, cholinergic and cervical activities have been reported.

Chemical tests

1. Ispaghula seeds form red colour with ruthenium red solution.
2. On adding water, mucilage forming surrounding layer outside the seed is swelled.
3. *Determination of swelling factor* : The drug (1 g) is placed in a 25 ml graduated cylinder. Water is added up to 20 ml mark and left for 24 hours with occasional shaking. The seeds are allowed to settle for 1-2 hours and the total volume occupied by the swollen seeds is noted. The swelling factors for the seeds are as : 14 ml for *P. psyllium*; 10 ml for *P. ovata* and 8 ml for *P. indica*.

Adulterants and substitutes

P. lanceolata Linn., occurring wild in India, is adulterated in Ispaghula. Its seeds are oblong elliptical in shape with yellowish brown colour. The seeds of *P. asiatica*, (syn. *P. major* L.), found in Andhra Pradesh and Tamil Nadu, are substituted to Ispaghula. It is also adulterated with the seeds of *P. arenaria*. The seeds of *Salvia aegyptica* are frequently mixed which also yield copious mucilage. The seeds of *P. media* L. have different colour and swell very little in water.

   P. asiatica contains mucilage which is composed of β-1,4-linked D-xylopyranose residues having three kinds of branches.

BAEL

Synonyms

Bel, Bengal quince, Fructus belae, Bael fruit.

Biological source

Bael consists of the entire unripe fruit or its slices of *Aegle marmelos* Corr. (Family : Rutaceae).

Habitat

Bael plant is found all over India in sub-Himalayan forests, Bengal, central and south India and also in Burma and Sri Lanka.

Collection

Tree is slender, deciduous, nearly 12 m in height. Generally bael is propagated by seeds which are covered with earth and watered. The tree can be propagated by root-cuttings and layers. The unripe or half-ripe fruits are collected, epicarp is removed and cut into transverse slices or irregular pieces.

Morphology

The fruit is a woody, large berry with green colour when unripe and yellowish brown on maturing, diameter 10-20 cm. The fruit is sub-spherical in shape, epicarp is hard, woody, smooth, about 2 mm thick, slightly granular. A circular scar is left by the re-

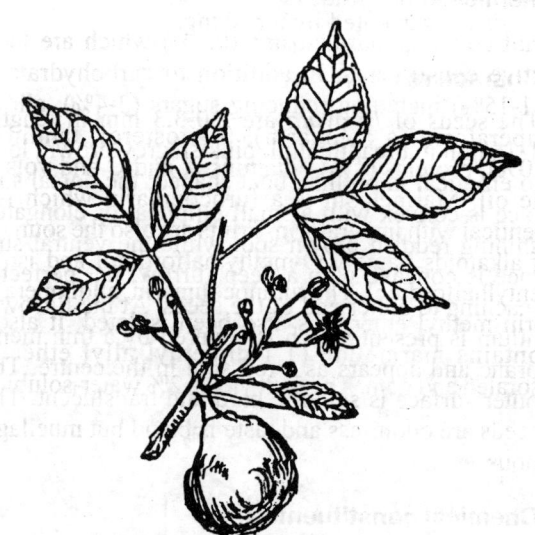

Fig. 14.4. *Aegle marmelos.*

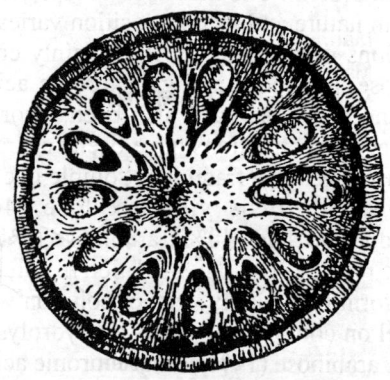

Fig. 14.5. Bael fruit. Transverse section.

moval of the stalk. Internally it consists of reddish-brown pulpy endocarp; mesocarp consists of 10-15 chambers, each containing several hairy, oblong, multicellular seeds surrounded by reddish mucilage. Odour is faint and aromatic and taste is mucilaginous and sweet.

The peripheral part just within the rind is fleshy and thick and has a pleasant resinous odour. The walls separating the chambers are yellow. The chambers are full of amber- or honey-coloured, viscous, very sticky or glutinous, translucent pulp.

Chemical constituents

Fruit contains marmelosins (0.4%) which are the active constituents, in addition to carbohydrates (11-15%) including reducing sugars (3-4%), allo-imperatorin (a coumarin), β-sitosterol, tannins (20%), proteins (1%), vitamins A and C and volatile oil. Marmelosin is a furocoumarin which is identical with imperatorin. Fruits are also the source of alkaloids namely O-methylhalfordinol and iso-pentylhalfordinol. The furanocoumarin, alloimperatorin methyl ether, has also been isolated. It also contains marmelide (1,1-dimethyl allyl ether), psoralen and gum. The fruit yields 2% water-soluble

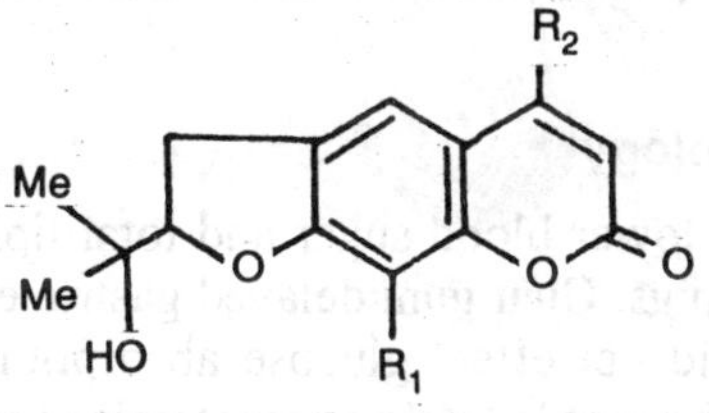

Marmelosin A : $R_1 = R_2 = H$
Marmelosin B : $R_1 = H; R_2 = Me$
Marmelosin C : $R_1 = Me; R_2 = H$

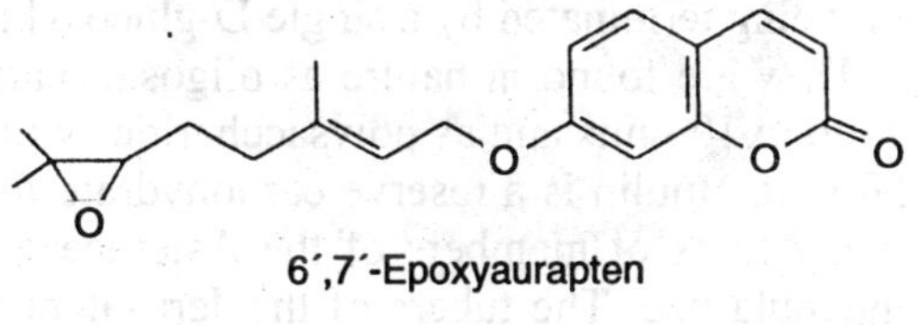

6′,7′-Epoxyaurapten

Fig. 14.6. Coumarins of Bael.

gum which on hydrolysis gives galactose, arabinose, D-galacturonic acid and rhamnose.

Uses

Unripe fruit is astringent, digestive, demulcent, stomachic and used in diarrhoea and dysentery. Ripe fruit is sweet, aromatic, cooling, alternative and nutritive. When taken fresh, it is useful in habitual constipation, chronic dysentery and dyspepsia. Fresh juice is bitter and pungent. Root and stem barks are used as antipyretic. Aegelin, a sterol isolated from the leaves, has been tried to treat bronchial spasm. The cathartic action is caused by the swelling of the mucilaginous seed coat, therefore, giving bulk and lubrication. The seed should be taken with a considerable amount of water. In combination with powdered anhydrous dextrose, sodium bicarbonate, monobasic potassium phosphate, citric acid and others, plantago husk is used as remedy for constipation.

GUAR GUM

Synonyms

Guar flour; Decorpa; Jaguar; Jaguar gum; Guaran; Gum cyamopsis; Cyamopsis gum; Burtonite V-7-E; Guar galactomannan.

Biological source

Guar gum is the ground endosperms of *Cyamopsis tetragonolobus* (L.) Taub. (Family: Leguminosae).

Habitat

The plant is cultivated in dry climates in India (Maharashtra, Gujarat, Karnataka and Rajasthan), Pakistan and USA (Texas).

It is a robust, erect, annual, 1-3 m high plant, bearing cluster of thick and fleshy pods.

The plant is hardy and drought-resistant. It grows well on deep alluvial soils and sandy loams. It is cultivated usually as a mixed crop. The seeds are sown broadcast in northern India in May-June and harvested in September-October.

Characters

Guar gum is a pale-yellow free flowing powder; completely soluble in cold and hot water; practically insoluble in oils, greases, hydrocarbons, ketones and esters. Water solutions are tasteless, odourless, nontoxic and neutral. It is stable to heat. It has five to eight times the thickening powder of starch. It forms thick colloidal solution in water and swells rapidly. The water soluble fraction (85%) is called guaran.

Chemical constituents

Guar gum contains mainly of a high molecular weight hydrocolloidal polysaccharide which is a galactomannan. Guaran consists of linear chains of $(1\rightarrow4)$-β-D-mannopyranosyl units; 1,6-linked α-D-galactopyranosyl units are attached to alternate mannose units. Ratio of D-galactose to D-mannose is 1 : 2. On hydrolysis Guar gum yields galactose and mannose. It also contains small amount of proteins (5-7%).

This molecular structure gives properties that are intermediate between those associated with branched and linear hydrocolloids. The gum hydrates in cold water and is stable in acidic formulations.

The drug also contains flavonol, glycosides 3-O-(2-glucosylrhamnosido)-7-O-β-(2-rhamnosyl glucosido) myricetin and kaempferol-3-O-(2-dirhamnosylglucosido)-7-O-glucoside and a saponin of 3β-hydroxy-12-en-29-oate (3-epikatonic acid). The lipid soluble compounds are palmitate, oleate, linoleate and some long chain fatty acids. Seed hydrolysate contains gallic acid, galactose and flavonoids. The seed coat pigment is composed of iron salts of galactose, gallic acid and 2,3, 4-trihydroxybenzoic acid.

Free fatty acids and their esters are also present.

Chemical tests

1. Powdered Guar gum on treatment with ruthenium red does not form pink colour (difference from Sterculia and Agar).
2. Aqueous solution of Guar gum is converted to a gel by small amount of borax.
3. Aqueous solution of Guar gum is precipitated with 2% solution of lead acetate.
4. Aqueous solution of Guar gum does not produce any colour with iodine solution.
5. TLC analysis of the gum shows the presence of mannose and galactose.

6. The gum must pass a limit test for total viable aerobic count (not more than 10^3 micro-organisms/g) and tests for *E. coli* and *Salmonella* species.

Uses

Guar gum is used as a bulk-forming laxative, binder and disintegrator; as an emulsifying agent, as a protective colloid, stabilizer, thickening and film forming agent for cheese, salad dressings, ice creams and soups; in pharmaceutical jelly formulations; in suspensions, emulsions, lotions, creams, toothpastes; in the mining industry as a flocculent, as a filtering agent; and in water as a coagulant aid. Guar gum is also used to cure colopathies with constipation.

Guar gum is used recently as a possible oral hypoglycaemic drug. It can produce changes in gastric emptying and in the gastrointestinal transition time, which can delay absorption of sugars and oligosaccharides from the gut. It lowers LDL and cholesterol levels, possibly by binding bile salts in the gut without affecting other lipoproteins and without decreasing triglycerides. However, the contribution of guar gum to diabetic control 'remained unproven'. The gum has 5-6 times the thickening power of starch and is used in the food industry.

Pharmacology

The seeds lower blood sugar and total lipid levels in guinea pigs. Guar gum delayed gastric emptying rate but did not effect glucose absorption rate in glucose tolerance in total gastroectomised rats. Guar gum inhibited rapid increase in blood sugar levels. Both Guar gum and galactomannan delayed elimination of glucose from blood. The seeds depress growth in poultry and rat.

Fructans

Fructans are D-fructose polymers in which each chain being terminated by a single D-glucosyl residue. They are found in nature as oligosaccharides with up to 10 units and as polysaccharides with up to 50 units. Inulin is a reserve carbohydrate found in many roots of members of the Asteraceae and Campanulaceae. The tubers of the Jerusalem artichoke (*Helianthus tuberosus*) and roots of chicory

(*Cichorium intybus*) are rich sources. Other fructans are the phleins found in grasses, *e.g.*, in *Phleum pratense*, and sinistrin present in *Urginea maritima*.

Biosynthesis

Fructans are not produced by the conjugation of identical monosaccharide units. They originate with a molecule of sucrose (glucose + fructose) to which is added further molecules of furanofructose. No monosaccharide nucleotide (*e.g.*, glucose adenine diphosphate) is involved in the addition of the fructose and two fructose molecules occur in nature and the mode of the linkage of the second fructosyl unit to the sucrose and the extent of the addition of more fructosyl units to the trisaccharide determine the properties of the final polymer. Inulin biosynthesis proceeds via the enzymatic transfer of a fructosyl group from sucrose to another molecule of sucrose giving the trisaccharide 1-ketose and free glucose. A second enzyme (a fructan fructosyltransferase) then mediates the addition of further fructosyl units from other oligomeric fructans. The final molecule is terminated at one end by a glucosyl unit. However, for the formation of various fructans different fructosylsucrose trisaccharides are involved and elongation of the polymer chain may occur at either end of the trisaccharide so that the final fructan molecule has a glucosyl residue situated towards the middle of the chain.

PECTIN

Biological source

Pectin is a purified complex polysaccharide substance present in cell walls of all plant tissues which functions as an intercellular cementing material. It is a purified carbohydrate obtained from the dilute acid extract of inner portion of the peel of citrus fruits or from apple pomace. Lemon or orange rind is the richest source of pectin which contains about 30% of this polysaccharide. Other sources of pectin are papaya, guava, mangoes and roots (beets and gentian).

Geographical source

On commercial scale pectin is prepared in India, USA, Switzerland and some other European countries.

Preparation

Pectins are abundant in unripe fruits. At first they are insoluble and import rigidity to the tissues. Later on they are degradated to monosaccharides and acids during ripening. Pectin occurs in the middle lamellae of cell walls, and in an insoluble form it is called as protopectin. It is converted to the soluble form pectinic acids (pectins) by treating the fruit pulp with a 20 times its weight of dilute acid at high temperature (90°C) for 30 minutes at pH 3.4-4. The aqueous solution is filtered, and alcohol is added to the filtrate to precipitate pectin. The precipitated pectin is separated and dried under reduced pressure. On commercial scale, pectin is extracted from citrus waste (2-4% in fresh pulp) and residual pulp of apple left over after extracting juice. After inactivating the enzymes by boiling, pectin is dissolved in hot acidic aqueous solution. The extract is filtered, freed from starch and treated with isopropanol to precipitate pectin,

Characters

Pectin occurs as a coarse or fine powder, yellowish-white in colour, practically odourless, and taste is mucilaginous. It is almost completely soluble in 20 parts of water, forming a viscous opalescent and colloidal solution containing negatively charged, very much hydrated particles. Aqueous solution is acidic to litmus. It is insoluble in alcohol and in other organic solvents. It is stable under mildly acidic conditions. Depolymerization takes place in more strongly acidic or basic conditions.

Alkaline pectates are soluble in water; pectates of di- and trivalent cations are sparingly or not all soluble. In solutions, the carboxylic groups of the polyanion are ionized and the molecules repulse one another. Pectin hot solutions form gel upon cooling. Gelification is rapid in the presence of calcium by formation of junction zones of the egg-box type. In methylated pectins, gel formation takes place slowly in acidic medium and in the presence of sucrose.

Chemical constituents

Pectins are glycanogalacturonans in which mono-saccharides are linked to galacturanans. Pectins from different sources vary in their complex constitution; the principal components being blocks of D-galacturonic acid residues linked by α-1,4-glycosidic linkages and interspersed with rhamnose units; some of the carboxyl groups are methylated. These molecules are combined with small amounts of neutral arabinans (branched polymers of α-1,5-linked L-arabofuranose units) and galactans (linear chains of β-1,4-linked D-galactopyranose units). Pectin occurs naturally as partial methyl ester of α-(1 → 4) linked D-poly-galacturonate sequences interrupted with (1 → 2)-L-rhamnose residue. On hydrolysis it produces D-galactose, L-arabinose, D-xylose and L-fucose.

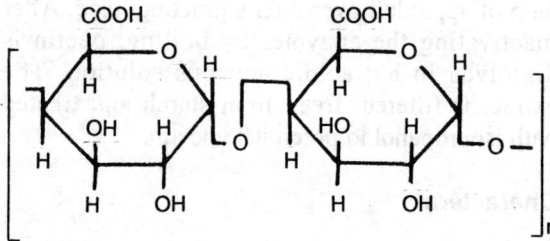

Fig. 14.7. Pectic acid.

Chemical tests

1. Pectin (1 g) is dissolved in water (10 ml). A stiff gel is produced.
2. To 1% aqueous solution of pectin add 2% aqueous solution of sodium hydroxide (5 ml). Within 20 minutes a transparent gel is produced. On shaking the gel with dilute hydrochloric acid gelatinous precipitates are formed which turn white on boiling.

Uses

Pectin is used in the treatment of vomiting in infants and diarrhoea due to property of colloidal absorption of toxins. It is also used as haemostatic for haemorrhage, as emulsifying agent, gelling agent, as a plasma substitute, for preparation of cosmetics, jellies and as a thickening agent in food industry for the sauces, jams and ketchup. As a colloidal solu-

tion, it has the property of conjugating toxins and enhancing the physiological action of the digestive tract through its physical and chemical properties. In the upper intestinal tract, pectin has a surface area composed of ultramicroscopical particles. These particles, called micelles, have the property of colloidal absorption of toxins. Pectins are efficacious in the control of blood cholesterol levels and to prevent cardio-vascular diseases.

ALGIN

Synonyms

Alginic acid sodium salt; Sodium alginate; Sodium polymannuronate; Kelgin; Minus; Protanal.

Biological source

Algin is a gelling polysaccharide of a mixture of polyuronic acids extracted with dilute alkali from giant brown seaweed, *Macrocystis pyrifera* (giant kelp), Family Lessoniaceae; or from *Laminaria digitata* (horsetail kelp), Family Laminariaceae, or from *Laminaria saccharina* (sugar kelp). Other sources are the species *Ascophyllum, Ecklonia* and *Nereocystis*. It contains not less than 19% and not more than 25% of carboxylic groups (COOH), calculated with reference to the dried substance.

Geographical source

USA (California), Norway, Chile, China, Canada, Iris Republic, Australia, Iceland, UK (Scotland), and South Africa.

Preparation

The dried milled seaweed is macerated with dilute sodium carbonate solution. The resulting paste-like mass is diluted with soft water to separate the insoluble matter by modern super-decanters or continuous-setting devices. The resulting clear liquor contains most of the alginate originally present in the algae. It is poured into dilute sulphuric acid or dilute calcium chloride solution, when the insoluble alginic acid or its salt, calcium alginate, is precipitated as a bulky, heavily hydrated gel from which liquor is separated by roller or expeller presses. Wood pulp-like product is obtained which is agitated against a stream of hydrochloric acid. Then calcium is removed and the highly swollen pulp of alginic acid is roller-pressed and then neutralized with sodium carbo-nate to give sodium alginate. In an another procedure the sodium alginate may be precipitated from the clear liquor by addition of ethyl alcohol directly or after partial evaporation.

Characters

Algin is a cream-coloured powder, soluble in water, forming a viscous and colloidal solution, insoluble in alcohol and in hydro-alcoholic solution in which the alcohol content is >30% v/v. It is in-soluble in chloroform, ether and in aqueous acid solutions when the pH is below 3. It liberates carbon dioxide from carbonates. With compounds containing ions of alkali, metals, or ammonium or magnesium, it reacts to give salts (alginates) which are water soluble. The salts of most other metals are water-insoluble.

Chemical constituents

Alginic acid is composed of residues of D-mannu-ronic and L-glucuronic acids; the chain length is long and varies with the method of isolation and the source of algae. The sugar units are joined by β-1, 4-glycosidic linkages.

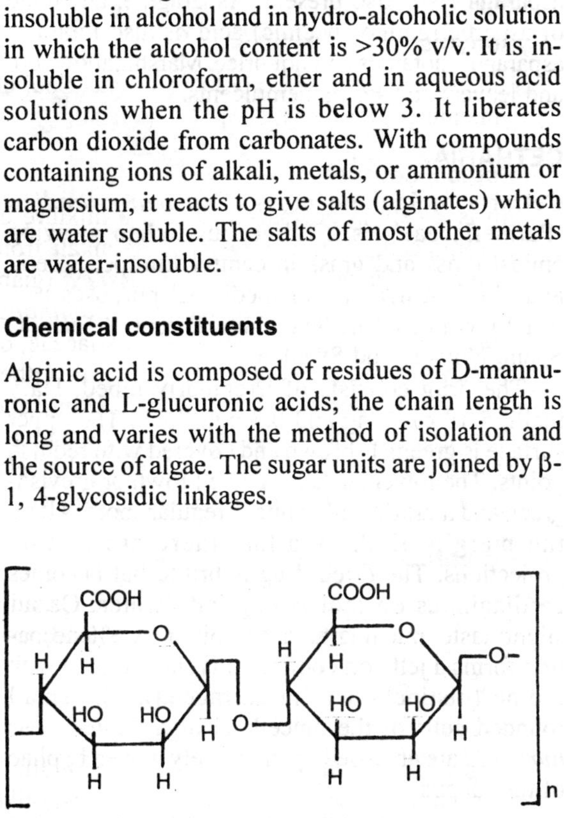

Fig. 14.8. Algin.

The composition varies according to the biological source, thus providing a range of properties which are exploited commercially. It is a hetero-polyuronide consisting of chains of β-1,4-linked D-mannuronic acid units interspersed with lengths of α-1,4-linked L-guluronic acid units together with sections in which the two monouronide units are regularly interspersed. In alginic acids from differ-ent sources the ratios of the two uronic acids vary

from 2 : 1 to 1 : 2. The chain length varies with the method of preparation and molecular weight. Its molecules vary from 220 to 860 units.

Uses

Alginates are used as stabilizing, digestant, thick-ening, emulsifying, deflocculating, gelling and film- and filament-forming agents in the rubber, paint, textile, food (including as stabilizing colloid), cos-metics and pharmaceutical industries. It is also used in drilling muds; in coatings, in flocculation of sol-ids in water treatment; as sizing agent, thickener, emulsion stabilizer, suspending agent in soft drinks and in dental impression preparations. Alginate fi-bres are used as absorable haemostatic dressings.

Algin is metabolized in the body. It has a ca-loric value of about 1.4 calories per gram. Alginic acid is relatively less soluble in water. It is used as a tablet binder and thickening agent. Gel-forming properties are associated with salts of different poly-valent cations and alginic acid. The propylene gly-col ester of Algin has been prepared. It is useful in formulations that require greater acid stability than that of the parent hydrocolloid.

Alginates are combined with sodium bicarbo-nate and aluminium hydroxide and taken after meals. Gastric acidity frees alginic acid which forms a foamy gel and forms a floating barrier over the gas-tric contents. The gel protects the mucosa of the esophagus against aggression by the gastric juice. Alginates are incorporated into antacids prepara-tions. Calcium alginate is used as a hemostatic wool or gauze. In contact with blood and exudates, it forms a fibrillar gel resulting in a rapid hemostasis. The alginate wool is used for bleeding of wounds or epistaxis, in stomatology (tooth extraction) and for as a dressing for cutaneous ulcers.

Alginates are also used for disintegrating prop-erties; for slow-release formulations and for formu-lations resistant to gastric acidity. Due to their film-forming, emollient and hydrating properties, they are added in skin preparations.

QUINCE SEEDS

Quince seeds are obtained from *Cydonia oblonga* (Rosaceae), a tree cultivated in South Africa, Cen-tral Europe and the Middle East. Iran is the main producer of Quince seeds, supplying about 75% of the total world production.

The seeds are separated from the pear-shaped fruits and dried. They adhere together in masses due to their surface coating of dried mucilage. The mucilage (20%) is derived from the outer epidermis of the testa. The mucilage is composed of units of arabinose, xylose and uronic acid derivatives. The seeds also contain 15% of fixed oil and a small quantity of cyanogenetic glycoside and an enzyme which effects its hydrolysis. The seeds are used as a demulcent, and emulsifying agent and in the preparation of hair-fixing lotions.

SLIPPERY ELM BARK

Slippery elm bark is obtained from *Ulmus rubra* (*Ulmus fulva*) (Ulmaceae), a tree 15-20 m in height found in the USA and in Canada. In the spring, old bark is stripped from the trees. The outer part of the bark is removed. The inner part, which forms the commercial drug, is dried.

The drug occurs in broad, flat strips, about 50-100 cm in length and from 1 to 4 mm in thickness. A few reddish-brown patches of the imperfectly removed rhytidome is present. The bark consists only of secondary phloem. The outer surface is brownish-yellow and striated, the inner surface yellowish-white and finely ridged. The bark is identified by the characteristic, fenugreek-like odour and the strongly fibrous fracture.

The chief constituent of the bark is mucilage, which is a mixture of two or more polyuronides. The mucilage has demulcent, emollient and nutritive properties.

MARSHMALLOW ROOT

Marshmallow root is derived from *Althaea officinalis* (Malvaceae), a perennial herb, which is found wild in moist situations in southern England and Europe.

The plant has a woody root-stock with the numerous roots up to 30 cm in length. The drug is collected from cultivated plants 2 years old. The roots are dug up in the autumn, scraped free from cork and dried.

The drug occurs in whitish, fibrous pieces,

15-20 cm long and 1-2 cm in diameter, or in small transverse slices. Odour slight; taste sweetish and mucilaginous. The bark is about 1-2 mm thick, separated by a greyish, sinuate cambium from the white, radiate wood. There are numerous mucilage cells, the contents of which are coloured a deep yellow by a solution of sodium hydroxide.

Marshmallow root contains about 10% of mucilage. It, on hydrolysis, gives a number of sugars. Starch, pectin and sugars and about 2% of asparagine are also present. Asparagine, an amide of aspartic (amino-succinic) acid, is also found in asparagus, potatoes and liquorice. Marshmallow root and leaves are used as demulcents.

CETRARIA

Cetraria or Iceland moss, *Cetraria islandica* (Parmeliaceae), is a foliaceous lichen growing amidst moss and grass in central Europe, Siberia and North America. For medicinal purposes it is usually collected in Scandinavia, central Europe, Spain, Norway and Sweden.

The drug consists of irregularly lobed, leafy thalli, 5-10 cm long and 0.5 mm thick. The upper surface is greenish-brown and covered with reddish points. The lower surface is pale brown or greyish-green and marked with white, irregular spots. Along the margin of the thallus, there are minute projections. The dried drug is brittle but becomes cartilaginous on moistening with water. Odour slight; taste, mucilaginous and bitter. A 5% decoction forms a jelly on cooling. It is stained blue with iodine (distinction from carrageen). The small rounded cells of the unicellular alga *Cystococcus humicola* are enclosed by the closely woven hyphae of the fungus.

The lichen contains mucilage and is utilized in cosmetic preparations and in sizing textiles. It is a source for glucose and used for the production of alcohol.

The lichen is tough when damp, but brittle when dry. It has a slight odour and a bitter, mucilaginous taste. It is used as a tonic in convalescence and exhausting diseases and haemoptysis. The bread prepared from it is given to diabetics. The lichen possesses demulcent property and its decoction is given as tea or as pastille in chronic catarrh, bronchitis and cough. In jelly form, it improves appetite and digestion. Its excessive use may cause loose bowels. It is also used for the care of skin and hair, as a substitute for salve-bases in the preparation of emulsions and in distinguishing the bitter taste of certain drugs. It is also used for the preparation of culture-medium for bacteria.

Lichenin is soluble in hot water and is not coloured blue by iodine containing sodium bicarbonate. Isolichenin is soluble in cold water and gives a blue colour with iodine. Both on hydrolysis give glucose. Cetraria also contains a very bitter depsidone, cetraric acid, and other acids such as lichestearic and usnic acids. The gum from the powdered plant appears to be hemicellulose containing uronic acid, galactose, mannose and glucose. The latter compound is an antibiotic. Iceland moss is used as a bitter tonic and for disguising the taste of nauseous medicines. It is used in hair-setting lotions and other cosmetics. Sea biscuits prepared from cetraria are more resistant to weevil infestation than when wheat flour alone is used.

Chemical constituents .

The lichen contains lichenin (40%), isolichenin (10%), glucose, glycerol, umbilicin, cetraric, protocetraric, fumarprotocetraric, lichesteric, protolichesteric, dl-usnic and fumaric acids, friedelin, cetrarin, fatty acids, ribonuclease; flavanones, flavones, quinones and iodine. The lichen polysaccharide contains D-galacto-D-mannans. The soluble proteins are albumin, glutelins, prolamines and globulins.

Lichenin and isolichenin are effective against sarcoma 180 in mice. Cetrarin promotes the flow of bile and pancreatic juices on intravenous administration. The usnic acid and protolichesteric acid in the lichen and its crude, aqueous extract show antibacterial activity against several pathogenic bacteria. Lichenin or moss-starch is insoluble in cold water but soluble in hot water and forms gelatin on cooling. A light-coloured transparent and high-grade gelatin, isinglass, is prepared from Iceland moss. A hemicellulose gum, similar to locust-bean gum, is also extracted. Glycerol is extracted from the lichens which is used in cold creams. The lichen is used to dye woollens.

INULIN

Inulin was first obtained from the dahlia, *Inula helenium* (Asteraceae). It is particularly abundant in taraxacum, inula (elecampane), lappa (burdock root) echinacea (cone flower), and chicory (succory or blue dandelion root). Inulin is obtained by immersing the fresh rhizome or root in alcohol for some time, the inulin usually crystallizes in sphaerite aggregates. It occurs either in solution in the cell sap or in alcohol-preserved material as sphaero-crystalline masses. It is hygroscopic, sparingly soluble in cold water but readily dissolves at around 70°C without gelatinizing. It is not stained by iodine solution and not hydrolysed by mammalian enzymes.

Chemically inulin consists of a chain of 35-50 1,2-linked fructofuranose units terminated by one glucose unit. The furanose ring systems render the molecules much less rigid in comparison to cellulose or starch. In a sample of inulin there is a mixture of molecular species, the smaller molecules being probably intermediates in the polymerizing chain. Its molecular weight is about 5,000. It forms spherical crystals from water.

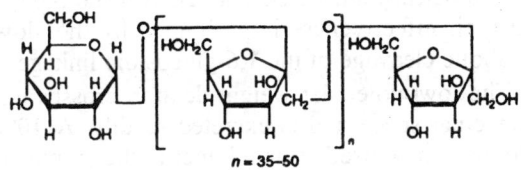

Fig. 14.9. Inulin

Inulin is a D-fructo-furanose polymer whose residues are linked in linear fashion by β-2,1 bonds. Inulin is used in culture media as a fermentative identifying agent for certain bacteria and in special laboratory methods for the evaluation of renal function. It is filtered only by the glomeruli and is neither excreted nor reabsorbed by the tubules. The usual dose is 10 g dissolved in 100 ml of sodium chloride injection by intravenous infusion.

Inulin is not metabolized by the body and is excreted unchanged making it a useful reagent for the testing of renal efficiency. It has potential use in the food and drinks industry as a source of fructose.

DEXTRAN (INN)

Dextran is an α-1,6-linked polyglucan that is formed from sucrose by the action of a transglucosylase enzyme system (dextran sucrase) present in *Leuconostoc mesenteroides.*

$$\text{nSucrose} + \underset{\text{Primer}}{\text{(Glucose)}} \rightarrow \underset{\text{Dextran}}{\text{(Glucose)}_{x+n}} + \text{nFructose}$$

These molecules are branched, of high molecular weight and are synthesized by an exocellular enzyme present in various bacteria of the genera *Leuconostoc, Lactobacillus* and *Streptococcus.* The enzyme dextransucrase polymerizes α-glucopyranosyl moieties by transfer from sucrose.

Dextrans of the desired size are prepared by controlled depolymerization (acid hydrolysis, fungal dextranase, or ultrasonic vibration) of native dextrans or by controlled fermentation. Dextrans with clinical utility have average molecular weights of 40,000, 70,000, and 75,000. The two large dextrans are used in 6% solutions as plasma expanders in shock or pending shock caused by hemorrhage, trauma, or severe burns. Dextran is not a substitute for whole blood. Osmolarity and viscosity of Dextran preparations resemble those of plasma, they are serologically indifferent and relatively non-toxic, and their effectiveness is prolonged by the slow metabolic cleavage of the 1,6-glucosidic linkage.

The low-molecular-weight dextran crosses extravascular space and is excreted readily. A 10% solution can be used as an adjunct in the treatment of shock. It reduces blood viscosity and improves microcirculation at low flow states. Dextrans interfere with some laboratory tests and many significantly increase clotting time.

Iron dextran injection is a sterile, colloidal solution of ferric hydroxide in complex with partially hydrolyzed dextran of low molecular weight in water for injection. It is a hematinic preparation that is administered by intramuscular or intravenous injection. Iron dextran injection is useful when oral iron preparations are not well tolerated.

Dextran is non-toxic, serologically neutral, of prolonged action and completely eliminated. It is a plasma substitute used for plasma volume expansion in shock due to hemorrhage, trauma and toxic infection and for preoperative hemodilution. It inferferes with hemostasis. In combination with sorbitol, it is used to treat edema of serious cerebral infarctions. Dextran formulation of eye drops is prescribed to cure lacrymal insufficiency and to improve the comfort of contact lens bearers by maintaining a lubricating film on the cornea. Dextran sulphate formulation is used as anti-inflammatory in traumatology (sprains, dislocation, contusions), phlebology and rheumatology (tendinitis, small joint arthropathy). Dextranomer (INN) is used to cleanse wounds and ulcers through absorption of exudates and tissue debris.

CARRAGEENAN (Iris moss, Chondrus, Carrageen, Carragenin)

It is a mixture of closely related hydrocolloids obtained from red algae or seaweeds. *Chondrus crispus* (L.) Stack and *Gigartina mamillosa* Agardh (Family : Gigartinaceae) are major sources of corrageenan.

These plants are common along the north-western coast of France, the British Islands, the coast of Nova Scotia and from Norway to North Africa. The name carrageenan is derived from the Irish coastal town of carragheen.

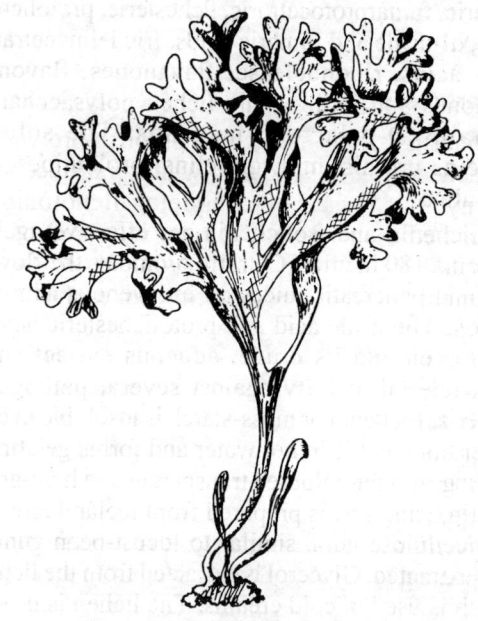

Fig. 14.10. *Chondrus crispus.*

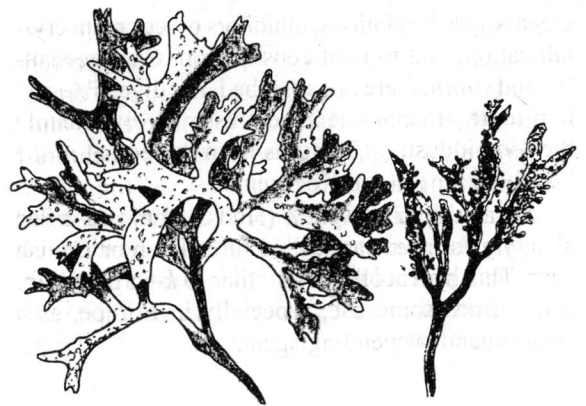

Fig. 14.11. *Gigartina* species.

Collection and preparation

The algae grow on rocks just below low-water mark. In Ireland collection takes place during the autumn; in America, during the summer. Carrageen is bleached by spreading it on the shore and submitting it for some weeks at suitable intervals. After drying in sheds, the drug is packed in bales weighing up to 300 kg. World production of Irish moss is around 20,000 tonnes.

Carrageenan is obtained from red seaweeds by extraction with water or aqueous alkali and recovered by alcoholic precipitation, drum drying or by freezing.

Characters

Chondrus is purplish-red to purplish-brown. The bleached drug is yellowish-white, translucent and horny. It consists of complete, dichotomously branched thalli about 5-15 cm long and of very variable form, some thalli having broad fan-like segments, others having ribbon-like ones. Many samples of Chondrus contain large quantities of the related alga *Gigartina mamillosa*. These algae may be distinguished from one another by the form of their large compound cytocarps, which contain carpospores. Chondrus has oval cystocarps about 2 mm long which are sunk in the thallus, while *G. mamillosa* has peg-like ones about 2-5 mm long. *G. pistillata* is rare round the coast of Britain, and its presence would indicate a drug of French origin.

Chondrus is sometimes covered with calcareous matter which effervesces with hydrochloric acid.

The drug has a slight odour and a mucilaginous and saline taste.

Chondrus swells in cold water, about 47% slowly dissolving, while on boiling about 75% passes into solution. A 5% decoction forms a jelly on cooling. A cooled 0.3% solution gives no precipitate with solution of tannic acid (distinction from gelatin) and gives no blue colour with iodine (distinction from Iceland moss and absence of starch). Dilute aqueous solutions are viscous. The viscosity increases almost logarithmically with increased concentrations. Aqueous solutions for gel on addition of hydrophobic cations such as potassium and ammonium. It is soluble in anhydrous hydrazine, sparingly soluble in formamide and methyl sulphoxide. It swells but does not dissolve in N,N-dimethylformamide. It is insoluble in oils and organic solvents. It precipitates proteins when pH of the solution is below the isoelectric point of the protein. A low concentrations, it causes agglomeration of milk proteins. Carrageenan undergoes depolymerization in acid solution. Solutions at pH 9 are most stable.

Constituents

The constituents of Carrageenan resemble those of Agar. It contains about seven galactans, known as carrageenans. Three important ones are κ-, t- and λ-carrageenans, which differ in the amount of 3,6-anhydro-D-galactose they contain and in the number and position of the ester sulphate groups. *C. crispus* produces different carrageenans in the two phases of its life cycle; κ-carrageenan predominates in the gametophyte generation and λ-carrageenan in the diploid tetrasporophyte generation. The drug is rich in halogen salts, and the extract differs from that of Agar in that it has a higher sulphate and ash content. Its structure consists of alternating copolymers of β-(1 → 3)-D-galactose and (1 → 4)-3,6-anhydro-D or L-galactose.

There are some differences in the specific properties and applications of the individual carrageenans. For example, *k*- and *i*-carrageenans tend to orient in stable helices when in solution, but λ-carrageenan does not. Consistent with these properties, *k*- and *i*-carrageenans are good gelating agents, and the nongelling λ-carrageenan is a more useful thickener.

Uses

Carrageenans are widely used to form gels and to give stability to emulsions, pastes, creams and suspensions. The firm texture and good rinsability of these hydrocolloids are particularly desirable in toothpaste formulations. They are also used as a demulcent, a bulk laxative, and an ingredient in many food preparations.

Chondrus is used as an emulsifying for cod liver oil and other oils, as a gelling and stabilizing agent, and as a binder in toothpastes, shampoos, ointments, creams, gels and lotions; inhibitors of ice cream crystallization; and to treat constipation. Carrageenans (k- and t-forms) are not absorbed, not digestible and non-toxic. Its many technical uses involve mainly the food industry. Chondrus is an ingredient in the laxative preparation, Kondremul.

Furecellaria fastigiata (Huds.) Lamour., a red alga, yields an extract called furcellaran or Danish agar. This hydrocolloid is similar to k-carrageenan, and it finds some use, especially in Europe, as a gelating and suspending agent.

Glycosides

Glycosides are compounds which upon hydrolysis give rise to one or more sugars (glycones) and a compound which is not a sugar (aglycone or genin).

In a glycosidic compound a sugar residue is linked to C-1 through oxygen (O-glucoside), nitrogen (N-glucoside) or sulphur (S-glucoside) moiety. β-D-Glucose is the most common sugar found in glycosides. The other sugars detected are rhamnose, digitoxose and cymarose (deoxysugar). The glycosides from individual sugars are called glucoside, rhamnoside, galactoside, fructoside, etc.

In glycosides the hydroxyl of a sugar is condensed with the hydroxyl of the non-sugar component. The secondary hydroxyl within the sugar molecule is condensed to form an oxide ring. Thus, they may be considered as acetals or sugar ethers. By acid or base catalyzed or enzymic hydrolysis glycosides yield the parent sugar together with the non-sugar compound. The sugar component is known as the *glycone*; while the nonsugar residue is called as *aglycone*. The aglycone may be an alcohol, phenol, cyanohydrin or complex fused ring or heterocyclic hydroxy compounds. More than one molecule of sugars may be present in glycosides which are formed by either separate linkages or stepwise substitution of the sugars to the aglycone. In plants only β-forms of glycosides are formed, although the α-linkage is detected in nature in some carbohydrates such as sucrose, glycogen and starch. In α-strophanthoside, the outer glucose molecule occurs in α-linkages and the inner glucose possesses β-linkage.

Most of the glycosides are colourless, crystalline compounds. Anthracene glycosides are red or orange coloured compounds and flavone glycosides are yellowish in colour. They are soluble in water and alcohol, but insoluble in other organic solvents like petroleum ether, solvent ether, chloroform and carbon tetrachloride. Glycosides are optically laevorotatory.

Classification

Various types of classifications of glycosides have been mentioned. On the basis of linkage of sugar molecules to aglycones, they are divided as follows:

1. *O-glycosides* : In these glycosides, the sugar is combined with alcoholic or phenolic hydroxyl function of aglycone; *e.g.,* digitoxin.
2. *N-glycosides* : In these glycosides, nitrogen of amino group ($-NH_2/-NH-$) is condensed with a sugar, *e.g.,* nucleoside.
3. *S-glycoside* : These glycosides contain a sugar moiety attached to a sulphur of the aglycone, *e.g.,* isothiocyanate glycosides.
4. *C-glycosides* : Condensation of a sugar directly to a carbon atom gives C-glycosides, *e.g.,* aloin and cascaroside. These glycosides are not hydrolyzed with acids, alkalies or enzymes.

On the basis of the chemical nature of aglycone the glycosides are classified as follows :

1. *Steroidal glycosides* : These glycosides contain a sterol as an aglycone, *e.g.,* diosgenin.
2. *Flavonoid glycosides* : A flavonoid aglycone is present in these glycosides, *e.g.,* rutin.

3. *Anthraquinone glycosides*: In these, glycosides, sugar moiety is attached to an anthracene aglycone, *e.g.*, frangulin, barbaloin.

4. *Cyanophoric glycosides* : Cyanogen is the aglycone part. They yield hydrocyanic acid on hydrolysis, *e.g.*, amygdalin, prunasin.

5. *Triterpenic glycosides* : A triterpene molecule is condensed with a sugar component, *e.g.*, glycyrrhizin.

6. *Alcohol glycosides*, *e.g.*, Salicin.

7. *Lactone glycosides*, *e.g.*, Hydroxycoumarin glycosides.

8. *Isothiocyanate glucosides*, *e.g.*, Sinigrin, sinalbin.

9. *Saponin glycosides*, *e.g.*, Dioscin.

Pharmacological classification of glycosides is dependent on their activities. For example, cardiac glycosides exhibit their action on the heart. Glycosides possessing bitter taste are called bitter glycosides, *e.g.*, glycosides of Gentianceae.

Glycosides are used for the treatment of various illness. Digitalis and Strophanthus contain glycosides and are used as cardiac stimulant drugs. Anthraquinone glycosides, present in Senna, Cascara, Rhubarb and Aloe, are used as laxative. Picrorhiza roots and rhizomes possess picroside glycosides and are utilized as bitter tonic and to protect damaged liver. Wild Cherry bark and Scilla glycosides have expectorant properties. Dioscin is a saponin glycoside found in the tubers of *Dioscorea* species and its hydrolysis furnishes diosgenin aglycone. Various steroidal drugs have been synthesized from diosgenin. Some glycosides are less effective in original form, but produce active compounds on hydrolysis. For example, sinigrin, a glycoside of black mustard, is non-irritating in its natural form, but on hydrolysis a powerful irritating substance, allylisothiocyanate, is formed.

Cardiac glycosides

These are steroidal glycosides and show highly specific and powerful action upon the cardiac muscles. The sugar part is attached at C-3 position of the steroidal nucleus. The steroid aglycone or genins are of two types :

(i) Cardenolides which are C_{23} steroids having an α, β-unsaturated five-membered lactone ring attached at 17β position. These compounds are present in Digitalis, Strophanthus, Oleander, Calotropis and Convallaria.

(ii) Bufadienolides which are C_{24} steroids having double unsaturated six-membered lactone ring at the 17α position. The name bufadienolides has been derived from the generic name for the toad, *Bufo*, since the compound bufalin was isolated from the skin of toads.

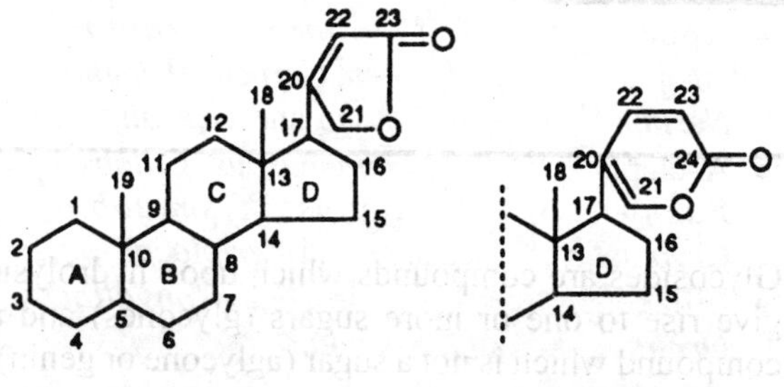

Cardenolide   Bufadieolide

Fig. 15.1. Cardiac glycoside aglycones.

For maximum cardiac activity the aglycone should possess an α, β-unsaturated lactone ring attached β-position at 17-carbon of the steroid nucleus and the A/B and C/D ring junctions should have the cis-configuration. The sugar portion of the glycoside helps in its absorption and distribution in the body. Oxygen substitution on the steroid nucleus also affects the distribution and metabolism of the glycosides. When number of hydroxyl groups is increased on the molecule, the more rapid is the action in the body. The heart-arresting properties of these glycosides render them most effective as arrow poisons.

Cardiac glycosides increase the force of systolic contraction and decrease the heart rate.

The sugar units, attached at C-3 of the steroid, are composed of up to three sugar molecules. Glucose, rhamnose, digitoxose and cymarose are the sugars usually attached to the aglycone. Cardiac glycosides containing cyclic sugars have been isolated from *Calotropis* species.

Distribution in nature

In plants cardiac glycosides are present in the Angiosperms. Cardenolides are more common in the Apocynaceae, Asclepiadaceae, Liliaceae (*e.g.*,

Convallaria), Ranunculaceae, Moraceae, Brassicaceae, Sterculiaceae, Euphorbiaceae, Tiliaceae, Celastraceae, Leguminosae and Scrophulariaceae. The bufanolides occur in some Liliaceae (*e.g.*, *Urginea*) and in some Ranunculaceae (*e.g.*, *Helleborus*). In toad venomes the genins are partly free and partly conjugated with suberylarginine.

Some of the main genera containing cardiac glycosides are :

- Apocynaceae : *Adenium, Acokanthera, Strophanthus, Apocynum, Cerbera, Tanghinia, Nerium, Thevetia, Carissa* and *Urechites.*
- Asclepiadaceae : *Gamphocarpus, Calotropis, Pachycarpus, Asclepias, Xysmalobium, Cryptostegia, Merabea* and *Periploca.*
- Liliaceae : *Urginea, Bowiea, Convallaria, Ornithogalum* and *Rohdea.*
- Ranunculaceae : *Adonis* and *Helleborus.*
- Moraceae : *Antiaris, Antiaropsis, Naucleopsis, Maquira* and *Castilla.*
- Brassicaceae : *Erysimum* and *Cheiranthus*;
- Sterculiaceae : *Mansonia.*
- Tiliaceae; seeds of *Corchorus* spp.
- Celastraceae : *Euonymus* and *Lophopetalum.*
- Leguminosae : *Coronilla.*
- Scrophulariaceae : *Digitalis.*

Structure of glycosides

Two types of genin with a five- or six-membered lactone ring, are present in cardiac glycosides, represented as cardenolides (*e.g.*, digitoxigenin) and bufanolides or bufadienolides (*e.g.*, scillarenin).

The sugar moieties, attached to the aglycone by a C-3,β-linkage, are composed of up to four sugar

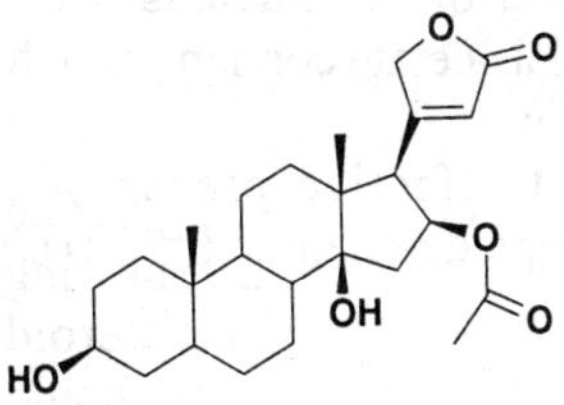

Oleandrigenin

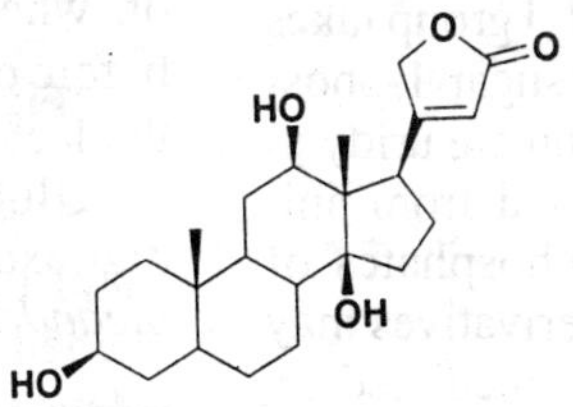

Digoxigenin

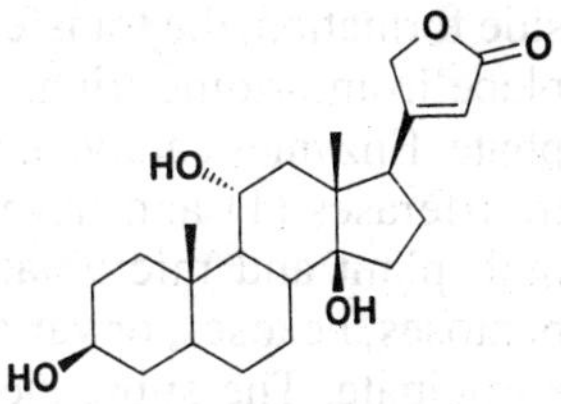

Sarmentogenin

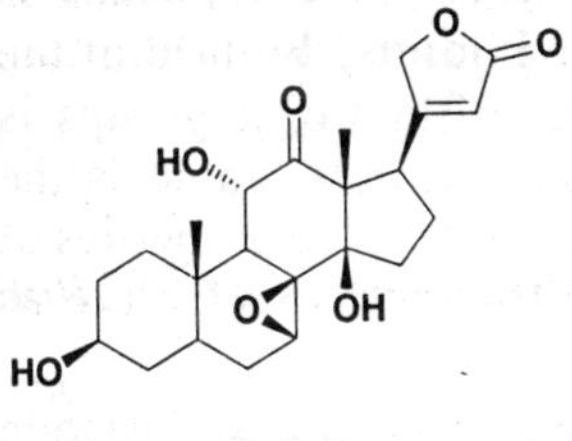

Sarverogenin

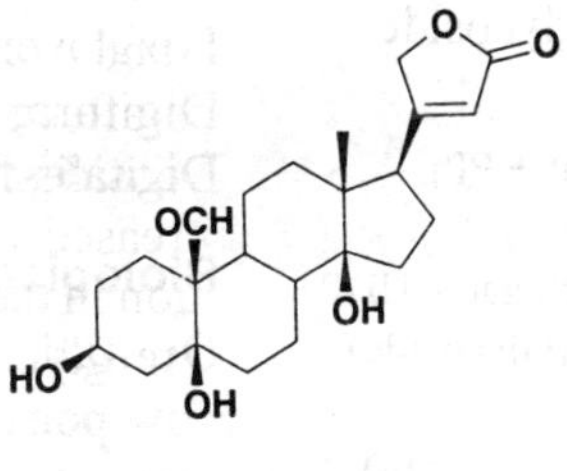

k-Strophantidin = cymarigenin

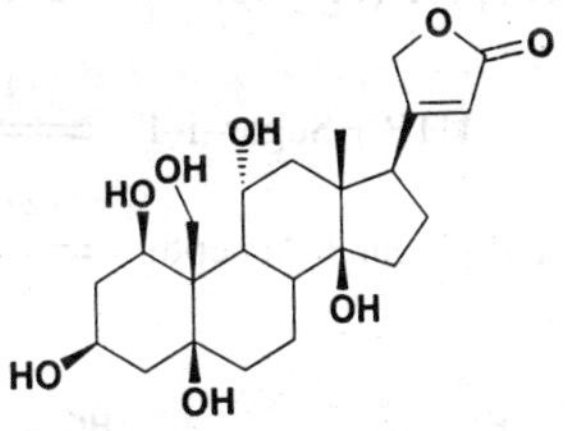

Ouabaigenin

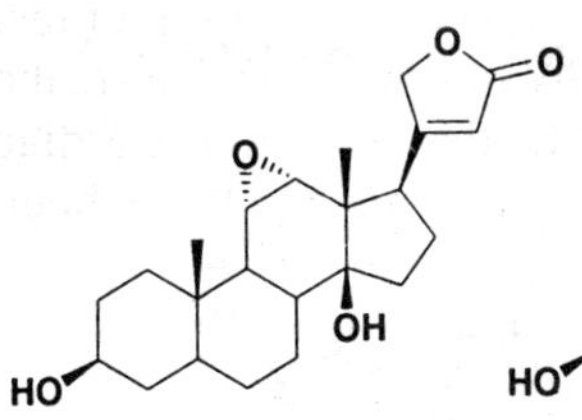

Cerbertigenin

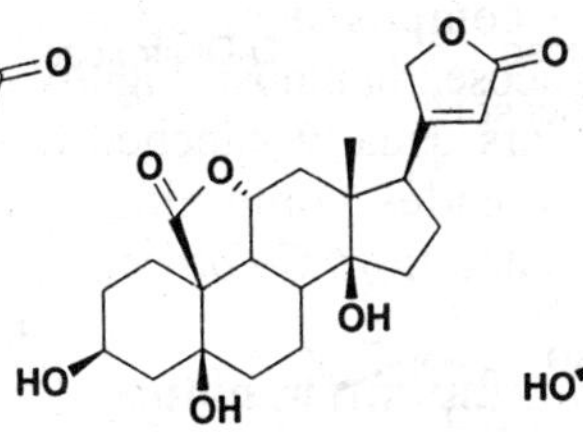

Strogogenin

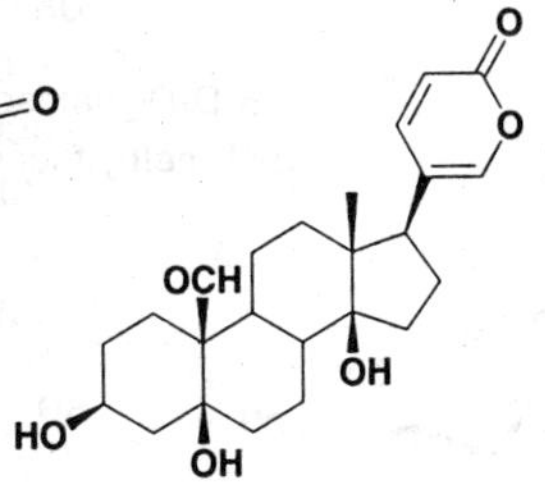

Hellebrigein

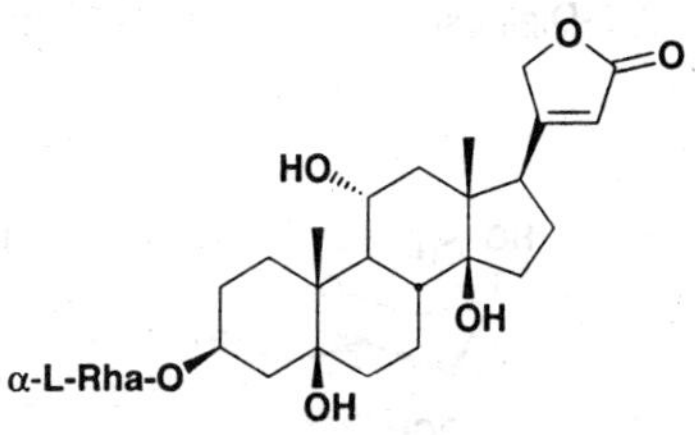

Lokundjoside

Fig. 15.2. Cardenolides.

units which may include glucose or rhamnose together with other deoxy-sugars whose natural occurrence is associated only with cardiac glycosides. The deoxy-sugars are 2,6-dideoxy-hexoses (*e.g.*, digitoxose) or their 3-*O*-methyl ethers (*e.g.*, cymarose). In addition to rhamnose and fucose, a number of other 6-deoxy-hexose derivatives are present together with 2-*O*-methyl and 2-*O*-acetyl sugars. In fucose, the D-form is known only in cardiac glycosides, where the L-form is widely distributed in nature. Cardiac glycosides involving cyclic sugars are present in *Calotropis* spp.

Biogenesis of cardiac glycosides

Consideration of glycoside (heteroside) biosynthesis consists of 2 parts. The general reactions couple a sugar residue to an aglycone. This transfer reaction is similar in all biologic systems. In glycoside formation, the transfer of a uridylyl group takes place from uridine triphosphate to a sugar 1-phosphate. Enzymes catalyzing this reaction are uridylyl transferases (1) and have been isolated from animal, plant and microbial sources. Phosphates of pentoses, hexoses, or various sugar derivatives may participate. The subsequent reaction, mediated by glycosyl transferases (2), involves the transfer of the sugar from uridine diphosphate to a suitable acceptor (aglycone), thus forming the glycoside.

$$\text{UTP} + \text{Sugar--i--P} \underset{(1)}{\rightleftharpoons} \text{UDP--Sugar} + \text{PPi}$$

$$\text{UDP--Sugar} + \text{Acceptor} \underset{(2)}{\rightleftharpoons} \text{Acceptor--Sugar} + \text{UDP}$$
$$\text{(Glycoside)}$$

When a glycoside is formed, other enzymes may transfer another sugar unit to the monosaccharide moiety, converting it to a disaccharide. Enzymes occur in various glycoside-containing plants that are capable of producing tri- and tetrasaccharide moieties of the glycosides by similar reactions.

Aglycones of the cardiac glycosides are derived from mevalonic acid but the final molecules arise from a condensation of a C_{21} steroid with a C_2 unit. Bufadienolides are condensation products of a C_{21} steroid and a C_3 unit.

Progesterone, formed with cardiac glycosides in *Digitalis lanata* as a result of feeding pregnenolone, is itself a precursor of the cardiac glycosides. In *Strophanthus kombe,* the cardenolides are formed as progesterone → 5β-pregnanolone → 5β-hydroxy-pregnanolone → cardenolides.

The alternative pathways may exist depending on whether hydroxylation of the nucleus occurs before or after the essential acetate condensation for the lactone ring formation.

Glucose is the most effective precursor of digitoxose and of the sugar side-chain of the *Nerium oleander* glycosides.

DIGITALIS

Synonyms

Foxglove; Purple foxglove; Fairy gloves; Digifortis; Digitora; Neodigitalis; Pildigis; Folia digitalis; Digitalis folium.

Biological source

Digitalis consists of dried leaves of *Digitalis*

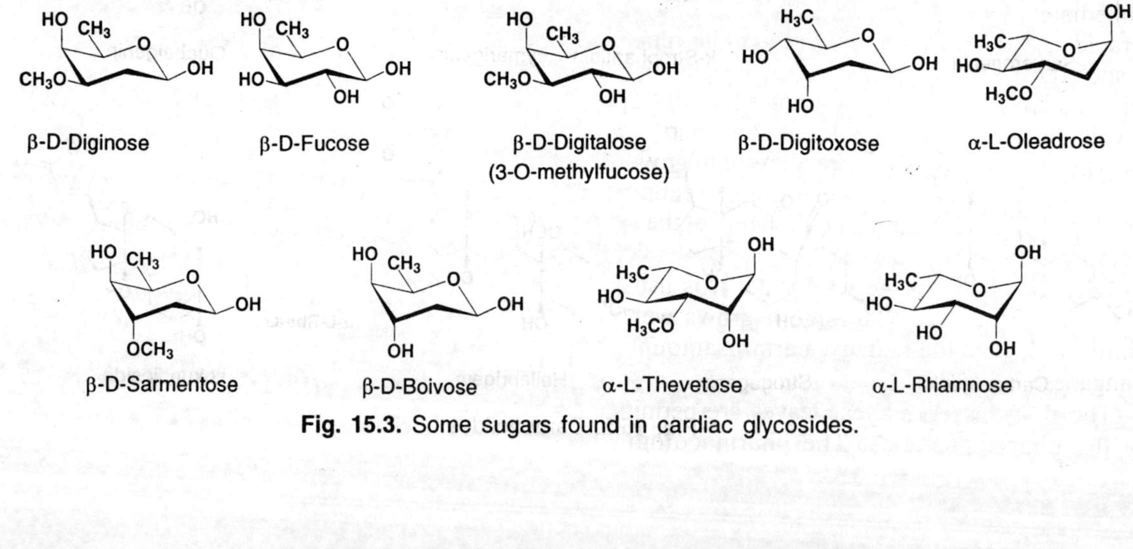

β-D-Diginose β-D-Fucose β-D-Digitalose (3-O-methylfucose) β-D-Digitoxose α-L-Oleadrose

β-D-Sarmentose β-D-Boivose α-L-Thevetose α-L-Rhamnose

Fig. 15.3. Some sugars found in cardiac glycosides.

purpurea Linn. possessing not less than 0.3 per cent of total cardenolides calculated as digitoxin. The collected leaves are immediately dried at a temperature below 60° and stored in a water proof container. The moisture should not be less than 5 per cent (Family : Scrophulariaceae).

Habitat

Southern and Central European countries, England, Germany, Holland, France, Northern USA and in Kashmir. In India it is cultivated in Kashmir at Tangmarg and Kishtwar at 2000-2300 m; Darjeeling and the Nilgiris.

Collection

Digitalis is a biennial herb occurring wildly. For its cultivation especially stained seeds are sown in a soil consisting of equal parts of clean sand, garden soil, manure and leaf mould in March. After about two months the seedlings are transferred in fields. In the first year the plant forms a rosette of leaves and in the second year an 1-1.5 m tall aerial stem. The inflorescence is a raceme of bell-shaped flowers of the floral formula K(5), C(5), A4 didynamous, G(2). The common wild form of the plant has a purple corolla about 4 cm long, the ventral side of which is whitish but bears deep purple eyespots on its inner surface. The fruit is a bilocular capsule which contains numerous seeds attached to axile placentae. The leaves are collected in the early afternoon from September to November by hand. Leaves of the first year crop contain maximum amount of active constituents. The leaves are dried immediately after collection below 60°C. If drying is rapidly, then characteristic green colour remains as such. Dried leaves are packed in airtight containers. Usually a desiccating substance like silica gel or calcium oxide is placed in the container to absorb moisture. Some plants are allowed to grow for the next year during flowering and seeds are developed which are used for cultivation of the next crop.

Digitalis grows in the wild state. It is usually found in semi-shady positions. It grows well in sandy soil, provided that a certain amount of manganese is present.

The first- or second-year leaves are permitted by the pharmacopoeias. The pharmacological activity of leaves increases during the course of a day to reach a maximum in the early afternoon. First-year leaves collected in July-August have the highest content of total glycosides and that after a fall during the winter months.

Characters

The leaves are linear or oblong-lanceolate, with obtuse or rounded apex, size 10-10 cm long and 4-8 cm wide. The margin is crenate to dentate with water pores on many teeth. Lamina is decussate at the tapering base. Upper surface is pubescent, dark green and little wrinkled and veins are depressed. The lower surface is greyish-green and veins are more prominent. Both the surfaces are hairy, but the lower surface is more hairy in comparison to upper one. Venation is pinnate, the veins are less prominent on the upper surface, lateral veins leave the mid-rub at an acute angle and anastomose on the margin. Petiole is winged, 2.5-10 cm in length. Odour is distinct and taste is bitter.

Microscopical characters

A transverse section of the leaf shows a typical bifacial structure and a midrib strongly convex on the lower surface. Stomata and hairs are present on both surfaces, but are more prominent on the lower one. The palisade tissue is absent at the midrib. A zone of collenchyma underlies both epidermis in the midrib region. The crescent-shaped midrib bundle is enclosed in an endodermis one or two cells thick developed as a starch sheath. The pericycle is parenchymatous above and collenchymatous below. Sclerenchymatous fibres and calcium oxalate are absent.

The upper epidermis consists of polygonal, straight-walled cells, with both clothing and glandular hairs. The cells of the lower epidermis are waxy. The stomata and hairs are more numerous on the lower side than on the upper surface of the leaf. The stomata are small and slightly raised above the surrounding cells. The clothing hairs are uniseriate, two- to seven-celled, bluntly pointed, smooth or finely warty, with cells often collapsed alternatively at right angles. The glandular hairs are unicellular with a short uniseriate pedicel and a unicellular or bicellular terminal gland. The cuticle of the hairs and epidermal cells may be stained red with a solution of Sudan Red in glycerin.

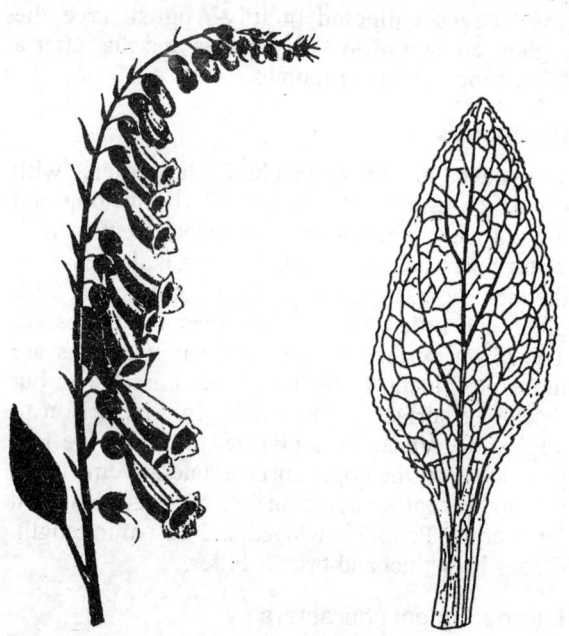

Fig. 15.4. *Digitalis purpurea* leaf.

Prepared Digitalis

This is a standardized powder; the strength is adjusted with weaker powdered digitalis or with powdered grass.

Chemical constituents

Digitalis contains about 35 glycosides. The most important compounds of medicinal importance are digitoxin, gitoxin and gitaloxin which are secondary glycosides. These glycosides possess a linear chain of three deoxy sugars at C-3 of the aglycone and not the terminal glucose as in purpurea glycosides A and B. These two glycosides are the prominent active components of the fresh leaves. When the drug is dried, enzymatic degradation takes place resulting the removal of terminal glucose to give digitoxin, gitoxin and gitaloxin.

Purpurea glycosides A and B and glucogitaloxin are the primary glycosides which contain a linear chain of three digitoxose sugar moieties terminated by the fourth sugar glucose at C-3 of the aglycone residue.

The other cardiac glycoside of Digitalis are glucodigitoxigenin-digitoxoside, acetyl glucogitoroside, glucoevatronoside, glucogitoroside, digitalinum verum, stropeside, glucogitaloxin, glucogitaloxigenin-bis-digitoxoside, gluco-lanadoxin, glucoverodoxin, verodoxin, digoxigenin-glucosylbis-digitoxoside, digitoxigenin-O-glucosyl-6-deoxyglucoside, glucodigifucoside, acetyl digitalinum verum and purlanosides A and B.

Digitoxin and gitoxin are the main active components of the dried drug. Poor storage conditions will lead to further hydrolysis and complete loss of activity. The gitaloxigenin series with its formyl group at C-16 is less stable than the other two series. The glycosides of this series have similar or greater activities than those of the digitoxigenin group. The aglycones digitoxigenin and gitoxigenin are produced by acid hydrolysis of the respective glycosides but they are not found in quantity in the fresh or dried leaves. The aglycones are formed in the plant via the acetate-mevalonate pathway common to other steroids; cholesterol, pregnenolone and progesterone serve as intermediates.

Other glycosides, present in small proportions, contain digitalose and glucose. They exist as mono- and diglycosides. In this group verodoxin has toxicity of three times that of gitaloxin.

In addition to cardiac glycosides tannins, inositol, luteolin, fatty matters, antirhinic acid, digitalosmin, digitoflavone and pectin have been reported in the drug. It also contains anthraquinone derivatives such as 1-methoxy-2-methylanthra-quinone, 3-methoxy-2-methyl-anthraquinone, digitolutein (3-methyl-alizarin-1-methyl ether), 3-methylalizarin and 1,4,8-trihydroxy-2-methyl-anthraquinone.

Saponins have also been isolated from the leaves, the sapogenins being produced more readily than cardenolides towards the end of the growing season. A number of leaf flavonoids have been isolated.

The plant also contain digogenin, digitonin, digipronins (sterol glycosides), isodigipronin, purpnigenin (aglycone purpnin), trihydroxy pregn-5-en-20-one, purpragenin, allodigitalinum verum, digacetigenin, odorobioside G, purlanosides A and B, digipurpurogenin, alloneogitostin, digicitrin (flavone), purpnin, purpronin, digiprogenins, degalactotigonin, F-gitonin (gitogenin-3β-lycote-

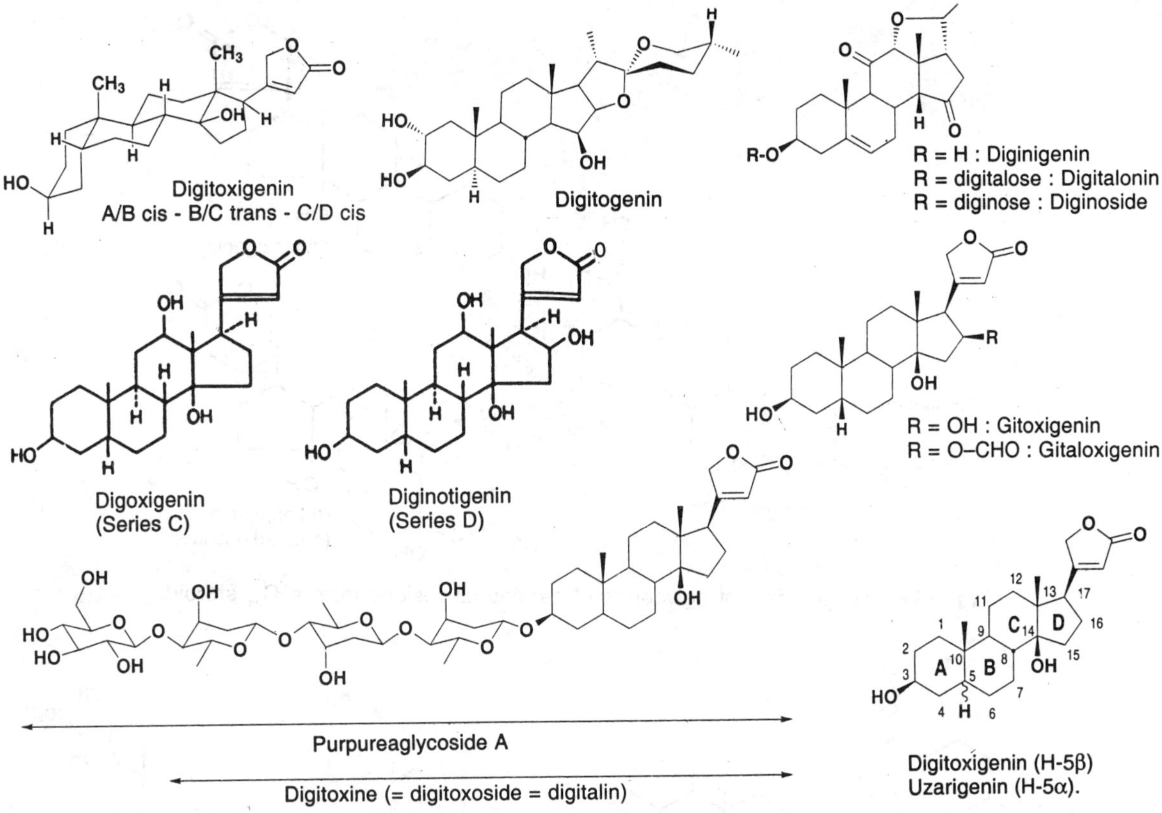

Digitoxigenin
A/B cis - B/C trans - C/D cis

Digitogenin

R = H : Diginigenin
R = digitalose : Digitalonin
R = diginose : Diginoside

Digoxigenin
(Series C)

Diginotigenin
(Series D)

R = OH : Gitoxigenin
R = O–CHO : Gitaloxigenin

Purpureaglycoside A

Digitoxine (= digitoxoside = digitalin)

Digitoxigenin (H-5β)
Uzarigenin (H-5α).

Fig. 15.5. Cardenolides.

traoside), digalonin, deglucodigitonin, digiprolac-tone, 1-methoxy- and 3-methoxy-2-methylanthra-qinone, digitolutein, digitopurpone, phomarin, isochrysophanol, cycloeucalenol, obtusifoliol, 24-ethylene-lophenol, β-sitosterol, stigmasterol, iso-fucosterol, campesterol, cholesterol, 24-methyl-enecholesterol, cycloartenol, 24-methyllo-phenol, 24-ethyllo-phenol, purpureagitoside, apigenin, dinatin, chrysoeriol, nepetin, derhamnosyl acteoside, forsythiaside and purpureasides A, B and C.

Uses

Digitalis is used as a cardiac stimulant and tonic. The drug stimulates cardiac muscles, increases the systole of heart ventricle and normalizes the heart frequency. The drug is useful in congestive heart failure, atrial flutter and atrial fibrillation.

They act by increasing cardiac output, relieving pulmonary congestion and peripheral edema.

Intoxication with *Digitalis* glycosides is common and hazardous. Toxic symptoms include anorexia, ventricular ectopic beats and bradycardia. In severe intoxication, symptoms are characterized by blurred vision, disorientation, diarrhoea, ventricular tachycardia and sinoatrial block.

Chemical tests

Digitalis glycosides respond to the following tests due to five-membered lactone ring present at C-17.

1. *Keller-Kiliani test for digitoxose* : Powdered digitalis leaf (1g) is boiled with 10 ml of 70% alcohol for 2-3 min., filter; dilute the filtrate with 10 ml of water and add 0.5 ml of strong solution of lead acetate; shake and filter. Shake the filtrate with 5 ml of chloroform, allow to separate, pipette off the chloroform and remove the solvent by gentle evaporation in a porce-

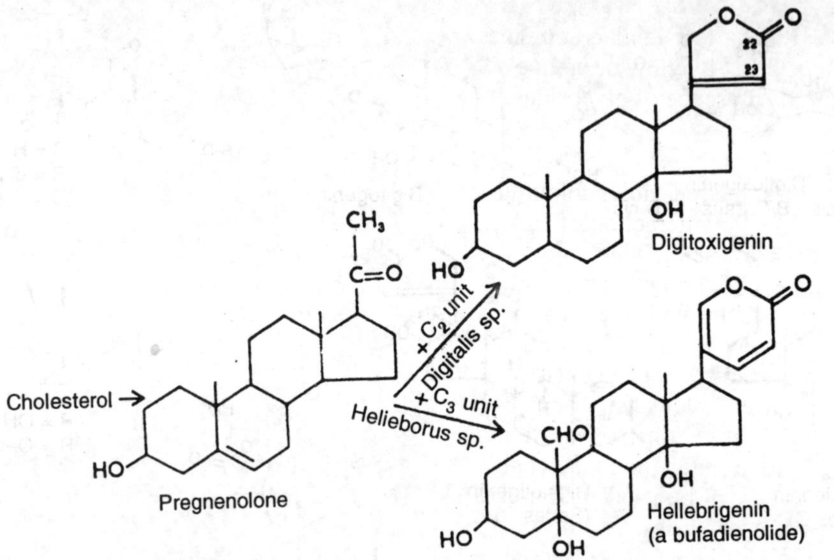

Fig. 15.6. Biosynthesis of aglycones of cardiac glycosides from a C_{21} steroid.

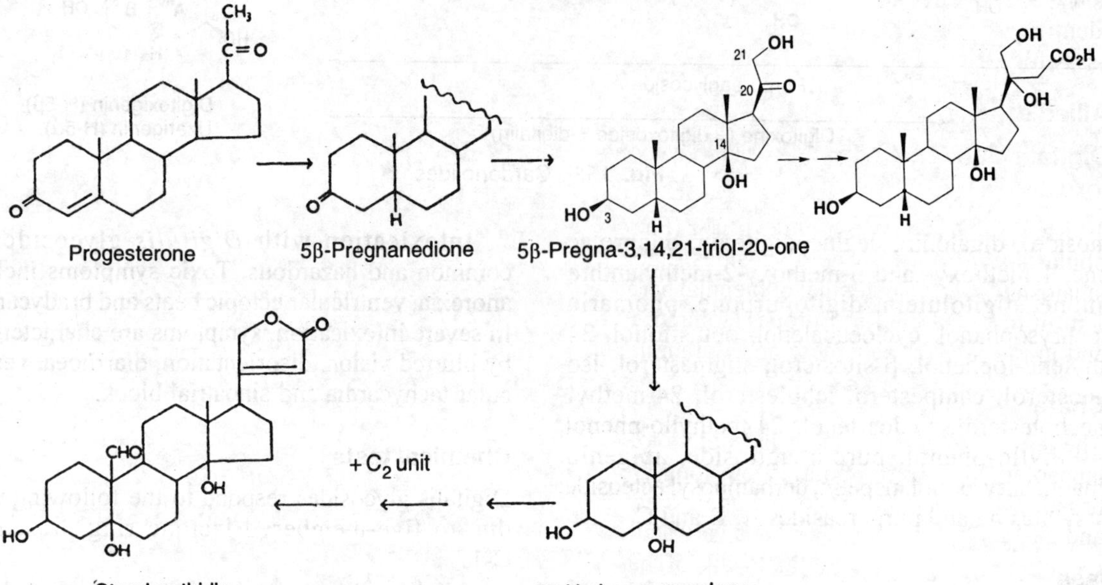

Fig. 15.7. Conversion of progesterone to cardiac glycosides.

lain dish. Dissolve the cooled residue is glacial acetic acid (3 ml) containing two drops of 5% ferric chloride solution. Transfer this solution to the surface of 2 ml of concentrated sulphuric acid; a reddish-brown layer forms at

the junction of the two liquids and the upper layer slowly becomes bluish-green, darkening with standing.

2. *Legal test* : To a solution of glycoside in pyridine, sodium nitroprusside solution and sodium

hydroxide solution are added. A pink to red colour is formed.

3. *Baljet test* : To a leaf lamina sodium picrate reagent is added. A yellow or orange colour is formed in the presence of glycosides.

Assay

For digitalis leaves, the red-violet colour (λ_{max} 540 nm) is produced by the interaction of cardenolides and 3,5-dinitrobenzoic acid. Other colour reactions based on the butenolide moiety are the red-orange (λ_{max} 495 nm) produced with the alkaline sodium picrate reagent (assay for digitoxin and digoxin), the red colour with xanthydrol reagent (test for digitalis leaf) and the red colour (λ_{max} about 470 nm) produced with sodium dinitroprusside. In the ultraviolet region the butenolide side-chain shows λ_{max} 217 nm which can be used for rapid evaluation. These spectroscopic tests do not distinguish between glycosides and their corresponding aglycones.

A colour test specific for the digitoxose moiety is the Keller-Killiani test. The test is used for the identification of digitoxin and digoxin and as an assay for digoxin injection and tablets (λ_{max} 590 nm).

Allied drugs

Digitalis lanata (Greecian Foxglove, Wooly foxglove

The leaves of *Digitalis lanata* Ehrh. (Fam. Scrophulariaceae) contain the glycosides digoxin and lanatoside C. It is a perennial or biennial herb, nearly 1 m in height, found in Europe, Holland, Ecuador and in Kashmir at Tangmarg and Baramulla.

Characters

The leaves are sessile, linear-lanceolate to oblong-lanceolate and up to about 30 cm long and 4 cm broad. The margin is entire, the apex is acuminate and the veins leave the midrib at a very acute angle. It contains the beaded anticlinal walls of the epidermal cells, the 10-14-celled nonglandular trichomes which are confirmed almost exclusively to the margin of the leaf, and the glandular hairs found on both surfaces; some have bicellular heads and unicellular stalks, while others have unicellular heads and 3-10-celled, uniseriate stalks. The pericyclic fibres and calcium oxalate are absent.

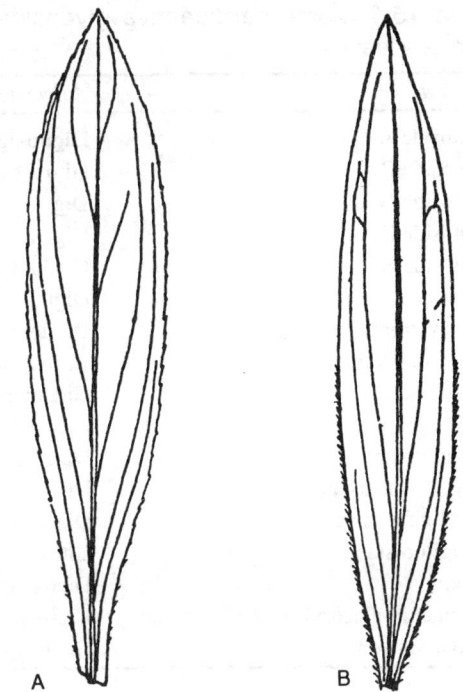

Fig. 15.8. Typical leaves of *Digitalis lutea* (A) and *D. lanata* (B).

Chemical constituents

D. lanata contains lanatosides A, B, C, D and E, acetyldigitoxin, digitoxin, glucogitoroside, digitalinum verum, deacetyl-lanatoside C, digoxin, glucolanadoxin and glucoverodoxin. The aglycone parts of lanatosides A-E are given in Table 15.1. Some flavone derivatives, *e.g.*, scutellarein, luteolin and dinatin have also been reported from *D. lanata*.

Partial hydrolysis of the glycosides occurs during the drying and storage of leaves, and deacetylation will produce the same products as in *D. purpurea*. The glycosides, involving digoxigenin and diginatigenin are found in the leaves. Digoxigenin glycoside levels is not influenced by collection date or by time of collection. However, total glycoside levels are higher in first-year leaves but the important medicinal glycosides (*e.g.*, lanatoside C) attain their highest levels in the second-year plants. The primary glycosides are stored exclusively in the vacuoles of cells.

Anthraquinone derivatives, similar to those found in *D. purpurea*, have been identified in the

Table 15.1. Some cardioactive glycosides of *D. lanata* leaves

Glycoside	Aglycone
Lanatoside A	Digitoxigenin
Lanatoside B	Gitoxigenin
Lanatoside C	Digoxigenin
Lanatoside D	Diginatigenin
Lanatoside E	Gitaloxigenin
Digitoxin	Digitoxigenin
Glucoevatromonoside	Digitoxigenin
Digitalinum verum	Gitoxigenin
Glucolanadoxin	Gitaloxigenin
Acetyldigitoxin	Digitoxigenin
Acetyldigoxin	Digoxigenin
Deacetyl-lanatoside C	Digoxigenin
Glucodigifucoside	Digitoxigenin
Glucogitoroside	Gitoxigenin
Digoxin	Digoxigenin
Digoxigenin-glucosyl-bis-digitoxoside	Digoxigenin
Glucoverodoxin	Gitaloxigenin

leaves and a number of flavonoid glycosides characterized.

The plant also contains 25β-tigogenin, digalogenin, 25α-gitogenin, lanatigonin I, lanadigalonins I and II, 5,7,4'-trihydroxy-3',6-dimethoxyflavone, 3-epi-digitoxigenin, digifolein, digoxoside, neo-digoxoside, 1-methoxy-2-methy-lanthraquinone, 3-methoxy-2-methylanthraqui-none, digitolutein, 3-methyl-alizarin, scutellarein, luteolin; cholesterol, campesterol, stigmasterol, sitosterol, cycloartenol, 24-methylene cycloar-tenol, hispidulin, jaceosidin, chrysoeriol, nepetin, jaceoside, hispidulin-7-glucoside, nepitrin, luteolin-7β-D-glucoside, pectolinarigenin, desmethoxy-centaureidin apigenin.

The other cardioglycoside isolated from *D. lanata* are digitoxigenin, 3-epidigitoxigenin, odorobioside G, acetyl-gitorin, neo-odorobioside G, neo-digitalinum verum, digitoxigenin-O-glucosyl-6-deoxyglucoside, digitoxigenin-β-D-glucoside, dihydrodigoxin, digoxigenin digitaloside, digoxigenin-3-O-β-D-digitoxosido-β-D-2,6-dideoxyglucoside, digoxigenin-3-O-β-gluco-digoxoside, digitoxigenin-3-O-β-D-digitoxosido-β-D-xyloside, digoxigenin-3-O-β-D-digitoxosido-β-D-digitoxosido-β-D-xyloside.

Uses

The leaves are used for the preparation of the lanatosides and digoxin. Digoxin is most widely used in the treatment of congestive heart failure. In long-term treatments patients require about 1 mg day^{-1}. The worldwide use of the drug now amounts to several thousand kilograms per year. Digoxin is more rapidly absorbed from the gastrointestinal tract than are the purpurea glycosides, which renders it of value for rapid digitalization in the treatment of atrial fibrillation and congestive heart failure. Lanatoside C is less absorbed than digitoxin but it is less cumulative. For rapid digitalization the deacetyl derivative is preferable.

Cell and organ culture

Green hairy roots produced by light exposure give a 600-fold increase in cardenolide accumulation over roots cultivated in the dark.

Pharmacology

An extract of *D. lanata* is more cardiotoxic than *D. purpurea* extract. The molar toxic activity of digitoxin was found to be 5.2 and that of digoxin 10, compared with digoxigenin as 1. An extract of leaves of *D. purpurea*, injected into carotid artery of cat, markedly increased action of potentials of carotid sinus nerve which was followed by bradycardia. Noncardiotonic glucoside, digitonoside, increased toxicity of cardiotonic glycoside mixture in mice. It increased toxicity of K-strophanthin when administered separately by venous route. It showed haemolytic effect in mice. 16-Acetyl derivative of digitarium verum was about 5 times as lethal as digitarium verum. Digitoxin, lanatoside A and C and strophanthoside augment the response of isolated guinea pig uterus to oxytocin. Digitalin, ouabain and K-strophantho-side induced contraction of perfused guinea pig ileum, followed by relaxation. Digoxin increased lysophosphatidylcholine and phosphatidylethano-lamine concentrations in blood plasma of healthy men. In cat, digoxin showed neuroexcitatory effect and increased systemic vascular resistance in man. Digoxin produced satisfactory clinical response in neonates with heart failure. Cardiac glycosides affected total serum calcium levels in patients with cardiac insufficiency but all increased ionic Ca^{2+} levels. Digitoxin normalized myocardial

ATP, AMP and cytochrome C oxidase and significantly increased myocardial contractility in healthy human without significant changes in heart rate and blood pressure. Digoxin and deslanoside produced marked cardiotoxic activity.

Nepitrin increased survival time of irradiated mice and inhibited increase in capillary permeability caused by histamine in mice. Lanatoside C decreased heart rate and modified profoundly ECG and VCG pattern. Digoxin induced immuni-sation in guinea pigs and rabbits resulting in protection from digoxin toxicity. Anticonvulsant activity of digoxin is due to its influence on membrane Na^+. K^+-ATPase and K^+-concentration. Flavonoid saponoside complex from seeds of *D. purpurea* exhibited immunostimulant effects in animals.

Digitalis seeds

The seed of *D. purpurea* consist of the physiologically active 'digitalinum verum', with other water-soluble glycosides, including the saponins digitonin and gitonin.

Other allied drugs

Digitalis thapsi is found in Spain and Italy. The leaves have a crenate margin and decurrent lamina, nonglandular hairs are absent, glandular hairs of two types are present, some consisting of a bicellular gland and unicellular stalk; others having a unicellular gland and a three- to four-celled stalk. A striated cuticle, pericyclic fibres and small prisms of calcium oxalate are also present. The vein-islet number is higher than the other Digitalis species, varying from 8.5 to 16. *D. lutea* has a potency similar to those of *D. purpurea* and *D. ferruginea* and is cultivated in Russia.

Adulterants

Digitalis is adulterated with the leaves of mullein (*Verbascum thapsus* Linn.), comfrey (*Symphytum officinale* Linn.), primrose (*Primula vulgaris* Huds.), elecampane (*Inula helenium* Linn.), ploughman's spikenard (*Inula conyza DC*) and nettle (*Urtica dioica*).

Digoxin

Digoxin is used as the cardiotonic glycoside. It is obtained from the leaves of *D. lanata*. On hydro-lysis digoxin yields 1 molecule of digoxigenin and 3 of digitoxose. It is a highly potent drug. Digoxin occurs as a white, crystalline powder.

Digoxin tablets are 60 to 80% absorbed. Because of the low therapeutic index of the drug, a patient should not be changed from one brand of tablet to another after a reasonable therapeutic effect has been achieved with one preparation. Otherwise, either a toxic or nontherapeutic effect may result owing to a change in the bioavailability of the drug.

Upon oral administration, the onset of action is 30 minutes to 2 hours, with a peak at 2 to 6 hours. Digoxin is also administered parenterally for a more rapid effect. The major route of elimination is the kidneys, and with a plasma half-life of 30-40 hours. A drug-serum level of 0.5-2 µg/ml is required for full therapeutic effect, and levels exceeding 2.5 µg/ml may produce symptoms of toxicity.

Digoxin has the same uses and precautions as digitalis. It is relatively short-acting and rapidly eliminated when compared with digitoxin. However, digitoxin may be indicated in patients with impaired renal function.

Digitoxin

Digitoxin is a cardiotonic glycoside obtained from *D. purpurea*, *D. lanata*, and other species of *Digitalis*. On hydrolysis, digitoxin yields 1 molecule of digitoxigenin and 3 of digitoxose. Digitoxin occurs as a white or pale buff, odourless, microcrystalline powder. It is a bitter substance that is practically insoluble in water and slightly soluble in alcohol. It is the most lipid-soluble of the cardiac glycosides used in therapeutics.

The major pharmacokinetic parameters for digitoxin include complete oral absorption, which distinguishes it from other cardiac glycosides. Upon oral administration, the onset of action is 1 to 4 hours with a peak at 8 to 14 hours. Approxi-mately 50 to 70% of the glycoside is converted by the liver to inactive genins, which are excreted in the kidneys. Because of a long plasma half-life (168 to 192 hours), it may take from 3 to 5 weeks for complete dissipation of the drug from the body following discontinuation of therapy. A drug-serum level of 14 to 26 µg/ml is required for full therapeutic effect, and levels exceeding 35 µg/ml may produce symptoms of toxicity.

It has the same uses and precautions as Digitalis.

Deslanoside

Deslanoside is desacetyllanatoside C, which on hydrolysis yields 1 molecule of digoxigenin, 3 of digitoxose, and 1 of glucose. Deslanoside occurs as a white, crystalline powder. It is hygroscopic, absorbing about 7% of moisture when exposed to air, and is highly potent.

Deslanoside is used to attain rapid initial loading by parenteral administration. Onset of action is 10-30 minutes; maximal effects occur in 2-3 hours, with dissipation in 3-6 days.

STROPHANTHUS

Synonyms

Strophanthus seeds; Semina strophanthi.

Biological source

Strophanthus is the ripe seeds of *Strophanthus kombe* Olive, or *S. hispidus* DC. (Fam. Apocyanaceae).

Habitat

East and central Africa.

Collection

Seeds are collected usually from wild plants. The plants are large climbers. Fruits are many-seeded, dehiscent and consist of two divergent follicles. Mature fruits are collected in June-July, epicarp and mesocarp are separated and seeds are removed. The seeds are washed and dried.

Chemical constituents

Strophanthus contains a cardiac glycoside strophanthin-K (2-5%), kombic acid, choline, trigonelline, fixed oil (30%), resin and mucilage. Strophanthin-K is a mixture of K-strophanthoside, K-strophanthin-β and cymarin and the genin part of all these glycosides is strophanthidin. The genin strophanthidin is coupled to a trisaccharide consisting of cymarose, β-glucose and α-glucose.

The enzyme α-glucosidase removes the terminal α-glucose to yield K-strophanthin-β and the enzyme, strophanthobiase, present in seeds, converts this to cymarin and glucose.

S. kombe also contains periplocymarin, cymarol, helveticoside, strophanthidin digitoxosido-glycoside, erysimoside, erysimosol, gluco-cymaral, glucoerysimoside, helveticoside (strophanthidin digitoxoside), periplocin, K-strophan-thol-γ, strophanthoside-19-carboxylic acid, 17β-H-strophanthidine and neoglucoerysimoside.

Uses

Strophanthus is used as cardiac tonic, diuretic and arrow poison.

Allied drugs

Strophanthus gratus contain 4-8% of ouabain (G-strophanthin), a rhamnose glycoside more stable than those present in other species. It can be isolated in a pure crystalline form, and has been used as a standard in biological assays and for the preparation of ouabain injections. Ouabain is also the principal glycoside of the wood of the African *Acokanthera schimperi* (*A. ouabaio*).

S. gratus also contains sarmentoside A and K, acolongifloroside K, strogoside and dambonitol (in leaves).

Seeds of *S. sarmentosus* contain a number of glycosides with sarmentogenin as the aglycone.

Oleander glycosides

These glycosides have an action similar to that of Digitalis and are present in the oleander plant (*Nerium oleander*) and its relatives. The principal constituents of the leaves are oleandrin and digitalinum verum. Oleandrin is the monoside, comprising oleandrigenin (16-acetylgitoxigenin) and L-oleandrose. The uzarigenin glycosides have a *trans*-fusion of the A/B rings at C-5 (uzarigenin - 5α-digitoxigenin) and have a lowered activity. The adynerigenin and Δ^{16}-dehydroadynerigenin glycosides having diginose and digitalose are inactive. Adynerigenin is digitoxigenin in which the 14-OH group has been substituted with a 8,14-β-epoxy group.

The leaves also contain gitoxigenin and digitoxigenin glycosides. The glycosides isolated from *N. odorum* are oleandrigenin-β-D-glucosyl-β-D-diginoside and gentiobiosyloleandrin.

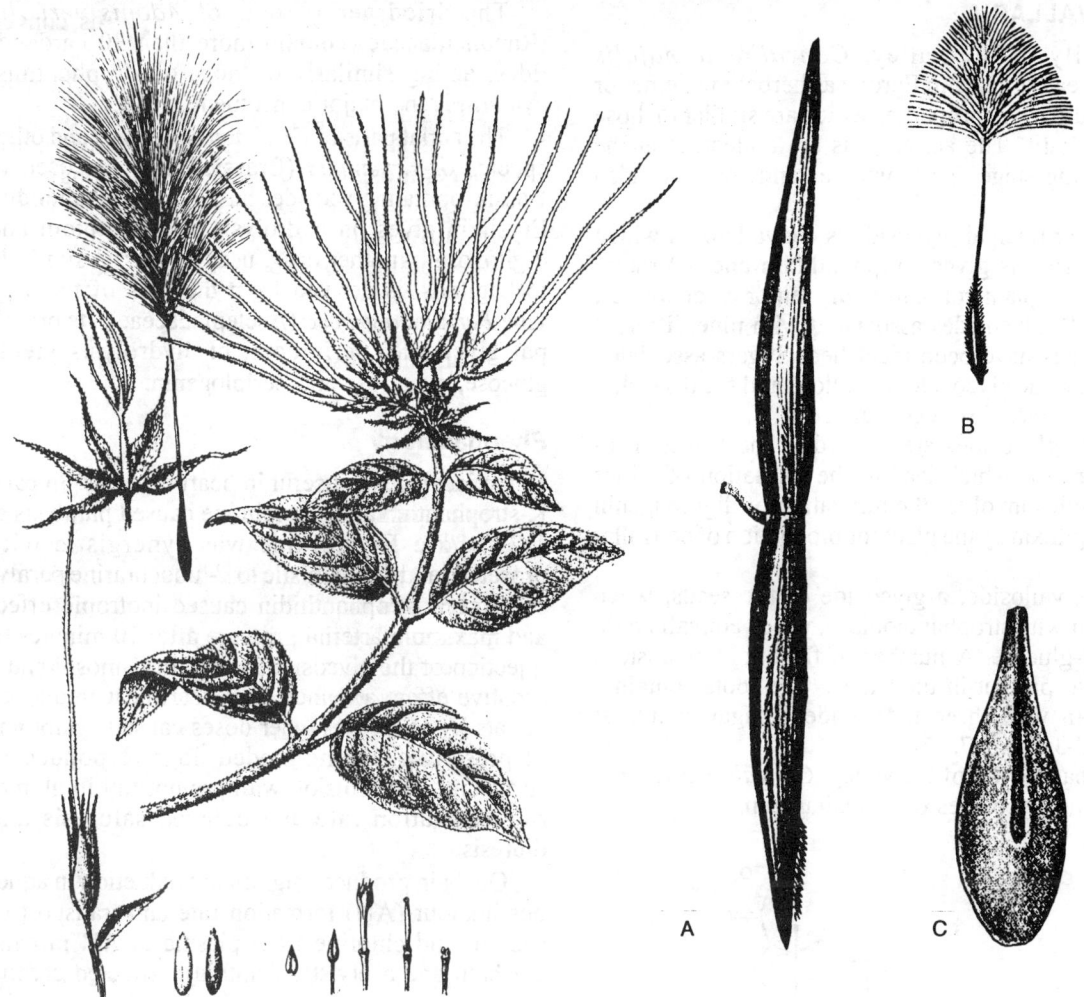

Fig. 15.9. Seed of *Strophanthus hispidus.*

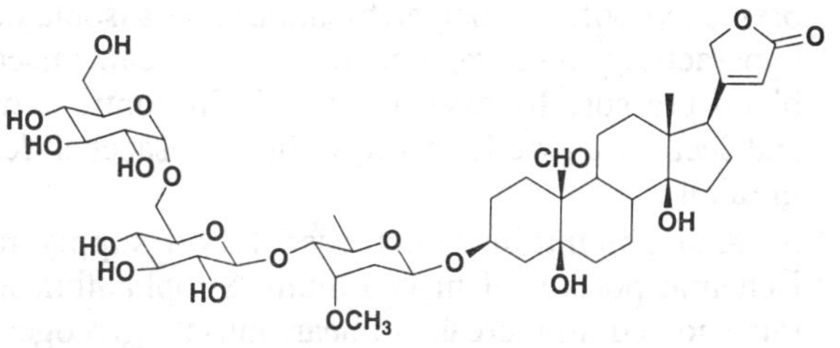

Fig. 15.10. K-Strophantoside.

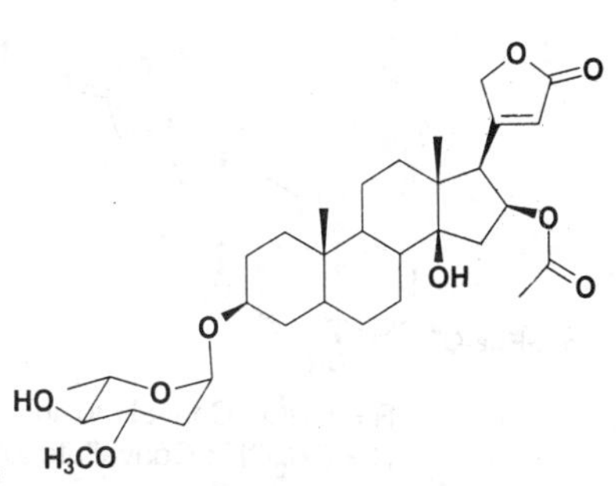

Fig. 15.11. Oleandrin.

CONVALLARIA

The lily of the valley, *Convallaria majalis* (Liliaceae) is used in Europe as herbal medicine for its cardioactive properties which are similar to those of Digitalis. The aerial parts are collected at the flowering stage. The rhizomes and roots are also used.

The principal glycoside is convallatoxin which on hydrolysis gives strophanthidin and (–)-rhamnose. The plant contains many minor cardenolides, about 40 glycosides associated with nine different aglycones have been identified. Sugars associated with cardiac glycosides are allose and the disaccharide rhamnosido-6-deoxyallose.

The glycosides are formed in the leaves. Bioconversions which lead to the formation of minor glycosides involves the utilization of digitoxigenin and digitoxin by the plant for production of convallatoxin.

Convalloside, a glycoside of the seeds, when reacted with strophanthobiase, yields convallatoxin and D-glucose. A number of flavonoid glycosides are also present in the leaves. The roots contain a saponin with three independent sugar chains at C-1, C-3 and C-7.

Japanese lily of the valley, *Convallaria keiskei*, contains glycosides of convallagenin.

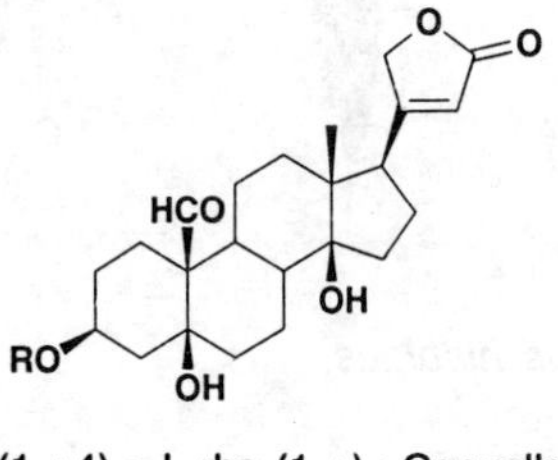

R = β-D-glc-(1→4)-α-L-rha-(1→) : Convalloside
R = α-L-rha-(1→) : Convallatoxin

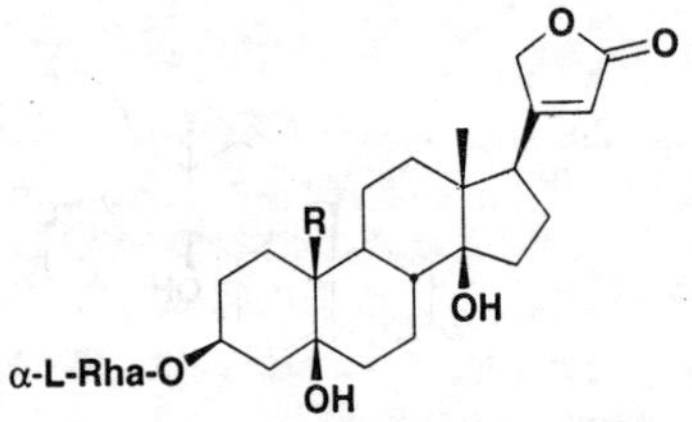

R = CHO : Convallatoxin
R = CH₂OH : Convallatoxol

Fig. 15.12. Chemical constituents of convallaria.

The dried aerial roots of *Adonis vernalis* (Ranunculaceae) contain more than 30 cardenolides, acting similarly to those of strophanthus; cymarin is the major constituent.

The aerial parts of *Erysimun conescens* and other species of *Erysimum* (Brassicaceae) are used in Russia, contain glycosides based on strophanthidin. Erysimin gives on hydrolysis strophanthidin and digitoxose. Another drug, used in Russia similarly to Digitalis, is derived from the bark of the silkvine *Periploca graeca* (Asclepiadaceae). Its principal glycoside, periplocin, on hydrolysis yields glucose, cymarose and periplogenin.

Pharmacology

Helveticoside was useful in heart diseases. In cats, K-strophanthin and erysidimine caused paralysis at 1-2 mg/kg. Erysidinine was synergistic with proserine and antagonistic to *d*-tubocurarine paralysis. Acetyl strophanthidin caused inotropic effect and maximum arterial pressure after 10 minutes of injection of the glycoside in dog. Erysimosol had a sedative effect and increased heart-beat frequency in cats by 15-20%; higher doses caused symptoms of poisoning. Saline loaded dogs responded to strophanthidin infusion with prompt fall in glomerular filtration rate and delayed saluresis and diuresis.

Ouabain produced significant reduction in aqueous humour (AH) formation rate and transport of sodium and chlorine from plasma to AH in cats. Ouabain and acetylstrophanthidin affected carotid sinus baroreceptors in cats. Ouabain increased the apparent volume of calcium distribution in heart, antagonized contractile response of intestinal smooth muscle, ehnanced electrical activity in vagus, sympathetic and phrenic nerves of cats, caused increase in force of cardiac contraction in dog, prolonged pentobarbitone sleeping time in rats, prevented both cardiac arrhythmias and associated hyperactivity on sympathetic nerves in cat, raised blood pressure by over 50 mm Hg in control rats and decreased pyretic activity of lipopolysaccharides in rabbit.

K-strophanthin-β increased blood supply to ischemic portion of myocardium. Strophanthin in rats showed an increase in heart muscle glycogen, rise in myocardial hexokinase and a drop in glucose-6-phosphate. It lowered total lipids by 6-15% and lipoproteins by 22-37% and increased lipolytic activity by 10-19% in myocardium of intact rats. K-strophanthin decreased blood pressure in patients with hypertonicity.

Ouabain increased the developed tension in strips of human atrial and ventricular muscle. It had no direct effect on calcium binding of isolated dog or pig cardiac sarcoplasmic reticulum. It exeted both inhibitory and stimulatory effects on Ca^{2+} current in frog ventricular cells, and increased phospholipase C activity 5-fold in rat pinealocytes. It caused constriction of tracheal smooth muscle. Ouabain showed inotropic effect in hypertrophied rat heart. Ouabain injection was associated with fall in plasma angiotensin II level and rise in plasma adrenaline level, but plasma noradrenaline level remained unchanged.

THEVETIA

Peela-kaner, Kaner zard, Yellow oleander.

Biological source

It consists of the seeds, latex, roots and other parts of *Thevetia peruviana* (Pers.) Schum., (syn. *T. neriifolia* Juss). (Family : Apocynaceae).

Habitat

It is a shrub or or small tree, native of tropical America and West Indies, cultivated in gardens in the plains throughout India.

Morphology

The plant is a large, evergreen shrub, 4-6 m tall; leaves simple, glabrous, lanceolate, acute at both ends, 10-15 cm long, shining green, flowers large, bright yellow or pinkish yellow, funnel shaped, scented, in terminal cymes, drupes triangular, fleshy with 2-4 seeds.

The stem bark is greyish brown, rough, longitudinally wrinkled, recurved with horizontal lenticels. The inner surface is dark brown, odour typical, taste bitter and acrid.

Chemical constituents

The seeds contain glycosides of digitoxigenin, cannogenin, and cannogenic acids. These glyco-

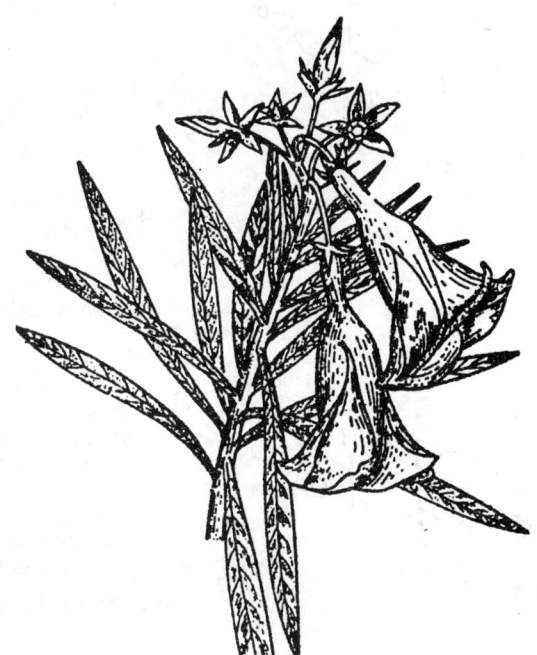

Fig. 15.13. *Thevetia peruviana.*

sides are known as cerberoside (thevetin B), 2'-acetylcerberoside, neriifolin, 2'-O-neriifolin (cerberin), thevefolin, theveside, theviridoside, viridoside, thevetin A (19-oxo-cerberoside), peruvoside (19-oxo-neriifolin), theveneriin (ruvoside) and peruvosidic acid (perusitin). The yellow seed oil (58%) is composed of palmitic (15%), stearic (11%), oleic (61%), linoleic, linolenic, behenic and crucic acids.

The leaves contain flavonols thevefolin, quercetin-3-galactoside, kaempferol, its 3-glycoside; viridoside, bornesitol, iridoids theviridoside, theveside (from roots), syntheviridoside, and 10-O-β-D-fructosyl theviridoide. The leaves also contain amino acids glutanic acid, aspartic acid, leucine, glycine, isoleucine, arginine, valine, alanine, proline, phenylalanine, cystine, lysine, sesine, tyrosine, histidine, threonine, methionine and tryptophan; C-nor-D-homocardenolide glycosides thevetiosides A, B, C, D, D, F and G; digitoxigenin α-L-acofrioside, neriifoside, peruvoside; lupeol acetate, oleanolic acid, ursolic acid, α- and β-amyrin acetates, 4,16-pregnadien-12β-hydroxy-3,30-dione, 3β-hydroxy-11α-12α-epoxyurs-13β,28-olide,

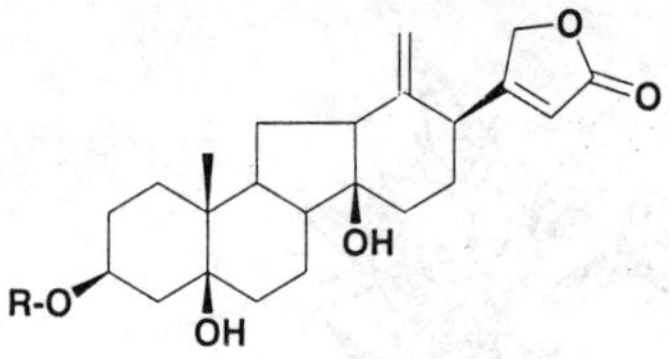

Thevetioside

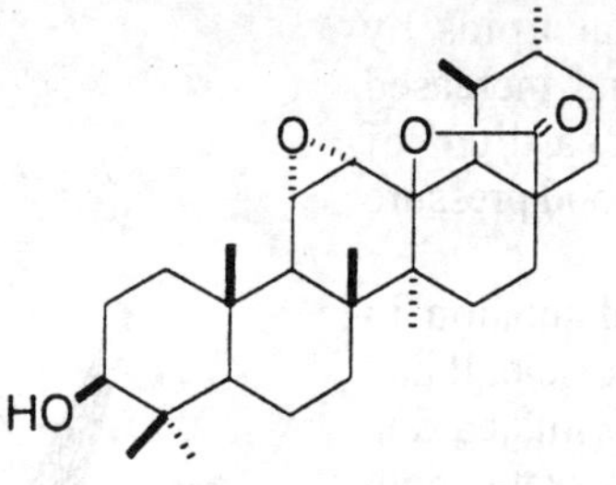

3β-Hydroxy-11α, 12α-epoxy-urs-13β, 28-olide

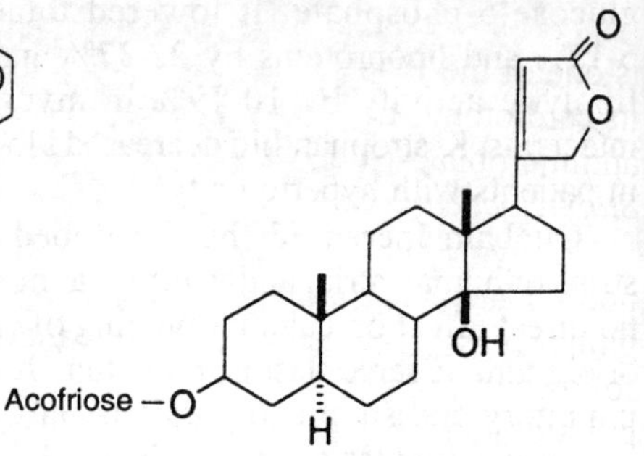

Neriifoside

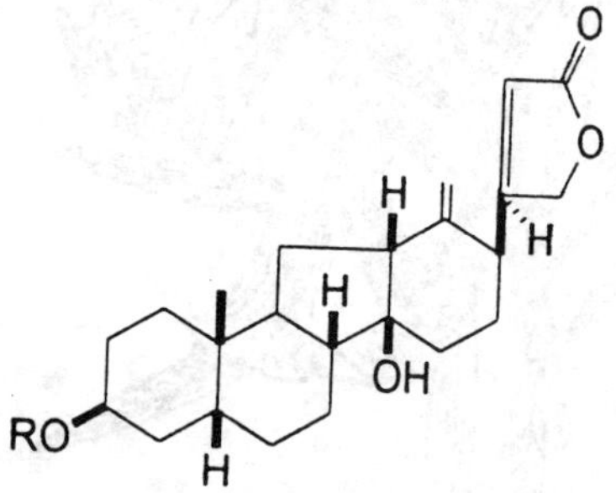

Thevetioside A, R	= Thevetose
Thevetioside B, R	= Acofriose
Thevetioside C, R	= Thevetose (4→1) Glu
Thevetioside D, R	= Acofriose (4→1) Glu
Thevetioside E, R	= Thevetose (2-Ac) (4→1) Glu
Thevetioside F, R	= Thevetose (4→1) Gentiobiose
Thevetioside G, R	= Thevetose (2-Ac) (4→1) Gentiobiose

Fig. 15.14. Cardenolides of Thevetia.

3β-O-thevetose-3β,14β-dihydroxy-14-abeo-.5β,12β,14β- carda-13(18), 29(22)-dienolide.

The stem bark contains ursene-type triterpenes peruvian ursenyl acetates A, B and C; isolupenyl acetate, lupedienyl acetate, peruvianursenyl glucoside, α-amyrin acetates and lupenol acetate.

The flowers yield phenylpropanoloids. β-(2-hydroxy-4-carboxy) phenyl acetic acid and its methyl ester, α- and β-amyrins, epiperuviol acetate, hesperitin-7-glucoside, kaempferol, quercetin, thevefolin (tamarixetin-3-O-digalactoside), lupeol acetate, β-(2-hydroxy-4-carboxyl) phenyl lactic acid and its methyl ester, quercetin-3-galactoside and -3-digalactoside.

The fruit pericarp yields hesperitin-7-glucoside, α- and β-amyrins, epiperuviol acetate, kaemferol and quercetin. Viridoside is present in the stem bark.

Apigenin-5-methyl ether is reported from the seed shells.

The roots contain lupeol, α- and β-amyrins, and taraxasterols.

Uses

The seeds are used as cardiotonic, abortifacient, purgative, alexiteric, insecticidal and to treat dropsy and rheumatism.

The plant latex is applied to sores and is placed in the cavities of the teeth to relieve toothache. A tincture of the bark is used as a bitter, cathartic, emetic and febrifuge. A root paste is applied to tumors. An aqueous extract of the plant is applied to boils, blisters and skin diseases. The stem bark acts as bitter cathartic, emetic, purgative, abortifacient, bactericidal, cardiotonic, alexiteric and rotenticide and is useful to cure dropsy, rheumatism, skin diseases, boils, blister and cancer.

Yellow-oleander poisoning is treated by washing stomach and administration of atropine to counteract the effect of the poison.

Pharmacology

Oral administration of peruvoside produces digitalization in congestive cardiac failure. All forms of cardiac insufficiency can be successfully treated with peruvoside. It is well tolerated and the side effects include gastrointestinal irritation. In Germany, peruvoside is marketed under the trade name 'Endocordin' and used to treat as a cardiotonic agent in congestive heart failure.

Peruvoside has a strong positive inotropic action in experimental animals. Thevetin has a digitalis-like effect, identical with ouabain. Cerberoside is one of the weakest of the *Thevetia* glycosides in its cardiotonic effect. The seed oil possesses strong antimicrobial activity against *Bacillus subtilis* and *Staphylococcus aureus*.

Peruvoside evoked vomiting by stimulation of nodose ganglion. It showed bradycardia in dogs and guinea pigs. It also showed positive inotropic effect followed by cardiac arrest in guinea pig heart, musculotropic activity on smooth muscles and marked cardiotonic effect in isolated heart-lung preparation of dog. It was as potent as ouabain. Among thevetin, neriifolin, peruvoside and its 2'-monoacetate, peruvoside showed the strongest cardiotonic effect and the highest therapeutic activity.

Table 15.2. Glycosides isolated from the seeds of *T. peruviana*

Glycosides	Aglycone	Sugars
Cerberoside (Thevetin B)	Digitoxigenin	L-Thevetose + D-Glucose (2 mols)
2'-O-Acetyl cereberoside	Digitoxigenin	L-Thevetose + D-Glucose
Neriifolin	Digitoxigenin	L-Thevetose
2'-O-Neriifolin (Cerberin)	Digitoxigenin	L-Thevetose
Thevetin A (19-Oxo-cerebroside)	Connogenin	L-Thevetose + D-glucose
Peruvoside (19-Oxo-neriifolin)	Cannogenin	L-Thevetose + L-Thevefose
Theveneriin (Ruvoside)	Cannogenin	L-Thevetose
Peruvosidic acid (Perustin)	Connogenic acid	L-Thevetose

Bufadienolides

The bufadienolides are less widely distributed in nature than are the cardenolides; they are found in some Liliaceae and Ranunculaceae. In the toad venoms, the genins are partly free and partly combined with suberyl arginine. Therapeutically they are less used as cardioactive drugs due to their low therapeutic index and their production of side-effects.

SQUILL

Synonyms

Sea onion; Bulbus Scillae; Meerzwiebel, Scilla bulb; White Squill; European Scilla; Radix scillae.

Biological source

Squill consists of the dried sliced scales of the fleshy inner bulb of the white variety of *Urginea maritima* (L.) Baker (*Scilla maritima* L.). The central part of the bulb is removed during its preparation. (Family Liliaceae).

Habitat

It grows in Mediterranean seacoasts of Spain, France, Italy, Greece, Algeria, Morocco; Algiers and Cyprus.

The white variety of *U. maritima* is grown in Malta and Italy and also from Indian squill. Red squill, which is also derived from a variety of *U. maritima*, is collected in Algiers and Cyprus, and differs from the white form in containing red anthocyanin pigment and the glycoside scilliroside.

Collection

The bulbs grow half-immersed in the sandy soil. It is collected in August during flowering stage. Outer membraneous scales, fibrous roots and central portion are removed. Then the bulbs are cut transversely into thin slices, dried in the sun or stove heated and packed in bags or in barrels. On drying about 80% weight is lost.

Morphology

Squill bulbs are pear-shaped, tapering at both ends, diameter 15-30 cm. Surface contains longitudinal furrow. Colour is yellow, fracture is short and brittle. The slices of the drug are nearly 0.5-5 cm long, tapering at both ends. The odour is slight and taste is bitter, mucilaginous and acrid. The drug is hygroscopic and should be stored carefully in airtight containers.

Microscopical characters

Squill shows abundant large polygonal parenchymatous cells of the mesophyll, containing mucilage, under the microscope and raphides of calcium oxalate. The mucilage sheath is stained by corallin soda. In mesophyll cells, small, rounded starch grains, about 10 μm diameter, are present. The epidermis is composed of rectangular cuticularized, polygonal and axially elongated cells. Stomata are absent or very rare on the adaxial surface;

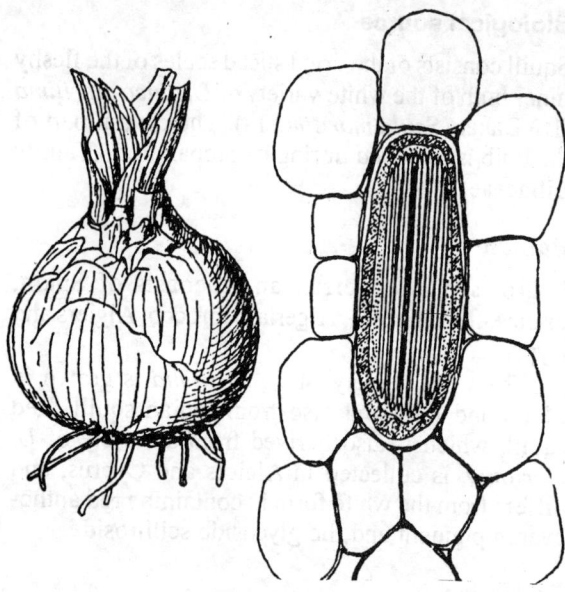

Fig. 15.15. Squill.

a few are constantly present on the abaxial surface. They are circular, with wide guard cells. The mesophyll is traversed by numerous small vascular bundles with small spiral & annular xylem vessels.

Chemical constituents

The drug contains about a dozen of cardioactive glycosides scillaren A, scillaren B, glucoscillaren A, proscillaridin A, scillaridin A, scilliglaucoside, scillipheoside, glucoscillipheoside, scillicyanoside, scillicoeloside, scilliazuroside and scillicryptoside.

Scillaren A is hydrolyzed by an enzyme scillarenase or by acids.

Other glycosides with 12α- and 12β-OH substitution have similar sugar side-chains at C-3.

Two-third amount of the total glycosides is of scillaren A. On hydrolysis it forms the aglycone scillarenin (bufadienolide), rhamnose and glucose. In addition to glycosides the drug also contains various flavonoids, like quercetin derivatives and kaempferol polyglycosides; sinistrin, mucilage and calcium oxalate.

The drug also contains *C*-glycosides such as vitexin and isovitexin, sinistrin and a fructan resembling inulin; it is composed largely of β-D-fructofuranosyl residues.

Idioblasts contain calcium oxalate crystals embedded in mucilage consisting mainly of glucogalactans. Anthocyanins are present in small amount.

Uses

Squill is used as expectorant, diuretic, and cardiotonic, but it shows emetic action.

The glycosides are poorly absorbed from the gastrointestinal tract. They are of short-action duration and they are not cumulative. In small doses the drug promotes mild gastric irritation causing a reflex secretion from the bronchioles. It is used as an expectorant. In larger doses it causes vomiting.

Allied drugs

Indian Squill or Urginea

It consists of dried longitudinal slices of the bulb of *Drimia indica* (syn. *Urginea indica* Kunth). (Family Liliaceae). The drug is found in western Himalaya, Bihar, Chota Nagpur, Konkan and Coromandel Coast. It is a small glabrous herb, bulb diameter is about 1.5 cm, flowers appearing before the leaves drooping or spreading. Surface of the bulb is fleshy and longitudinally ribbed, fracture is brittle, with yellow colour, odour is slight and taste is bitter and acrid.

It is cultivated is sandy soils near the sea-shore in southern India. The bulb prefers a sandy soil and average temperature of 15°C. The plants are grown from seeds and in 5-6 years the bulb develop. Bulbs are also raised from the bulblets. Planting is generally done in rows. The bulbs are collected in the early autumn when the leaves wither after flowering. The bulbs are cleaned of the soil, the dry outer scales separated and cut into four parts. The core is cut out and the quarters are finally sliced. The slices are dried in the sun, or on slow fire to lose 80% of their weight and packed in bags or barrels.

Indian Squill occurs in the form of curved or irregularly shaped strips, 3-6 cm long, 3-8 mm broad and 1-3 mm thick. They are thickened in the middle, but tapering towards the ends, translucent or yellowish white, and slightly darker in colour than the European Squill. They are brittle when dried, but become tough when moistened; fracture is brittle. It is odourless and has a slight bitter, mucilaginous and acrid taste.

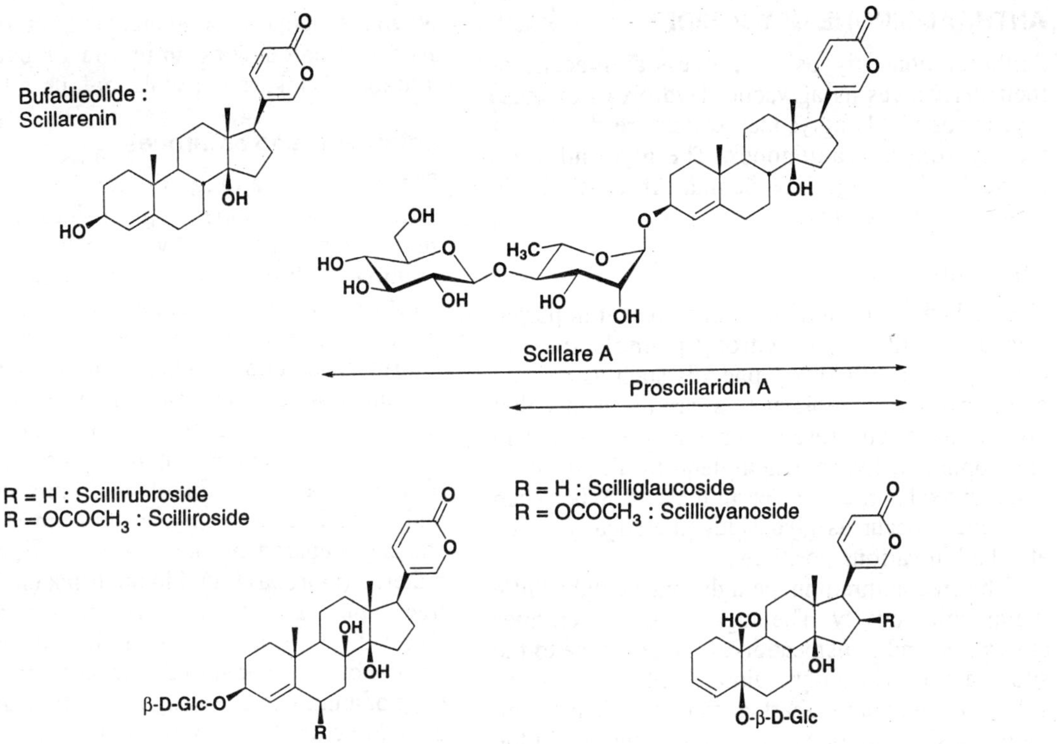

Fig. 15.16. Cardenolides of squill.

Indian Squill contains scillarens A and B and mucilage is consisted of mannose, glucose and xylose. Scillaren A yields on hydrolysis proscillaridin A and then scillaridin A. With iodine water a reddish purple colour is formed and this test is negative with European Squill. Indian squill also contains scillarenin, scillarenin-3-O-α-L-rhamnoside, scillarenin-3-O-α-L-rhamnosido-β-D-glucoside, scillipheosidin-3-O-α-L-rhamnoside, scilliglaucosidin-3-O-α-L-rhamnoside, scilliglaucosidin-3-O-β-D-glucoside and 6-desacetoxys cillirosidin.

Uses

Indian Squill has a digitalis-like action on the heart and in small doses is used as an expectorant.

In large doses it is emetic and cathartic and may cause cardiac depression. It is used to treat cough, dropsy, rheumatism, skin troubles; to remove warts and corns; as cardiac conic, expectorant and diuretic.

Red Squill

Red Squill is a variety of *Urginea maritima* (Fam. Liliaceae). It contains cardiac glycoside scillaren A, an enzyme scillarenase composed of proscillaridin and glucose and glycosides scilliroside and scillirubroside. Red Squill is used as a rodenticide to kill rodents. When taken by rodents, convulsions, respiratory failure and death occur.

Black hellebore rhizome

Black hellebore rhizome is obtained from *Helleborus niger* (Ranunculaceae), a perennial herb indigenous to Central Europe. It contains three crystalline cardiac glycosides : helleborin, helleborein and hellebrin. The last two glycosides have a digitalis-like action, hellebrin being approximately 20 times more powerful than helleborein. The aglycone hellebrigenin is the bufadienolide analogue of strophanthidin. It has abortifacient and cardiotonic properties.

ANTHRAQUINONE GLYCOSIDES

Anthraquinone glycosides possess anthracene or their derivatives as aglycone. Hydrolysis of these glycosides yields aglycones which are di-, tri- or tetrahydroxyanthraquinones. The glycosides are found in the drugs like Senna, Aloe, Rhubarb, Cascara and Cochineal.

Anthraquinones

The derivatives of anthraquinone present in purgative drugs may be dihydroxy phenols such as chrysophanol, trihydroxy phenols such as emodin or tetrahydroxy phenols such as carminic acid. Other groups are often present, for example, methyl in chrysophanol, hydroxymethylene in aloe-emodin and carboxyl in rhein and carminic acid. When such substances occur as glycosides, the sugar may be attached in various positions.

The free anthraquinone aglycones exhibit little therapeutic activity. The sugar residue facilitates absorption and translocation of the aglycone to the site of action. The anthraquinone and related glycosides are stimulant cathartics and exert their action by increasing the tone of the smooth muscle in the wall of the large intestine. Glycosides of anthranols and anthrones elicit a more drastic action than do the corresponding anthraquinone glycosides, and a preponderance of the former constituents in the glycosidic mixture can cause discomforting griping action.

Anthraquinone derivatives are usually orange-red compounds, soluble in water or dilute alcohol.

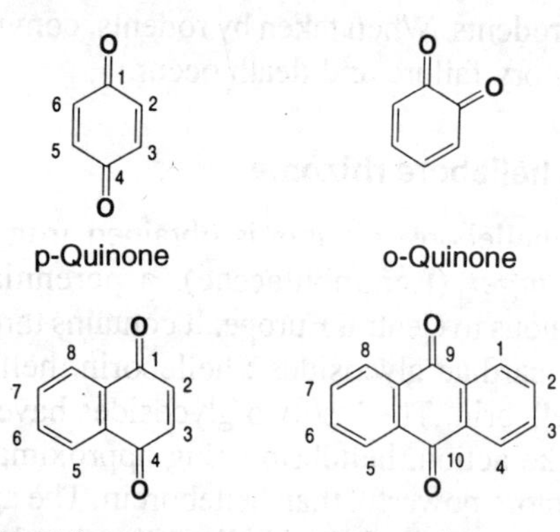

p-Quinone   o-Quinone

Naphthoquinone   Anthraquinone

Fig. 15.17. Quinones.

When the alcoholic or ethereal extract of powdered drug is treated with ammonia or caustic soda solution, a pink, red or violet colour is formed.

Anthranols and anthrones

These reduced anthraquinone derivatives occur either free or combined as glycosides. They are isomeric and may be partially converted to the other in solution. Anthrone, is a pale yellow, nonfluorescent substance which is insoluble in alkali; its isomer, anthranol, is brownish-yellow and forms a strongly fluorescent solution in alkali. Anthranol derivatives, present in aloes, have similar properties, and the strong green fluorescence which aloes give in borax or other alkaline solution is used as a test for its identification. Antranols and anthrones are the main constituents of chrysarobin, a mixture of substances prepared by benzene extraction from the material (araroba) found in the trunk cavities of the tree *Andira araroba*. If chrysarobin is treated on a white tile with a drop of fuming nitric acid, the anthranols are converted into anthraquinones. A drop of ammonia allowed to mix gradually with the acid liquid produces a violet colour. This modification of Borntrager's test had been used to identify these compounds.

They are converted to other compounds in solution. They are pale yellow, non-fluorescent substances, and insoluble in alkali. They contain significant therapeutic action of the crude drugs.

Oxanthrones

These are intermediate products between anthraquinones and anthranols. They give anthraquinones on oxidation and Fairbairn's modification of the Borntrager test accomplishes this by means of hydrogen peroxide. An oxanthrone is present in cascara bark. They produce anthraquinone on oxidation.

Dianthrones

These are compounds derived from two anthrone molecules, combined at C-10, which may be identical or different. They are formed by oxidation of the anthrone or mixed anthrones (*e.g.*, a solution in acetone and presence of atmospheric oxygen). They are important aglycones in species of *Cassia, Rheum* and *Rhamnus*; e.g., the sennidins, aglycones of the sennosides. Reidin A, B and C of Senna and Rhubarb are heterodianthrones, *i.e.*, composed of unlike anthrones, and involve aloe-emodin, rhein, chryophanol or physcion.

Two chiral centres (at C-10 and C-10') are present in the dianthrones, and for a compound having two identical anthrone moieties, *e* , sennidin A, two forms (the 10*S*, 10'*S* and 10*R*, 10'*R*) are possible together with the *meso* from (sennidin B). These compounds are present in the plant as their 1,1'-diglucosides.

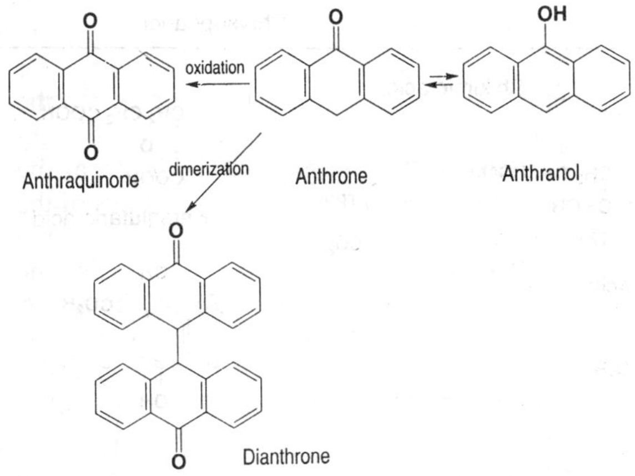

Fig. 15.18. Interrelationships of anthraquinone derivatives.

Aloin-type or *C*-glycosides

The aloin obtained from species of *Aloe* is strongly resistant to normal acid hydrolysis but may be oxidized with ferric chloride. The sugar is joined to the aglycone with a direct C-C linkage (a *C*-glycoside). Two aloins (A and B) are known and arise from the chiral centre at C-10.

The anthraquinone aglycones in free state exhibit little therapeutic activity. The anthraquinone and related glycosides act as stimulant cathartics and increase the tone of the smooth muscle in the wall of large intestine. Glycosides of anthranols and anthrones exhibit more drastic action than the related anthraquinone glycosides.

The action of anthraquinone laxatives is restricted to the large bowel; hence their effect is delayed for up to 6 h or longer. The common anthraquinone

and anthranol derivatives influence the ion transport across colon cells by inhibition of Cl channels.

Biosynthesis of anthraquinone glycosides

Natural anthraquinones are synthesized either via the acetate-malonate pathway or they are derived from shikimate and mevalonate. The anthraquinones are formed by the former route and all have a 1,8-dihydroxy substitution. The compounds such as alizarin which have one of the rings substituted arise by the second pathway. The 1,8-dihydroxyanthraquinone derivatives occur with 1,8-dihydroxynaphthalene glycosides.

Feeding of labeled acetate to *Penicillium islandicum*, a species that yields several anthraquinone derivatives, showed the distribution of radioactivity in these compounds in consistent with formation via a head-to-tail condensation of acetate units. A poly-β-ketomethylene acid intermediate is first produced and then gives rise to the various oxygenated aromatic compounds following intramolecular condensations. Anthranols and anthrones are likely intermediates in the formation of anthraquinones. Presumably, the emodin-like anthraquinones are formed in higher plants by a similar pathway. The transglycosylation reaction, which creates a glycoside, probably occurs at a late stage in the pathway after the anthraquinone nucleus has been formed.

SENNA

Synonyms

Alexandrian Senna; Egyptian Senna; Tinnevelly Senna; Indian Senna; Senna Leaves; Folia sennal.

Biological source

Senna consists of dried leaflets of *Cassia acutifolia* Delile (*C. senna* L.) known as Alexandrian Senna, and of *C. angustifolia* Vahl, known as Tinnevelly Senna. It contains about 2.5% of hydroxyanthracene glycosides calculated as sennoside B. (Family: Caesalpiniaceae).

Habitat

Egypt and neighbouring region for Alexandrian Senna; Tinnevelly Senna is cultivated in South India in Tinnevelly, Madurai, Trichinopoly, Mysore; in N.W. Pakistan and Jammu.

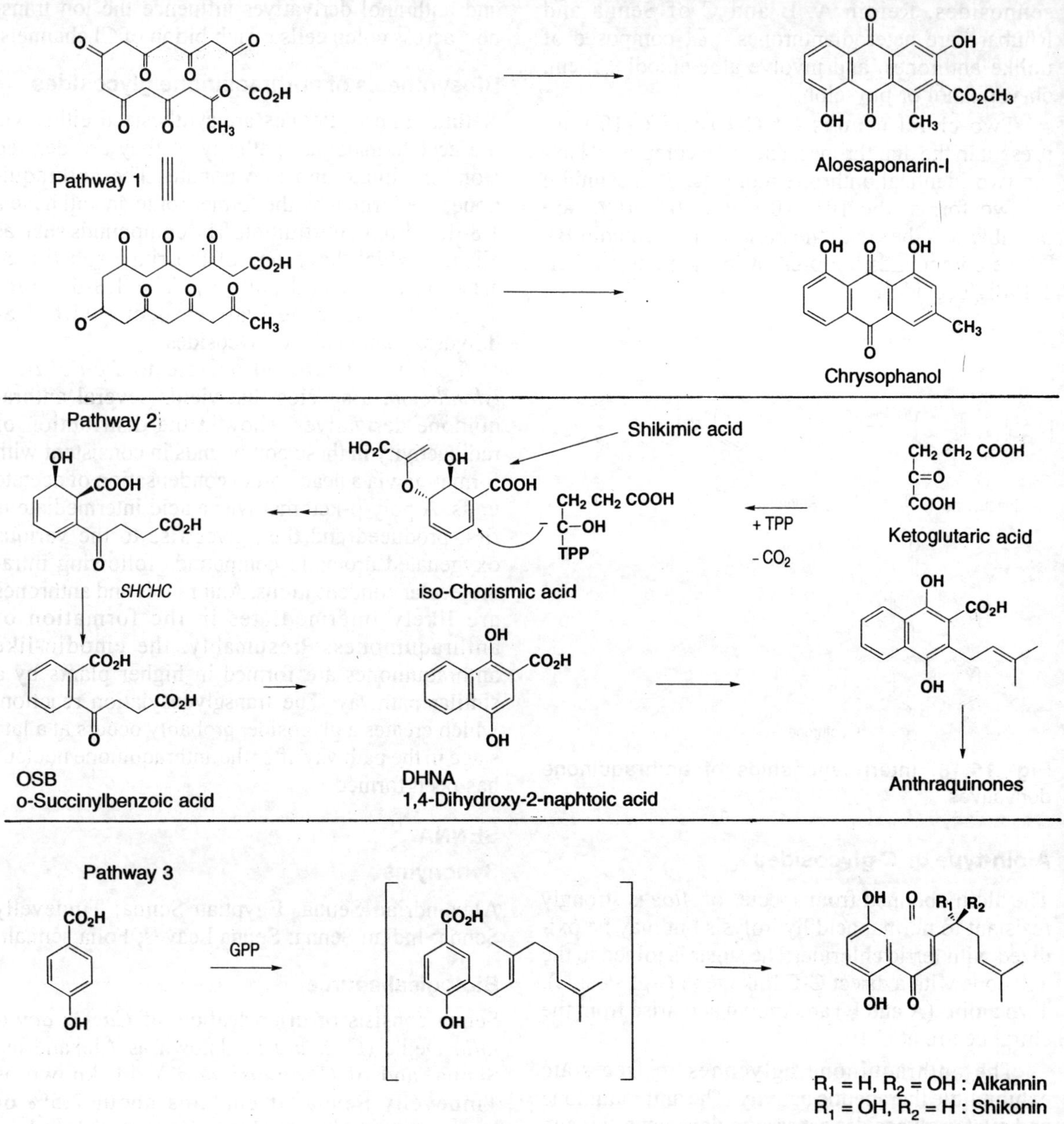

Pathway 1

Aloesaponarin-I

Chrysophanol

Pathway 2

Shikimic acid

iso-Chorismic acid

SHCHC

Ketoglutaric acid

+ TPP
− CO$_2$

OSB
o-Succinylbenzoic acid

DHNA
1,4-Dihydroxy-2-naphtoic acid

Anthraquinones

Pathway 3

GPP

R$_1$ = H, R$_2$ = OH : Alkannin
R$_1$ = OH, R$_2$ = H : Shikonin

Fig. 15.19. Biosynthetic origin of quinones.

Collection

The plant is a small shrub bearing paripinnate compound leaves.

When the leaves are fully grown and are thick and bluish in colour, they are stripped off by hand before flowering. The leaves are spread out on a hard floor to dry in shade. The pods and large stalks are separated by means of sieves. The color changes to yellow. They are graded and packed under hydraulic compression into balls and sent to the market.

Alexandrian Senna is collected mainly in Sept., from both wild and cultivated plants. The branches bearing leaves and pods are dried in the sun. The pods and large stalks are first separated by means of sieves, shaken in shallow trays, the leaves are gathered to the surface and heavier stalk fragments and sand to the bottom. The leaves are graded, partly by means of sieves and partly by hand-picking into whole leaves. The whole leaves are those usually sold to the public, while the other grades are used for making galenicals. The drug is packed loosely in bales and exported.

Tinnevelly Senna plants are more luxuriant than Alexandrian Senna. It is grown on dry or wet conditions as a successor to rice. The leaves are gathered by hand and dried in the sun.

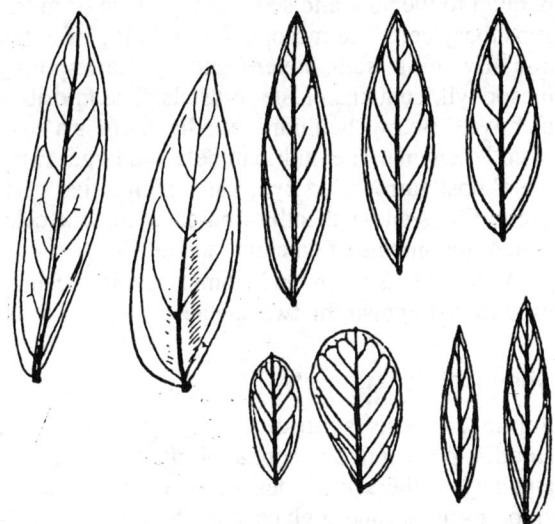

Fig. 15.21. Senna leaves.

Tinnevelley Senna differs slightly from the Egyptian Senna. Its leaflets are 2.4-6 cm long, shape is lanceolate and colour is yellowish green.

Epidermal trichomes are present on the leaflets which are unicellular, conical, thick-walled and with a warty cuticle. Lamina is isobilateral.

Microscopical characters

Senna leaflets have an isobilateral structure. The epidermal cells have straight walls, and many contain mucilage. Both surfaces bear scattered, unicellular, nonlignified warty hairs, curved at the base. The stomata have two cells with their long axes

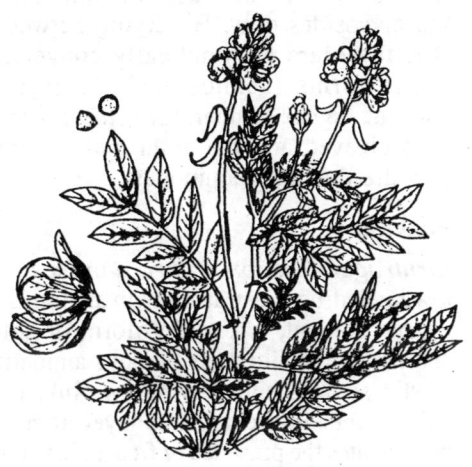

Fig. 15.20. Senna twig.

Morphology

Senna occurs in leaflets. The leaflets of Alexandrian Senna are less entire and more broken, 2-4 cm long, about 1 cm wide; margin is entire, curled, apex is acute with sharp spine at apex, base is asymmetrical, surface is pubescent, venation is pinnate, veins are anastomosing towards margin, texture is thin, brittle; colour is greyish green, odour is faint, taste is mucilaginous and slightly bitter. Senna leaflets bear stout petiolules. The surfaces are pubescent. Odour, slight but characteristic; taste, mucilaginous, bitterish and unpleasant.

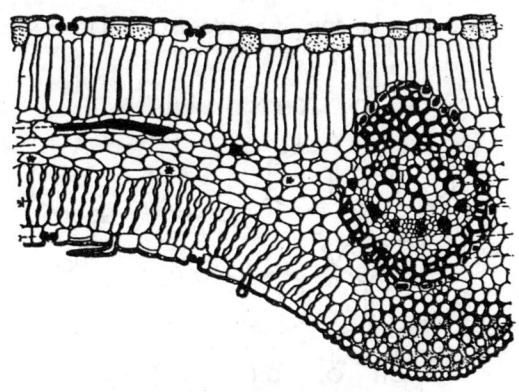

Fig. 15.22. T.S. of senna leaf.

parallel to the pore and sometimes a third or fourth subsidiary cell. The mesophyll consisting of upper and lower palisade layers and median spongy mesophyll, contains cluster crystals. The midrib is biconvex. Below the midrib bundle, there is a zone of collenchyma. The midrib bundle and larger veins are almost surrounded by a zone of lignified pericyclic fibres and a sheath of parenchymatous cells containing prisms of calcium oxalate.

Vein-islet numbers and stomatal indices can be used to distinguish the two species.

Chemical constituents

Senna contains sennidin, chrysophanic acid, emodin, physcion, chrysophanol, rhein, dianthrone glycosides, the sennosides A, B, C and D, aloe-emodin-dianthrone-diglycoside, rhein-anthrone-8-glycoside, rhein-8-diglycoside; rheinemodin, aloe-emodin-8-glucoside and aloe-emodin-anthrone diglucoside. Sennoside A and sennoside B both hydrolyse to give two molecules of glucose and the aglycones sennidin A and B. Sennidin A is dextrorotatory and B is its mesoform formed by intramolecular compensation.

Sennosides C and D are the glycosides of heterodianthrones involving rhein and aloe-emodin. The other compounds reported are palmidin A; rhein-1-glucose, and a primary glycoside having greater potency than sennosides A and B and distinguished from them by the addition of two glucose molecules. An anthraquinone glycoside, emodin-8-*O*-sophoroside (a diglucoside), has been isolated in 0.0027% yield from dried Indian senna leaves.

Two naphthalene glycosides isolated from senna leaves and pods are 6-hydroxymusizin glucoside and tinnevellin glucoside. The former is found in Alexandrian senna and the latter in Indian senna. Senna also contains the yellow flavonol colouring matters kaempferol (3,4',5,7-tetrahydroxyflavone), its glucoside (kaempferin) and isorhammetin; also a sterol and its glucoside, mucilage, calcium oxalate and resin. Water soluble polysaccharides and a lignan are also present.

In young senna seedlings anthraquinone formed are in the sequence of chryophanol, aloe-emodin and finally rhein. In the presence of light glycosylation follows and later the glycosides are translocated to the leaves and flowers. During fruit development the amounts of aloe-emodin glycoside and rhein glycoside fall markedly, and sennosides accumulate in the pericarp.

The fresh leaves of *Cassia senna* contain anthrone glycosides only. By drying between 20 and 50°C these are enzymatically converted to dianthrone forms (sennosides). If drying is conducted at higher temperature, the glycosidic linkage is cleaved and the anthrones are immediately oxidized to anthraquinones.

Chemical test

1. *Borntrager test for anthraquinones* : The powdered drug is extracted with an immiscible organic solvent, *e.g.*, chloroform or solvent ether, and after filtration aqueous ammonia or caustic soda is added, when a pink, red or violet colour in the aqueous layer after shaking indicates the presence of free anthraquinone derivatives. If glycosides are present, the test should be modified by first hydrolysing with alcoholic potassium hydroxide solution of 2 M

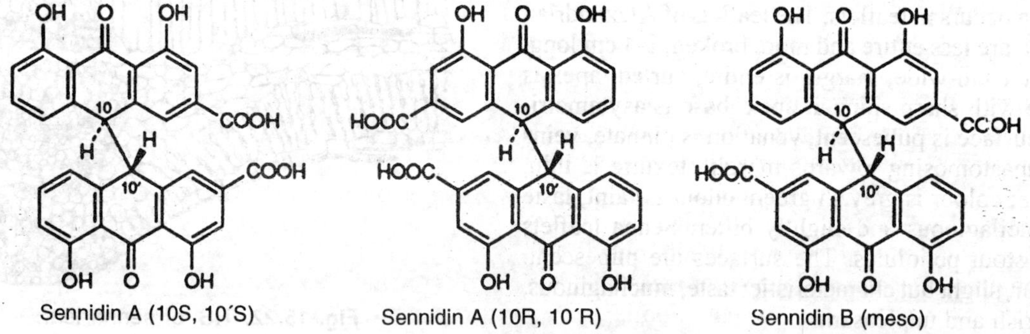

Sennidin A (10S, 10'S)   Sennidin A (10R, 10'R)   Sennidin B (meso)

Fig. 15.23a. Sennidins from Senna.

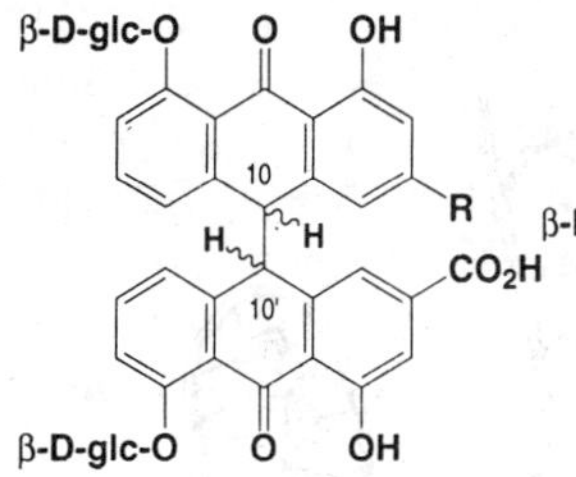

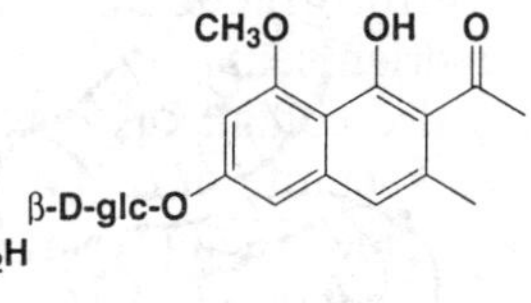

Fig. 15.23(b). Chemical constituents of Senna.

R	C-10	C-10'	
CO$_2$H	R	R	Sennoside A
CO$_2$H	R	S	Sennoside B
CH$_2$OH	R	R	Sennoside C
CH$_2$OH	R	S	Sennoside D

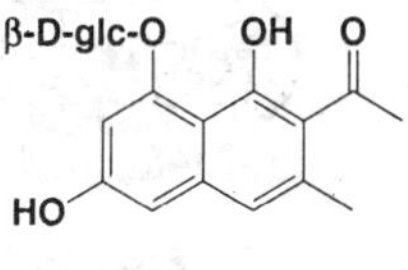

Tinevellin (glucoside)

6-Hydroxymusizin (glucoside)

acid. When alkali is added to powdered drugs or to sections, the red colour produced serves to locate the anthraquinone derivatives in the tissues. If the drug contains either very stable anthraquinone glycosides or reduced derivatives of the anthraquinone glycosides or reduced derivatives of the anthranol type, Borntrager's test will be negative.

Anthraquinones containing a free carboxylic acid group (*e.g.*, rhein) can be separated from other anthraquinones by extraction from an organic solution with sodium bicarbonate solution.

2. A little drug extract is treated with 5 N sodium hydroxide and sodium hyposulphite. On heating red colour appears.

Senna leaf must contain foreign parts (43%), foreign matter (41%), total ashes (< 12%) and HCl-insoluble ash (< 2.5%).

Assay

Senna leaves are extracted with hot water. Sennosides are liberated by treating the aqueous extract with an acid. After neutralization and centrifugation to break the emulsion, ferric chloride is added to the anthraquinone glycoside solution for oxidation which is refluxed and then acidified. The aglycones are extracted with ether, and redissolved in a solution of magnesium acetate. After measurement of the UV absorbance, the concentration is calculated and expressed as sennoside B (2.5%).

TLC analysis is conducted with an aqueous alcoholic (50%) extract. Spots are visualized by spraying a solution of sodium hydroxide and by oxidation with HNO$_3$.

Uses

Senna is used as purgative and cathartic. It is a stimulant laxative. The drug is used in acute constipation and in all cases in which defaecation with a soft stool is required; *e.g.*, with haemorrhoids, after anal-rectal operations, before and after abdominal operations, with anal fissures and for the evacuation of X-ray contrast media from intestines. The sennosides are first hydrolyzed by the intestinal bacteria and then reduced to anthrone stage, the actual active form.

There may be reddening of urine (harmless) and passage of some of the anthracene derivatives into mother's milk which may cause diarrhoea in infants. Overdose may lead to colicy abdominal pains and the formation of thin, water stools.

Allied drugs

Bombay, Mecca and *Arabian Sennas* are the leaves of *Cassia angustifolia* found in Saudi Arabia and used as a substituent. The leaflets resemble those of Tinnevelly Senna but are more elongated and narrower, and of a brownish-green colour. They may be distinguished microscopically from other sennas by their vein islet number.

Dog Senna is obtained from the leaves of *Cassia obovata*. The leaves are ovate and it contains about 1% anthraquinone derivative. The plant is indigenous to Upper Egypt. The leaves are obovate and quite different in appearance from the official leaflets. When in powder they may be distinguished by the papillose cells of the lower epidermis. They contain 1.0-1.15% of anthraquinone derivatives. It is used in France.

Palthe Senna is obtained from *Cassia auriculata*. This adulterant does not contain any sennosides. It can be examined with a hand lens by the dense pubescence on the lower surface of the leaf, and by the trichomes, which are very long, slightly wirty, and more sharply covered towards the tips. With 80% sulphuric acid, palthe senna gives a carmine-red colour due to conversion of leucoanthocycinidin to the oxonium salt. In addition to these, leaves of other senna are substituted.

In Nigeria, the leaves of the local *Cassia podocarpa* are used as a substitute for the official Senna.

Substituents

Argel leaves are derived from *Solenostemma arghel* (Asclepiadaceae), and mixed in a definite proportion with Alexandrian Senna. The plant occurs in the Sudan. In senna powder, it may be distinguished by the two- or three-celled hairs, each of which is surrounded by about five subsidiary cells.

Coriario myrtifolia leaves (Coriariaceae), are used as an adulterant of cut and powdered senna. The adulterant gives positive tests for tannin and microscopically shows an absence of trichomes and crystal idioblasts.

SENNA FRUIT

Senna pods (*Sennae Fructus*) are the dried, ripe fruits of *Cassia acutifolia* (*C. senna*) and *C. angustifolia* (Caesalpiniaceae), which are known as Alexandrian and Tinnevelly senna pods, respectively.

Collection

The pods are collected with the leaves and dried. After separation from the leaves they are handpicked into various qualities. the finer pods are sold in cartons and the inferior ones used for making galenicals.

Characters

The Tinnevelly pods are longer and narrower than the Alexandrian and the brown area of pericarp surrounding the seeds is greater. The remains of the style are distinct in the Tinnevelly but not in the Alexandrian.

The pods are readily opened after soaking in water and about six wedge-shaped seeds are disclosed, each attached to the dorsal surface of the pod by a thin funicle. Under a lens the testas of the Tinnevelly shows a general reticulation and wavy, transverse ridges; the Alexandrian has a general reticulation only. The pericarp of the pod bears unicellular hairs and stomata of a type similar to those found on Senna leaves.

Constituents

The active constituents of the pods are located in

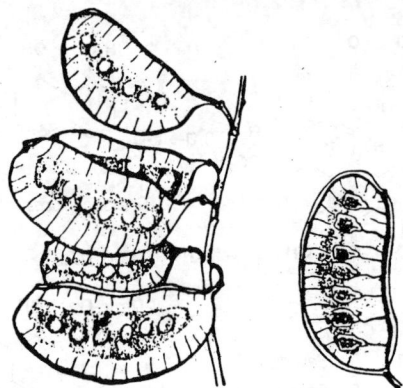

Fig. 15.24. Senna fruits.

the pericarp; they are similar to those of the leaves, together with sennoside A (15%). The seeds contain very little sennoside, 1.2 to 2.5% in the Tinnevelly and from about 2.5 to 4.5% in the Alexandrian.

Cassia pods

Cassia pods are the dried ripe fruits of *Cassia fistula* (Caesalpiniaceae), a large tree indigenous to India and widely cultivated in the tropics, the West Indies (Dominica and Martinique) and Indonesia.

The fruit is a cylindrical indehiscent pod about 25-30 cm long and 20-25 mm diameter. It is dark chocolate brown to black in colour and contains from 25 to 100 oval, reddish-brown seeds separated by membranous dissepiments. In the fresh pods the seeds are completely embedded in black pulp. The pulp has a prune-like odour and a sweetish taste.

The pulp is dissolved from the crushed fruit by percolation with water. The percolate is strained and evaporated to a soft extract. The most important anthraquinone derivatives of the pulp is rhein and combined sennidin-like compounds. Cassia pulp also contains about 50% of sugars, colouring matter and a trace of volatile oil. The leaves of *C. fistula* contain free and combined rhein, sennidins and sennosides A and B. The heartwood contains barbaloin and rhein together with a leucoanthocyanidin.

Pharmacology

Calcium sennoside A and calcium sennoside B produced contraction of rat colon which was blocked by piperazine citrate but not by atropine. Sennoside C showed much purgative activity as sennoside A in mice. Oral administration of a pod extract produced an increase in number of soft faeces in rats. It increased prostaglandin production in colonic lumen of normal rats by about four times. Oral administration of sennosides to fasted dogs induced strong and long-lasting inhibition of myoelectrical colon activity after 6-10 hours. Rhein and emodin had greater antitumor activity than aloe-emodin and showed immunosuppressive effect in mice. Rhein and emodin inhibited DNA and RNA formation. Sennosides A and B inhibited bovine serum monoamine oxidase activity. Rhein anthrone induced diarrhoea in rats 20 minutes after intracaecal administration but pretreatment with prostaglandin biosynthesis inhibitor, indomethacin, suppressed onset of diarrhoea. Rhein anthrone stimulated PGE2 release into rat colonic lumen which was depressed by indomethacin.

RHUBARB

Synonyms

Rheum, Rhizome Rhei, Rhei Radix, Revandchini (Hindi); Rhubarb rhizome; Turkey Rhubarb, Radix rhei.

Biological source

Rhubarb is the dried rhizome and roots of *Rheum officinale* Baill, *R. palmatum* L. or other species of *Rheum* (excepting *R. rhaponticum* L.), deprived of most of its bark. It contains about 2.5% of hydroxyanthracene derivatives, calculated as rhein. (Family : Polygonaceae).

Habitat

China, Tibet, Nepal, Central Asia; cultivated in Europe, southern Siberia and North America.

Collection

Rhubarb grows at a high altitude of 3000 m. The plant is perennial bearing large and vertical rhizome and thick-branched roots.

The drug is collected in autumn or spring from 6-10 years old plant by digging out. Roots are cut and outer bark is separated by peeling. The big rhizomes are cut longitudinally into small pieces, dried and exported.

The best grade of the drug is known as Shensi rhubarb. Some inferior drug is exported, much of which fails to give the pink fracture characteristic of good quality rhubarb.

The grades commonly listed are: 'flat', 'common round', 'small round', 'extra small round', 'sticks', 'third grade' and lower qualities. The flat and round are further categorized on a percentage basis (*e.g.*, 'flat, 90%' or 'common round 80%'), depending on the pinkness and quality of the fracture.

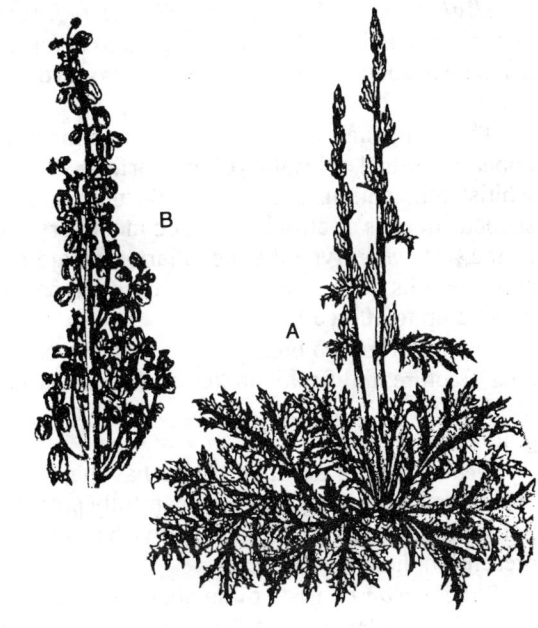

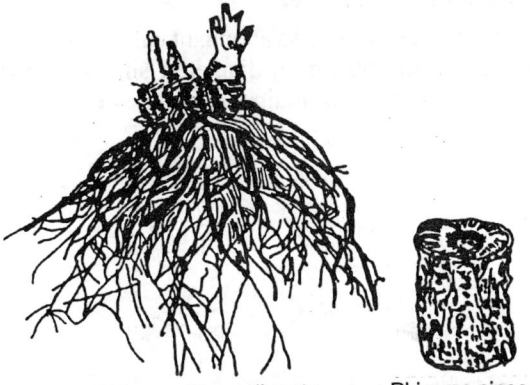

Rhizome with small roots   Rhizome piece

Fig. 15.25. *Rheum palmatum* plant and rhizome.

Morphology

The drug occurs as round or flat pieces, 5-15 cm long, diameter is 3-8 cm; shape is cylindrical; surface is smooth, firm, non-shrunken and bright yellow showing white reticulations due to fusiform or lozenge-shaped cut ends. Fracture is irregular and granular. Odour is characteristic and aromatic; taste is bitter and astringent. Holes in pieces of the drug may be caused by insect attack or made for hanging the drug up to dry.

High-grade, Chinghai or *Shensi-type* drug occurs in rounds or flats weighing up to about 200 g and up to about 15 cm long, obtained from younger plants.

The drug has a firm texture, nonshrunken appearance and a bright yellow surface showing whitish reticulations due to the fusiform or lozenge-shaped cut ends of closely arranged medullary rays. In the *palmatum* type the medullary rays are only about 6 cells deep, but in the *officinale* type they may be up to 200 cells deep.

The best rhubarb breaks with a marbled or 'nutmeg' fracture, the fleshy broken surface showing a bright pink colour—this is one character used in grading.

Medium-grade or Canton-type has the general characters of the drug but is less carefully prepared. Some pieces are badly trimmed, greyish patches are present on the outer surface.

Third grade consists of smaller pieces than in the higher grades. Only a small percentage of the fractured surfaces show a good pink fracture.

Microscopy of powder

Powdered rhubarb shows abundant calcium oxalate rosettes up to 200 μm in diameter; simple two to five compound starch grains; reticulate vessels and other wood elements which give no reaction for lignin. The yellow contents of the medullary ray cells (anthraquinone derivatives) become reddish-pink with ammonia solution and deep red with caustic alkalies.

Chemical constituents

Rhubarb contains free anthraquinones and their glycosides (3-12%) such as chrysophanol, aloe-emodin, physcion and rhein. Anthrones or dianthrones of chrysophanol, emodin, aloe-emodin, or physion are reported. The dianthrone glucosides of rhein (sennosides A and B) and the oxalates of these (sennosides E and F) are isolated. Heterodianthrones are derived from two different anthrone molecules; for example, palmidin A (aloe-emodin anthrone and emodin anthrone); palmidin B (aloe-emodin anthrone and chrysophanol anthrone), palmidin C (emodin anthrone and chrysophanol anthrone), sennidin C, rheidin B and rheidin C.

The dianthrone glucosides of rhein (sennosides A and B) and the oxalates of these (sennosides E and F), have been isolated. Sennosides A and B have been identified in callus cultures of a *R. palmatum* hybrid.

Heterodianthrones derived from two different anthrone molecules are palmidin A from aloe-emodin anthrone and emodin anthrone; palmidin B from aloe-emodin anthrone and chrysophanol anthrone. Rhein anthrone occurs combined with aloe-emodin anthrone (sennidin C and as sennoside C), chrysophanol anthrone (reidin B) and physcion anthrone (reidin C). These dianthrones may be oxidized into their two components by means of ferric chloride.

Besides these, Rhubarb contains glucogallin, free gallic acid, (−)-epicatechin gallate, catechin, rheotannic acid, erythroretin, methylchrysophanic

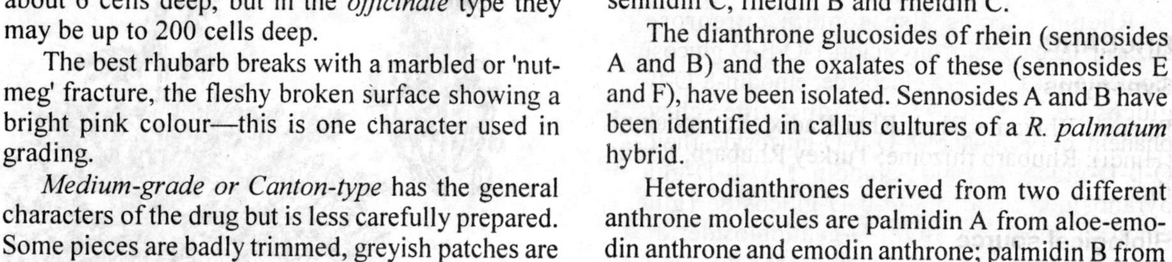

R_1=H R_2=CH$_3$: Chrysophanol
R_1=H, R_2=CH$_2$OH: Aloe-emodin
R_1=H, R_2=CO$_2$H: Rhein
R_1=OH, R_2=CH$_3$: Emodin

Fig. 15.26. Anthraquinones of Rhubarb.

acid, rhubarberon, cinnamic acid and calcium oxalate glycerol gallate, gallic acid glucoside gallates and isolindleyin (a methyl p-hydroxyphenyl-propionate derivative of a glycogallate). A new class of gallototannins has a sucrose core and chromone glucosides have also been identified.

Rhubarb also contains starch and calcium oxalate. The total ash is very variable, as the amount of calcium oxalate varies from about 5 to 40%. The acid-insoluble ash should not exceed 1%.

The anthraquinones are the major components of the anthracene mixture in the summer months and the reduced forms, the anthrones, in winter. The conversions occur within a time lapse of about 3 weeks, & just before each, the anthrone diglycoside content increases markedly. The anthraquinone → anthrone conversion could be artificially induced by decreasing the ambient temperature. The age of the rhizome also affects the ratio of reduced and oxidized glycosides.

Rheum species also contain citreorosein, alizarin, laccaic acid, physicion-1-O-β-D-glucoside, aloe emodin 1-O-β-D-glucoside, emodin-8-O-β-D-glucoside, emodin -1-O-β-D-glucoside, chrysophanein, chrysophanol-8-O-β-D-glucoside, rhein-1-O-β-D-glucoside, aloe-emodin 1'-O-β-D-glucopyranoside, emodin-3-O-β-D-glucoside (gluco-emodin), physcion-8-O-β-D-gentiobioside; dianthrones like chrysophanol dianthrone, aloe emodin dianthrone, sennidins A, B, C, rheidins A, B, C; sennosides D, E and F; rheinosides A, B, C and D; tannins 3,3'-di-O-galloylprocyanidin B-2, 3-O-galloylprocyanidin B-1, 1,2,6-tri-O-galloyl-glucose, lindleyin, 3-O-galloyl-epicatechin, gallic acid, 1-O-galloyl-glycerol, gallic acid -3-O-β-D (6'-O-galloyl) glucoside, gallic acid 4-O-β-D (6'-O-galloyl)-glucopyranoside, 1,6-di-O-galloyl-D-glucose, 6-O-galloyl glucose, isolindeyin, catechin-5-O-β-D-glucoside, catechin-7-O-β-D-glucopyranoside, 2-O-cinnamoyl-D-glucose, 2-O-cinnamoyl-1,6-di-O-galloyl-D-glucose, 2-O-(p-coumaroyl)-1-O-galloyl-D-glucose, 1-O-galloyl-fructose, 2-O-cinnamoyl-1-O-galloyl-D-glucose, 1-O-galloyl-D-glucose, 2,6-di-O-galloyl-D-glucose, 3,5-dihydroxyphenol-1-O-D-(6'-O-galloyl)-glucoside, procyanidin B2 6-C-β-D-glucoside, procyanidin B2 8-C-β-D-glucoside, catechin 3'-O-β-D-glucoside, catechin 4'-O-β-D-glucoside, catechin 7,3'-di-O-β-D-glucoside, catechin 5,3'-di-O-β-D-glucoside, catechin 3',4'-di-O-β-D-glucoside, catechin 5,4'-O-β-D-glucoside, catechin 6-C-β-D-glucopyranoside, catechin 6-C-β-D-glucopyranoside, procyanidin B3 7-O-β-D-glucopyranoside, procyanidin B3 7-O-β-D-glucopyranoside, procyanidin B1 8-C-β-D-glucopyranoside, procyanidin B1 6-C-β-D-glucopyranoside, 4-(4-hydroxyphenyl)-2-butanone-4'-O-β-D-glucopyranoside, gallic acid 4-O-β-D-gluco-pyranoside, 6-galloylisolindleyin, 6-cinnamoylisolindleyin, 6-p-hydroxyphyscionin, cinnamoylisolindleyin, pulmatin and chrysophanein. The chromone derivatives isolated from Rhubarb are 2,5-dimethyl-7-hydroxychromone, 2-methyl-5-carboxy-methyl-7-hydroxy chromone, 2-(2-hydroxypro-pyl)-5-methyl-7-hydroxy-chromone, 2-(2-hydroxy-propyl)-5-

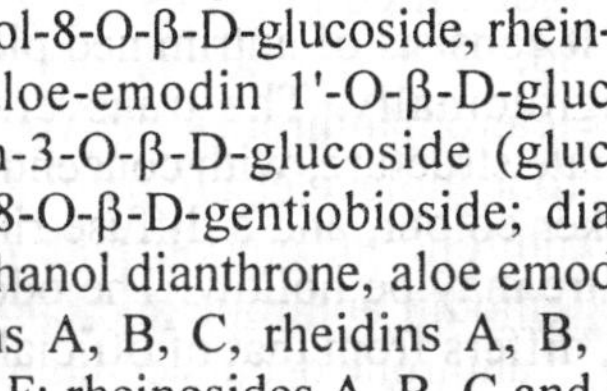

Chrysophanol-8-glucoside

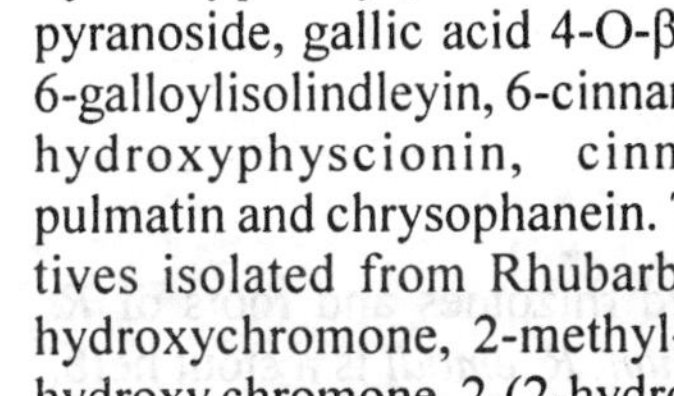

Aloe-emodin-8-glucoside

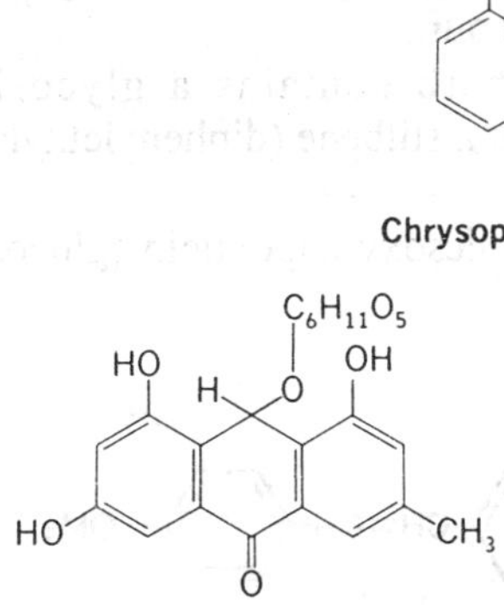

(±)-Emodin-oxanthrone glucoside

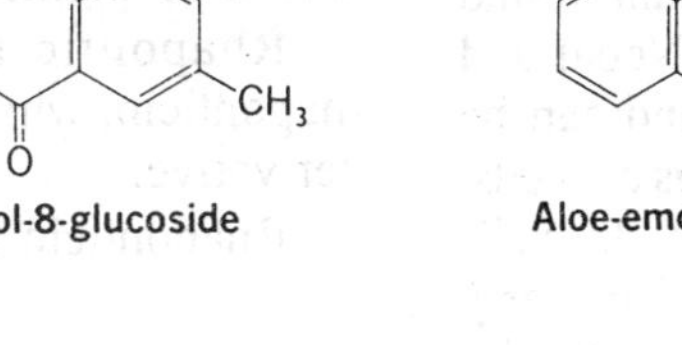

Rhein-8-glucoside

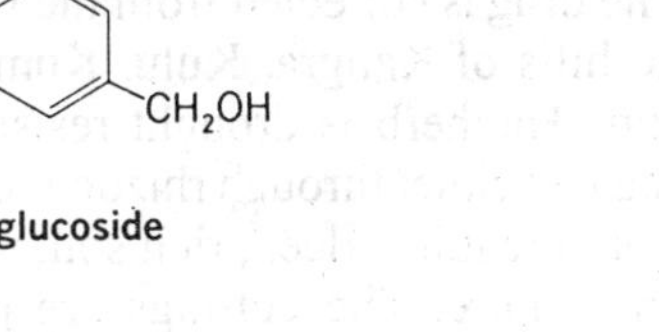

4´-O-Methylpiceid

Fig. 15.27. Chemical constituents of Rhubarb.

methyl-7-hydroxy-chromone 7-O-β-D-glucopyra-noside, 2-methyl-5-carboxymethyl-7-hydroxy-chromanone and torachrysone 8-O-β-D-glucopyra-noside.

The stilbene isomers isolated from Rhubarb ar⁻ piceid, 3,5,4'-trihydroxy-stilbene-4'-O-β-D-glucopyranoside, 3,5,4'-trihydroxystilbene 4'-O-β-D-(6"-O-galloyl)-glucopyranoside and 3,5,4'-tri-hydroxystilbene 4'-O-β-D-(2"-O-galloyl)-glucopyranoside. Two polysaccharides, DHP1 and DHP2, are present in roots and rhizomes.

Chemical tests

1. Borntrager's test described under Senna is positive due to anthraquinone derivatives.
2. It gives pink colour with ammonia.
3. A blood red colour is formed on treating Rhubarb powder with 5% KOH solution.

Uses

Rhubarb is used as a laxative; in larger doses as a purgative. It is valued as a bitter stomachic and to treat diarrhoea. Purgation is followed by an astringent effect. It is not suitable for the treatment of chronic constipation.

Other Rhubarbs

Indian rhubarb

It consists of the dried rhizomes and roots of *R. emodi* and *R. webbianum*. *R. emodi* is a stout herb, 1.5-3.0 m in height, distributed in the Himalayas from Kashmir to Sikkim at altitudes of 3,300-5,200 m. It is also cultivated in Assam for its leaves consumed as vegetable. Roots are very stout.

The drug is collected from the wild plant, found in the hills of Kangra, Kulu, Kumaun, Nepal and Sikkim. The herb is drought resistant, and can be propagated either through rhizome-cuttings or seeds. The plant requires deep, rich soil, mixed with well-rotten manure. The cuttings are planted in early spring at a spacing of 1.2-1.5 m beneath the surface. Aerial portions wither away during winter and die, but the rhizomes regenerate during the ensuring spring. Rhizomes and roots are dug up in September from 3 to 10 years old plants. They are washed and cut into pieces of proper size, kiln- or sun-dried, stored in air-tight containers and protected from sunlight.

Indian rhubarb contains a number of anthraquinone derivatives based on emodin, emodin-3-monomethyl ether (physcion), chrysophanol, aloe-emodin and rhein. These occur free and as quinone, anthrone or dianthrone glycoside. The astringent principle consists of gallic acid, present as gluco-gallin, along with tannin and catechin. The drug also contains cinnamic and rheinolic acids, volatile oil, starch and calcium oxalate. Free chrysophanic acid, sennoside A and sennoside B are also present. The characteristic odour of the essential oil is due to the presence of eugenol.

R. webbianum contains 1,8-dihydroxy-3-methyl-1,8-dihydroxy-3-hydroxymethyl- and 1,6,8-trihydroxy-3-methyl-anthraquinones and 3',5-dihydroxy-4-methoxystilbene.

Indian rhubarb is used as a purgative and astringent tonic, in atonic dyspepsia, and for cleaning teeth. Powdered roots are sprinkled over ulcers for quick healing.

Chinese rhapontic (Rhapontic rhubarb)

It is obtained from *Rheum rhaponticum*. Its odour is sweet.

It consists of untrimmed pieces sometimes split longitudinally. The transverse surface shows a radiate structure, with concentric rings of paler and darker colour, and a diffuse ring of star spots. The centre may be hollow. The odour, which is sweetish, differs from that of official rhubarb. Rhapontic rhubarb gives a positive test for anthraquinone derivatives. When the test for absence of rhapontic rhubarb is applied, it gives a distinct blue fluorescence, which may be further intensified by exposure to ammonia vapour.

Rhapontic rhubarb contains a glycoside, rhaponticin, which is a stilbene (diphenylethylene) derivative.

Rhaponticin and desoxyrhaponticin (glucoside

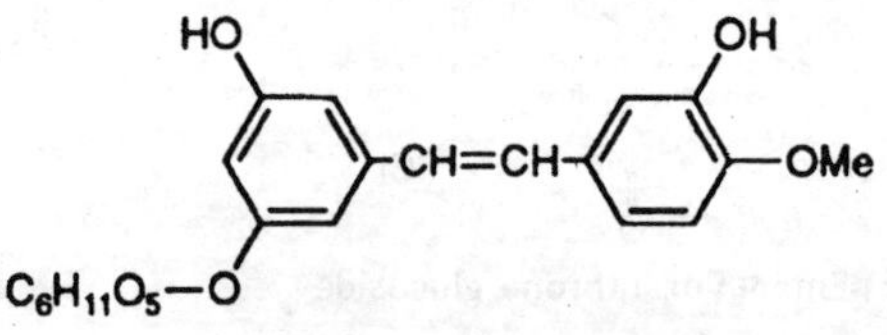

Fig. 15.28. Rhaponticin.

of 3,5-dihydroxy-4'-methoxystilbene) show the difference in fluorescence between official and rhapontic rhubarbs. Rhapontic rhubarb does contain anthraquinone derivatives, although these differ from those in the official drug. One is the glucoside glucochrysaron. It also contains 3,3',4'-5-tetrahydroxystilbene.

Chemical tests

1. *Test for anthraquinone derivatives* : A powder is shaken with 10 ml of ferric chloride solution mixed with 5 ml of hydrochloric acid and heated on a water-bath for 10 min. After filtration and cooling the filtrate is extracted with 10 ml of carbon tetrachloride. The organic layer is separated, washed with 5 ml of water and shaken with 5 ml of dilute solution of ammonia. Official and Rhapontic rhubarbs give a rose-pink to cherry-red colour.

2. *Test for Rhapontic rhubarb* : An extract of 0.5 g of powder with 10 ml of 45% alcohol for 20 min is prepared. Place one drop of the filtrate on a filter paper. When examined in ultraviolet light, the spot shows no blue colour with official Rhubarb but a distinct blue fluorescence if Rhapontic rhubarb is present. The colour is intensified by exposure to ammonia vapour.

Its alcoholic extract on filter paper shows a distinct blue fluorescence in U.V. light due to rhaponticin.

Japanese rhubarb

It is a hybrid of *R. coreanum* and *R. palmatum* and contains anthraquinone derivatives, naphthalene glycosides, stilbene glycosides and *d*-catechin.

English rhubarbs : These are cultivated forms of *R. officinale* and *R. rhaponticum*.

Pharmacology

The anthraquinones aloe-emodin, emodin and rhein inhibited the growth of *Bacillus subtilis* and *Staphylococcus aureus*, with rhein being the most effective compound. Rhein showed antimicrobial activity against *Escherichia coli, Micrococcus luteus, Candida albicans, Clostridium perfringens, Fuso-bacterium varium* and *Bacteriodes fragilis*.

Rhein and sennosides in *R. palmatum* are responsible for purgative activity. In mice, sennoside C had a stronger laxative activity than sennoside A. Sennosides act predominantly on large intestine motility after their degradation of colonic microorganisms. Sennosides are hydrolyzed by microbial β-glycosidase to the corresponding sennidins via 8-monoglycosides.

Oral administration of emodin and rhein provoked marked diuretic, natriuretic and kali-uretic effects in rabbits. The plasma corticosterone level was increased in rats suffering from diarrhoea induced by feeding rhubarb anthraquinones. A decoction of Rhubarb showed antipyretic effect in rabbits.

Plant extract of *R. officinale* is a strong and effective scavenger of oxygen radicals in xanthine/xanthine oxidase and it may probably contribute to anti-ageing and health protection through scavenging of oxygen radicals and depressing lipid peroxidation.

Chrysophanol and emodin exhibited mild spermicidal activity against human spermatozoa. Rhein exhibited antibacterial activity against *Bacillus fragilis*. 4'-O-methylpiceid and rhapontin exhibited moderate α-glucosidase inhibited activity. Pulmatin, physionin and chrysophanein showed moderate cytotoxic activity against several types of carcinoma cells.

ALOE

Synonyms

Aloes; Ghrit kumari (Sansk).

Biological source

Aloe is dried juice of the leaves of *Aloe barbadensis* Mill. (*A. vera* L.), *A. ferox* Mill and *A. africana* Mill. or their hybrids. It contains about 28% of hydroxyanthracene derivatives, calculated as anhydrous barbaloin.

The liquid is obtained from the transversely cut leaves which is concentrated by boiling and solidifies on cooling. (Family : Liliaceae).

Habitat

There are about 180 species of Aloe and most of them are found in South Africa and West Indies. *A. barbadensis* is a native of Northern Africa but it is planted in Indian gardens and many other tropical countries. Aloe plant is a typical xerophyte with thick, fleshy, strongly cuticularized spiny margined leaves arranged in rosette formation. Erect unbranched flower rises after rainy season in winter. It flourishes on poorest soil and can be propagated easily by means of a sucker.

The official varieties of aloes are the Cape from South Africa and Kenya, and the Curacao from the West Indian Islands of Curacao, Aruba and Bonaire. Socotrine and Zanzibar varieties are not official at present.

Commercial varieties of Aloe

1. *Aloe barbadensis* (Syn. *A. vulgaris, A. officianalis*) : This is known as Curacao Aloe or Barbados Aloe. It is native of northern Africa. At present it is cultivated in Aruba, Bonaire and Curacao islands near West Indies. It is a coarse-looking perennial plant with a short stem, found in semi-wild parts; leaves 30-60 cm, erect, crowded in basal rosette, full of juice, glaucous - green, narrow-lanceolate, long-acuminate, smooth; flowers yellow, in dense racemes terminating the scapes. The juice of the Aloe is collected by a thin vessel. It is packed in gourds. The Aloe is also known as Hepatic Aloe or Liver Aloe. The plant of *A. barbadensis* is of herbaceous type.

2. *Aloe ferox and its hybrids* : This drug is called as Cape Aloe and occurs wildly on the Islands of Socotra, South Africa, Kenya and neighbouring mainland of East Africa. The juice of the plant is collected in canvas or goat skin. Cape Aloe is exported from the Republic of South Africa and largely used in veterinary practice. The plant of *A. ferox* is of the arborescent type.

3. *Aloe perryi* : This Aloe is known as Socotrine and Zangibar Aloes. This is cultivated in Socotra and Zangibar Islands. It has simple stem, 2.5 cm in diameter, scarcely rising above the ground, and crowded leaves much shorter than those of *A. succotrina*. The plant is much shorter than those of *A. succotrina*. The plant is suitable to grow in the limestone-tract and can be cultivated in the driest situation and poorest soil. Zangibar Aloe is packed in skins of carnivorous animals. This Aloe is also called

as Monkey skin Aloe. The juice of Socotrine Aloe is collected in goat or sheep skin.

Leaf structure

Transverse sections of an *Aloe* leaf usually show a strongly cuticularized epidermis with numerous stomata on both surfaces; a region of parenchyma containing chlorophyll, starch and needles of calcium oxalate; a central region three-fifths of the diameter of the leaf consisting of large, mucilage-containing parenchymatous cells; a double row of vascular bundles which lie at the junction of the two previous zones and have a well-marked pericycle and endodermis. The aloetic juice, from which the drug is prepared, is present in the large, pericyclic cells and sometimes in the adjacent parenchyma. When the leaves are cut, the aloetic juice flows out. No pressure should be applied otherwise the aloes will be contaminated with mucilage. The mucilage is used in the cosmetic and herbal industries in 'aloe vera' preparations.

Preparation of Curacao Aloe

The Aloe leaves contain spines at the margins. For collection of juice of *A. barbadensis*, (Curacao Aloe) the leaves are cut in March-April in V-shaped and a vessel is kept under the incision. The juice is evaporated in copper vessel on open fire, poured into cans or tins, allowed to solidify and exported. The methods of preparation of aloes from different varieties are varied slightly. The juice of *Aloe perryi* (Scotorine Aloe) is collected in goat's or sheep's skin container which is evaporated itself without applying heat.

The temperature used is generally lower than in the case of Cape aloes and the product is usually opaque. Its semi-transparent product is known in commerce as 'Capey Barbadoes'. The drug is exported in cases each including about 58.5 kg.

Characters of Curacao Aloe

Curacao aloe varies in colour from yellowish-brown to chocolate-brown, or almost black. The drug is opaque and breaks with a waxy fracture. The semi-transparent 'Capey Barbados' becomes more opaque on keeping. Curacao has a nauseous and bitter taste and a characteristic iodoform like odour. It shows small acicular crystals, when mounted in lacto-phenol.

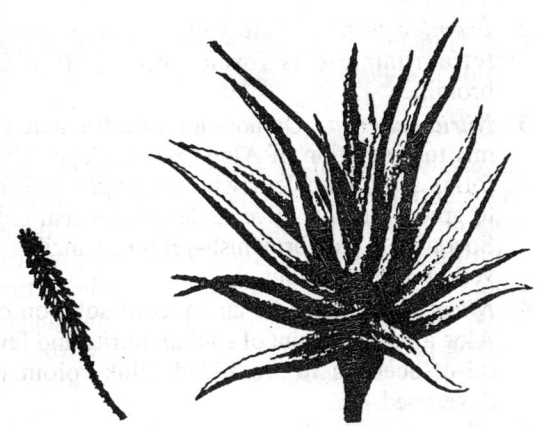

Fig. 15.29. *Aloe vera.*

Preparation of Cape Aloe

Cape aloe is prepared from wild plants of *A. ferox* and its hybrids. The leaves are cut transversely near the base and about 200 of them are arranged round a shallow hole in the ground, which is lined with plastic sheeting or a piece of canvas or a goatskin. The leaves are arranged so that the cut ends overlap and drain freely into the canvas. After about 6 h all the juice has been collected and it is transferred to a drum or paraffin tin in which it is boiled for about 4 h on an open fire. The product is poured while hot into tins, each holding 25 kg, where it solidifies. For export the tins are placed in cases holding either two, four or eight tins.

Characters of Cape Aloe

The drug occurs in dark-brown or greenish-brown, glassy masses. This fragments are deep olive colour and semitransparent. The powder is greenish-yellow, and when pieces of the drug have rubbed against each other, patches of powder are found on the surface. It has a very characteristic, sour odour. Taste, nauseous and bitter. The powder under the microscope in lactophenol is usually amorphous.

Chemical constituents

Aloe contains a mixture of crystalline glycosides known as 'aloin' (4-5% in Cape Aloe; 18-25% in Curacao Aloe), resin (16-63%), emodin and volatile oil. It also possesses the anthraquinone glycosides like barbaloin (aloe-emodin anthrone C-10 glucoside); chrysophanic acid, β-barbaloin, and iso-

barbaloin. Barbaloin is a C-glycoside and it can not be hydrolyzed easily. Barbaloin can be decompoed by oxidative hydrolysis, with ferric chloride, to yield glucose, aloe-emodin anthrone and aloe-emodin.

Aloin A is (10S)-barbaloin and aloin B the (10R)-epimer. The two are interconvertible via the corresponding anthranol form. All varieties of aloes give a strong greenish fluorescence with borax, a characteristic of anthranols, which are readily formed from anthrones by isomeric change.

Small quantities of aloe-emodin are present in aloes. Cape aloe also contains aloinosides A and B, which are *O*-glycosides of barbaloin. Aloinside B has rhamnose attached via an oxy-methyl group at C-3. In *A. barbadensis* free and esterified 7-hydroxyaloins A and B are characteristic 10-C glucosyl-anthrones which are responsible for the violet-purple colours given in various specific tests for Barbados aloes.

5-Methylchromones isolated from Cape aloes include aloeresin A and C which are *p*-coumaroyl derivatives linked via a hydroxyl of the glucose. A glycosidic 6-phenylpyran-2-one derivative (aloenin A) is present in *A. arborescens* leaves. Aloenin B has been obtained from Aloe found in Kenya.

Three new naphtho [2,3-*c*] furan derivatives have been isolated from a commercial sample of Cape aloes.

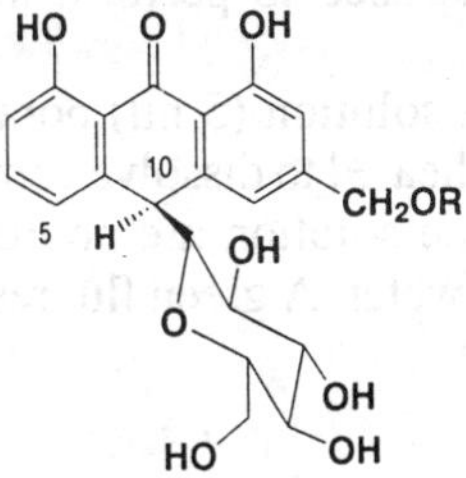

R = H, *Aloin A*
R = α-L-Rha, *Aloinoside A*

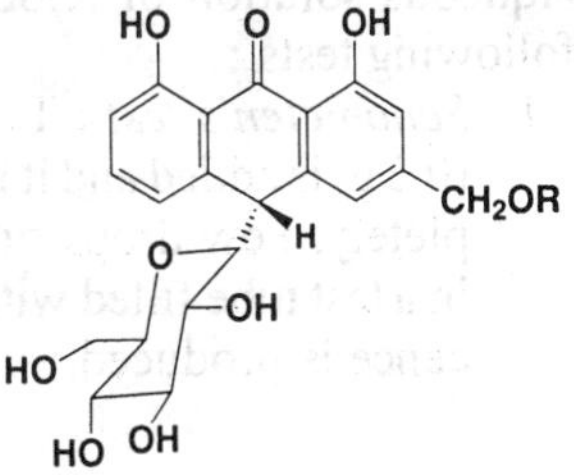

R = H, *Aloin B*
R = α-L-Rha, *Aloinoside B*

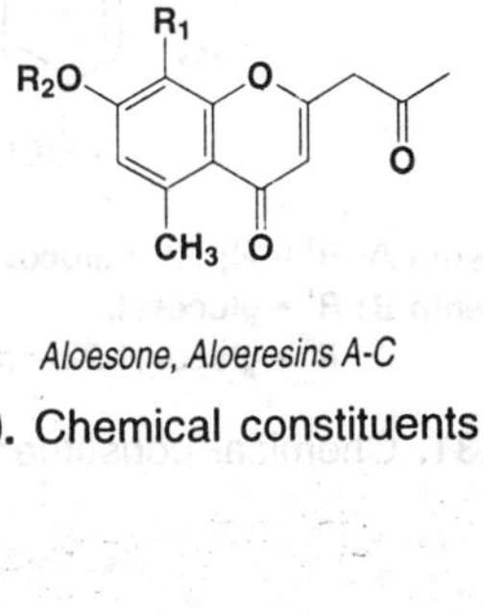

Aloesone, Aloeresins A-C

Fig. 15.30. Chemical constituents of Aloe.

The O-glycosides present in the Aloe are aloe-emodin-8-glucoside and emodin oxanthrone glucoside. Aloe resin is the ester of *p*-coumaric acid or *p*-hydroxycinnamic acid with aloe resinotannol.

Aloe *perryi* contains aloinoside B, aloesin and aloesone.

A. barbadensis also contains glucomannan, galactomannan and isoaloesin.

The principal constituents of aloin are barbaloin, isobarbaloin, β-barbaloin, aloe-emodin and resins. Phenolic glucosides identified are isoeleu-theraol β-D-glucopyranoside, aloesaponol II-6-O-D-glucopyranoside, aloesaponol III-8-O-β-D-glucopyranoside, aloenin and aloesin. During storage of aloin the content of aloe-emodin increases. In addition to these, flavonoids, oxanthra-quinones, coumarins, amino acids, monosaccharides, polysaccharides, oils, sterols, triterpenes, vitamin C and group B vitamins, citric, L-malic and formic acids are present in all aloes. Cholesterol, compesterol, β-sitosterol and lupeol are found in lipid fraction. The presence of minerals B, P, Al, Mg, Cu, Ni, Ca, K, Si, Fe, Pb, Cr, Ba, Ag, Zn and Sr have been confirmed. A bitter C-glucoside, aloe resin D, has also been isolated from Kenya aloe. Some aloes also contain polysaccharides "aloeferon" and "aloeulcin".

Chemical tests

Aqueous solution of Aloe is used to perform the following tests :

1. *Schonteten's test* : To a solution (5 ml) borax (0.2 g) is added and it is heated to dissolve completely. Few drops of the solution are poured in a test tube filled with water. A green fluorescence is produced.

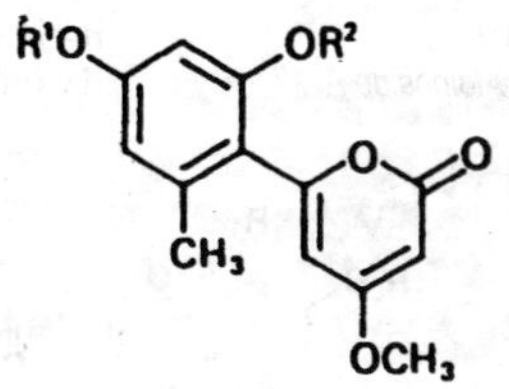

Aloenin A: R^1 = H; R^2 = glucosyl
Aloenin B: R^1 = glucosyl;
$\quad\quad\quad R^2$ = glucosyl-2-*p*-coumarate

Fig. 15.31. Chemical constituents of Aloe.

2. *Bromine test* : A pale yellow precipitate of tetrabromaloin is formed on addition of bromine.

3. *Nitric acid test* : On addition of nitric acid (2 ml) to a solution of Aloe (5 ml), Cape Aloe forms a brown colour which changes rapidly to green; Curacao gives a deep brownish-red; Socotrine a pale brownish-yellow; Zanzibar a yellow-brown colour.

4. *Nitrous acid test* : To an aqueous solution of Aloe a small amount of sodium nitrite and few ml of acetic acid are added. Pink colour is developed.

5. *Klunge's isobarbaloin test* : To an aqueous solution (20 ml) copper sulphate solution (1 drop) is added followed by sodium chloride (1 g) and 90% alcohol (10 ml). A purple colour is formed due to the presence of isobarbaloin. This test is sensitive in case of Curacao Aloe. Zanzibar and Socotrine aloes give no colour. The appearance of the red colour is rapid by warming.

6. *Modified Borntrager's test* : Aloe (0.1 g) is boiled with dil. HCl (5 ml) and 5% solution of $FeCl_3$ (5 ml) for 5 minutes. The solution is cooled, filtered and the filtrate is shaken with benzene. The benzene layer is separated, ammonia solution added to this when a pink colour is formed. Ferric chloride and dilute hydrochloric acid to bring about oxidative hydrolysis, can be used.

Uses

Aloe is used as purgative and given in constipation. It is one of the ingredient of Compound Benzoin Tincture. Ointment of aloe gel is used to cure burns caused by heat, sun or radiation, for cracks, abrasions, frostbite, chaps, insect bites, diaper rash and skin irritations. The plant is valued to cure many skin diseases, ulcerative skin conditions, wounds, burns, snake bite, as hair tonic, to treat enlarged spleen; tonic for stomach and brain, as a febrifuge and emmenagogue to relieve buring sensation. Its activity is increased when it is administered with small quantities of soap or alkaline salts, while carminatives moderate its tendency to cause griping.

In Congo, mucilage from the leaves is rubbed on the body to reduce perspiration and to eliminate human scent. Indians use pulp of the leaves mixed with burnt alum for healing sore eyes. The pulp is valued as a cooling application on inflammatory joints. In the form of lotion, it is recommended in catarrhal and purulent ophthalmia. Aloe dissolved in spirit, is used as a hair dye to stimulate hair growth. Pulp mixed with honey and Turmeric is given in coughs and colds. The juice of the leaves is useful in painful inflammation and chronic ulcers. Aloe gel is used in radiation burns to get relief from pain and itching and to keep down keratosis and ulceration.

Aloe powder and aloin are official in I.P. as purgative. Aloin is a mixture of crystalline compounds obtained from Aloes. It is yellow coloured powder with a faint odour of Aloes and intensely bitter taste. On exposure to light and air, it turns dark. It is soluble in water and alcohol (90%) and sparingly soluble in chloroform, solvent ether and benzene.

A. vera gel is useful in eczema, ulcers, poison ivy and burns. Application of fresh Aloe pith relieves pain, burning and itching, has antiseptic action and stimulates rapid granulation and formation of new tissues. *Aloe vera* gel has stimulating effect on the healing of leg ulcers, hair growth and drying of seborrheic skin. The action is believed to be due to the presence of mucopolysaccharides in the gel which may be aided by enzymatic removal of necrotic tissue. Aloe penetrates tissue injury, relieves pain, is an anti-inflammatory, dilates capillaries and increases the blood supply to the injured area by inhibiting TxA_2 and maintaining the PGE_2 and PGE_{2a} ratio without causing a collapse of the injured blood vessels. Aloe extracts reverse the degenerative skin changes seen with ageing by stimulating the synthesis of collagen and elastic fibres.

Allied drug

Indian Aloe

It is obtained from *Aloe vera* var. *officinalis*. It is found on the coasts of Bombay, Gujarat and Tamil Nadu. The colour of the Aloe is dark. It contains aloin but *iso*-barbaloin is almost absent. It is widely used in cosmetic products.

Aloe is substituted by Socotrine and Zangibar varieties from *Aloe perryi* and Natal Aloe (*A. candelabrum*). Socotrine Aloe occurs as yellowish-brown to blackish brown, opaque masses and breaks with a porous fracture. Zanzibar is identical but has a waxy fracture. Natal Aloe grows near Pietermaritzburg. It contains nataloin, homonataloin, and a resin consisting of natalores-inotannol and paracoumaric acid. Mocha Aloe is imported from Bombay. It is black, brittle, glassy aloe with strong odour and is of inferior quality, Jafferabad Aloe is nearly black.

'Aloe vera' products

The mucilaginous gel has been used for the treatment of numerous conditions. Its use in the herbal and cosmetic industries has become very big business in the USA and Europe. It is largely composed of a mucilaginous polysaccharide consisting of glucomannans and pectic substances together with a range of other organic and inorganic compounds. Prostanoids have been isolated.

Chrysarobin

Chrysarobin is prepared from araroba or Goa powder by extraction with hot benzene. Araroba is extracted from cavities in the trunk of *Andira araroba* (Papilionaceae). Chrysarobin contains chrysophanol anthranol, the corresponding anthrone and other similar constituents; it gives a strong green fluorescence in alkaline solutions. Chrysarobin is used for skin disease.

CASCARA BARK

Synonyms

Sacred bark; Chittem bark; Chittim bark; Purshiana bark; Persian bark; Bearberry bark; Bearwood; Cascara sagrada; Rhamnus purshiana; Cortex rhamni.

Biological source

Cascara is the dried bark of *Rhamnus purshiana* DC., syn. *Frangula purshiana* (DC.) A. Gray usually collected one year before its use.

It should be aged for at least 1 year prior to use in medicinal preparations. Reduced forms of emodin-type glycosides are present in the fresh bark; during the minimum 1-year storage period, these glycosides are converted to monomeric oxidized glycosides, which exhibit a milder cathartic activity. (Family : Rhamnaceae).

Habitat

Cascara is grown on the Pacific coast of North America, British Columbia, Oregon, Washington, California and Kenya.

Collection

The bark is collected during April-August from 6-12 meters high tree. The bark is removed from the tree by making longitudinal incisions. The trees are often felled and the bark is separated from larger branches. It is dried in the shade or in sun by keeping cork upper side. The bark is stored by protecting from rain and damp. The dried bark is cut into small pieces.

The inner surface is not exposed to the sun in order to retain the yellow colour. After the large quills are dried, they are run through a "breaker" and broken into small transversely curved pieces.

Such material is referred to as 'natural' cascara. The commercial supplies contain small fragment known as 'evenized', 'processed' or 'compact' ca cara. During preparation and storage the bark m be protected from rain and damp, to check pa: ual extraction of the constituents or the bark may become mouldy. The bark appears to increase in medicinal value and price until it is about 4 years

old. Many companies prefer to use bark which has been stored for considerably more than 1 year. To reduce freight and handling charges on the bark, large quantities of the extract are used directly.

Macroscopical characters

The bark occurs in quills, or channelled or nearly flat pieces, 20 cm in length and are 1-4 mm thick, the thinner bark is valued. The flat strips from the trunk are usually much wider (up to 10 cm) than the quills or channelled pieces (about 5-20 mm) obtained from the branches.

Cascara possesses patchy, silvery-grey coat of lichens. Pieces bearing moss are also quite common. Between the patches of lichen there is a smooth, dark purplish-brown cork marked with lighter-coloured, transversely elongated lenticels. On scraping the cork, no bright purple inner cork is disclosed (distinction from *R. alnus*). The inner surface is dull purplish-brown to black, striated longitudinally and corrugated transversely. The fracture is short and granular in the outer part, but fibrous in the phloem. In the yellowish-brown cortex and phloem lighter groups of sclerenchymatous cells and phloem fibres are present. They become more distinct by staining with phloroglucinol and hydrochloric acid. The medullary rays are well seen in sections mounted in potash. Odour slight but characteristic; taste bitter.

Microscopical characters

A transverse action of Cascara bark shows a partial coat of whitish lichen, 10-15 layers of flattened cork cells with reddish-brown contents and a cortex composed of collenchyma, parenchyma and groups of sclereids. The collenchymatous cells show thickened pitted walls and contain chloroplasts filled with starch. Some of the parenchymatous cells contain chloroplasts, starch; a yellow substance coloured violet by alkalis and rosette crystals of calcium oxalate. The parenchymatous cells present on the groups of sclereids contain prisms of calcium oxalate. The sclereids are irregular or ovoid in shape, variable in size and have thick lignified walls with stratification and traversed by funnel-shaped pits. A pericycle is not clearly delimited. The phloem is composed of elongated groups of phloem fibres, enclosed in a sheath of parenchymatous cells con-

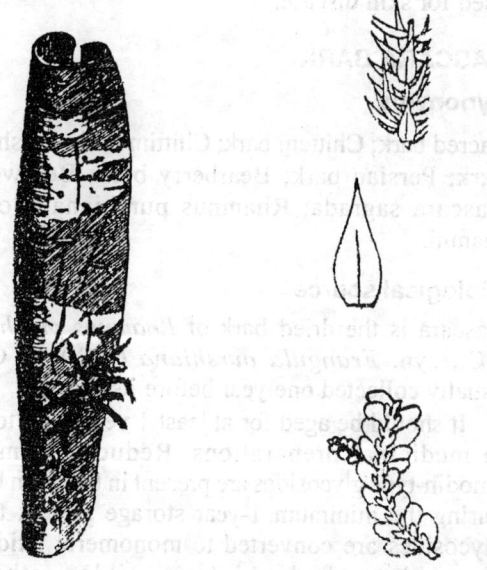

Fig. 15.32. Cascara sagrada.

taining prisms of calcium oxalate which alternate with sieve tubes and phloem parenchyma. The individual fibres are yellow in colour, 8-15 μm in diameter, and have thick lignified walls showing stratification and pit canals. The sieve tubes show sieve plates, each with several sieve fields. The sieve plates are usually covered with a deposit of callus and can be identified after staining with alkaline solution of corallin. The phloem parenchyma contains plastids, starch, material coloured violet by alkali, and rosettes of calcium oxalate. The medullary rays are 1-5 cells wide and 15-25 cells deep. The medullary rays are parenchymatous, radially elongated and with similar contents to those of the parenchyma; their content of material stained violet by alkali is often high. Fragments of moss leaves and liverworts are present in the powder.

Chemical constituents

Cascara contains anthracene derivatives which are normal O-glucosides (10-20%) and C-glucosides (80%) and free anthraquinones. Cascarosides A, B, C and D contain both O- and C-glucosidic linkages.

Two aloins, namely barbaloin derived from the aloe-emodin anthrone and chrysaloin derived from chrysophanol anthrone, are the C-glycosides. Cascara possesses O-glycosides derived from emodin, emodin oxanthrone, aloe-emodin and chrysophanol. Various dianthrones such as those of emodin, aloe-emodin and chrysophanol and the heterodianthrones palmidins A, B and C have been reported in Cascara bark. It also contains aloe-emodin, chrysophanol and emodin in the free state.

Cascara bark stored at least 1 year gave galenicals which were better tolerated that as effective as those prepared from more recently collected bark.

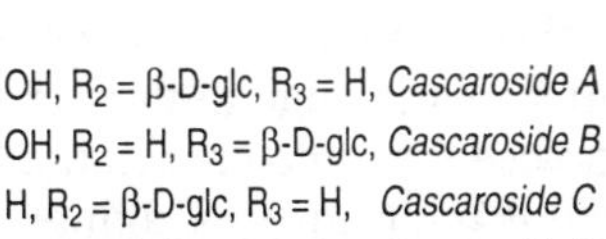

R$_1$ = OH, R$_2$ = β-D-glc, R$_3$ = H, *Cascaroside A*
R$_1$ = OH, R$_2$ = H, R$_3$ = β-D-glc, *Cascaroside B*
R$_1$ = H, R$_2$ = β-D-glc, R$_3$ = H, *Cascaroside C*
R$_1$ = H, R$_2$ = H, R$_3$ = β-D-glc, *Cascaroside D*

Fig. 15.33. Cascarosides.

This is due to hydrolysis or other changes during storage. The bitter taste of Cascara is reduced by treating extracts with alkalis, alkaline earths or magnesium oxide.

The primary glycosides are more active than the aloins whereas the cascarosides have a sweet and more pleasant taste than the aloins. The bark should contain not less than 8.0% of hydroxyanthracene glycosides of which not less than 60% consists of cascarosides, calculated as cascaroside A. A two-point spectrophotometric assay is employed with absorbance measurements at 515 nm and 440 nm.

The free anthraquinones are formed in the leaves which are stored in the bark mainly as C-glycosides, the older bark containing the most C-glycosides. *Rhamnus purshianas* cell suspension cultures will produce anthracene derivatives in which the accumulation of these compounds, particularly emodin, is significantly raised by a 12 h light/dark cycle, continuous illumination of the cultures suppresses anthraquinone formation.

Substitutes

These include *R. alnifolia*, which is too rare to be a likely substitute; *R. crocea*, whose bark bears little resemblance to the official drug. *R. californica* is very closely related to *R. purshiana*. It has a more uniform coat of lichens and wider medullary rays than the official species, but resembles the latter in having sclerenchymatous cells. The bark of *R. fallax* has been recorded as a Cascara substitute.

Uses

Cascara is a purgative resembling senna in its action. It is mainly used in the form of liquid extract or elixir or as tablets prepared from a dry extract. It is also used in veterinary medicine.

Allied drugs

Frangula bark

Frangula bark, alder buckthorn, is obtained from *Rhamnus frangula* L. (*Frangula alnus* Mill) (Rhamnaceae). It is a shrub 3-5 m high and found in Britain and Europe. It bears dark-purple berries.

The bark is required to contain not less than 6% of hydroxyanthracene derivatives calculated as glucofrangulin A.

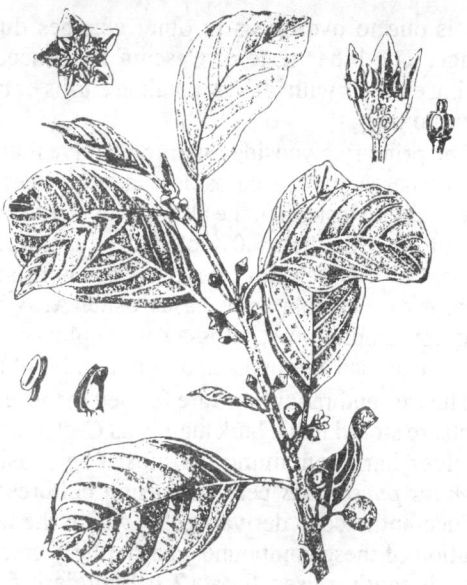

Fig. 15.34. *Rhamnus frangula.*

The bark occurs in single or double quills which are usually of smaller size than those of Cascara and about 0.5-2 mm thick. It has a purplish cork and transversely elongated, whitish lenticels. On removing the outer cork cells by scraping, a dark crimson inner cork is exposed. The transverse section closely resembles that of Cascara but groups of sclerenchymatous cells are absent.

Frangula contains anthraquinone derivatives present mainly in the form of glycosides. Frangulosides A and B are formed by partial hydrolysis of the corresponding rhamnoglucosides, glucofrangulins A and B. The fresh bark also contains anthranols and anthrones, emodin-dianthrone, palmidin C, palmidin C monorhamnoside and emodin-dianthrone monorhamnoside, frangulin B as 6-O-(D-apiofuranosyl)-1,6,8-trihydroxy-3-methyl-

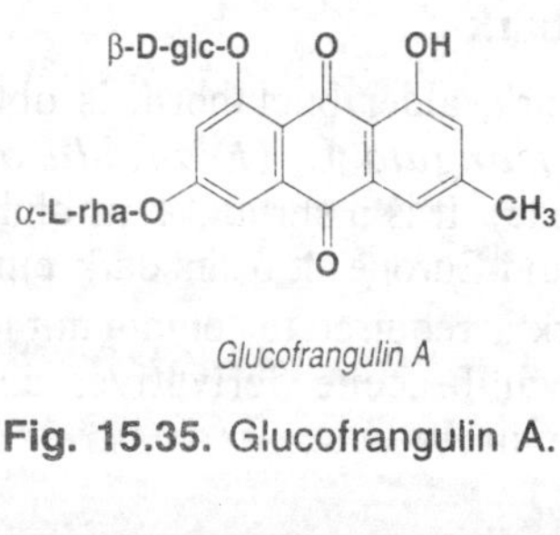

β-D-glc-O

α-L-rha-O

OH

CH_3

Glucofrangulin A

Fig. 15.35. Glucofrangulin A.

anthraquinone and another glycoside emodin-8-*O*-β-gentiobioside. It is used as a laxative.

Buckthorn

The common buckthorn, *Rhamnus cathartica*, has a glossy reddish- or greenish-brown cork and does not possess sclereids. It contains frangula-emodin and a glycoside, rhamnicoside, which yields on hydrolysis rhamnicogenol (an anthraquinone derivative), glucose and xylose, the anthraquinone glycoside alaternin; 1,2,6,8-tetrahydroxy-3-methyl-anthraquinone; physcion; chrysophanol; and fragulaemodin, blue-fluorescent substances which in the chromatograms produced by the tests of identity for Cascara and Frangula serve to distinguish this adulterant. The fluorescent substances have been identified as naphtholide glycosides of the sorigenin type.

The bark of *R. carniolica* has a dull reddish cork and differs from Frangula bark in that it possesses sclerenchymatous cells and has wider medullary rays. The barks of Turkish species of Rhamnus have been systematically examined for their anthraquinone and flavonoid contents.

Hypericum

The dried, flowering, aerial parts of *Hypericum perforatum* (Guttiferae), act as a sedative and astringent. It has antibacterial properties and is used in the treatment of infections, and as a food preservative. Dark-coloured glands visible in the leaves and petals contain the red dianthrone pigment hypericin which acts as a photosensitizing agent in mammals. The narrow-leaved varieties, both in Europe and Australia, are the most poisonous and contain hypericin. The plant also contains the acyl-phloroglucinol, hyperforin, which is antibacterial. Alkanes in the series C_{16}-C_{29} are present.

Saponin glycosides

Saponins are highly complex glycosides which are widely distributed in the higher plants. The drugs like Quillaia, Sarsaparilla and Senega have their medicinal properties due to the saponins they contain. Saponins form colloidal solution in water which give a soap-like froth on shaking. They have the property of causing haemolysis of red blood corpuscles, even at great dilution. Most of the saponins are highly toxic when injected into the body, and when taken orally. They are very toxic to fish. Sarsaparilla is rich in saponins but is widely used in the preparation of nonalcoholic beverages.

Saponins have a high molecular weight and a high polarity and their isolation in pure form is difficult. Often they occur as complex mixtures with the components differing only slightly from one another in the nature of the sugars present, or in the structure of the aglycone. Various chromatographic techniques are used for their isolation. On hydro-lysis they yield an aglycone known as 'sapogenin' which may be a steroid or a triterpene and the sugar moiety may be glucose, galactose, a pentose or a methylpentose.

According to the structure of the aglycone or sapogenin, two kinds of saponin are known, e.g., steroidal (commonly tetracyclic triterpenoids) and the pentacyclic triterpenoid types. Both of these have a glycosidal linkage at C-3 and have a common biogenetic origin via mevalonic acid and isoprenoid units.

Steroidal saponins of the steroidal alkaloids are present in many members of the Solanaceae. They possess a heterocyclic nitrogen-containing ring, giving the compounds basic properties.

Steroidal saponins

The steroidal saponins are less widely distributed in nature than the pentacyclic triterpenoid type. They are present in many monocotyledonous families, particularly the Dioscoreaceae (e.g., Dioscorea spp.), Amaryllidaceae (e.g., Agave spp.) and Liliaceae (e.g., Yucca and Trillium spp.). In the dicotyledons the presence of diosgenin in Fenugreek (Papilionaceae) and of steroidal alkaloids in Solanum (Solanaceae) is of importance. Some species of Strophanthus and Digitalis contain both steroidal saponins and cardiac glycosides.

Steroidal saponins are related to compounds such as the sex hormones, cortisone, diuretic steroids, vitamin D and the cardiac glycosides. Some are used as starting materials for the synthesis of these compounds. Diosgenin is the principal sapogenin. Most yams contain a mixture of sapogenins in the glycosidic form. Natural sapogenins differ only in their configuration at carbon atoms 3, 5 and 25, and in the spirostane series the orientation at C-22. Mixtures of the C-25 epimers diosgenin (Δ^5, 25α-spirosten-3β-ol) and yamogenin (Δ^5,25β-spirosten-3β-ol) are of normal occurrence and their ratio is dependent upon morphological part and stage of development of the plant. The side-chain forms ring F of the sapogenin is kept open by glycoside formation as in the bisdesmosidic saponin sarsaparilloside of Smilax aristolochiaefolia.

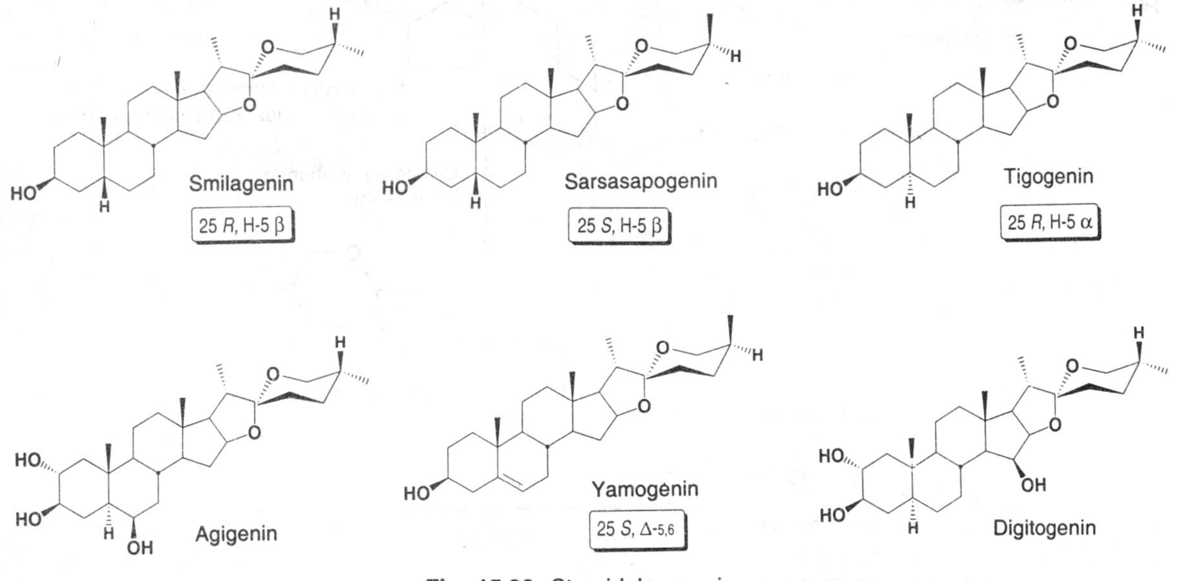

Fig. 15.36. Steroidal saponins.

Biogenesis of steroidal saponins

Steroidal saponins arise via the mevalonic acid pathway. A scheme for the subsequent cyclization of squalene gives cholesterol. Cholesterol can be incorporated into a number of C_{27} sapogenins without side-chain cleavage. The steroidal saponins exist in plants in a form where the side-chain is held open by glycoside formation. Such open-chain saponins are formed from cholesterol. In *Dioscorea* homogenates, such compound is converted to dioscin (a diosgenin glycoside).

Biosynthesis of saponin glycosides

The main pathway leading to sapogenins is similar and involves the head-to-tail coupling of acetate units. However, a branch occurs, probably after the formation of the triterpenoid hydrocarbon, squalene, that leads to steroids in one direction and to cyclic triterpenoids in the other.

DIOSCOREA

Synonyms

Wild yam; Colic root; Rheumatism root.

Biological source

Dioscorea is the dried rhizome of several species of *Dioscorea* like *D. villosa, D. prazeri* Prain & Burk; *D. composita, D. spiculiflora; D. deltoidea* and *D. floribunda.* (Family : Dioscoreaceae).

Habitat

North America and Mexico. In India the plants grow wild in western Himalayas up to an altitude of 3000 m.

Dioscorea plants are climbing; roots tuberous; tubers large; stem leafy.

Dioscorea species are distributed throughout India except in the dry north-western region. These plants are cultivated mostly as garden crops or subor-

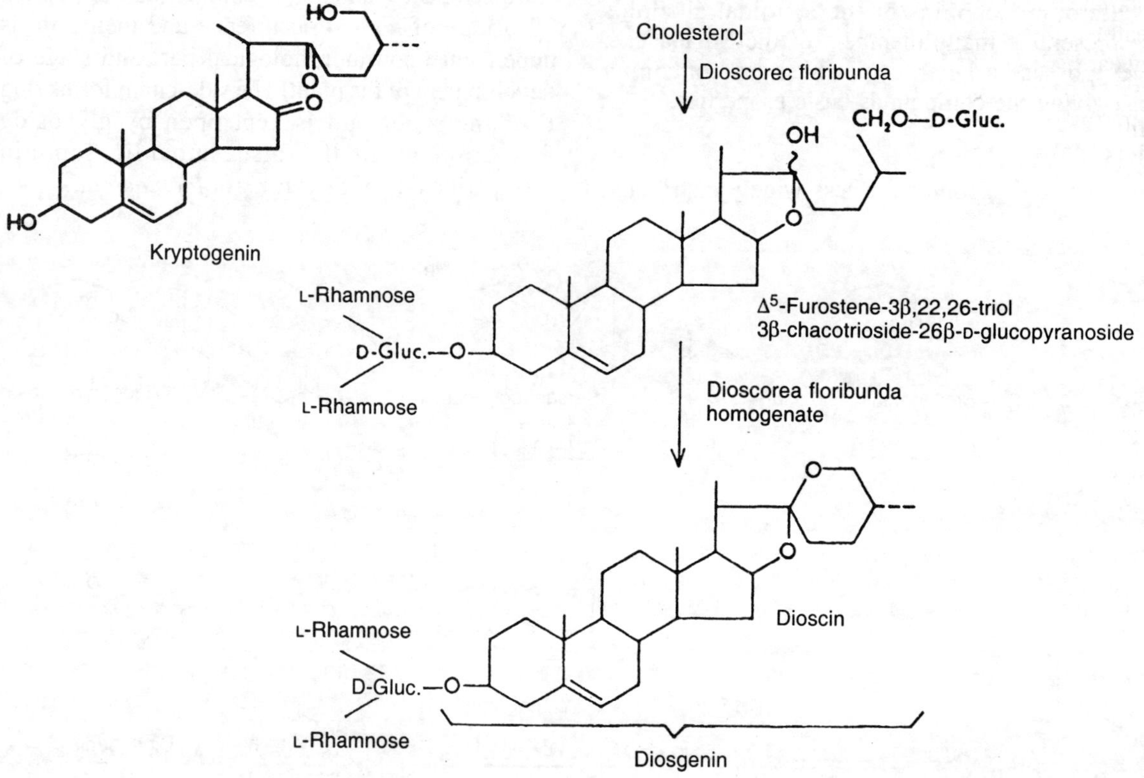

Fig. 15.37. Biosynthesis of an open-chain saponin in Dioscorea.

dinate crops with ginger, turmeric, brinjal, sweet potato or maize. They thrive best in deep sandy loams with adequate moisture and good drainage. The field should be well prepared by digging to considerable depth and manuring liberally. Farmyard manure is usually applied. Both tuber tops and aerial tubers borne on the stems are used for propagation. The planting period is generally April-June before the onset of the monsoon, but it may vary according to local condition and the species. Vines are allowed to trail on ground or are trailed over stakes or trees nearby. The crop is ready after 5-8 months of planting. During this period, the field is hoed and weeded and earthed up round the stems.

Tubers are variable in shape and size. Some species produce large cylindrical tubers penetrating deep into the ground while others produce globose tubers, close to the soil surface. Tubers are either solitary-one from each plant - or several of them are clustered together at the base of the plant. The yield ranges from 2 to 14 tons per acre depending upon the variety cultivated, the soil and the cultural treatment. Discoreas are stored in cool sheds under dry earth or sand for about 6 months.

The yams of several species are soft, fleshy and edible.

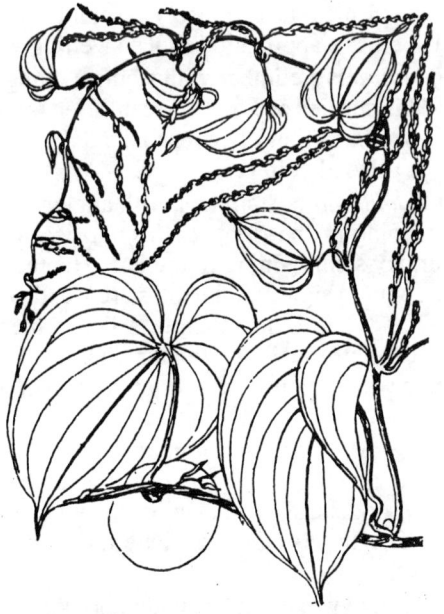

Fig. 15.38. *Dioscorea bulbifera.*

Chemical constituents

Dioscorea is a source of saponin glycoside diosgenin. Botagenin and diosgenin are obtained from the root of *Dioscorea spiculiflora*. Diosgenin is obtained by hydrolysis of dioscin. Dioscorea also contains small quantities of hecogenin having keto group at 12 position of diosgenin; and an acrid resin. Dioscin on acidic hydrolysis yields dios-genin, rhamnose and glucose.

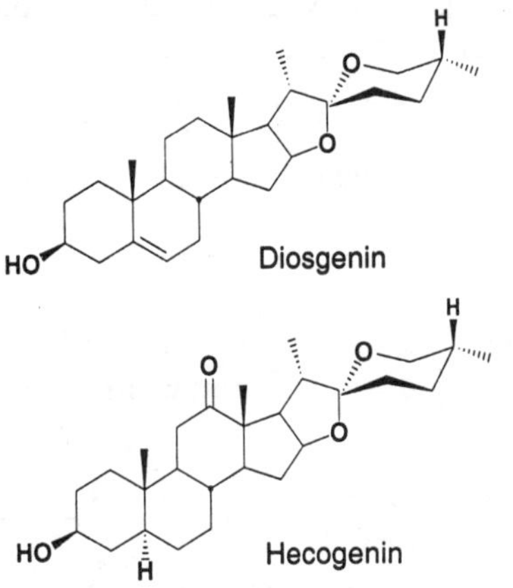

Fig. 15.39. Sapogenins.

Besides the steroid components, furanoid norditerpenes, *viz.*, diosbulbins A, B, C, D, E, F, G and H were isolated. *D. bulbifera* also contains glycosides diosbulbinosides D and F, acetophenone derivatives 4-hydroxy-2-(*trans*-3,7-dimethylocta-2,6-dienyl)-6-methoxyacetophenone and 4,6-dihydroxy-2-(4-hydroxybutyloxy)-acetophenone.

D. floribunda contains steroidal saponins floribundasaponins A, B, C, D, E, F, amino acids, zeatin and its riboside diosgenin.

The alkaloid, dioscorine, and the saponin, dioscin, occur in varying quantities in different species. American species contain the steroidal sapogenins, diosgenin, yamogenin and kryptogenin. Botogenin, obtained from *D. mexicana*, is a starting material for the synthesis of cortisone, used in the treatment of rheumatoid arthritis and rheumatic fever.

Uses

Diosgenin is used for the production of various steroidal drugs like progesterone, and as a cheap source of carbohydrate food. Some species, *e.g.*, *D. alata*, are used for the extraction of starch. Some of them are rich in vitamins B_1, B_2 and B_6.

Allied species

D. alata, a native of south east Asia, is the most important cultivated species throughout the tropics. The tubers are starchy and used as vegetable, anthelmintic, in leprosy, piles and gonorrhoea. *D. alata* contains cyanidin-3-gentiobioside, (+)-catechin, procyanidins B_1 and B_3, alatanins 1 and 2, A, B and C.

D. bulbifera is a large unarmed climber with stems twining to the left. The tubers are used mostly as famine food, to prepare starch, for washing wool, as fish bait in Kashmir and to treat ulcers, piles, dysentery and syphilis. *D. bulbifera* tuber possesses furanoid diterpenoids diosbulbins A, B, C, D, E, F, G and H, dihydro-phenanthrene, 2,4,5,6-

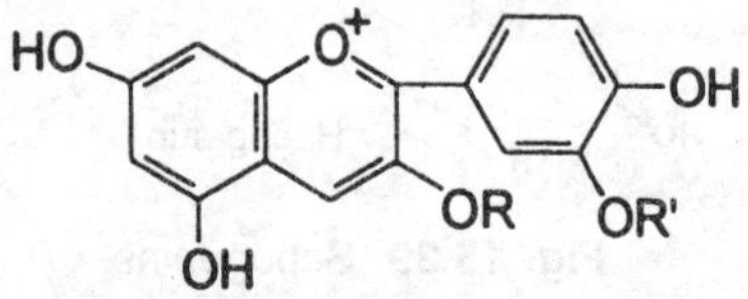

Alatanin 1
R = Gentiobiose(4"-O-sinapoyl), R' = H
Alatanin 2
R = Gentiobiose(4"-O-sinapoyl), R' = Me

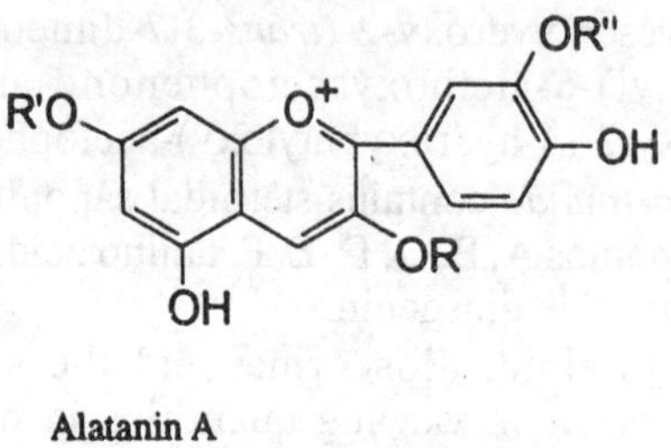

Alatanin A
R = X-(3→1)Glu, R' = Glu(6-O-(E)
sinapoyl), R" = Glu
Alatanin B
R = X, R' = Glu(6-O(E)sinapoyl),
R" = Glu
Alatanin C
R = X, R',R" = H

X = Glu(6→1)Glu(6-O-(E)sinapoyl)

Fig. 15.40. Anthocyanidins.

tetrahydroxy phenanthrene, D-sorbitol, 4-hydroxy-2-(*trans*-3',7'-dimethyl-octa-2'-6'-dienyl)-6-methoxyacetophenone, 4,6-dihydroxy-2-O-(4'-hydroxybutyl) acetophenone, 2,4,6,7-tetrahydroxy-9,10-dihydrophenanthrene, and diosbulbins B, D, E, F, G and H.

An acetone extract of rhizomes of *D. bulbifera* inhibited food intake in rats.

D. deltoidea is an extensive climber with unarmed stem twining to the left. The tubers are rich in saponin and are used for washing silk, wood and hair, and in dyeing. They kill lice. The *D. deltoidea* rhizome contain total sapogenins (1.87%), diosgenin, yamogenin, deltonin, deltoside and diosgenin-3-O-β-D-glucosyl-(1→3)-glucosyl-(1→4)-glucopyranoside. Deltofolin is present in the leaves. It also contains smilagenone, epismilagenin, diosgenin acetate, trioside and tetraoside of furostanol, deltofolin, cholesterol, β-sitosterol, stigmasterol and dioscin.

The maximal biliary cholesterol output significantly increased by 500% in diosgenin-fed animals.

D. esculenta is a prickly climber; tubers 4 to many stalked, produced in branches close to the surface of the ground. The tubers are starchy and free from dioscorine. They have a sweetish taste; in flavour and mealiness, closely resemble potatoes. The Tubers are applied to reduce swelling.

D. glabra is a climber with stems twining to the right. This species occurs in Assam, Bengal, Bihar, Orissa, Andaman and Nicobar Islands. The tubers are used as food edible.

D. hamiltonii is a climber with angled glabrous stem twining to the right. *D. hispida* is a climber with pricky stem twining to the left. The tubers are large, contain high amount of starch and used as famine food. The toxic principle is dioscorine which is distributed throughout the plant. The milky juice of tubers with the juice of *Antiaris toxicaria* is used as arrow poison.

D. oppositifolia is a climber with glabrous or finely pubescent stem. The tuber is usually single with few rootlets; skin reddish; flesh white, soft and edible. The tubers are used externally to reduce swellings.

D. pentaphylla is a tall, slender, prickly climber. Tubers are almost invariably single; texture and shape variable, skin brown, yellow or purplish. They are used to disperse swellings and as tonic.

D. prazeri is a climber with smooth or slightly ridged, unarmed stem. The tubers contain saponin and used for hair wash for killing lice and as fish poison. *D. prazeri* contains steroidal sapogenins prazerigenins A, B, C and D, 9,10 dihydrophenanthrenes, diosgenin glycosides, prazerol, smilagenone, epismilagenin, diosgenin, 9,10-dihydrophenanthrenes, prazerigenin A glycoside.

D. puber is a large unarmed climber. The tubers are edible.

GLYCYRRHIZA

Synonyms

Liquorice; Licorice; Liquorice root; Mulethi (Hindi), Sweetwood; Radix glycyrrhizae.

Biological source

Glycyrrhiza consists of the dried unpeeled roots and rhizome of *Glycyrrhiza glabra* L. var. *typica* or of *G. glabra* var. *glandulifera* or of other varieties of *G. glabra* yielding a yellow and sweet wood. It contains not less than 4% of glycyrrhizinic acid. (Family : Papilionaceae).

Habitat

The drug is found from southern Europe to central Asia in Iran, Iraq, Russia, Saudi Arabia, Afghanistan, Turkestan, Asia Miror, Greece and Siberia. The plant is cultivated in Punjab, sub-Himalayan tracts from Chenab eastwards, Sind, Peshawar valley, to Burma and in Andaman Islands.

Glycyrrhiza glabra var. *typica* is about 1.5 m high bearing typical papilionaceous flowers of a purplish-blue colour. The underground portion consists of long roots and thin rhizomes or stolons. The principal root divides just below the crown into several branches which penetrate the soil to a depth of 1 m or more. A considerable number of stolons are also given off, which attain a length of 2 m but run nearer the surface than the roots. The plant is grown in Spain, Italy, England, France, Germany and the USA.

G. glabra L. var. *glandulifera* is abundant in the wild state in Galicia and central and southern Russia. The underground portion consists of a large root-stock, which bears numerous long roots but no stolons.

G. glabra var. β-*violacea* is a source of 'Persian' liquorice, which is collected in Iran and Iraq in the valleys of the Tigris and Euphrates; it bears violet flowers.

Cultivation and collection

The plant is a 1 m high perennial herb. It is cultivated by planting rhizome or stolon cuttings in well moist sandy soil in March or from seeds. It grows better near the banks of river in sunny climate. Manure is added for favourable growth. Drug is collected from 3-4 years old plants during autumn. Roots and rhizomes are dug out, rootlets and buds are removed, washed in water and cut into small pieces.

Propagation of the variety *typica* is generally done by rhizome cuttings that are planted in rows about 1.3 meters apart. At the end of the third or fourth year, the rhizome and roots are dug in the autumn and from plants that have not borne fruit, for maximum sweetness of the sap. The washed material is air-dried (4 to 6 months) and packed into bales or cut and tied into short cylindric bundles. The large thick roots of Russian licorice are peeled before drying. In Turkey, Spain, and Israel, a considerable amount of the crop is extracted with water, the liquid is clarified and evaporated, and the resulting extract is molded into sticks or other forms.

In some parts a large proportion of the crop is made into stick or block liquorice. This is prepared by the process of decoction, the liquid being subsequently clarified and evaporated to the consistency of soft extract. The latter is made into blocks or sticks, stamped with the maker's name dried, and exported in cases. Chinese blocks weighing 5 kg each are exported. It is available in bundles of stolons, each bundle being about 15 cm long, 15 cm diameter, and bound with wire. The bundles are packed in plaited wood containers. Generally, the stolons have a smaller diameter than the Europe drug.

Morphology

The drug occurs in peeled or unpeeled stolons and roots, length 5-30 cm, diameter 1-2 cm, cylindrical, branche or unbranched. Unpeeled drug is longi-

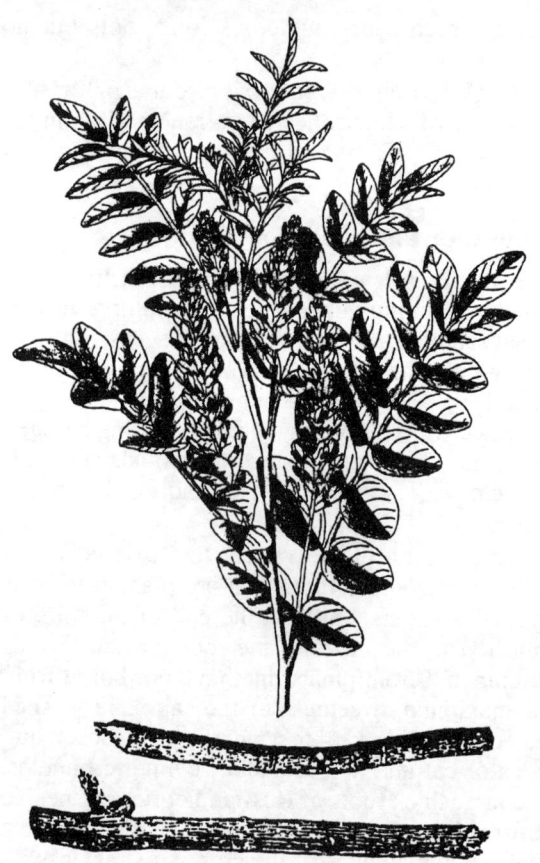

Fig. 15.41. Glycyrrhiza.

tudinally wrinkled; contains dark, reddish-brown bark. The peeled drug has yellow colour. Fracture is fibrous; odour faint and typical; taste, sweet.

Unpeeled 'Russian' liquorice occurs in tapering pieces up to 30 cm long and 5 cm in diameter. It consists of rootstock and roots. The surface is covered with a scaly, purplish cork. The pieces of rootstock often bear buds and have a pith, but the roots may be distinguished from the stolons of the Spanish drug by the absence of buds. Fracture is very fibrous, the strands of fibres tending to separate from one another. This variety is sometimes peeled. The taste is sweet with some bitterness or acridity. 'Persian' liquorice from Iran closely resembles the Russian variety and is generally unpeeled. Anatolian or Turkish liquorice may be peeled or unpeeled and some pieces may have a diameter of up to 8 cm.

Microscopical characters

The roots show secondary thickening and the absence of a medulla in the root. The epidermis and most of the cortex are absent, being thrown off by the development of cork. The outer surface of the unpeeled drug is bounded by some 10 rows of narrow cork cells. Within the cork is a phelloderm or secondary cortex composed of parenchymatous cells, some of which may become collenchymatous. These cells contain simple starch grains and prisms of calcium oxalate. The secondary phloem is composed of alternating zones of groups of fibres and sieve tissue. The phloem fibres are very thick-walled, are lignified and occur in cylindrical bundles surrounded by a sheath of parenchymatous cells each of which contains a single prism of calcium oxalate. The cambium is an incomplete line composed of about three layers of flattened cells. The secondary xylem is composed of large vessels, wood fibres and wood parenchyma. The vessels show reticulate or pitted walls. The pits are slit-like bordered pits.

The vessels occur singly in small groups and alternate with bundles of wood fibres. They resemble the phloem fibres in form and are enclosed in a sheath of parenchyma containing calcium oxalate. The parenchyma of the xylem has lignified pitted walls. The secondary tissues are divided by radial medullary rays in the xylem and funnel-shaped in the phloem.

Chemical constituents

Glycyrrhiza contains 6-14% of glycyrrhizin (the glycoside of glycyrrhetic acid), sugars and resin. The saponin-like glycoside, glycyrrhizin, is 150 times as sweet as sugar. On hydrolysis the glycoside is converted into the aglycone glycyrrhetic acid and two moles of glucuronic acid. Glycyrrhetic acid is a pentacyclic triterpene of β-amyrin series. Other hydroxy- and deoxytriterpenoid acids related to glycyrrhetic acid and 20-epimer of glycyrrhetic acid (liquiritic acid) have been reported in the drug. The yellow colour of Glycyrrhiza is due to the presence of more than 30 flavonoids like isoliquiritin (a chalcone), liquiritin, liquiritigenin, isoliquiritigenin, rhamnoliquiritin and various 2-methylisoflavones. The other constituents are a coumarin named as liqcoumarin (6-acetyl-5-hydroxy-4-methyl-

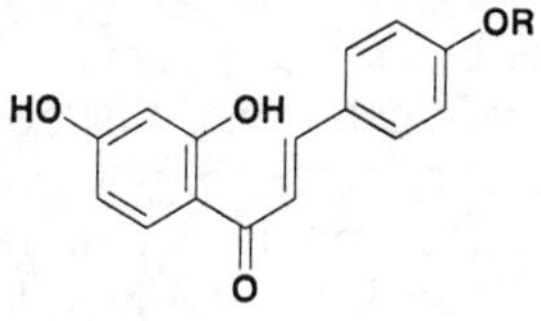

1 : Isoliquiritigenin (R = H) and Isoliquiritin (R = glucose)
2 : Liquiritigenin (R = H) and Liquiritin (R = glucose)

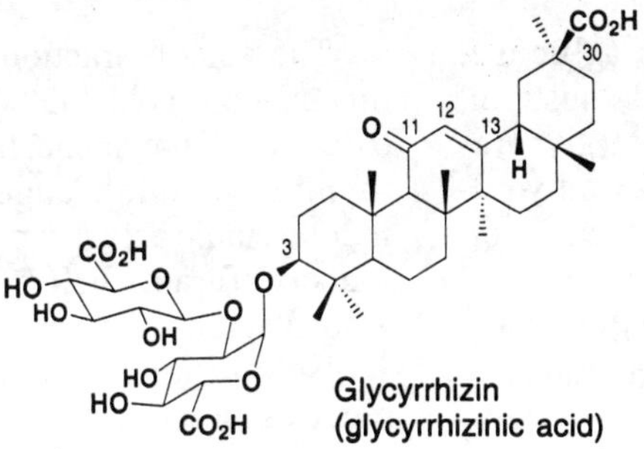

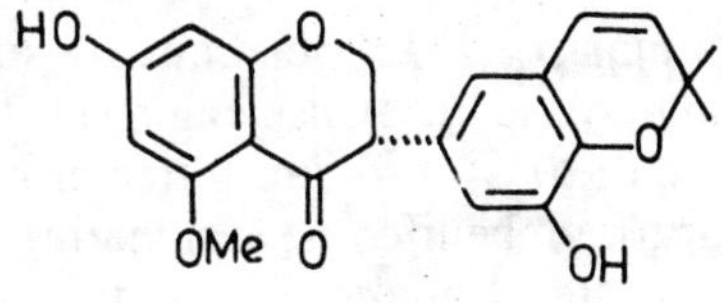

Glycyrrhizin
(glycyrrhizinic acid)

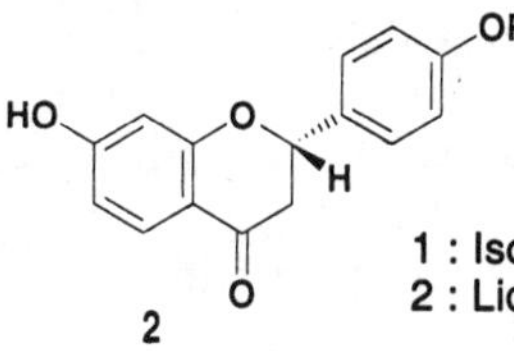

Glycyrrhisoflavanone

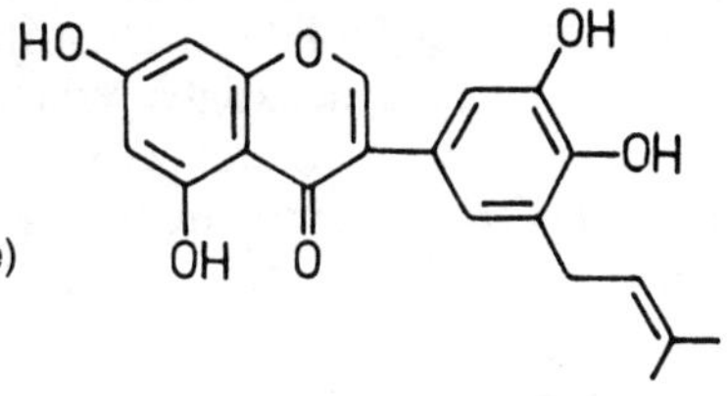

Glycyrrhisoflavone

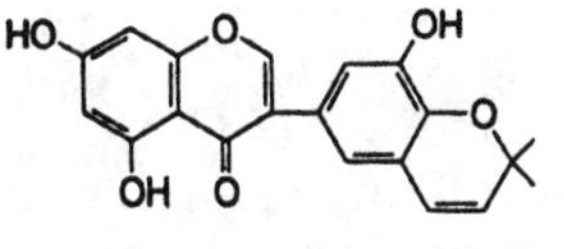

Semilicoisoflavone

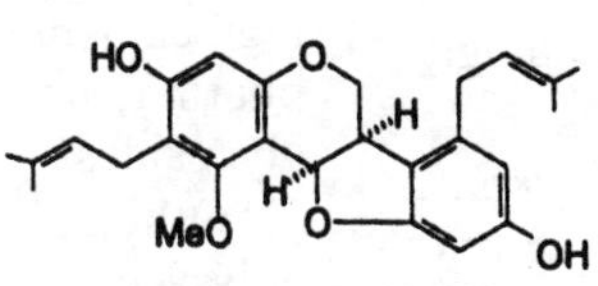

1-Methoxyficifolinol

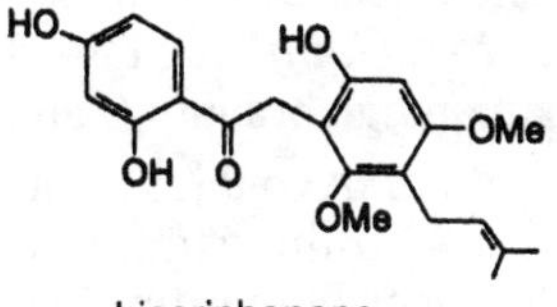

Licoriphenone

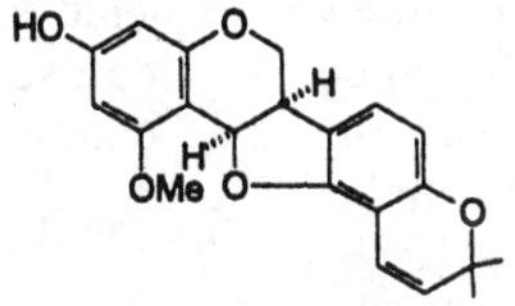

1-Methoxyphaseolin

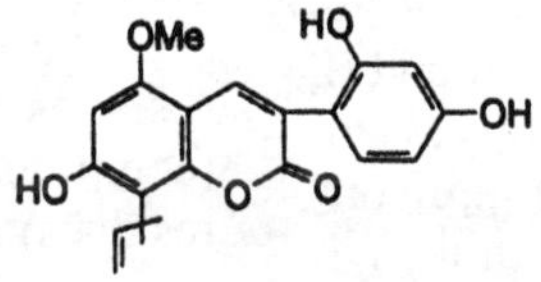

Licoarylcoumarin

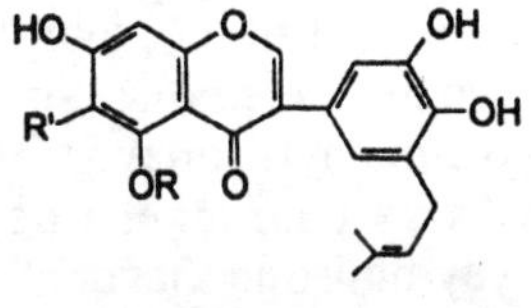

Glisoflavone
R = Me, R′ = H
Isoangustone A
R = H, R′ = Isopentenyl

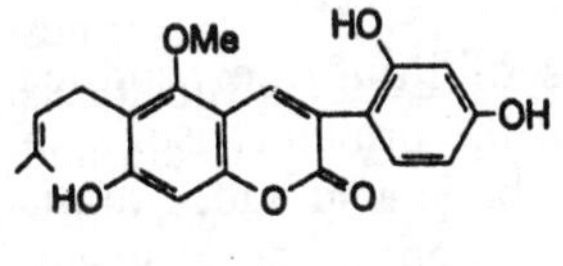

GU-12

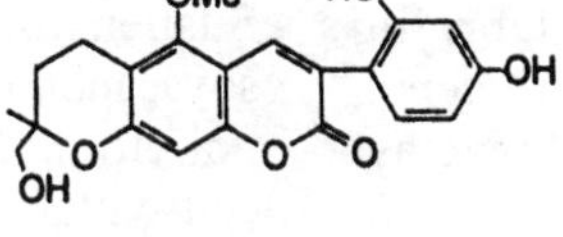

Licopyranocoumarin

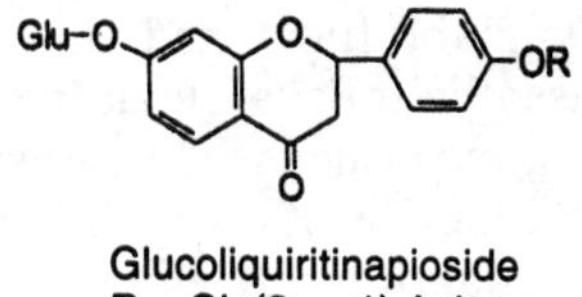

Glucoliquiritinapioside
R = Glu(2 → 1) Apiose

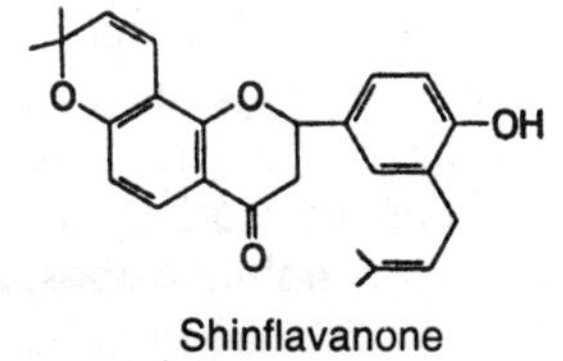

Shinflavanone

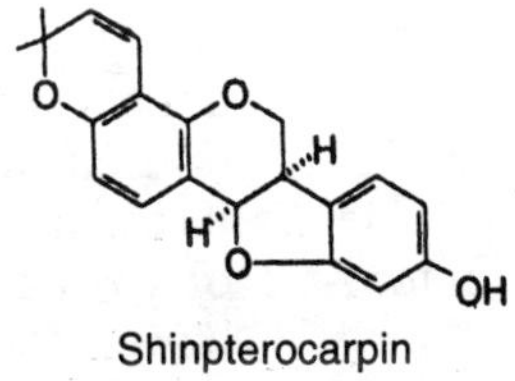

Shinpterocarpin

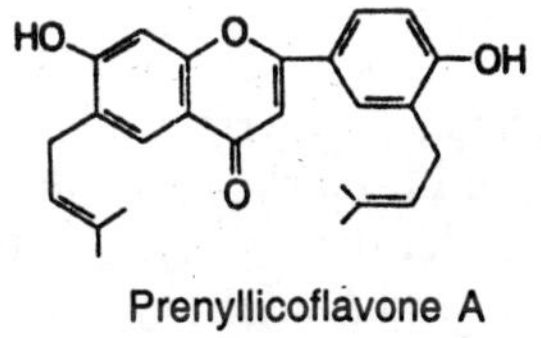

Prenyllicoflavone A

Fig. 15.42. Chemical constituents of Glycyrrhiza.

coumarin), 5-15 per cent of sugars (glucose, mannitol, sucrose), asparagine (1-2%), β-sitosterol, starch (20%), protein, bitter principles (glycyramarin), umbelliferone (coumarin), 22, 23-dihydrostigmasterol, malic acid and resin. Liquiritin on hydrolysis affords liquiritigenin and glucose.

Oleanane-type minor constituents of Glycyrrhiza are liquiritic acid, glabrolide, isoglabrolide, deoxoglabrolide, glabric acid, deoxoglycyrrhetic acid, 18α-glycyrrhetic acid, glycyrrhetol, 21α-hydroxyisoglabrolide, 23-hydroxyglycyrrhetic acid, 24-hydroxyliquiritic acid, liquiridiolic acid, and 28-hydroxyglycyrrhetic acid.

The Chinese species G. uralensis yields methyl -3β, 24-dihydroxyolean-11, 13(18)-diene-30-oate, 24-hydroxyglabrolide, uralsaponins A and B, uralenolide licorice-saponins A3, B2, C2, D3 and E2 and from G. inflata araboglycyrrhizin, apioglycyrrhizin and glabranins A and B.

The minor flavonoids isolated from Glycyrrhiza species are isoliquiritin, neoliquiritin, rhamnoliquiritin, neoisoliquiritin, licuroside, saponaretin, vitexin, isovitexin, pinocembrin, prunetin, licoricone, glabranine, formononetin, glabrone, glabrene, glabridin, glabrol, 7-acetoxy-2-methylisoflavone, 7-methoxy-2-methyl-isoflavone, 7-hydroxy-2-methyl-isoflavone, licochalcones A and B, 4-hydroxy-chalcone, liqcoumarinm, glycyrol, isoglycyrol, isolicoflavonol; glycycoumarin, licoricidin, liconeolignan, 4'-O-β-D-apio-D-furanosyl-(1 → 2) β-D-glucopyranosyl-liquiritigenin, ononin, neolicuroside, licoflavanone, glycyrrhisoflavone, licocoumarone, licoflavonol, kumatakenin, glycyrol, licoricone, glyzaglabrin, licoisoflavones A and B, licoiso-flavanone, 4'-7-dihydroxyflavone, echinatin, hispaglabridin A and B, 4'-O-methylglabridin, phaseollinisoflavan, liquiritigenin, isoliquiritigenin, 4-hydroxychalcone, 3-hydroxyglabrol, 4'-O-methyl glabridin, 3'-methoxyglabridin, phaseolinisoflavin, hispaglabridins A and B, galangin, naringenin, genistein, pinocembrin, glycyrrhisoflavanone, glycyrrhiso-flavone, licochalcone B, licuroside, neolicuroside, semilicoisoflavone B,1 methoxyficifolinol, isoangustone A, licoriphenone, echinatin, licoricone, glycyrin, isoliginritigenin, coumarin GU-12, pino-cembrin, prunetin, glucoliquiritin apioside, phenylicoflavone A, shinoflavanone, shinpterocarpin and 1-methoxyphaseolin.

The volatile fraction of G. glabra is composed of hexanoic acid (32%), γ-nonalactone, linalool, α-terpineol, p-cymene, thujone, fenchone, guaiacol, thymol, geraniol, eugenol, estragole, anethole, indole, cumic acid, propionic acid, 2-acetyl-pyrrole, 2-acetyl-furan, furfuryl alcohol, hexanoic acid, γ-nonalactone and cumic alcohol.

Isoliquiritigenin is reported to be an aldosereductase inhibitor and may be effective in preventing diabetic complications. Rhamnoliquiritin was isolated from the roots. Various 2-methylisoflavones have been isolated from indigenous Indian roots together with an unusual coumarin (liqcoumarin), 6-acetyl-5-hydroxy-4-methylcoumarin. The flavonoid contents vary only in the relative proportions of constituents. Japanese traditional (kampo) extracts prepared by boiling show a high content of flavonoid aglycones which may be pharmacologically more active than the parent glycosides.

Other active constituents of liquorice are polysaccharides with a pronounced activity on the reticuloendothelial system. Glycyrrhizan GA has been characterized as the representative polysaccharide with immunological activity. It has an estimated mass of 85000 with a core structure which includes a backbone chain of β-1,3-linked D-galactose residues 60% of the units carrying side chains (composed of β-1,3- and β-1,6-linked D-galactosyl residues) at position 6.

A TLC test is used to identify the quality in the water-soluble extractive (not less than 20.0%) and content of glycyrrhizinic acid (not less than 4.0%).

Cell cultures

Suspension cell cultures of liquorice produce soyasaponins I and II, and the principal isoflavonoid formononetin. Glycyrrhetic acid added to the cell culture undergoes a different mode of glycosylation so that normally occurring in the roots.

Uses

Glycyrrhiza possesses tonic, laxative, demulcent, diuretic, emmenagogue and emollient properties and is used in genito-urinary diseases, coughs, sore throat, in scorpion-sting, in inflammatory affections or irritable conditions of the bronchial tubes, bowels and catarrh; and to relieve peptic ulcer pain.

Glycyrrhiza is added to chewing gums, chocolate candy, cigarettes, smoking mixtures, snuff and chewing tobacco. Glycyrrhetinic acid is used to cure rheumatoid arthritis, Addison's disease and various inflammatory conditions.

Glycyrrhiza root extract is used to treat asthma, laryngitis and bronchitis. It shows an inhibitory effect on smooth muscle contraction in the gastro-intestinal tract. Successive use of Glycyrrhiza root extract for long time might cause side effects such as edema and hypertension, which disappear after withdrawal. A flavanone rhamnoglycoside, isolated from roots, is used as a depressor of smooth muscle fibres.

Due to deoxycorticosterone effects of liquorice extracts and glycyrrhetenic acid, it is used for the treatment of rheumatoid arthritis, Addison's disease and various inflammatory conditions. The flavonoid component of the root, which possesses antimicrobial properties, also exerts spasmolytic and anti-ulcerogenic activity. The formulation of a liquiritin cream is used, with no adverse effects, for the removal of skin stains in patients with chloasma, senile melanoderma in Japan.

Liquorice may give symptomatic relief from peptic ulcer pain. Glycyrrhizin gel can act as a useful vehicle for various drugs used topically; due to its anti-inflammatory and antiviral effects. Glycyrrhizin enhances skin penetration by the drug. Most of the liquorice is used in the tobacco trade and in confectionery.

Substituents and adulterants

Glycyrrhiza uralensis is a source of Manchurian Liquorice. It resembles Russian Liquorice in appearance. The bark is pale chocolate-brown in colour and exfoliates readily. It contains only a small percentage of sugar and gives a pungent extract. It contains about as much glycyrrhizin as the other varieties, together with a number of new oleanane-type triterpene oligosaccharides called licorice saponins. Only traces of sugars are present and it gives an unpleasantly pungent extract. As with *G. glabra* the yellow colouring matter contains the flavonoid glycoside liquiritin, a glycoside involving liquiritigenin, apiose and glucose, and a new chalcone oligoglycoside isoliquiritin apioside.

Like *G. glabra*, *G. uralensis* contains poly-saccharides showing immunological activities; glycyrrhizin UA is composed of L-arabinose, D-galactose, L-rhamnose and D-galacturonic acid.

Other species which have been investigated include *G. aspera*, *G. echinata*, *G. hirsuta*, *G. inflata*, *G. macedonia*, *G. pallidiflora* and *G. yunnanensis*.

G. glabra var. *typica* is the source of Spanish Liquorice collected chiefly in Sicily and Spain. The drug consists of pieces of underground roots. Unpeeled pieces are dark reddish or purplish brown in colour and longitudinally wrinkled. The fracture is fibrous in the bark and splintery in the wood. Peeled pieces are smooth and yellow. The drug has a faint characteristic odour and a sweet taste free from bitterness.

Russian Liquorice is derived from *G. glabra* var. *glandulifera*. It is collected in southern Russia chiefly from wild plants. It consists mainly of roots and some pieces of rootstock. Bigger pieces are longitudinally split. Unpeeled pieces are purplish; taste is sweet accompanied by a perceptible, bitterness and acridity. It is usually exported in peeled form.

Persian Liquorice is derived from *G. glabra* var. *violacea* and is collected chiefly from the Tagris and Euphrates valley in Iraq. It is usually thicker than other varieties and is marketed in an unpeeled state.

Pharmacology

Glycyrrhiza fractions, given intraduodenally to pylorus-ligated rats, inhibited gastric secretion and prevented the formation of ulcer. Administration of pure glycyrrhizin showed no effect on the ulcer. Glycyrrhetic acid showed mineralocorticoid-like effects and inhibited 5β-reduction of cortisol, aldosterone and testosterone by rat liver preparations. Glycyrrhizin completely inhibited growth and cytopathic effects of vaccinia, herpes simplex type 1 and other viruses. Glycyrrhizin completely inhibited human immunodeficiency virus - induced plaque formation, and inhibited the passive cutaneous anaphylaxis response in rats indicating anti-allergic activity. Glycyrrhizin and glycyrrhetic acid prevent the development of experimental cirrhosis. After oral administration of glycyrrhizin, glycyrrhetic acid was detected in blood due to absorption of glycyrrhizin in the small intestine in the form of glycyrrhetic acid.

The Glycyrrhiza flavonoids inhibited the passage of $BaSO_4$ suspension from the rat stomach into the intestine by reducing stomach mobility. They showed a spasmolytic action on isolated rat and guinea pig ileum preparations and an inhibitory effect on the development of exudative processes in inflammation caused by formalin, albumin and dextran in rats.

Glycyrrhizin showed significant antidiuretic effect in rats and rabbits. Glycyrrhetic acid aluminium salt showed protective effect in rats with ulcers. Hispaglabridins A and B, 4'-O-methyl-glabridin, glabridin, glabrol and 3'-hydroxyglabrol showed antimicrobial activity. Sodium glycyrrhetinate, ursolic acid and its acetate showed hypo-lipidaemic and antiatherosclerotic activity in rabbits. Glycyrrhetinic acid inhibited oedema in rat paw and leucocyte migration in pleural space. Aqueous extract is effective in conjunctivitis and showed anti-inflammatory activity like cortisone. Glycyrrhizine increased weight of spleen and thymus of mice. It has immunostimulant and hepatoprotective properties, decreased intracellular Ca^{2+}-aequorin luminescence in diaphragm muscles of mouse, showed antiviral action on Varicella-zoster virus, increase proliferation of human fibroblasts, inhibited passive cutaneous anaphylaxis response in mice, inhibited contraction of rabbit ileum and guinea pig trachea, inhibited granuloma formation in guinea pig and suppressed production of platelet-activating factor from rat peritoneal exudate cells.

Licochalcone B showed highest binding activity to haemoglobin. Plant extract inhibited melanogenesis and tyrosinase activity. Glycyrrhetinic acid increased amplitude of cochlear microphonic potential and auditory nerve action potential in guinea pig. Sodium glycyrrhizate possess anti-ulcer activity and stimulated re-generation of the skin. Glycyrrhizin was effective against DHBV virus, reduced pancreatic cell damage due to hereditory action, affects fibroblasts to suppress granuloma formation and suppressed pulmonary granulomes. Glycyrrhetinic acid topically applied to female mice inhibited TPA- and DMBA- induced skin tumor initiations. Isoliquiritigenin inhibited rat lens aldose-reductase and sorbitol accumulation in human red blood cells and suppressed sorbitol accumulation in red blood cells. Licochalcone A possesses potent anti-malarial activity.

QUILLAIA BARK

Synonyms

Quillaia; Soap bark, Quillary bark, Panama bark; China bark, Murillo bark, Panama wood; Cortex quillaiae.

Biological source

Quillaia bark is the inner dried bark of *Quillaia saponaria* Molina and other species of *Quillaia*. (Family : Rosaceae).

Habitat

Q. saponaria is about 18 m high evergreen, graceful tree found in Peru, Chile, Bolivia, South America and California.

The bark is collected from the stem; outer, dark-coloured rhytidome is removed, dried and graded. It consists mainly of saponaceous inner bark (phloem).

Morphology

Quillaia bark occurs in flat pieces, about 1 m long, 20 cm wide, and 3-10 cm thick. Outer surface is brownish-white, smooth and contains reddish- or blackish-brown patches of rhytidome adhere to the outer surface. The rhytidome is made of dead secondary phloem. The inner surface is yellowish-white and smooth. Fracture is splintery. Large crystals of calcium oxalate are present. Odour is sternutatory and taste is acidic and astringent (Fig. 15.44a).

Microscopical characters

A transverse section of quillaia bark shows alternating bands of lignified and non-lignified phloem. The medullary rays are usually 2-4 cells wide. The phloem fibres are tortuous and often accompanied by small groups of rectangular sclereids. The parenchyma contains numerous starch grains and calcium oxalate prism.

Chemical constituents

Quillaia bark contains saponins (10%), quillaic acid, calcium oxalate, starch, sucrose and tannin. Quillaia saponin on hydrolysis forms pentacyclic triterpenoid, quillaic acid (Quillaia sapogenin), a sugar glucuronic acid and gypsogenin.

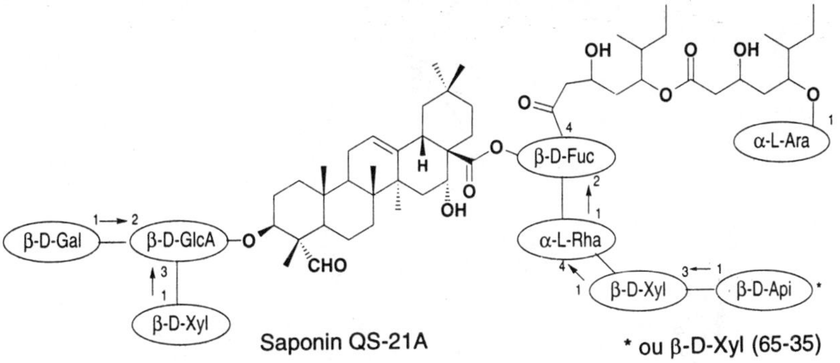

Fig. 15.43. Saponin QS-21A.

Quillaia saponin is a mixture of acylated triterpenoid oligoglycosides (acylated saponins). Mild alkaline hydrolysis gives two deacyl saponins (quillaic acid 3.28-*O*-bisglycosides) together with less polar compounds (the eliminated acyl groups). These acyl moieties, together with the deacyl saponins, constitute the parent quillaia saponins.

Quillaia contains about 10% of saponins, ethanol (45%) soluble extractive not less than 22.0%, and also sugars, starch and calcium oxalate.

Quillaia also contains quercetin, kaempferol, leucocyanidin, caffeic and *p*-coumaric acids, saponins quillinin A, quillajasaponins, DS-1, DS-2, QS-7, QS-17, QS-18 and QS-21.

Chemical tests

1. Powdered drug on shaking with water produces soap like froth which persists for some time.
2. On addition of a small portion of drug or its alcoholic extract in a drop of blood on a microscopic slide, a haemolytic zone surrounding the drug is formed.

Uses

Quillaia bark is used as an emulsifying agent, for coal tar emulsion, cleaning industrial equipments, washing delicate fabrics, to prepare tooth powders, tooth pastes, hair shampoos, hair tonics, tar solutions and metal polishes. It is added in topical preparations for skin disorders, and as a protective agent for cracks, bruises, frostbite and insect bites. The drug is highly irritating and causes nausea and is expectorant on internal consumption. It is diuretic and a cutaneous stimulant.

SENEGA
Synonyms

Senega snake root; Seneca snake root; Rattle snake root; Radix senegae.

Biological source

Senega consists of the dried roots and rootstocks of *Polygala senega* Linn. or *P. senega* var. *latifolia*. (Family : Polygalaceae).

Habitat

North America, Canada and Japan.

Collection

The plant is a perennial herb, 20-30 cm in height consisting of yellow twisted, branched roots with crown. Roots are dug out, aerial parts are removed, washed and dried.

Senega thrives in the open and also in partial shade. It grows in any type of soil, containing a fair amount of leaf-mould. It can be propagated either by seed or rootstocks. The seedlings cannot withstand frost in the first year and need protection. The plants grow slowly and nearly 4-year old plants yield roots of the required size. They are cleaned and dried.

In market foreign Senega (*P. senega*), Indian Senega (*P. chinensis*), Nowshera or Pakistan Senega (roots of *Andrachne aspera*), Delhi Senega, Kulu Senega, Tuticorin yellow (*Glinus oppositifolius*) and Tuticorin Brownish green are available.

Macroscopical characters

The roots are twisted, curved, tapering, lonti-

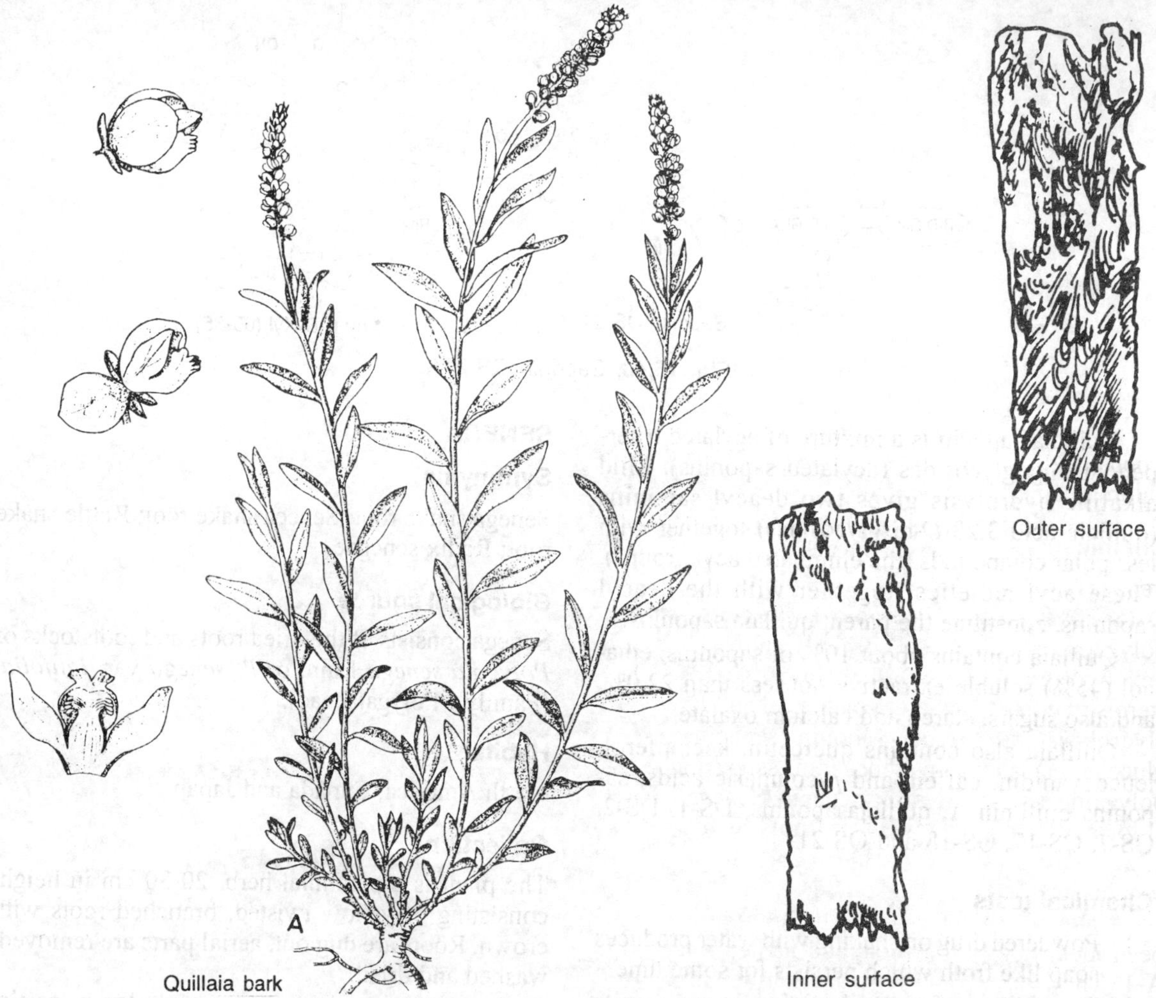

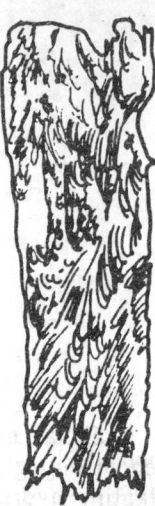

Outer surface

Inner surface

Quillaia bark

A

Fig. 15.44. Polygala senega plant and Quillaia bark (a).

tudinally striated, colour-brown, odour is methyl salicylate-like, taste is first sweet and then acrid.

The rootstocks are yellowish orange to brownish conical pieces, 5-20 cm long and 2-12 mm in diameter. They are sweetish and acrid in taste. The odour is characteristic, resembling that of methyl salicylate. Powdered Senega causes sneezing.

The lower part is yellowish, the crown is darker. The lower part is knotty and bears numerous, purplish buds and the remains of aerial stems, which should not exceed about 2%. The tapering and curved root divides into two or more branches. Some of the pieces bear a keel or ridge in the form of a rapidly descending serial. The drug has a marked odour of methyl salicylate. Taste, at first sweet, afterwards acrid. The saponins present cause the drug to have stemutatory properties and to froth when shaken with water.

Transverse sections of different senega roots have widely different appearances. Some have a normal bark, which occupies nearly half the radius and a uniform central wood with narrow medullary rays. In others, an abnormal local development of phloem gives rise to the keel, V-shaped, medullary rays give a very characteristic appearance to the

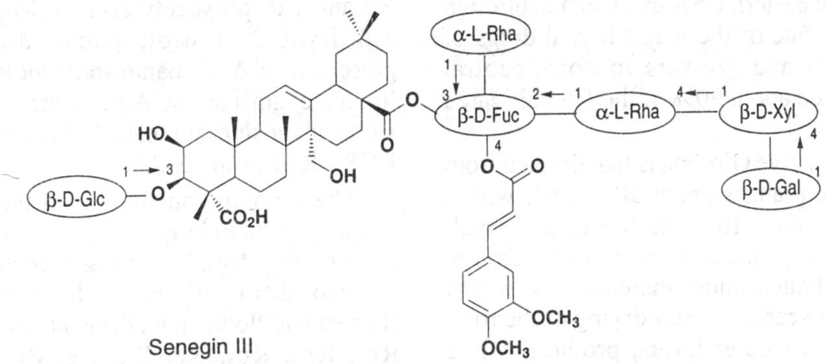

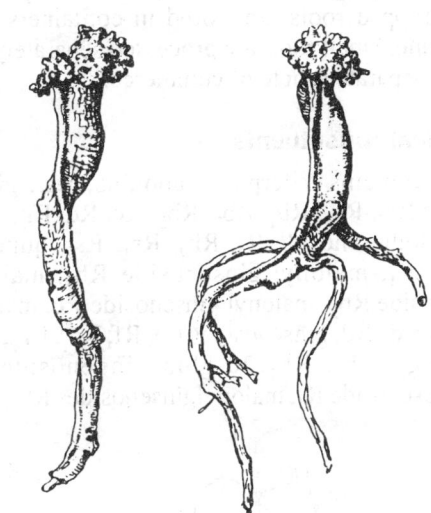

Senegin III

Fig. 15.45. Chemical constituent of Senega.

wood. This is well observed in sections stained with phloroglucinol and hydrochloric acid.

Chemical constituents

Senega contains a mixture of saponins A, B, C and D (8-10%), polygallic acid (senegenic acid), polygalitol (1, 5-anhydro-sorbitol), anhydride of the hexahydric sugar alcohol sorbitol, sucrose, fat, sterols, methyl salicylate, volatile oil and fixed oil. Hydrolysis of the crude saponin (senegin) yields glucose, presenegenin, senegenin, senegenic acid, polygallic acid and hydroxysenegin. Senegenin is a chlorinated triterpenoid. The roots also contain 2, 3, 27-trihydroxy-12-oleanene-23, 28-dioic acid, α-spinasterol and free fatty acids.

A number of oligosaccharide multi-esters have been identified in the roots and named senegoses A-1. They are di- and tetra-saccharides involving glucose and fructose esterified with acetic, benzoic, and *trans-* and *cis-*ferulic acids. A further series, senegoses J-O, are pentasaccharides. These compounds are structurally similar to the tenuifolioses isolated from *P. tenuifolia.*

Uses

Senega is used as a stimulant, expectorant in chronic bronchitis and as emetic.

Side effects include nausea, diarrhoea, stomach upsets and dizziness.

Allied species and substitutes

P. tenuifolia is used in China and Japan as an expectorant, tonic and sedative. It contains constituents similar to those of *P. senega,* includ-

Fig. 15.46. Senega roots.

ing saponins, xanthones, phenolic glycosides (tenuifolisides A-D) and oligosaccharides (tenuifolioses A-F). *Southern* or *white senega* is collected in the southern USA from *P. alba* and *P. boykini.* The roots are smaller than those of *P. senega* and have a normal wood. Some Indian senega consists of the roots of *Glinus oppositifolius* (Arizoaceae) and is easily distinguished by the presence of several rings of vascular tissue.

GINSENG

The roots of *Panax ginseng* (Araliaceae) are produced in China, Korea and Siberia, and considerable quantities, derived from *P. quinquefolium,* are exported from the eastern USA and Canada through Hong Kong. It is one of the major herbal drugs of US foreign trade and growers in north-central Wisconsin produce about 90% of the US cultivated drug.

The most expensive Ginseng is that derived from Korean root. The plant is about 50 cm tall with a crown of dark green verticillate leaves and small green flowers giving rise to clusters of bright red berries. It is cultivated under thatched covers and harvested when 6 years old. Sun-drying of the root, after removal of the outer layers, produces white Ginseng, whereas the red ginseng is obtained by first steaming the root, followed by artificial drying and then sun-drying. The roots are graded and packed. The wrapped roots are stored in containers with quicklime. Small roots are processed separately and form a separate article of commerce.

Chemical constituents

Panax contains triterpene saponins, *viz.*, ginsenosides Ra_2, Ra_3, Rb_1, Rb_2, Rb_3, Rc, Rd, Rg_3, Rh_1, Ro; notoginsenoside R_4, Rh_2, Rs_1, Rs_2, quinquenoside R_1, malonyl ginsenoside Rb_1, malonyl ginsenoside Rb_2, malonyl ginsenoside Rc, malonyl ginsenoside Rd, ginsenosides Re, Rf, Rg_1, Rg_2, Rg_3, Rg_4, Rg_2, Rh_1, Rh_2 20-glucosingenoside Rf, notoginsenoside R_1, malonylginsenosides Rb_1, Rb_2,

Rc and Rd, polyacetylenes, 1,8-hepta-decadiene-4,6-diyne-3,10-diol, panaxydol, panaxynol, ginsenoynes A-K, panaxynol linoleate, panaxydol linoleate, ginsenoyne A linoleate, denichin, daucosterin adenosine, sucrose, β-sitosterol, polypeptides RGPI, RGPII and S-2A.

The saponin constituents of the aerial parts of *P. ginseng* include ginsenosides Rb_1, Rb_2, Rc, Rd, Re, Rg_1, Rg_2, Rg_3, 20-glucoginsenoside, Rf, Rg, and ginsenosides F_1, F_2 and F_3 from the leaves. From flowers and flower bud, the isolation of sinsenosides Rb_1, Rb_2, Rb_3, Rc, Rd, Re, Rg_1, Rg_2 and 20-glucoginsenoside Rf was reported. The fruits yield ginsenosides Rb_1, Rc, Rd, Re, Rg_1, Rg_3, protopanaxatriol, daucosterol and β-sitosterol.

The stem and leaves of American Ginseng afforded ginsenosides Rb_2, Rb_3, Rd, Re, F_2, Rg_1, Rh_2 and Rh_2 and pseudoginsenoside F_{11}.

The volatile component of ginseng root con-tains eremophilane, β-gurjunene, *cis-* and *trans-* caryophyllene, ε-muurolene, γ-patchoulene, β-eudesmol, β-farnesene, β-bisabolene, aromadendrene, β-guaiene, alloaromadendrene, γ-elemene, mayurone, pentadecane, 2,5-dimethyltridecane, palmitic acid, 3-*sec*-butyl-2-methoxy-5-methylpyrazine, 3-isopropyl-2-methoxy-5-methylpyrazine, 3-isopropyl-2-methoxy-5-methylpyrazine, acetylene compounds panaxynol, panaxydol,

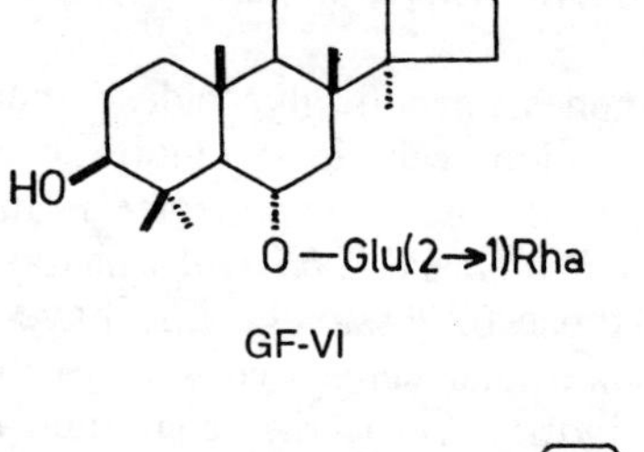

GF-VI

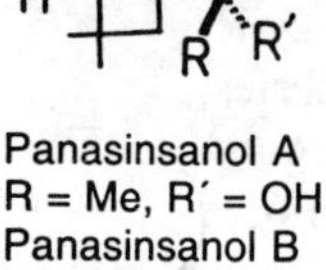

Panasinsanol A
R = Me, R′ = OH
Panasinsanol B
R = OH, R′ = Me

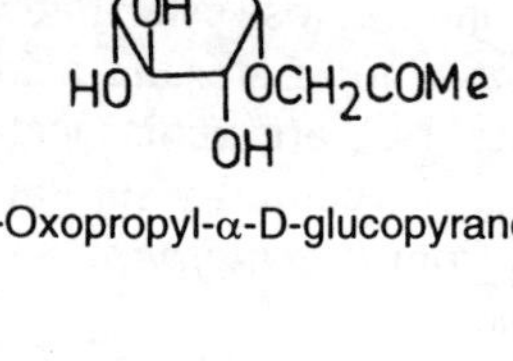

2-Oxopropyl-α-D-glucopyranoside

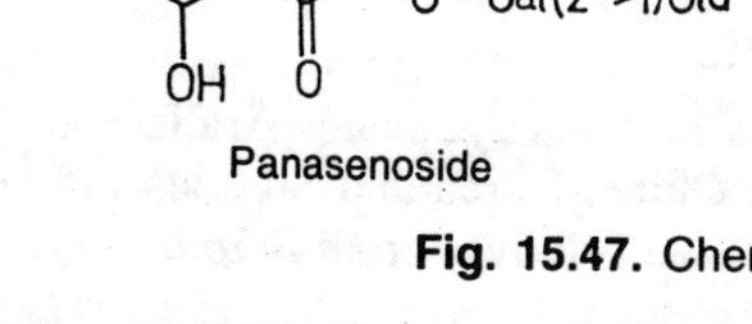

Panasenoside

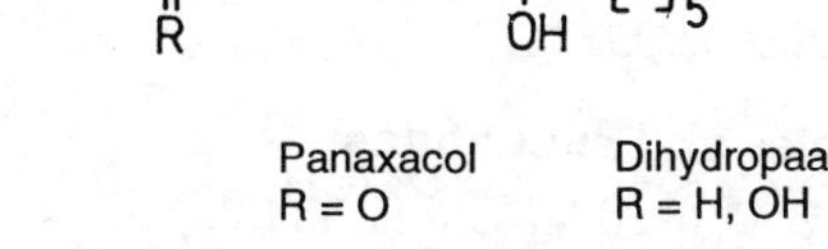

Panaxacol
R = O

Dihydropaaxacol
R = H, OH

Fig. 15.47. Chemical constituents of Ginseng. *(contd.)*

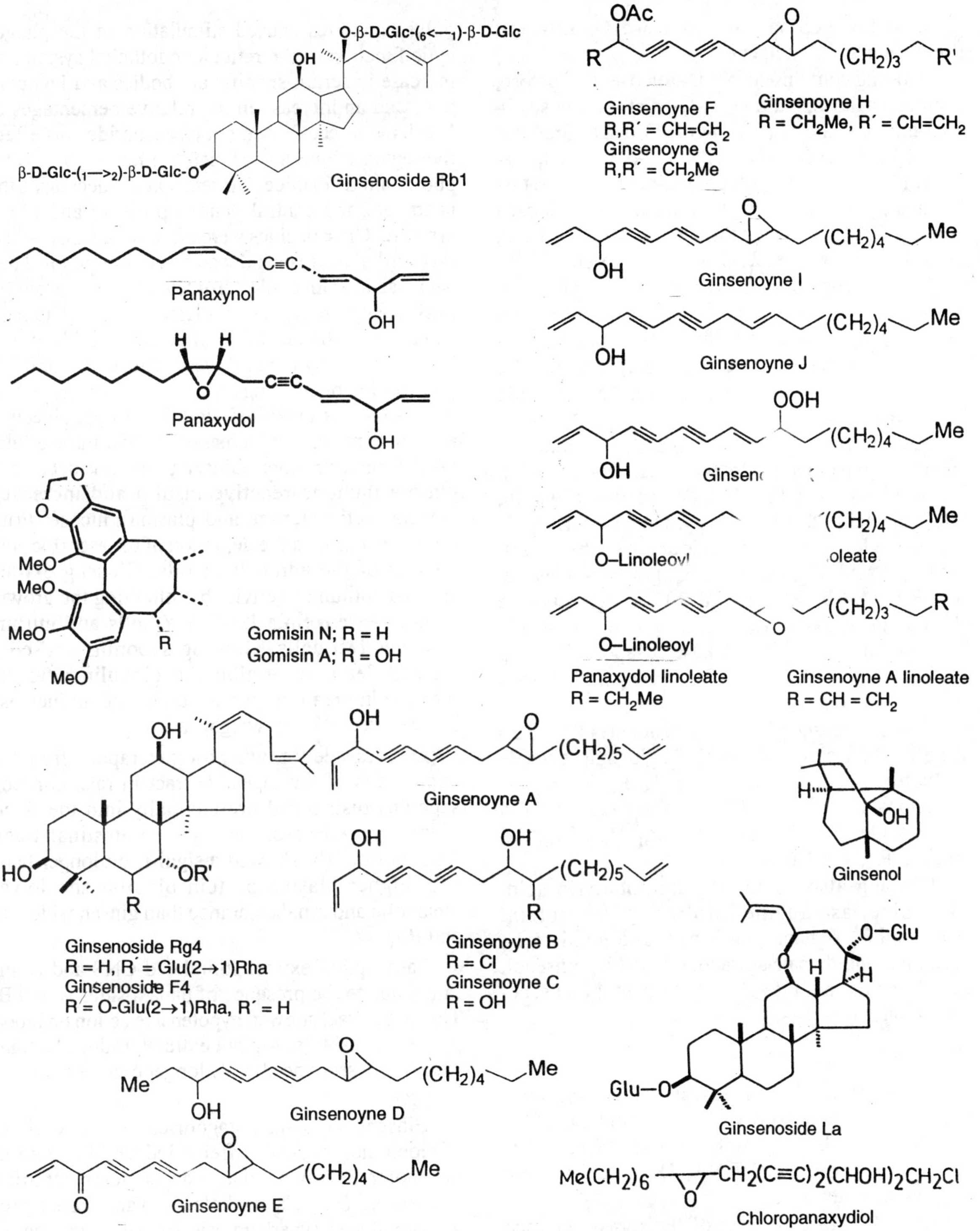

Ginsenoside Rb1

O-β-D-Glc-(6←—1)-β-D-Glc

β-D-Glc-(1—>2)-β-D-Glc-O

Panaxynol

Panaxydol

Gomisin N; R = H
Gomisin A; R = OH

Ginsenoyne F
R,R′ = CH=CH₂
Ginsenoyne G
R,R′ = CH₂Me

Ginsenoyne H
R = CH₂Me, R′ = CH=CH₂

Ginsenoyne I

Ginsenoyne J

Ginsenc

O–Linoleoyl   oleate

O–Linoleoyl
Panaxydol linoleate
R = CH₂Me

Ginsenoyne A linoleate
R = CH = CH₂

Ginsenoside Rg4
R = H, R′ = Glu(2→1)Rha
Ginsenoside F4
R′ = O-Glu(2→1)Rha, R′ = H

Ginsenoyne A

Ginsenoyne B
R = Cl
Ginsenoyne C
R = OH

Ginsenol

Ginsenoside La

Ginsenoyne D

Ginsenoyne E

$Me(CH_2)_6$ —CH₂(C≡C)₂(CHOH)₂CH₂Cl

Chloropanaxydiol

Fig. 15.47. Chemical constituents of Ginseng.

panaxytriol, heptadeca-1-en-4,6-diyn-3,9-diol; β-elemene and β-selinene.

Ginseng contains sugars D-glucose, D-fructose, sucrose, maltose, maltosyl-β-D-fructofura-nose, O-α-D-glucopyranosyl (1→2)-O-β-D-fructofuranosyl (1 → 2)-β-D-fructofuranose and O-α-D glucopyranosyl (1 → 6)-O-α-D-glucopyra-nosyl-(1 → 4)-α-D-glucopyranose. Hypoglycemic peptide glycans isolated from Ginseng root are panaxans A, B, C, D, E, F, G, H, I, J, K, L, Q, R, S, T and U.

Red ginseng affords 3-hydroxy-2-methyl-pyran-4-one, its glucoside, hydroxy-acetone glucoside and α-D-glucopyranoside of dihydroxy-pyran-3-one.

Three flavone constituents, kaempferol, trifolin and panasenoside were isolated from the leaves and stems of *P. ginseng*.

Japani Ginseng, *Panax japonicum*, contains saponins ginsenoside Ro (chikusetsusaponin V), chikusetsusaponin IV, IVa, IVa methyl ester, Ib, oleanolic acid 28-β-D-glucopyranosyl ester, Pjs-2, 3-O-β-D-glucopyranosiduronic acid-(methyl ester)-oleanolic acid, zingiberoside R_1, ginseno-sides Re, Rg_1, Rg_2, F_1, Rb_1, Rb_3, Rc, Rd, 20-glucoginsenoside Rf, notoginsenoside R_2, Rd, 20-glucoginsenoside Rf, notoginsenoside R_2, chikusetsusaponin L_5, L_{10}, Ia, III, majorosides F_1, F_2, F_3, F_4 and 24(S)-pseudoginsenoside.

P. notoginseng contains ginsenosides Rb_1, Rb_2, Rb_3, Rc, Rd, Re, Rg_1, Rg_2-Rh_1, F_2, glucoginsenoside Rf, notoginsenosides R_1, R_2, R_3, R_6, R_4. Fa, Fc, Fe, gypenoside XVII and IX. Ginseng leaves yield ginsenosides F_4, Rh_1, Rh_2, Rh_3, Rg_1, Rg_2, Rg_3, Re, Rd, Rc, Rb_1 and Rb_2.

Ginseng also contains γ-aminobutyric acid, glutamine, asparagine, proline, glycoprotein, tetrapeptide, lignans gomisin A and gomisin N, sesquiterpenoids panasinsanols A and B, ginsenol, 20(R)-dammaran-3, 6, 12, 20, 25-pentol and senecrassidol.

Pharmacology

Ginsenosides of Ginseng stem and leaves showed a marked increase in body weight and contents of the protein and RNA of muscles in liver of rats. The root extract stimulated RNA, DNA and protein synthesis of rats.

A total aqueous extract of the roots increased the primary IgM response and IgG. Ginseng polysaccharides caused stimulation of the phagocytic function of the reticuloendothelial system, an increase in serum-specific antibodies and IgG contents and an increase in the relative percentages of B cells in mice. Ginseng polysaccharide was effective against immunodeficiency induced by cyclophosphamide in mice. Ginseng extract decreased the heart rate, the central venous pressure and blood pressure. Ginsenosides were effective against mouse myocardial necrosis induced by isoproterenol. They decreased serum cholesterol level in rats and serum low-density lipoprotein cholesterol level. The liver damage and the elevation of enzyme and bilirubin levels caused by ethanol were reduced by oral administration of Ginseng saponins. Ginseng saponins and pana-xans exhibited significant hypoglycemic actions in mice, and increased adrenal intracellular cAMP concentrations. Ginseng saponins decreased plasma immuno-reactive insulin and increased plasma corticosterone and plasma glucose. Fruit saponins inhibited the depletion of the ascorbic acid content of the adrenals in rats. Ginseng extract showed antitumor activity by inhibiting the growth of murine leukemia L517-8 Y cells and murine sarcoma 180 cells. Ginseng saponins caused a marked decrease in albumin; globulin ratio, an increase in urea nitrogen in serum and an increase in liver weight/body weight ratio.

Ginsenoside Rg_1 was absorbed rapidly from the upper parts of the digestive tract in rats. Ginseng saponins distributed preferentially into the liver, kidney, blood serum and gastrointestinal tract. Ginsenoside Rb_2 showed a significant longer half-life, higher plasma protein binding and lower metabolic and renal clearance than ginsenosides Re and Rg_1.

Panax plant extract stimulated CNS and respiration due to the presence of panaxosides A and B. The root extract showed hypotensive action on blood pressure in rabbits. A plant extract produced a transitory depressor and slightly longer pressor response in dogs.

Ginseng saponins antagonised analgesic effect of clonidine, reduced caffeine-induced increase in locomotor activity in mice, reduced norepinephrine and dopamine levels in whole brain and cortex, prevented induced hyperkeratosis, showed antimutation effect, suppressed lesion of cultured cells, exhibited antiviral activity and protection against herpes simplex 1 virus. Ginsenosides, increased cerebral blood flow, reduced Ca^{2+} accumulation and K^+ loss in cerebral cortex, showed antiarrhythmic activity in rats and inhibited rat kidney microsome Na^+, K^+-ATPase activity. Ginseng peptide GPP decreased levels of blood sugar and hepatic glycogen in rats. Ginseng polysaccharides reduced levels of blood glucose and liver glycogen in mice, increased content of pyruvic acid but decreased that of lactic acid, accelerated oxidative phosphorylation, stimulated release of insulin and resulted in increase of interleukin-2 and of interferon production. The polysaccharide restored levels of interleukin-2 and antagonized cobra venom factor. Dencichin enhanced histamine-induced contraction of guinea pig aorta.

Saponin fraction accelerated absorption of α-tocopherol and, thereby, stimulated its antioxidant activity. Ginseng aqueous extract and diolsaponins markedly inhibited lipid photooxidation and decreased lipid hydroperoxides in total lipids of serum. Ginseng inhibited hepatic cytosolic xanthine oxidase activity in mice. Administration of Ginseng extract for 7 days to rats inhibited development of tolerance of analgesic and hyperthermic effects of morphine. Ginseng markedly reduced serum triglycerides and cholesterol in hyperlipidaemic monkeys; HDL-cholesterol/total cholesterol ratio was increased. The drug may have beneficial effects as antiatherogenic. It acutely increased diurnal slow wave sleep and chronically decreased nocturnal locomotor acti-vity. The root extract produced rapid reversible reduction of Ca^{2+} current by 22% suggesting that the extract acts on sensory neurons through a similar pathways as that of u-type opioids. Total saponins promoted hematopoesis in mice after phenylhydrazine treatment or cobalt 60 iradiation. Saponins showed nonspecific enzyme stimulatory effect. Ginseng volatile oil inhibited tumor growth by interfering with metabolism of carbohydrate and nucleic acid.

Water-soluble fraction of a leaf extract and an alkali-soluble polysaccharide fraction obtained therefrom prevented HCl/ethanol-induced ulcerogenesis in mice. It also inhibited formation of gastric ulcers induced by water immersion stress. It significantly reduced both gastric acidity and pepsin activity in gastric juice. Ginseng root saponins

or ginsenoside Rb completely antagonized immunosuppression induced by cold water swim stress in rats and inhibited increase of serum corticosterone in animals. Ginsenosides brought down increased cholesterol level to normal and increased cAMP level which was usually reduced to 55% of that of control group due to the presence of LDL in medium. Ginseng fruit saponin decreases haemorrhagic stock. An aqueous extract of the root stimulated proliferation of hamster kidney-21 cells. An aqueous extract of wild Ginseng showed mitogenic activity. A nerve growth factor-like immunoreactive substance, *Panax ginseng* NGK, is present in the roots. Ginsenosides alleviated increase of platelet aggregation, and plasma PG12 levels and reduce increase in pulmonary vascular permeability in trachea and lung of rabbits.

Use of ginseng may cause Stevens-Johnson syndrome with painful erosions in the mouth and urogenital mucosa, corneal ulceration and widespread purpuric macules. Korean ginseng is considered as a general tonic with antifatigue and anti-stress properties. Adverse reactions of ginseng may include hypertension, dizziness and inability to concentrate.

Allied species

Eleutherococcus senticosus (*Acanthopanax senticosus*), Siberian Ginseng, is used in Russia, as an abundant and inexpensive substitute for Ginseng. It is also cultivated in China for the roots which are used as a tonic and sedative. The roots contain active saponins (eleutherosides), different to those of *Panax ginseng*, and a series of glucans (eleutherans A-G) and a heteroxylan with 'adaptogenic' properties. The eleutherans show hypoglycaemic activity. The isolation and structure determination of glycosides of protoprimulagenin A from the root have been reported.

Panax pseudoginseng ssp. *himalaicus* var. *augustifolius* (Himalayan Ginseng). The roots con-

Oleanolic acid$^{(3\rightarrow1)}$glucuronic acid$^{(2\rightarrow1)}$xylose

Oleanolic acid$^{(3\rightarrow1)}$glucuronic acid$^{(2\rightarrow1)}$xylose

phthalic acid

Fig. 15.48. Pseudoginsenoside-RI$_2$.

tain active saponins and ginsenosides R_0 and R_{b1}, chikusetsusaponins IVa and VI, pseudoginsenoside-RI_2 which consists of oleanolic acid, phthalic acid, glucuronic acid and xylose moieties.

Panax notoginseng roots (Sanchi-ginseng) contain several dammarane saponins, identical or similar to those of Ginseng, and a polysaccharide (sanchinan-A) having a branched structure with a galactose backbone and side-chains containing arabinose and galactose; this glycan contains a small amount of protein and possesses reticulo-endothelial activating properties.

Panax japonicum and *P. japonicum* var. *major* contain chikusetsusaponins, ginsenosides and glycans.

Panax vietnamensis (Vietnamese Ginseng). The roots are used as a secret remedy of the Sedang ethic minority and contain a number of known and new ginsengosides.

Cell culture

Five saponins, differing from those of the cultivated plant, are isolated from the cell cultures of *P. notoginseng*. The production of diol- and triol-type ginsenosides by the culture of *Agrobacterium rhizogenes*-transformed Ginseng roots is reported. The glycosylation and malonylation biotransformation abilities of hairy root cultures have also been studied. In callus and cell suspension cultures of *P. quinquefolium* the R_b and R_g groups of ginsenosides reach maximum yields at different ages of the culture.

Uses

The drug is used for the treatment of anaemia, diabetes, gastritis, sexual impotence, many conditions arising from the onset of old age, and for the improvement of stamina concentration, resistance to stress and to disease. The action of the drug is described as 'adaptogenic'.

Many Ginseng products are available as OTC products either for oral administration or as cosmetic preparations.

Ruscus aculeatus, Butcher's broom (Liliaceae)

The rhizomes of this plant contain saponins related to those of *Dioscorea*, *e.g.*, 1β-hydroxydiosgenin (ruscogenin). The plant glycosides involve up to three sugars attached at the C-1 hydroxyl with glucose terminating an uncyclized side chain at C-26.

Both the alcoholic extract of the roots and the ruscogenins show anti-inflammatory activity, produce diminished capillary permeability and exert a vasoconstrictor effect in the peripheral blood vessels. The ointments and suppositories containing the active constituents are for the treatment of relative diseases.

CYANOGENETIC OR CYANOPHORE GLYCOSIDES

Cyanogenetic glycosides on hydrolysis yield hydrocyanic acid as one of the products. The glycoside amygdalin is most widely distributed in nature.

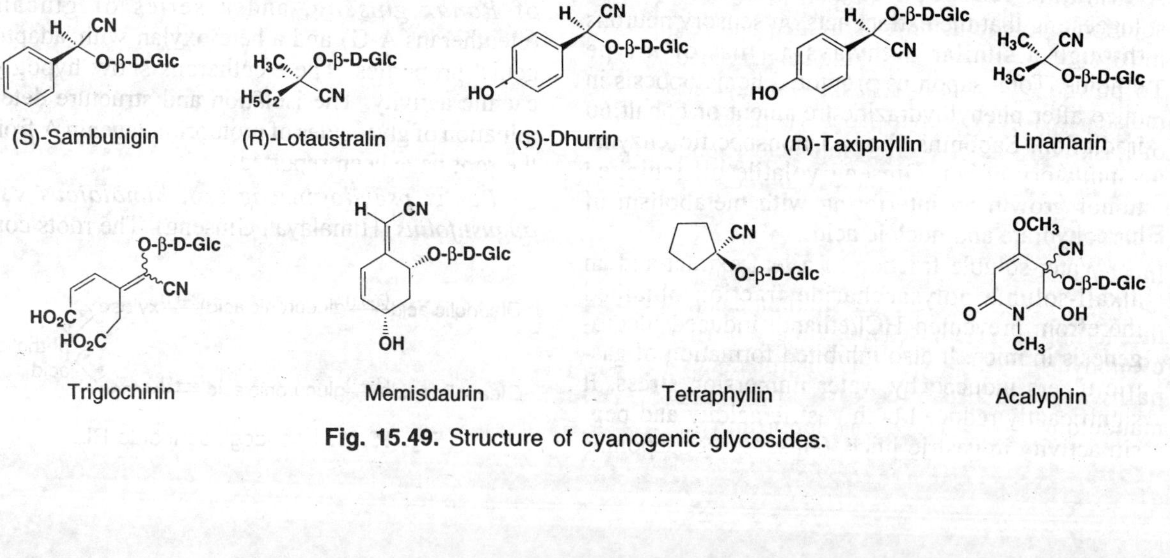

Fig. 15.49. Structure of cyanogenic glycosides.

Usually these glycosides are derived from the nitrile of mandelic acid. The group is represented by amygdalin which is the major component of bitter almonds and in kernels of apricots, cherries, peaches, plums and many other seeds of the Rosaceae. Prunasin is found in *Prunus padus* and yield d-mandelonitrile on hydrolysis as the aglycone. Other cyanogenetic aglycosides are prulaurasin from cherry laurel leaves and sambunigrin from *Sambucus nigra*.

Cyanogenetic glycosides contain nitrogen, but the sugar moiety is attached to oxygen and not to nitrogen. The sugar residue of the molecule may be a monosaccharide or a disaccharide as gentio-biose or vicianose. Amygdalin on hydrolysis yields two molecules of glucose. The enzyme emulsin, found in almond kernels, consists of two enzymes, amygdalase and prunase. The first enzyme breaks the molecule to liberate one of mandelonitrile glucoside. The latter enzyme liberates the remaining glucose forming benzaldehyde-cyanohydrin known as mandelonitrile.

Drugs containing cyanogenetic glycosides are widely used as flavouring agents and as anticancer agents.

They have a helpful sedative and relaxant effect on the heart and muscles in small doses. Wild cherry bark contains cyanogenic glycosides, which contribute to plant's ability to suppress and soothe irritant dry cought.

Chemical tests

Sodium picrate test

A strip of filter paper is dipped in 10% aqueous solution of picric acid. It is drained and re-dipped in 10% sodium carbonate solution and drained again. To powdered drug in a flask, water is added to moisten it. Sodium picrate paper is kept on the mouth of flask with cork. Hydrocyanic acid vapours turn the paper brick red or maroon-coloured.

Biogenesis

In a cyanogenic glucoside, the amino acid phenylalanine, which arises from the shikimate pathway, is the starting precursor. An aldoxime, a nitrile, and a cyanohydrin are involved as intermediates in the pathway. The presence of a chiral center in mandelonitrile provides the opportunity for 2β-

glucosides to occur. In wild cherry, *Prunus serotina*, prunasin (D-mandelonitrile glucoside) is formed. The isomeric sambunigrin (L-mandelo-nitrile glucoside) is formed in *Sambucus nigra*. Apparently, these compounds do not occur in the same species, further confirming the stereo-specificity of the glycosyl transferases that catalyze their formation.

The aglycones of cyanogenetic glycosides are derived from nitrogen intermediates. Feeding phenol [3-^{14}C]alanine, phenyl[2-^{14}C]alanine and phenyl[1-^{14}C]alanine to the leaves *Prunus laurocerasus*, three labelled precursors obtained were active benzaldehyde and inactive hydrocyanic acid; inactive benzaldehyde and active hydrocyanic acid; and inactive hydrolytic products consistent with the following incorporation :

$$C_6H_5 - \overset{*}{C}H_2 - \underset{\underset{H}{|}}{\overset{\overset{NH_2}{|}+}{C}} - COOH \xrightarrow{\text{P. laurocerasus}} C_6H_5 - \underset{\underset{OH}{|}}{\overset{\overset{\overset{+}{CN}}{|}}{\overset{*}{C}}} - H$$

Formation of α-hydroxynitrile

Similarly, phenyl[2-^{14}C]alanine fed to *P. amygdalus* gives amygdalin with most activity in the carbon atom of the nitrile. The nitrile nitrogen of the cyanogen is derived from the nitrogen atom of the amino acid. Similar results have been obtained with dhurrin isolated from sorghum seedlings fed with labelled tyrosine.

BITTER ALMOND

Synonyms

Badam (Hindi); Amygdala amara.

Biological source

Bitter almond is the dried ripe seeds of *Prunus amygdalus* Batsch var. *amara* or *P. amygdalus* var. *dulcis*. (Family : Rosaceae).

Habitat

Italy, Spain, southern France, North America and Kashmir.

Cultivation

The almond requires a cold and dry climate, but a fairly warm weather during its ripening period. The

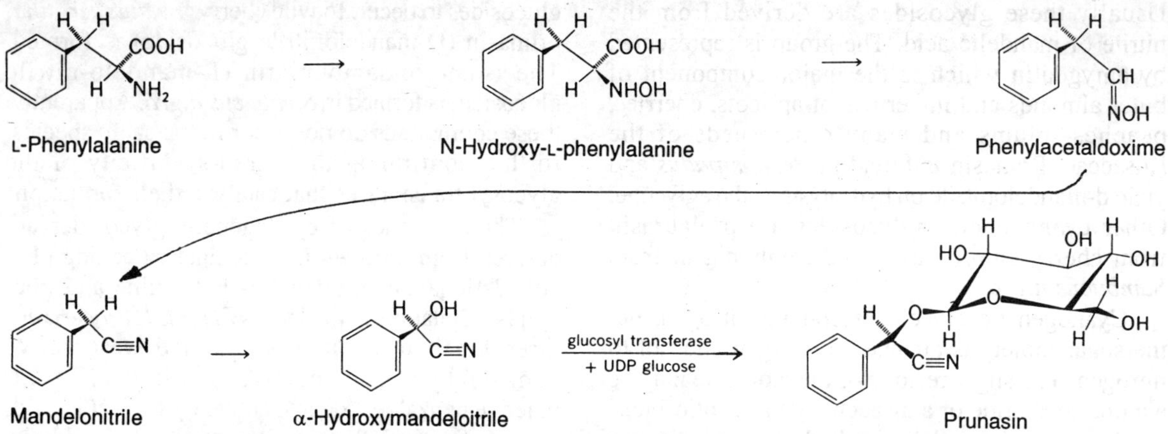

Fig. 15.50. The biosynthetic pathway for cyanogenic glycoside, prunasin.

trees are raised from seeds which are sown in nurseries and seedlings transplanted after one year. The trees are planted 6-8 m apart in circular pits. The trees tend to grow large with long branches. The fruit is borne largely on short-spurs. The almond crop comes to harvest from July to September. Almonds are graded into several classes to meet the demand for specific purposes. Unshelled almonds are stored in a cool, dry and well-ventillated place.

Characters

Almond tree is about 5 m in height. The bitter almond is 1.5-2 cm long, rounded at one end and pointed at the other. Cinnamon-brown coloured testa is present which is removed by soaking in hot water. The oil kernel consists of two large, oily planoconvex cotyledons. A small plumule and radicle are present. Some almonds possess cotyledons of unequal sizes. The presence of bitter almonds in sweet almonds can be detected by the sodium picrate test for cyanogenetic glycosides.

Chemical constituents

Bitter and sweet almonds con-

tain fixed oil (40-55%), proteins (20%), mucilage and emulsin. The bitter almonds contain a colourless, crystalline, cyanogenetic glycoside amygdalin (about 3%). In the presence of water the enzyme emulsin acts upon amygdalin and decomposes it into a volatile oil which is a mixture of benzaldehyde and hydrocyanic acid. A casein like protein, amandin, is also present in bitter almond.

It also contains prunasin, daucosterin, β-sitosterol, a biflavone, coumaric acid, Z-methylnonacosan-3-one, *n*-octacosanol, n-triacontane, procyanidin dimer, (+)-catechin, and (-)-epicatechin. The oil is composed of glycosides of myristic, palmitic, stearic, oleic and linoleic acids.

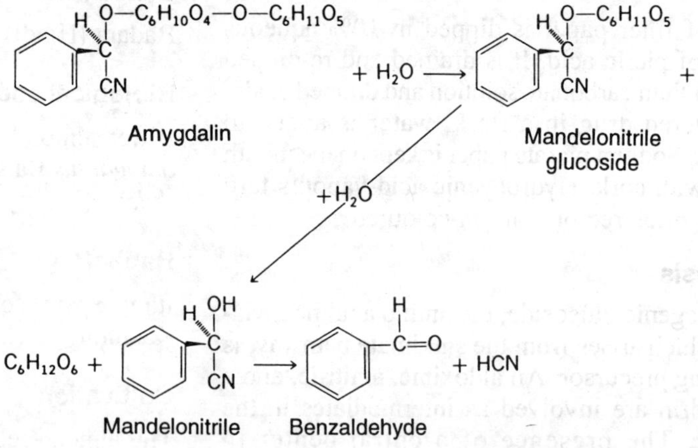

Fig. 15.51. Hydrolysis of amygdalin.

Uses

Bitter Almond seeds have demulcent, mild laxative, stimulant and nervine tonic properties. Almond oil is used as a flavouring agent in the preparation of toilet articles, as a vehicle for oily injections and in manufacture of liquors. Due to the presence of hydrocyanic acid in the volatile oil, it gives relief in bronchitis and cough.

WILD CHERRY BARK

Synonyms

Wild black cherry, Cherry bark; Virginian Prune bark; Prune bark, Cortex Pruni Virginianae; Prunus Virginiana; Prunus serotina.

Biological source

Wild Cherry bark is the dried stem bark of *Prunus serotina* Ehrh. (Family : Rosaceae).

Habitat

United State and Canada.

Collection

Wild Cherry plant is a tree, 30 m high or more. The bark is collected in autumn from young branches & stem, cork & cortex are removed by peeling to get 'rossed bark', dried and preserved in containers.

Morphology

The drug occurs in curved or channelled pieces, length up to 10 cm, width 5 cm, thickness 0.3-1.4 mm. Outer surface of unpeeled bark (unrossed bark) is reddish-brown, covered with thin papery, glossy, exfoliating cork cells and bears very conspicuous whitish lenticles. The outer surface of the bark is rough with pale buff-coloured lenticels. Inner surface is reddish-brown with striated and reticulately furrowed appearance. Patches of wood adhering to the inner surface are sometimes present. The branch bark is covered with a thin, glossy, easily exfoliating, reddish-brown to brownish-black cork, which bears very conspicuous whitish lenticels. In the rossed bark pale buff-coloured lenticel scars are present and the other surface is rough. The fracture is a granular and short. Slightly moist drug contains benzadehydic odour. Taste is bitter and astringent. The microscopic characters include sclereids,

prismatic and cluster crystals of calcium oxalate, cork cells with brown contents and starch granules.

Chemical constituents

Wild Cherry bark contains a cyanogenic glycoside, prunasin (d-mandelonitrile glucoside), the enzyme prunase, benzoic acid, trimethylgallic acid, *p*-coumaric acid, starch, tannin and volatile oil.

The enzyme emulsin hydrolyzes prunasin to benzaldehyde, glucose and hydrocyanic acid. The bark possesses resin which yields the fluorescent compounds, *e.g.*, scopoletin, on hydrolysis.

Uses

Wild Cherry is used in cough preparations as sedative, expectorant and as a flavouring agent.

Cherry-laurel leaves

Cherry-laurel leaves are obtained from *Prunus laurocerasus* (Rosaceae), an evergreen shrub common in Europe.

The leaves have some odour when entire, but when crushed an odour of benzaldehyde is apparent and a positive test for cyanogenetic glycoside is obtained. The cyanide content of small young leaves is as 5%, rapidly decreases to about 0.4-1.0% as leaf-size increases.

Isothiocyanate glycosides

Isothiocyanate glycosides contain sulphur and present in many Cruciferous plants. On hydrolysis, they produce isothiocyanate aglycones which may be aliphatic or aromatic. Sinigrin from Black Mustard, sinalbin from White Mustard and gluconapin from Rapeseed are isothiocyanate glycosides. Sinigrin on hydrolysis in the presence of the enzyme, myrosin, yields allyl isothiocyanate, glucose and potassium acid sulphate. The activity of the fixed oil content of these seeds is due to allyl isothiocyanate. These glycosides are irritant and employed as counter-irritant externally in neuralgia and rheumatism.

MUSTARD

Synonyms

Black Mustard, Brown Mustard, Red Mustard, Sinapis Nigra; Semina Sinapis Nigrae.

Biological source

Mustard is the dried ripe seed of *Brassica nigra* (L.) Koch or of *B. juncea* (L.) Czern. et Coss or of these varieties. (Family : Brassicaceae).

Habitat

Europe, USA, southwestern Asia, India. *B. juncea* is abundantly cultivated in upper Indian region.

Collection

The plant is an annual herb with erect slender stems and yellow flowers. Leaves are large, pinnatifid, without basal lobes, terminal lobe much larger. The aerial parts of the plant are cut after maturation. Seeds are removed by thrashing or beating of the dried parts and then sieving.

Characters

Seeds are small, about 1 mm diameter, brown to red colour, globular in shape, testa is minutely pitted, embryo is oily, yellow in colour, consisting of two cotyledons, folded along their midribs to enclose the radicle. Powdered mustard shows a brighter yellow colour on treatment with alkali.

Chemical constituents

Mustard contains fixed oil (30-35%), proteins (20%), sinigrin (potassium myronate), myrosin, sinapine sulphocyanate, erucic acid, behenic acid and sinapolic acid. Sinigrin is the active constituent of the drug and its amount varies from 0.7 to 1.3%. In the presence of water myrosin activates the hydrolysis of sinigrin and yields allyl isothiocyanate, potassium hydrogen sulphate and glucose. It also contains phenylacetonitrile, 3-phenylpropionitrile, brassicasterol, compesterol, β-sitosterol, 5-dehydro-arvenasterol, quercetin-3-glycoside and verbenone.

Uses

Mustard is used in the form of plasters, as rubefacient, vesicant, counter-irritant and as condiments. It acts as emetic in large doses.

Allied drugs

White Mustard or *Sinapsis alba* Bois. is the dried ripe seed of *Brassica alba* Bois. (Fam. Brassicaceae). The seeds are globular in shape, 1.5-2.5 mm in diameter. It contains the glucoside sinalbin

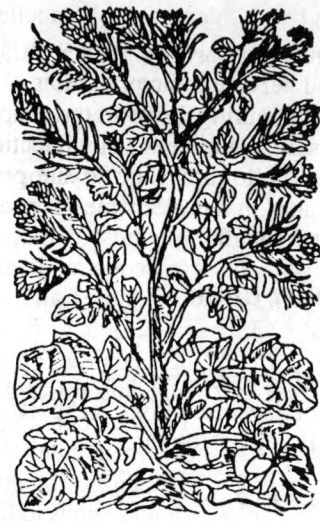

Fig. 15.52. *Brassica nigra.*

and myrosin. In the presence of moisture, sinalbin is hydrolyzed into sinapin hydrogen sulphate, acrinyl isothiocyanate and glucose. The isothiocyanate is an oily liquid with pungent taste. Sinapine hydrogen sulphate is the salt of an unstable alkaloid. The seeds also contain fixed oil (30%), protein (20-25%) and mucilage.

The isothiocyanate is an oily liquid with a pungent taste and rubefacient. It has the pungent odour of allylisothiocyanate. Sinapine hydrogen sulphate, which is also found in black mustard, is the salt of an unstable alkaloid. The seeds also contain about 30% of fixed oil, 25% of proteins and mucilage. Ash is about 4%.

White Mustard is used as counter-irritant, emetic and carminative.

Biosynthesis

The suitable amino acids are converted to thio-

$$CH_2-NCS$$

OH

Fig. 15.53. Acrinyl isothiocyanate.

glucosides by the plant. Doubly labelled (^{14}C, ^{15}N) amino acids afforded glucosides with ^{14}C : ^{15}N ratio consistent with direct incorporation.

All intermediates in this conversion are nitrogenous compounds giving a similar situation to that found in the biosynthesis of cyanogenetic glycosides. The appropriate aldoximes were effective precursors of these compounds in flax (linamarin), *Cochlearia officinalis* (glucoputran-jivan), *Lepidium sativum* (benzylglucosinolate) and *Tropaeolum majus* (benzylglucosinolate).

Sinigrin, the thioglucoside found in horseradish leaves and in black mustard seeds, is the most effective precursor of the carbon chain is homomethionine rather than allyglycine. Homomethionine arises by chain lengthening of methionine with acetate by a mechanism analogous to the formation of leucine from valine. Although the sulphur atom on the thioglucoside moiety may be introduced by feeding with methionine, the sulphur of DL-[^{35}S]cysteine is a more efficient precursor. The sulphur of the bisulphite portion of the molecule is more readily introduced from inorganic sources.

LACTONE GLYCOSIDES (Coumarin)

Coumarin is the lactone of *o*-hydroxycinnamic acid. It occurs as colorless, prismatic crystals and has a characteristic fragrant odour and a bitter, aromatic, burning taste. It is soluble in alcohol. Coumarin can be synthesized readily.

Coumarin is widely distributed in nature; mainly in tonka beans (1 to 3%), sweet vernal grass (*Anthoxanthum odoratum* Linn., Fam. Poaceae), sweet clover [*Melilotus albus* Medicus and *M. officinalis* (Linn.) Lamarck, (Fam. Papilionaceae), sweet-scented bedstraw (*Galium triflorum* Michaux, Fam. Rubiaceae), and red clover (*Trifolium pratense* Linn., Fam. Papilionaceae).

Several glycosides of hydroxylated coumarin derivatives occur in plant materials; these glycosides include skimmin in Japanese star anise, aesculin in various parts of the horse chestnut tree, daphnin in mezereum, fraxin in ash bark, scopolin in belladonna and limettin in citrus trees. None of the hydroxycoumarin glycosides is of particular medicinal importance.

Coumarin of *tonka beans*, coumarin-containing seeds of *Dipteryx odorata* (Aublet) Willdenow and *D. oppositifolia* (Aublet) Willdenow (Fam. Papilionaceae), were formerly used pharmaceutically as flavoring agents. Some coumarin derivatives still find application for their anticoagulant properties. The antispasmodic activity of the barks of *Viburnum prunifolium* Linn. (black-haw) and *V. opulus* Linn. (true cramp bark) (Fam. Caprifoliaceae) has been attributed to scopoletin (6-methoxy-7-hydroxy-coumarin) and other coumarins. Preparations of these plant drugs are used as uterine sedatives. Other lactone-containing natural products include cantharidin and methoxsalen which are used for dermatologic purposes, and *santonin*, which is obtained from the unexpanded flowerheads of *Artemisia cina* Berg, *A. maritima* Linn. and several other *Artemisia* species (Fam. Asteraceae). Santonin was formerly used as an anthelmintic, but its use has been discontinued due to its potential toxicity.

Bishydroxycoumarin or dicumarol is a drug related to coumarin. It was obtained originally from improperly cured leaves and flowering tops of *Melilotus officinalis* but it is now prepared synthetically. Dicumarol is an anticoagulant. A number of synthetic analogs of bis-hydroxycoumarin also are used in anticoagulant therapy; these include warfarin salts.

GENTIAN

Synonyms

Yellow Gentian, Pale Gentian, Gentian root, Bitter root; Radix Gentianae.

Biological source

Gentian is the dried rhizome and roots of *Gentiana lutea* Linn. It contains about 33% of water-soluble extractives. (Family : Gentianaceae).

Habitat

Central and southern Europe and Asia Minor.

G. lutea requires a moist situation, good drainage and a suitable soil consisting of loam, peat and grit. Seeds are slow to germination, seedlings frequently taking several years to appear. The roots and rhizomes are collected from the 2-5 years old plants during May-October and allowed to ferment in heaps. They are then washed, dried in the open and cut into variable length.

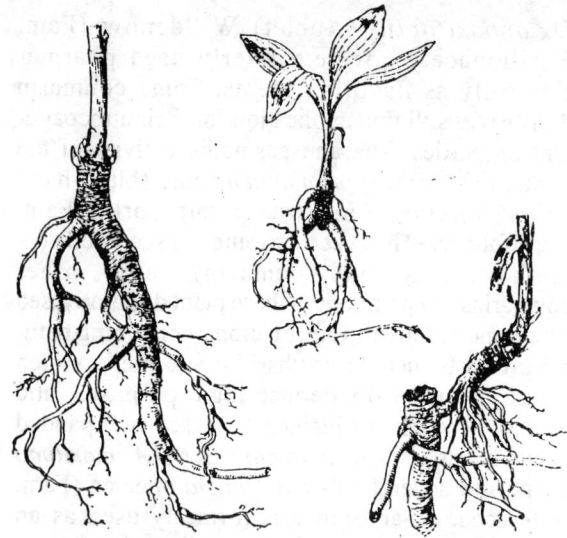

Fig. 15.54. Gentian rootstock and roots.

Collection

The plant is a large perennial herb. The drug is collected from a 2-5 years old plant in the autumn. Turf is stripped and the rhizomes are dug up. It is cut into pieces of different length and dried quickly first in air and then in sheds. The drug becomes much darker in colour, loses some of its bitterness and acquires a very distinctive odour.

Morphology

Gentian consists of brownish, subcylindrical, entire or longitudinally split pieces of rhizomes and roots, 15-20 cm or more in length and 2.5 to 8 cm in thickness at the crown. The root is longi-tudinally wrinkled and the rhizome, which is sometimes branched, frequently terminates in one or more buds and bears numerous encircling leafscars, which appear as transverse annulations. The drug is brittle and breaks with a short fracture. It has a characteristic odour and the taste is sweet at first and intensely bitter afterwards.

Microscopical characters

A transverse section shows an orange-brown bark separated by a darker cambium line from the porous, very indistinctly radiate wood. The rhizomes show a pith, about 4-6 rows of thin-walled cork cells between which and the cambium is a thick-walled

phelloderm and wide zone of brown, thin-walled parenchyma containing oil globules and minute needles of calcium oxalate. Small groups of soft phloem are present but phloem fibres are absent.

The wood and pith contain abundant parenchyma having similar cell contents to those of the bark. The vessels occur either isolated or in small groups and show mainly reticulate or scalariform thickening. There are a few spiral and annular vessels. Groups of soft phloem ('phloem islands', 'interxylary phloem') occur in the xylem. The drug contains some starch granules and no sclerechymatous cells or fibres.

Chemical constituents

Gentian contains the bitter glycoside gentiopicrin (~2%) as a principal active constituent. On hydrolysis it yields the aglycone mesogentiogenin and glucose. Gentiopicrin is a secoiridoid, gentiopicroside, and it is decomposed on fermentation and drying of the drug. Other bitter compounds are gentisin, amaropanin, amarogentin and amaroswerin. Gentian also contains gentiin, gentiamarin, gentisic acid, tannins, pectin and calcium oxalate.

On hydrolysis gentiopicrin yields a lactone (gentiogenin) and glucose. A biphenolic acid ester of gentiopicroside, amarogentin, occurs in small amount (0.025 to 0.05%). It has a bitterness value some 5000 times greater than that of gentiopicroside and is an important constituent of the root; other bitters isolated are sweroside and swertiamarin.

The yellow colour of fermented Gentian root is due to xanthones and includes gentisin (gentiamarin), isogentisin and gentioside (1,3β-prime-verosidoisogentisin). Gentian also contains gentisic acid (2,5-dihydroxybenzoic acid) and about 0.03% of the alkaloids gentianine and gentialutine, which may be artefacts of the preparation process.

Gentian is rich in sugars, which include the trisaccharide gentianose, the disaccharides gentiobiose and sucrose. During the fermentation process these are partially hydrolysed into glucose and fructose. If fermentation is allowed to proceed for long time, the hexose sugars are converted into alcohol and carbon dioxide. Gential should yield 33-40% of water-soluble extractive but highly fermented root yields much less.

Gentiopicroside showed anti-inflammatory

activity in carrageenin-induced foot edema in rats. Gentianine reduced the swelling of the ankle joint in rat hind leg. It also showed hypotensive activity in cats.

Uses

Gentian is used as a bitter tonic and stomachic for increasing appetite and to cure debility.

Allied drugs

The roots of other species of *Gentiana* (*e.g.*, *G. purpurea*, *G. pannonica* and *G. punctata*) are also used. They have similar medicinal properties to the official drug but are usually of smaller size. In India the roots of *G. kurroa* and *Picrorhiza kurroa* are used as Gentian substitutes under the name of 'kathi roots'.

Adulterants

Adulteration occurs due to careless collection. The rhizomes of *Rumex alpinus* give the test for anthraquinone derivatives. It is a dangerous but easily detected admixture with the rhizomes of *Veratrum album*.

QUASSIA

Synonyms

Bitter wood, Bitter ash; Quassia wood; Lignum quassiae.

Biological source

Quassia is the dried stem wood of *Picrasma excelsa* (Swartz) Planchon (syn. *Picroena excelsa* or *Aeschrion excelsa*) which is known in commerce as Jamaica Quassia, or of *Quassia amara* Linn. which is known in commerce as Surinam Quassia.

The plant is propagated by seeds, cuttings or layers. (Family : Simarubaceae).

Habitat

P. excelsa inhibits in West Indies, Jamaica and the Caribbean Islands. *Quassia amara* Linn. is a native of Brazil and Guiana and is cultivated in Colombia, Panama and the West Indies.

Collection

P. excelsa is a 25 m high tree; *Q. amara* is a branch-ing, 2-3 m high shrub or small tree. The stem is cut and small branches are separated. Bark is removed from the stem and big branches are cut into logs of up to 30 cm length or chips and dried to check mould's growth.

Morphology

Quassia is found in logs, chips or rasping. The logs are up to 30 cm in length, covered with a dark grey cork. The colour of wood is white in beginning and becomes yellow on exposure. The drug is odourless but the taste is intensely bitter.

It shows blackish markings due to the presence of a fungus. The logs split readily and the chips break very readily into smaller fragments.

A small piece of Quassia wood should be smoothed and the transverse, radial and tangential surfaces examined with a lens.

The commercial chips usually contain bark in addition to the wood. The cork shows blue and yellow patched on a velvety brown background in U.V. light, the phloem fluoresces an intense grey-ish-white, the regions attacked by fungus become violet, and the false annual rings become very distinct and fluoresce a much brighter yellow than the remainder of the wood.

Microscopical characters

A transverse section of Quassia shows two to five cells wide medullary rays with 6-8 per millimetre of arc. In longitudinal section the medullary rays are mostly 10-15 cells high. The medullary ray cells are radially elongated and have slightly thickened pitted walls. The xylem is composed of vessels, wood fibres and wood parenchyma. The vessels are large and occur singly or in groups of 2-11 which often extend from one medullary ray to the next. In longitudinal sections, the vessels show minute bordered pits. The wood parenchyma occurs in concentric rings, often irregular and interrupted, with false annual rings. Wood parenchyma also occurs in small amounts around the vessels. The wood parenchyma cells are elongated longitudinally, are square or polygonal in transverse section and have moderately thickened pitted walls. The ground mass of the xylem is composed of the thick-walled, longitudinally elongated wood fibres having finely pointed ends and showing fine oblique pits. Single prisms of calcium oxalate, enclosed in a delicate membrane, occur scattered in the medullary ray cells and wood parenchyma cells. Starch grains are few; occasionally two-compound, mostly simple and spherical.

Chemical constituents

Quassin and neoquassin are the bitter terpenoid principles of Surinam Quassia while picrasmin (isoquassin) is the active constituent of Jamaica Quassia. These bitter principles are obtained in 2% yields and appear commercially under the name of quassin. Other compounds reported from Quassia are 18-hydroxyquassin, scopoletin (coumarin) and cathine-6-one (alkaloid).

The quassins are estimated by sensory means separation, by TLC, HPLC and circular chromatography, followed by absorption measurements.

Uses

Quassia is used as a bitter tonic, as an insecticide in the form of fly poison on fly-paper, and as an enema for the expulsion of thread worms.

GINKGO

The leaves of Ginkgo are obtained from the dioeceous tree *Ginkgo biloba* (Maidenhair-tree) (Ginkgoaceae).

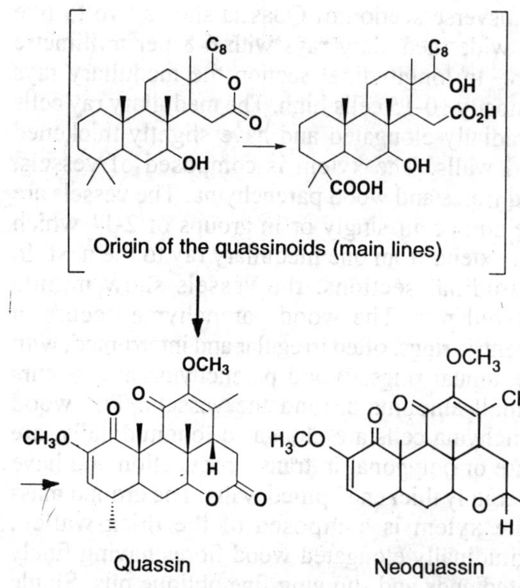

Fig. 15.55. Biosynthesis of quassin.

The leaves are bilobed, each lobe being triangular in outline with a fine radiating, fan-like venation. The leaf is glabrous, petiolate and has an entire margin.

It is a native to China and Japan and cultivated ornamentally in many temperate regions.

In Europe it is now estimated to have a turnover of about Rs. 25000 million. The standardized extracts of the drugs are used for the treatment of circulatory diseases resulting from older age.

Chemical constituents

The diterpene lactones and flavonoids possess therapeutic activity. Five diterpene lactones (ginkgolides A, B, C, J, M) have been characterized; these have a cage structure involving a tertiary butyl group and six 5-membered rings including a spirononane system; a tetrahydrofuran moiety and three lactonic groups. These com-pounds are platelet-activating factor (PAF) anta-gonists and as they do not react with any other known receptor, their effect is very specific. A tertiary butyl group is present in the sesquiterpene bilobalide; no PAF-antagonist activity has been demonstrated for this compound.

About 40 flavonoids have now been isolated from the leaves including glycosides of kaempferol, quercetin and isorhamnetin derivatives. The tree also synthesizes a number of biflavonoids based on amentoflavone.

Other compounds isolated from the leaves include long-chain hydrocarbons and derivatives, and long-chain phenols with anti-tumour, antimicrobial and toxic properties.

With the flavonoids there is a higher concentration of flavonol glycosides in spring leaves and of biflavones in autumn leaves.

Ginkgolides have been detected in Ginkgo cell cultures.

Uses

Ginkgo is used as an antiasthmatic, bronchio-dilator and for the treatment of chilblains. Extracts of the leaf containing selected constituents are used for improving peripheral and cerebral circulation in those elderly with symptoms of loss of short-term memory, hearing and concentration; it is also claimed that vertigo, headaches, anxiety and apathy are cured.

FLAVONOL GLYCOSIDES

The flavonol glycosides and their aglycons are called flavonoids. A large number of different flavonoids are found in nature. These are yellow pigments of higher plants. The important flavonoids are rutin, quercitrin, hesperidine, hesperetin, diosmin and naringen. Rutin and hesperidine are known as vitamin P or permeability factors. They are used in the treatment of different disorders such as capillary bleeding and increased capillary fragility. Bioflavonoids are reported to treat symptoms of the common cold.

Rutin

Rutin, the rhamnoglucoside of quercetin, is found in many plants, and commercial suppliers are made from tobacco residues, *Sophora* and *Eucalyptus* spp. or buckwheat (*Fagopyryum esculentum*), which yields about 3-4%. The flowers of *Sambucus nigra* (elder) have long been used in domestic and veterinary medicine, particularly in the form of ointment. They contain *p*-coumaric acid, rutin and kaempferol.

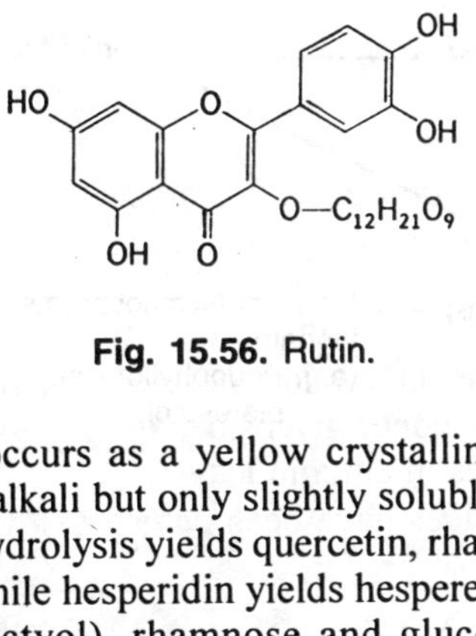

Fig. 15.56. Rutin.

Rutin occurs as a yellow crystalline powder, soluble in alkali but only slightly soluble in water. Rutin on hydrolysis yields quercetin, rhamnose and glucose, while hesperidin yields hesperetin (or methyl eriodictyol), rhamnose and glucose. Rutin gradually darkens on exposure to light. It contains three moles of water. Anhydrous rutin is hygroscopic; recrystallizes as pale yellow needles from water.

ALCOHOL GLYCOSIDES

Salicin is an alcoholic glycoside obtained from *Salix purpurea* and *S. fragilis*. Salicin is hydrolyzed into D-glucose and saligenin by emulsin. Salicin has

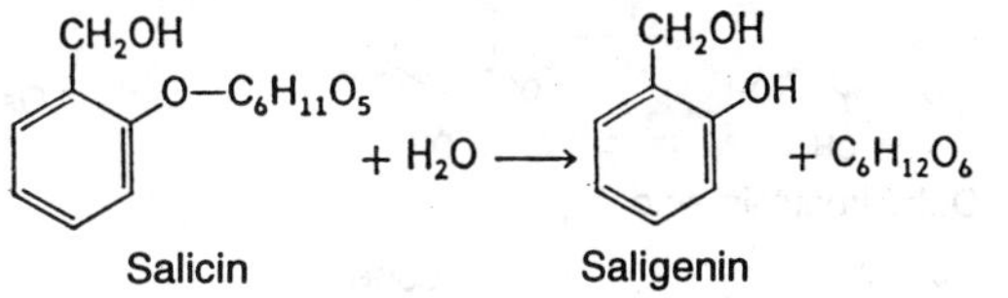

Fig. 15.57. Hydrolysis of salicin.

antirheumatic properties. Its actions are similar to that of salicylic acid.

ALDEHYDE GLYCOSIDES

Vanilla contains an aldehydic aglycone, vanillin, Vanilla is the cure, full grown unripe fruit of *Vanilla planifolia* or of *V. tahitensis* (Family Orchidaceae). The plants are perennial, climbing, dioecious epiphytes attached to the trunks of trees and found in eastern Maxico. The plant is propagated from cuttings. The fruits are collected, cured by dipping in worm water and repeated sweating between woolen blankets in the sun for two months. Green Vanilla contains two glycosides, glucovanillin and glucovanillic alcohol. Vanilla is used as flavouring agent and as a pharmaceutical aid. It is a source of vanillin.

PHENOL GLYCOSIDES

The aglycone groups of many of the naturally occurring glycosides are phenolic in character. Thus, arbutin, found in uva ursi, chimaphila, and other ericaceous drugs, yields hydroquinone and glucose upon hydrolysis. Hesperidin, which occurs in various citrus fruits and is included with the flavonol group, may be classified as a phenol glycoside. Phloridzin, found in the root bark of rosaceous plants, baptisin from baptisia, and iridin from *Iris* species are phenol glycosides.

UVA URSI

Uva ursi or Bearberry is the dried leaf of *Arctostaphylos uva-ursi* (Linn.) Sprengel or its varieties *coactylis* or *adenotricha* (Fam. Ericaceae). The plant is a procumbent evergreen shrub indigenous to Europe, Asia, the northern United States and Canada.

In addition to the glycoside, arbutin (6-10%), the leaves contain corilagin, pyroside, several esters of arbutin, quercitin, gallic acid, elagic acid,

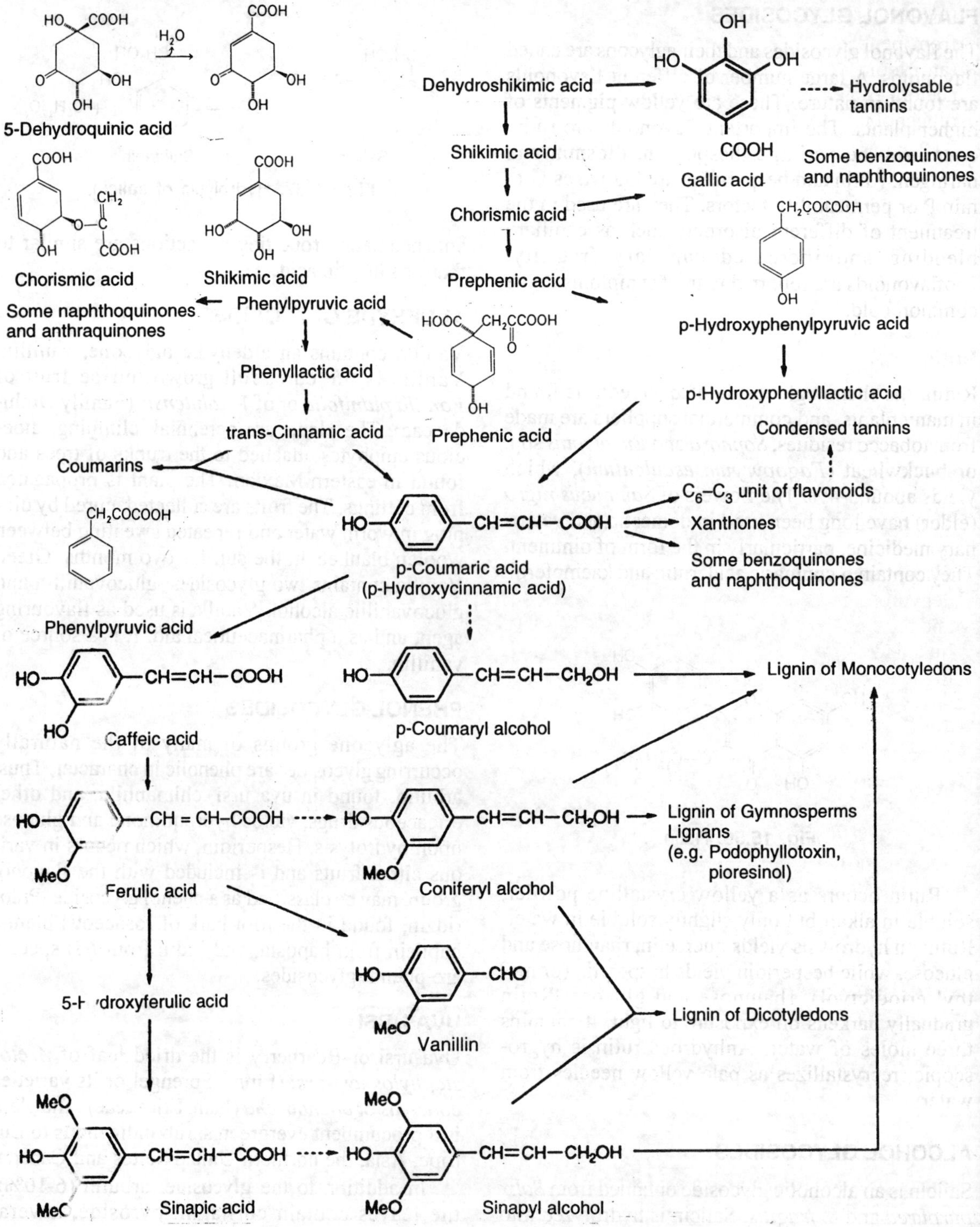

Fig. 15.58. Phenolic compounds originating from shikimic acid.

ursolic acid, methylarbutin, gallotannins derived from pentagalloylglucose (15-20%), monotropein (an iridoid) and picein (a glycoside of 4-hydroxy-acetophenone). Upon hydrolysis, arbutin yields a diphenol which is readily oxidized to hydroquinone.

Uva ursi has diuretic and astringent properties. Uva ursi and other diuretic materials are added in various products intended for weight reduction. It is prescribed to enhance the renal excretion of water. Bearberry leaf can cause nausea and vomiting in some persons with delicate stomach.

Steroidal alkaloidal glycosides

These glycosides are predominant in the families Solanaceae and Liliaceae. Like saponins, they show haemolytic properties. Examples are α-solanin (potato, *Solanum tuberosum*), soladulcin (bitter-sweet, *S. dulcamara*), tomatin (tomato, *Lycopersicon esculentum*) and rubijervine (*Veratrum* spp.). The sugar components are attached in the 3-position. They may be glucose, galactose, rhamnose or xylose one to four in number. Solasodine and 5-dehydrotomatidine are stereoisomeric spirosolanes and the configuration of the nitrogen atom is always linked to that at C-25. Solasodine, the nitrogen analogue of diosgenin is $\Delta^5,22\beta,25\alpha$-spirosolen-3β-ol and 5-dehydrotoma-tidine is $\Delta^5,22\alpha,25\beta$-spirosolen-3β-ol.

Tomatidine

Solanidine

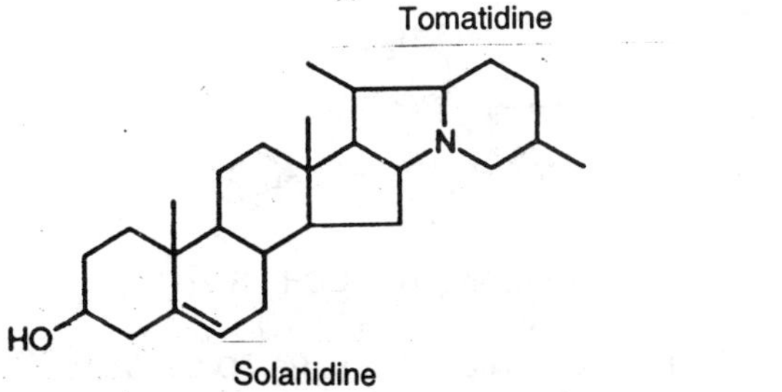

Fig. 15.59. Steroidal alkaloids.

Solanum species

Some of the steroidal alkaloids are the nitrogen analogues of the C_{27} sapogenins (*e.g.*, solasodine and diosgenin). Another series of C_{27} compounds contain a tertiary nitrogen in a condensed ring system (*e.g.*, solanidine). These compounds are also used in the partial synthesis of steroidal drugs. Species so exploited are *Solanum laciniatum*, *S. khasianum and* S. *aviculare*.

Glycosidal resins

The complex resins of the Convolvulaceae found in Jalap and Scammony are glycosidal; they yield on hydrolysis sugars such as glucose, rhamnose and fucose together with normal fatty acids and the hydroxyl derivatives.

Glycosidal bitter principles

Many glycosides have a bitter taste, *e.g.*, gentiopicrin or gentiopicroside of Gentian root; picrocrocin or picrocroside of Saffron; and cucurbitacins of the Cucurbitaceae (*e.g.*, Colocynth).

Betacyanins and betaxanthins

Some plant pigments contain nitrogen and termed 'nitrogenous anthocyanins'. Betacyanins and betaxanthins are red-violet and yellow, respectively. These compounds are present in *Beta vulgaris* (the red beet) and the anthocyanin and are anthoxanthin pigments. These compounds contained nitrogen, but they are not flavonoid derivatives. Betanin, on hydrolysis, gives the aglycone betanidin; indicaxanthin, is not a glycoside. These compounds are used as food colourants.

Antibiotic glycosides

Certain antibiotics are of glycosidal nature. Streptomycin is formed from the genin streptidin (a nitrogen-containing cyclohexane derivative) to which is attached the disaccharide streptobiosamine. The latter contain one molecule of the rare methylpentose streptose and one molecule of *N*-methylglucosamine.

Nucleosides or nucleic acids

These substances have three components; a sugar unit (either ribose or 2-desoxyribose), a purine or pyrimidine base (*e.g.*, adenine, guanine and cytosine) and phosphoric acid. These are *N*-glycosides. When conjugated with proteins they form nucleoproteins.

SOYA BEAN

The soya (soy, soja) plant, *Glycine max* (*G. soya*) (Papilionaceae) is extensively cultivated for its seeds, which are rich in oil and protein. The seeds also contain appreciable quantities of the phytosterols stigmasterol and sitosterol. They are obtained as by products of soap-making, being components of the unsaponifiable matter of the fixed oil. Pure stigmasterol, with its unsaturated side-chain is subjected to chemical conversion to suitable starting materials and can replace diosgenin. Sitosterol, has saturated side-chain which could not be removed chemically. Similar phytosterols are found in other products, *e.g.*, cotton-seed oil, tall-oil (from the wood-pulp industry) and sugarcane wax.

SARSAPARILLA ROOT

Sarsaparilla consists of the dried roots and of the rhizomes of the species of *Smilax* (Smilacaceae).

The plants produce numerous roots, 3 m or so long, which are attached to a short rhizome. The roots are cut. Sometimes the rhizomes and the roots are collected. After drying in the sun the drug is tied into bundles and the bundles into bales.

Sarsaparilla is imported in large bales bound with wire. Each bale usually contains numerous bundles of uniform size. These consist of long roots, with or without pieces of rhizome and aerial stems. The commercial varieties differ from one another in colour, ridges and furrows; in the presence or absence of rhizome and aerial stems; in the relative proportions of cortex, wood and pith. The drug is nearly odourless but has a sweetish and acrid taste. Due to the presence of saponins, aqueous extractives form froth readily.

Different species contain one or more steroidal saponins. Two isomeric genins are known : smilagenin and sarsasapogenin. These differ only in their configuration at C-25 and correspond to the reduced forms of diosgenin and yamogenin, respectively. The principal crystalline glycoside of *Smilax aristolochiaefolia* is parillin (sarsasaponin, sarsasa-

ponoside). On hydrolysis it gives sarsasapogenin, three molecules of glucose and one of the rhamnose. Sarsaparilloside is a bisdesmosidic saponin.

Uses

Sarsaparilla is used to treat syphilis, rheumatism and certain skin diseases, like psoriasis and eczema, and rheumatoid arthritis due to the presence of steroid content of the roots. It is used as a vehicle, and large quantities are processed for the manufacture of non-alcoholic drinks. The genins are used in the partial synthesis of cortisone and other steroids.

VISNAGA (Khella)

The drug consists of the dried ripe fruits of *Ammi visnaga* (Apiaceae), an annual plant about 1-1.5 m high. It grows in the Middle East, Morocco and Egypt. The greyish-brown mericarps are usually separate but are sometimes attached to the carpophore. Each mericarp is broadly ovoid and about 0.5 mm long. It has five prominent primary ridges and six vittae. Odour, slightly aromatic; taste, very bitter.

Khellin, the most important active constituent, is crystalline and has been synthesized. It is 2-methyl-5,8-dimethoxyfuranochrome. It occurs in the immature fruits (1%), and is accompanied by two other crystalline compounds, visnagin (about 0.1%) and khellol glucoside (about 0.3%) of volatile oil. It also contains khellol, khellinol, visnadin, samidin, dihydrosamidin, lipids (~ 18%), furano-acetophenone, flavonoids and angular pyrano-coumarins vismadin, samidin and dihydro-samidin. The furanochromones are present in the large secretory canals of the primary ribs and in the endosperm.

It is used in the treatment of angina pectoris and

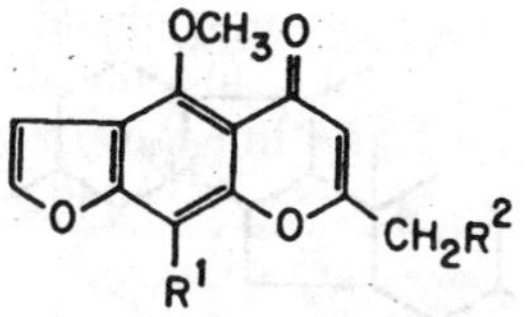

Khellin : $R^1 = OCH_3$, $R^2 = H$
Visnagin : $R^1 = R^2 = H$
Khellol glucoside : $R^1 = H$, $R^2 = O$-Glucoside

Fig. 15.60. Chemical constituents of Visnaga.

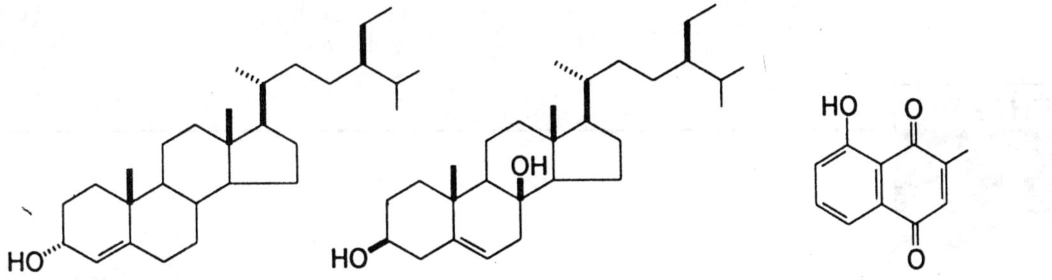

Fig. 15.61. Chemical constituents of Henna.

bronchial asthma. Khellin is a spasmolytic agent and used in the preventive therapy of *angina pectoris* and as a coronary vasodilator.

HENNA

It consists of the dried leaves of *Lawsonia inermis*, (Lythraceae), a shrub cultivated in north Africa including Egypt, Pakistan, India and Sri Lanka. The leaves are greenish-brown to brown and about 2.5-5 cm long. The apex is mucronate, the margin entire and revolute, and venation pinnate. Henna contains a colouring matter, lawsone (a hydroxy-naphthoquinone), various phenolic glycosides, coumarins, xanthones, quinoids, β-sitosterol gluco-side, lansaritols, isoplumbagin, flavonoids including luteolin and its 7-O-glucoside, fats, resin and henna-tannin. Henna is used as a dye for the hair and wool.

LITHOSPERMUM

It consists of the seeds of the European *Lithospermum officinale* (gromwell).

It contains shikonin, a naphthoquinone deriva-tive; scyllitol, a cyclitol; a cyanoglucoside-litho-spermocide; caffeic, chlorogenic and ellagic acids; and catechin-type tannins. Shikonin, the enantiomer of alkannin is also a constituent of *L. erythrorhizon* root and is produced for the cosmetic and pharma-ceutical industries in Japan by cell culture of the

plant. The preparations of the purple roots are used for the treatment of burns, inflammations, wounds and ulcers.

ALKANNA ROOT

Alkanet or Anchusae Radix is the dried root of *Alkanna tinctoria* (Boraginaceae), a herb found in Hungary, southern Europe and Turkey. It consists of reddish-purple roots about 10-15 cm long and 1-2 cm diameter near the crown. The surface is deeply fissured and readily exfoliates. Alkanna is used for colouring oils and tars and in the form of a tincture for the microscopical detection of oils and fats. The pigments are naphthoquinone derivatives.

Alkanin itself may be an artefact arising from various esters. Most of the pigment compounds produced in cell culture give alkannin on KOH hydrolysis.

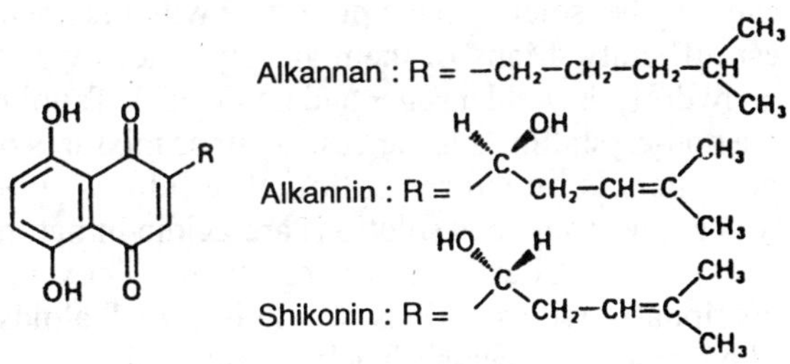

Fig. 15.62. Chemical constituents of Alkanna root.

Tannins

Tannins are complex organic, non-nitrogenous derivatives of polyhydroxy benzoic acids which are widely distributed in the vegetable kingdom. They are the active constituents of materials like oak bark, which are used in the tanning of skins. They are present in aerial parts, *e.g.*, leaves, fruits, barks or stem; generally occur in immature fruits, but disappears during ripening process. New leaves of deciduous plants contain high concentration of tannins. Tannins occur in many crude drugs. They probably serve as a protective to the plant during growth and are destroyed or deposited as end products of metabolism in some dead tissues of the mature plant, *i.e.*, outer cork, heartwood and galls. Some phenolic substances, such as gallic acid, catechins and chlorogenic acid often occur with tannins and are called as 'pseudotannins'. Most of the true tannins have the molecular weight between 1000 to 5000.

Most tannins are very complex substances which can only be isolated in the pure state with the greatest difficulty. Many of them are glycosides which on hydrolysis yield a sugar and gallic acid. Tannins are non-crystalline substances, occur as mixtures of polyphenols and form colloidal solutions with water. Their aqueous solutions are acidic in nature and possess sharp 'puckering' taste. They are precipitated with solutions of gelatin and alkaloids. They produce greenish black or blue colour with ferric chloride and deep red colour with potassium ferricyanide and ammonia. They form precipitate with salts of copper, lead and tin and by strong aqueous potassium dichromate or 1% chromic acid.

A tannin is a substance which is detected qualitatively by a tanning test (the goldbeater's skin test) and is determined quantitatively by its absorption on standard hide powder.

To be effective for tannage the polyphenol molecule must be neither so large as to be unable to enter the interstices between the collagen fibrils of the animal skin nor so small that it is unable to cross-link between the protein molecules of adjacent fibrils at several points.

Tannins precepitate and combine with proteins. The protein tannin complex is resistant to proteolytic enzymes. This property is known as astringent action and many tannin-containing drugs are used in medicine as astringent. During healing process of burns, the proteins of the exposed tissues are precipitated producing a mildly antiseptic, protective layer under which the new tissues are regenerated. Tannins are used in the tanning process of animal hides to convert them into leather. Aqueous solutions of tannins are used to precipitate gelatin, proteins and alkaloids in the laboratory. They are used as healing agents in inflammation, leucorrhoea, gonorrhoea, burns, piles and diarrhoea. Tannin-containing drugs are used traditionally as styptics and internally for the protection of inflamed surfaces of mouth and throat. They act as antidiarrhoeals and as antidotes in poisoning by heavy metals, alkaloids and glycosides. Anti-HIV activity has also been demonstrated. Absorbed tannic acid can cause severe central necrosis of the liver. Tannins exhibit a strong anti-tumour activity. Ellagitannin monomer units having galloyl groups at the O-2- and O-3-positions on the glucose cores, as in the tellimagradins, are required. Their deep red coloured complexes with iron salts are used to manufacture inks. Tannins are classified as :

1. *Hydrolysable tannins* : These tannins are esters of a sugar, usually glucose with one or more trihydroxybenzene carboxylic acid (gallic acid) and hexahydroxydiphenic acid. They are hydrolyzed by acids or enzymes to yield several molecules of phenolic acids such as gallic and ellagic acids. The phenolic acids are combined to a central glucose residue by ester linkages. The tannins derived from gallic acid are known as gallitannins and from that of ellagic acid as ellagitannins. Gallitannins occur in Rhubarb, Cloves, Chestnut, Rose petals, Bearbery leaves, Chinese leaves, Turkish galls, Maple and Chestnut, The sources of ellagitannins are Myrobalans, Pomegranate bark and rind, Eucalyptus leaves, Chestnut and Oak bark. These tannins form blue or black colour with ferric chloride, and pyrogallol on heating. They do not give blue colour with bromine solutions.

Ellagic acid can arise by lactonization of hexahydroxydiphenic acid during chemical hydrolysis of tannins.

Agromoniin, an oligomeric hydrolysable tannins, was isolated from *Agrimonia*. These tannins are composed of two, three or four monomeric units. About 20 of these units including geraniin and tellimagrandins 1 and 2 are involved in the production of over 150 compounds. C-glucosidic ellagitannins are common in the Myrtaceae, Hamamelidaceae, Punicaceae and Rosaceae and several have also been recorded as moieties of more than 10 oligomeric ellagitannins.

β-D-Glucogallin acts as both donor and acceptor of the galloyl group in the enzymatic formation of 1,6-digalloyl-D-glucose; the responsible enzyme is β-glucogallin; β-glucogallin 6-*O*-galloyltransferase.

2. *Condensed tannins* (*Proanthocyanidins*) : Condensed tannins are resistant to hydrolysis and they are derived from the flavanols, catechins and flavan-3, 4-diols. On treatment with acids or enzymes they are decomposed into phlobaphenes. On dry distillation condensed tannins produce catechol. Therefore, these tannins are also called as catechol tannins. Condensed tannins are found in bark (Cinnamon, Cinchona, Wild Cherry, Willow, Acacia, Oak and Hamamelis), roots and rhizomes (Krameria and Male fern), flowers (lime and hawthorn), seeds (Cacoa, Kola, Areca and Guarana), leaves (Hamamelis and Tea) and extracts (Catechu, Acacia and Butea gum). These tannins give green colour with ferric chloride solution, produce catechol on heating, yield phloroglucinol with conc. HCl or vanillin-HCl and phlobaphene on oxidation.

On treatment with acids or enzymes condensed tannins are converted into red insoluble compounds known as phlobaphenes. Phlobaphenes give the characteristic red colour to many drugs such as red Cinchona bark,

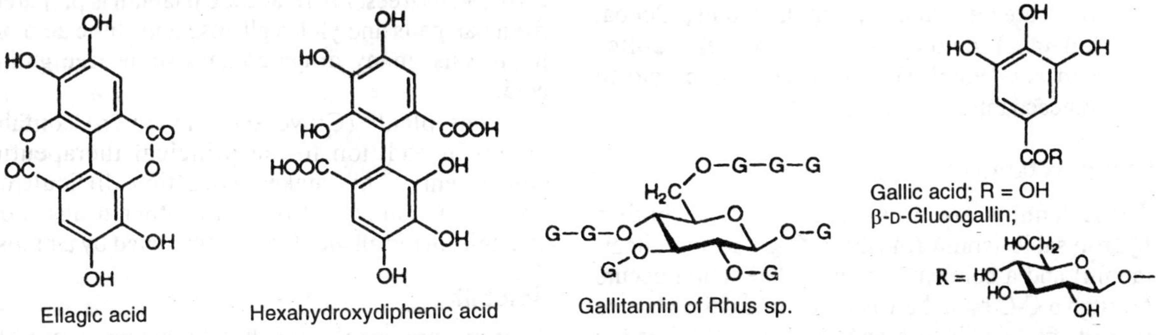

Ellagic acid Hexahydroxydiphenic acid Gallitannin of Rhus sp. Gallic acid; R = OH β-D-Glucogallin;

Fig. 16.1. Hydrolysable tannins.

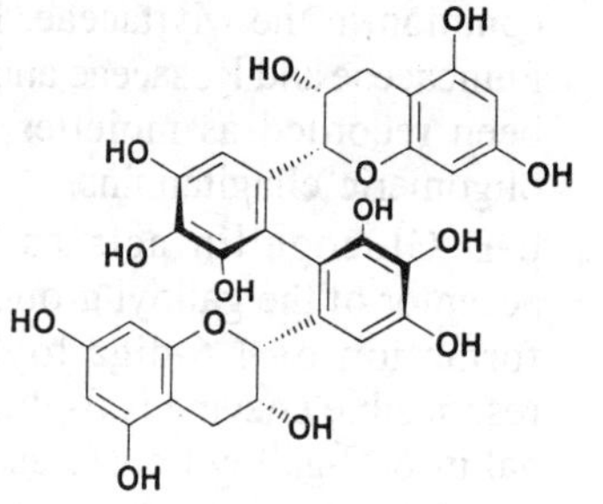

Theasinensin C

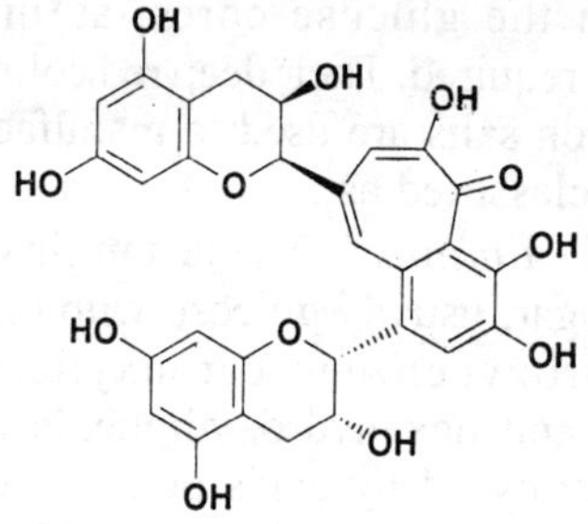

Theaflavin

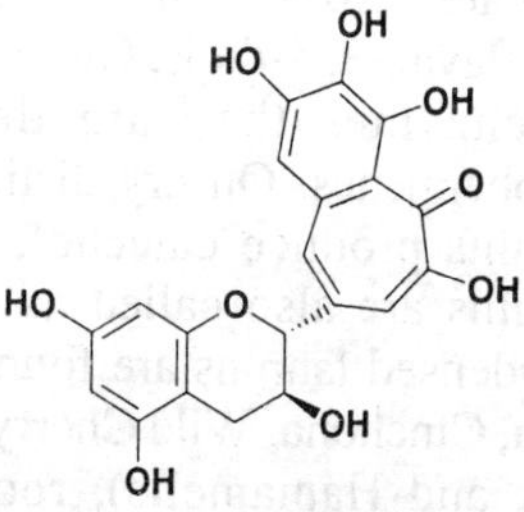

Theaflagallin

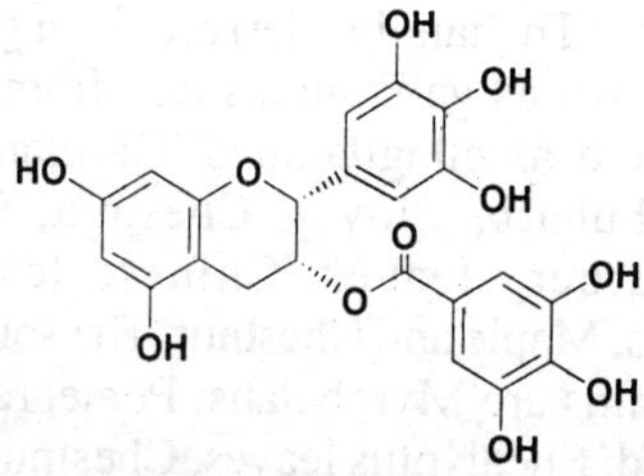

(–)-Epigallocatechin 3-O-gallate

Fig. 16.2. Condensed tannins.

which contain these phlobatannins and their decomposition products. Catechins, which also occur with the tannins and flavan-3,4-diols (leucoanthocyanidins) are inter-mediates in the biosynthesis of the polymeric molecules. Stereochemical variations add to the variety of possible structure.

3. *Pseudotannins* : Pseudotannins are phenolic compounds of lower molecular weight and they do not show the goldbeater's skin test. They occur as gallic acid (in Rhubarb), catechins (in Catechu, Acacia, Cutch, Kinos, Cocoa, Guarana), chlorogenic acid (in Mate, Coffee and Nux vomica) and ipecacuanhic acid in Ipecacuanha.

Complex tannins

These tannins are biosynthesized from both a hydrolysable tannin (mostly a C-glucoside ellagitannin) and a condensed tannin. The union occurs through a C-C bond between the C-1 of the glucose unit of the ellagitannin and the C-8 or C-6 of the flavan-3-ol derivative. The monomers take part in oligomer formation. Complex tannins have been isolated from the Combretaceae, Papilionaceae (*Quercus, Castanea*), Myrtaceae, Polygonaceae (*Rheum*) and Theaceae (*Camellia*).

Tannins are usually found in greatest quantity in dead or dying cells. They exert an inhibitory effect on many enzymes due to protein precipitation. Therefore, they may contribute a protective function in barks and heartwoods. Commercial tannins, are used in the leather industry and are obtained from quebracho, wattle, chestnut and myrobalans trees. Pharmaceutical tannin is prepared from oak galls and yields glucose and gallic acid on hydrolysis; many drugs contain some free gallic acid.

Some plants (Clove and Cinnamon) contain tannin in addition to the principal therapeutic constituents. This makes extraction difficult or produce incompatibilities with other drugs. For example, many alkaloids are precipitated by tannins.

Solubility

Tannins are freely soluble in water, alcohol, glycerol, acetone and dilute alkalies. They are

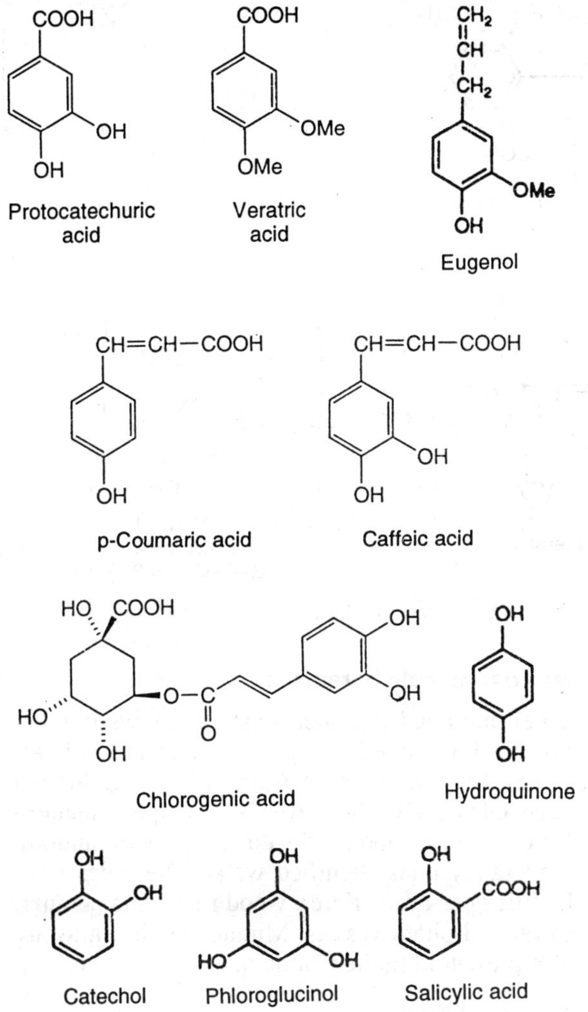

Fig. 16.3. Pseudotannins.

sparingly soluble in chloroform, ethyl acetate and some other organic solvents.

Phlobaphenes are soluble in alcohol but practically insoluble in water. Phlobaphenes result from phlobatannins in many ways. They are slowly deposited from a cold aqueous solution of a phlobatannin, and rapidly if the solution is subjected to prolonged boiling, or if boiled with sulphuric acid. Glycerine minimizes conversion of phlobatannins to phlobaphenes.

Chemical tests

1. *Goldbeater's skin test* : A small piece of gold-beater's skin (a membrane prepared from the intestine of an ox) is soaked in 2% hydrochloric acid, rinsed with distilled water and placed in a solution of tannin for 5 minutes. The skin piece is washed with distilled water and kept in a solution of ferrous sulphate. A brown or black colour is produced on the skin due to the presence of tannins.

2. *Gelatin test* : To a solution of tannin (0.5-1%) aqueous solutions of gelatin (1%) and sodium chloride (10%) are added. A white buff-coloured precipitate is formed.

3. *Phenazone test* : A mixture of aqueous extract (5 ml) of a drug and sodium acid phosphate (0.5 g) is heated, cooled and filtered. A solution of phenazone (2%) is added to the filtrate. A bulky coloured precipitate is formed.

4. *Catechin test* (*Matchstick test*) : A matchstick is dipped in aqueous plant extract, dried near burner and moistened with concentrated hydrochloric acid. On warming near a flame the matchstick wood turns pink or red due to formation of phloroglucinol.

5. *Chlorogenic acid test* : An extract of chlorogenic acid containing drug is treated with aqueous ammonia. A green colour is formed on exposure to air.

6. *Vanillin-hydrochloric acid test* : (Vanillin 1 g, alcohol 10 ml, concentrated hydrochloric acid 10 ml). When a drug is treated with vanillin-hydrochloric acid reagent, pink or red colour is formed due to formation of phloroglucinol.

PALE CATECHU

Synonyms

Gambier; Catechu; Gambier Catechu; Terra japonica.

Biological source

Pale Catechu is the dried aqueous extract of leaves and twigs of *Uncaria gambir* (Hunter) Roxb. (Fam. Rubiaceae).

Habitat

The plant is indigenous to Malaya and cultivatved in Indonesia, Malaya and Borneo.

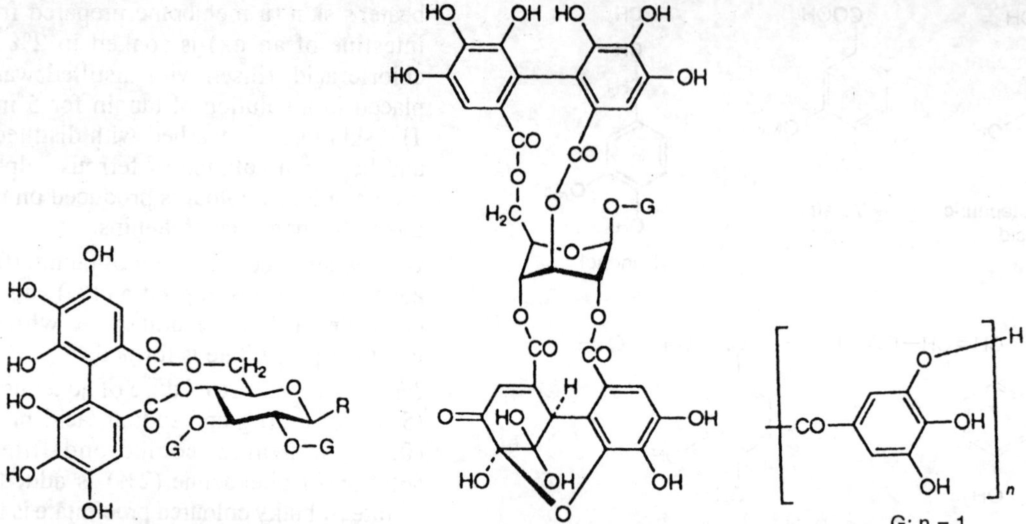

Fig. 16.4. Hydrolysable tannins and their component acids.

Tellimagrandin 1; R = OH
Tellimagrandin 2; R = (β)-OG

Geraniin

G; n = 1
G–G; n = 2
G–G–G; n = 3

Preparation

Plant is a climbing shrub and grown from seeds. The leafy twigs up to 50 cm in length are cut at an interval of 4-6 months from 2 to 10 years old plant. The leaves and twigs are boiled with water for 3 hours in a large pan. The leaves and twigs are removed and the extract is concentrated to form a yellowish green pasty mass. It is cooled in shallow wood tubs, put into trays or tin containers and cut into cubes of uniform size. The cubes are dried in sun, packed and exported. Sometimes semisolid mass is packed into bales. It contains more water, less tannins and is of inferior quality.

Many different forms of catechu are used in the East, which frequently has 20-50% of fine rice husks added as the liquid coagulates in the tubs. Such catechu is unofficial and contains starch.

Characters

Pale catechu occurs as cubes of 2.5 cm length and breadth. Sometimes cubes are broken and adhere to each other. Colour is dark reddish-brown; internal surface is pale brown, porous and dull. Cubes break easily and are friable. The fractured surface appears porous internally. The drug is odourless and taste is astringent followed by bitterness in the beginning and sweetish afterwards.

Microscopical characters

When mounted in water, catechu shows minute, branched and interlacking acicular crystals of catechin. They dissolve on warming leaving behind vegetable debris. The leaves bear simple, unicellular hairs up to about 350 μm long, with smooth, moderately thick, lignified walls. The twigs have lignified pericyclic fibres, wood fibres and annular, spiral and pitted vessels. Minute starch grains are also present in limited amount.

Chemical tests

1. *Gambir-fluorescin test* : A mixture of alcoholic extract of Pale Catechu (1 g), sodium hydroxide solution (5 ml), and petroleum ether (5 ml) is shaken and kept for sometimes. The petroleum ether layer shows green fluorescence.
2. Catechin or matchstick test is positive in Pale Catechu.
3. Vanillin-hydrochloric acid test is positive in Pale Catechu.
4. *Chlorophyll test* : Powdered drug (0.5 g) is heated with chloroform (5 ml) on a water bath for 1-2 minutes. The organic layer is filtered in a white China dish and evaporated on the water. A greenish residue is remained due to the presence of chlorophyll.

Chemical constituents

Pale Catechu contains catechins (7-33%), catechu-tannic acid (22-50%), catechu red, quercetin, pyrogallol, Gambhir fluorescein, fixed oil and wax. It contains not less than 70% water-soluble substance and not less than 60% alcoholic soluble portion. It should show a loss on drying not more than 15.0% and a water-insoluble matter not more than 33.0% with reference to the dried material.

It readily yields the phlobaphene catechu-red. If the drug is carefully prepared, it will contain a high proportion of catechin and correspondingly smaller amounts of catechutannic acid and catechu-red.

Catechin is crystallized into white, acicular crystals which are water soluble. Removal of one mole of water from catechin gives catechutannic acid which is an amorphous phlobatannin.

It also contains gambirine, mitraphylline, isogambridine, indole alkaloids roxburghines A, B, C, D and E, 7α-acetoxy dihydronomilin; proanthocyanidin dimer gambiriin, mexicanolide (in seeds), chalcone-flavon dimers gambiriins A1, A2, A3, B1, B2 and B3.

Uses

Pale Catechu has astringent action and is used in diarrhoea, in lozenges, for tanning and dyeing fabrics brown or black.

BLACK CATECHU

Synonyms

Cutch, Catechu; Cachou; Peru Catechu; Cashoo; Catechu nigrum; Kattha (Hindi).

Biological source

Black Catechu is a dried aqueous extract prepared from the heartwood of *Acacia catechu* Willd. (Fam. Mimosaceae).

Habitat

The tree is a native of India and found in Burma.

Preparation

The tree is felled and bark as well as sapwood are removed, cut into small pieces and boiled with water in earthenware or stainless steel vessels. The decoction is filtered and concentrated to get a viscous mass. The thick syrup is poured into wooden frames on papers, cooled and the solidified product is cut into small pieces.

Characters

Black Catechu occurs in black, irregular mass. Outer surface is rough and dull and rarely glossy. Fracture is hard and brittle and the broken surface is dark brown with a dull gloss and porous. It is partially soluble in cold water and alcohol and completely soluble in hot water. The drug is odourless and taste is bitter in the beginning and astringent afterwards.

Chemical constituents

Black Catechu contains a mixture of catechin isomers, acacatechin (2-12%), catechutannic acid or phlobatannin (25-35%), gum (20-30%), quercitrin, quercetin, catechu red and water. Acacatechin contains (-)-epicatechin which is the *trans*- form of acacatechin. During the extraction of heartwood chips with boiling water epicatechin undergoes epimerization and recemization to *dl*-acacatechin. Isomers of acacatechin present in Black Catechu are *l*-acacatechin (m.p. 230°) and *d-iso*-acacatechin (m.p. 226-228°).

Acacatechin is insoluble in cold water but soluble in hot water. It undergoes oxidation to catechutannic acid in the presence of water.

A. catechu also contains kaempferol, dihydrokaempferol, faxifolin, isorhamnetin and (+)-afzelechin.

Uses

Black Catechu possesses cooling and digestive properties. It is used in relaxed condition of throat, mouth and gums and in cough and diarrhoea. Externally as an astringent medicament, it is applied to ulcers, boils and skin eruptions and used in a number of medicinal preparations.

Black Catechu is mainly used as an ingredient of betal leaf (Paan) and *Paan masala*.

Allied drug

Cutch is an extract prepared from the heartwood of *Acacia catechu* (Mimosaceae). Cutch occurs in black, porous masses. The taste resembles that of gambir. Microscopical examination of the water-soluble residue shows wood fibres and large

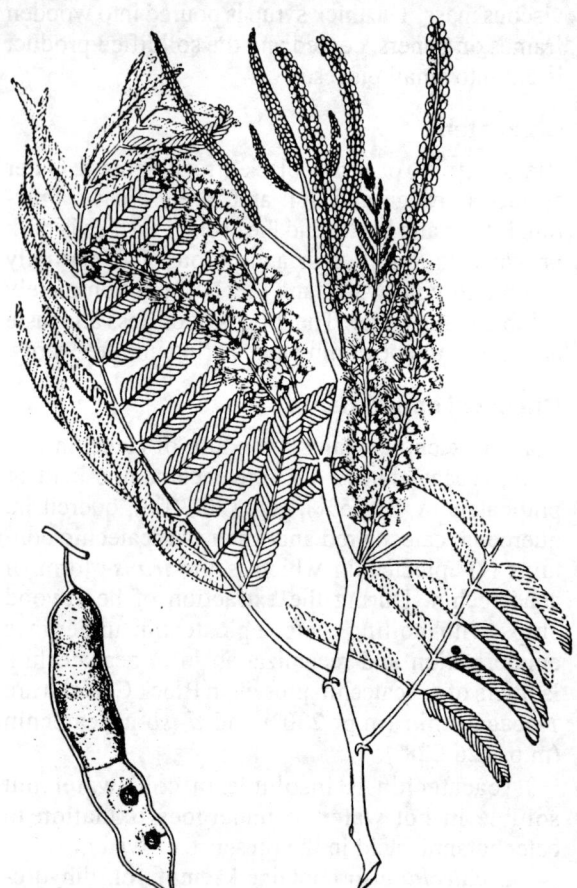

Fig. 16.5. *Acacia catechu*—flowering branch and fruit.

vessels and sometimes fragments derived from the leaves on which the drug is spread.

Cutch contains 2-12% of catechins, 25-33% of phlobatannin, 20-30% of gummy matter, quercitrin, quercitin and moisture. It yields 2-3% of ash. The catechin (acacatechin) is not identical with that in gambir. The drug may be distinguished from gambir as it gives no reaction for gambir fluorescein.

Kinos

Kino consists of a number of dried juices, rich in phlobatannins and formerly used for their astringent properties. They include Malabar kino from *Pterocarpus marsupium* (Papilionaceae), butea gum or Bengal kino from *Butea frondosa* (*B. monosperma*) (Papilionaceae) and eucalyptus kino or red gum from *Eucalyptus rostrata* (Myrtaceae).

Croton lechleri

The bark of this tree (Fam. Euphorbiaceae) yields a blood-red sap commonly known in South America as Sangre de Grado, Sangre de Drace, or dragon's blood (not to be confused with the dragon's blood obtained from species of *Daemonorops* palms). It is used locally for its anti-infective, antitumour and wound healing properties. Proanthocyanidins are the principal constituents (*c.* 90%). Minor components isolated are phenols, alcohols, sterols and diterpenoids. An alkaloid, tapsine, has been ascribed as the wound healing constituent.

Chemical tests

1. Catechin (match-stick) test is positive.
2. Vanillin-hydrochloric acid test is positive.
3. Gambir-fluorescin test is negative distinguishing it from Pale Catechu.
4. Chlorophyll test is also negative distinguishing Black Catechu from Pale Catechu.
5. Add a few drops of a fresh aqueous extract to lime water (10 ml); a brown colour is produced and on standing for three minutes a red precipitate is formed.
6. To an aqueous solution (2%), add solution of ferric ammonium sulphate; a dark green colour is formed. Add sodium hydroxide solution, the colour changes to purple.

GALLS

Synonyms

Turkey galls, Galla, Nutgall, Aleppo galls, Blue galls, Gallae ceruleae.

Biological source

Galls are vegetable outgrowths formed on the twigs of dyer's oak, *Quercus infectoria* (Fam. Papilionaceae) due to deposition of eggs of the gall-wasp *Adleria gallaetinctoriae* Olivier (Fam. Cynipidae).

Habitat

The plant is found in Turkey, Syria, Persia, Cyprus and Greece.

Preparation

The plant is a 2 m high small tree or shrub. The gall-wasp lays eggs on the twigs in early summer.

Larvae come out from the eggs and enter into the soft epidermis near the growing point of the twigs. The larvae secrete an enzyme from its mandible which stimulates abnormal development of vegetable tissues around the larvae. During this process their is rapid conversion of starch in the surrounding tissues into sugars which stimulates cell division. Shrinkage of tissue takes place due to disappearance of starch and a central cavity is formed in which development of larvae and pupae takes place. The larva remains in the galls for 5 to 6 months. The mature insect bores the covering of the galls and escapes. The colour of galls changes from bluish-grey to white during this process. The galls are collected before escaping the insect. They are graded according to colour into three grades, blue, green and white.

Several stages in the development of the gall correspond to the development of the insect :

1. When the larva begins to develop and the gall begins to enlarge, the cells of the outer and central zones contain numerous small starch grains.
2. When the chrysalis stage is reached, the starch near the middle of the gall is replaced in part by gallic acid, but the peripheral and central cells contain masses of tannic acid.
3. As the winged insect develops, nearly all of the cells contain masses of tannic acid with a slight amount of adhering gallic acid.
4. When the insect emerges from the gall, a hole to the central cavity is formed. Thus, the tannic acid, owing to the presence of moisture and air, may be oxidized in part into an insoluble product, and the gall becomes more porous, thereby producing the so-called *white gall* of commerce.

Characters

Galls are globular or subspherical in shape, 1-2.5 cm in diameter with short basal stalk. Numerous rounded projections are present on the outer surface. 'White galls', from which the insects have emerged, contain circular holes, 2-3 mm in dia-meter, on the lower part on one side. Colour is grey or white and the projections are dark brown in colour. Gall are hard and heavy and shrink in water. Taste is very astringent.

The 'blue' variety are grey or brownish-grey in colour. These, and the olive-green 'green' galls, are preferred to the 'white' variety, in which the tannin is partly decomposed. White galls also differ from the other grades in having a circular tunnel through which the insect has emerged. Galls without the opening have insect remains in the small central cavity.

Microscopial characters

A transverse section of a gall shows a very large outer zone of thin-walled parenchyma, a ring of sclerenchymatous cells, and a small, inner zone of thick-walled parenchyma surrounding the central cavity. The parenchymatous tissues contain abundant starch, masses of tannin, rosettes and prisms of calcium oxalate, and the rounded 'lignin bodies', which give a red colour with phloroglucinol and hydrochloric acid.

Chemical constituents

Galls contain tannin known as gallotannic acid (50-70%), gallic acid (2-4%), ellagic acid, β-sitosterol, methyl betulate, methyl oleanolate, starch, calcium oxalate, nyctanthic acid, roburic acid and syringic acid. Gallotannic acid is prepared by fermenting the galls and extracting with water-saturated ether.

The fruits contain amentoflavone hexamethyl ether, isocryptomerin and β-sitosterol.

Pharmacology

Methanol extract of galls showed analgesic activity in rats, significantly reduced blood pressure in rabbits, exhibited CNS-depressant activity due to syringic acid and moderate antitremorine activity. It showed anaesthetic action due to complete blockade of isolated frog sciatic nerve conduction.

Uses

Galls are used as astringent, for tanning and dyeing, and in the manufacture of inks and tannic acid. Syringic acid has been identified as the CNS-active component of the methanolic extract of galls.

Allied drugs

Chinese and Japanese galls

They are produced on the petioles of the leaves of *Rhus chinensis* (Anacardiaceae) by an aphis,

Schlectendalia chinensis. The galls on breaking show a large, irregular cavity and contain tannin (57-77%). The galls contain gallic acid ester, quercitrin, 7-hydroxy-6-methoxy coumarin, ethyl gallate, 3,7,4'-trihydroxy- and 3,7,3',4'-tetrahydroxy-flavones, salicylic acid derivatives semialatic acid, 3-heptadecylcatechol and β-sitosterol.

The plant is used to treat heart disease and bronchitis. They are used as astringent and to treat haemorrhoids. In China, these tannins are valued as astringent and styptic.

Crowned aleppo galls

They are about globular, 0.5 cm in diameter, stalked and contained a crown of projections near the apex. They are produced by an insect, *Cynips polycera.* These galls are added as an adulterant in the samples.

Hungarian galls

They are formed on a tree, *Quercus robur*, growing in Yugoslavia, by an insect *Cynips lignicola. Q. robur* contains friedelin, 3α-friedelanol, quercetin, leuco-anthocyanidins, and leucopelargonidin in the heartwood.

It is introduced into India in hills of Nilgiris and Himachal Pradesh. They are used in tanning.

English oak galls

They are produced by *Adleria kollari* on *Quercus robur* and contain tannins (15-20%).

TANNIC ACID AND GALLS

Synonyms

Tannin, Gallotannin, Gallotannic acid.

Biological source

Tannic acid occurs in nutgalls of *Quercus infectoria* Oliv, bark of the oak species, in Sumac and Myrobalan. It is produced from Turkish or Chinese nutgalls, the former containing 50-60%, the latter about 70%. Galls are produced by an aphis, *Schlectendalia chinensis*, on the petioles of the leaves of *Rhus chinensis* (Fam. Anacardiaceae).

Preparation

Tannic acid is obtained by extracting powdered galls with a mixture of ether, alcohol and water. Two layers are formed; the aqueous layer contain gallotannin and the free gallic acid is present in the ethereal layer which is evaporated to get the gallic acid. Tannic acid is purified by various procedures.

Previous to extraction the galls are exposed to a moist atmosphere for some time, during which fermentative changes occur and the yield is increased.

Chemical composition

The chemistry of the tannic acid is most complex and non-uniform. Tannic acid is not a single homogenous compound but a mixture of esters of gallic acid with glucose. Chinese Galls on hydrolysis yield methyl gallate and 1, 2, 3, 4, 6-pentagalloyl glucose.

Turkish tannin, which is a mixture of hexa- or heptagalloylglucoses, hydrolyzes to form methyl gallate and a mixture of 1,2,3,6- and 1,3,4,6-tetragalloylglucose. On milder treatment, both types of tannic acid yield methyl *m*-digallate, indicating the presence of a *m*-trigalloyl group in each.

Tannic acid is yellowish white to light brown, amorphous; bulky powder or flakes, or spongy masses; faint characteristic odour, astringent taste, gradually darkens on exposure to air and light, mp 210-215°, decomposes mostly into pyrogallol and CO_2. It gives insoluble precipitates with albumin, starch, gelatin, most alkaloidal and metallic salts and produces a bluish-black colour or precipitate with ferric salts. One gram of tannic acid is dissolved in 0.35 ml water, 1 ml warm glycerol; very soluble in alcohol & acetone, practically insoluble in benzene, chloroform, ether, petroleum ether, carbon disulphide and carbon tetrachloride.

Tannic acid is a hydrolysable tannin yielding gallic acid and glucose and having the minimum complexity of pentadigalloyl glucose. Solutions of tannic acid tend to decompose on keeping with formation of gallic acid, a substance which is also found in many commercial samples of tannic acid. It may be detected by the pink colour formed on the addition of a 5% solution of potassium cyanide.

Uses

Tannic acid is astringent and styptic. It is used as haemostatic, in solution for burns, as a heavy metal antidote and for alkaloidal poisoning. It is also used as mordant in dyeing, manufacturing ink; sizing paper and silk; printing fabrics, with gelatin and albumin for manufacturing of imitation horn and tortoise shell, tanning, clarifying beer or wine, in photography, as coagulant in rubber manufacturing, for commercial preparation of gallic acid and pyrogallol and as a reagent in analytical chemistry.

Utilization of certain tannin-rich plant materials for long time may be harmful due to their carcinogenic activity. The habitual chewing of betal nut (*Areca catechu*) produces oral and esophageal cancers. The drug contains piperidine-type alkaloids like arecoline, arecaidine, guvacine and guvacoline and is also rich in condensed tannins. Utilization of ordinary tea (leaves of *Camellia sinensis*) without milk causes esophageal obstruction. Milk binds tannins of the tea and it becomes less harmful.

The property of precipitation of proteins by tannins is also utilized in the process of vegetable tanning. It converts animal hides to leather. The tannin affects the pliancy and toughness of the leather and acts as a preservative due to its antiseptic action. Different types of tannins produce a variety of leather. Certain hydrolyzable tannins form a *bloom leather* whereas the nonhydrolyzable tannins give the *tanner's red leather*. Solution of tannins are used in the laboratory as reagents for the detection of gelatin, proteins and alkaloids due to their precipitating properties.

HAMAMELIS

Hamamelis (*Witch hazel leaves*) consists of the dried leaves of *Hamamelis virginiana* (Hamamelidaceae), a shrub or small tree, 2-5 m high, which is widely distributed in Canada and the USA.

Macroscopical characters

The leaves are shortly petiolate, 7-15 cm long, broadly oval to ovate; base asymmetrically cordate, apex acute. The lamina is dark brownish-green, very papery in texture. The venation is pinnate and the margin crenate or sinuate-dentate. The veins are very conspicuous on the lower surface; they leave the mid-rib at an acute angle and non straight to the margin, where they terminate in a marginal crenation. Odour, slight; taste, astringent and bitter.

Microscopical characters

The drug has characteristic stomata present on the lower surface only; very large lignified idioblasts crystal cells accompanying the pericyclic fibres, tannin-containing cells and, in young leaves, stellate hairs. The calcium oxalate is in monoclinic prisms, 10-35 μm long.

Constituents

Hamamelis contains gallitannins, ellagitannins, free gallic acid, polygalloyl glucose, hamamelitannin, epicatechin gallate, proanthocyanidins, bitter principles and traces of volatile oil. With ferric chloride solution the gallitannins and the free gallic acid give a blue colour and the ellagitannins, green.

The leaves contain about 7.0% tannins.

Allied drugs

Hamamelis bark occurs in curved or channelled pieces; up to 10 cm long or 2 cm wide; silvery grey and smooth, or dark grey and scaly. The inner surface is pinkish and often bears fragments of whitish wood. Sections show a cortex containing prismatic crystals of calcium oxalate, a complete ring of sclerenchymatous cells, and groups of phloem fibres. The bark contains a mixture of hamamelitannin and condensed tannin; the former is a potent oxygen scavenger. Three separate hamamelitannins, α-, β- and γ-, are present. The most important, β-hamamelitannin, is formed from two gallic acid molecules and one molecule of the sugar hamamelose. A series of new galloylhamameloses has been reported.

Uses

Hamamelis has astringent, anti-inflammatory and haemostatic properties due to the presence of the tannins. These are widely applied to sprains, bruises and superficial wounds, as an ingredient of eye lotions, for phlebitis, piles, skin diseases, diarrhoea, and inflammation of the gums and mucous membranes of the mouth. It contains safrole and other volatile components.

RHATANY

Rhatany is the dried root of *Krameria triandra* (Krameriaceae), a small shrub with decumbent branches about 1 m long. The drug is collected in Bolivia and Peru and is known in commerce as Peruvian rhatany.

The root has a knotty crown and gives off numerous branch roots up to a length of 60 cm. The roots are nearly cylindrical and are covered with a reddish-brown cork, which is scaly. A reddish-brown bark occupies about one-third of the radius and encloses a yellowish, finely radiate wood. A small, deeply coloured heartwood is present in the larger species. The bark is astringent and readily separates from the wood.

The tannins (10-15%) of krameria root (krameria-tannic acid) are condensed (proanthocyanidin) type having a 'polymeric' flavin-3-ol structure. A phlobaphene (krameria-red), starch and calcium oxalate are also present. Two benzofuran derivatives, ratanhiaphenols I and II, are separated from the root. Both compounds are effective UV light filters and could be useful in sun-protection preparations. The drug is used as an astringent and antimicrobial to treat mouth and throat infections, cutaneous capillary fragility, piles, gingivitis and stomatitis.

Allied species

The Peruvian drug, *Krameria cystisoides* of Mexican origin, contains over 20 compounds of the lignan, neolignan and norneolignan type. Similar constituents are reported for *K. lanceolata*.

Pomegranate rind

This consists of the dried pericarp of the fruit of *Punica granatum* (Punicaceae). It occurs in thin, curved pieces, about 1.5 mm thick. The outer surface is brownish-yellow or red. The inner surface bears impressions left by the seeds. Pomegranate rind, used in India as a herbal remedy for non-specific diarrhoea, is very astringent and contains about 28% of tannin (ellagitannins) and colouring

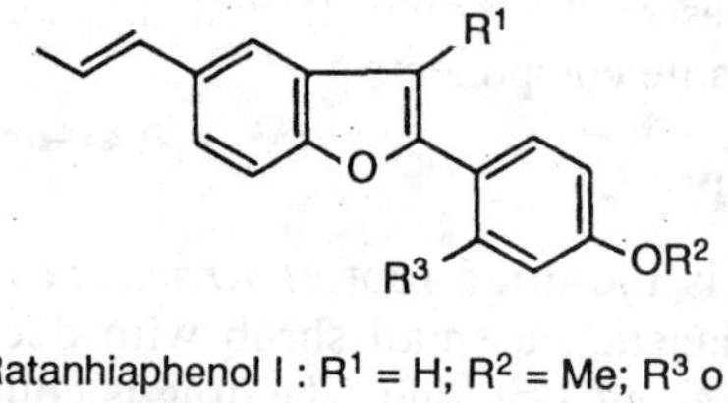

Ratanhiaphenol I : R^1 = H; R^2 = Me; R^3 o OH
Ratanhiaphenol II : R^1 = Me; R^2 = R^3 = H

Fig. 16.6. Ratanhiaphenols.

matters. It should be distinguished from the root bark, which contains alkaloids.

Aspidosperma barks

The bark of *Aspidosperma quebracho-blanco* (Apocynaceae), is used as a tanning material.

KATTHA INDUSTRY

With an annual turn over of Rupees 40 crores, a Kattha industry yields very high revenue to the forests and provides employment to thousands of workers both in the factories and forests.

Kattha is a solidified water extract of the heartwood of trees of Khair (*Acacia catechu*; family : Mimosoideae). Three distinct varieties of *A. catechu* are recognized, namely, *A. catechu* proper, var. *catechunoids* and var. *sundra.*

These trees are extensively found in Uttar Pradesh, Himachal Pradesh, Bihar, Madhya Pradesh, Gujarat and other Indian States; also in Nepal and Burma. In Uttaranchal and Gujarat it is also being grown as a plantation crop because of the high commercial value that the tree fetches.

The aqueous extract of heart wood of *A. catechu* trees gives two fractions when concentrated and cooled. A less soluble fraction separates out on cooling giving a pale product rich in *catechu*–this being called Kattha; the highly soluble fraction when evaporated to dryness gives the Cutch of commerce.

Methods of manufacture

(a) Traditional method

Considerable quantities of Kattha are manufactured by the crude method (the traditional method) in the forests.

The manufacturing season is during winter (November to March). Mature trees are felled and sometimes sawn to suitable length. The bark and sap wood is peeled off leaving behind the heart wood. The heartwood is reduced to fairly uniform chips (2 to 4 cm long and 0.5 to 1.5 cm thick). Earthen pots, which are egg shaped and which can hold about 6 to 9 kg of chips, are placed in long rows over a tunnel-like hearth (or *bhatti*) which is fired by the sap wood, bark and extracted chips. Usually 32-35 pots are handled in one furnace and the number of "bhattis" (hearths) in one establishment (known as "*Jhala*") is between 2 in very small units to as high as 50 in big establishments.

Each "bhatti" processes about 444 qunital chips per season (60 days) and there are establishments working in Uttaranchal, which processed as much 22,200 quintals of chips per season.

The chips in earthen pots are covered with water and boiled a number of times till they are nearly exhausted of the solubles. Sometimes three to five changes of water are given, the extraction being carried out for nearly three to four hours. The extract after straining through muslim cloth is concentrated in earthen pots to a particular consistency and then set aside for natural cooling for several days, when the less soluble portion separates out. Both the consistency and colour of the liquor changes and the liquor turns into a semi-solid mass. The mass, which contains Kattha and cutch, is then processed in a very crude way to separate the less soluble fraction that is Kattha. One practice is to transfer the mass to baskets strewn with ash while the other method is to transfer it to rectangular pits with bed of sand and clay covered with jute hessian or muslin. The idea is to remove the soluble cutch portion. The mass is left undisturbed for several days during which time the cutch portion oozes out or is absorbed by the ash or the clay, leaving behind the solid mass of Kattha in the basket or the pit. This mass is now scooped out by hand and made into blocks (30 cm × 30 cm × 22.5 cm). These blocks are set aside for drying in the shade. As they lose moisture, they are reduced in size systematically by cutting to evolve the tablets. This process is carried out over a period of days. The final tablets still contain between 20 to 25% moisture and have to be further dried for 20 to 30 days depending on the humidity in the atmosphere.

The yield of the final product which is called as "Bhatti Kattha", "Crude Kattha", and "Desi Kattha" is 6 to 7% of the heart wood processed and depends to a great extent on the quality of wood and the experience of the "Jhala" staff.

From technical and economic point of view there are various drawbacks in this method; however, each "Jhala" is a very well knitted organization sometimes managing as many as thousand labourers. The Jhala gives employment to a large number of workers, generally forest tribe who work as family.

In certain States as in Maharashtra, it gives employment to certain agricultural labour from coastal belt who are otherwise idle during these months. They leave their village soon after Diwali festival (November/December) and return to their village for Holi (March/April).

The traditional method is not at all sound since the total recovery is hardly 50% of what could be achieved under controlled conditions of factory working. Naturally this is a waste of the precious raw material.

The Kattha obtained by this method contains besides catechin the other soluble components of Khair wood together with wood fragments, sand, dust and other accidental impurities. Sometimes there is intentional adulteration with agents like soap, stone powder and clay.

Attempts to refine this crude Kattha have not always been successful because of the cost involved in refining and, hence, all this crude Kattha directly goes to the consumer.

(b) Factory method

Indian Wood Products Limited, Izatnagar (UP) was the first Kattha factory which started functioning in 1920. In the factory method, mechanical appliances are used in converting wood into chips. The extraction of the chips is done in a scientific way in extractors using steam as heating medium ensuring better extraction efficiency. The extract so obtained is concentrated in evaporators working under vacuum. The concentrated liquor is then cooled to desired temperature by the use of refrigeration. The cooled liquor which contain the crystallized or separated kattha is filtered or centrifuged to remove the soluble portion. The cakes obtained on the centrifuge or filter are pressed in hand or hydraulic presses and then cut in improvised gadgets to get the tablets of suitable size. These tablets are then dried in controlled atmosphere over a period of days to get the final product for the market. The highly soluble portion, that is the mother liquor, is concentrated in evaporators so that on cooling it solidifies to give the cutch. All the "Unit Operations" in this process are exactly the same as those in the traditional method except that each unit operation is mechanical as far as possible and performed in a scientific way.

(c) Unit operations in manufacture of kattha

The process of manufacture of Kattha and Cutch consists of a series of "Unit Operations". Due to high soaring prices of Khair wood, the efficiency of each operation has to be maintained and this could be achieved only by scientific means and experienced hands.

(i) *Debarking-desapping* : The bark and the sap wood from the logs is removed by manual labour working with the axe. No high technique is required for this operation and a man who can use an axe can peel the wood. Certain tribes can do this job much more efficiently than the others.

The recovery of the heartwood from the khair trees depends on various factors. The important ones being the birth of the tree and the quality of the tree. The tree which grows in the dry lands have very thin bark and sap wood, while the trees near the river beds have thick bark and sap wood.

The overall yield of the heartwood is of the order of 60% on weight of the Khair wood. Machines are used in well advanced countries for debarking lumber, but they are very expensive.

(ii) *Chipping* : The heartwood after cutting into logs of suitable size is converted into chips in powerful chippers. A number of designs of chippers are available and the one which gives chips of uniform size and thickness is preferable. In some factories the chips are further reduced by passing them through the disintegrator. But generally they are worked as such preferably after screening, the oversize being further reduced in disintegrators.

The size and shape of the chips depend on the individual working of the factory. Pulverized chips do not burn efficiency in Lancashire boilers unless they are provided with special furnaces for burning the chips.

The size is not as critical as the thickness for efficient extraction. Very fine chips or saw dust do not give good extraction efficiency. Probably it tends to form solid mass in the extractors, thus not allowing proper penetration of water through the mass.

Very fine chips do not give good final product due to two reasons, firstly due to oxidative changes that set up as more surface is exposed to atmosphere during handling and secondly fine dust finds its way in the leach and is difficult to remove and consequently it increases the non-soluble solids in kattha.

(iii) *Extraction* : The equilibrium aspect and the rate aspect of extraction have to be considered. The available extractive present in the wood can be economically obtained with a fast speed.

In the simple multiple extraction, which is necessarily of batch type, the chips are boiled in water until no more of the extractives present in the chips are transferred to water, *i.e.*, an equilibrium between the soluble solids present in the chips and extracted by water is reached. When this stage is reached the water extract is drained off. To recover the soluble solids still present in the chips fresh water is added to the charge and the boiling continued till the degree of extractive reaches maximum, the extract is drained off again. This process is repeated many times. Theoretically, at no stage the chips will be completely exhausted of its solubles, but the process is discontinued when the cost of concentrating the liquor is more than the additional revenue expected from extractive. Hence, proper balance has to be struck on the equilibrium stage.

With water thrice the weight of the chips, the first equilibrium is reached when the specific gravity of the liquor reaches about 1.014 (2.8° Tw). After this the specific gravity of extract nearly touches one, but still the leaches are coloured.

In the counter current extraction, the fresh water contacts the poorest chips and the outgoing liquor contacts the fresh chips. The important feature of this process is that fresh water reduces the soluble solids in the chips to the minimum while the outgoing liquor reaches a very high concentration, thus the final liquor obtained is of low volume depending on the ratio of chips to water and further processing of the liquor is eased.

Most of the factories follow the counter current extraction method, five stages, using a battery of three extractors. Research work has also been carried out for extraction of kattha by solvents like alcohol. But its commercialization has not been feasible due to high cost of the solvent involved.

Some factories use copper or bronze low pressure autoclaves for extraction. Most of the factories use open wooden vats and the boiling is done at atmospheric pressure; this is achieved either by live steam or indirectly by the use of suitable heating coils (copper).

The efficiency of extraction by autoclaves (2 to 5 lbs. sq. inch pressure) is slightly higher to atmospheric boiling. Though in the autoclaves the equilibrium is reached much early and extraction period is shortened, but as it extracts certain linings, the quality of kattha obtained with the autoclaves is slightly different to that obtained in the open vats. The high temperature in the autoclaves seems to have a deleterious effect on the Kattha.

Their is a consideration for the solubility of the various components present in the chips—catechins, tannins, sugary matter, pentosans and mineral matter. The solubility of catechins is much lower to that of tannins. In fact catechin is sparingly soluble in cold water; water is the specific solvent.

(iv) *Evaporation* : The density of the extract from the extractors depends on the running conditions, but usually the liquor contains an average of 4 to 6.5% total solids. This liquor has to be concentrated to a liquor containing between 16 to 25% total solids—the degree to which the liquor is concentrated is a variable and individual factories determine the optimum degree most beneficial for their process. The best equipment for evaporation should be the one which minimizes any chemical change in the liquor due to heat and other factors.

Some evaporators work with single or multiple effect standard. Basket type evaporators work under vacuum, while some work with climbing and falling film, the long tube evaporators working at atmospheric pressures. The quality of kattha from liquor concentrated under vacuum is, better to the one obtained in the long tube evaporators. The evaporators should be made of copper since the liquors are very susceptible to iron or its alloys.

(v) *Crystallization* : The concentrated liquor from the evaporators containing 16 to 25% solids is cooled to requisite crystallisation temperature which varies between 4.5 to 15.5°C. The cooling is affected in stages which are carefully controlled and every factory has its own technique of cooling. Generally in the first stage, cooling is done by means of cold water while in the second stage cooling is done by refrigerated brine. After the liquor is cooled to requisite temperature, it is stored in cold rooms for conditioning wherein sufficient time is allowed for the kattha to solidify or crystallize out.

During the cooling stage the liquor goes on changing its colour and viscosity, as the kattha starts separating out. In the cold room it becomes semi-solid mass which has to be scooped out from the tanks.

Crystallization is a technique and the recovery of kattha and the quality of recovered kattha depends on the factors involved in crystallization such as the percentage of total solids in the mother liquor, the gradient of cooling and the time allowed for conditioning of the crystals, besides the quality of the wood itself. Good recovery and best qualities are obtained when the crystallization is affected slowly allowing the crystals to grow as big as possible. Bigger crystals allow better removal of the tannin portion during the subsequent stage. The ratio of kattha to total solids present in wood has an important bearing on crystallization; kattha crystallizes out with difficulty where the ratio is high.

(vi) *Filtration* : The most used process of filtration is the plate and frame type. The crystallized liquor is pumped through the filters to drain the cutch portion. With well crystallized liquors filtration is much easy and not much technique is required, while with badly crystallized liquors filtration becomes a problem and rate of pumping the liquor to filters has to be carefully controlled.

The filter cake is the wet kattha while the filtrate is cutch liquor.

(vii) *Pressing of kattha* : The cake is taken on filter cloth and properly wrapped into a plate. A number of such plates are heaped on the platform of a hydraulic press and sufficient pressure is given so that the cutch portion accompanying the cake is oozed out and kattha having 30 to 35% moisture is obtained. The pressed liquor is allowed to drain into the filtrate.

(viii) *Cutting of the cake* : The cake obtained from the presses is cut into suitable sizes on cutting machines much the same way the soap is cut into cakes.

(ix) *Drying* : Kattha is very sensitive to both heat and air. Heat redissolves the kattha crystals and softens the tablets. The air sets oxidative changes deleterious to the external appearance of kattha and makes them blackish-brown. The oldest method was atmospheric drying, and it is still followed in some factories. This is a very lengthy process and during the rainy season it becomes problematic as the conditions are favourable for the fungus growth on the tablets. The modern method followed by many of the factories is low temperature drying in dehumidified atmosphere. The dehumidification is done by refrigeration. Though this method of drying is quite costly, the quality of kattha obtained is superior and the process pays itself.

(x) *Sorting and packing* : The dried kattha tablets are taken out from racks and graded based on external appearance and other factors which decide the quality of kattha. The graded tablets are then packed in wooden cases (generally 20 kg in a case).

Each factory has its own standards for grading and there is no uniformity. Initially the gradation was marked as A-1, A, B, C, D, etc. or 1, 2, 3, 4 (the best quality being either A-1 or 1). Later on the grades are marked differently as, for example, GS, CR, CR-R and MR. The Indian Standard Institute recognizes two grades of kattha based on ISI specifications, *i.e.*, Grade I and Grade II. But so far none of the factories have adopted these specifications.

(xi) *Processing of filtrate* : The filtrate from filter presses is processed for Cutch. It contains between 15 to 20% total solids and is concentrated to 85 to 90% solids to give the Cutch of commerce. The concentration is done in evaporators. Any evaporators could be used but test product is obtained in climbing and falling film type evaporators known as Finishers.

To manufacture certain grades of cutch sometimes the liquor is processed in open kettles, directly fired on steam heated, but only a part of the production is processed thus.

Solidified cutch is either packed in wooden cases (50 kg each) or in hessian bags (40 kg each). Many a times it is packed in various other forms and shapes. It is also marketed in pulverized form.

Quality and standards

The trade recognizes kattha by their own standards, these standards are mostly empirical and not at all scientific.

The two criteria which are recognized as determining the value of kattha are colour and freedom from impurities. The more the white. more it is valued and commands a higher price. Pale coloured kattha is more expensive than the dark coloured kattha produced in certain States. Kattha when wet is liable to oxidative changes and during the process of drying changes its appearance. Unless the drying is controlled, this external appearance is one of the recognized specifications of the trade and consumer.

Internal appearance

The appearance of the good grade kattha tablet when broken open in two halves known as "Tod" in the trade should be pale-yellow with smooth uniform surface. Poor qualities of kattha show ununiform surface on breaking and the surface is blackish-white to brown in colour. Indigenous kattha shows alternate layers of pale and dark brown.

Unfortunately, the colour standards are far from standardized and, hence, in the trade the external appearance and the "Tod" are generally compared with the contracted sample, in case of any disputes arising in the supplies.

The water absorption power of kattha

This is the property much valued in the trade. Kattha after coarse powdering is boiled with 4-5 times its weight of water and after the kattha has dissolved, it is allowed to cool down for at least 6-8 hours or sometimes overnight. On cooling, the solution turns into a thick paste. This paste is taken on a muslim cloth kept on a heap of wood ash when the tannin portion drains out into the ash, leaving behind a semisolid paste. In the laboratory the paste could be filtered on a Buchner funnel till the mass is of a particular consistency. The wt. of this mass which contains varying amount of moisture is determined.

The solid mass is known as "Londi". Very good quality of kattha gives as high as three times its weight of "Londi" while poor grade of kattha gives its own weight or sometimes even less.

The taste

It is a general practice in trade to taste kattha, for bitterness, astringency, besides the feel in the mouth which it gives when macerated with saliva. Good quality kattha gives a bitter taste which is not very sharp, besides it is smooth in the mouth. While inferior katha gives a taste which is bitter and not so astringent. Like tea tasters and wine tasters, there are persons in this trade who are very accurate in their assessment of kattha quality.

ISI standards

The Indian Standards Institution after extensive collaborative work, carried out on a large number of samples in different laboratories, have formulated the specifications for Kattha. The methods for testing have been given in IS : 2962-1964 and standards in IS : 4359-1967. Two grades of kattha have been recognized based on the following values :

	Grade I	Grade II
Loss on drying	15	15
Catechin content (% weight)	55	40
Extractives in cold water (% wt. on dry basis)	45	60
Matter insoluble in rectified spirit	25	25
Insolubles in boiling water (% wt., maximum)	3	6
Total ash (% wt.)	1.5	4

Kattha is generally adulterated or contaminated unavoidably with sand, dust, ashes, fillers like China clay, soap stone powder and starch. This free use of the adulterants is a serious menace to the trade and to the health of the community.

Indian Pharmacopoeia standards for Black Catechu (Synonym Kattha)

Indian Pharmacopoeia gives specifications for Black Catechu prepared from the heartwood of *Acacia catechu*. Willd and *Acacia chundra* Willd.

1. Water insoluble residue — Not more than 25%
2. Alcohol insoluble residue — Not more than 30%
3. Loss on drying residue — Not more than 12%
4. Ash — Maximum 6%

A 10% w/v filtered solution give a dark green colour with 5% w/v solution of ferric chloride; on making slightly alkaline with solution of sodium hydroxide, the colour should change to purple.

In prevention of Food Adulteration Act the Standards laid down for Catechu are as follows :

1. 5% ml of 1 aqueous solution, and 0.1% solution of ferric ammonium sulphate shall give a dark green colour, which on the addition of sodium hydroxide solution shall change to purple.
2. When dried to constant weight at 100°C, it shall not lose more than 12% of its weight.
3. Water insoluble residue (dried at 100°C) shall not be more than 25% by weight (water insoluble matter shall be determined by boiling water).
4. Alcohol insolubles residue in 90% alcohol dried at 100°C—not more than 30% by weight.
5. Total ash on dry basis—not more than 8% by weight.
6. Ash insoluble in HCl—not more than 0.5% on dry weight basis.

Uses

Kattha possesses cooling and digestive properties and is used in relaxed condition of throat, mouth and gums and in cough and diarrhoea. Externally as an astringent medicament it is applied to ulcers, boils and skin eruptions. Kattha includes all varieties of solidified extract of Khair wood, whether refined or crude. However, the market recognizes two distinct qualities *White Kattha* or catechu and the *Dark Kattha* or cutch. Kattha contains large portion of catechu while cutch consists of non-crystalline tannins. Kattha is commonly sold in the market in the form of small blocks or tablets. Its major use is as an ingredient in *Paan* (betal leaf). It is generally pained to Paan after making a thin paste of Kattha in water. It is also an ingredient of *Pan Masala*.

Cutch is available in various forms—there are at least a dozen marketed varieties of Cutch varying in shape and form. For some markets it is wrapped in *Tad* (*Borassus flabellifer*) leaves while for some others in *Sal* (*Shorea robusta*) but for industrial use it is packed in 40 or 50 kilo blocks or bags, either solid or in powder form.

Cutch is used as a cheap substitute for Kattha; its consumption being more in the rural population and in undeveloped villages and tribes. Industrial uses for cutch are wide and varied. It is used for dyeing and colouring. It produces browns and olives with different mordants and imparts excellent fastness and resistance to mildew attack. It is applied as a protective agent to fishing nets and sails which are constantly exposed to water. It is used for colouring certain varieties of chewing tobacco. Though it contains above 55% tannin, it is not a very useful tanning agent as it produces harsh leather and causes discolouration. As a tannin it is used in water softening, but by far its greatest industrial use is for reducing the viscosity of drill mud. Other uses are for ore floatation and in the removal of mercaptans from gasoline and manufacture of iron exchange resins.

Chemistry of kattha and cutch

Kattha does not consist of a single substance. It has been separated by extraction with various solvents into fractions with different physical and chemical properties. The principal fraction in Kattha has been identified as mixtures of catechin isomers.

Acacia catechu contains (–)-epicatechin which is a diastereo isomer of 5,7, 3',4', tetrahydroxy flavan-3-ols. It is a white crystalline substance and is obtained by cold acetone extraction of the shavings of the chips of the heart wood. Epicatechin is the *trans* form of acatechin, it is readily soluble in cold ether and acetone. During the extraction of heart wood chips with boiling water, epicatechin undergoes epimerization and racemization to *dl*-acacatechin ($C_{15}H_{14}O_6.3H_2O$). Isomers of *dl*-acacatechin present in Kattha are *l*-acacatechin (mp 230) and *d*-iso-acacatechin (m.p., 226 to 228°).

Acacatechin is insoluble in cold water but soluble in hot water. It undergoes oxidation to catechutannic acid in the presence of water.

Naturally occurring catechins are converted into high molecular weight products as water soluble non-crystalline condensed tannins. Catechins are thus the building units for the formation of condensed tannins.

Cutch

The chemistry of Cutch is little known. It consists of highly complex mixture of polyphenolic compounds known as tannins. They are complex polyhydric phenols having a molecular size and degree of hydroxylation which permits suitable solubility in water. They precipitate gelatin and alkaloids from solutions, are astringent, give colour reaction with iron salts, form precipitate with many metallic ions and are rather unstable in the presence of moisture and light. Tannins are easily oxidized in alkaline solutions. They are soluble in alcohol, acetone, dioxane and ethyl acetate provided the solvent contains at least small amounts of water. For the most part they are insoluble in ether, benzene and similar solvents. They are amorphous, non-crystalline materials. Tannins in general act on skin to form leather. Tannins acting as negatively charged colloid neutralize the positively charged proteins in the skin (when in acidic medium) whereby coprecipitation or combination of tannins with proteins occurs. Other complex processes also take place during tanning.

The kattha trade

The scattered nature of the kattha manufacture in small units in remotest places in the forests has led to a rather complex system of dealers, stockists, brokers, merchants who handle the trade of indigenous kattha. Most of the factories have their selling agents who have their own well developed marketing organizations having contact with consuming centres.

Kattha trade is subject to keen competition and speculative activity. Because of the diverse interests represented, there is very little organization in the trade. Though there are three associations (Delhi Kattha Dealers Association, Delhi; Bhartiya Kattha Vyavasaik Seva Sangh, Kanpur (UP) and Kattha Manufacturers' Association, Najibabad], but there being no coordination and cooperation between the various interests there was no follow up for good of the industry. It is only of late that Kattha Manufacturers' Association has taken up with respective authorities some of the problems.

Kattha is almost entirely consumed in the country and very little of it is exported. The consumption of kattha is entirely for Paan chewing, a very small fraction of the production finding its use in Ayurvedic and Unani medicines. The States of Bihar, West Bengal, Orissa, Uttar Pradesh, Gujarat and Northern Maharashtra are the major consumers. Though Paan chewing is common in other States also like Karnataka, Tamil Nadu, Andhra Pradesh, Kerala, it is generally without the addition of kattha and hence very little kattha finds its way to the Southern States.

Fats, Oils and Waxes

Fixed oils and fats are neutral substances and esters of glycerol with higher long-chain fatty acids such as palmitic, stearic, oleic and linoleic acids. Fats are solid or semi-solid at 15.5-16.5°C while oils occur as liquid at this temperature. These compounds are obtained from plants (Arachis oil, Castor oil) or animals (Lard, Cod liver oil). There is no chemical difference in fats and oils. The fatty acids may be saturated (*e.g.*, palmitic acid, stearic acid) or unsaturated (*e.g.*, oleic acid), but usually they contain unbranched carbon chains and have an even number of carbon atoms.

Most of the saturated glycerides are solid at ordinary temperature, but most unsaturated glycerides are viscous liquids. Therefore, vegetable oils contain larger proportions of unsaturated glycerides than the solid animal fats. The identity, quality and purity of fatty substances are determined by finding out their acid value, saponification value, Reichert-Meissl number, iodine number, melting point, specific gravity and refractive index.

If the fatty acid present in a glyceryl ester is the same, then it is known as 'simple' glyceride. For example, tripalmitin, tristearin, and triolein are simple glycerides. If different fatty acids are present in a glyceride, then it is called as mixed glyceride, *e.g.*, 2-oleodipalmitin and 1-oleo-2-palmitostearin. In mixed glycerides two or sometimes three different acid groupings are present. Animal fats, such as Lard and Suet, and 'fixed' or fatty vegetable oils, such as Olive oil, Almond oil, and Theobroma oil, are mixtures of glycerides. On hydrolysis they yield

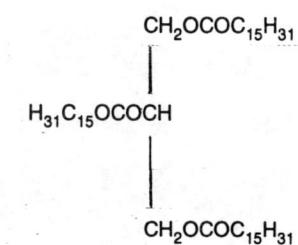

Fig. 17.1. A simple lipid or triacylglycerol (tripalmitin).

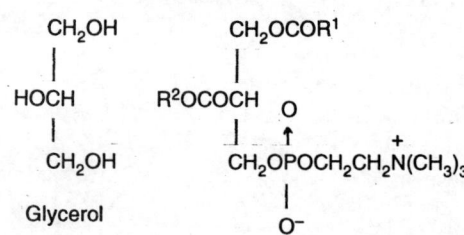

Fig. 17.2. A complex lipid (a 1,2-diacyl-*sn*-glycero-3-phosphorylcholine).

both saturated and unsaturated fatty acids. In addition to glycerides, the oils and fats contain other substances like phosphatides, phytosterols, hydrocarbons, fat-soluble vitamins A, D and E, some volatile substances and glycolipids. They play a fundamental role in living organisms.

Seeds are the principal source of fats and oils. The oil containing seeds are Sesame seed, Coconut, Arachis and Castor. The compounds are also present in Olive fruits, Cod liver and Shark. The fats and oils are important products used as pharmaceutically, industrially and as articles of food. They are constituents of cell membrane phospho- and glycolipids, coating elements (waxes or cutins), reserve substances and energy sources for the cell.

Fixed oils and fats are separated from plant parts by hot or cold expression in hydraulic press or by extraction with an organic solvent. Animal fats are isolated by heating the animal tissues with steam. The fat melts which floats on the top and is separated by decantation.

Fats and oils have certain common characteristics. They are hydrophobic or amphophilic, greasy substances and are lighter than water. They are insoluble in water, sparingly soluble in alcohol, and freely soluble in solvent like petroleum ether, chloroform and benzene. Their specific gravity is always less than water and, therefore, they float on the aqueous surface. When a drop of fats or oils is placed on a paper, they form a permanent translucent stain on it. Due to this property they are called as fixed oils. They cannot be distilled and on heating they are decomposed producing an odour of scorched fat due to formation of acraldehyde (CH_2=CH-CHO). Many fats and oils become rancid on long exposure to air, give acidic reactions and develop very disagreeable odour. In moist conditions the hydrolysis of fats is affected with lipase enzyme and free fatty acids are formed. In the presence of light and microorganisms keto-, keto acid-, oxide- and peroxide-derivatives of fatty acids are produced and all these substances are responsible for rancidity of fats.

The oil obtained by expression contains water, mucilaginous matter and ground seed tissues in suspension. It may also has a strong odour and a dark colour. The presence of a very small proportion of fatty acid affects the taste and flavour of oils. The oils are purified and refined by removing free fatty acids, decolourization, deodourization and demargination. Free fatty acids are removed by adding sodium hydroxide solution and the resulting sodium salts are separated by suitable means. For decolourizing, the oil is heated to about 200°C for about 30 minutes with 2-4% fuller's earth or diatomaceous earth and 0.2-1.0% of animal charcoal, followed by filtration. For deodourization, the oil is placed in an autoclave, vacuum is created in the apparatus and then superheated for a very short time to remove aldehydes and ketones responsible for unpleasant odour. In demargination process, the solid glycerides are removed at room temperature. Cod-liver oil is to be demarginated and this is accomplished by cooling it to about 0°C; at which temperature a portion solidifies and is separated by filtration, the filtrate constituting non-freezing Cod Liver oil.

Wax present in sunflower, corn and cotton oils is removed by cooling (winterization) and then filtering the crystallized wax. *Degumming* (mucilage removal) is done to eliminate lacithins, proteins and other constituents present in the colloidal suspension. The hot oil is hydrated, whereupon the colloids forms a dense gel which separates from the lighter oil.

Catalytic reduction of unsaturated fatty acids in the presence of hydrogen and a catalyst (*e.g.*, Raney Nickel or Pd-C) yields saturated compounds which are solid at normal temperature. Vegetable ghee is prepared by hydrogenation of the fixed oils.

A thin layer of Linseed oil is dried and forms a hard transparent film. This oil is, therefore, called as drying oil and used in paints and varnishes. Cottonseed oil resinifies and dries without forming a thin film. Such oils are called semi-drying oils. Some oils, like Olive oil, neither dry nor form a thin layer. Such oils are called as non-drying oils.

Sulfated or sulfonated oils are obtained by reacting sulfuric acid with the oil at low temperature. The oil is then washed and neutralized. If the oil contains an olefinic linkage, the acid molecule adds onto the double bond. The compound formed is a sulfate of the fat. These materials have surfactant properties that find industrial application.

Fixed oils and fats are used in pharmaceuticals for their emollient properties. They serve, either in their natural form or in emulsions, as vehicles for other medicaments regimens.

Sodium morrhuate, the sodium salts of fatty acids obtained from cod liver oil, is used as a sclerosing agent to obliterate varicose veins. Other fatty acids are used as topical antifungal agents, dietary supplements and agents of pharmaceutic requirement.

The oil-soluble vitamins are lipids by nature. Fats and oils are used in the manufacture of soaps (sodium and potassium salts of the fatty acids), as drying oils in the manufacture of paints and varnishes, and as lubricants. Lipids also form an important class of foods. They have high caloric value and low osmotic pressure. Some plant oils are used as parenteral nutrients in hyperalimentation regimens.

Fatty acids are used to treat skin lesions (lino-lenic and linoleic acids), wounds, burns, sunburns, eczema and dandruff; as emollient, laxative (Castor oil), in the preparation of ointments, liniments and suppositories, as a source of vitamins A, D and E; as cholesterol suppressant, antifungal agent, and in the manufacture of soaps, glycerine, paints, varnishes and lubricants. Chaulmoogra oil is utilized to cure leprosy.

Fats are required nutrients and they must constitute 30-35% of the daily caloric intake in a normal diet. Some polyunsaturated fatty acids are called essential fatty acids (EFA), since they are not synthesized by the human body in sufficient amounts. They are constituents of the phospho-lipids of cell membrane and they may contribute to ensuring their fluidity. They are precursors of prostaglandins, leukotriens and thromboxanes (eicosanoids) which act as cellular mediators and as agents in platelet aggregation or in the inflam-matory process. The EFA are biosynthesized from arachidonic acid which normally arises from the desaturation of linoleic acid to linolenic acid in the presence of Δ^6-desaturase, followed by chain elongation and by a new desaturation yielding arachidonic acid. This acid is converted to eicosanoids due to action of cyclo-oxygenase and lipoxygenase. Linoleic acid provides 6-8% of the caloric ration. Deficiency of linoleic acid causes dermatitis, *e.g.*, eczema, impetigo and erythema; delayed growth, hypertension and poor platelet aggregation.

The activity of Δ^6-desaturase is mainly decreased by stress, ageing, alcoholism, nicotine addiction, hepatic insufficiency and diabetes mellitus. The polyunsaturated fatty acids are present in eggs and livers.

Saturated fatty acids detected in oils and fats

Butyric	$CH_3 (CH_2)_2 COOH$
Isovaleric	$(CH_3)_2 CHCH_2 COOH$
Caproic	$CH_3 (CH_2)_4 COOH$
Caprylic	$CH_3 (CH_2)_6 COOH$
Capric	$CH_3 (CH_2)_8 COOH$
Lauric	$CH_3 (CH_2)_{10} COOH$
- Myristic	$CH_3 (CH_2)_{12} COOH$
Palmitic	$CH_3 (CH_2)_{14} COOH$
Stearic	$CH_3 (CH_2)_{16} COOH$
Arachidic	$CH_3 (CH_2)_{18} COOH$
Behenic	$CH_3 (CH_2)_{20} COOH$
Lignoceric	$CH_3 (CH_2)_{22} COOH$

Unsaturated fatty acids detected in oils and fats

Palmitoleic	$CH_3 (CH_3)_5 CH=CH (CH_2)_7 COOH$
Oleic	$CH_3 (CH_2)_7 CH=CH (CH_2)_7 COOH$
Ricinoleic	$CH_3 (CH_2)_5 CHOH\text{-}CH_2 CH=CH (CH_2)_7 COOH$
Linoleic	$CH_3 (CH_2)_4 CH=CHCH_2 CH=CH (CH_2)_7 COOH$
Linolenic	$CH_3 CH_2 CH=CHCH_2 CH=CHCH_2 CH=CH\text{-}(CH_2)_7 COOH$
Eleostearic	$CH_3 (CH_2)_3 (CH=CH)_3 (CH_2)_7 COOH$
Licanic	$CH_3 (CH_2)_3 (CH=CH)_3 (CH_2)_4 CO(CH_2)_2 COOH$
Parinaric	$CH_3 CH_2 (CH=CH)_4 (CH_2)_7 COOH$
Tariric	$CH_3 (CH_2)_7 C \equiv C (CH_2)_7 COOH$
Gadoleic	$CH_3 (CH_2)_9 - CH=CH (CH_2)_7 COOH$
Arachidonic	$CH_3 (CH_2)_4 (CH=CHCH_2)_4 (CH_2)_2 COOH$
Cetoleic	$CH_3 (CH_2)_9 CH=CH (CH_2)_9 COOH$
Erucic	$CH_3 (CH_2)_7 CH=CH (CH_2)_{11} COOH$
Selacholeic or nervonic	$CH_3 (CH_2)_7 CH=CH (CH_2)_{13} COOH$

Fatty acids with less than 12 carbon atoms are less abundant in plants. Glycerides of caproic acid and caprylic acids are present in palm. Lauric acid glyceride occurs in bay butter and Nutmeg butter. Palmitic acid is the major saturated constituent of vegetable oils.

BIOSYNTHESIS OF LIPIDS

Biosynthesis of fats are triglycerides involving long-chain saturated or unsaturated acids and constitute an important food reserve for animals and plants (in seeds). Related to the simple fats are the complete lipids, most of which are diesters of orthophosphoric acid; they have the status of fundamental cellular constituents.

The fatty acids, on liberation from the fat, are available for the production of acetyl-CoA by the removal of C_2 units. In this β-oxidation sequence one turn of the spiral involves four reactions—two dehydrogenations, one hydration and a thiolysis liberating a two carbon unit of acetyl-CoA. All these reactions are reversible. The biosynthetic route of fatty acids operates in the reverse direction, starting from acetyl-CoA.

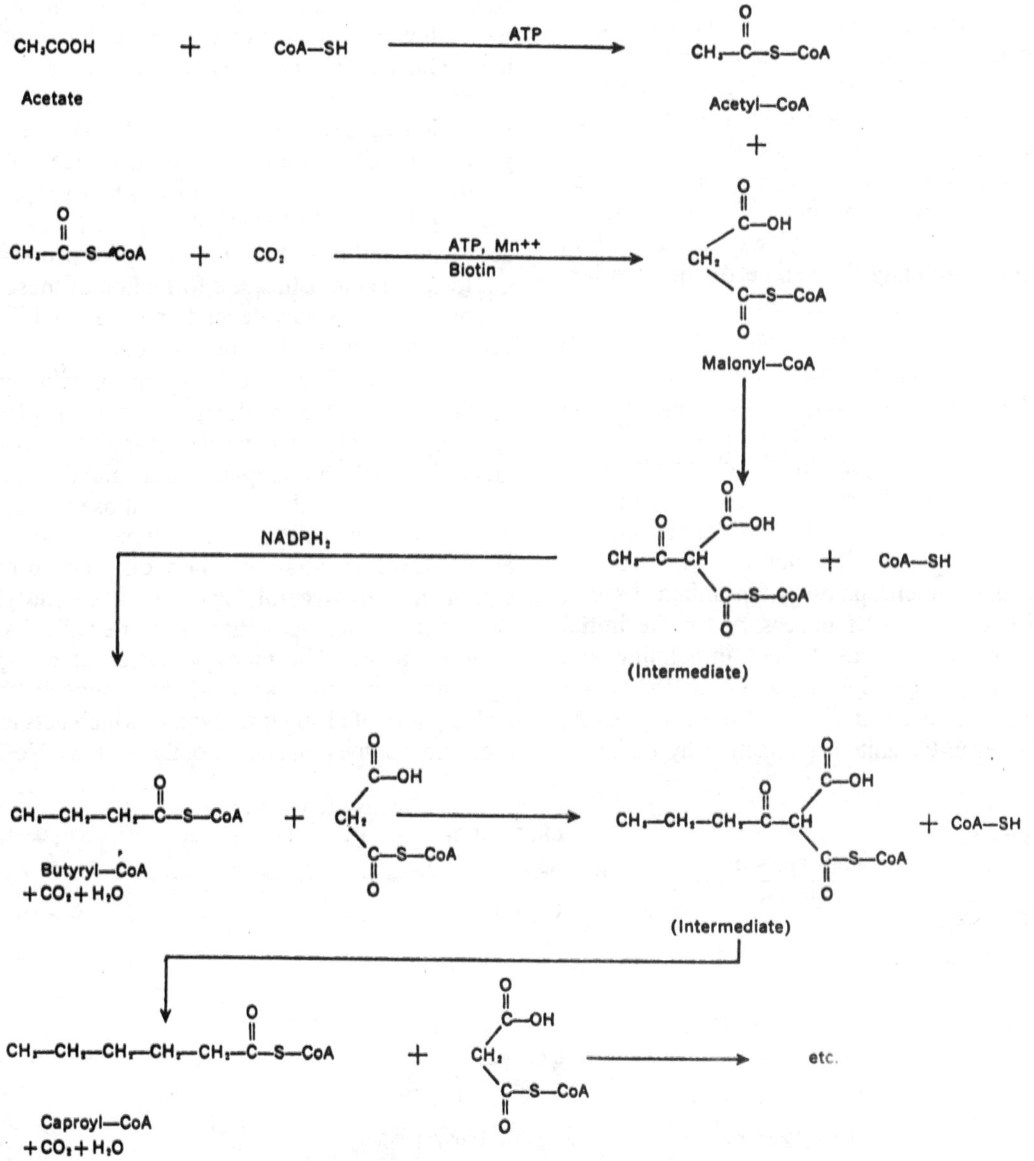

Fig. 17.3. Biosynthesis of fatty acids.

Biosynthesis of saturated fatty acids

The biosynthesis of the fatty acid moieties is carried out by a series of reactions involving 2 enzyme complexes plus ATP, $NADPH_2$, Mn^- and carbon dioxide.

Acetate first reacts with CoA, and the acetyl-CoA thus formed is converted by reaction with carbon dioxide to malonyl-CoA. This, in turn, reacts with an additional molecule of acetyl-CoA to form a 5-carbon intermediate, which undergoes reduction and elimination of carbon dioxide to produce butyryl-CoA. Malonyl-CoA again reacts with this compound to form a 7-carbon intermediate, which is reduced to caporyl-CoA. Repetition of the reaction results in a fatty acid containing an even number of carbon atoms in its chain. Thus, the malonyl portion of malonyl-CoA, a 3-carbon compound, is actually the source of the 2-carbon biosynthetic units of the fatty acids.

The biosynthetic route for fatty acids operates in the reverse direction to the β-oxidative sequence for the degradation of these acids and started with acetyl CoA. However, the unfavourable equilibrium of the initial thiolase reaction in such a pathway.

The poor yield of long-chain fatty acids obtained with purified enzymes of the β-oxidation pathway suggested the possibility that this was not the principal biosynthetic pathway. In animal tissues, malonyl coenzyme A is necessary for the initial condensation with acetate. In fact, in palmitic acid (C_{16}) only one of the eight C_2 units (*i.e.* the C15 + C16 carbons) is derived directly from acetyl-CoA; the other seven C_2 units are attached by malonyl-CoA, which is formed by carboxylation of acetyl-CoA.

The involvement of the acyl carried protein (ACP) takes place to produce fatty acyl thioesters of ACP. This conversion serves (1) to activate the relatively unreactive fatty acid and (2) to provide a carrier for the fatty acid acyl group. Thus, these ACP thioesters are the obligatory intermediates in fatty acid synthesis, whereas it is fatty acid thioesters of coenzyme A which operate in the catabolic oxidation pathway. Reactions are repeated for lengthening the fatty acid chain by two carbons (derived from malonyl-S-ACP) at a time. Each enzymes have been identified as being involved in the synthesis of palmitoyl-ACP and stearoyl-ACP from acetyl-CoA.

In purified enzyme systems, when propionyl-CoA replaced acetyl-CoA, the product was a C_{17} acid and, similarly, butyryl-CoA gave primarily a C_{18} (steatic) acid. Thus, the formation of these C_{16}, C_{17} and C_{18} acids may depend on the availability of acetyl-, propionyl- and butyryl-CoA.

In animals, fatty acid biosynthesis takes place in the cytosol, but in plants it occurs in plastids (chloroplasts in green tissue, proplastids in non-green tissue). In higher plants and animals, the predominant fatty acid residues are those of the C_{16} and C_{18} species, palmitic oleic, linoleic, and stearic acids. However, there are many different forms of combination of glycerol, fatty acids, and hydrophilic compounds such as serine, choline, inositol, or various sugars. The many varieties of phospholipids and glycolipids are made from phosphatidate, a phosphorylated sugar derivative which acts as the precursor for the polar heads of these lipids. Vesicles

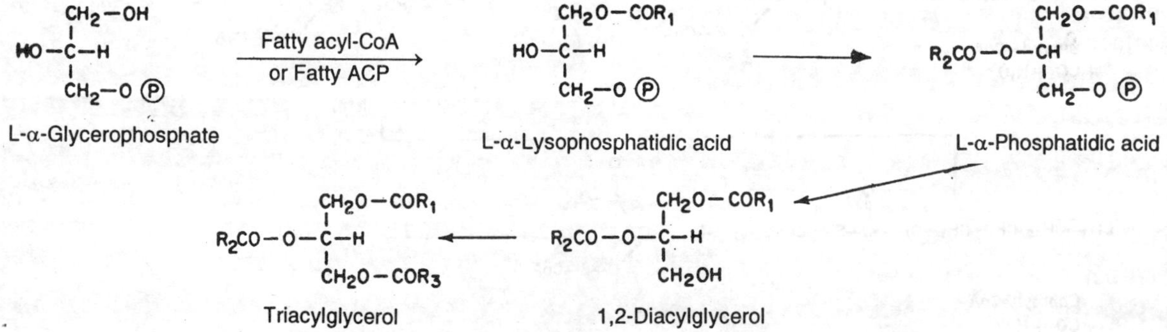

Fig. 17.4. Formation of acylglycerols.

that bud off of the ER or Golgi apparatus carry specific phospholipids to their proper location in the plasma membrane or organelles. Plants also have different metabolic pathways that produce waxes which make up the protective cuticle of epidermal cells and terpenes which are lipids synthesized from acetyl CoA via the mevalonic acid pathway.

Biosynthesis of fatty acids in plants operates in the same way as in animal tissues, but whereas in the latter the enzymes are located in the cytoplasm, in plants they are found in the mitochondria and chloroplasts. The mitochondria derived from the mesocarp of the avocardo fruit have been used to demonstrate the incorporation of [^{14}C] acetate into esterified long-chain fatty acids.

Biosynthesis of unsaturated fatty acids

The first step in the production of a mono-unsaturated acid is the formation of the acyl-CoA derivative of its saturated analog. This is followed by enzymatic desaturation. Hydroxylation appears to be independent or to follow desaturation. Apparently, hydroxylation is not involved as an intermediate step in the desaturation process. The saturated acyl group of the acyl-CoA derivative is transferred to the 2-position of phosphatidyl glycerol before the desaturation and additional reactions.

In aerobic organisms, monoenoic acids with the double bond in the 9,10-position arise by direct dehydrogenation of saturated acids. In higher plants, for this reaction, coenzyme A may be replaced by the acyl carried protein (ACP). Stearoyl-S-ACP is an effective enzyme substrate of the desaturase system of isolated plant leaf chloroplasts. The reduced forms of nicotinamide adenine dinucleotide (NADH) or nicotinamide adenine dinucleotide phosphate (NADPH) and molecular oxygen are cofactors.

$$CH_3(CH_2)_{16} Co-S-ACP + O_2 + NADPH \rightarrow$$
$$CH_3(CH_2)_7 CH=CH(CH_2)_7-Co-S-ACP + H_2O + NADP$$

The position of the vinylic bond in respect to the carboxyl group is governed by the enzyme; hence, chain length of the substrate acid is most important. The hydrogen elimination is specifically *cis* but a few unusual fatty acids such as that in the seed oil of *Punica granatum* (9c, 11t, 13c) have *trans* bonds. Further double bonds may be similarly introduced to give linoleic and linolenic acid.

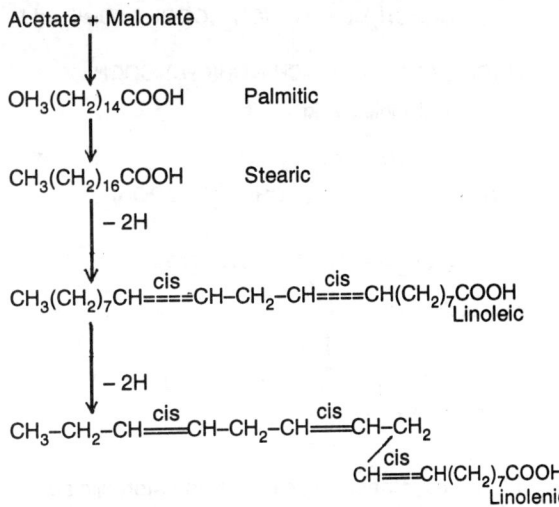

Fig. 17.5. Formation of olefinic fatty acids in plants.

Unsaturated fatty acids can also be formed in plants by elongation of a medium-chain-length unsaturated acid by the formation of an intermediate, β, γ-unsaturated acid rather than the α,β-unsaturated acid normally produced in saturated fatty acid biosynthesis. The β,γ-bond is not reduced and more C_2 units are added in the usual way.

Sterculic acid, a component of seed oils of the Malvaceae and Sterculiaceae, is a cyclopropene and is also derived from oleic acid, with methionine supplying the extra carbon atom to give, first, the

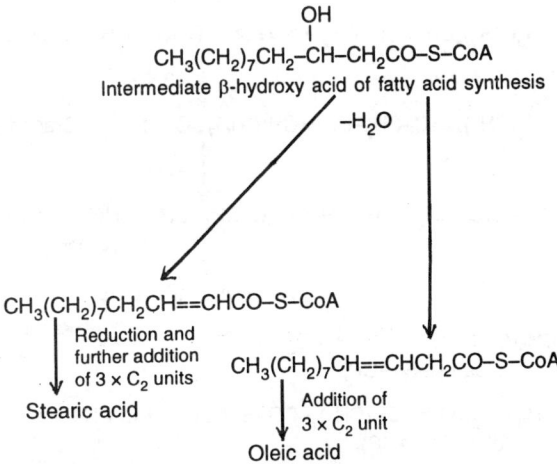

Fig. 17.6. Biosynthesis of unsaturated fatty acids.

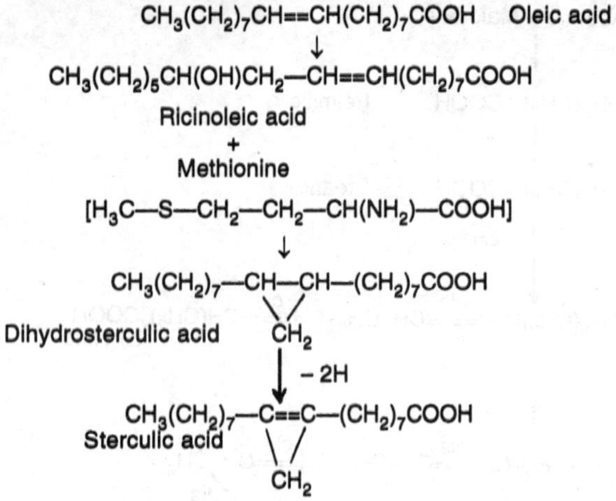

$$CH_3(CH_2)_7CH{=}CH(CH_2)_7COOH \quad \text{Oleic acid}$$
$$\downarrow$$
$$CH_3(CH_2)_5CH(OH)CH_2{-}CH{=}CH(CH_2)_7COOH$$

Ricinoleic acid

+

Methionine

$$[H_3C{-}S{-}CH_2{-}CH_2{-}CH(NH_2){-}COOH]$$
$$\downarrow$$
$$CH_3(CH_2)_7{-}CH{-}CH{-}(CH_2)_7COOH$$

Dihydrosterculic acid $\qquad CH_2$

$$\downarrow \; {-}2H$$

$$CH_3(CH_2)_7{-}C{=}C{-}(CH_2)_7COOH$$
Sterculic acid

$$CH_2$$

Fig. 17.7. Biosynthesis of ricinoleic and sterculic acids from oleic acid.

cycloprepane. Ricinoleic acid is a hydroxy fatty acid found in castor seed oil is again biosynthesized from oleic acid.

Enzymes present in certain fractions of unripe castor seeds can hydroxylate oleic acid to produce ricinoleic acid.

The triple bonds are formed from double bonds by a mechanism analogous to that for the formation of double bond. The range of acetylenes found in Basidiomycetes and in the Asteraceae, Araliaceae and Apiaceae can be derived from linoleic acid via its acetylenic 12,13-dehydroderivative, crepenynic acid, an acid present in the seeds of *Crepis* species.

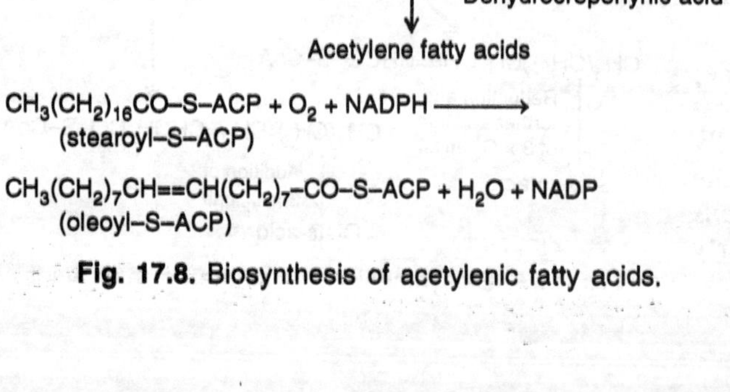

$$CH_3(CH_2)_4CH{=}CH{-}CH_2{-}CH{=}CH(CH_2)_7COOH \quad \text{Linoleic acid}$$

$$\downarrow \; {-}2H$$

$$CH_3(CH_2)_4{\equiv}C{-}CH_2{-}CH{=}CH(CH_2)_7COOH \quad \text{Crepenynic acid}$$

$$\downarrow \; {-}2H$$

$$CH_3{-}CH_2{-}CH_2{-}CH{=}CH{-}C{\equiv}C{-}CH_2{-}CH{=}CH(CH_2)_7COOH$$
Dehydrocrepenynic acid

$$\downarrow$$

Acetylene fatty acids

$$CH_3(CH_2)_{16}CO{-}S{-}ACP + O_2 + NADPH \longrightarrow$$
(stearoyl–S–ACP)

$$CH_3(CH_2)_7CH{=}CH(CH_2)_7{-}CO{-}S{-}ACP + H_2O + NADP$$
(oleoyl–S–ACP)

Fig. 17.8. Biosynthesis of acetylenic fatty acids.

L-α-Glycerophosphate, which are derived either from free glycerol or from the glycolysis intermediate, dihydroxyacetone phosphate, reacts successively with 2 molecules of fatty acyl-CoA to form first L-α-lysophosphatidic acid and then L-α-phosphatidic acid. The latter compound is converted to an α, β-diglyceride, which can either cycle back to the phosphatidic acids or react with another fatty acyl-CoA to form a triglyceride.

Extractions

Fixed oils and fats are obtained by expression of seeds or fruits in a hydraulic press. If the expression is carried at low temperature in cold, the oil is known as a 'virgin oil' or a 'cold-pressed oil'. When the oil is expressed in heat, it is known as a 'hot-pressed oil'. Sometimes organic solvents, *e.g.*, petroleum ether or chloroform, are used for the isolation of a fixed oil. Animal fats are separated from other tissues by heating them with steam. The melted fat rises to the top and may be removed by decanation.

The initial steps involved before extraction depends on the biological sources. The cotton seeds require delinting and castor seeds and ground nuts require decorticating with special machines. Removal of the oil may take the form of cold or hot expression, centrifuging or solvent extraction, again depending on the commodity. With seeds the remaining cake usually forms a valuable cattle feed and for this reason complete removal of the oil is not always necessary. The crude oil requires refining. Cold-drawn oils usually require filtration; castor oil requires steaming to inactivate lipase; the addition of a determined amount of alkali may be required to remove free acid; and washing and decolorization may be performed.

Quantitative chemical tests

Some quantitative tests are commonly used to evaluate fixed oils and fats.

Acid value refers to the number of mg of potassium hydroxide required to neutralize the free acids in 1 g of the oil; high acid values arise in rancidified oils.

Saponification value : the hydrolysis reaction of lipids can be used to determine the saponification value of the oil and is expressed as the number of mg of potassium hydroxide required to neutralize the free acids in, and to hydrolyse the esters in, 1 g of the substance.

Ester value is the difference between the saponification and acid values.

Iodine value gives a measure of the unsaturation of the oil. Oils which partially resinify on exposure to air are known as semidrying or drying oils. Such oils (*e.g.* linseed oil) have high iodine values. In animal fats such as butter, the determination of *volatile acidity* is useful, since the lower fatty acids such as butyric acid are volatile in stream and this may be used for their separation and estimation.

Unsaponifiable matter, consists of compounds such as sterols which remain after saponification of the acylglycerols and removal of the glycerol and soaps by means of solvents.

Acetyl value is the number of milligrams of potassium hydroxide required to neutralize the acetic acid freed by the hydrolysis of 1 g of the acetylated fat. The oil is first acetylated with acetic anhydride, which combines with any hydroxyl groups present. Because these are absent from most fatty acids, the small acetyl values usually obtained are due to relatively small amounts of sterols. In an oil such as castor oil, however, the acetyl value is high (146-150), due to the large amounts of the hydroxy acid ricinoleic acid. Certain physical constants of fixed oils and fats are significant: specific gravity, melting point, refractive index and sometimes optical rotation (*e.g.* castor oil).

CASTOR OIL

Synonyms

Castor bean oil; Castor oil seed; Ricinus oil; Oil of Palma Christi; Tangantangan oil; Neoloid; *Oleum Ricini*, Cold-drawn Castor oil.

Biological source

Castor oil is a fixed oil obtained by cold-expression from the seeds of *Ricinus communis* Linn. (Family: Euphorbiaceae).

Habitat

The plant is extensively cultivated in temperate climate such as India, South America, African countries, Brazil, China, East and West Indies and Thailand. The plant is an annual, soft-wooden, 15 meters high tree. The fruit is a three-celled spiny capsule, each cell has an ovoid albuminous seed.

Cultivation

Castor is an essential crop of the tropics and to some extent of subtropics. It is grown on sandy or clayey deep red loams and on good light alluvial loams. Generally seeds are sown in September-October. Application of organic manures such as farmyard manure, groundnut or castor cake, and inorganic fertilizers is beneficial. The harvesting period varies between 4 and 9 months. The harvested spikes are stacked in heaps till the capsules blacken. They are dried in the sunlight. The seeds are beaten out of the capsules by sticks, or thrushed under the feet of bullocks.

Characters of seeds

The seeds are oval, anatropous, compressed, 0.8-1.8 cm long, 0.4-1.2 cm broad with variable size and colour. The testa is smooth, thin and brittle. The colour is grey, brown or black with brown or black mottled. At one end there is a small yellowish caruncle from which the raphe extends on the flat or ventral side, to the chalazal at the opposite end. The testa is easily removable exposing the large white and oily endosperm bearing thin, flat foliaceous cotyledons, one on either side of a central, lenticular cavity, and connected with the short caulicle and radicle.

Castor oil preparation

The seed coat is removed by passing the seeds through a decorticator. The rollers with sharp

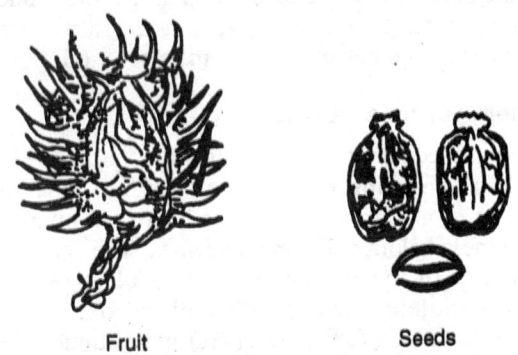

Fruit   Seeds

Fig. 17.9. Castor (*Ricinus communis*).

cutting edges break testa but do not injure the kernel. The testa are removed with sieves and compressed air. The kernels are cold expressed with 1-2 pressure per sq. inch to get about 30% oil. The oil is filtered and steam is passed through the oil to destroy toxic proteins albumins (ricin). The oil is bleached and sold. About 33% of the oil is obtained by cold expression.

The cake left after expression of the castor oil is unfit as a cattle food. It contains poisonous proteins, known as ricins (toxins) which produce an antiricin (antitoxin) in the body. Ricin D is a sugar protein which contains 493 amino acids and 23 sugar molecules. It has a strong lethal toxicity. Acidic ricin and basic ricin show similar actions. Ricin and abrin (from Abrus seeds) display anti-tumour properties. The seeds also contain lipases, ricinine (a non-toxic alkaloid), which is structurally related to nicotinamide.

Characters

Castor oil is a colourless or pale yellow viscous liquid. It has slight somewhat characteristic (nauseating) odour. The crude oil tastes slightly acrid with a nauseating after-taste. It has excellent keeping qualities, and does not turn rancid unless subjected to excessive heat. When exposed to the air, it gradually thickens, darkens in colour and develops more intense odour and taste. It is dextro-rotatory, $[\alpha]_D$ 0.96, viscosity 6-8 poises, acid value <4, saponification number 176-187, iodine number 81-91, acetyl value 144-150, hydroxyl value 161-169. It is miscible with alcohol, ether, chloroform and glacial acetic acid. It dissolves in its own volume of petroleum ether and in 95% alcohol due to the presence of hydroxyl group in ricinoleic acid. When heated to 300° for several hours, it polymerizes and becomes miscible with mineral oil.

Chemical constituents

Castor seeds contain fixed oil (45-55%), proteins (20%) consisting of globulin, albumin, nucleo-albumin, glycoprotein and ricin (a toxalbumin), ricinine alkaloid and some enzymes. The fixed oil consists of the glycerides of ricinoleic (87%), iso-ricinoleic, stearic (1%), dihydroxystearic (traces), linoleic (3%), oleic (7%) and palmitic (2%) acids. The purgative nature of the oil is due to free

ricinoleic acid and its stereoisomers which are produced by hydrolysis of triricinolein by lipases in the duodenum.

The seed coat contains lipids and phosphatides. A glycoprotein and two hemicelluloses are present in endosperm. 30-Norlupan-3β-ol-20-one was isolated from the bean coat.

The flowers yield hyperoside, rutin and ricinine. Ricinine is derived from nicotinic acid or other participants of the pyridine nucleotide cycle; hence, glycerol and succinic acid proved to be good precursors.

Uses

Castor oil is purgative and emollient. It is used as an ointment base, for the preparation of flexible collodion, to prepare undecylenic acid which is a fungistatic preparation and to manufacture lipsticks, perfumed hair oil and hair fixers. Nonionic surfactants (polyethoxylated castor oils) are prepared by treating castor oil with ethylene oxide and used for the administration of some drugs with low aqueous solubility in the forms of intravenous preparations. Hydrogenated castor oil is used as a stiffening agent. As an industrial raw material it is used in coating, urethane derivatives, surfactants, dispersants, cosmetics, lubricants, paints, varnishes, grease, polishes, soaps, plasticizers and Turkey red oil. It is the chief raw material for the production of sebacic acid. Undecylenic acid, heptanal (a raw product for textile polyamides and polypol esters) and electrical insulation coatings.

Castor oil produced large amounts of platelet activating factor in duodenum and jejunum but not in ileum and colon in rats. Intraluminal release of acid phosphatase was also increased in these rats.

Allied drugs

Croton seeds are obtained from *Croton tiglium* (Euphorbiaceae), a small tree producing similar capsules to those of castor but devoid of spines. The seeds are identical to castor seeds in size and shape but have a dull, cinnamon-brown colour and readily lose their caruncles. They yield about fixed oil (50%) which contains croton resin; 'crotin', a mixture of croton-globulin and croton-albumin comparable with ricin, diesters of the tetracyclic diterpene phorbol; acids involved are acetic as a

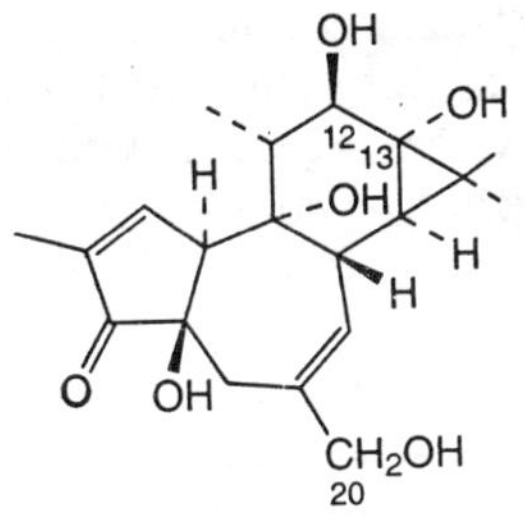

Phorbol

Fig. 17.10. Phorbol of croton oil.

short-chain acid, and capric, lauric and palmitic as long-chain acids. These compounds are cocarcinogens and also possess inflammatory and vesicant properties. Also present are phorbol-12,13,20-triesters (R^1, R^2 and R^3 are all acyl groups). These are 'cryptic irritants'. They are not biologically active as such but become so by removal of the C-20 acyl group by hydrolysis. The plant also contains alkaloids. Croton oil acts as a violent cathartic.

Physic nuts or *Purging nuts* are the seeds of *Jatropha curcas*, (Euphorbiaceae). The seeds are black, oval and 15-20 mm in length. They contain about 40% of fixed oil and curcin. Both seeds and oil are powerful purgatives.

Abrus seeds (prayer beans) are red and black, but poisonous seeds of *Abrus precatorius* (Papilionaceae). They contain a toxic glycoprotein (abrin) and another non-toxic peptide having haemagglutinating properties. Various alkaloids (abrine, hyaphorine, precatorine) of the indole type, sterols and lectins have been reported. The seeds are used to treat many ailments, also to procure abortion and to hasten labour. In India they are employed as an oral contraceptive and as they are remarkably uniform, and each weighs about 1 carat (*c.* 200 mg), have been used traditionally as weights.

SHARK LIVER OIL

Synonyms

Oleum selachoide.

Biological source

Shark liver oil is the fixed oil obtained from the fresh and healthy livers of shark fish, *Hypoprion brevirostris*. (Order : Selachii).

Habitat

Shark is found on seacoasts of many European countries and in India in Tamil Nadu, Maharashtra and Kerala.

Preparation

Livers are removed from the fish, cleaned thoroughly, freed from fatty substances and attached tissues like gall-bladders. Then the livers are heated in water at about 80°C. The oil exudes, floats on the top, and is separated, washed and water is removed. The dehydrated oil is cooled to separate stearin. The suspended materials are removed by centrifugation. The oil is supplemented with vitamins A and D in desired amount.

Characters

Shark liver oil is pale yellow to brownish yellow, viscous liquid with fishy odour and bland taste. It is insoluble in water, sparingly soluble in alcohol and freely miscible in non-polar solvents such as petroleum ether, chloroform and benzene. Its acid value is about 2, saponification value 150-200 and iodine value 160-350.

Chemical constituents

The active principle of Shark liver oil is vitamin A which varies from 15,000-30,000 I.U. per g of the oil. It contains glycerides of saturated and unsaturated fatty acids.

Chemical tests

1. A solution of Shark liver oil (1 drop) in chloroform (1 ml) is treated with sulphuric acid (1 drop). A violet colour changing to purple or brown is formed due to the presence of vitamin A.
2. Shark liver oil (1 ml) is dissolved in chloroform (10 ml). Few drops of saturated solution of antimony trichloride in chloroform are added to the solution. A blue colour is formed due to the presence of vitamin A.

Uses

Shark liver oil is used to treat xerophthalmia (abnormal dryness of the surface of conjunctiva) occurring due to deficiency of vitamin A. The oil is nutritive and used as a tonic.

Storage

The oil is sensitive to light and air. It should be stored in air tight, completely filled, coloured containers.

ARACHIS OIL

Synonyms

Groundnut oil; Monkeynut oil; Peanut oil; Katchung oil; Earth-nut oil.

Biological source

Arachis oil is obtained by expression of shelled and skinned seeds of *Arachis hypogaea* Linn. (Family : Papilionaceae).

Habitat

South America (Brazil) is the original home of ground nut and now found in South and Central America, Peru, Argentina, Nigeria, Australia, Gambia and other reasonably warm regions of all countries.

Groundnut plant is a small, prostrate, diffuse, erect, branched, annual herb, 30-60 cm in height, leaves alternate with adnate stipules and yellow papilionaceous flowers. After fertilization, the pedicel elongates rapidly and enters the ground, where the ovary begins to develop into a pod maturing in about two months. Pods or nuts are cylindrical, hard, reticulated, indehiscent and inflated, 2.5-5.0 cm long, 1-3 seeded, with pericarp constricted between the seeds. The seeds are covered by a light or deep reddish brown seeds coat, and consisting of two white fleshy cotyledons rich in oil and proteins.

Fruits are dug out by raking the plants from the soil, seeds are separated by machine and expressed in a hydraulic press at ordinary temperature. The remaining oil of cakes is removed by solvent extraction. The two oil fractions are combined and purified.

Cultivation

Groundnut is predominantly a crop of the tropical and subtropical countries, up to an elevation of 1,160 m. It requires plenty of sunlight, timely and evently distributed rainfall (50-125 cm) during its growth and a long season for its maturation and harvesting. It also requires a high temperature (21-26°) parti-cularly during the nights to induce early flowering. The plant does not stand frost, long and severe drought and water stagnation. Groundnut seeds are sown from April-May to June-July. It requires light, well-drained, loose, friable soil. No regular manuring is done by the growers and the plant is bene-fitted from green manuring.

Groundnut is susceptible to infection by several fungi, bacteria and viruses. Some important diseases in India are tikka leaf spot, collar rot, dry root rot, stem rot, rust, bud necrosis and yellow mould.

Groundnut oil is a non-drying oil belonging to the oleolinoleic acid group of oils. It is pale-yellow in colour or almost colourless liquid with a nutty odour and bland taste. Clouds are formed in the oil at low room temperature. It has acid value 0.08-6, saponification value 188-195, iodine value 84-102; thiocyanogen value 67-73 and hydroxyl value 2.5-9.5. It is very slowly thickens and becomes rancid on prolonged exposure to air. It is miscible with solvent ether, petroleum ether, chloroform, carbon disulphide, benzene; very slightly soluble in alcohol.

Chemical constituents

The important constituents of the glycerides of groundnut oil are the fatty acids palmitic (8.3%), stearic (3.1%), oleic (56%), linoleic (26%), arachidic (24%), eicosenoic, behenic (3.1%) and lignoceric (1.1) acids. Myristic, hexacosanoic, erucic, caprylic, lauric and trace amounts of odd carbon fatty acids are also present.

The principal glycerides of the oil are triolein (11%), dioleolinolein (21%), saturated oleolinoleins (22%), dilinoleoolein (12%), saturated diolein (15%) and saturated dilinoleoolein (6%).

The yellow colour of the oil is due to the presence of carotenoid pigments, chiefly β-carotene and lutein. The unsaponifiable matter consists of sterols, (campesterol, stigmasterol, β-sitosterol and choles-terol), sterol glycosides (β-sitosterol-D-glycoside and others), and triterpenoid alcohols (β-amyrin, cycloartenol and 24-methylene cycloartenol). Tocopherols occur free in groundnut oil. Squalene, an unsaturated hydrocarbon, occurs in extremely small amounts in the unsaponifiable fraction. Two other unsaturated hydrocarbons, hypogene and arachidene, have also been reported.

The kernels contain fixed oil (40-50%), proteins (26.2%), water (1.8%), carbohyorates (20.6%), ash and high concentration of thiamine. The chief proteins are arachin and conarchin, both are globulins of different solubility. The vitamin content of groundnut is moderate, the largest being in the episperm.

The seeds also contain α-resorcylic, *p*-hydroxybenzoic, *cis*- and *trans*-*p*-coumaric, phloretic, protocatechuic and chlorogenic acids, luteolin, daucosterol, stilbene, phytoalexins, vanillic acid, dancosterin, 5,7-dihydroxy-chromone, pratensein, chrysoeriol, eriodictyol, apigenin, soyasaponin I, 5,7-dihydroxychromone, eriodictyol, and N^6-methyl agmatine.

Uses

Groundnut oil is used as an edible oil, in control of pasture bloat, as a substitute for Olive oil, as a solvent in pharmaceutical aid, in hydrogenated state as shortening, in mayonnaise, in confections; for the manufacture of margarine, soap, points, liniments, plasters and ointments, as vehicle for intramuscular medication and in the laboratory as heat transfer medium in melting point apparatus.

SESAME OIL

Synonyms

Benne oil; Teel oil; Gingelli oil; Sesamum seed oil.

Biological source

Sesame oil is obtained by refining the expressed or extracted oil from the seeds of cultivated varieties of *Sesamum indicum* Linn. (Family : Pedaliaceae).

Habitat

The plant is widely cultivated in India, China, Japan, East Indies, West Indies and in the southern United States.

Cultivation

The plant is an annual herb, 1 m in height. Sesamum is cultivated in the plains and on elevations up to 1,200 m at temperature of 21° and above. It requires a warm climate and cannot withstand frost, continued heavy rain or prolonged drought. It grows on a light well-drained soil which is capable of retaining adequate moisture. It thrives best on typical sandy loams.

The seeds are sown broadcast. In northern India, the crop is sown in June-July and harvested in October-November. The crop is not generally manured.

The seeds are small, flat, oval, smooth and shiny, whitish, yellow or reddish brown; sweet and oily taste; odour is slight. They are pointed at one end where hilum is located, raphe runs as a line from hilum, along the centre of one flat face to the broader end. The endosperm is present as a thin layer around the embryo. The seeds contain fixed oil (45-55%), proteins (aleurone, 22%) and mucilage (4%).

Preparation

The oil is expressed by hydraulic or low and medium-powered screw presses. A good yield of the oil is obtained by three successive expression. Prior to processing in the screw press, the seed is subjected to a cooking process. If live steam is used for cooking, the cuticles separate partly from the kernels and the mixture of kernels, cuticles and seed slips in the cage and lumpy material is obtained instead of a firm cake. If the seed is heated in cooker without the addition of steam or water, and water is added at the point of entry of dried seed into the screw press cage, the efficiency of oil extracton is greatly enhanced. Alkali refining, bleaching, hydrogenation and decolourization of Sesame oil can be effected with very little loss.

The sesame oil (40-50%) is pale yellow liquid, almost odourless, bland taste, saponification no. 188-193, iodine no. 103-122, soluble in chloroform, solvent and petroleum ethers, carbon disulphide; slightly soluble in alcohol and insoluble in water.

Chemical constituents

Sesame oil consists of a mixture of glycerides of oleic (43%), linoleic (43%), palmitic (9%), stearic (4%), arachidic, hexadecenoic, lignoceric and myristic acids. It also contains the lignan sesamin (1%), the related sesamolin and vitamins A and E. During industrial refining, sesemolin is readily converted into antioxidant phenols sesamol and sesamolinol.

Sesamol forms pink colour when the oil (2 ml) is shaken with concentrated hydrochloric acid

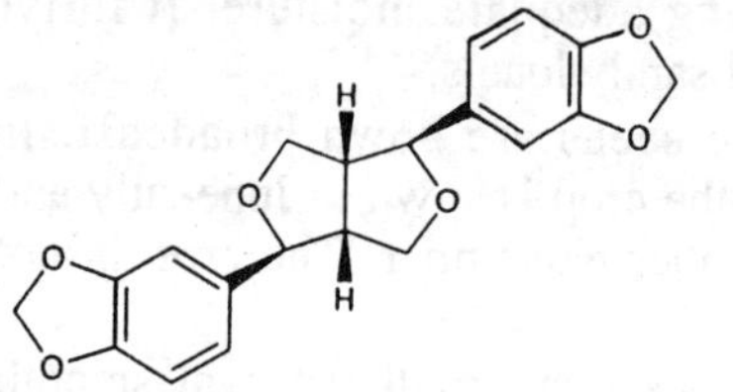

Fig. 17.11. Sesamin.

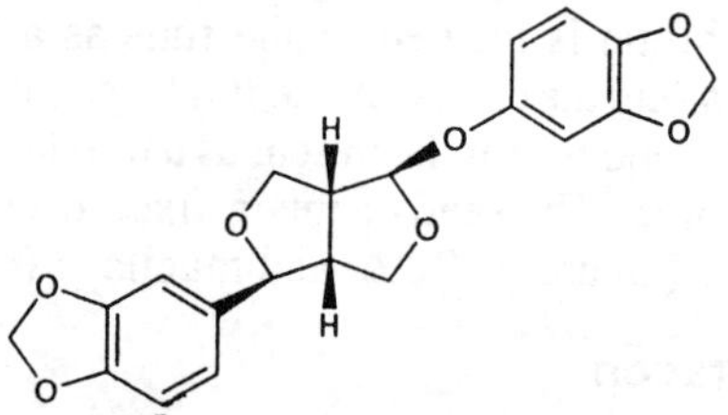

Fig. 17.12. Sesamolin.

(1 ml) containing 1% sucrose (Bandouin's test). Furfural may be used in place of sucrose and this modified test (Villavecchia test) is widely used to detect Sesame oil in other oils and fats. The presence of sesamolin or free sesamol is responsible for this colour which are not found in other vegetable oils.

The seeds also contain a lignan sesamolinol, γ-tocopherol, sesaminol, pinoresinol, its glycosides, sesaminol glucosides VI, VII and VIII, triglucoside KP3, carbohydrates (20%), proteins (20-25%), sterols (campesterol, stigmasterol, β-sitosterol and Δ^5-avenasterol), γ- and δ-tocopherols.

Sesamolinol exhibited stronger antioxidative activity than vitamin E. Lignan glycoside KP3 prevented oxidation of linoleic acid in aqueous solution.

Uses

Sesame oil is used as demulcent, in dysentery and urinary complaints, as a solvent for injection of steroids, antibiotics and hormones, as mild laxative, nutritive, emollient, pediculicide, in manufacture of oleomargarine, cosmetics, iodized oil, anti acids and ointment. It is injectable as a vehicle for fat soluble substances. The oil is also used in insecticidal sprays. Sesamolin, present in the unsaponifiable fraction of the oil, is an effective synergist for pyrethrum insecticides. An extract enriched in lignans as an antioxidant and radical scavenger is used in cosmetic industry.

LINSEED AND LINSEED OIL

Synonyms

Flax seed, Alsi (Hindi), Linum; Semina Lini.

Biological source

Linseed is the dried, ripe seed of *Linum usitatissimum* Linn. Linseed oil is obtained by expresson of linseeds. (Family : Linaceae).

Habitat

Linseed is cultivated in many sub-tropical countries such as South America, India, USA, Canada, England, Russia, Greece, Italy, Spain and Algeria.

Collection

Linseed in an erect annual herb, 60-120 cm high with sky-blue flowers and a globular capsule. The plant is cultivated for its seeds and fibre (flax). A moderate rainfall is best suited for its growth. It grows in almost all types of soils where sufficient moisture is available, but thrives best in heavy soils with high moisture retaining capacity. As a mixed crop it is sown either on the margins of fields or in rows alternating with the other crop. Nitrogenous fertilizers yield better crop. The crop is harvested in February and March before the capsules are dried. Plants are cut close to the ground, dried in the field and threshed to separate seeds.

Morphology of seeds

The seeds are oval, flattened, elongated, 4-6 mm long, and 2-3 mm wide. Testa is glossy, smooth, reddish-brown with minutely pitted surface. Seeds are rounded at one end. The other end is obliquely pointed where the hilum and micropyle are present in a slight depression. Raphe is present along one edge. Endosperm is narrow and encircles the embryo. It consists of two thick flattened, planoconvex cotyledons and a radicle. The seeds are odourless but possess an oily and mucilaginous taste.

Microscopical characters

Under microscope the testa shows a mucilagecontaining outer epidermis; one or two layers of collenchyma or 'round cells'; a single layer of sclerenchyma; the hyaline layers or 'cross-cells' composed in the ripe seed of obliterated parenchymatous cells; and an innermost layer of pigment cells. The outer epidermis is composed of cells, rectangular or five-sided in surface view, which swell up in water and become mucilaginous. The outer cell walls, when swollen in water, show an outer solid stratified layer. The radial layers or 'round cells' are cylindrical in shape and show distinct triangular intercellular air spaces. The sclerenchymatous layer is composed of elongated cells, up to 250 μm in length, with lignified pitted walls. The hyaline layers are attached to portions of the sclerenchymatous layer in the powdered drug. The pigment layer is composed of cells with thickened pitted walls and containing amorphous reddish-brown contents. The cells of the endosperm and cotyledons are polygonal with thickened walls, and contain numerous aleurone grains and globules of fixed oil.

Chemical constituents

Linseed contains fixed oil (30-40%), mucilage (6-10%), protein (25%) (linin and colinin), small amount of enzyme lipase and linamarin which is a cyanogenetic glycoside. The carbohydrates present are sucrose, raffinose, cellulose and mucilage. Linamarin is a glucose either of acetone cyanohydrin and is identical to phaseolunatin. Unripe seeds contain starch which is converted to mucilage on ripening the seeds. The mucilage can be fractionated into a neutral fraction a remified, arabinoxylan composed of D-xylose, L-arabinose, D-glucose and D-galactose; and an acidic fraction mainly composed of L-rhamnose and D-galactose. Mucilage swells with water and forms red colour with ruthenium red. Linamarin on hydrolysis yields acetone, hydrocyanic acid and glucose. The other consti-

tuents are phytin, lecithin, wax, resin, pigments, malic acid, cyanogenic glycosides linustatin neolinustatin and secoisolariciresinol and phenylpropanoid glucoside linusitamarin.

LINSEED OIL

Preparation

The dried seeds are crushed in rollers, moistened and heated to 80-90°C in steam to soften the seed tissues. They are then pressed through hot hydraulic press at a high pressure. The oil so obtained is treated with alkali to separate free fatty acids and bleached with fuller's earth or charcoal. On cooling the oil waxy substances are removed.

Linseed oil is a yellowish liquid, with a peculiar odour and bland taste. On exposure to air it gradually thickens, becomes darker and acquires a more pronounced odour and taste. On drying it forms a hard varnish. It has a high iodine value (~170) which indicates the presence of excess amount of glycerides of unsaturated fatty acids. The oil is slightly soluble in alcohol, miscible with chloroform, ether, petroleum ether, carbon disulphide and terpentine oil. It has density 0.925-0.935, viscosity 1.47, congealing point –20°C, saponification number 187-195, refractive index 1.47-1.48, and unsaponifiable matters not over 1.5%. A water-soluble resinous matter with antioxidant properties has been isolated from the oil.

On hydrolysis Linseed oil produces unsaturated acids like linolenic acid (30-50%), linoleic acid (23-24%), oleic acid (10-18%) together with saturated acids-myristic, stearic and palmitic (5-11%).

Uses

Linseed is used as demulcent and in form of poultices for gouty and rheumatic swellings. Internally

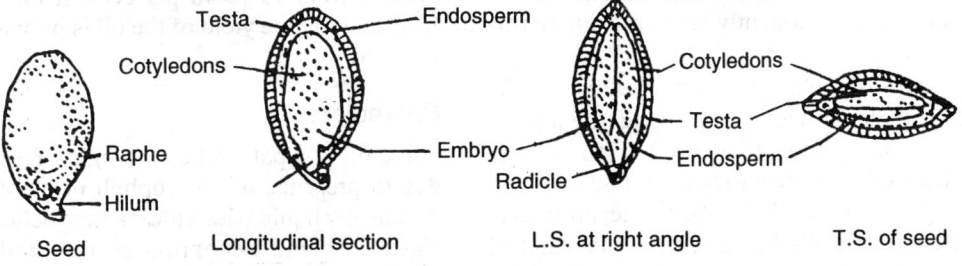

Seed   Longitudinal section   L.S. at right angle   T.S. of seed

Fig. 17.13. Linseed.

it is used for gonorrhoea and irritation of the genito-urinary system. Linseed oil has emollient, expectorant, diuretic, demulcent and laxative properties and is utilized externally in lotions and liniments. Non-staining iodine ointment soap, linoleum, greases, polishes, polymers, varnishes, paints, putty, oil cloths, printing inks, artificial rubber, tracing cloth, tanning and enamelling leather, are prepared from Linseed oil. It is applied to paper and fabrics to render them waterproof and tough. The mucilaginous infusion is used internally as a demulcent in colds, coughs, bronchial affections, inflammation of the urinary tract, gonorrhoea and diarrhoea.

Linseed stimulates persistalsis and protects the mucous membrane in case of inflammation (colitis). Obese patients should swallow the seeds without chewing them, to avoid releasing the fixed oil, a source of calories (1 g seeds = 4.7 kcal)

Hydrolysed Linseed oil has potentially useful antibacterial properties as a topical preparation in that it is effective against *Staphylococcus aureus* strains resistant to antibiotics. Linseed cake is a valuable cattle food.

For use in paint linseed oil is boiled with 'driers' such as litharge or manganese resinate which, by forming metallic salts, causes the oil to dry more rapidly. Such 'boiled oils' must not be used for medicinal purposes.

Enterodiol and enterolactone are formed by degradation of the glycoside of secoisolarici-resinol by the flora of the colon. These lignans show anti-tumor effect.

Adulterants

When market price is high, Linseed oil is adulterated with vegetable oils, such as rape, cottonseed, soyabean, sunflower, safflower and candlenut, as well as with rosin and mineral and fish oils. Boiled Linseed oil is more frequently adulterated than raw oil. Adulteration is rather difficult.

Admixture of rape and mustard oils may be detected by the presence of erucic acid; the adulterants lower the saponification value. Fish oil may be detected by the odour produced on heating and by melting points of ether - insoluble bromides. Rosin and mineral oils increase the proportion of unsaponifiable matter.

OLIVE OIL

Synonyms

Salad oil; Sweet oil; Oleum olival.

Biological source

Olive oil is a fixed oil obtained by expression of the ripe fruits of *Olea europoea* Linn. (Fam. Oleaceae).

Geographical source

Olive is a native of Palestine and produced extensively in the countries adjoining the Mediterranean sea, Spain being the largest producer. It is also grown in the south western United States and many other subtropical localities.

The tree is propagated by cuttings; grafting and budding of *O. europoea* or Indian olive (*O. ferruginea*).

For proper growth the plant needs deep fertile soil and a temperature average to 13° not dropping to below –10°.

Collection and preparation

The olive is an evergreen tree, up to 12 m in height which produces drupaceous fruits about 2-3 cm in length, purplish in colour when ripe. The fruits are collected from November to April. After grinding, the pulp is introduced into coarse, grass baskets and placed in a screw press. The oil coming out is collected into tubes containing water and the upper layer is skimmed off. The product is called as *Virgin oil* obtained by gently pressing the peeled pulp freed from the endocarp. The marc is then treated with water and again expressed to yield second grade of edible oil. Finally, the pulp is mixed with hot water and pressed again for technical oil. The pulp may be extracted with carbon disulphide to obtain "sulphur" olive oil of inferior quality. The yield is from 15 to 40 per cent. If the fruit is not fully mature, the yield of the oil is poor and its taste is bitter.

Characters

Olive oil is a pale yellow or light greenish-yellow due to presence of chlorophyll or carotenes, non-drying oily liquid with a pleasanting delicate flavour. Taste is bland becoming cloudy and at 0°C it usually forms a whitish granular mass. It becomes faintly acrid. It is miscible with ether, chloroform and carbon disulphide and is slightly soluble in alcohol. Upon cooling at +5 to 10° it becomes cloudy and at 0°C usually forms a whitish granular mass. It becomes rancid on exposure to air. It has specific gravity of 0.914-0.919, acid value 0.2-2.8, saponification value 187-196 and iodine value 79-90.

Chemical constituents

Olive oil contains mixed glycerides of oleic acid (56-85%), palmitic (7-20%), linoleic (3-20%), stearic (1-5%), arachidic (0.9%), palmitoleic (3%), linolenic, eicosenoic, gadoleic and lignoceric acids. The minor constituents are squalene up to 0.7%, phytosterol and tocopherols about 0.2%. Italy-Spain type olive oil is higher in oleic acid and Greece-Tunisia type oil has higher levels of linoleic acid.

The seeds contain a triterpenic acid, oleanolic acid and 2,6,10,15,19,23-hexamethyl-tetracos-3,6,10,14,18,22-hexaen-2-ol.

Uses

Olive oil is used in the manufacture of pharmaceutical preparations, soaps, textile lubricants, sulphonated oils, liniments, cosmetics, plasters; as food in salads, and for cooking and baking. It has demulcent, emollient, choleretic or cholagogue and laxative properties. It is a good solvent for parenteral preparations.

CHAULMOOGRA OIL

Synonyms

Hydnocarpus oil; Gynocardia oil.

Biological source

Chaulmoogra oil is the fixed oil obtained by cold expression from ripe seeds of *Taraktogenos kurzii* King, (syn. *Hydnocarpus kurzii* (King) Warb.), *Hydnocarpus wightiana* Blume, *H. anthelmintica* Pierre, *H. heterophylla* and other species of *Hydnocarpus* (Family : Flacourtiaceae).

Habitat

The plants are tall trees, up to 17 m high, with narrow crown of hanging branches; native to Burma, Thailand, eastern India and Indo-China.

The tree bears irregular fruits which are collected once in 2-3 years when a full crop is expected. The seeds resemble brown pebbles in appearance and are of varying size and shape. Commercial oil obtained by the expression of kernels. They contains large amounts of free fatty acids which are of poor quality.

Characters

The oil is yellow or brownish yellow. Below 25°C it is a soft solid. It has peculiar odour and sharp taste. It is soluble in benzene, chloroform, ether, petrol; slightly soluble in cold alcohol; almost entirely soluble in hot alcohol and carbon disulphide.

Chemical constituents

Chaulmoogra oil contains glycerides of cyclopentenyl fatty acids like hydnocarpic acid (48%), chaulmoogric acid (27%), gorlic acid with small amounts of glycerides of palmitic acid (6%) and oleic acid (12%). The cyclic acids are formed during last 3-4 months of maturation of the fruit and are strongly bactericidal towards the Micrococcus of leprosy.

The seeds of *H. wightiana* contain a flavonolignan hydnocarpin; isohydnocarpin, methoxy hydnocarpin, apigenin, luteolin, chrysoeriol,

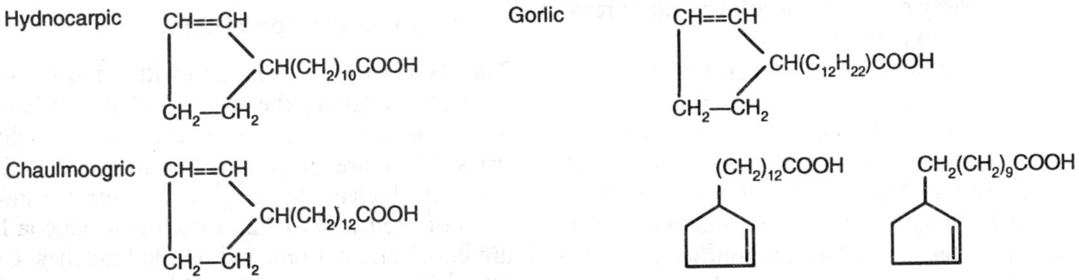

Fig. 17.14. Cyclopentenyl fatty acids.

hydnowightin, neohydnocarpin, epivolkenin, taraktophyllin and cyclopentenoid cyanohydrin glycosides.

Uses

The oil is useful in leprosy and many other skin diseases. The cyclopentenyl fatty acids of the oil exhibit specific toxicity for *Mycobacterium leprae* and *M. tuberculosis*. The oil has now been replaced by the ethyl esters and salts of hydnocarpic and chaulmoogric acids. At present organic sulphones have replaced Chaulmoogra oil in therapeutic use.

KOKUM

Synonyms

Kokum butter; Kokum oil.

Biological source

Kokum is the fat obtained by expression of the ripe seeds of *Garcinia purpurea* Roxb. (syn. *G. indica* Chois). (Family : Guttiferae; Clusiaceae).

Habitat

The trees are slender evergreen with drooping branches found in tropical rain forests in Konkan, western ghats of Maharashtra, Malabar and Karnataka.

Seeds are separated from the ripe fruits. The dried pericarp is composed of fat which is known as Kokum. Its taste is sweet-sour. Seeds are expressed to get solid wax-like 'Kokum butter' (30%). Kokum butter is also obtained by extracting the seeds with boiling water and skimming off the fat from the top or by churning the crushed pulp with water. It is greyish-white fat having slight odour or taste, mp. 39-42°C.

Kokum butter consists of egg-shaped lumps or cakes of light grey or yellowish colour with a greasy feel and a bland oily taste.

It contains a mixture of glycerides of stearic, oleic, palmitic, arachidic and linoleic acids. It has about 75% of mono-oleodisaturated glycerides. The glyceride components are as : tristearin (1.5%), oleodistearin (68%), oleopalmitostearin (8%), stearodiolein (20%), palmitodiolein and triolein. The Kokum butter has mp. 49-42°, saponification value 299.5 and iodine value 37.4.

Uses

Kokum has emollient, nutritive, demulcent and astringent action and is used to treat skin diseases, dysentery, mucous diarrhoea, and phthisis pneumonia. Externally, it is applied to cure ulcers, fissures of lips and hands, chapped skin, wounds and sores. It is used as a base in ointments, suppository, for the preparation of pomades, to give an acid flavour to curries and for preparing cooling syrups during hot months.

THEOBROMA

Synonyms

Cacao butter; Cocoa butter; Cacao seeds; Cacao beans; Semina Theobromatis; Cocao seeds.

Biological source

Theobroma oil is obtained by expression of the ground kernels of *Theobroma cacao* Linn. (Family Sterculiaceae).

Geographical distribution

The Cocoa tree (Chocolate tree) is a native of tropical America (Mexico), and cultivated in Ecuador, Curacao, Mexico, Trinidad, Central America, Brazil, West Africa (Nigeria and Ghana), Sri Lanka, the Philippine Islands, South India and Orissa.

Good growing conditions for Cacao require high humidity, temperature range from 18-32° and clay-loams, sandy loams and loam soils. It is reproduced by seeds. Seedlings may be raised in nursery beds. The seeds germinate within a week. Transplanting is done when seedlings are 4-5 months old. Adequate shade is necessary for the establishment of young trees.

Collection and preparation

The plant is a small evergreen with a dense rounded crown tree attaining the height of about 6-12 meters. The small flowers arise from the older branches or trunk. They are succeeded by large ovoid, fleshy red fruit which has ten longitudinal furrows and five rows of seeds, 10 or 12 in each row. Cocoa fruits are borne on the trunk and on the branches. Cocoa plantations are very vulnerable to pest attack. A pheromone technology is used to control the cocoa pod borer, also known as the cocoa moth (*Conopomorpha cramerella*), the most serious pest of the crop in S.E. Asia. Collection is done throughout the year, but the larger quantities are obtained in the spring and autumn. About 40-50 colourless, fleshy seeds embedded in a scanty, mucilaginous pulp are present. The seeds are separated from the pod and packed in boxes, in which they undergo a process of fermentation at 42°C. They are then dried in the sun. At the end of these processes the seeds acquire a reddish-brown colour, and the taste, at first astringent and bitter, and becomes mild and oily. They are then roasted (140°C), lossing water and developing distinct odour and taste. The roasted seeds are passed through a "nibbling" machine to crack the seed coats which are separated from the kernels by air. The broken kernels (nibs) are ground between hot rollers to yield a paste containing up to 50% of fat, called *Cacao Butter*. At room temperature the paste is congealed to yield *Bitter Chocolate*. When sugar and flavouring substances, like vanilla, are added to the *Bitter Chocolate* it is known as *Sweet Chocolate*. After expressing Cacao butter, the marc, retaining some oil, is powdered which is called as *Prepared Cacao* or *Breakfast Cocoa*.

Fermentation occurs in tubs, boxes or cavities in the earth for 3-9 days, and the temperature is not allowed to rise above 60°C. In Jamaica, fermentation is allowed to proceed for 3 days at a temperature of 30-43°C. During this process a liquid drains from the seeds, which change in colour from white or red to purple, and also acquire a different odour and taste. After fermentation the seeds are roasted at 100-140°C, when they lose water and acetic acid and acquire their distinct odour and taste. The seeds are cooled and the testa removed by a 'nibbling' machine. The nibs or kernels are separated from the husk by winnowing. Sometimes the seeds are simply dried in the sun but these are not as highly regarded owing to their astringent and bitter taste.

Plain or *bitter chocolate* is a mixture of ground cocoa nibs with sucrose, cocoa butter and flavouring. Milk chocolate contains in addition milk powder.

Microscopical characters

Cocoa seeds are flattened-ovoid, about 20-30 mm long, 15 mm wide and 7 mm thick. The seed-coat is chocolate brown in colour, brittle and thin. The kernel consists of two irregularly folded, chocolate-coloured cotyledons.

The embryo is surrounded by a thin membrane of endosperm. The cotyledons form the greater part of the kernel and are planoconvex and irregularly folded. Each shows on its plane face three large furrows, which account for the readiness with which the kernel breaks into angular fragments. Both testa and kernel are reddish-brown in colour.

Theobroma oil is yellowish-white solid, brittle below 25°; chocolate odour and taste. m.p. 30°-35°C; insoluble in water; slightly soluble in alcohol; soluble in boiling alcohol, very soluble in chloroform, ether and benzene.

Chemical constituents

Cocoa butter consists of the glycerides of stearic (34%), palmitic (26%), arachidic, oleic (37%) and other acids. These glycerides are present in the form of simple and mixed glycerides. Mono-oleo-disaturated glycerides, oleo-palmitostearin, are the major constituents.

The seeds contain 35-50% of a fixed oil, 15% of starch, 15% of proteins, 1-4% of the alkaloid theobromine and 0.07-0.36% of caffeine. Cocao-red is formed by the action of a ferment on a glyceride and gives red colour to the seeds. It also contains tyramine and procyanidins.

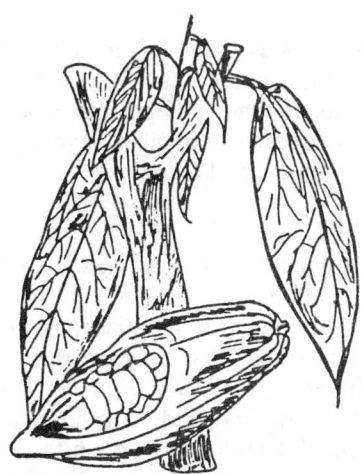

Fig. 17.15. *Theobroma cacao.*

Theobromine is present in the kernel (1-1.7%) and the shell (0.19-2.98%).

During the fermentation and roasting, much of the theobromine originally present in the kernel passes into the husk. The constituents other than fat and theobromine are extremely complex. The fresh seeds contain about 5-10% of water-soluble polyphenols (epicatechol, leucoantho-cyanins and anthocyanins) which are largely decomposed during processing, forming the coloured complex known as 'cocoa-red'. Condensed tannins are also present, and some 84 different volatile compounds, including glucosinolates, are present in the aroma.

Theobromine is produced on the commercial scale from cocoa husks. The process consists of decocting the husks with water, filtering, precipitating 'tannin' with lead acetate, filtering, removing excess of lead and evaporating to dryness. Theobromine is extracted from the residue by means of alcohol and purified by recrystallization from water.

Theobromine is 3,7-dimethylxanthine, the lower homologue of caffeine (trimethylxanthine). It is isomeric with theophylline (1,3-dimethylxanthine), which occurs in small quantities in tea. Theobromine crystallizes in white rhombic needles. It gives the murexide reaction. It is precipitated from a dilute nitric acid solution by silver nitrate. Theobromine sublimes at 220°C, caffeine at 178-180°C.

Callus and suspension cultures of cocoa both produce caffeine, theobromine and theophylline.

Uses

Theobroma oil is used as lubricant in massage, base for suppositories and ointments, in manufacturing chocolate, toilet soaps and creams. Cocoa, called "breakfast Cocoa", is a popular beverage, used as nutritive, stimulant and diuretic.

Allied drugs

Kola seeds (*Bissy* or *Gooroo nuts*) : Commercial kola consists of the dried cotyledons of the seeds of various species of *Cola* (Steruliaceae), trees found in West Africa, the West Indies, Brazil and Java. The fresh seeds of *C. acuminata* are white or crimson, *C. astrophora* red, *C. alba* white and *C. vera* (*C. nitida*) either red or white. The dried cotyledons are usually dull, reddish-brown and broken. They are usually graded as 'halves' and 'quarters'. The whole seeds are 2-5 cm long, odourless; taste, slightly astringent.

Kola seeds contain caffeine (1-2.5%) and theo-bromine, about 5-10% of tannoids ('kolatin'), particularly catechol and epicatechol. During preparation, oxidation and polymerization of these, the insoluble phlobaphene 'kola-red' is produced. The differences in the stimulatory action between fresh and dried seeds may be due to the formation of a caffeine-catechin complex in the latter.

Guarana (*Pasta Guarana* or *Brazilian cocoa*) is a dried paste prepared from the seeds of *Paullinia cupana* (Sapindaceae). The seeds are collected from plants in the upper Amazon basin. The kernels are separated from the shell, broken and made into a paste with water, along with starch and other substances. The paste is then made into suitable shapes and dried in the sun or over fires.

The drugs usually occurs in cylindrical rolls 10-30 cm long and 2.5-4 cm diameter. Portions of broken seeds are the dark chocolate at brown outer surface. The drug has no marked odour but an astringent bitter taste.

Guarana contains 2.5-7.0% of caffeine, other xanthine derivatives, tannins about 12% ('guarana red') and other constituents similar to those of cola and cocoa. Guarana resembles tea and coffee in its action and the powder grated from the masses is used in South America with water to make a drink. In the West it is used for combating fatigue, for slimming, and for the treatment of diarrhoea. The fat content of the drug effects a slow but steady release of the alkaloids.

Coffee consists of the seeds of *Coffea arabica* and other species of *Coffea* (Rubiaceae). It contains caffeine (1-2%), tannin and chlorogenic or caffeotannic acid, fat, sugars and pentosans.

Prepared coffee is the kernel of the dried ripe seeds of various species, including *C. arabica* (Arabica coffee), *C. liberica* and *C. canephora* (Robusta coffee) (Rubiaceae), deprived of most of the seed coat and roasted. The kernels are dark brown, hard and brittle, elliptical or planoconvex and about 1.0 cm long. Coffee has a distinct odour and taste. A decoction is used as a flavouring agent in Caffeine Iodide Elixir. Prepared coffee contains about 1-2% of caffeine, nicotinic acid, fixed oil and carbohydrates caramelized during roasting.

C. arabica is used to study purine alkaloid variations and biosynthesis.

Tea consists of the prepared leaves of *Thea sinensis* (*Camellia thea* Link.), a shrub belonging to the Ternstroemiaceae (Theaceae) which is cultivated in India, Sri Lanka, East Africa, Mauritius, China and Japan. The leaves contain thease, an enzymic mixture containing an oxidase, which partly converts the phlobatannin into phlobaphene. This oxidase may be destroyed by steaming for 30 seconds. Tea contains caffeine 1-5% and tannin 10-24%; small quantities of theobromine, theophylline and volatile oil. The alkaloid content of the leaves is dependent on age and season.

COTTONSEED OIL

Biological source

Cottonseed oil is a refined fixed oil obtained by expression of seeds of *Gossypium harbaceum* Linn. in hydraulic or other presses. The process is one of hot expression and a pressure of about 10000 kPa is used. (Family : Malvaceae).

Preparation

The cottonseed, after ginning off the fibers, is decorticated and cleaned of hulls. The kernels are steamed and pressed at about 1500 lb pressure to yield about 30% of oil which is turbid and reddish in colour. It is refined by filtering, decolorizing, and "winter chilling," which removes the stearin.

Characters

The crude oil is amber to deep red or black in colour with a characteristic odour, sp. gr. 0.92, saponification value 192-200, iodine value 100-115 and unsaponifiable matter 0.6-2.0 per cent. Refined Cottonseed oil is pale yellow in colour with a bland nutty taste and nearly odourless. The oil is a semi-drying substance. On cooling a sediment of olein or liquid glycerides separates out which may be collected by the filtration in the cooled condition. When used to adulterate other oils its presence may be detected by the test for semidrying.

Cottonseed oil is graded on the basis of its acidity; refining loses flavour. Refined oil is graded according to the colour, odour and flavour.

Chemical constituents

The important constituents of the glycerides of

Cottonseed oil are linoleic (45-50%), oleic (23-29%), palmitic (20-33%), myristic (1.5-3.5%), stearic (1.1-2.7%) and arachidic acids (1.0%). The glycerides present are palmito-oleolinoleins (35-40%), palmitodioleins (20%) and trioleo- or lineo-disaturated (12-13%). The unsaponifiable fraction contains β-sitosterol, ergosterol, vitamin E and tocopherols. The phosphatides present are lecithin (29%) and cephalins (71%). The minor constituents present in the oil are free fatty acids (0.3-5.6%), gossypol (0.05%), raffinose, pentosans, resins, wax, proteoses, peptones, phospholipids, inosite phosphates, phytosteroline, xanthophyll, chlorophyll and mucilage substances.

Cottonseed cake contains about 0.6% of a toxic principle, gossypol, which occurs in secretory cavities in all parts of the plant. It is present in cold-pressed oil and can be removed by treatment with alkalies.

Uses

Cottonseed oil is used as a solvent for injections and for edible purposes. The oil possesses emollient properties and is used in liniments, in several pharmaceutical preparations, as a substitute of Olive oil and in large doses as lubricant cathartic. Low grade oil is used in the manufacture of soaps, lubricants, sulphonated oils and protective coatings.

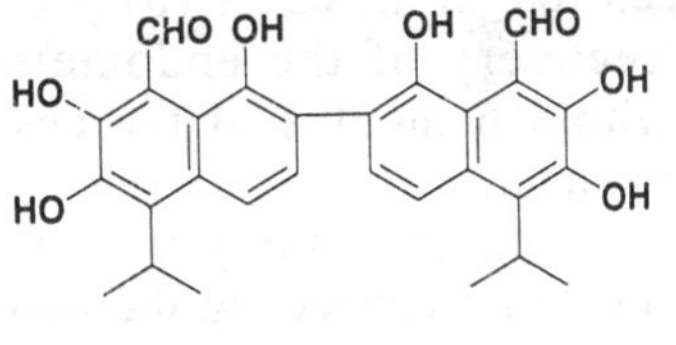

Gossypol

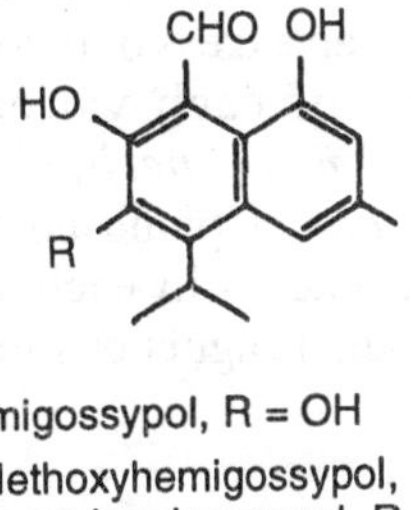

Hemigossypol, R = OH
6-Methoxyhemigossypol, R = OMe
6-Deoxyhemigossypol, R = H

Fig. 17.16. Phenol constituents of Cottonseed oil.

Cottonseed oil is detected when present in admixture with other oils by the Halphen colour test. The oil (1 ml) is dissolved in equal volume of amyl alcohol. A 1% solution of flowers of sulphur (1 ml) in carbon tetrachloride is added and the mixture heated for two hours on water bath. A red colour indicates the presence of Cottonseed oil.

Pharmacology

Gossypol, present in seeds and other parts, prolonged survival time of Ehrlich ascites tumor bearing mice. At higher dose, it caused loss of body weight and mortality. Gossypol produced marked negative inotropic and arrhythmogenic effects in guinea pig heart muscle. It markedly inhibited contractile responses of guinea pig lung parenchyma strip. Gossypol induced loss of K content of left ventricular myocardium together with depression of its contractility in isolated rabbit heart. Gossypol showed antitumor activity in SW-13 tumor-bearing nude mice and inhibited activity of aldose reductase from human placenta.

In addition to having insecticidal and various pharmacological properties, in humans it functions as a male antifertility agent. In China it was tested experimentally as a contraceptive with 12000 men. Drug is active in the therapy of menorrhagia, leimoyoma and and endometriosis. Endometrial atrophy occurred in all cases (67 women) and complete recovery of the endometrium was observed within 6 months of the cessation of gossypol treatment.

Gossypol acquires chirality by the restricted rotation of the bond connecting the two naphthyl moieties and so a pair of atropisomers exist. The compound isolated from the cotton plant was racemic, and this was used in the Chinese clinical trial. The gossypol enantiomer ratio appears to be species related. Thus, an excess of (+)-gossypol was found in the seeds of each variety tested of *Gossypium arboreum*, *G. herbaceum* (Asiatic cotton) and *G.hirsutum* (Upland cotton) whereas (−)-gossypol was in excess in each variety of *G. barbadense* (Egyptian, Tanguis or Pima cotton).

ALMOND OIL

Almond oil is a fixed oil obtained by expression from the seeds of *Prunus amygdalus* (Rosaceae) var. *dulcis* (sweet almonds), or *P. amygdalus* var. *amara* (bitter almonds). The oil is mainly produced from almonds grown in the countries bordering the Mediterranean (Italy, France, Syria, Spain and North Africa) and Iran.

Characters of plants and seeds

Almond trees are about 5 m in height. The young fruits have a soft, felt-like pericarp, the inner part of which gradually becomes sclerenchymatous as the fruit ripens to form a pitted endocarp or shell. The shells, consisting mainly of sclerenchymatous cells, are sometimes ground and used to adulterate powdered drugs.

The sweet almond is 2-3 cm in length, rounded at one end and pointed at the other. The bitter almond is 1.5-2 cm in length but of similar breadth to the sweet almond. Both varieties have a thin, cinnamon-brown testa which is easily removed after soaking in warm water. The oily kernel consists of two large, oily planoconvex cotyledons, and a small plumule and radicle, the latter lying at the pointed end of the seed. Some almonds have cotyledons of unequal sizes and are irregularly folded. Bitter almonds are found in samples of sweet almonds; their presence may be detected by the sodium picrate test for cyanogenetic glycosides.

Chemical constituents

Both varieties of almond contain 40-55% of fixed oil, about 20% of proteins, mucilage and emulsin. The bitter almonds contain in addition 2.5-4.0% of the colourless, crystalline, cyanogenetic glycoside amygdalin.

Almond oil is obtained by grinding the seeds and expressing them in canvas bags between slightly

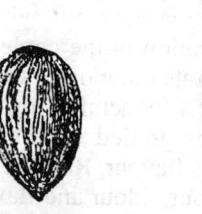

Bitter almond   Sweet almond

Fig. 17.17. Sweet almond.

heated iron plates. The oil is clarified by subsidence and filtration. It is a pale yellow liquid with a slight odour and bland nutty taste. It contains olein, with smaller quantities of the glycosides of linoleic and other acids. Bitter almonds, after maceration on hydrolysis of amygdalin yield a volatile oil that is used as a flavoring agent. Sweet almonds are extensively used as a food, but bitter almonds are not suitable for this purpose.

Essential or volatile oil of almonds is obtained from the cake left after expressing bitter almonds. This is macerated with water for some hours to allow hydrolysis of the amygdalin to take place. The benzaldehyde and hydrocyanic acid are then separated by stem distillation.

Almond oil consists of a mixture of glycerides of oleic (62-86%), linoleic (17%), palmitic (5%), myristic (1%), palmitoleic, margaric, stearic, linolenic, arachidic, gadoleic, behenic and erucic acid. Bitter almond oil contains benzaldehyde and 2-4% of hydrocyanic acid. Purified volatile oil of bitter almonds has all its hydrocyanic acid removed and, therefore, consists mainly of benzaldehyde. The unsaponifiable matter contains β-sitosterol, Δ^5-avenasterol, cholesterol, brassicasterol and tocopherols.

Uses

Expressed almond oil is an emollient and an ingredient in cosmetics. Almond oil is used as a laxative, emollient, in the preparation of toilet articles and as a vehicle for oily injections. The volatile almond oils are used as flavouring agents.

COCONUT OIL

It is the expressed oil of the dried solid part of the endosperm of the coconut, *Cocos nucifera* L. (Palmae). The plant is widely distributed throughout the tropics.

This tall tree rises to a height of 30 meters, has a tuft of leaves at the top, and bears 100 or more fruits (coconuts) each year. The fruit is a large drupe with hard endocarp and fibrous pericarp. The seed and its endocarp are termed as coconut in the commerce. The seed albumen is consisted of liquid (coconut milk) and solid (copra). Dry copra contains up to 65% lipids.

Coconut oil is a white, tasteless, odourless semisolid, melting at about 24°C and consisting of the triglycerides of mainly lauric and myristic acids, together with smaller quantities of caproic, caprylic, oleic, palmitic and stearic acids. This constitution gives it a very low iodine value (7.0-11.0) and a high saponification value. The oil consists of a mixture of glycerides in which 80 to 85% of the acids are saturated; it is a semisolid at 20°C. Lauric (43-51%) and myristic (16-21%) are the major fatty acids in addition to caprylic (~10%), capric, palmitic (~10%) and oleic (~10%) acids. The unsaponifiable matter contains carotenes and tocotrienols (80%).

The high proportion of medium chain-length acids means that the oil is easily absorbed from the gastrointestinal tract, which makes it of value to patients with fat absorption problems.

These low-molecular-weight acids give the oil a high saponification value, and coconut oil yields quality soaps and shampoos.

Coconut oil also contains glycerides of caprylic and capric acids (C_8 and C_{10} saturated fatty acids). A lipid fraction containing these medium chain triglycerides (MCT) is used when conventional food fats are not well digested or absorbed. Coconut oil and medium-chain triglycerides are ingredients in a number of combination products for oral administration as a balance dietary supple-ments.

Fractionated coconut oil

Fractionated and purified endosperm oil of the coconut contains triglycerides containing only the short and medium chain-length fatty acids (*e.g.*, octanoic, decanoic). It maintains its low viscosity until near the solidification point (about 0°C) and is useful as a nonaqueous medium for the oral administration of some medicaments.

PALM OIL

Palm oil is obtained by steaming and expression of the mesocarp of the fruits of *Elaeis guineensis* (Palmae); half of which is produced in Malaysia.

Palm oil is yellowish-brown in colour, of a buttery consistency (m.p. 30°C) and of agreeable odour. Palmitic (41-47%) and oleic (36-44%) acids are the principal esterifying acids, along with myristic, linoleic (6-12%) and stearic (~6%) acids.

Fractionated palm kernel oil

Palm kernel oil is obtained by heating the separated seeds for 4-6 hours to shrink the shell, which is then cracked and the kernels removed whole. The oil is then obtained by expression. It differs chemically from palm oil (above) in containing a high proportion (50%) of the triglycerides of lauric acid, a saturated, medium chain-length fatty acid. Fractionated Palm Kernel Oil is palm oil which has undergone selective solvent fractionation and hydrogenation. It is a white, brittle solid, odourless, m.p. 31°-36°C, used as a suppository base.

Evening primrose oil

The fixed oil from the seeds of *Oenothera* spp. (Onagraceae) contains esterified γ-linolenic acid (GLA), a $C_{18}6,9,12$-triene.

O. biennis yields an oil containing 7-9% GLA, higher yields for the oils of some other species are as *O. acerviphilla nova* (15.68%), *O. paradoxa* (14.41%) and an ecotype of *O. rubricaulis* (13.75%).

In animal tissues, the prostaglandins are formed from dietary linoleic acid by conversion to GLA which undergoes C_2 addition and further desaturation to give acids such as arachidonic acid, an immediate precursor of some prostaglandins.

The oil is now widely marketed as a dietary supplement, for cosmetic purposes, and for the treatment of atopic eczema and premenstrual syndrome.

Allied sources of GLA

A number of other seed oils contain appreciable quantities of GLA, these include those of *Ribes nigrum* and *R. rubrum* (the black and red currant), *Borago officinalis* (starflower) and *Symphytum officinale* (comfrey). *B. officinalis* yields an oil containing 25% GLA.

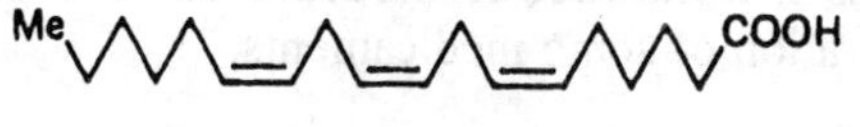

SOYBEAN OIL

Soybean is the ripe seed of *Glycine soja* (*G. max*) (Fam. Papilionaceae) an important food crop. The plant is an annual with trifoliate, hairy leaves, pale blue to violet flowers, and broad pods containing 2 to 5 seeds. The seeds are compressed, spheroidal or ellipsoidal, and vary in colour from white to yellow-green or brownish black. The seeds contain carbohydrates (35%), protein substances (50%), fixed oil (20%), and the enzyme, urease.

Soybeans are used medicinally as a food in diabetes and as a general food for humans and livestock.

Soybean oil is the refined, fixed oil obtained from the seeds of the soya plant. The oil is obtained by pressure, up to 10%. It consists of a mixture of glycerides of linoleic (50%); oleic (30%); linolenic (7%); saturated acids, chiefly palmitic and stearic (14%). It is a drying oil with an iodine value between 120 and 141 and is not useful as a cooking oil. The unsaponifiable matter contains β-sitosterol stigmasterol, campesterol, Δ^5-avenasterol and tocpherols.

Soybean oil is an ingredient in parenteral nutrients and is a source of lecithin.

Lecithin is an ingredient in a number of proprietary products that are useful in controlling deranged lipid and cholesterol metabolisms. Stigmasterol, obtained from the lipid fraction of soybeans, can be used as a precursor for steroidal hormones. The oil is used in the manufacture of varnishes, insulators and other products.

Partially hydrogenated soybean oil is an ingredient in a number of combination products for oral administration used as balanced dietary supplements.

Soybean cake, the residue after pressing out the oil, has a high value as a livestock food and contains a large amount of protein, some oil, and the 5% of ash consists largely of potassium and phosphorus.

Soybean meal is the flour prepared from the decorticated, ground seed of *Glycine soja* deprived of fat. It can be used for the detection of urea

γ-Linolenic acid (GLA)

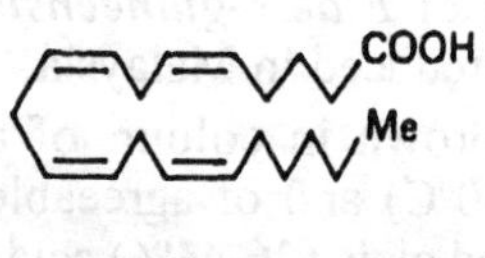

Arachidonic acid

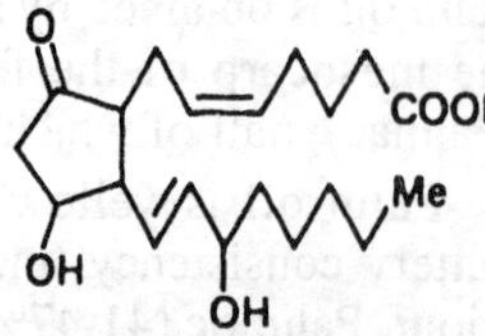

Prostaglandin E₂ (PGE₂)

Fig. 17.18. Unsaturated fatty acids.

nitrogen in blood serum by the enzymatic action of the urease in the soybean meal.

CORN OIL

Corn oil is the refined oil obtained from the embryo of *Zea mays* Linn. (Fam. Poaceae).

The oil-rich embryos (called germs) are separated by a flotation process during the preparation of corn starch. After the embryos are washed free of starch and gluten, they are subjected to pressure and heat to express the oil. The *germ oil cake* is used as cattle feed (*oil cake meal*). The crude oil is clarified by filtering and settling and refined by removing the fatty acids, refrigerating, filtering, and sterilizing. Corn oil is a clear, light yellow, oily liquid with a faint characteristic odour and taste.

The oil consists of a mixture of the tri-glycerides of linoleic (50%), oleic (37%), palmitic (10%), linolenic, arachidic, gadoleic, behenic, erucic and stearic (3%) acids. Due to high unsaturation (iodine value 110-128), it is a valuable diet factor and it lowers blood cholesterol levels.

The unsaponifiable matter contains β-sitosterol, compesterol and γ- and α-tocopherols.

Corn oil is used as a solvent for injections; for irradiated ergosterol. It is an edible oil and is used in salads and in the preparation of food. An emulsion containing 67% of corn oil is used as a high-calorie dietary supplement. Corn oil is also an ingredient in a number of combination products for oral administration that are used as balanced dietary supplements. When hydrogenated, the oil becomes semisolid and is used as a shortening for baking.

The oil should be protected from light and oxygen and stored at a temperature not exceeding 25°C.

SAFFLOWER OIL

Safflower seed oil is the fixed oil obtained from the seeds of *Carthamus tinctorius* Linn. (Fam. Asteraceae).

The oil consists of a mixture of glycerides linoleic acid (75%), oleic acid (18%) and a mixture of saturated acids (about 6%).

An emulsion containing 50% of Safflower oil is used orally as a high-calorie dietary supplement. Safflower oil is an ingredient in products that are balanced dietary supplements.

SUNFLOWER OIL

Sunflower oil is the fixed oil obtained from the seeds of cultivated varieties of *Helianthus annuus* Linn. (Fam. Asteraceae).

The oil consists of a mixture of glycerides that are rich in unsaturated acids. The poly-unsaturated acid content of sunflower oil is influenced by climate and genetics. The linolenic acid content ranges from 50 to 75%, the higher percentages occurring in oils from seeds grown in the cooler or northern temperate regions. Oleic acid is present up to 23% Glycerides of palmitic (3-10%), stearic and linoleic are also presents. Trilinoleate and oleodilinolein each represent about 1/3 of the triacylglycerols. The unsaponifiable matter contains β-sitosterol (60%), Δ^7-stigmasterol, Δ^5-avenasterol and α-tocopherol. The oil is used as an alternative to Corn oil and Safflower oil for culinary purposes, and it is an ingredient in a number of dietary supplements.

Ethiodized oil injection

Ethiodized oil is an iodine addition and steriled product of the ethyl ester of the fatty acids of poppy seed oil. It contains not less than 35.2% and not more than 38.9% of organically combined iodine. It decomposes when exposed to air and sunlight, becoming dark brown in colour.

Ethiodized oil is radiopaque and is used as a diagnostic aid in hysterosalpingography and lymphography.

WAXES

Waxes are the esters of higher straight-chain fatty acids with long-chain or high molecular weight monohydric alcohols, some containing more than 30 carbons in the chain. Waxes may be of plant origin such as Carnauba wax or of animal origin such as Beeswax, Wool-fat and Spermaceti.

In many ways, waxes are identical to fats, but they are more difficult to saponify. Fats may be saponified by aqueous or alcoholic alkalies but waxes are only saponified by alcoholic alkalies. Waxes are distinguished from fats and oils by their low saponification values and very low iodine value due to the presence of saturated acids.

Waxes usually contain esters of the free acids, hydrocarbons, free alcohols and sterols. The hydrocarbons and sterols are unsaponifiable. In plants, waxes are present on the outer cell walls of epidermal tissue. They protect the loss of water or its penetration to the inner part. Waxes are used in pharmaceuticals for hardening cosmetic creams and ointments and in preparation of cerates.

An important practical difference between fats and waxes is that fats may be saponified by means of either aqueous or alcoholic alkali but waxes are only saponified by alcoholic alkali. This fact is used for the detection of fats when added as adulterants to waxes, *e.g.*, for detecting the fat 'Japan wax' as an adulterant in beeswax. Saponification of the wax ester cetyl palmitate yields cetyl alcohol and potassium palmitate.

$C_{15}H_{31}COOC_{16}H_{33}$+alcoholic KOH $\rightarrow$ $C_{16}H_{33}OH$
Cetyl palmitate   Cetyl alcohol
                                   + $C_{15}H_{31}COOK$
                                   Potassium
                                   palmitate

The fats consist almost entirely of esters. Waxes are esters of the cetyl palmitate type and contain appreciable quantities of free acids, hydrocarbons, free alcohols and sterols. The hydro-carbons and sterols are unsaponifiable and both spermaceti and wool fat have high saponification values. The acid values of waxes are higher. The beeswax contains about 15% of free cerotic acid $C_{26}H_{53}COOH$. In most waxes, iodine values are relatively low and unsaponifiable matter is high.

LANOLIN

Synonyms

Wool fat; Oesipos; Agnin; Alapurin; Agnolin; Lanum; Lanain; Lanalin; Lanesin; Lanichol; Anhydrous lanolin; Adeps lanae; Laniol.

Biological source

Lanolin is the fat-like purified secretion of the sebaceous glands of sheep, *Ovis aries* Linn. (Fam. Bovidae) which is deposited into the wool fibres. It contains about 25-30% water.

Preparation

Wool is cut and washed with a soap or alkali. An emulsion of wool fat, called as wool grease, takes place in water. Raw lanolin is separated by crack-

ing the emulsion with sulphuric acid. Wool grease floats on the upper layer and fatty acids are dissolved in the lower layer. Lanolin is purified by treating with sodium peroxide and bleaching with reagents.

Characters

Lanolin is a yellowish white, tenacious, unctuous mass; odour is slight and characteristic. Practically, it is insoluble in water, but soluble in chloroform or ether with the separation of the water. It melts in between 34-40°. On heating it forms two layers in the beginning, continuous heating removes water. Lanolin is not saponified by an aqueous alkali. However, saponification takes place with alcoholic solution of alkali.

Anhydrous lanolin is a yellowish tenacious, semisolid fat with slight odour, mp 38-42°. Practically it is insoluble in water but mixes with about twice its weight of water without separation. It is sparingly soluble in cold, more in hot alcohol, freely soluble in benzene, chloroform, ether, carbon disulphide, acetone and petroleum ether.

Chemical constituents

Lanolin is a complex mixture of esters and polyesters of 33 high molecular weight alcohols, and 36 fatty acids. The alcohols are of three types: aliphatic alcohols, steroid alcohols, and triterpenoid alcohols. The acids are also of three types: saturated nonhydroxylated acids, unsaturated nonhydroxylated acids and hydroxylated acids. Liquid Lanolin is rich in low molecular weight, branched aliphatic acids and alcohols while waxy Lanolin is rich in high molecular weight, straight-chain acids and alcohols.

The chief constituents of Lanolin are cholesterol, isocholesterol, unsaturated monohydric alcohols of the formula $C_{27}H_{45}OH$, both free and combined with lanoceric ($C_{30}H_{60}O_4$), lanopalmitic ($C_{16}H_{22}O_3$), carnaubic and other fatty acids. Lanolin also contains esters of oleic and myristic acids, aliphatic alcohols, such as cetyl, ceryl and carnaubyl alcohols, lanosterol and agnosterol.

Uses

Lanolin is used as an emollient, as water absorvable ointment base in many skin creams and cosmetic and for hoof dressing. Wool fat is readily absorbed through skin and helps in increasing the absorption of active ingredients incorporated in the ointment. However, it may act as an allergenic contactant in hypersensitive persons.

BEESWAX

Synonyms

Yellow beeswax, White beeswax; Cera flava; Cara alba.

Biological source

Beeswax is obtained by purifying the honeycomb of *Apis mellifica* or *A. mellifera* and other bees. (Family : Apidae).

Geographical source

The beeswax is prepared in West Indies, California, Chile, Africa, Jamaica, Madagascar and India.

Preparation

Yellow Beeswax : Wax is secreted in cells on the ventral surface of the last four segments of the abdomen of worker bees. The wax comes out through pores in the chitinous plates and is used to form the comb for storing the honey. After separation of the honey, the honeycomb is melted in water and cooled. The water-soluble impurities are removed, stained and allowed to solidify in suitable moulds to get yellow beeswax.

White beeswax

It is prepared from the yellow beeswax by bleaching with charcoal, potassium permanganate, chromic acid and chlorine or slow bleaching with sunlight, air and water. For slow bleaching the melted wax is fell on a revolving moist cylinder. Ribbon-like strips of wax are formed which are exposed to sunlight and air. The strips are frequently moistened and turned until the outer surface is bleached.

Characters

The beeswax is yellowish to brownish-yellow or white pieces or plates, translucent when thin, soft to brittle, honey-like odour, slight balsamic taste, density 0.95-0.96, mp 62-65°. It is practically insoluble in water, slightly soluble in cold alcohol, soluble in hot alcohol, chloroform, benzene, ether, and carbon disulphide. It is soft and brittle, but becomes plastic on warming. On cooling it hardens and breaks with a flaky granular surface.

Chemical constituents

Beeswax consists mainly of myricyl palmitate (myricin) (~80%), myricyl stearate, free cerotic acid (15%) and its homologues, an aromatic substance cerolein, hydrocarbons (~12%), lactones, moisture, cholesteryl ester, pollen pigments, and propolis (bee glue). The colour of the wax is due to the presence of pollen pigments and propolis. The esters consist of straight-chain monohydric alcohols with even-numbered carbon chains from C_{24} to C_{36} esterified with straight-chain acids also having even number of carbon atoms up to C_{36}. The other examples of esters are triacontanol hexadecanoate and hexacosanol hexacosanoate. These esters are mixed with about 20% of hydrocarbons having odd numbered straight carbon chains from C_{21} to C_{33}.

The other constituents are 1,3-dihydroxyflavone, ω-myristolactone, lacceryl palmitate, myricyl cerotate, myricyl hypogaeate and ceryl hydroxypalmitate. The main alkane components are hentriacontane and nonacosane. The unsaturated hydrocarbon, melene, is also present. The free acids present are lignoceric, cerotic, montanic and psyllic acids; cerotic acid being the predominant saturated free acid. Palmitic, hydroxypalmitic and hypogaeic (7-hexadecenoic) acids are also reported.

Uses

Beeswax is used to prepare plasters, ointments, cerates, face creams, wax paper, candles, modelling artificial fruits and flowers, in process engraving and shoe polish.

Yellow wax is a stiffening agent and is an ingredient in yellow ointment. It is also used as a base for cerates and plasters. Commercially, it is contained in a number of polishes.

White wax is employed pharmaceutically in ointment and in cold creams.

A beeswax and vegetable oil mixture is used as a vehicle for the administration of respiratory forms of certain medicaments such as penicillin and curare. It is used in the formulation of medicinal preparations for treating skin cracks. A combination containing of tallow, olive oil, camphor, beeswax and common salt is used for ulcer and external tumour treatment.

$$C_{15}H_{31}COOC_{30}H_{61} \qquad C_{26}H_{53}COOH$$
Myricin   Cerotic acid

Adulterants

Beeswax is adulterated with solid paraffin, ceresin, carnauba wax, Japan wax (Fat of the fruits of *Rhus* species; family Anacardiaceae), stearic acid and colophony. Japan wax is not a true wax but a fat and may be saponified by means of boiling aqueous sodium hydroxide. Waxes are saponified by strong alcoholic potash, but are practically unaffected by aqueous alkali.

Detection of adulteration

1. On heating the wax with aqueous sodium hydroxide, cooling and acidifying, there should be no turbidity. Beeswax is a true wax and on saponification the cerotic acid does not form soap. The adulterated substances form water soluble components on treatment with alkali.
2. Wax is hydrolyzed with alcoholic alkali by heating, and cooled by stirring. It should be cloudy between 59-61°C and not above 61°.

CARNAUBA WAX

Carnauba wax is obtained from the leaves of *Copernicia cerifera* (Palmae). It is removed from the leaves by shaking and purified to remove foreign matter.

The wax is hard, light brown to pale yellow in colour and is supplied as a moderately coarse powder, as flakes or irregular lumps. It is usually tasteless with a slight characteristic odour and free from rancidity. Esters, chiefly myricyl cerotate, are the principal components, with minor consti-tuents. The acid value is low, the saponification value 75-95 and iodine value 7-14. Carnauba wax is used in pharmacy as a tablet-coating agent and in other industries for the manufacture of candles and leather polish. It has been suggested as a replacement for beeswax in the preparation of phytocosmetics.

It is used in the manufacture of candles, varnishes, leather and furniture polishes and in place of beeswax.

PROSTAGLANDINS

Prostaglandins are C_{20} lipid metabolites formed in the body from essential, unsaturated fatty acids of the diet. prostaglandins occur in nearly all mammalian tissues in low concentrations. The major prostaglandins are grouped into 4 main classes designated as prostaglandins A, B, E, and F. All prostaglandins (PG) have a cyclopentane ring with 2 aliphatic side chains. Subscripts indicate the number of double bonds in the side chains and the stereochemistry of members of each group.

Constituents in human semen could produce contraction and relaxation of the human uterus. Mammalian cells and tissues may respond differently (stimulation or inhibition of a biologic process) to individual prostaglandins; in some cases, this response may be a concentration factor. Prostaglandins act at the level of the cell membrane, and they may modulate the transmission of hormonal or other extracellular stimuli into cyclic AMP for the internal regulation of cellular stimuli into cyclic AMP for the internal regulation of cellular functions. Pharmacologic effects of these compounds involve contraction or, in some cases, relaxation of smooth muscles of the female reproductive system, the cardiovascular system, the intestinal tract, and the bronchi. They also influence gastric secretion and renal function.

The prostaglandins have diverse pharmacologic effects, and their therapeutic potential transcends that of the steroids. The PGE_2, PGF_{2a}, or 15-methyl PGF_{2a} are used for termination of second trimester pregnancies and PGE_1 for palliative therapy to maintain temporarily neonates with patent ductus arteriosus. Various prostaglandins are used to induce labor at term (PGE_2), to prevent premature labor (PGE), to induce menstruation (PGE), to increase fertility in certain conditions (PGE), to manage some types of hypertension (PGA_1 and PGE_2), to control certain cardiac arrhythmias (PGF_{2a}), to correct some defects in red blood cells (PGE), to exert antithrombogenic and thrombolytic activity (PGE_1), to control asthmatic seizures (PGE_1), to inhibit gastric secretions in the treatment of peptic ulcers (PGE) and to treat several other conditions.

Prostaglandin F$_{2a}$

Prostaglandin F1$_{2a}$, PGF$_{2a}$, or dinoprost is available as the tromethamine salt for use in terminating second trimester pregnancy. It stimulates contractions of the gravid uterus that are similar to the contractions of the term uterus at labor. Side effects are usually related to the contractile effect of PGE$_{2a}$; the action may extend to smooth muscle of the gastrointestinal tract, producing vomiting and diarrhoea, and to smooth muscle of the vascular system, causing elevation in blood pressure.

PGE$_{2a}$ is rapidly inactivated in the lungs and other body tissues. Two metabolic processes have been identified as participating in the inactivation of this prostaglandin: reduction of the unsaturated bond at position 13 and oxidation of the 15-hydroxyl group to a keto function. A short duration of action is usually considered desirable for oxytocic agents, but it could present a problem in other potential therapeutic applications.

The usual dose of PGF$_{2a}$ is 40 mg by slow injection into the amniotic sac. If the abortion process has not been established or completed with 24 hours, an additional dose of the drug may be administered.

15-methylprostaglandin F$_{2a}$

15-Methylprostaglandin F$_{2a}$, 15-methyl PGF$_{2a}$, or carboprost is the 15-methyl analog of PGF$_{2a}$. The 15-methyl substituent precludes metabolic inactivation via oxidation of the 15-hydroxyl group and permits a substantially different dosage regimen. It is available as the tromethamine salt, it elicits pharmacologic responses similar to those of PGF$_{2a}$, and it is used in terminating second trimester pregnancy.

The usual initial dose of 15-methyl PGF$_{2a}$ is 200 µg by deep intramuscular injection; the dosage may be repeated at 1.5 to 3.5 hour intervals, depending on uterine response. The total dose should not exceed 12 mg, and the therapeutic duration should not exceed 2 days.

Prostaglandin E$_2$

Prostaglandin E$_2$, PGE$_2$, or dinoprostone is another uterine stimulant used for termination of second trimester pregnancy. PGE$_2$ differs from PGF$_{2a}$ only in that the 9-oxygen substituent is a keto group. PGE$_2$ is available as a vaginal suppository that should be stored at a temperature below –20°C.

A 20 mg suppository is inserted intravaginally every 3 to 5 hours until abortion occurs, but the maximum dose should not exceed 240 mg. The pharmacologic effect of PGE$_2$ are similar to those of PGF$_{2a}$. There is the lack of vasoconstriction and resulting hypertension with high doses of PGE$_2$. The adverse reactions are vomiting, pyrexia, diarrhoea, nausea, headache and chills.

Prostaglandin E$_1$, *PGE$_1$, or alprrostadil* differs from PGE$_2$ only in the reduction of the unsaturated bond at position 5. PGE$_1$ produces vasodilation, inhibits platelet aggregation, and stimulates intestinal and uterine smooth muscle. It is used for palliative therapy to maintain temporarily neonates with patent ductus arteriosus and congenital heart defects that restrict the pulmonary or systemic blood flow. The dilated ductus arteriosus facilitates blood oxygenation and body perfusion pending surgical correction of the congenital defects.

PGE$_1$ is metabolized rapidly by oxidation of the 15-hydroxyl group, and the drug is administered by continuous intravenous infusion of the lowest dosage that maintains the desired response. The initial infusion rate is usually 0.1 µg per kg of body weight per minute. It is available in 1 ml ampules containing 500 µg of the drug.

CHAPTER

18

Volatile Oils

Volatile or essential oils are mono- and sesquiterpenes obtained from the sap and tissues of certain plants. They are flavouring compounds and have been used in perfumery from the ancient times. On exposition to air at room temperature they evaporate. Chemically, they are composed of hydrocarbons of the general formula $(C_5H_8)_n$ and their oxygenated, hydrogenated, and dehydrogenated derivatives. All the volatile oils are of vegetable origin.

The thermal decomposition of volatile oils gives isoprene as one of the products. Therefore, essential oils are built up of isoprene units. These units are joined 'hand-to-tail' in natural terpenoids.

In most instances the volatile oil pre-exists in plant. Volatile oils may be present in particular secretory parts such as glandular hairs, parenchyma cells, vittae or oil tubes, in mesophyll (Eucalyptus leaves), sub-epidermal tissues of Lemon and Orange, in lysigenous or schizogenous passages, in all tissues (Conifers), in petals (Orange, Rose), in bark and leaves (Cinnamon), in pericarp (Umbelliferous fruits), in glandular hairs of the stems and leaves (Mint), and in rind (Orange). Plants containing essential oils usually have the greatest concentration at some particular time, e.g., jasmine at sunset. In some cases volatile oil does not pre-exist, but is formed by the decomposition of a glycoside (in Black Mustard).

Four general methods of extraction of volatile oils are as :

1. steam distillation,
2. expression,
3. extraction by means of volatile solvents and
4. adsorption in purified fat.

Steam distillation is one of the most widely used method. In this method the plant is macerated and then steam distilled to get the oil. If some compounds are decomposed under these conditions, they may be extracted with light petrol at 50° and the solvent is removed by distillation under reduced pressure. Adsorption in fat is the alternate method used for isolation of volatile compounds. In this method, the fat is heated to 50°C and the flower petals are spread on the surface until it becomes saturated with essential oils. Then the petals are removed to dissolve the oils present in fat. Fat is removed by cold alcohol at 20°C. The alcoholic extract is fractionally distilled under reduced pressure to remove the solvent.

Volatile oils are colourless liquids and are lighter than water. They possess distinct odours, have high refractive indices, generally are optically active. They are immiscible with water, but the water shaken with an essential oil possesses its flavour due to slight solubility of the oil. Volatile oils are freely soluble in ether, alcohol, chloroform and acetone.

Each volatile oil differs widely in chemical composition. Usually hydrocarbons, alcohols, ketones, aldehydes, ethers, oxides and esters are present in volatile oils. Some of the essential oils possess high percentage of a particular compound e.g., eugenol in Clove oil (85%), allylisothiocyanate in Mustard oil (93%), menthol in Peppermint oil (~70%), and α-terpineol in Pine oil (~65%).

Volatile oils differ from fixed oils in various ways. The former oils are evaporated at room temperature, and can be distilled from their natural sources. They are not glyceryl esters of fatty acids and, therefore, cannot be saponified with alkalies. Volatile oils are not rancidified like fixed oils. On exposure to air and light, they oxidize and resins are formed.

Volatile oil containing drugs are used in perfumery, cosmetic, as insect repellents and as flavouring agents to mask the taste and smell of unpleasant medicines. They act as counter-irritants in inflammation and rheumatism. They have carminative, digestive, spasmolytic, stimulant, bacteriocidal, antiseptic, disinfectant, diuretic, expectorant and anthelmintic properties.

A volatile oil may contain hydrocarbons which are usually devoid of aroma. The other constituents of the oil are monoterpenes which are isomeric substances of the formula $C_{10}H_{16}$, but they vary considerably in structures. All terpenes are optically active. The important terpenes are pinenes, limonene, phellandrene and camphene. Sesquiterpenes of the general formula are also present in an essential oil. They are usually the highest-boiling fraction of the oil. The principal sesquiterpenes are caryophyllene and cadinene.

Volatile oils are mixtures of a number of biologically active constituents. They generally consist of an *eleoptene*, the hydrocarbon portion of the oil, which is liquid, and one or more *stearoptenes*, the oxidized hydrocarbon portions of the oil, which are usually solid. Thus, peppermint herb shows its activity to the volatile oil due to the stearoptene, menthol. Peppermint oil is used for different purposes than is menthol since the oil also contains menthyl acetate, menthone, cineole and other components. Stearoptenes are generally obtained by freezing the oil or by other methods. Menthol, thymol, and anethole are solid stearoptenes, whereas eucalyptol, eugenol, and methyl salicylate are liquids.

Chemistry of volatile oils

In most cases, volatile oils are mixtures containing different types of compounds. These compounds may be separated by low temperatures, fractional distillation; fractional crystallization from solvents; different forms of chromatography and removal by chemical action. Chemically, compounds with free acidic groups may be removed from the oil with sodium carbonate, basic compounds may be removed with hydrochloric acid, phenols with sodium hydroxide and aldehydes with sodium bisulphite.

There are chemical separation techniques based on capillary-column gas chromatography and high-pressure liquid chromatography, coupled with computerized instruments that combine gas chromatography with mass spectrometry (GC-MS), have led to the precise identification of the components of volatile oils.

Many volatile oils consist mainly of *terpenes*. Terpene units arise from acetate via mevalonic acid and are branched-chain, 5-carbon units containing 2 unsaturated bonds.

$$CH_3$$
$$|$$
$$CH_2{=\!=}C{-}CH{=\!=}CH_2$$
$$\text{Isoprene, } C_5H_8$$

Monoterpenes are composed of 2 isoprene units and have the molecular formula. $C_{10}H_{16}$. Sesquiterpenes, $C_{15}H_{24}$, contain 3 isoprene units. Diterpenes, $C_{20}H_{32}$, have 4 isoprene units, and triterpenes, $C_{30}H_{48}$, are composed of 6 isoprene units. The terpenes found most often in volatile oils are monoterpenes. They can occur in acyclic, monocyclic, and bicyclic forms as hydrocarbons and as oxygenated derivatives, such as alcohols, aldehydes, ketones, phenols, oxides and esters.

Another major group of volatile oil consti-tuents are the *phenylpropanoids* which contain the C_6 phenyl ring with an attached C_3 propane side chain. Many of the phenylpropanoids found in volatile oils are phenols or phenol ethers. In some cases, the carbon side chain has been linked to give a C_6-C_1 structure, such as in methyl salicylate and vanillin.

The physiologic responses elicited by each isomer can differ. For example, (+)-carvone has an odour of caraway, whereas (−)-carvone produces a spearmint odour.

Different kinds of olfactory receptor sites are present in the nose. Odourant molecules could lodge on these sites and would have shapes and sizes (varying stereochemistry) that were complementary to the shape and size of the particular receptor. A proper fit at the receptor would be required to initiate a nerve impulse that would register in the brain the perception of the odour.

The various constituents of volatile oils are responsible for the characteristic odours, flavours, and therapeutic properties of the oils. A chemical classification of the oils is based on their principal chemical constituents. Unoxygenated terpenes sometimes account for a large percentage of the oil. The stearoptene, which is present in smaller quantities, represents the constituent that is responsible for imparting the characteristic odour or flavour. The following are the divisions in which volatile oils and volatile oil containing drugs are placed : (1) hydrocarbons, (2) alcohols, (3) aldehydes, (4) ketones, (5) phenols, (6) phenolic ethers, (7) oxides and (8) esters.

The *stereochemistry* of the volatile consti-tuents determines the type of olfactory response evoked by the compounds. Geometric isomers, whether *ortho/meta/para* or *cis/trans*, are in most cases distinguished both as to quality and strength of odour. Both *enantiomers* (optically active isomers) exist in nature. In some cases, a plant species produces only one of the enantiomers, whereas a different species may produce both. Among the monoterpenes that occur as the (+) form in certain species and as the (–) form in others are limonene, α-terpineol, α-fenchol, borneol, menthone, carvone and linalool. In addition, limonene, α-terpineol, α-fenchol, carvone and camphor can be found in plants as the racemic mixture.

Hydrocarbon volatile oils

Hydrocarbons are present in all volatile oils. Limonene is the most widely distributed of the monocyclic terpenes. It occurs in Citrus, Mint, Myristica, Caraway, Thyme, Cardamom, Coriander, and many other oils. Another monocyclic hydrocarbon monoterpene is *p*-cymene, present in Coriander, Thyme, Cinnamon, and Myristica oils. Pinene, a dicyclic monoterpene, is also widely distributed. It occurs in many conifer oils and in Lemon, Anise, Eucalyptus, Thyme, Fennel, Coriander, Orange flower and Myristica oils. Sabinene, a dicyclic monoterpene of the thujane class, present

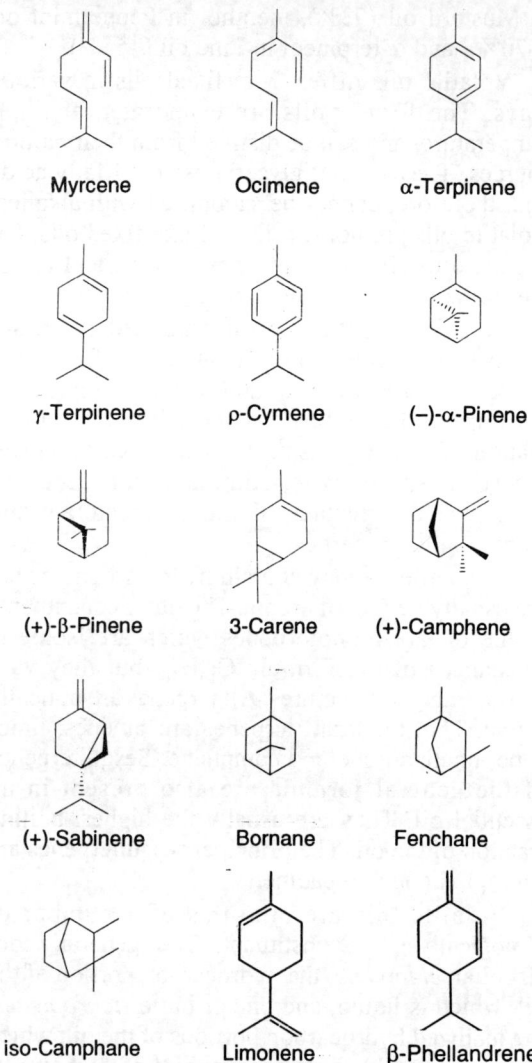

Fig. 18.1. Monoterpene hydrocarbons.

in cardamom and lemon oils. Acyclic monoterpene myrcene occurs in Myricia, Lemon, and Myristica. Cadinene occurring in juniper tar, is a sesquiterpene hydrocarbon. β-Caryophyllene is a sesquiterpene found in Wormwood, Peppermint, Cinnamon and Clove oils.

A volatile oil drug composed mainly of hydrocarbons is turpentine oil.

Alcohol volatile oil

Alcohols found in volatile oils are classified as : (1)

acyclic alcohols, (2) monocyclic alcohols and (3) dicyclic alcohols. Methyl, ethyl, isobutyl, isoamyl, hexyl and the higher aliphatic alcohols occur in volatile oils. They are soluble in water, hence, they are washed away in the process of steam distillation. Many natural oils contain acyclic alcohols, geraniol, linalool and citronellol. The important monocyclic alcohols are menthol (from Peppermint) and α-terpineol; borneol is a dicyclic terpene alcohol from Borneo camphor. Sesquiterpene alcohols include zingiberol santalols and artemisin..

The important alcohol volatile oil containing drugs are Peppermint, Cardamom oil, Coriander oil, Rose oil, Orange flower oil, Juniper oil and Pine oil.

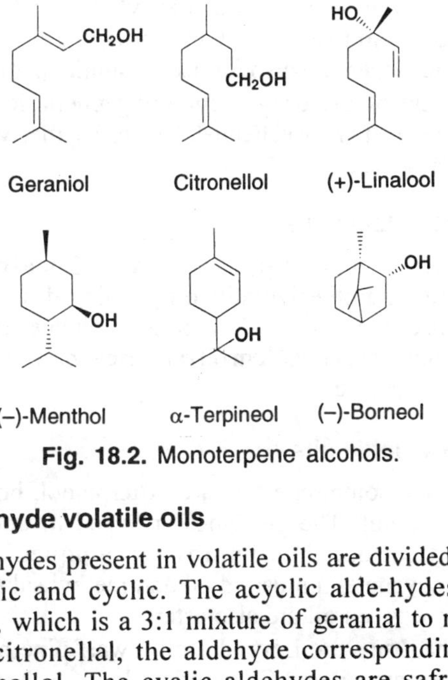

Geraniol   Citronellol   (+)-Linalool

(–)-Menthol   α-Terpineol   (–)-Borneol

Fig. 18.2. Monoterpene alcohols.

Aldehyde volatile oils

Aldehydes present in volatile oils are divided into acyclic and cyclic. The acyclic alde-hydes are citral, which is a 3:1 mixture of geranial to neral, and citronellal, the aldehyde corresponding to citronellol. The cyclic aldehydes are safranal,

Citral   Geranial   Neral   (+)-Citronellal

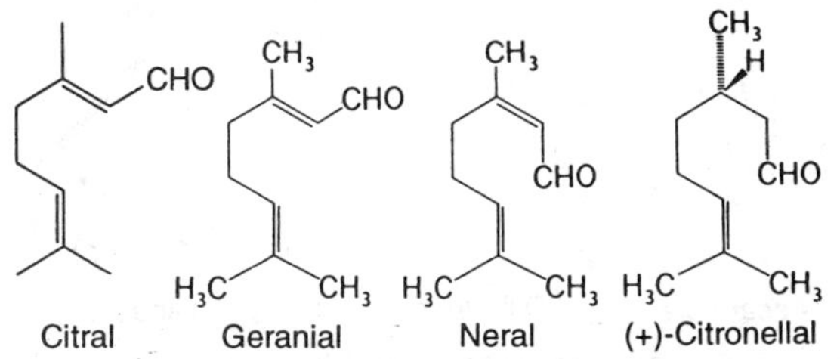

Fig. 18.3. Monoterpene aldehydes.

phellandral, photocitral A and myrtenal. The aromatic aldehydes include cinnamaldehyde and vanillin (vanilla, Benzoin, Tolu and Peru balsams).

Biosynthesis of aromatic aldehydes as benzaldehyde and vanillin takes place from phenylpropanoid precursors. These compounds constitute the aglycones of certain glycosides.

The terpene aldehydes are formed by acetate metabolism.

The important drugs in this class are Cinnamon, Cinnamon oil, Orange oil, Lemon peel, Lemon oil, Hamamelis water and Citronella oil.

Ketone volatile oils

Ketones present in volatile oils are divided into (1) monocylic terpene ketones, e.g., menthone, carvone, piperitone, pulegone and diosphenol; (2) dicyclic ketones, including camphor, fenchone, and thujone and (3) acyclic ketone, e.g., artemisia ketone and tagetone..

The important drugs in this category are Camphor, Spearmint, and Caraway.

Phenol volatile oils

Two kinds of phenols occur in volatile oils: those that are present naturally and those that are produced as the result of destructive distillation of certain plant products.

Eugenol, thymol and carvacrol are important phenols found in volatile oils. Eugenol occurs in Clove oil, Myrcia oil and other oils; thymol and carvacrol occur in Thyme oil, Ajowan oil and

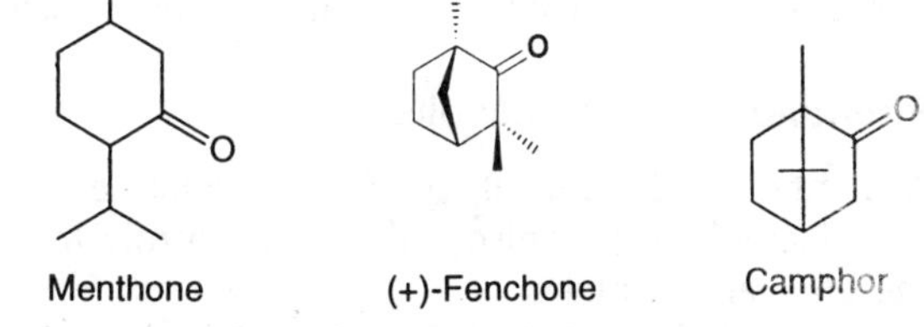

Tagetone   (+)-3-Thujone   (–)-Carvone

Menthone   (+)-Fenchone   Camphor

Fig. 18.4. Monoterpene ketones.

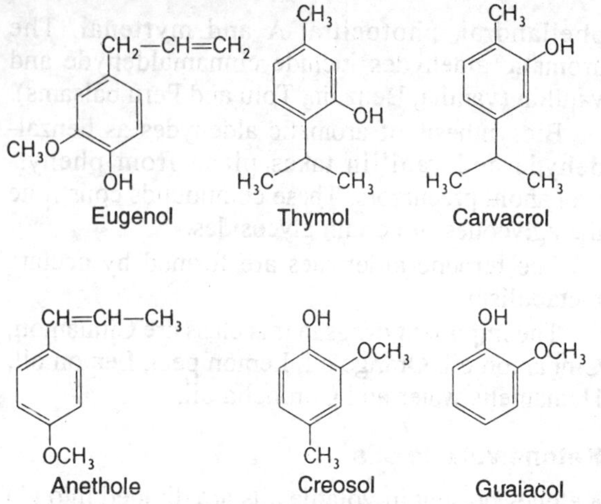

Eugenol Thymol Carvacrol

Anethole Creosol Guaiacol

Fig. 18.5. Phenols.

creosol and guaiacol are present in creosote and pine tar.

The more important drugs containing phenol volatile oils are Thyme, Clove, Myrcia oil, Creosote, Pine tar and Juniper tar.

Thymol is a phenol obtained from Thyme oil (*Thymus vulgaris*), from horsemint oil (*Monarda punctata*), from *Monarda didyma* oil, from ajowan oil (*Carum copticum*), or it may be prepared synthetically from *m*-cresol or *p*-cymene. The oil is freeze-cooled to crystallize thymol, or it is treated with sodium hydroxide solution, the aqueous solution of sodium thymol being separated and decomposed with acid, thus liberating the thymol, which is subsequently purified.

Thymol occurs as large colourless crystals or as a white crystalline powder. It has an aromatic thyme-like odour and a pungent taste. Thymol is micro-sublimed.

Thymol is an antifungal and antibacterial agent. It is used topically in lotions, creams, and ointments in concentrations ranging from 0.1 to 1%, in the feminine hygiene products, in the otic products, in the external analgesics; and in mouthwash.

Phenolic ether volatile oils

A number of phenolic ethers occur in volatile oils, e.g., anethole from Anise and Fennel, safrole from sassafras and Nutmeg.

Derivatives of safrole are also often found in

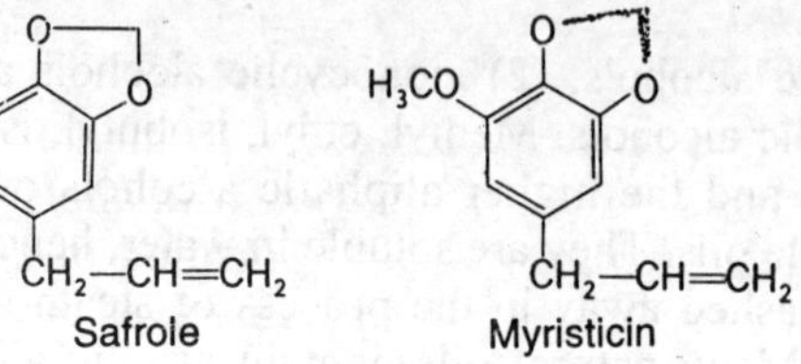

Safrole Myristicin

Fig. 18.6. Phenolic ethers.

volatile oils; *e.g.,* myristicin (methoxysafrole) in nutmeg.

Biosynthesis of phenolic ethers

In *Foeniculum vulgare* formation of anethole takes place from phenylalanine (shikimic acid-phenyl-propanoid pathway) via a number of intermediates. Methionine serves as a methyl donor for the methoxylation reaction. Other structurally related phenolic ethers are also formed by similar pathways.

Some of the drugs containing phenolic ether volatile oil are Anise, Fennel, Clove, Thyme, Myrcia and Myristica.

Oxide volatile oils

Cineole (eucalyptol) is found in Eucalyptus, Cajuput and other volatile oil-yielding drugs. The presence of limonene-1,2-epoxide, pinene oxides, ascaridole (chenopodium oil) and ascaridole epoxide is also reported.

Ester volatile oils

The most common esters are of terpineol, borneol and geraniol. The perfumes are aged to undergo esterification, thus improving bouquet. Allyl isothiocyanate in mustard oil and methyl salicylate in wintergreen oil are also esters.

The drugs are Lavender oil, dwarf pine needle oil, Mustard oil and Gaultheria oil.

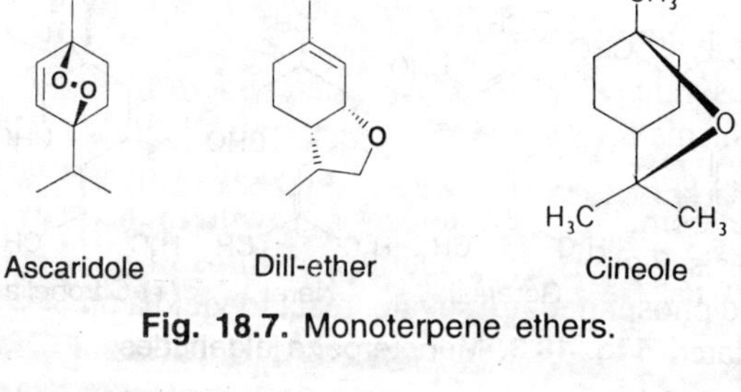

Ascaridole Dill-ether Cineole

Fig. 18.7. Monoterpene ethers.

Biosynthesis of esters

Terpene esters are generally formed from the respective alcohols by reaction with aliphatic acid moieties, *e.g.*, acetic acid. Formation of aromatic esters, *e.g.*, methyl salicylate, involves the reverse process; that is, the aromatic acid reacts with an aliphatic alcohol (commonly methanol) to form the ester.

Labeled cinnamic acid has been incorporated into methyl salicylate by *Gaultheria procumbens*. The reactive form of cinnamic acid is presumably an ester of coenzyme A. The biosynthetic pathway involves *o*-hydroxylation of the cinnamic acid and subsequent side-chain degradation.

Biosynthesis of volatile oil constituents

The biosynthetic building blocks for *terpenes* are isoprene units which are isopentenyl pyrophos-phate and dimethylallyl pyrophosphate. These compounds arise from acetate via mevalonic acid. Geranyl pyrophosphate is the C-10 precursor of the terpenes and plays a key role in the formation of mono-terpenes. It is formed by the condensation of one unit each of isopentenyl pyrophosphate and dimethylallyl pyrophosphate. Geranyl pyrophosphate is the direct precursor to acrylic monoterpenes. It is isomerized to neryl pyrophosphate before the cyclic monoterpenes can be formed since the *trans* isomer does not have the correct stereochemistry for cyclization. Another possibility is the formation of neryl pyrophosphate from isopentenyl pyrophosphate and dimethylallyl pyrophosphate independent of a geranyl pyrophosphate step. The intermediates in the formation of the cyclic terpenes occur as carbonium ions.

Cinnamic acid and *p*-hydroxycinnamic acid, (*p*-coumaric acid) are the principal precursors for *phenyl-propanoid* compounds. In plants, these compounds arise from the aromatic amino acids phenylalanine and tyrosine, respectively, which in turn are synthesized via the shikimic acid pathway. This biosynthetic pathway has been shown in microorganisms by using auxotrophic mutants of *Escherichia coli* and *Enterobacter aerogenes* that require the aromatic amino acids for growth. In the biosynthesis, 2 glucose metabolites, erythrose 4-phosphate and phosphoenolpyruvate, react to yield a phosphorylated 7-carbon keto sugar, DAHP. This compound cyclizes to 5-dehydroquinic acid, and is then converted to shikimic acid. Shikimic acid, through a series of phosphorylated intermediates, yields an important branch-point intermediate, chrismic acid. One branch leads to anthranilic acid and then to tryptophan. The other branch is converted to prephenic acid, the last nonaromatic compound in the sequence. Prephenic acid can be aromatized by dehydration and simultaneous decarboxylation to yield phenylpyruvic acid, the direct precursor of phenylalanine or by dehydrogenation and decarboxylation to yield *p*-hydroxyphenylpyruvic acid, the precursor of tyrosine.

Cinnamic acid is formed by the direct enzymatic deamination of phenylalanine, and *p*-coumaric acid can originate similarly from tyrosine or by hydroxylation of cinnamic acid at the *para* position.

Umbelliferous plants (Family Apiaceae)

Volatile oils are most frequently present in the pericarp of Umbelliferous fruits. The plants are erect and possess alternate, undivided or divided leaves, base of stalks often dilated and sheathing the stem. Flowers are small, usually less than 1.2 cm diameter, regular, polygamous, in umbels, rarely in heads. Umbels are compound or simple, with or without bracts and bracteoles at the base of the primary and secondary rays, respectively.

Medicinal fruits derived from plants of the family Apiaceae all of one type, are known as a *cremocarp*. The cremocarp is a variety of schizocarp or splitting-fruit which divides into one-seeded portions each corresponding to one carpel; the carpel itself does not open to liberate the seed, hence these schizocarps are indehiscent fruits. The cremocarp consists of two carpels, each containing one seed, and is derived from an inferior ovary. At the summit of the fruit there may be five small inconspicuous sepals or a slight rim representing the calyx and in the centre are the two styles surrounded below by the disc-like nectary and forming the *stylopod*. When the fruit splits, it divides vertically along the septum between the carpels, the two halves being termed mericarps. Each mericarp, therefore, has a flat surface, the commissural surface, and a rounded surface, the dorsal surface. From the central line of each commissural surface of a fine thread separates, being attached basally to the

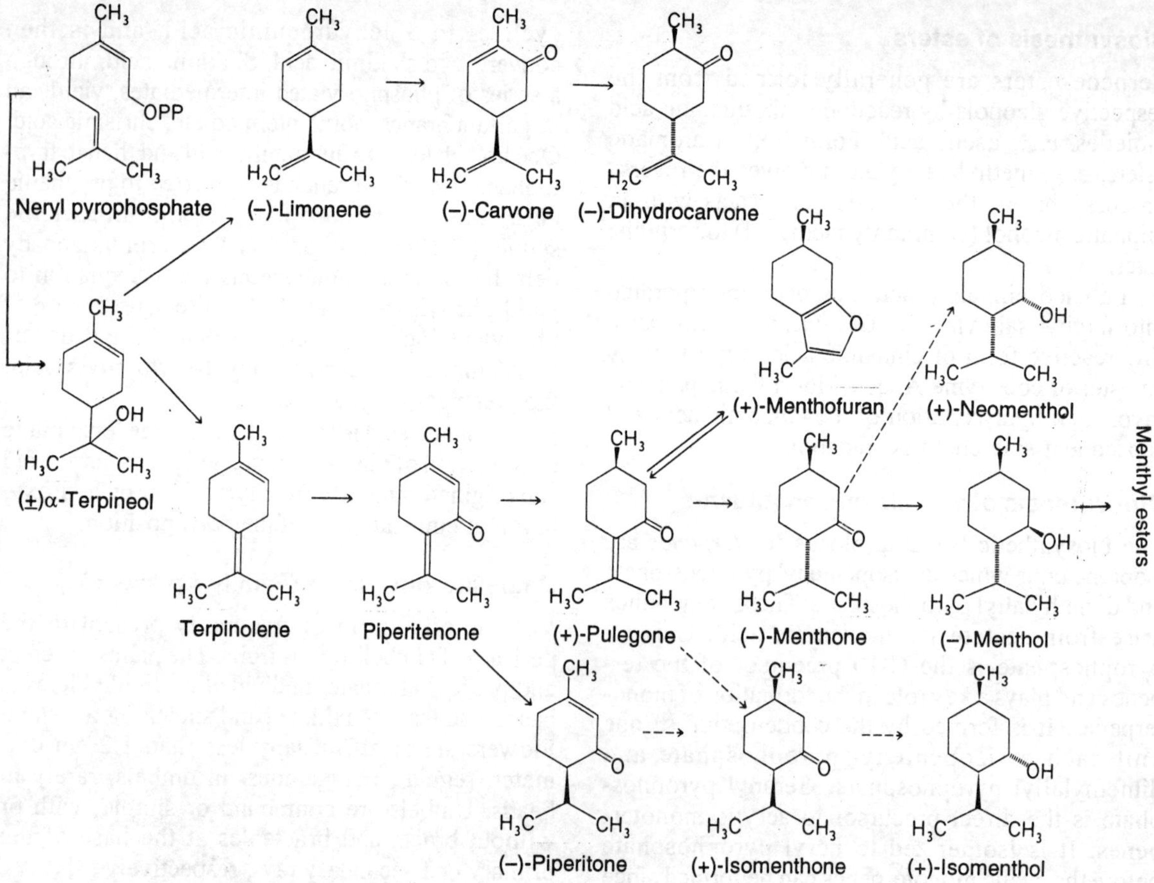

Fig. 18.8. Biosynthesis of monoterpenes.

pedicel and apically to the upper end of the mericarp; this thread is termed a *carpophore*. By the action of the wind or other disturbance the mericarps break loose from the carpophores and are scattered.

The Umbelliferous fruits are schizocarps (splitting), dried, consisting of two one-seeded, indehiscent carpels, which separate from a very slender, simple or forked, central axis. They have transversed longitudinal five ridges or wings, the central ridge being called the dorsal, two marginal the lateral and the remaining two the intermediate ridges.

The seed in each mericarp is attached by its testa to the pericarp so that it completely fills the loculus. The seeds contain a small embryo at the apical end, embedded in an abundant oily endosperm. In the majority of these fruits there are schizogenous

ducts extending through the mesocarp from base to apex; each duct is termed a *vitta* and the number and position of the vittae are often characteristic of individual fruits. Usually there are two vittae on the commissural surface and four on the dorsal surface. The ovules are anatropous and consequently on the commissural surface of each seed a fine vascular strand, the raphe, extends from base to apex in the central line of the testa, which is wider in that region than elsewhere. The number, distribution and arrangement of the vittae and ridges afford valuable characters for the identification of individual fruits.

The carpels are also often furnished with internal, longitudinal oils-canals or vittae, which are best seen in cross sections.

Schizocarps are simple dry indehiscent fruits.

They split into partial fruits possessing seeds in each part. Umbelliferous fruits are cremocarps in which the fruits split into two partial fruits, called mericarps, and is derived from inferior bicarpellary biocular ovary. Each mericarp possesses a stylopod at it apex. Stylopod is a disc-like nectary with style and remains of calyx. There are two surfaces of mericarps - the outer dorsal or curved surface and the inner, ventral or commisural surface. On the surface of mericarp five longitudinal, straight or wavy, conspicuous or inconspicuous ridges are present which join apex to the base. These ridges are called primary ridges due to the presence of vascular bundles below the ridges. In Coriander, secondary ridges are present alternatively with primary ridges. Vascular bundles are not present under the secondary ridges.

Coriander, Fennel, Caraway, Dill and Anise, are the important drugs belonging to Apiaceae family.

CORIANDER

Synonyms

Coriander fruit, Dhaniya (Hindi); Fructus coriandri.

Biological source

Coriander is the dried, ripe fruits of *Coriandrum sativum* Linn. (Family : Apiaceae).

Geographical source

Coriander is indigenous to Italy. It is extensively cultivated in Holland, central and eastern Europe, Morocco, Malta, Egypt, China, India and Bangladesh.

Collection

Coriander is an annual herb, about 0.7 m high with small white or pinkish flowers. Fruits are collected when ripe and dried. Aromatic odour is developed on drying the fruits.

Coriander is generally grown as a rain-fed crop. The time of sowing varies in different localities. Before sowing the fruits are rubbed till the two mericarps are separated and sown either broadcast or in rows. The crop requires 2 or 3 weedings and the field is irrigated whenever required. The crop matures in about 3 months after sowing. The plants are then pulled out by the roots and after drying, the fruits are threshed out. They are further dried in the sun, winnowed and stored in bags.

Morphology

The drug consists of entire cremocarps, 2.3-4.3 mm in diameter, shape sub-spherical. Cremocarps consist of two hemispherical mericarps united by their margins. On the surface there are ten primary ridges which are wavy and inconspicuous. Alternating to primary ridges there are eight more prominent, straight, secondary ridges. The colour is straw-yellow, odour is aromatic and taste is spicy. Fresh plant emits a very disagreeable odour on rubbing.

The Indian variety is oval. The spherical varieties vary in size.

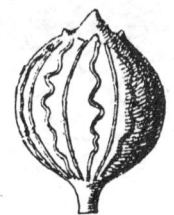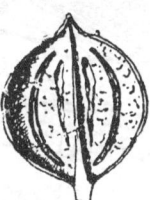

Fig. 18.9. Coriander.

Microscopical characters

A transverse section of a fully ripe fruit shows only two mature vittae in each mericarp on the commissural surface. The numerous vittae present in the immature fruit on the dorsal surface of each mericarp gradually join and are compressed into slits. The outer part of the pericarp possesses stomata and prisms of calcium oxalate. Within the mesocarp a thick layer of sclerenchyma is formed, which consists of pitted, fusiform cells. These sclerenchymatous fibres tend in the outer layers to be longitudinally directed and in the inner layers to be tangentially. Near primary ridges more of the fibres are longitudinally directed; in the secondary ridges all are tangentially directed. In position to the primary ridges there are small vascular strands composed of a small group of spiral vessels. The mesocarp within the sclerenchymatous band is composed of irregular polygonal cells with lignified walls. The inner epidermis of the pericarp is

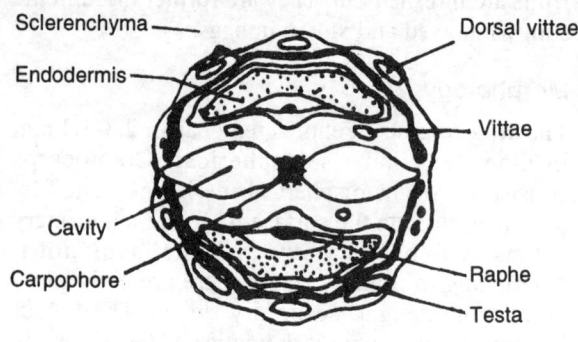

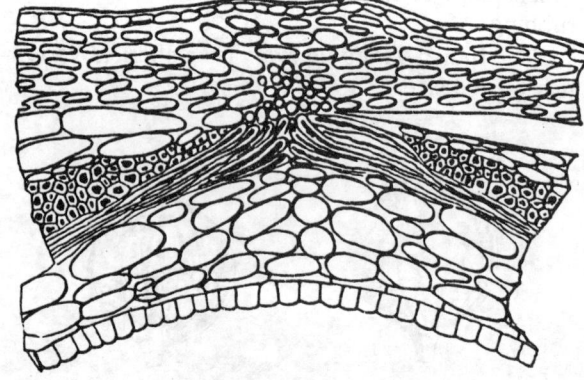

Fig. 18.10. T.S. coriander.

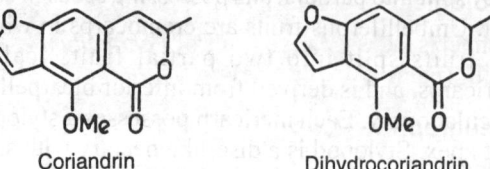

Fig. 18.11. Lectones of coriander.

composed of 'parquetry' cells, which in the powder are often seen united to the cells of the inner mesocarp. The testa is composed of brown flattened cells. The endosperm is curved and consists of parenchymatous cells containing fixed oil, aleurone grains and rosettes of calcium oxalate.

Chemical constituents

Coriander fruits contain volatile oil (2%). The prominent constituents of the volatile oil are (+)-linalool (65-70%) and pinene. Small amounts of geraniol, borneol, *p*-cymene, dipentene, phellandrene, terpinolene, α-and β-terpinenes, geraniol, *n*-decylic aldehyde, limonene, β-phellandrene, 1,8-cineol, β-caryophyllene, citronellol, thymol, linalyl acetate, geranyl acetate, caryophyllene oxide, elemol, methylheptenone, fixed oils, malic acid, esters of acetic and decylic acids, tannins, and mucilage are also present. Coriander oil is a colourless, pale yellow liquid, having characteristic odour

and taste. The fruits also contain fatty oil (~28%) which is a mixture of glycerides of palmitic, oleic, linoleic, petroselinic, lauric, myristic, myristoleic and palmitoleic acids.

The high content of fats (16-28%) and protein (11-17%) in the fruits make a distillation residues suitable for animal feed. The fruits yield 5-7% of ash.

The unripe plants and their volatile oils have an unpleasant, mousey odour due to the presence of aldehydes such as *n*-decanal contained in peripheral vittae. Marked changes occur in volatile oil composition during ontogenesis; the peripheral vittae flatten, lose their oil, and is then produced by the commissural vittae.

The seeds also contain β-sitosterol, D-mannitol, chlorogenic and caffeic acids, umbelliferone, scopoletin, triacontane, triacontanol, tricosanol, psoralen, angelicin, β-sitosterol glucoside, neocnidilide, Z-ligustilide, coriandrinonediol, gnaphalosides A and B, quercetin, isorhamnetin, rutin, luteolin, coriandrin, dihydrocoriandrin, coriandrones A and B.

Uses

Coriander is aromatic, stimulant, carminative, antibilious, diuretic, tonic, stomachic, refrigerant and aphrodisiac. It is used as flavouring agent to conceal the odour of other medicines and to correct the griping qualities of Rhubarb and Senna. Linalool is isolated from the oil as a starting material for other derivatives. Pharmaceutically coriander and its oils are used as a flavouring agent and carminative.

FENNEL

Synonyms

Large Fennel, Sweet Fennel, Fennel fruit, Saunf (Hindi); Fructus Foeniculi.

Biological source

Fennel is the dried, ripe fruits of *Foeniculum vulgare* Mill. (Family : Apiaceae).

Geographical source

Fennel is indigenous to Mediterranean region of Asia and Europe. It is widely cultivated in Russia, India, Japan, southern Europe, China and Egypt.

Cultivation

Fennel is a stout, glabrous, aromatic herb and cultivated as a garden or homeyard crop at all altitudes up to 2,000 m. It grows in any good soil, but thrives best in rich, well-drained loam or black sandy soil containing sufficient lime. It is propagated readily by seeds, but can also be grown by root or crown division. Seeds are sown broadcast by hand or by shallow drill in October-November in the plains and March-April on the hills.

The plants are thinned out to about 30 cm apart. Occasional weeding and irrigation once a week are done. The crop is harvested before the fruits are fully ripe. The stems are cut with the sickle and spread out loose to dry in the sun. The dried fruits are threshold out and cleaned by winnowing.

Fennel plant is a stout, glabrous, aromatic herb, about 2 m high, leaves pinnately decompound; flowers small, yellow, in compound terminal umbels.

Morphology

The drug consists partly of whole cremocarps and partly of mericarps. The fruit is 0.5-1.0 cm long, 2-4 mm broad. Shape is slightly curved and oval.

Surface is glabrous with 5 straight prominent straw-coloured primary ridges and bifid stylopod at the apex. Colour is greenish-brown, odour is aromatic and taste is distinct, sweet and aromatic.

Microscopical characters

Transverse section of Fennel mericarp shows commisural and dorsal surfaces. The commisural surface is flat containing two pronounced ridges and carpophore in the middle. The dorsal surface has five ridges. Mericarp is divided into pericarp, testa and bulky endosperm. The epicarp (exocarp) of the pericarp encircles the entire mericarp and consists of a layer of polygonal, tangentially elongated cells with smooth cuticle.

The mesocarp is made of parenchyma and bicollateral vascular bundles below the primary ridges. Vascular bundles are surrounded by reticulate and lignified parenchyma. Yellowish brown and elliptical vittae (schizogenous ducts), four on the dorsal surface and two on the commissural surface, are present in the mesocarp.

Endocarp contains cells in a single layer between mesocarp and testa. The testa is single layered and yellowish brown in colour.

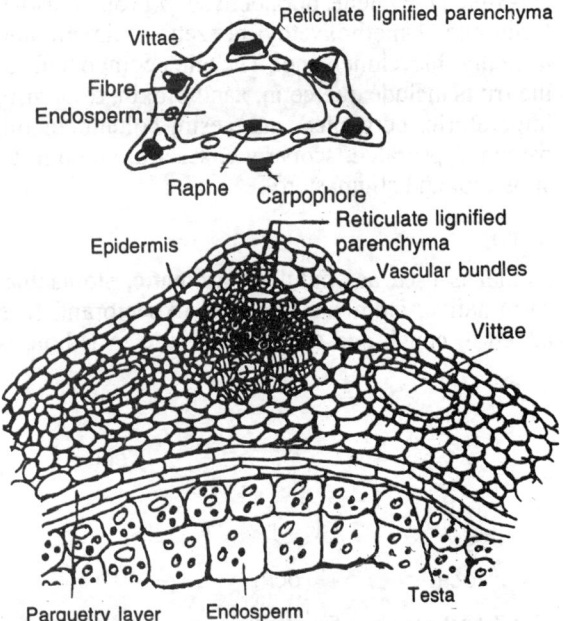

Fig. 18.13. Transverse section of Fennel fruit. (a) Mericarp (diagrammatic), (b) Cellular.

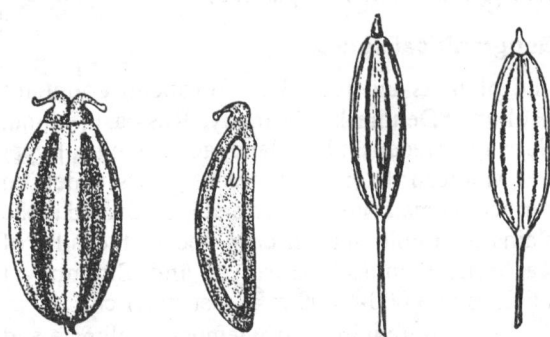

Fig. 18.12. Fennel fruit.

Endosperm consists of thick-walled, polygonal, colourless parenchyma. It contains aleurone grains and oil globules. A crescent shaped embryo is seen in sections through the apical region of mesocarp. Raphae is present in the middle of commissural surface in front of carpophore.

Chemical constituents

Fennel contains volatile oil (2-6.5%) and fixed oil (12%). The main constituent of the volatile oil are phenolic ether, anethole (50-60%) and the ketone, fenchone (18-20%) which give the fruit its distinct odour and taste; the other constituents of volatile oil are anisic aldehyde, anisic acid, α-pinene, dipentene and phellandrene. Minor constituents include monoterpene hydrocarbons such as limonene; anisaldehyde and estragole (methyl chavicol). Anethole is derived via the shikimic acid pathway and fenchone (a bicyclic monoterpene) is formed from fenchol by the action of a dehydrogenase.

The essential oil also contains camphene, feniculin, C_{27}-C_{33} paraffin, C14:0-C18:3 fatty acids petroselinic acid, C_{24}-C_{30} free alcohols, anisoxide, γ-terpinene, *p*-allyl-anisole, γ-cadinene, thujene, car-3-ene, *p*-cymene, duraldehyde, *p*-propylanisole, farnesene, 1-methoxyethyl-benzene, ocimene and trimethyl-bicycloheptanol. The other components of the fruits include quercetin, xanthotoxin, α-amyrin, imperatorin, bergapten, marmesin, columbianetin, osthenol, psoralen, scoparone, seselin, vanillin, β-sitosterol and stigmasterol.

Uses

Fennel is used as stimulant, aromatic, stomachic, carminative, emmenagogue and expectorant. It is added to cough and stomach mixture. Anethole is used in mouth and dental preparations. Fennel is used in diseases of the chest, spleen and kidney.

Pharmacology

Oral administration of a seed extract to male rats decreased total protein concentration in testes and vas deferens but increased it in seminal vesicles and prostate gland. In female rats, there was increase in weight of mammary glands, oviduct, cervix and vagina.

Adulterants

Fennel is generally adulterated with exhausted Fennel. The alcohol-exhausted Fennel looks like fresh Fennel and contains 1-2% volatile oil. The steam-exhausted Fennel fruits are darker in appearance. They contain little volatile oil and are heavier than water. It is also adulterated with undeveloped or mould-attack fruits.

Sweet Fennel is derived from *F. vulgare*, subsp. *vulgare*, var. *dulce*. The fruits resemble those of the bitter variety but have a sweet taste and lower volatile oil content (not less than 2.0%) of different composition. Not less than 80% of the oil is required to be anethole, not more than 7.5% fenchone, and not more than 10% estragole.

CARAWAY

Synonyms

Caraway fruit; Caraway seed, Carvi, Carum, Zira (Hindi), Fructus carvi.

Biological source

Caraway consists of the dried, ripe fruits of *Carum carvi* Linn. (Family : Apiaceae).

Geographical source

The plant is cultivated in European countries (Holland, Denmark, Germany, Russia, Finland, Norway, Sweden and England) and in China, Egypt and Morocco. In India the plant grows widely in northern Himalayan regions, and is cultivated in the plains as a cold season crop and in the hills of Kashmir, Kumaon, Garhwal and Chamba at altitudes of 3,000-4,000 m as a summer crop.

The plant requires a dry temperate climate and thrives well in soils rich in humus. The fruits may

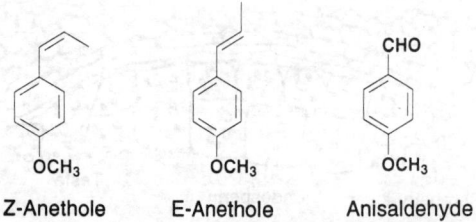

Z-Anethole   E-Anethole   Anisaldehyde

Fig. 18.14. Volatile constituents of Fennel.

be sown either broadcast or in rows. The fruits are collected before ripening. The plants are dried, the fruits threshed out, cleaned and stored in bags.

Morphology

Caraway is a perennial or biennial herb, about 1 m high with thick tuberous roots and compound leaves. The fruits consist of mericarps without pedicels. They are 4-7 mm long, 1 mm broad, slightly curved, smooth and tapering at both ends. There are five primary ridges, stigma is attached and a stylopod at the apex. The colour is brown, odour and taste are characteristic and spicy.

Microscopical characters

A transverse section of a caraway mericarp shows five primary ridges, in each of which is a vascular strand along with pitted sclerenchyma and with a single secretory canal at the outer margin of each. There are six flattened and elliptical vittae which extend from the base of the fruit to the base of the stylopod. They are lined with small, dark reddish-brown cells and contain a pale yellow or colourless oleoresin. The raphe lies on the inner side of the endosperm, which is nongrooved. The endosperm contains thickened cellulose walls deposits of a β-(1,4)-mannan as a reserve polysaccharide, fixed oil, aleurone grains and one or two microrosettes of calcium oxalate. The embryo, which is situated near the apex of the mericarp, is only be seen in sections passing through that region.

The outer epidermis of the pericarp is glabrous and has a striated cuticle. The mesocarp consists of collapsed parenchyma and lacks the reticulated cells of fennel. The endodermis consists of a single layer of elongated cells, arranged parallel to one another and without the 'parquetry' arrangement of coriander.

Chemical constituents

Caraway contains volatile oil (3-7%), fixed oil (8-20%), proteins, calcium oxalate, colouring matter, resins, sugar, tannins and mucilage. Monoterpenes identified in the volatile oil are carvone (50-60%), dihydrocarvone, limonene, carveol and dihydrocarveol.

The major constituents in fruit oil of Israeli plant are β-pinene, myrcene, 3-carene, γ-terpinene, p-cymene, myristicin, carveol-acetate, 4-terpineol, perillyl alcohol, cuminaldehyde; germacrene-D and β-elemene.

The seed lipids contain hydrocarbons, triglycerols, waxes, free fatty acids, alcohols, sterols and petrosetinic acid.

Uses

Caraway is used as aromatic, carminative, antispasmodic, stomachic, lactagogue, flavouring agent and as a spice.

CUMIN (Jira)

Cumin consists of the dried ripe fruits of *Cuminum cyminum* (Apeaceae), a small, annual plant indigenous to Egypt. It is cultivated in England, Sicily, Malta, Mogadore and India. Spain and Egypt are the major cumin oil producers.

Cumin fruits are about 6 mm long and resemble caraway. The mericarps are straighter than those of caraway and are densely covered with short, bristly hairs. Whole cremocarps are attached to short pedicels and isolated mericarps. Each mericarp has four dorsal vittae and two commissural ones. The odour and taste are coarser than those of caraway.

Cumin yields 2.4-4.0% of volatile oil. This contains 25-35% of aldehydes (cuminic aldehyde), pinene and α-terpineol.

DILL

Synonyms

Dill fruit, Fructus Anethi.

Biological source

Dill is the dried, ripe fruits of *Anethum graveolens* Linn. Indian Dill consists of dried ripe fruits of *Anethum sowa* Kurz. (Family : Apiaceae).

Source

Dill is cultivated in England, Germany, Rumania and USA. Indian dill is grown throughout India.

Cultivation

A. graveolens is an annual, erect, glabrous herb, 1 m in height, cultivated to a small extent in the plains. It prefers sandy loam soil of moderate fertility and avoids low lying damp areas. It is grown as a cold weather crop in Indian plains. The seeds are sown in October in rows and the seed crop is harvested by the end of April. Germination takes in 7 to 9 days. Flowering commences between 40-67 days after germination. Application of nitrogenous and phosphatic fertilizers increases yield on medium fertile lands. The crop is given 4 to 6 irrigations. The harvested umbels are dried in shade for 2 to 3 days and threshed. The dried seeds are stored in gunny bags lined with polythene to reduce storage loss of volatile oil.

Morphology

The drug consists of separate, broadly oval mericarps, 3-4 mm long, 2-3 mm wide, 1 mm thick. The fruit is dorsally compressed and has 5 primary yellow-coloured ridges. The two lateral ridges are extended as thin wings, the remaining three are inconspicuous. Stylopod is present at the apex of each mericarp. The colour is brown; odour and taste are aromatic and spicy.

Microscopical characters

Each mericarp has four vittae on the dorsal surface and two on the commissural. The outer epidermis has a striated cuticle and the mesocarp contains lignified, reticulate parenchyma. The endosperm is much flattened.

Chemical constituents

Dill contains volatile oil (3-4% and the principal constituent of the oil is carvone (50-60%). The other components of the oil are dihydrocarvone, d-limonene and phellandrene. The Indian variety contains essential oil from 2.5 to 6.0%, which consists of carvone (22-46%), dihydrocarvone (5-25%), dillapiole (12-15%), limonene (22-45%), isoeugenol, d-phellandrene, α-terpinene, carveol, α-pinene, anethofuran, carvacrol, methyl benzoate, 1,5-cineole, p-cymene, safrole, α-terpinene, dillapional, isodillapiole, 8-dehydro-p-cymene and linalyl acetate.

Isodillapiole tribromide showed fungicidal activity against *Helminthosporium oryzae* and *Aspergillus niger*. The plant showed appetite stimulating property.

In addition to volatile oil, the other compounds isolated from the fruits are myristicin, coumarins (bargapten, umbelliprenin scopoletin, esculetin), flavonoids (quercetin, isorhamnetin kaempferol, kaempferol-3-glucuronide, glucoflavone, dillanoside), phenolic acids (caffeic, ferulic and chlorogenic acids), sterols (γ-sitosterol, β-sitosterol glucoside), phytofluene, piperine, piperitone and dihydrobenzofuran.

Uses

Dill is used as carminative, stomachic, diuretic, anthelmintic, antiflatulant and flavour, to cure gastric disturbances of children and for preparation of dill water and gripe water.

ANISE

Synonyms

Anise fruit, Anise seed, Star anise; Fructus Anisi.

Biological source

Anise is the dried ripe fruit of *Pimpinella anisum* Linn. (Family : Apiaceae).

Geographical source

The plant is native to Asia Minor, Egypt and Greece and widely cultivated in Spain, Germany, Italy, Russia, Bulgaria, Chile and Mexico. In India the drug is grown in north-west region, U.P., Punjab and Orissa.

Morphology

The plant is an annual herb. The fruit is ovoid or pyriform, entired, compressed cremocarps attached to pedicles, 2-12 mm in length. Cremocarps are 3-6 mm long and 2-3 mm broad. There are five wavy ridges on each mesocarp. Outer surface contains short, numerous, conical epidermal trichomes (papillae). Odour is aromatic and taste is sweet.

Microscopical characters

Microscopically the epidermis bears numerous papillae and unicellular hairs. On the dorsal surface of each mericarp are 15-45 branched vittae. A small amount of vascular tissue and reticulated parenchyma is present. The endosperm is slightly concave on the commissural surface and contains protein and fixed oil.

The oil is a clear, colourless or pale yellow

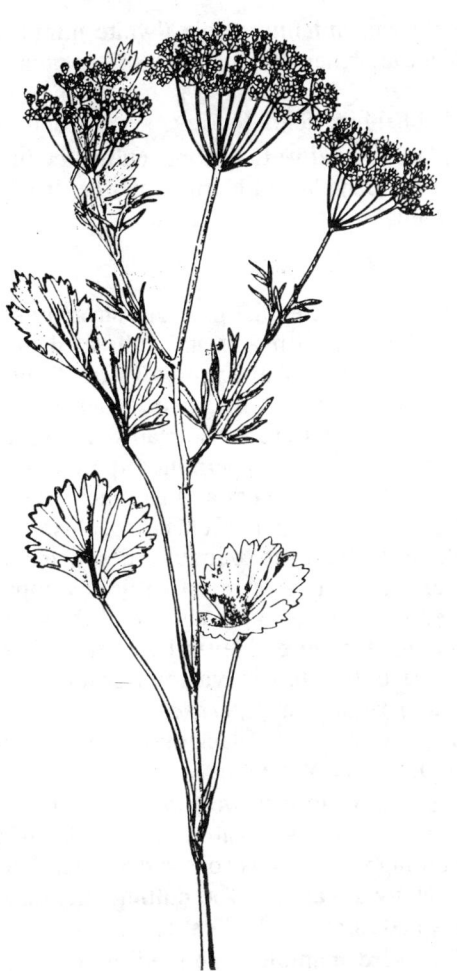

Fig. 18.15. *Pimpinella anisum.*

liquid, free from water, crushed fruit like odour and sweet and aromatic taste. It crystallizes on cooling.

Chemical constituents

Anise fruit contains volatile oil (1.5-3.5%), starch protein and fixed oil (30%). The principal constituent of the volatile oil is anethole (90%), rest being *p*-methoxyphenyl acetone, methyl chavicol, chavicol, terpenic hydrocarbons, carvone, β-caryophyllene, dihydrocarvyl acetate, estragole, limonene, α-pinene, comphene, phellandrene, anisketone, cinnamic aldehyde, β-elemene, *trans*-α-bergamotene and cinnamyl alcohol.

The fruits also contain mannitol, luteolin, its

7-O-glucoside and xyloside, 4-O-β-D-glucosylbenzoic acid and phenylpropenyl esters.

Anethole exhibited antibacterial activity. Phenylpropenyl ester inhibited germination of tested seeds, *e.g.*, carrot, ryegrass and lettuce.

Uses

Anise fruit is diuretic and carminative and used to prevent flatulence colic, as flavouring agent and in mouth and dental preparations. Anethole is employed as expectorant, aromatic, carminative and flavouring agent.

STAR-ANISE OIL

Biological source

It is a volatile oil obtained from the fruits of the Chinese Star-anise, *Illicium verum* (Family : Illiciaceae).

Habitat

The Star-anise is an evergreen tree, about 4-5 m in height, indigenous to the south-west states of China and other tropical countries. The fruits are collected and the oil distilled locally in China and Vietnam.

The fruits consist mostly of eight one-seeded follicles. Each follicle is about 1.5 cm in length. The pericarp is reddish-brown, woody and slightly wrinkled. Each carpel has the seed which has a brittle, shining testa and oily kernel. The beak of each carpel is not turned upwards and the fruit stalk, which is about 3 cm long, is curved (distinction from *I. religiosum*). The oil, present in both seed and pericarp, gives the drug an aromatic odour and spicy taste.

Bastard star-anise or *shikimi fruits* are derived from *I. religiosum*, a species cultivated in Japan. The carpels are equal in number to those of *I. verum*

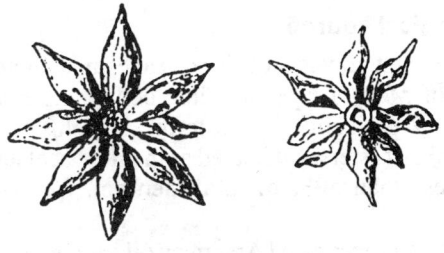

Fig. 18.16. Star-anise fruits.

but are smaller, wrinkled and have a curved-up apex. The stalk is shorter than the genuine fruit, are poisonous and contain toxic substances sikimitoxin and sikimin, sesquiterpene lactones (anisatin-like compounds).

Chemical constituents

The fruits yield a volatile oil (2.5-5%) which contains anethole (80-90%) as the main component. The other compounds present in the oil are chavicol methyl ether, *p*-methoxy-phenyl acetone, safrole, anisoxide, α- and β-pinenes, β-myrcene, α-phellandrene, car-3-ene, *p*-cymene, limonene, cineole, (4(10)-thujene, linalool, 4-terpineol, α-terpineol, estragole, anisaldehyde, copaene, anisketone, sesquicitronellene, caryophyllene, β-bergamotene, methyl 3-methoxy-benzoate, farnesene, methylisoeugenol, β-bisabolene, nerolidol, *m*-methoxy-α-methylbenzene acetic acid and feniculine.

The fruits also contain kaempferol, its 3-rutinoside and 3-galactoside, quercetin and its rhamnoside, 3-rutinoside and 3-xyloside, fixed oil composed of glycerides of myristic, palmitic, stearic, oleic and linoleic acids; veranisatins A and B (convulsant compounds).

The oil is liable to atmospheric oxidation and both anisic aldehyde and anisic acid are normally present. This change is said to diminish the tendency of the oil to solidify, which is normally does on cooling to about 15°C.

Uses

The oil is used as a flavouring agent and carminative.

PEPPERMINT

Synonyms

Brandy mint; Lamb mint.

Biological source

Peppermint consists of dried leaves and flowering tops of *Mentha piperita* Linn. containing not less than 1.2 per cent of volatile oil. It yields not less than 5% of esters, calculated as menthyl acetate, and not less than 50% of total menthol, free and as esters.

The European and American oil are derived from *M. piperita* var. *vulagris* Sole ('black mint') and *M.*

piperita var. *officinalis* Sole ('white mint'). (Fam. Lamiaceae).

Geographical source

The plant is a native to Europe; cultivated in Asian countries, Canada and North America. It is grown in gardens.

Cultivation

The plant is a perennial glabrous strongly scented herb, 40-70 cm in height and cultivated in fertile soil having capacity of holding water. If rainfall is unsufficient, water is irrigated. Much sunlight is required for better crop. The plants are propagated by rhizome cutting. Peppermint requires a daytime length of 15 to 16 hours and as much sunlight as possible. To obtain good field crops, clean planting stock must be used because disease control measures have not yet been fully developed. At flowering stage plants are cut, dried for sometime in sunlight and stored. Several varieties of peppermint are cultivated in various countries, e.g., *Mentha arvensis* var. *piperascens* (Japan mint), *M. piperita* var. *vulgaris* (Black mint) and *M. piperita* var. *officinalis* (White mint).

Peppermint thrives well in humid and temperate climates and is sensitive to drought. It grows well on high calcareous soil or deep rich loams in open sunny situations. The cuttings of rootstocks are planted in rows 30-90 cm apart.

Farmyard manure is applied as a basal dose before planting. Planted in February or March, the plants flower in July of the second year, when the crop is harvested; a second flush may be taken in September after the rain.

Macroscopical characters

The mints have square stems and creeping rhizomes. The black mint, has purple stems and dark green petiolate leaves which are tinged with purple. The leaf blades are 3-9 cm long and have a grooved petiole up to 1 cm long. They have a pinnate venation with lateral veins leaving the midrib at about a 45° angle, acuminate apex and sharply dentate margin. Glandular trichomes are seen as bright yellowish points. The leaves are broader than those of *M. spicata* (spearmint), but narrower than those of *M. aquatica* (water mint).

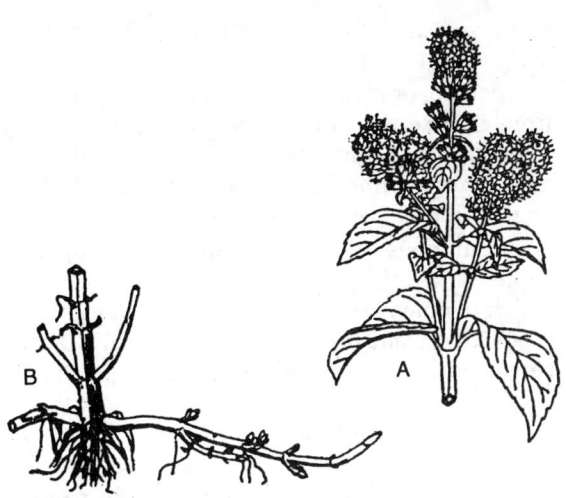

Fig. 18.17. Peppermint.

Microscopical characters

Under microscope the peppermint leaves show numerous diacytic stomata on the lower surface, three- to eight-celled clothing trichomes with a striated cuticle, and two types of glandular trichome, one with a unicellular base and small single-celled head and the other with a multi-cellular head. Calcium oxalate is absent.

There is a 5% limit of stems over 1 mm in diameter for the official leaves. The mints are very susceptible to most diseases, there is a 10% limit of leaves infected by *Puccinia menthae*.

Characters of volatile oil

Peppermint oil is colourless, pale yellow or greenish yellow liquid with a strong aggreable odour and a powerful aromatic taste, followed by a cooling sensation when air is drawn into the mouth. On ageing, the oil darkens in colour and becomes viscous. When chilled, menthol separates out.

Chemical constituents

Peppermint contains volatile oil, resin, tannins and gum. The predominant constituent of the oil is menthol (50-90%), the other compounds identified are *l*-and *d*-menthone (10%), menthyl acetate, menthyl valerate, menthofuran, (+)-isomenthone, (+)-neomenthone, menthyl isovalerats, jasmone, phellandrene, α-pinene, cineole, *l*-limonene, terpinene, cadinene, amyl alcohol, acetic acid, isovaleric acid, acetaldehyde, isovaleric aldehyde and piperitone. American peppermint also contains acetaldehyde, isovaleraldehyde, acetic acid, isovaleraldehyde, acetic acid, valeric acid, limonene, cadinene, amyl alcohol and dimethyl sulphide.

The oil also contains sesquiterpenes β-elemene, (-)-caryophllene, (-)-γ-muurolene, (+)-γ-muurolene, (+)-ε-muurolene, (+)-γ-cadinene, (+)-δ-cadinene, calamene, aromadendrene, ylangene, cubebene, α- and β-bourbonenes, bicycloelemene, ε-furgurene, α-maaliene and viridiflorol.

It also contains isomenthol, neomenthol, neoisomenthol, pulegone, piperitone, β-pinene, carvone, mintlactone, isomintlactone, thymol, carvacrol, eugenol and limonene.

Plants of the same species and geno type may produce oils of different quality when grown in different areas. The long days of northern latitudes favour the production of a peppermint oil that contains relatively small amounts of menthone and menthofuran and large amounts of menthol, whereas plants subjected to short day illumination produce an oil that contains small amounts of menthol and relatively large amounts of menthofuran.

Pulegone is the predominant terpene in young tissues of peppermint. Menthone, which is found in older tissues, gradually disappears while menthol accumulates and is replaced by menthyl acetate.

Peppermint oils obtained from plants containing relatively large amounts of young tissue are inferior. High concentrations (up to 30%) of menthofuran in such oils impart a disagreeable odour to products in which they may be incorporated. The oils of good quality can be obtained only from plants containing a high percentage of mature tissues.

Uses

The herb is considered aromatic, stimulant, counter-irritant, and carminative, and used for allaying nausea, flatulence and vomiting, to relieve nasal congestion in common cold; as an analgesic for diseases of the mouth and pharynx, in mouthwashes; as an adjunctive, emollient and itch-relieving in skin diseases and as a tropical protective agent for cracks, bruises, frost bite and insect bite. Bruised leaves are employed externally for relieving local pain and headache. A hot infusion in taken to allay stomachache and diarrhoea. The drug is frequently adulterated with spearmint, which is difficult to detect.

Oil of peppermint

The oil is required to contain 4.5-10% of esters calculated as menthyl acetate, not less than 44% of free alcohols calculated as menthol and 15-32% of ketones calculated as menthone.

The limits for individual compounds are : limonene 1.0-5.0%, cineole 3.5-14.0%, menthone 14-32%, menthofuran 1.0-9.0%, isomenthone 1.5-10.0%, menthyl acetate 2.8-10.0%, menthol 30.0-55.0%, pulegone >4.0%, carvone >1.0%. The ratio of the cineole to limonene contents exceeds 2.

A basic fraction of the oil contains pyridine derivatives such as 2-acetyl-4-isopropenyl pyridine which has a powerful grass-like minty odour. High resolution GC has been used to identify over 85 components of the oil.

The oil composition of *M. piperita* is greatly influenced by genetic factors and seasonal variations.

Peppermint oil is used for flavouring in pharmaceuticals, dental preparation, mouth washes, cough, drops, soaps, chewing gums, candies, confectionery and alcoholic liquers. It is widely used in flatulence, nausea and gastralgia. The oil has mild antiseptic and local anaesthetic properties. It is used externally in rheumatism, neuralgia, congestive, headache and toothache.

Menthol is antipruritic and used on the skin or mucous membrane as a counter-irritant, antiseptic and stimulant. Internally it has a depressant effect on the heart. Its chief commercial importance is as a flavor for confections, especially for chewing gum.

The use of peppermint oil in USA was as follows: chewing gum, 55%, toothpaste, mouthwash, and pharmaceuticals, 34%; confectionary products, 10%; and other products, 1%. Peppermint oil is used as a flavoring agent in mouthwash and as a carminative and flavoring agent in the antacid products.

Japanese peppermint oil or *Mentha arvensis oil* is obtained by steam distillation from *Mentha arvensis* Linn. var. *piperascens*. This oil is considerably higher in menthol content but is inferior in flavour to peppermint oil. It is, therefore, solely employed as a source of menthol. The plant is indigenous to Japan.

Menthol or menthan-3-ol is an alcohol obtained from diverse mint oils or prepared synthetically. Menthol may be levorotatory [(−)-menthol], from natural or synthetic sources, or racemic [(±)-menthol], produced synthetically.

Menthol is usually prepared from Japanese peppermint oil by refrigeration (−22°C), during which the menthol crystallizes. The liquid portion is poured off, and the crystallized menthol is present between filter papers and subsequently purified by recrystallization. Synthetic racemic menthol is produced by hydrogenation of thymol. Menthol is also prepared from pinene.

Menthol occurs as colourless, hexagonal crystals or needlelike, as fused masses, or as a crystalline powder. It has a pleasant, peppermint-like odour.

Menthol is a topical antipruritic. It has been used on the skin or mucous membranes as a counter-irritant, antiseptic and stimulant; internally, menthol has a depressant effect on the heart. Menthol is topically applied as 0.1 to 2% preparations for use on the skin.

Menthol is used as an antipruritic in burn and sunburn preparations, to treat poison ivy rash, in douche powders, and in preparations to treat athlete's foot. It is used as a counter-irritant in external analgesic preparations.

Biogenesis of peppermint monoterpenoids

The essential oils of the Lamiaceae are synthesized in the cells of the glandular trichomes, techniques such as cell and root culture are of little value as experimental tools. New procedures, using gentle abrasion of leaf surfaces with glass beads, have been developed for isolating in high purity and excellent yield the peltate glandular trichomes of peppermint which retain their biosynthetic activity.

The hydrolase system involving (−)-limonene-3-hydroxylase in the formation of the alcohol (−)-*trans*-isopiperitenol is cytochrome-P450-dependent. The remaining steps are catalysed by soluble enzymes of the oil cells. (+)-Pulegone is a branching point for the formation of menthol stereoisomers.

Japanese peppermint oil, derived from *M.*

canadenis var. *piperascens*; contains 70-90% menthol.

Cell-free extracts from *Mentha* leaves with pulegone-^{14}C have confirmed the pulegone → menthone → menthol portion of the pathway and have established that $NADPH_2$ is an essential cofactor in these reduction reactions. An enzyme preparation from *Mentha* leaves reduces the isopropylidene double bond of piperitenone to yield piperitone. Small amounts of menthone and menthol were also formed with piperitone as the substrate, due to reduction of the cyclohexene double bond.

A key step in the biosynthesis of the *p*-menthane monoterpenes is the dehydration of α-terpineol to terpinolene and limonene. The steps leading to the formation of α-terpineol from mevalonic acid are common to several different species of mints. The pathways then diverge when α-terpineol is dehydrated to limonene in spearmint and to terpinolene in peppermint. The next step is hydroxylation and subsequent dehydrogenation to produce either the carvone series of monoterpenes found in spearmint or the piperitenone series of monoterpenes found in peppermint. A single dominant gene produces the carvone series, whereas the homozygous recessive genotype produces the piperitenone series. The gene that differentiates between these series may be the gene that governs the enzyme that dehydrates α-terpineol to either limonene or terpinolene.

Pharmacology

Peppermint oil relaxed carvachol-contracted guinea pig tenia coli and inhibited spontaneous activity in guinea pig colon and rabbit jejunum. It relaxes gastrointestinal smooth muscle by reducing calcium influx and reduced gastric emptying time in dyspeptics.

CINNAMON BARK

Synonyms

Ceylon Cinnamon; Dalchini (Hindi); Saigon Cinnamon; Chinese Cassia; Cortex Cinnamoni.

Biological source

Cinnamon is the dried bark of *Cinnamomum loureirii* Nees or *C. zeylanicum* Nees. (Family : Lauraceae).

Geographical source

Cinnamon is a native of China, Japan and Formosa

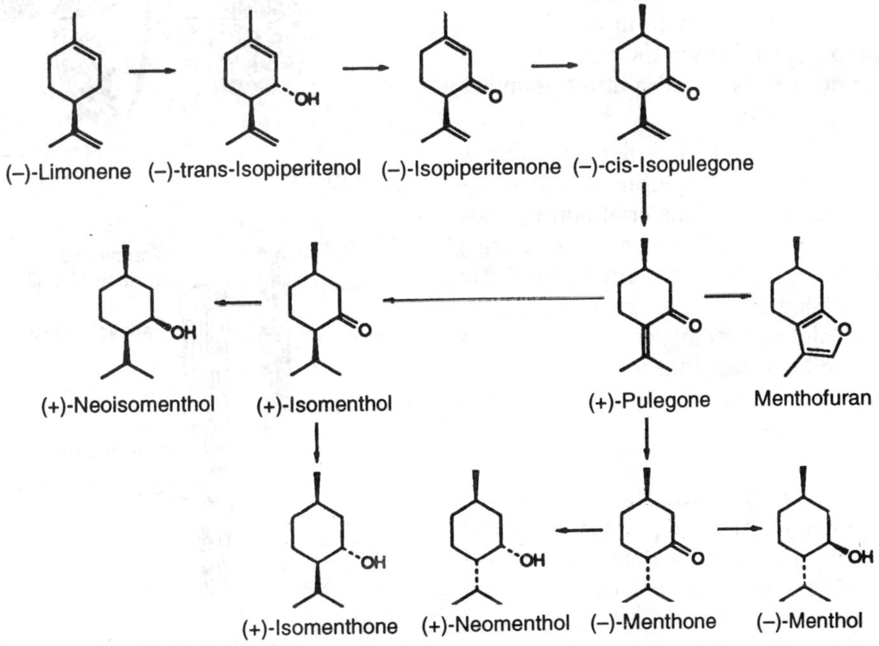

(−)-Limonene (−)-trans-Isopiperitenol (−)-Isopiperitenone (−)-cis-Isopulegone

(+)-Neoisomenthol (+)-Isomenthol (+)-Pulegone Menthofuran

(+)-Isomenthone (+)-Neomenthol (−)-Menthone (−)-Menthol

Fig. 18.18. Biosynthesis of some monoterpenoids of *Mentha piperita*.

and found in Sri Lanka, Java, Vietnam, Sumatra, West Indies, Jamaica, Laos, Indonesia, Brazil and Seychelles. In India the plant occurs widely in the southern coastal regions up to an altitude of 2,000 meters.

Collection

Cinnamon is a large handsome, evergreen, 6-10 meter high tree. It is grown in rich but light soil. It requires a rainfall of nearly 200-300 cm and temperature 32°C. The fresh seeds are sown in seed beds. The plants are transplanted at a distance of 2-3 meter apart. Two or three years old trees are coppiced few inches above the ground. From each plant 5 to 6 straight shoots are allowed to grow. After about 18 months of growth, and when some 3 m long and 2 cm diameter, shoots are harvested, trimmed and, following a few hours 'fermentation', the bark is removed with a nonferrous knife. The peeled bark is then stretched over a suitable stick and the outer cork and cortex scraped off with a curved scraper. Bark separated from shoots is about 1 cm thick. Bark is collected from April to July after heavy rainy season. The shoots and twigs are removed with a brass knife-like instrument (Catty). Leaves and twigs are separated and bark is stripped off from shoots. The bark is kept in the shade for about 24 hours and then kept in the open air wood frames. The dried bark is sorted, put into bundles and enclosed in jute cloth.

The grades of cinnamon are designated: 00000, 0000, 000, 00, 0, 1, 2, 3, 4, quillings, featherings and chips. Most commercial material corresponds to Nos. 1-4 grades. Quillings and featherings consist of small pieces, the latter often containing some outer bark; they are used for grinding and for oil distillation. Chips consist mainly of outer pieces of bark, and the oil derived from them has a lower specific gravity and a lower aldehyde content than that from the inner bark.

The bark as it dries, contracts and forms a quill. During the drying process, which takes about 3 days, the quills are rolled by hand and pressed to prevent swelling and splitting. The bark obtained from the central branches is superior to that from the outer shoots. The quills are graded on the basis of appearance and aroma.

Macroscopic characters

Cinnamon occurs in single or double compound quills. Length of quill is up to 1 meter, 6-10 mm in diameter and 0.5 mm thick. The external surface is yellowish brown and shows longitudinal wavy lines (pericyclic fibres) and occasional scars and holes. The inner surface is dark brown longitudinally striated. Fracture is short and splintery. Odour is aromatic; taste is warm, sweet and aromatic.

Microscopy

Transverse section of Cinnamon bark under microscope indicates that except occasional patches of cork and underlying parenchyma, cork and cortex are absent. The outermost layer consists of a continuous band, three or four cells wide, of peri-

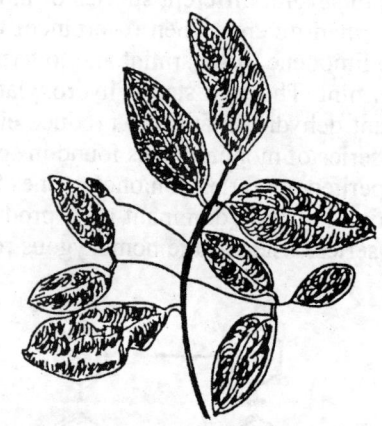

Fig. 18.19. *Cinnamomum zeylanicum* twig.

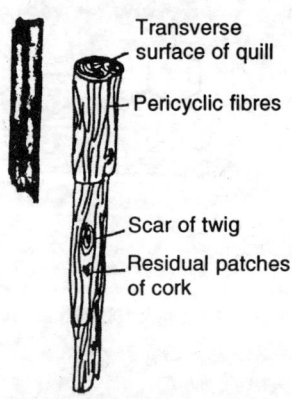

Transverse surface of quill

Pericyclic fibres

Scar of twig

Residual patches of cork

Fig. 18.20. Cinnamon bark.

cyclic lignified sclerenchyma. On the outer margin there are small group of about six to fifteen peri-cyclic fibres occurring at intervals. The sclereids have thickened lignified walls, showing well-defined pit canals. The thickening on the outer walls is often less pronounced than on the radial and inner tangential walls. The lumen is clearly visible and contains a few starch grains. The pericycle fibres have strongly thickened lignified walls showing stratification and pit canals. Primary phloem can not be differentiated. The secondary phloem is consisted of phloem parenchyma, containing oil and mucilage; phloem fibres and medullary rays. The *sieve-tubes* are arranged in tangenital bands which are completely collapsed in the outer layers. The sieve plates are on the trans-verse walls. The phloem parenchyma is composed of thin-walled cells, with yellowish-brown cells and contains starch grains. These cells are sub-rectan-gular in shape. Some cells contain scattered minute needles of calcium oxalate. Some of the phloem parenchyma cells contain tannins. The secretary cells, containing volatile oil or mucilage, are two or three times the diameter of the phloem fibres, and are axially elongated. The phloem fibres, which

occur isolated or in tangential rows, are more abundant towards the inner part of the bark. The secondary phloem is divided up by the radial medullary rays, which are uni- or biseriate near the cambium but become broader towards the outside by tangenital growth of the cells. The rays are 7-14 cells in height. The medullary ray cells are radially elongated, thin walled with yellow-brown cell contents possessing numerous acicular crystals of calcium oxalate.

Chemical constituents

Cinnamon contains volatile oil (1-6%), phloba-tannin, mucilage, calcium oxalate, sugar and starch. The principal constituent of the volatile oil is cinnamic aldehyde, C_6H_5 CH=CH-CHO (60-75%). The other components identified are eugenol (4%), pinene, phellandrene, caryophyllene, cinnamyl acetate and small quantities of ketones and alcohols (benzaldehyde, methyl amyl ketone, cumic alde-hyde), esters of isobutyric acid, p-cymene, linalool, α-terpineol, benzyl acetate, eugenyl acetate, benzyl benzoate, caryophyllene, cinnamyl alcohol, hydroxy-cinnamaldehyde and salicylaldehyde.

The drug also contains pentacyclic diterpenes cinnzeylannin and cinnzeylanol, glucosides cinncas-siol C1, C2, C3, D1, D2 and D3, and pro-anthocyanidins. Cinncassiol D1 and its glucoside exhibited anticomplement activity.

Chemical tests

1. Volatile oil (1 ml) is dissolved in alcohol (5 ml) and then a drop of $FeCl_3$ is added. Ferric chloride on reaction with cinnamic aldehyde and phenolic compound, eugenol, produces pale green colour.
2. Alcoholic extract of the bark (1 g) or volatile oil (1 ml) on treatment with phenylhydrazine hydrochloride forms red coloured phenylhydra-zone of cinnamic aldehyde.

Uses

Cinnamon is pungent, aromatic, astringent, stimu-lant and carminative. It is useful for checking nausea and vomiting. It is valued as flavouring agent and it has antiseptic and antidiarrhoeal properties and is a powerful germicide. It is employed as a

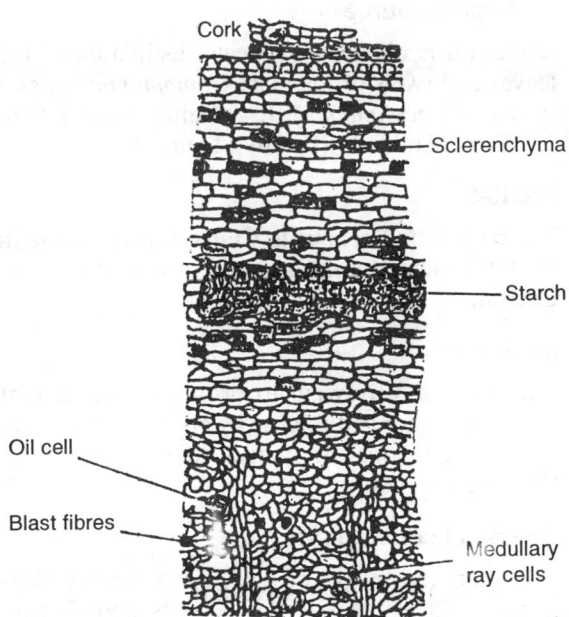

Fig. 18.21. Transverse section of Cinnamon bark.

counter-irritant in the treatment of muscular strains, rheumatism and inflammations.

Allied drugs

Saigon Cinnamon is obtained from wild trees of *C. loureirii* Nees grown in Annam. It contains numerous starch grains and volatile oil. It is used as flavouring agent and mild astringent.

Cassia or Chinese cinnamon

Cassia bark is obtained from *Cinnamomum cassia* Blume (Fam. Lauraceae). The plant is grown in south eastern provinces of China and Cochin. Bark is removed from 6 years old tree.

The cork and cortex are partly removed by planting, the bark tied into bundles and exported in boxes, via Hong Kong.

Cassia bark occurs in channelled pieces or single quills up to 40 cm long, 1-2 cm wide and 1-3 mm thick. The outer surface is darker than that of Ceylon cinnamon and shows patches of grey cork. The odour is coarser than that of cinnamon and the taste more astringent.

Transverse sections resemble cinnamon and exhibit the starch grains and phloem fibres which are somewhat larger. Outside the sclerenchymatous ring are the cortex and cork layer.

Cassia bark contains about 10% mucilage. Ceylon cinnamon is an inner bark, whereas with cassia bark outer cortex and cork are present.

Cassia yields 1-2% of volatile oil which contains no eugenol but about 85% of cinnamic aldehyde. Cinnamon oil is required to contain not less than 80% by volume of aldehydes. High yields of oil are distilled from the leaves, twigs and bark. It is inferior in flavour to the oil of *C. zeylanicum* but it is cheaper.

Cassia contains the tannin complex. Three flavan-3-ol glucosides identified are (–)-epi-catechin 3-*O*-, 8-*C*- and 6-*C*-β-D-glucopyranosides. Three oligomeric procyanidins (named cinnamatannins A_2, A_3, A_4) were tetra-, penta- and hexameric compounds respectively, consisting exclusively of (–)-epicatechin units linked linearly through C-4–C-8 bonds. Free (–)-epicatechin and procyanidins are present. Procyanidins occur also in dimeric form and as *C*-glucosides.

Cassia volatile oil also contains caryophyllene, methyl O-cumin aldehyde and coumarin.

An arabinoxylan of cassis bark activates the reticulo-endothelial system. This neutral polysaccharide, named cinnaman AX contains L-arabinose and D-xylose.

Callus and suspension cultures of *C. cassia* yields condensed tannins, the precursors (–)-epicatechin and procyanidins B2, B4 and C1.

Cassia 'buds', are the dried immature fruits of *C. cassia*. The yield about 20% of volatile oil having a cinnamaldehyde (80%).

Java or Indonesian cinnamon is derived from *C. burmanii* Blume, and is used in Holland. The tree is found in Sumatra, Java and Timor. Its powder has tabular crystals of calcium oxalate. The oil contains cinnamic aldehyde (75%).

Oliver bark or *black sassafras* is obtained from the 'white sassafras' tree, *C. oliveri*, found in Queensland. It is used locally as a cinnamon substitute. It occurs in flat strips about 20 cm long, 4 cm wide and 1 cm thick. The outer surface is brownish and warty, and bears patches of greyish cork. It has about 1-2.4% of volatile oil.

CASSIA OIL (CINNAMON OIL)

Biological source

Cassia oil is obtained by steam distillation of the leaves and twigs of the plant *Cinnamomum cassia* Blume (*C. zeylanicum*). It contains not less than 1.0% of volatile oil. (Family : Lauraceae).

Habitat

The plant is indigenous to China. It also occurs in Sri Lanka and Burma. In India, it is cultivated in Cochin.

Characters

The oil is a yellowish to brownish liquid that becomes darker and thicker by age or by exposure to air. It contains the typical odour and taste of Cassia Cinnamon.

Chemical constituents

The main constituent of the oil is cinnamic aldehyde (80-95%); the other components identified are limonene, *p*-cymene, linalool, β-caryophyllene, eugenol, pinene, phellandrene, ketones, alcohol and esters.

Oil distilled from fresh bark samples collected in Ghana contained a high proportion of cinnamyl acetate. Phenylalanine is a precursor of both cinnamic aldehyde and eugenol in the living plant.

Uses

Cassia oil is used as a flavouring agent. It has carminative, pungent, antiseptic and aromatic properties. It is a powerful germicide.

It should be stored in well-filled, tight, light-resistant containers and protected from excessive heat.

Adulteration

The oil is adulterated with cinnamon leaf oil and with oil of cassia. Cinnamon leaf oil contains 70-95% of eugenol and an alcoholic solution yields a blue colour with solution of ferric chloride. Oil of cassia contains about 80-95% of aldehydes and a similar test with ferric chloride gives a brown colour. Oil from the root-bark contains much camphor and other monoterpenes but negligible phenylpropanes.

Allied drugs

Cayenne cinnamon consists of the bark of cultivated plants of *Cinnamomum zeylanicum* planted in French Guiana, Brazil and the islands of the West Indies. It is inferior in quality.

C. loureirii grows in Vietnam, in districts of Annam, China and Japan. It resembles cassia bark more closely than cinnamon, and occurs in quills up to 30 cm long, 4 cm wide and 0.7-7.0 mm thick. The outer surface is greyish-brown, warty and ridged. The odour is coarser than that of Ceylon cinnamon and the taste sweeter.

LEMON PEEL

Synonym

Fructus Limonis.

Biological source

Lemon peel is obtained from the fresh ripe fruit of *Citrus limon* (L.) Burm. f. (*C. medica* var. *limon* Linn.). (Family : Rutaceae).

Geographical habitat

It is cultivated in California. West Indies, Italy, Spain, Sicily, Portugal, Florida, California, Jamaica and Australia; grown all over India, particularly in home gardens and small-sized orchards.

Collection

Lemon plant is a small, 3-5 m high, evergreen thorny tree with shining leaves. Fruits are collected before their green colour changes to yellow in January, August and November. The outer dark yellow peel is removed with a sharp knife. Dried lemon peel is spiral, 20 cm long, 1.5 cm wide, 2-3 mm thick, outer surface is rough and yellow, inner surface is pithy and white. Odour is strong and aromatic, taste is aromatic and bitter.

Chemical constituents

Lemon peel contains volatile oil (2.5%), vitamin C, hesperidin and other flavone glycosides, mucilage, pectin and calcium oxalate. The important constituents of the volatile oil are limonene (90%), citronellal, geranyl acetate, α-pinene, camphene, linalool, terpineol, methyl heptenone, octyl and nonyl aldehydes, γ-terpinene, β-pinene, bergamotene, neral and geranial.

The peels also contain flavonoids eriocitrin, epigenin, luteolin, chrysoeriol, quercetin, isorhamnetin, limocitrin, limocitrol, isolimocitrol, hespe-

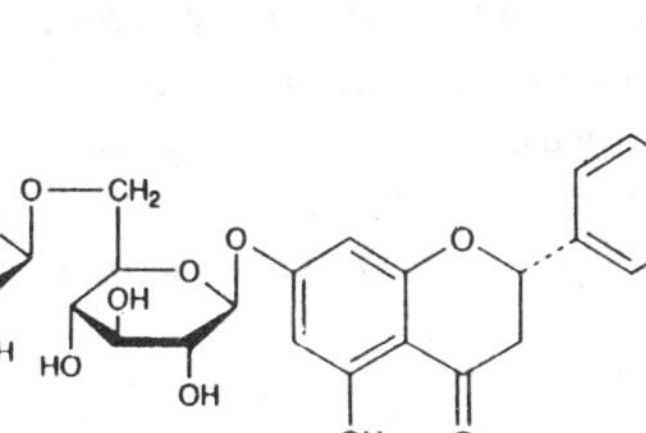

Fig. 18.22. Hesperetin.

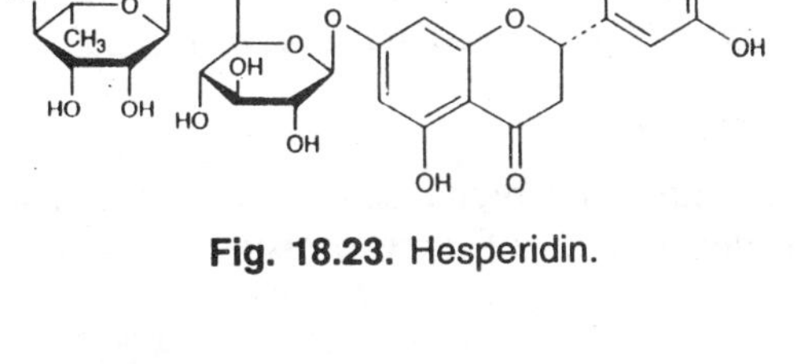

Fig. 18.23. Hesperidin.

ridin; coumarins scopoletin and umbelliferone; sinapic acid and *p*-coumaric acid.

Uses

Lemon peel is stomachic stimulant and carminative. It is used as a flavouring agent in medicine, also in beverages, confectionery and cooking.

Lemon oils

Lemon volatile oil is prepared around the Mediterranean, North and South America, in Australia and in parts of Africa. *Citrus* oils are best extracted by means other than distillation. Lemon oil is separated from the peel by distillation without deterioration in quality, and some expressed oil of lemon is fractionally distilled to make terpeneless oil of lemon. The oil prepared from the peel by steam distillation is inferior. Distilled oil of lemon is cheaper than that prepared by expression and used for nonpharmaceutical purposes.

The lemon peel is candied with sugar. The pulp of the fruit yields on expression lemon juice, which may be canned or used for the preparation of citric acid and citrates. Pulp residues are used for pectin manufacture and as cattle food.

The following processes are used for the production of oil.

Machine processes

The quality of machine-produced oil is inferior. The machines are designed to set free the oil by puncture, rasping or cutting and by gentle squeezing action of the sponge method. There is virtually no conduct between the oil and the inner white part of the peel (*albedo*). Deterioration in odour results from enzyme action in the finely divided albedo.

The *sfumatrice machines* (squeezing machines) exert a gentle pressing action on the peel passing on a stainless-steel hand against stationary protrusions. Spray water is used to remove the oil, which is separated by a centrifuge. The *sfumatrice* machine has fine knives which cut into the outer peel (*flavido*), but partly also in the *albedo*.

Distilled oil

Some lemon oil is produced by distillation, mainly from the residues of the expression processes. It fetches a much lower price than either 'hand-pressed' or 'machine-made' oil.

Constituents

Lemon oil contains terpenes (about 94% (+)-limonene), sesquiterpenes, aldehydes (citral, 3.4-3.6%, and citronellal) and esters (1% geranyl acetate). Limonene is a liquid, b.p. 175°C. Citral or geranial, a liquid, b.p. 230°C, is an aldehyde. Lemon oil shows a marked tendency to resinify and should be protected from air and light. Principal reactions which cause these changes are oxidations of monoterpenes, aldehydes and esters, peroxide formation, polymerizations and isomerizations (e.g., limonene → α-terpinene).

Adulteration

Oil of lemon is adulterated with oil of turpentine, 'terpeneless oil of lemon', and the cheaper distilled oil of lemon. The value of the oil is judged on the citral content, but a normal citral content alone is not a sure indication of purity since citral may be added from a cheaper source such as oil of lemon grass, which contains 75-85% of this aldehyde.

Uses

Oil of lemon is used for flavouring and in perfumery.

Terpeneless lemon oil

Terpeneless lemon oil is prepared by concentrating lemon oil in *vacuo* until most of the terpenes have been removed, or by solvent partition. The concentrate has a citral content of 40-50%. Terpeneless lemon oil is equivalent in flavour to about 10-15 times its volume of lemon oil; Lemon Spirit is a 10% solution in ethanol (96%).

Preparation

The outer portion of the rind containing the volatile oil is removed by grating. The raspings so obtained are placed in canvas bags and a pressure is applied. The resultant turbid oil is kept to separate sediment. The oil is decanted leaving behind the sediments.

In Sicily, the lemon is peeled and pieces of the peel are pressed flat to rupture the oil cells. The oil is absorbed by a sponge. On saturation, it is squeezed out and the process is separated.

In another procedure used in West Indies, the entire fruit is rotated in a saucer-shaped container having several rows of sharp metal pins. The pins rupture the oil cells, and the exuding oil is collected in a long narrow depression in the bottom of the saucer.

In California, the cold-pressed oil is obtained by applying very high pressure to the lemons to remove the juice and oil rapidly. The juice and oil mixture are separated by high-speed centrifugal separation at the lowest feasible temperature and in minimum time.

BITTER ORANGE PEEL

Synonyms

Fructus Aurantii; Seville Orange.

Biological source

Bitter orange peel is the dried rind of nearly ripe fruit of *Citrus aurantium* var. *amara* L. and *C. aurantium* var. *sinensis* L. (Family : Rutaceae).

Geographical source

Bitter orange is native to India. It is grown near Mediterranean Sea, Spain, West Indies, Florida, California, Sicily and Malta.

Collection

Fruits are collected when they are about to ripe. The peel is removed in four 'quarters' or in a spiral band.

Characters

The bitter orange peel occurs as spiral or irregular ribbons, 2-6 mm thick, brittle and hard, breadth is 6-12 mm. Outer surface is dark orange red, rough due to raising over oil glands, various small pits and reticulate ridges. Inner surface is yellowish white, pithy, fracture is hard and short. Odour is aromatic and taste is aromatic and bitter. Fine slicing causes the rupture of a large number of oil glands and some loss in aroma.

Microscopically the peel contains a small-celled epidermis with characteristic stomata; parenchyma with prismatic crystals of calcium oxalate, or sphaerocrystalline masses of hesperidin; small anastomosing vascular bundles; and large oil filled cavities arranged in two irregular rows.

Chemical constituents

Bitter Orange peel contains volatile oil (1-2.5%), vitamin C, flavonoid glycosides hesperidine (vitamin P-factor), neohesperidine, naringin, aurantiamaric acid, aurantiamarin (1.5-2.5%); acrid resin, gum and tannin. The bitter taste of the peel is due to the presence of flavonoids aurantiamarin, aurantiamaric acid, naringin, hesperidine and isohesperidine. The dominant component of the volatile oil is limonene (90%) in addition to citral, citronellal and methyl anthranilate. Conifer has been reported in *C. sinensis* and may add to effect of limonin and naringen.

The flavones tangeretin, tetra-O-methyl-scutellarin, 3, 5, 6, 7, 8, 3', 4'-heptamethoxy-flavone, nobiletin, sinensetin, auranetin and 5-hydroxy-auranetin were found in the peel of *C. aurantium*. An active alkaloid, synephrine, identified as 4-hydroxy-α-[(methylamino)-methyl] benzenemethanol, is present in the peel of *C. reticulata*.

Most of carotene pigments identified from the peel of *Citrus* species are cryptoxanthin, 5,5', 6, 6'-tetrahydo-β, β-carotene, luteoxanthin, mutato-chrome, auroxanthin, zeaxanthin, phytoene, phytofluene, sintaxanthin and β-apo-10'-carotenal.

The volatile oil of *C. aurantium* 'Valencia' is composed of limonene (93%), linalool, β-caryophyllene, α- and β-humulenes, myrcene, nootkatene, α-pinene, sabinene, *epi*-α-selinene, valencene, *cis*- and *trans*-carveol, citronellol, decanol, dodecanol, elemol, geraniol, intermedeol, 1-8-*p*-menthadien-9-ol, *cis*- and *trans*-2, 8-*p*-methadien-1-ol, nerol, nonanol, octanol, α-terpineol, undecanol, acetaldehyde, decanal, dodecanal, geranial, octanal, perillaldehyde, α- and β-sinensal, acetone, carvone, ethyl vinyl ketone, nootkatone, piperitone, ethyl acetate, ethyl butyrate, ethyl propionate, methyl butyrate, 1,8-*p*-menthadien-9-yl acetate, octyl acetate, 1,1-ethoxyethone, *trans*-linalool oxide, *cis*- and *trans*- 4,7-dimethyl-bicyclo [3.2.1] oct-3-one. *C. aurantium* also contains limonin, ichangin, deacetylnomilin, nomilinic acid, deacetylnomilinic acid, hesperidin, poncirin, 6,7-dimethoxy-coumarin, 5-hydroxyauranetin, 5-O-demethyl-nobiletin and nobiletin.

Chemical test

Concentrated hydrochloric acid is put on a thick

section of the drug. A dark green colour is obtained. This test is absent in sweet orange peel.

Uses

Bitter orange peel is used as flavouring agent, stomachic, carminative and bitter tonic. Hesperidin in the soluble form in the fresh fruit functions as vitamin P.

SWEET ORANGE PEEL

Biological source

Sweet orange peel is the fresh rind of fruit of *Citrus aurantium* L. var. *sinensis* (Fam. Rutaceae). The plant is about 8 m in height and found where the bitter orange grows.

The volatile oil from the orange may be extracted by methods other than by distillation, e.g., mechanical expression of the fresh peel; although chemically almost identical with the bitter orange oil, it does not have the bitter taste or odour of the latter. These oils contain the terpene (+)-limonene and smaller quantities of citral, citronellal and methyl anthranilate. Libyan fresh orange peel oil contains 62 components.

Lemon oil and orange oil, often develop a terebinthinate odour during storage. A considerable amount of these terpenes may be removed by distillation under reduced pressure. A terpeneless lemon oil with a citral content of 40 to 50% may be prepared. In terpeneless orange oil, about 95% of the terpenes have been removed. They are higher in price than the natural oils. One part of the terpeneless oil is equivalent to about 15 parts of the sweet orange oil. The oil is required to contain not less than 18% of aldehydes calculated as decanal.

Chemical constituents

The volatile oil of sweet orange peel contains limonene (90%), citral (5%), methyl anthranilate, decyclic aldehyde, linalool and terpineol, Other constituents isolated from the peel are flavonoids aurantin, hesperidine, 5-hydroxyaurantin and 5-O-desmethyl nobiletin. The colour originates from a complex mixture of carbonyl carotenoids, the principal components being violaxanthin (9-*cis*-violaxanthin), di-*cis*-violaxanthin and all-*trans*-violaxanthin, together with a number of other

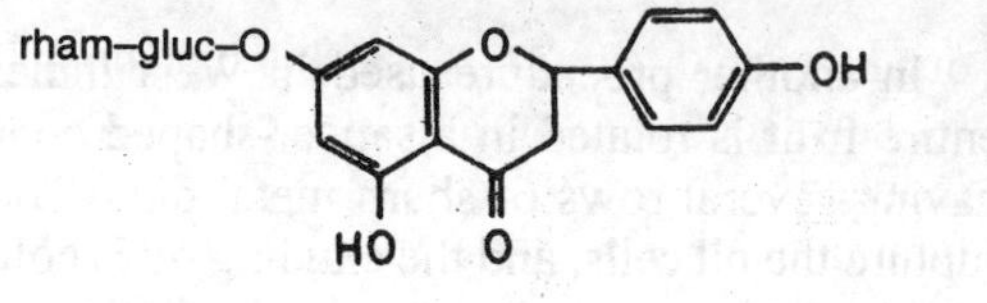

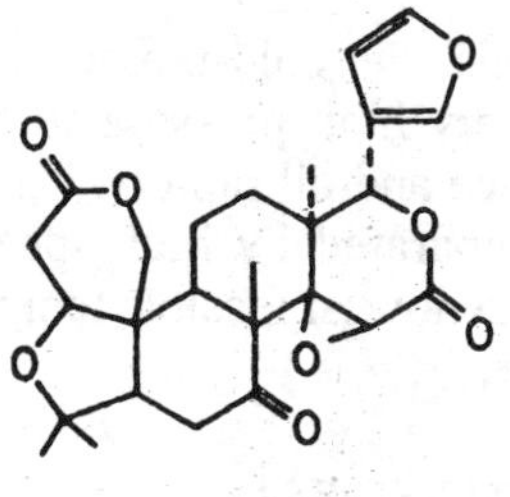

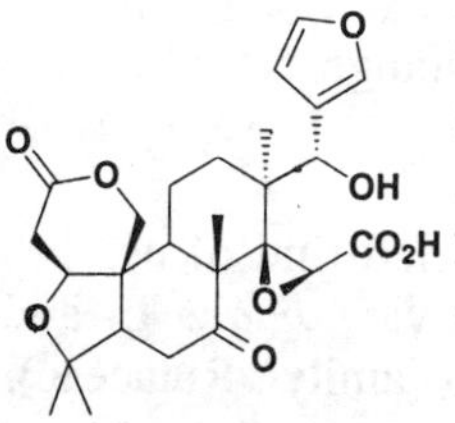

Fig. 18.24. Chemical constituents of orange peel.

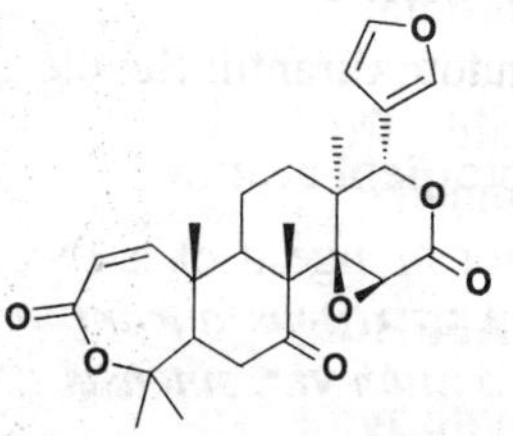

carotenoids, auranetin, 5-hydroxyauranetin, 5-O-demethylnobiletin and umbelliferone.

The other compounds present in the peel are β-sitosterol, ergosterol, desmosterol, limonoids isolimonoic acid, its methyl ester, limonin, deacetylnomilinic acid, nomilinic acid, ichangin and deacetylnomilin.

Uses

The peel is aromatic and used as carminative, tonic and flavouring agent. Fresh rind is rubbed on the face as remedy for acne.

The bitter orange oil is known as *Essence de Bigarde* and that from the sweet orange is called *Essence de Portugal*.

Pharmacology

Naringin showed anti-inflammatory and capillary-strengthening activities. Naringin and naringenin selectively inhibited growth of cancer cells. Naringin strongly inhibited DNA formation in human cancer tissues. Hesperidin decreased rat paw oedema induced by dextran by 33%, inhibited pleurisy induced by carrageenin and slightly reduced hyperthemia induced by yeast in rats. Synephrine and N-methyl-tyramine increased blood pressure and rate of blood circulation in brain, kidney and coronary artery in dogs. In guinea pig, it increased heart contraction, decreased heart rate and caused changes in ECG.

Intraperitoneal injection of maringin to rats caused a depression of cardiac action and reduced blood pressure. Intravascular infusion of 4 mg/min synephrine into healthy volunteers significantly increased the systolic and mean arterial blood pressure, but did not affect the diastolic pressure and heart rate.

5-Methyl-tyramine inhanced contractility and automaticity in isolated papillary muscle from endotoxin-shocked cats. Polymethoxylated flavonoids from pericarp inhibited sedimentation of human erythrocytes.

SAFFRON

Synonyms

Crocus, Spanish, Saffron, French Saffron.

Biological source

Saffron is the dried stigma and styletops of *Crocus sativus* Linn. (Family : Iridaceae).

Geographical source

The plant is native of south Europe and is found in Spain, France, Macedonia, Italy, Austria, China, Germany, Switzerland and Iran. In India the plant is cultivated in Kashmir.

Cultivation and collection

The plant is a small, perennial herb, 6-10 cm high. The corms are planted in July-August in well-prepared soil. In the following year flowering takes place. Each corm is replaced by daughter corms. The flowers are collected early in the morning. The style of each flower is separated just below the stigma and dried by artificial heat for 30-45 minutes. The drug is cooled and stored in dry place. About 1 kg of dried drug is collected from nearly 100,000 flowers.

Saffron thrives well in cold regions with warm or subtropical climate. It requires a rich, well-

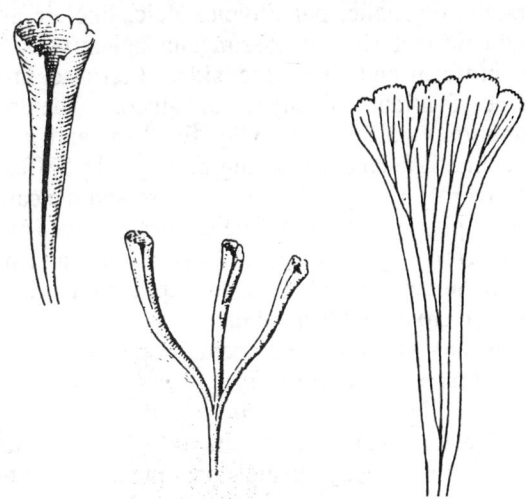

Fig. 18.25. Saffron.

drained, sandy or loamy soil. The plant is propagated by bulbs. No manure is applied or irrigation given once the plants are established. The bulbs continue to live for 10 or 15 years, new bulbs being produced annually and the old ones rotting away.

The plants flower in October-December, heavy rains during this period are harmful. Styles and stigmas are separated and dried in the sun or over low heat on sieves in earthen pots.

The tripartite stigmas plucked from fleshly collected flowers and dried in the sun constitute Saffron of the best quantity.

Characters

Saffron is flattish-tubular, almost thread like stigmas which are about 3 cm long with slender funnel having dentate or fimbricate rim. Colour is reddish-brown with some yellowish pieces of tops of styles. Odour is strong, peculiar and aromatic; taste is aromatic and bitter.

Chemical constituents

Saffron possesses a number of carotenoid coloured compounds such as ester of crocin (a coloured glycoside), picrocrocin (a colourless bitter glycoside), crocetin (an aromatic compound), gentiobiose, α- and γ-carotenes, lycopene, zeaxanthin, crocin-1, crocin-2, crocin-3, crocin-4, mono- and di-gentiobiosyl and glucosyl esters of crocetin; β-sitosterol, ursolic, oleanolic, palmitoleic, oleic, linoleic and linolenic acids (in bulbs); astragalin, helichrysoside, kaempferol and its diglucosides. Picrocrocin is made of safranal (aldehyde) and glucose. The drug contains volatile oil (1.3%), fixed oil and wax. Crocin is the chief colouring principle in Saffron. On hydrolysis, it yields digentiobiose and the carotenoid pigment crocetin. The colourless glycoside, picro-crocin, gives on hydrolysis glucose and the aldehyde, safranal. Stearoptene (m.p. 106°) has been isolated from the essential oil.

About 34 more components, especially terpenes, terpene alcohols and esters, have been identified in the essential oil.

The important components of volatile fraction are safranal, phenylethanol, naphthalene, 2-butenoic acid lactone, palmitic, stearic, oleic and linoleic acid, 2,6,6-trimethyl-4-hydroxy-1-cyclohexen-1-carboxyaldehyde, 2,4,4-trimethyl-3-formyl-6-hydroxy-2,5-cyclohexadien-1-one, isophorone, 3,5,5-trimethyl-4-hydroxy-2-cyclo-hexen-1-one, 3,5,5-trimethyl-1,4-cyclohexadione, 3,5,5-trimethyl-2-cyclohexene-1,4-dione and 3,5,5-trimethyl-2-hydroxy-2-cyclohexene-1,4-dione.

A novel xanthone-carotenoid glycosidic conjugate, named mangicrocin, is present in saffron. The petals contain astragalin, helichrysoside, kaempferol

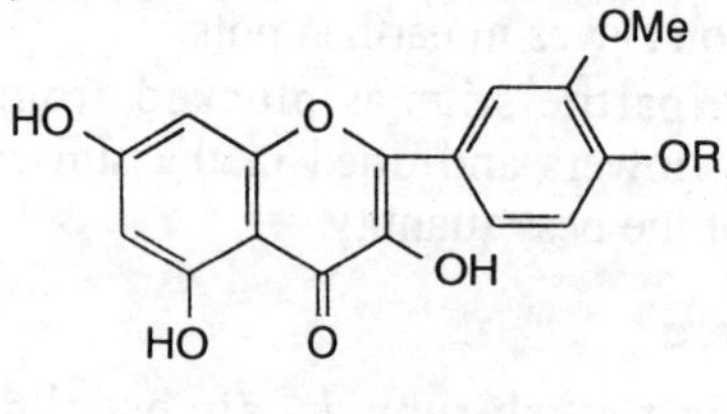

Crosatoside A
R = Glu(2→1)Rha

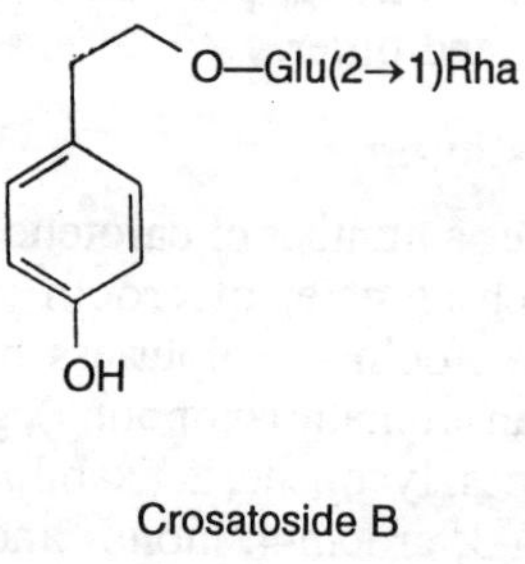

Crosatoside B

Fig. 18.26. Chemical constituents of Saffron.

and its glycosides. Crosatosides A and B occur in pollen grains.

Uses

Saffron is used in fevers, cold, melancholia and enlargement of the liver; as colouring and flavouring agent, catarrhal, snake bite, cosmetic pharmaceutical preparations, and as spice. Saffron has stimulant, stomachic, tonic, aphrodisiac, emmenagogue, sedative and spasmolytic properties.

Pharmacology

Various extracts of saffron showed stimulating action on uteri of guinea pigs, rabbits and dogs. Intramuscular injection of crocetin into rabbits reduced severity of atherosclerosis. Serum cholesterol levels were reduced by 50 per cent. Malignant cells were more sensitive than normal cells to inhibitory effect of the plant extract on both DNA and RNA synthesis.

Adulterant

Saffron is frequently adulterated with styles, anthers and parts of carolla of Saffron. Exhausted Saffron, flowers and floral parts of some *Compositae* like *Calendula* species and *Carthamus tinctorius*, corn silk, and various materials coloured with coal tar dyes, are also used as adulterants. Water, oil or glycerine is added to increase the weight. Coke Saffron of commerce often contains safflower florets with adhesive sugary substances.

CAMPHOR

Synonyms

2-Bornanone, 2-Comphanone, Gum Camphor, Japan Camphor.

Biological source

Camphor is a solid ketone, $C_{10}H_{16}O$, obtained from the volatile oil of *Cinnamomum camphora* (L.) Nees et Eber (Family : Lauraceae).

Synthetic camphor, which is optically inactive, is prepared from turpentine and would probably have completely replaced the natural product.

Geographical source

The plant is a big tree native to Eastern Asia. It is

found widely in Mediterranean region, Sri Lanka, Egypt, South Africa, Java, Sumatra, Brazil, Jamaica, Florida, Formosa, Japan, South China and California. In India the tree is planted in gardens up to 1300 meters height in the N.W. Himalayas. It is successfully cultivated at Dehradun, Saharanpur, Calcutta, Nilgiris and Mysore.

The plant is cultivated at elevations of 1,500-2,000 m provided the temperature does not fall below 15°F. A fertile, well-drained, sandy loam is needed for its successful cultivation. Manuring is recommended. The plants can be raised from seeds, layers, branch cuttings, root cuttings, and root-suckers. For obtaining good seeds, ripe fruits should be collected directly from the tree. Seed should be sown immediately after collection. Germination takes place in about 3 months after sowing. Careful weeding is necessary. After six months of germination, the seedlings are transplanted into seeds baskets.

Preparation

Old trees possess high concentration of Camphor. The small wood chips are treated with steam. Camphor is sublimed and liquid volatile oil passed away into the receiver. Excess of Camphor is obtained from the volatile oil. Camphor is purified by treating it with lime and charcoal and resublimation into large chambers to form 'flowers of camphor'. The collected Camphor is made into blocks by hydraulic pressure.

Synthetic camphor is prepared from American turpentine. By the action of hydrogen chloride the pinene is converted into bornyl chloride which, on treatment with sodium acetate, yields isobornyl acetate. Hydrolysis of this yields isoborneol and subsequent oxidation gives camphor.

The specific rotation of natural camphor is +41°-+43°. The synthetic camphor is optically inactive.

Characters

Natural Camphor is colourless translucent mass with crystalline fracture, rhombohedral crystals from alcohol, cubic crystals by melting and chilling. Odour is characteristic and taste is pungent and aromatic which is followed by cold sensation. It evaporates at room temperature and pressure, m.p. 180°, very volatile in steam. At 25°, one gram dissolves in about 800 ml water (giving a colloidal solution), in 1 ml alcohol, 1 ml ether, 0.5 ml chloroform, 0.4 ml benzene, 0.4 ml acetone, 1.5 ml of turpentine oil, and 0.5 ml glacial acetic acid. Camphor has a peculiar tenacity and cannot be powdered in a mortar unless it is moistened with an organic solvent.

Chemical constituents

Comphor oil contains camphor, cineole, pinene, camphene, phellandrene, limonene and diterpenes. Camphor is entirely a monoterpenic ketone, $C_{10}H_{16}O$. Its basic carbon framework is related to borneol.

Camphor oil also contains sesquiterpenes 1α-ylangene, 1-β-elemene, 1-β-caryophyllene, humulene, selinene, d-nerolidol, camphorenone, camphorenol, β-santalene, δ-guaiene, δ-cadinene, calamenene, calacorene, γ-patchoulene, 1,6-dimethyl-4-isopropyl-7,8-dihydronaphthalene, 9-oxonerolidol, 9-oxofarnesol, eugenol, methyl vinyl ketone, methylisobutyl ketone, mesityl oxide, hexanol, hexen-3-ol, myrcene, 1,8-cineole, p-cymol, ocimene, linalool oxide, terpinen-4-ol, α-terpineol, safrole, nerol, geraniol, β-selinene, carvacrol, cresol, alcanfor, borneol, cinnamaldehyde, benzyl benzoate, heliotropin and vanillin.

The leaves also contain lignans kusunokinin, cinnamonol, kusunokinol, dimethyl matairesinol, hinokinin and dimethyl secoisolariciresinol.

Uses

Camphor is used externally as a rubefacient, counter-irritant and internally as a stimulant, carminative and antiseptic. It is a topical anti-pruritic and anti-infective, used as 1-3% in skin medicaments and in cosmetic. It is also used to manufacture some plastics, celluloid, in lacquers, varnishes, explosives, pyrotechnics, as moth repellent and in embalming fluids.

Allied drugs

Borneo camphor, obtained from *Dryobalanops aromatica* (Dipterocarpaceae), and Ngai camphor, obtained from *Blumea balsamifera* (Asteraceae), are used in China and Japan. In California laevo-rotatory camphor is produced from species of *Artemisia* (Asteraceae).

SPEARMINT

Synonyms

Mint, Pudina (Hindi).

Biological source

Spearmint consists of the dried leaf and flower tops of *Mentha spicata* . (*M.viridis* L.) or *M. cardiata*. Gerard ex. Baker. (Family : Lamiaceae).

Geographical source

The plant is found in European and Asian countries and widely cultivated in USA.

Mentha is cultivated throughout the plains of India. It thrives best in heavy loams well supplied with farmyard manure. It is usually propagated by planting divisions of old plants in rows 30 cm apart. The field is weeded and watered during dry weather. The plants produce leaves for a number of years.

Character

Mint is a glabrous herb identical to peppermint, 30-90 cm high, with creeping rhizomes, but the stems are usually more purple, leaves are crumpled, opposite, ovate-lanceolate, 3-7 cm long. The apex is acute or acuminate, and the margin unequally serrate. The leaves are almost sessile with bright green colour free from purple. Inflorescence is slender, interrupted cylindrical spikes or crowded lanceolate spikes with 7-10 mm long bracts. Odour and taste are aromatic and characteristic without any cooling sensation.

Spearmint oil is a colourless, yellow or greenish yellow liquid that has the characteristic odour and taste of spearmint.

Chemical constituents

Spearmint contains volatile oil (0.5%), resin and tannin. The principal component is carvone (50-55%) along with some other monoterpenic constituents like limonene, phellandrene, dipentene, dihydrocarveol, dihydrocarveol acetate, cineole, α-pinene and linalool. The carvone is optically isomeric with the (+)-carvone found in oil of Caraway and oil of Dill.

5-Methyl-2(2-oxo-3-butyl) phenol, 5-methyl-2-(3-oxo-2-pentyl) phenol, 3-(5,5-dimethyl tetrahydrofuran-2-yl) 2-buten-1-ol, isomanthone, linalyl acetate, pulegone, neodihydrocarveol, dihydrocarveol, 3-octanol-β-D-glucoside, diosmetin, diosmetin-7-O-glucoside, luteolin-3'-glucoside, diosmin, and 3-octanol-β-D-glucoside are also present in the leaves.

Limonene is the precursor of the monoterpenoids. The action of a (–)-limonene-6-hydroxylase predominates to give the alcohol (–)-*trans*-carveol which is oxidized to carvone. Dihydrocarvone is formed later in the season.

Like peppermint, oil production is influenced by the age of plant, time of collection, chemical varieties and hybridization.

Uses

Spearmint is used as flavouring agent, spice and carminative. It has stimulant, digestive, spasmolytic and diuretic properties. It is given in fever, vomiting and bronchitis and employed as a lotion in aphthae.

Green leaves are used for making chutney and for flavouring food preparations, vinegar, jellies and cold drinks. The volatile oil is used in toothpastes (50%), chewing gums (47%) and mouth-wash.

A soothing tea is brewed from the leaves. A sweetened infusion of the herb is given as a remedy for infantile troubles, vomiting in pregnancy and hysteria.

LAVENDER OIL

Lavender oil is obtained by distillation from the fresh flowering tops of *Lavendula intermedia* Loisel (English oil) or of *L. angustifolia* P. Miller (foreign oil) (Lamiaceae). These oils differed markedly in composition. The English oil fetches a higher price. They have different 'ester value' (English oil, 25-45; foreign oil 100-170) and 'ester value after acetylation'.

The true lavender, *L. officinalis*, yields the best oil when grown at a high altitude. At a lower altitude it yields a less esteemed oil. 'Grande lavande', *L. latifolia* Villers (*L. spica* DC), yields a much coarser oil, which is sold as oil of spike. The above plant readily hybridizes with *L. officinalis* yielding a plant known as 'grosse lavande' or 'lavandin', the oil of which is an intermediate in character between that of the parent forms.

The plant flowers from July to September and the fresh flowering spikes yield about 0.5% of volatile oil. The lavender oil normally contains over 35% of esters. Oil of spike, which is largely used in cheap perfumery, contains little ester but a high proportion of free alcohols (about 23-41% calculated as borneol); 30 components have been identified. The Spanish oil contains 50 compounds, the principal ones being 1:8-cineole, linalool and camphor. In the oil of *L. angustifolia*, linalyl acetate was not present.

L. stoechas has a markedly different odour and fenchone, pinocaryl acetate, camphor, eucalyptol and myrthenol predominate, in its 51 volatile components.

Uses

Lavender oil is used in the toiletry and perfumery industries, in ointments, to mask disagreeable odours and pharmaceutically in the anti-arthropod preparation Gamma Benzene Hexachloride Application. Lavender flowers are used in treatment of flatulent dyspepsia and topically, as the oil, for rheumatic pain. The oil is extensively used in aromatherapy.

BUCHU LEAVES

Synonyms

Bucco; Bucku; Buku; Folia Buchu.

Biological source

Buchu is the dried leaf of *Barosma betulina* Barti et Wendl (short or round Buchu) or of *B. crenulata* (L.) Hook. (oval Buchu) or of *B. serratifolia* Willd (long Buchu) (Family : Rutaceae).

Geographical source

South Africa.

Characters

Leaves of *B. betulina* are small, 12-20 mm long, 4-5 mm broad, rhomboid-ovate in shape, with a blunt and recurved apex and numerous oil glands. The margin is dentate towards upper side and serrate towards the base. Dried leaves are brittle and coriaceous. Odour and taste are strong and characteristic.

Round or *short buchu* consists of the leaves and a small percentage of the stems, fruits and flowers

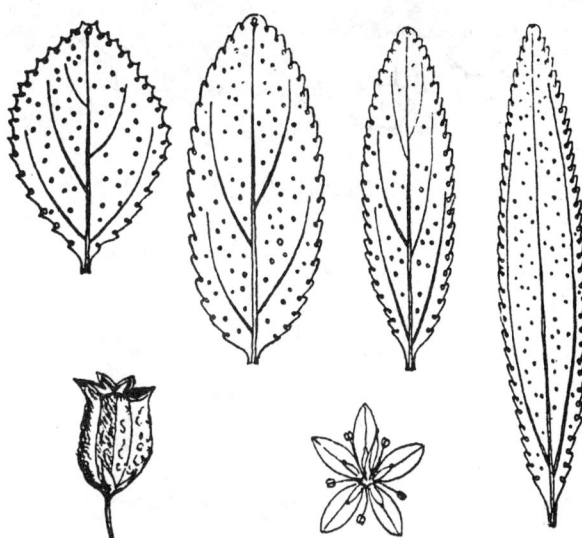

Fig. 18.27. Buchu leaf (*Barosma betulina*).

of *Barosma betulina*. A large oil gland is situated at the base of each marginal indentation and at the apex. Numerous smaller ones are scattered throughout the lamina. Reddish-brown fragments of stems, up to about 5 cm, brown fruits with five carpels and flowers with five whitish petals are usually present, but an excessive amount of these is considered as an adulteration.

Oval buchu is obtained from *Barosma crenulata* Hooker. The leaves are 15-30 mm long and 7-10 mm broad, oval; the apex is blunt but not recurved and possesses a terminal oil gland; marginal serration very minute.

Long buchu is obtained from *Barosma serratifolia* Willd. The leaves are 12-40 mm long, 4-10 mm broad, and linear lanceolate in shape; the apex is truncate and possesses a terminal oil gland; the margin is serrate.

Chemical constituents

Buchu leaves contain volatile oil (30%), diosmin (flavonoid), mucilage, resin and calcium oxalate. The important constituent of the oil is a phenolic camphor, diosphenol (buchu camphor), isomenthone, pulegone, *d*-limonene, dipentene, 1-menthone and *p*-menthane-8-thio-3-one. Diosmin on hydrolysis yielded diosmetin, glucose and rhamnose. The characteristic odour of the oil has been ascribed

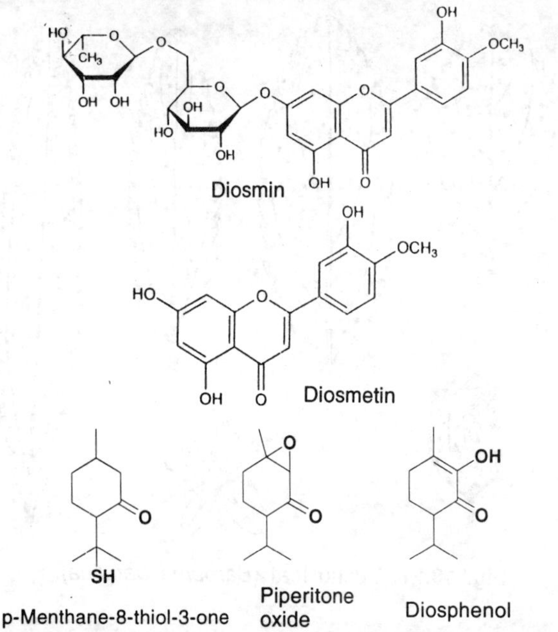

Fig. 18.28. Chemical constituents of Buchu leaves.

to sulphur compounds and *p*-menthane-8-thio-3-one has been characterized; it is present in quantities up to 0.5% of the oil and is probably derived from (–)-pulegone.

Uses

Buchu is used as a urinary antiseptic, diuretic and carminative.

CLOVE

Synonyms

Caryophyllus, Clove buds, Caryophyllum; Caryophylli; Laung (Hindi).

Biological source

Cloves are the dried flower buds of *Eugenia caryophyllata* Thumb (Syn. *Syzygium aromaticum* (L.) Merr. (Family : Myrtaceae).

Geographical source

The clove tree is native of Molucca Island. It is cultivated in Zanzibar, Sumatra, South America, West Indies, Brazil, Pemba, Ambon, Madagascar, Mauritius, Tanzania, Sri Lanka and South India.

Cultivation

Clove is pyramidal or conical evergreen plant, 10-20 meters in height, grown in well-drained soil. The plant is propagated from seeds sown during August-October. Dehusked seeds are immediately sown, as their viability deteriorates rapidly. Ripe fruits may be sown without removing the skin, but the germination is poor. Germination takes place in 4-5 weeks. Seedlings are transplanted when they attain a height of about 25 cm during rainy season.

It requires moist, warm and equable climate and suitable rainfall. The plants are protected from pests, diseases and direct sunlight. When seedlings are 9 months old, they attend the height of about 1 meter and then transplanted at a distance of 6 meters in the beginning of rainy season. The plants are shaded by banana planting up to 3 years.

Collections

Flower buds are collected when their base turns into crimson-red in colour in dry weather from August to December. Natives climb on the tree or put ladder for the collection. The cloves are dried in open air and their stalks are separated. On drying about 70% water is lost. Dried cloves are graded according to size, packed into bales and exported.

Morphology

Cloves are reddish-brown, 1-1.7 cm long, consisted of lower solid stalk called hypanthium and upper crown or cap. Hypanthium is swelling, subcylindrical, slightly flattened, tapering below, 10-13 mm long, 4 mm wide and 2 mm thick. A bilocular ovary containing numerous ovules attached to axile placentae is present above the stalk. Various schizolysigenous oil glands are present in the hypodermis.

The crown consists of calyx, corolla, stamens and style. Calyx contains four slightly projecting teeth. Corolla is dome-shaped, which is made of four pale yellow-coloured, imbricate, immature, membraneous petals. Many free, introse and tetradelphous stamens are enclosed in the crown.

The clove sttalk consists of a cylindrical hypanthium or swelling of the torus, above which is a bilocular ovary containing numerous ovules attached to axile placentae. The 'head' consists of four slightly projecting calyx teeth; four membra-

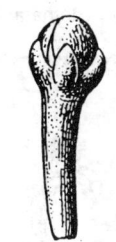

Fig. 18.29. Clove bud.

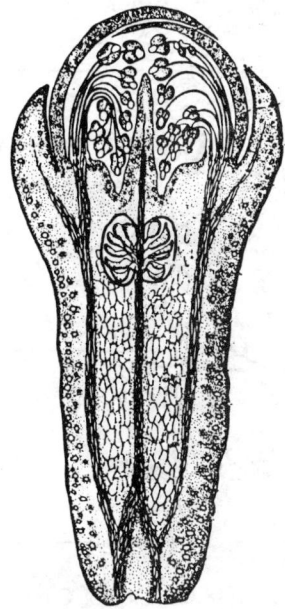

Fig. 18.30. Longitudinal section of clove.

nous, imbricated petals and numerous incurved stamens around a large style.

Ovary contains numerous ovules with axile placentation. A single, erect, firm style reaching up to corolla is present. A nectar-disc (nectary) is present at the base.

Clove has a strong fragrant and spicy odour and pungent, aromatic taste.

Microscopy

Transverse section of Clove hypanthium below the ovary shows epidermis, cortex and columella.

Epidermis is heavily cuticularized with straight walls in which occur ranunculaceous stomata.

There are three different regions in the cortex.

The peripheral region is composed of 2-3 layers of large, ellipsoidal, schizolysigenous oil glands arranged in two or three intermixed layers. The oil glands are ellipsoidal in shape, with the long axis radial and show an epithelium composed of two or three layers of flattened cells. Cluster of crystals of calcium oxalate occur in many of the parenchymatous cells. Within the oil gland layer there is a zone of cells with thickened walls embedding a ring of bicollateral vascular bundles. The ground tissue of this zone contains cluster crystals of calcium oxalate. The meristeles are enclosed in an incomplete ring of lignified fibres.

The middle region contains one or two rings of bicollateral vascular bundles with few pericyclic fibres. The xylem is composed of 3-5 lignified spiral vessels. Within the ring of vascular bundles is a zone of aerenchyma, composed of air spaces and columella. The ground tissue of the columella is parenchymatous and rich in calcium oxalate clusters. In the outer region of the columella is a ring of some 17 small vascular bundles. Numerous sphaeraphides are present scattered throughout the columella.

The hypanthium, in the region below the ovary, shows in transverse section, a heavy cuticularized epidermis, stomata, well-defined substomatal spaces and radially arranged parenchymatous cells containing numerous schizolysigenous oil glands. The oil glands are ellipsoidal in shape, with the long axis radial and show an epithelium composed of two or three layers of flattened cells. The contents of the oil glands are soluble in alcohol and are blackened with alcoholic ferric chloride or osmic acid. The ground mass of parenchyma also gives the blackening with ferric chloride. Within the oil gland layer is a zone of cells with somewhat thickened walls, embedding a ring of bicollateral vascular bundles. The ground tissue of this zone contains cluster crystals of calcium oxalate. The meristeles are enclosed in an incomplete ring of lignified fibres. The xylem is composed of 3-5 lignified spiral vessels. Within the ring of vascular bundles is a zone of aerenchyma composed of air spaces separated by lamellae one cell thick, which supports the central columella. The ground tissue of the columella is parenchymatous and it contains calcium oxalate clusters. In the outer region of the columella is a ring of some 17 small vascular bundles.

The hypanthium, in the region of the ovary, contains epidermis, oil gland layer and ring of bicollateral bundles. A zone of cells with very strongly thickened cellulose walls is present in this region. The dissepiment of the ovary is parenchymatous; the placentae are rich in cluster crystals and contain vascular bundles. The sections of the hypanthium mounted in a concentrated solution of potassium hydroxide show acicular and radiately aggregate crystals.

The sepals and petals are simple in leaf structure. The mesophyll parenchyma contains calcium oxalate and embeds numerous oil glands. The epidermis of the sepals show stomata. The epidermis of the petals is devoid of stomata and is composed of very irregular cells. The stamens are composed of filament, connective and anther.

The filament shows an epidermis of longitudinal elongated cells, a ground mass of parenchyma embedding numerous oil glands and a single vascular strand enclosed in a sheath of crystal cells. The vascular strand is continuous into the connective, which is terminated by an oil gland. The fibrous layer of the anther-wall is composed of cells with spiral bands of lignified thickening. The

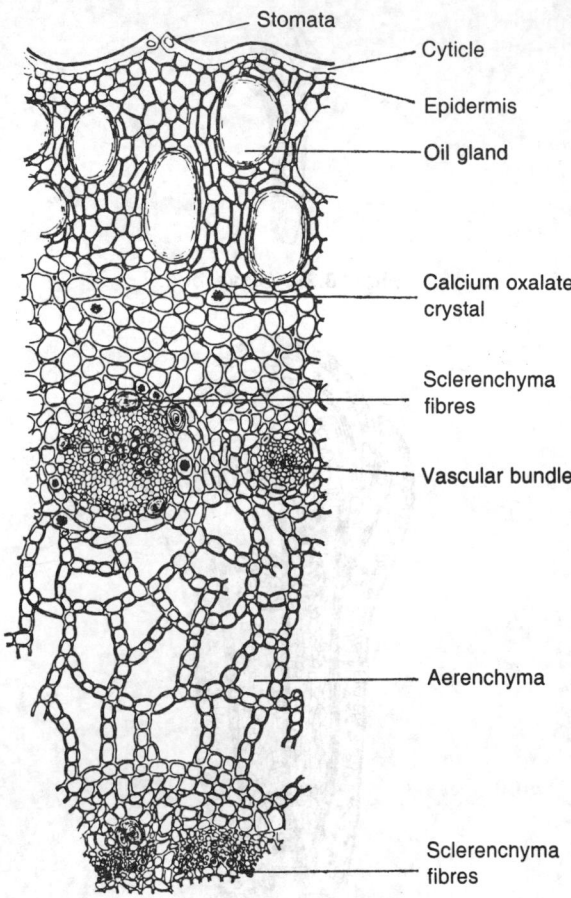

Fig. 18.32. L.S. of Clove.

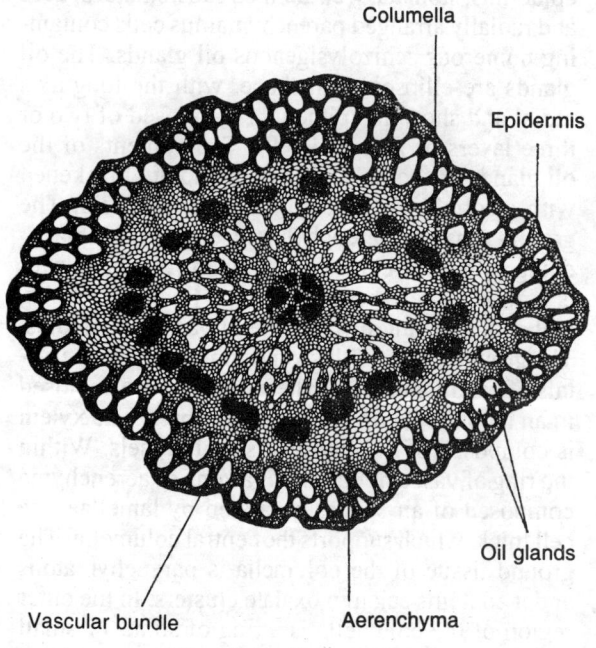

Fig. 18.31. T.S. of Clove.

pollen grains are triangular in outline and 15-20 mm diameter. The style and stigma have similar characters to those of the filament.

Starch, prisms of calcium oxalate and lignified sclereids are absent in powder of the flower buds. Clove stalks contain lignified sclereids and reticulately thickened xylem vessels. The starch is absent in the clove fruits.

Chemical constituents

Clove contains volatile oil (14-21%), tannins (10-13%), triterpenic acids (*e.g.*, oleanolic acid) and esters, glucosides of sitosterol, stigmasterol and campestrol, vanillin, chromone, eugenin, gum and resin. The important chemical constituents of the volatile oil are eugenol (85-90%), acetyl eugenol (3%), α- and β-caryophyllenes, methyl amyl ketone, methyl furfural, dimethyl furfural, carbinol, vanillin and methyl-*n*-heptyl ketone. Eugenol is a colourless or pale yellow liquid, b.p. 255°. It becomes dark and thick on exposure to air. It has the odour of cloves and spicy, pungent taste. Other substances present in traces are methyl salicylate, methyl benzoate, methyl alcohol, benzyl alcohol, furfuryl alcohol, furfural, methyl furfuryl alcohol, β-pinene, 2-heptanol, 2-nonanol, 2-hydroxy-4, 6-dimethoxy-5-methylacetophenone, naphthalene, caryophyllene oxide, caryophylla-3(12), 6-dien-4-ol, caryophylla-3(12), 8(13)-dien-6α-al, acetophenone, benzyl salicylate, α-cadinol, γ-decalactone, fenchone, hexanol, 2-hexanone, methyl palmitate, γ-muurolene, palustrol, propyl benzoate, β-salinene, α-thujene and α-humulene, Clove also contains ellagitannin eugeniin, eugenol-4-O-(6'-O-galloyl)-glucoside, 2-methyl-5,7-dihydroxychromone-8C-glucoside, its 6'-O-gallate, 2,4,6-trihydroxyacetophenone-3C-glucoside, its gallate derivatives, veloneic acid bislactone, gallic acid glucosides, strictinin, genin D, 1-desgalloyl eugeniin, 1-O-galloylpedunculagin, rugosin A, casuariin, pterocarinin A and rugosins.

Eugeniin showed antiviral activity against herpes simplex virus. β-Caryophyllene, its oxide, α-humulene, its epoxide and eugenol inhibited chemical carcinogenesis.

Uses

Clove has antiseptic, aromatic, counter-irritant, carminative and stimulant actions. It is used in flatulence, dyspepsia, throat infection, baking, confections and as flavouring agent. Clove oil is used in toothache, dental preparation and in mouth washes. The sesquiterpenes of clove are potential anticarcinogenic compounds.

CLOVE OIL

It is a colourless or pale yellow liquid, which is slightly heavier than water (relative density 1.047-1.060). It is soluble in alcohol (70%).

Clove oil contains 84-95% of phenols (eugenol with about 3% of acetyleugenol), sesquiterpenes (α- and β-caryophyllenes) and small quantities of esters, ketones and alcohols. It does not possess monoterpene derivatives. The phenols can be esti-mated by absorption with solution of potassium hydroxide in a graduated flask. The oils with low phenol content are known in commerce as 'opt' and are mainly used in pharmacy. The 'strong' oils are used for the manufacture of vanillin.

Clove oil is used as a flavouring agent, stimulant, aromatic and antiseptic.

Clove stem oil produced in Tanzania and in Madagascar is used in the flavouring and perfumery industries. *Clove leaf oil* is distilled in Madagascar, Tanzania and in Indonesia, and is used for the isolation of eugenol.

Eugenol or 4-allyl-2-methoxyphenol is a phenol obtained from clove oil and from other sources. It is prepared from clove oil by shaking with a 10% solution of sodium hydroxide to form sodium eugenolate. The mixture is washed with ether, and the sodium eugenolate is then decom-posed with sulfuric acid. The eugenol is separated by steam distillation. It is a colourless or pale yellow, thin liquid that has a strongly aromatic odour of clove and a pungent spicy taste.

Eugenol is used as a dental analgesic. It is applied topically to dental cavities and is incorporated in dental protectives. Eugenol is an ingredient in the toothache preparations, mouth-washes and ointments.

At high doses, clove oil is toxic in children. It causes CNS depression, hepatic necrosis, convulsions and hemostatic abnormalities. It is caustic for the skin and mucous membranes. Clove oil is an industrial source of eugenol which is the starting material for vanillin.

Chemical tests

1. Treatment of hypanthium of clove or clove oil with potassium hydroxide solution (50%) forms needle-shaped crystals of potassium eugenate.
2. To clove oil (1 ml) in alcohol (5 ml) add $FeCl_3$ solution (1 ml). The solution turns blue due to the presence of phenolic hydroxyl group.
3. Add $FeCl_3$ solution to aqueous extract of clove. Blue-black colour is formed due to the presence of tannins.

The assay of clove buds is carried out by determination of the amount of essential oil and TLC characterization of eugenol (75-88%), its ester (4-15%) and caryophyllene (5-14%) in a dichloromethane extract. The peduncle, petiole and fruits must be not more than 4% and foreign matter must be less than 0.5%.

Adulterants

1. *Exhausted clove* : Exhausted cloves are oilless, darker in colour, more shrunken and float on water surface. The volatile oil is removed by distillation.
2. *Clove stalks* : Clove stalks are subcylindrical, longitudinally wrinkled, jointed, sometimes branching, brown and less aromatic than clove. They contain 4-7% of volatile oil.

   During collection buds are collected along with stalks and some stalks remain attached to the buds after separation. Clove stalks contain calcium oxalate and stone cells which are not present in clove buds.
3. *Clove fruits* : Clove fruits are ripened fruits, about 2 cm long, ovate and tapering below, dark brown in colour with rough outer surface. Each fruit possesses a single firm seeds. It is slightly aromatic and contains starch. Small amount of volatile oil is present in the clove fruit and adulterated with clove buds.

NUTMEG

Synonyms

Jaiphal; Jayepatri; Myristica; Nux moschata; Nuces (Semen) nucistae; Myristicae semina.

Biological source

Nutmeg is the dried, ripe seeds of *Myristica fragrans* Houtt deprived of its seed coat and with or without a thin coating of lime. (Family : Myristicaceae).

Natural distribution

The plant is native of eastern Moluccas Island near Indonesia. Now it is cultivated in Malay, Sumatra, Java, Sri Lanka, West Indies and other tropical countries. In India it is found only as a specimen tree in southern region. Current world demand for nutmegs stands at about 10000 tonnes per annum of which about 75% originates from Indonesia and 15% from Grenada.

Cultivation and collection

Nutmeg is a dioecious or occasionally monoecious evergreen aromatic tree, usually 9-20 m high. It is grown from fresh seeds which are germinated in about one month. The 6-months old plants are transplanted to the fields. When the sex can be determined (5-8 years), the male trees are reduced to about 10% of the total. This method leads to irregularly spaced trees in the plantation. In some places vegetative propagation of the female trees is performed by *marcotting* or *air layering*. In this, female shoots are split but not detached, and by the use of hormone powder and suitable packing of the wound, are induced to root. This takes 4-18 months after which the rooted shoots are detached and brought on before planting out. Fruiting begins 8-9 years old trees and continues up to 20-30 years. Fruits are 5-7 cm long, 4-5 cm wide, light yellow, drupaceous, ovoid, peachlike berries, and dehisce longitudinally when ripe. The seeds are exposed with its lobed, red arillus. Fruits are collected in November and December or in April-June. The seeds are dried in oven by keeping them in trays. In the East the fruits are collected by means of a hooked stick. From mature plantations the annual yield per acre is about 250-500 kg of nutmeg and about 50-100 kg of mace. The nutmeg are dried in the shells. In Malaya sun-drying is used. Large quantities are dried in ovens and in brick buildings by placing the seeds on trays over low charcoal fires. When drying is completed, the kernel rattles within the brittle testa, which constitutes about one-quarter of the weight of the seed. The testa is cracked with a wooden truncheon, mallet or special machine, and

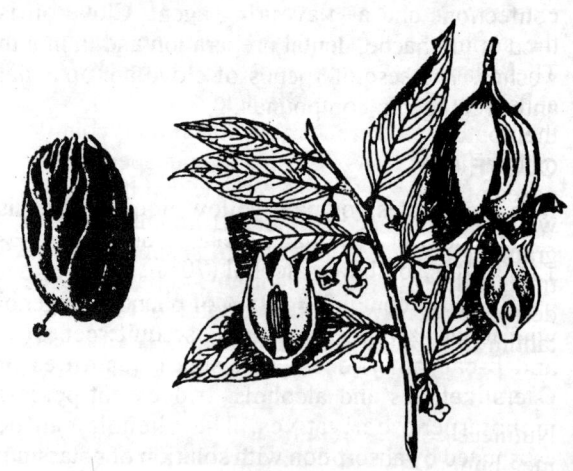

Fig. 18.33. Nutmeg.

the nutmeg extracted. The nutmegs are graded abroad into sizes represented by numbers per unit weight. Elongated nutmegs and small or damaged ones are kept separate. Nutmegs are exported in barrels or cases containing about 50 kg.

Morphology

The kernels consist of perisperm, endosperm and embryo. They are 2-3 cm long and about 2 cm in breadth. Shape is ovoid. Outer surface is rough, dark-brown with reticulate furrows. There is a light-coloured patch with brown lines radiating from the hilum and one end, which is surrounded by a raised ring. Micropyle and hilum are present near the projection. From hilum light furrow runs to chalaza which indicates the position of raphe. The odour is strong and aromatic, taste is pungent and slightly bitter.

A longitudinal section shows a lustrous appearance. The outer tissue, consists of dark brown perisperm, penetrates the light brown endosperm, the infoldings branching and giving rise to the marbled appearance. The perisperm possesses fibrovascular bundles with reticulate furrows found on the outer surface.

Microscopical characters

The outer perisperm cells are radially flattened, contain brownish contents and insoluble in potassium hydroxide or chloral hydrate. A few of the cells contain prismatic or disc-shaped crystals of potassium acid tartrate. The inner perisperm shows numerous extensive lamellae, corresponding to the furrows on the surface, and penetrating into the endosperm. These lamellae are composed of parenchymatous cells with thin brown walls and of oval oil cells. In their outer part there are vascular strands composed of lignified spiral vessels. The endosperm is composed of parenchymatous cells, with thin brown cell walls. It contains simple or 2-10 compound starch grains, globular or irregular in shape, with sometimes a slit-like hilum; aleurone grains, with a well-defined crystalloid; feathery crystals of fat; and some tannin cells, containing tannin and starch.

Chemical constituents

Nutmegs contain volatile oil (5-10%), fat or nutmeg butter (30-40%), proteins, phytosterin, starch, amylodextrin and colouring matter. The important

Methyl eugenol   Methyl iso-eugenol   Elemicin

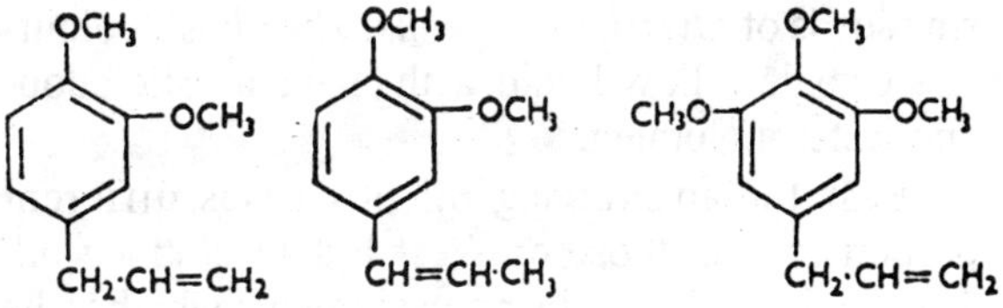

Fig. 18.34. Chemical constituents of Nutmeg.

constituents of volatile oil are myristicin, elemicin, eugenol, camphene (60-80%), dipentene, methyl eugenol, methoxy eugenol, methyl isoeugenol, iso-elemicin, safrole, *p*-cymene, isoeugenol, dehydrodi-isoeugenol, α-*p*-dimethyl-stryrene, *p*-menth-2-en-1-ol, *p*-menth-2-en-1, 4-diol, 3-methol-4-decen-1-ol, its acetate, limonene, α- and β-pinenes, α-terpineol, terpene-4-ol, 5-methoxy-dehydro- and dihydro-isoeugenol.

The seeds also contain dimeric phenyl propanoids, glyceryl trimyristate, dehydroisoeugenol, derivatives of 4-allyl-2, 6-di-methoxyphenoxy-propan-1-ol, guaiacin, macelignan, fragransols A, B, C and D, fragransins D1, D2, D3 and E1, austrobailignan-7, myristicanols A and B, licarin B and malabaricones B and C. The myristicin fraction of the volatile oil together with elemicin (>25%) may be responsible for the signified hallucinogenic properties of Nutmeg seed. Nutmegs contain 15% free myristic acid. Neolignans, polyphenols, tannins, epicatechin, cyanidin, thiamine, riboflavin and niacin have also been reported in Nutmegs. They yield about 3% of total ash and about 0.2% of acid-insoluble ash.

Uses

Nutmegs are carminative, astringent, aphrodisiac, and stomachic useful in flatulency, nausea and vomiting and as a source of myristica oil. The essential oil from *M. fragrans* showed antibacterial activity. Ingestion of large quantities causes drowsiness, stupor and death. In Indian medicine an aqueous extract of Nutmeg is used for the treatment of infantile diarrhoea.

NUTMEG OIL

Nutmeg oil or myristica oil is the volatile oil distilled with steam from the dried kernels of the ripe seeds of *Myristica fragrans*. The oil is a colourless or pale yellow liquid with characteristic odour and taste of Nutmeg.

East Indian Nutmeg oil possesses different properties than those of West Indian Nutmeg oil. The label of the container must indicate whether the oil is of East Indian or West Indian origin.

Nutmeg oil is distilled from the kernels imported into Europe and the USA, and is produced in Indonesia (about 120 tons annually), Sri Lanka (30 tons) and India (5 tons). There are differences in optical rotation, refractive index, weight per millilitre and solubility in alcohol between the West Indian and East India oils. Myristicin is 4-allyl-6-methoxy-1,2-methylene-dioxybenzene. It is crystalline and, due to its high boiling point, is mainly found in the last portions of the distillate. Myristicin is toxic to human beings and large doses of Nutmeg or its oil may cause convulsions. The seeds contain dimeric phenyl-propanoids from the seed; the units include isoeugenol, elemicin and myristicin. Similar dimeric compounds, shown to cause significant changes in hepatic enzyme systems, have been isolated from mace oil.

Pharmacology

Aril extract showed antibacterial activity against *Streptococcus mutans*, inhibited rat paw oedema and reduced the number of writhings induced by acetic acid. Phenylpropyl derivatives act as neoplasm inhibitors. Myristicin, licarin B and dehydrodi-isoeugenol prolonged hexabarbital-induced sleep and reduced liver aminopyrine N-demethylase and hexabarbital hydrolase activities, shortened duration of hypnosis and increased hepatic enzyme activities. Malabaricones B and C exhibited strong antifungal and antibacterial activities.

In recent years, Nutmeg is considered as a hallucinogenic agent. However, the relatively large amount (up to 15 g) causes the desired intoxication also produces flushing of the skin, tachycardia, absence of salivation, and other undesirable side effects. Myristicin and elemicin may be responsible for the effects on the central nervous system. Perhaps, there is *in vivo* biotransformation of these nutmeg constituents into amphetamine-like, nitrogen-containing metabolites.

Nutmeg oil is a flavouring agent. It possesses carminative properties.

MACE

Common mace consists of the dried arillus or arillode of *M. fragrans*. It is of a bright red colour and is removed either by the finger or a knife. After flattening under the feet or pressing between boards the mace is slowly dried. The volatile oil of mace resembles that of Nutmeg, the major phenolic compounds isolated being dehydrodi-isoeugenol and 5'-methoxydehydrodi-isoeugenol. Some lignans and neolignans have been isolated from mace.

Bombay mace is almost valueless as a spice. It is dark red in colour, lacking in aroma and yields about 30% of extractive to light petroleum (genuine mace yields about 3.5%). Papua mace has dull brownish surface with lack of aroma and acrid taste.

Allied drugs

Papua Nutmegs are derived from *M. argentea*, a tree grown in New Guinea and exported to Macassar and Papua. They are longer (about 3.5 cm) than the official Nutmegs, have a uniform, scurfy surface, some odour and a disagreeable taste.

Bombay Nutmegs are obtained from *M. malabarica*, grown in India. They are very long and narrow and lack the distinct aroma of the genuine drug.

CALAMUS

Synonyms

Sweetflag; Bach (Hindi); Calamus rhizome; Vaj, Godavaj; Rhizoma Acori Calami.

Biological source

Dried peeled or unpeeled rhizomes of *Acorus calamus* Linn. are called Calamus (Family Araceae).

Geographical source

The plant widely occurs in Asia, Europe and North America. It is found throughout India and Sri Lanka.

As a semi-aquatic, perennial, erect, aromatic herb with creeping rhizomes, it grows wild and also is cultivated. Rhizomes are horizontal, joined, and vertically compressed.

The plant is grown in clayey loams and light alluvial soils of river banks. The field is irrigated and ploughed with green manure before planting. The crop is ready for harvest in about a year. The plants are dug out, rhizomes removed and the tops kept for the next planting. The rhizomes are cut into pieces of 5-8 cm and all fibrous roots are removed. The pieces are washed thoroughly and dried in the sun. The dried material is put into rough gunny bags and rubbed to remove the leafy scales.

Morphology

The subcylindrical rhizome is up to 20 cm long and 2 cm in diameter, longitudinally furrowed on the upper surface with root scars on the lower surface.

Chemical constituents

Calamus contains volatile oil (2-4%) from which α-asarone, β-asarone, calamene, calamenol and calamenone have been identified. Glucoside acorin has also been reported in the rhizome. Other constituents of Calamus oil are methyl eugenol, eugenol, α-pinene and camphene. The presence of small amounts of palmitic, heptylic and butyric acids, asaronaldehyde, calamol, calamone and azulene has also been reported. Sesquiterpenic ketones like

Acorenone

γ-Asarone

β-Asarone
(cis-isoasarone)

Shyobunone

2,6-Di-epi-shyobunone

Acorone

Fig. 18.36. Chemical constituents of Calamus.

acorone, calarene, calacone, calacorene, acrorenone, calamusenone, isocalamusenone, acolamone, isoacolamone, epishyobunone, shyobunone, isoshyobunone, acoragermacrone and alcohols like isocalamendiol and preisocalamendiol are also present. The hydro-carbons present in the oil are elemene, caryo-phyllene, calamenene, cadalene, humulene, 9-aristolene, β-gurjunene, telekin, isotelekin, isocalamendiol, preisocalamendiol, cadala-1,4,9-triene, β-ocimene, 4,7-decadienal and calamen-sesquiterpinenol.

The rhizome also contain luteolin-6,8-C-diglucoside, acoradin, 2,4,5-trimethoxybenzaldehyde, 2,5-dimethoxybenzoquinone, galangin, β-sitosterol, fixed oil composed of linolenic (24.5%), palmitic (18.2%), palmitoleic (16.4%), stearic (7.3%), oleic (29.1%), arachidic and myristic acids; maltose, glucose, fructose; 3-(2,4,5-trimethoxyphenyl)-2-propenol, 3-(2,4,5-trimethoxyphenyl)-2-propenol and 3-(2,4,5-trimethoxyphenyl) indene derivative.

The composition of the oil from 2n, 3n and 4n varieties differs and the β-asarone content increases

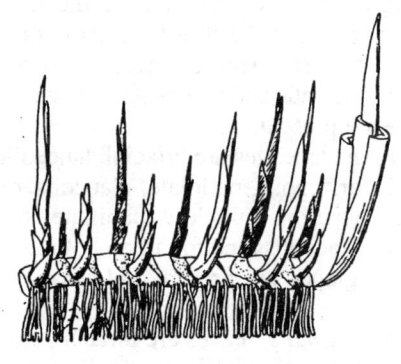

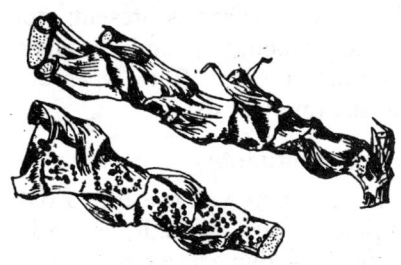

Fig. 18.35. Calamus rhizome.

with ploidy. The phenylpropane deriva-tives showed carcinogenic activity in animal tests.

The oil from the rhizome of the American $2n$ race contains no β-asarone but consists of shyobu-nones and acorones.

Uses

Calamus is an anthelmintic, insectifuge, nauseant, aromatic, antispasmotic, nervine stimulant, expectorant, carminative, emetic, stomachic, sedative drug and used to treat dyspepsia, colic, intermittent fevers, bronchitis, dysentery of children, kidney and liver troubles, rheumatism, eczema, snake-bite, mental ailments, diarrhoea, bronchial catarrh and glandular tumors. The powdered rhizome is used as an insecticide for the destruction of fleas, bedbugs, moths and lice.

The rhizomes are used in the form of powder, balms, enemas and pills.

Oil of calamus, administered as *Acorus calamus* rhizome in many preparations, is believed to be carcinogenic. Calamus oil is credited with carminative, anti-spasmodic and antibacterial properties. Asarone is a mild sedative, tranquilizer and hypotensive substance.

Substitution

Calamus rhizomes are sometimes substituted with the rhizomes of *Alpinia galanga* (Bach) and *Aconitum* species (Bish).

Pharmacology

The calamus essential oil showed spasmolytic activity in animals. Asarone and β-asarone prolonged β-hypnotic activity of anaesthetic agents. They caused significant reduction in rectal temperature of mice and showed cardiac depressant activity, moderate hypotensive action in dogs and anti-acetylcholine activity. Asarone caused atoxia, hypnosis and loss of righting reflex. The root extract excited antimicrobial activity. *cis*-Asarone showed antifungal activity against *Helmintho-sporium oryzae.*

EUCALYPTUS OIL

Synonyms

Gum wood oil; Australian fever tree oil; Blue-gum tree oil.

Biological source

Eucalyptus oil is a volatile oil obtained by steam distillation of the fresh leaves of various species of *Eucalyptus* such as *E. globulus* Labill, *E. citriodora*, *E. polybractea*, *E. smithii*, *E. viminalis*, and *E. australiana*. It contains not less than 65% of caneole (Family : Myrtaceae).

Habitat

E. globulus is a native of Australia and Tasmania. Now it is cultivated in South France, Spain, Portugal, Brazil, Zaire and India (Nilgiri hills).

E. globulus is a large tree attaining a height of 100 m or more with a clean straight bole under forest conditions.

It grows well in Nilgiris (1,700-2,700 m), Annamalai and Palni hills in South India. A cool, moist, equitable climate and deep fertile soil, which is not calcareous or saline, are favourable for the growth of *E. globulus*. It is propagated by seeds.

Morphology

In *E. globulus* leaves are bifacial, lanceolate, scythe-shaped, glabrous, sessile, thin and wax-coated. A coating of wax is present over the thin cuticle, stomata of ranunculaceous type occur on the lower surface and few round internal oil glands are present. Prismatic and rosette type crystals of calcum oxalate are present.

E. rostrata leaves are bifacial, lanceolar, sickle-shaped, coriaceous, petiolate, glaucous, ovate with distinct venation. Cuticle is papillate, stomata are of ranunculaceous type found on both the surfaces; many oil glands are present and also rosette crystals.

In *E. viminalis,* leaves are bifacial, elongated or falcate-lanceolate, glabrous, glaucous and sessile. Thick cuticle with minute papilla in upper and marked in lower surface is present; stomata are ranunculaceous occur on both surfaces and oil glands are also present. Both types of crystals, prismatic and rosette, exist.

Chemical constituents

Eucalyptus contains volatile oil (3-6%), resin, tannic acids, dihydroflavanol, aromadendrin-7-methyl ether, *p*-coumaric acid, cinnamic acid, eucalyptic acid and rutin.

Eucalyptus oil is a colourless or pale yellow liquid having a typical, aromatic, camphor-like odour and pungent, spicy cooling taste. The oil contains cineole (70-85%) as the predominent compound. Other components identified in the oil are pinene, camphene, butyric aldehyde, valerenic aldehyde, caproic aldehyde, aromadendrene, cuminaldehyde, pinocarveol, phellandrene, 1,8-cineole, *o*-cresol, *cis*- and *trans*-pinocarveol, α-pinocarvone, citronellal, d-myrtenal, carvone, citral, globulol, eudesmol, piperitone, geranyl acetate, S-guaiazulene, cinnamic acid, eudesmyl acetate, aromadendrone, alloaromadendrene, epiglobulol, ledol, viridifloral, α-, β- and γ-terpenes, terpinen-4-ol, linalool oxide, α-gurjunene, piperitone, eremophilene, γ-cadinene, fenchone, α- and β-thujone, verbenone, isoamyl alcohol, *trans*-verbenol, borneol, myrtenol, α-terpineol, thymol, bornyl acetate, caproic acid, farnesols and δ-guaiene.

The leaves also contain gallic, caffeic, ferulic and protocatechuic acids, quercitol, quercitrin, rutin, hyperoside, quercitol-3-glucoside, euglobals Ia$_1$, Ia$_2$, Ib, Ic, IIa, IIb, IIc, III, IV, V, VII, IVb, *n*-

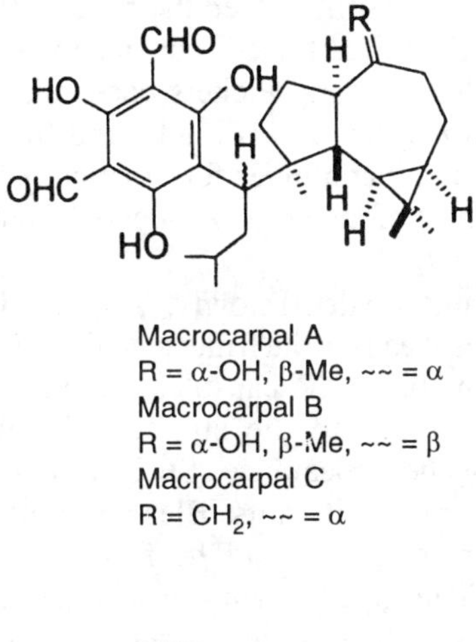

Macrocarpal A
R = α-OH, β-Me, ~~ = α
Macrocarpal B
R = α-OH, β-Me, ~~ = β
Macrocarpal C
R = CH$_2$, ~~ = α

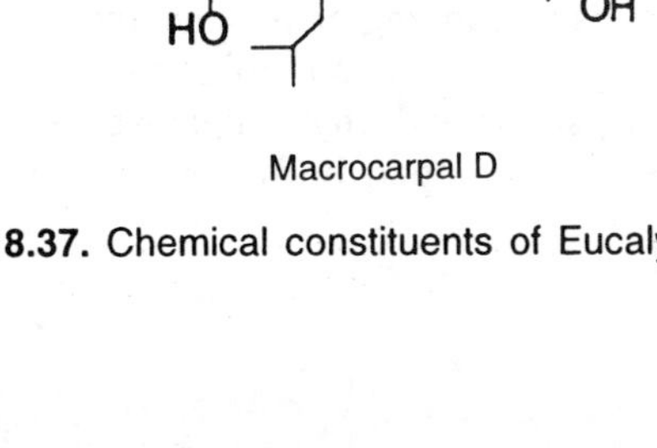

Macrocarpal D

Fig. 18.37. Chemical constituents of Eucalyptus.

triacontan-16,18-dione, oleanolic and maslinic acids, hydroxytritriacontan-16,18-dione, 16-hydroxy-18-tritriacontanone & macrocarpals A-E.

Uses

Eucalyptus oil is antiseptic, disinfectant, diuretic, diaphoretic, decongestant, expectorant and flavouring agent. It is used in infections of the upper respiratory tract, malaria, certain skin diseases, in ointment for burns and as mosquito repellent. Internally, it is used as a stimulating expectorant in chronic bronchitis and asthma. Eucalyptus increases the flow of saliva, gastric and intestinal juices and thus increases appetite and digestion. It increases the rate of heart beats, lowers the arterial tension and quickens respiration. In toxic doses it is a narcotic poison. It paralyses the respiratory centre in the medulla. Oil obtained from Indian species does not contain butyric and valerinic aldehydes; it is less likely to produce cough and other unpleasant side effects. Mixed with an equal amount of olive oil, it is useful as a rubefacient for rheumatism. The antimicrobial action of this oil is synergistic action of citrorallal and citronellol in the ratio of 90:75.

Cineole (encalyptol) is obtained from eucalyptus oil as a colourless liquid with a distinct, aromatic, camphoraceous odour and a pungent, cooling, spicy taste. It is obtained from eucalyptus oil by fractional distillation and subsequent freezing of the distillate or by treating the volatile oil with phosphoric acid and then decomposing the cineolephosphoric acid with water. Cineole is also obtained from terpin hydrate as a dehydration product on treatment with acids. It is used as a flavouring agent in nasal inhalares and sprays, as external analgesics and as mouth-washes.

Pharmacology

Euglobals showed granulation-inhibiting activity. *n*-Tritriacontan-16,18-dione showed marked antioxidant activity in water/alcohol system, but no antioxidant activity in oil system. Euglobal-III showed strong inhibitory activity followed by euglobals Ib, IIa, Ia1 and Ia2.

CHENOPODIUM OIL

Synonyms

American Wormseed oil, Mexican Tea oil, Spanish Tea oil, Jerusalem Tea oil, Ambrosia oil.

Biological source

Chenopodium oil is the essential oil collected by steam distillation of fresh aerial parts of *Chenopodium ambrosioides* L. variety *anthelmintica* (Family : Chenopodiaceae).

Habitat

Chenopodium plant is an erect, much-branched aromatic herb with glandular hairs, about 30-60 cm in height commonly found in eastern USA and cultivated in Maryland, Carroll Country and South India. It is indigenous to the West Indies. The oil is formed in glandular hairs occurring on the leaves, flowers, and fruits but it is found in excess on pericarp and ovary.

Chemical constituents

Chenopodium contains volatile oil (1-4%) which is light yellow in colour with a characteristic unpleasant odour and a bitter burning taste. The chief active constituent of the oil is ascaridol (70%) which is an unsaturated terpene peroxide. It explodes on heating or on treating with certain acids. Other constituents of the oil are limonene, myrcene, methyl salicylate, pinene, *p*-cymene, *l*-limonene, *d*-camphor, xylene isomers, pinocarveol, thymol, carvacrol, carvone, *trans*-carveol, *trans*-isocarveol, *p*-mentha-2,8-dien-1-ols and 1,4-diol, 1,4-epoxy-*p*-mentha-2,3-diol and menth-1(7), 8-dien-2-ol.

Chenopodium also contains triterpene glycosides chenopodosides A and B; kaempferol and its glycosides, isorhamnetin and quercetin.

Ascaridole exhibited analgesic and sedative activities.

Uses

Chenopodium oil is an anthelmintic, particularly for roundworms, hookworms and intestinal amoebae. It is generally used in veterinary practice.

CARDAMOM

Synonyms

Grains of Paradise, Cardamom Fruit, Ilayachi (Hindi).

Biological Source

Cardamom consists of the dried ripe seeds of *Elettaria cardamomum* Maton var. *minuscula*. (Family : Zingiberaceae).

Geographical Source

Cardamom is cultivated in Sri Lanka, south India (Mysore and Kerala) and Guatemala.

Cultivation

Plant is reed-like 3-4 meters high herbaceous perennial herb with long leaves arising from the rhizome. Seeds are planted in nurseries. After one year the young seedlings are transplanted in fields. Fruits are developed in 3-4 years old plants. The nearly ripe capsules, when their colour turns from green to yellow, are collected, washed to remove sand and dried quickly to get green Cardamom. Bleaching takes place when the fruits are dried for longer time in sunlight or by placing trays of the fruits over burning sulphur. Stalk, calyx and split fruits are removed and graded according to size and quality.

It is important to collect fruits when nearly ripe and before they split to shed their seeds. It is best to cut off each fruit at the correct stage with a pair of short-bladed scissors. Pickers can collect about 5 kg of fruit per day. In Sri Lanka and India flowering and fruiting continues for practically the whole year but most of the crop is collected from October to December.

The fruits are dried slowly. Very rapid drying is avoided, as it causes the fruits to split and shed their seeds. Sometimes the capsules are moistened and further exposed to the sun for bleaching and improving the appearance. Such drying increases the number of split fruits. Bleaching may also be done by placing trays of the fruits over burning sulphur. The green curing procedure is used in Guatemala. Enhanced colour retention is obtained by soaking the fruits for 10 min in 2% sodium carbonate solution before drying.

The capsules have the remains of the calyx at the apex and a stalk at the base. These are removed either by hand-clipping or by machines. The fruits are then graded by means of sieves into 'longs', 'mediums', 'shorts' and 'tiny'. Sulphur-bleached fruits are aired in the open before being packed for export.

Morphology

The Cardamom frui is an ovoid or oblong, trilocular capsule, 1-2 cm long, apex is beak-shaped, base is rounded with remains of stalk, surface is longitudinally striated, colour is light green. The seeds are up to 4 mm in length, irregularly angular, dark reddish brown. The odour is aromatic and taste is aromatic, pleasant and somewhat pungent.

Internally the capsule is three-celled, a double row of seeds attached to axial placentas occurring in each cell. The seeds in each loculus are tightly pressed together and usually separate in a single mass.

The testa is transversely wrinkled and is covered by a membranous aril. A groove on one side of the seed indicates the position of the raphe and a depression at one end of the hilum.

Seeds cut longitudinally and transversely and stained with iodine show the aril, testa, perisperm (containing starch) and the endosperm and embryo (both free from starch).

Microscopical characters

There is a very thin membraneous arillus, enveloping the seed and composed of several layers of

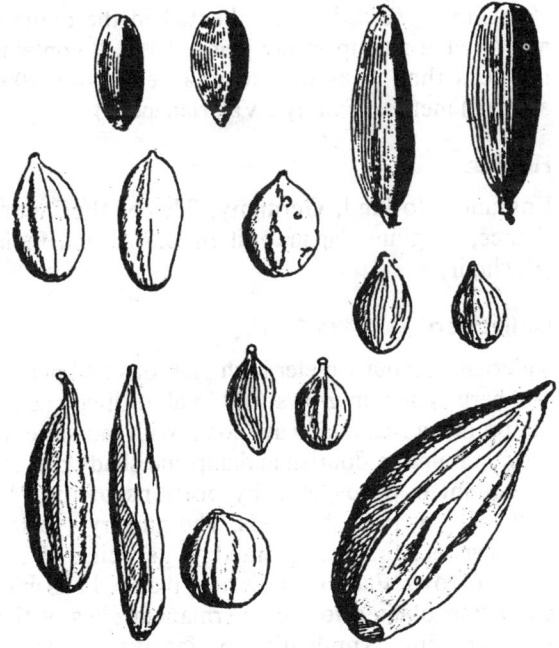

Fig. 18.38. Cardamom fruits.

collapsed cells, yellow in colour and containing oil. The brownish testa is composed of an outer epidermis consisting of a single layer of cells rectangular in transverse section, longitudinally elongated and with prosenchymatous end walls in surface view; light yellow in colour and having slightly thick end walls; a single layer of large parenchymatous cells containing volatile oil. In the region of the raphe there are two layers of oil cells separated by the raphe meristele; several layers of small flattened parenchymatous cells, and an inner epidermis of sclerenchymatous cells, radially elongated, with anticlinal and inner walls very strongly thickened and reddish-brown in colour. The operculum or embryonic cap is composed of two or three layers of these sclerenchymatous cells. The micropyle is a narrow canal passing through the operculum. Within the testa is a well-developed perisperm composed of parenchymatous cells packed with minute globular starch grains, and containing in the centre of each cell a small prismatic crystal of calcium oxalate. The perisperm encircles the endosperm and embryo, both composed of thin-walled cells rich in protein.

Cardamom pericarps or husks is identified in the form of powder by the pitted fibres and spiral vessels of the fibrovascular bundles and by the abundant, empty parenchymatous cells.

Chemical constituents

Cardamom contains volatile oil (3-8%), resin, fixed oil (1-2%), starch and calcium oxalate. The essential oil possesses eucalyptol (cineole) (50%), borneol, sabinene, terpineol and its acetate, limonene, terpinene, 1-terpinen-4-ol and its formate and acetate, dipentene, α-pinene, sabinene, myrcene, cineole, cymene, methyl heptenone, linalool, linalyl acetate, neryl acetate, geraniol, nerol, heptacosane, sabinene and nerolidol. The fixed oil consists of the glycerides of oleic, stearic, linoleic, palmitic, caprylic and caproic acids. The unsaponifiable matter from the fixed oil contains β-sitosterol. The seeds contain vitamin B_1.

The green seeds contain β-sitosterol, γ-sitosterol, phytol, n-alkanes and n-alkenes.

Uses

Cardamom is aromatic, stimulant, stomachic, carminative, diuretic and used as a flavouring agent for pharmeceutical syrups, curries and cake and for preparation of Compound Cardamom Tincture.

Allied drug

1. *Elettaria cardamomum* var. *major* : This species is the source of the long wild native Cardamom of Sri Lanka. They are 4 cm long, pericarp is dark brown and coarsely striated. Its volatile oil is used in liquors.

2. *Amomum aromaticum* and *A. subulatum* : *A. aromaticum* is obtained from Bengal and Assam and known as Bengal Cardamom. *A. subulatum* is obtained from Nepal, Bengal, Sikkim and Assam and known as Nepal or Greater Cardamom. *A. subutalum* contains petunidin-3,5-diglucoside, leucocyanidin-3-glucoside, cardamonin, alpinetin, and aurone glucoside subulin.

Malabar Cardamom is characterized by a short leafy shoot, 3 m in height, the fruit shape is roundish or elongated, smaller than the Mysore Cardamom.

Mysore Cardamom is a robust with leafy stem, up to 5 m high. Mysore Cardamom fruits are elongated, 2-5 cm long, yellowish green when ripe, slightly arched and darkish brown when dry; seeds are numerous, large and less aromatic.

Mangalore cardamom resembles the Malabar but are more globular and have a rougher pericarp. *Alleppy* fruits are narrower than the above varieties, have a markedly striated pericarp and colour varies from greenish-buff to green. *Ceylon greens* resemble Alleppy, but are generally greener and more elongated. The seeds of the above varieties resemble one another. The seeds of allied species resemble those of the true cardamom are : *A. cardamomum*, cardamom of Siam and Java; *A. xanthioides*, the bastard or wild Siamese cardamom; *A. maximum*, a Japanese plant; *Aframomum korarima*, the Korarima or Abyssinian cardamom; *A. mala*, the East African cardamom; *A. hanburii* and *A. danielli*, Cameroon cardamoms; *A. angustifolium*, Madagascar cardamom; *Costus speciosus*, Chinese cardamom.

Adulteration

Cardamom fruits are often adulterated with orange seeds and unroasted coffee grains. The adulterants of seeds are small pebbles and seeds of *Amomum* spp. Powdered seeds are adulterated with the powder of husks.

Grains of paradise, also known as Guinea grains or melegueta pepper, consists of the seeds of the West African reed-like herb *Aframomum melegueta* (Zingiberaceae), which has many of the characters of Cardamom. The seeds are hard, flat, triangular, reddish-brown, about 3 mm long; testa is papillose; aromatic odour; pungent taste. The seeds yield about 0.5% of volatile oil which contains principally β-caryophyllene, α-humulene and their epoxides. The pungency arises from paradol, a substance related to gingerol, and from small quantities of shogaol and gingerol. The seeds are used in alcoholic liquors and in veterinary medicine.

VALERIAN

Synonyms

Valeriana; Valerian rhizome; Valerian root; European Valerian; Rhizoma Valerianae.

Biological Source

Valerian is the dried roots, rhizome and stolons of *Valeriana officinalis* L., collected in the autumn and dried at a temperature below 40ºC. It contains not less than 15% of extractable (about 60% alcohol) metter. (Family : Valerianaceae).

Habitat

England, Holland, Germany, The Netherlands, France, Belgium, Japan, eastern U.S.A. and India (Kashmir).

Collection

Valerian is about 1 meter high glabrous and perennial herb. Valerian grows well in all ordinary soils, but prefers a rich and heavy loam with moisture. It is often found to flourish in damp and shady places. The plant is propagated by portions of the old rootstocks or from the seeds. The nursery - raised seedlings are first transplanted at a spacing of 18-20 cm in rows. Early in the spring, the seedings may be re-transplanted to their permanent sites at the same spacing. Application of farmyard manure favours the growth of the plants and roots.

The rhizomes and roots of the plants are harvested in the autumn, though the yield is low. The bud-raised plants do not attain a suitable size up to second year. Their tops are cut at the ground-level before the rhizomes are dug up. The rhizomes and roots are washed thoroughly, dried in the sun and the longer rhizomes are longitudinally cut into pieces. Fresh drug is odourless but dried drug becomes darker in colour and develops a typical smell of isovaleric acid produced by hydrolysis of borneol isovalerianate which is one of a constituent of the drug.

Morphology

The drug consists of rhizomes, stolons and roots. The rhizomes are 2-4 cm in length and 1-2.5 cm wide. The roots are up to 10 cm in length and 2 mm in diameter, usually matted and broken. Longitudinal slices are also present. Roots are longitudinally striated. The fracture is short and horny. The odour is characteristic valerianaceous and taste is camphoraceous and slightly bitter. The development of the characteristic odour during drying and storage results from a breakdown of the unstable valepotriates and the hydrolysis of esters of the oil to give isovaleric acid as a product.

Microscopical characters

A transverse section of the rhizome shows a thin periderm, a large parenchymatous cortex which is rich in starch and an endodermis containing globules of volatile oil. A ring of collateral vascular bundles contain a large pith with scattered groups of sclerenchymatous cells.

A transverse section of a root shows an epidermis with papillae and root hairs, and an exodermis containing globules of oil. The cortex and pith contain starch. The starch is present mainly in compound grains with two to four components, having 3-20 μm diameter.

Chemical constituents

Valerian contains volatile oil (~1%), alkaloids (0.05-0.1%) like chatinine, valerine, 2-acetyl-pyrrole ketone and valerianine; valeric, formic and malic acids, tannins, resin and epoxy-iridoids called as valepotriates (e.g., valtrate, didrovaltrate, acevaltrate, and isovaleroxyhydroxy didrovaltrate).

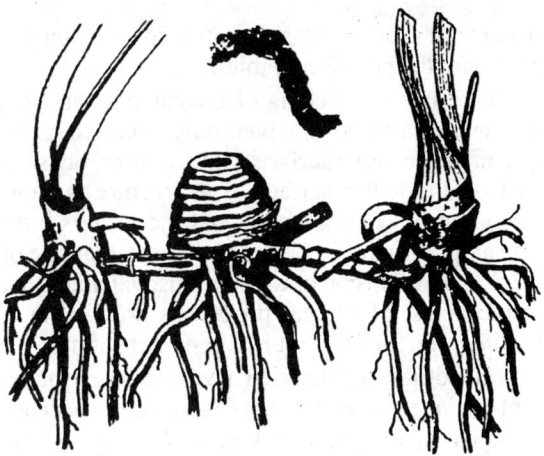

Fig. 18.39. *Valeriana officinalis* - Rootstocks with stolon.

On prolonged storage, hydrolysis of these valepotriates takes place to yield isovaleric acid and activity of the drug is changed. The composition of the valepotriate mixture differs greatly according to the variety. Valerenic and acetoxy-valerenic acids are the characteristic constituents of the official drug.

Volatile oil contains esters, like bornyl isovalerianate, bornyl acetate, bornyl formate, eugenyl isovalerate, isoeugenyl isovalerate, alcohols, eugenol, terpenes and a sesquiterpene alcohol (valerianol).

Uses

Valerian is carminative, antispasmodic, tranquillizer and sedative and used to cure hysteria, epilepsy, shell shock, neurosis, insomnia, nervous excitement and palpitation of the heart. Valepotriates possess mild but definite tranquillizing activity in animals. The drug is also utilized in the perfumery industry and to treat fevers and inflammations.

Allied drug

Indian Valerian (Syn. Mushkbala or Tagar in Hindi)

It consists of the dried rhizome and roots of *Valeriana wallichii* DC, syn. *V. jatamansii* Jones. It occurs in temperate Himalayas from Kashmir to Bhutan and Khasia Hills. It consists of yellow-brown rhizomes, size is 4-8 cm long, about 1 cm thick.

The size of roots is variable which may be up to 7 cm in length and 1-2 mm thick.

There is no branching of the rhizome and it is somewhat flattened dorsiventrally. Leaf scars are present on the upper surface while roots or root scars exist on the lower surface. The fracture is short. The odour is valerianaceous and the taste is bitter and camphoraceous. The drug possesses volatile oil (0.3-1.0%) which contains esters of isovalerianic and formic acids. Medicinal properties are similar to *V. officinalis* for which it is a good substitute.

Valepotriates of Valerian have also been isolated from *Centranthus ruber* root (Fam. Valerianaceae).

Japanese valerian or *Kesso (V. angustifolia)* contains about 8% volatile oil which is different from the oil of *V. officinalis.*

Harpagophytum (Devil's claw)

The dried, secondary roots of *Harpagophytum procumbens* (Pedaliaceae) are used to treat rheumatic disease. The plant is native to southern and eastern Africa near the Kalahari desert.

The drug consists of transverse, fan-shaped slices of the tuberous root with a brown, longitudinally wrinkled cork. It is odourless with very bitter taste.

The roots contain iridoid glycosides, flavonoids, various phenolic acids, triterpenes including oleanolic and ursolic acids, a quinone (harpagoquinone) and a high concentration of sugars, mainly trisaccharide stachyose.

The iridoids are involved in the anti-inflammatory and analgesic effects. The principal glycosides are harpagide, its cinnamoyl ester and the epoxyiridoid glycoside procumbide.

GARLIC

Synonyms

Allium; Lasan (Hindi).

Biological Source

Garlic is the ripe bulb of *Allium sativum* Linn. (Family Liliaceae).

Habitat

Garlic occurs in central Asia, southern Europe, and USA. It is widely cultivated in India.

Morphology

It is a perennial herb having bulbs with several cloves, enclosed in a silky white or pink membraneous envelop.

Cultivation

The cultivation of Garlic is similar to that of onion. It is generally grown as an irrigated crop throughout the year. It can be grown under a wide range of climatic conditions but it succeeds best in mild climates without extremes of heat and cold. It is grown on a wide variety of soils. It requires a rich well-drained clay loam to grow well. The land is well ploughed to a fine tilth, beds and channels are made. Garlic is planted during October-November in plains and during February-March in the hills. The cloves are separated and pressed lightly into the soil. Garlic requires heavy manuring.

Chemical constituents

Allicin, a yellow liquid responsible for the odour of garlic, is the active principle of the drug. It is miscible with alcohol, ether and benzene and decomposes on distilling. The other constituents reported in Garlic are alliin, volatile and fatty oils, mucilage and albumin. Alliin, another active principle, is odourless, crystallized from water-acetone and practically insoluble in absolute alcohol, chloroform, acetone, ether and benzene. Upon cleavage by the specific enzyme alliinase, an odour of garlic develops, and the fission products show antibacterial action similar to allicin. Essential oil (0.06-0.1%)

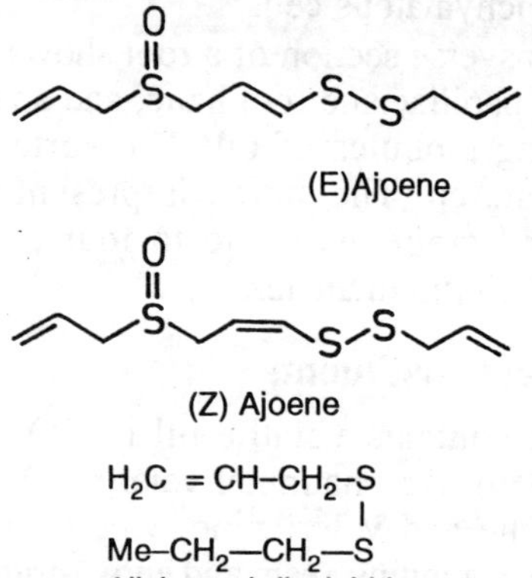

(E)Ajoene

(Z) Ajoene

$H_2C = CH–CH_2–S$
|
$Me–CH_2–CH_2–S$
Allylpropyl disulphide

Fig. 18.40. Chemical constituents of Garlic.

contains allyl propyl disulphide, diallyl disulphide and allicin. γ-Glutamyl peptides are isolated from the Garlic. The amino acids present in the bulb are leucine, methionine, S-propyl-L-cysteine, S-propenyl-L-cysteine, S-methyl cysteine, S-allyl cysteine sulphoxide (alliin), S-ethyl cysteine sulphoxide and S-butyl-cysteine sulphoxide.

The bulb also contain polypeptide scordinin A_1, saponins; polysaccharides, diallyl trisulphide, allyl methyl disulphide; gibberellins A3 and A7; ajoene, 4,5,9-trithiadodeca-1,6,11-triene-9-oxide, 3-vinyl-4H-dithiin, 2-vinyl-4H dithiin protoeruboside, steroid saponins I and II; sativoside B_1, protodesgalactotigonin, desgalactotigonin, F-gitonin, pyran-4-one derivative, methyl-2-propenyl thioether, 1,2-dithiocyclopent-3-ene, galacturonic acid, mannose, arabinose, palmitic, stearic, oleic, linoleic and linolenic acids lysolecithin, lecithin, phosphatidylinositol, phosphatidylserine, phosphatidylethanolamine and β-sitosterol in unsaponifiable matter.

Other cyclic sulfur compounds separated from the benzene fraction of the steam volatile oils from garlic are the trithiolane derivatives *cis*- and *trans*-3,5-diethyl-1,2,4-trithiolane and *cis*- and *trans*-3-methyl-5-ethyl-1,2,4-trithiolane.

In garlic, 2-vinyl-1,3-dithiin and allyl 1,5-hexadienyltrisulfide were also detected.

E and *Z* isomers of 4,5,9-trithiododeca-1,6,11-triene-9-oxide (ajoene) from garlic oil can be readily synthesized by decomposing allicin in acetone and water.

All of the sulfur containing products isolated from garlic are derived from allicin. β-elimination of allicin should yield 2-propene-sulfenic acid and thioacrolein. The latter compound is reported to dimerize to 3-vinyl-4H-1,2-dithiin and 2-vinyl-4H-1,3-dithiin. S-Allylthiolation of allicin should give a sulfonium ion, which could undergo β-elimination to a cation. Subsequent γ-addition of 2-propenesulfenic acid gives (E,Z)-ajoene. Hydrolysis of the sulfonium ion yields allyl alcohol and diallyl trisulfide. Hydrolysis of allicin should give 2-propenesulfinic acid; β, γ-unsaturated sulfinic acids are known to readily lose sulfur dioxide. Diallyl disulfide could arise via attack of 2-propenethiol on allicin. The absence of allyl 2-propenethiosulfonate could be explained if the rate of loss of sulfur dioxide from 2-propene-sulfinic acid is more rapid than its rate of nucleophilic attack on allicin.

In addition, some sulfur containing acidic peptides such as γ-glutamyl-S-methyl-cysteine and its sulfoxide derivative, γ-glutamyl-S-(2-carboxypropyl)-glycine, γ-glutamyl-S-allylcysteine, as well as γ-glutamylphenylalanine without sulfur are found in Garlic.

The cysteine sulfoxide fraction of garlic consists of 85% alliin along with 2% S-propylcysteine sulfoxide and 13% S-methylcysteine sulfoxide.

Allinase activity on the S-substituted cysteine sulfoxide fraction from garlic extract yields allyl methanesulfinothioic acid ester and other symmetrical or asymmetrical sulfinothioic acid esters with methyl, propyl and allyl substituents. The presence of S-allyl-L-cysteine, which may be a precursor of alliin, has also been reported.

Additional volatile components of garlic extract were identified as allyl alcohol, methyl allyl disulfide, diallyl disulfide, dimethyl trisulfide, allyl methyl trisulfide, diallyl trisulfide and sulfur dioxide.

Allicin decomposed nearly completely at 20°C within 20 h, giving diallyl disulfide as the major product and diallyl trisulfide, diallyl sulfide, sulfur oxide, and trace amounts of two 1,2-dithiin compounds: 3-vinyl-6H-1,2-dithiin and 3-vinyl-4H-1,2-dithiin.

Uses

Garlic is carminative, aphrodisiac, expectorant, stimulant and used in fevers, coughs, febrifuge in intermittent fevers, respiratory diseases such as chronic bronchitis, bronchial asthma, whooping cough and tuberculosis. It is also used in atherosclerosis and hypertension.

In Germany, Garlic is consumed as a complement in the diet of hyperlipemic patients and for the prophylaxis of the vascular changes induced by ageing. The Garlic can cause gastrointestinal distress and alters breath and skin odour.

Pharmacology

Garlic or its constituents exhibit various biological activities such as antibacterial, antifungal, antiviral, antitumor and antidiabetic effects. The greatest interest, however, has been focused on their anti-cholesterolemic and antithrombotic activities. Applied orally, garlic and its ethanol extract reduced plasma and liver cholesterol levels in male rats fed a diet containing 1% cholesterol. In particular, very low density lipoprotein and low density lipoprotein cholesterol fractions were reduced. The hypo-cholesterolemic principle of garlic was found in the ethanol extract and was stable when autoclaved at 120°C for 1 h. Oral administration of an aqueous extract of garlic to hypercholesterolemic patients for 2 months significantly reduced cholesterol levels. Withdrawal of treatment increased the cholesterol level again.

Garlic improves systolic and diastolic arterial tension in hypertensive and atherosclerotic patients and showed bactericidal effect on pathogenic microorganisms. Extracts of different parts exhibited a stimulating effect on the uterus of guinea-pigs. Blood cholesterol level was significantly decreased in human beings after two months of ingestion of garlic. Diallyl disulphide showed anti-microbial activity. An extract of the plant inhibited enhancement of phospholipid metabolism caused by a tumor promotor. It suppressed the first stage of tumor promotion in mouse skin carcinogenesis and inhibited platelet aggregation. Ajoene showed strong inhibition of platelet aggregation. Allicin inhibited human platelet aggregation without affecting cyclo-oxygenase or thromboxane synthase activity. It also inhibited ionophore A 23187 stimulated human neutrophil lysosomal enzyme release. Allicin dilated mesenteric circulation of cat. Garlic counteracted coagulability-enhancing and fibrinolysis lowering effects of cholesterol feeding rabbits. Feeding of garlic oil prevented cholesterol and triglycerides in serum, rise of total lipids in liver and accumulation of cholesterol in kidney and liver in rabbits. Garlic extract increased liver glycogen and decreased fasting blood sugar, serum triglycerides and liver and serum proteins in sucrose-fed rabbits.

Garlic powder given daily for 3 months to 40 humans aged 70 and above, caused significant reduction in serum cholesterol, phospholipids and triglyceride concentrations. Aqueous garlic extract significantly increased level of blood serum urea in rats. Garlic oil given to fed rats did not affect blood serum urea or enzymes. An acetone or chloroform extract showed antimutagenic activity. Plant extract inhibited 5-lipoxygenase, cyclo-oxygenase, thrombocyte aggregation and angiotensin I converting enzyme. Dialysate of garlic bulbs showed inhibition of cardiovascular functions in dogs. Application of allixin to mice inhibited tumor induced by DMBA. A polysaccharide SE-GPS inhibited human cytomegalovirus. Allixin suppressed tumor promoting stage of carcinogenesis. Allicin inhibited bacterial acetyl-CoA forming system.

Ajoene inactivated human gastric lipase which assisted digestion and absorption of dietary fats. S-Allylcysteine sulphoxide showed antidiabetic effect in rats. It decreased levels of serum lipids and blood glucose, activated serum enzymes and increased liver and intestinal HMG CoA reductase. Sulphur compounds showed virucidal effect against herpes simplex viruses, vaccinia viruses, stomatitis vesicular virus and para-influenza virus in order of ajoene > allicin > allyl methyl thiosulphinate. Fresh garlic extract was virucidal. Garlic oil and allyl methyl trisulphide inhibited platelet aggregation and inhibited production of thromboxane B2 and prostaglandin E2.

Garlic treatment did not alter concentrations of circulating thyroid hormones. Garlic significantly increased the fibrinolytic activity of blood from healthy individuals and from patients with acute myocardial infarction. Garlic reduced microflora in the intestine of rats.

Allicin, methyl allyl trisulfide, ajoene, diallyl trisulfide, 2-vinyl-1,3-dithiin and allyl 1,5-hexadienyl trisulfide all inhibited platelet aggregation. Allicin produced dose-dependent hypoglycemia, improved glucose tolerance and increased serum insulin effect and liver glycogen synthesis.

$$CH_2=CH-CH_2-S-S-CH_2\ CH=CH_2$$
$$||$$
$$O$$
Allicin

$$CH_2=CH-CH_2-S-CH_2\ CH-COOH$$

with O and NH$_2$ substituents shown above.

Alliin

PYRETHRUM FLOWERS

Synonyms

Dalmatian insect powder; Persian insect powder, Pyrethrum Insect flowers; Pyrethrum; Flower Heads; Flores pyrethri.

Biological source

Pyrethrum flowers are the dried flower heads of *Chrysanthemum cinerariifolium* Visiani or *C. coccineum* Willd. (*C. roseum* Weber et Mohr.) or *C. marschallii* Asch. (Family : Asteraceae).

Habitat

The plant is indigenous to the Dalmatia (Yugoslavia-Balkans). It is widely grown in Kenya, Japan, Ecuador, Yugoslavia, east central Africa, Brazil, Tanzania and Zaira. In India the plant is cultivated in Kashmir, Nilgiris and north-west Himalayas.

Cultivation and collection

Pyrethrum is a 1 meter long glaucous perennial herb with finely cut leaves and numerous flower heads. It is cultivated by planting seeds and transplating in calcareous soil. The plant grows better at an altitude of 1900-2700 m (as in Kenya) and annual rainfall of 76-180° cm. Pyrethrum thrives best in a dry climate on well-drained sandy soil. It can grow on mountain slopes and waste lands. Sowing is usually done in spring or in autumn in shade. Before sowing, the seeds are soaked in water, wrapped in cloth, and buried in damp sand. The seeds germinate in 10-15 days and the shading is removed after the shoots appear. The land must be well-drained. Application of excessive nitrogen manures suppresses flowering. The plants flower within one year of transplanting but the yield in poor. The flower heads are gathered when the last florets are about to open. The active principles in over-mature flowers decompose more rapidly than in immature or nearly mature flowers. A low night temperature (5-15°C) stimulates high bud production. Pyrethrum flowers are collected from 2-6 years old plants by hand. The flowers are immediately dried in sunlight or in ovens below temperature 55°C. Fresh flowers are not toxic to insects. Dried flowers are packed tightly in bales and sent to the market.

Morphology

The closed heads of Pyrethrum flowers are nearly 6-9 mm in diameter and open-heads are 9-12 mm in diameter. Peduncle is short, striated longitudinally, receptacle is 4-8 mm in diameter, flat and without paleae, surrounded by an involucre of two or three rows of yellowish or greenish yellow lanceolate, hairy bracts with a membraneous margin. The receptacle contains various tubular florets and a single row of 15 to 23 white, cream or straw-coloured ligulate florets which are 10-20 mm in length and have about 17 veins and three rounded teeth. The central teeth is very small and suppressed. Calyx is tubular and membraneous. Ovary is inferior, achenes are 5-ribbed, style is filiform and stigma is bifid. Calyx and gynaecium in tubular florets are identical to ligulate florets. The colour is rose-like of ray florets and ten-ribbed fruits. The odour is slightly aromatic and taste is bitter and acrid.

Chemical constituents

Pyrethrum contains volatile oil (1-1.5%), esters of chrysanthemic acid (chrysanthemum monocarboxylic acid), pyrethric acid (mono-methyl ester of chrysanthemum dicarboxylic aci), sesquiterpene lactones, the triterpene pyrethrol, resin, pyretol, pyrethrotoxic acid, pyrethrosin, chrysan-themine, chrysathemumic acids, chrysanthin, palmitic, caproic, lauric, oleic, isovaleric, protocatechuic and linoleic acids. Choline and stachydrine are also present. Pyrethrin I, jasmolin I and cinerin I are esters of chrysanthemic acid while pyrethrin II, jasmolin II and cinerin II are esters of pyrethric acid. The alcoholic group of the pyrethrins is the keto-alcohol pyrethrolone and that of the cinerins is the keto-alcohol cinerolone. The pyrethrin I includes the esters of pyrethrolone, dihydropyrethrolone and cinerolone with chrysanthemum dicarboxylic acid; flowers also contain pyrethrosin, pyrethrol, lupeol, α- and β-amyrol and taraxasterol; (+)-sesamin and β-cyclopyrethrosin; its dihydroderivatives are chrysanin and chrysanolide. Pyrethrins are readily oxidized and become inactive in air. They are yellowish in colour, insoluble in water, soluble in alcohol, petroleum ether and carbon tetrachloride.

Pyrethrum also contains, apigenin, luteolin, apigenin-4'-glucuronide, 11,13-dihydrotatridins A and B, 6β-glucosyl of 11,13-dihydrotatridin B, tatridins A, B, dihydro-β-cyclopyrethrosin, jaceidin, apigenin-7-galactapigenin, apigenin-7-galacturonic acid methyl ester and 7-glucuronic acid.

Uses

Pyrethrum flowers and pyrethrins are toxic and insecticidal and used as a contact poison for insects in the form of powder or spray. They can cause severe allergic reactions. Large amounts may cause nausea, vomiting, tinnitus, headache and other CNS disturbances.

Pyrethrins are practically non-toxic to warm blooded animals when ingested, but if introduced into the blood circulation, they have a marked toxic effect. The principal site of action is the spinal cord. Cases of dermitis and other skin affections are reported.

Pyrethrum is a contact poison, highly toxic to insects. It is used as a livestock spray against parasitic insects.

The efficacy of Pyrethrum compositions against specific organisms is greatly enhanced by certain additives. Sesome oil, sesamin, isosesamin and asarinin are effective activators against house flies. Derivatives of alkanamides, piperic and phthalic acids, and a number of other compounds function as synergists. Pyrethrum is effective as an external application in pediculosis and scabies.

Pyrethrum powder is adulterated with the stem and leaf of the pyrethrum plant, and powdered flowers of other members of Asteraceae, particularly *C. leucanthemum* Linn. Lead chromate, Turmeric and fustic are used for imparting a yellowish tinge to the powder.

Pyrethrum concentrates should be stored after the addition of antioxidants in sealed containers.

	R_1	R_2
Pyrethrin I	Me	$CH=CH_2$
Jasmolin I	Me	CH_2-CH_3
Cinerin I	Me	CH_3
Pyrethrin II	CO_2Me	$CH=CH_2$
Jasmolin II	CO_2Me	CH_2-CH_3
Cinerin II	CO_2Me	CH_3

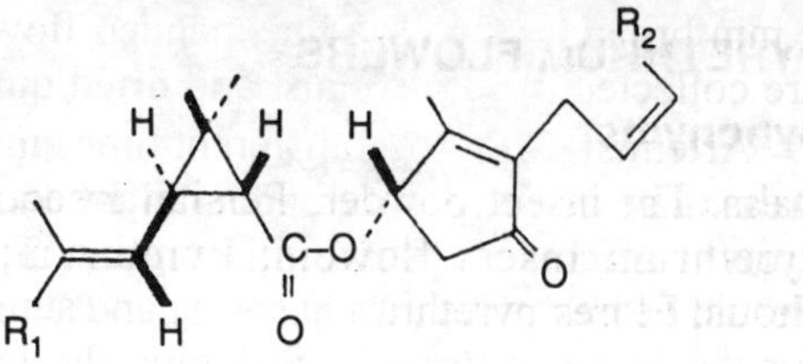

Fig. 18.41. Chemical constituents of Pyrethrum.

FEVERFEW

Feverfew *Chrysanthemum parthenium* (L.) Bernh., *Tanacetum parthenium* (L.) Schultz-Bip., *Maticaria parthenium* L. (Asteraceae) plant is used for the treatment of fever, arthritis, migraine, and menstrual problems. Feverfew yields sesquiterpene lactones, *e.g.*, parthenolide, 3β-hydroxy-parthenolide and other compounds with an α-methylene butyrolactone ring. The drug is standardized on its parthenolide content, 0.1% or 0.2% by HPLC. Different commercial products vary in their parthenolide contents.

Some commercial samples contain no parthenolide. The name 'feverfew' is applied to different species in different localities and countries. Its products undergo rapid deterioration on storage.

SANTONICA

Synonyms

Levant wormweed; Artemisia; Flores cinate; Santonica flowers; Semen cinae; Semen contra.

Biological source

Santonica consists of the dried unexpanded flower heads of *Artemisia maritima* (Berg) Willkomm. (Family : Asteraceae).

Habitat

Santonica is found in Turkestan, Pakistan, Iran, Tibet, Nepal and India (from Kashmir to Kumaon) at altitudes of 2,100-2,700 m.

Collection

Santonica is a small deciduous perennial shrub with much branched woody rootstalk, up to 100 cm in height. It is distinguished by its short, white-tomentose, 2-pinnatisect leaves with linear segments. Dried close flower heads are 2.4 cm long and nearly

1 mm broad, green. The unexpanded flower heads are collected in July-August and dried quickly.

Artemisias flower at different times in different areas. The age of the individual plant and stage of growth affects the santonin content. The plants should be harvested during spring and summer both for the luxuriant growth. Stripping the leaves and flower buds directly from the plant by hand is suggested. This enables the plants to put on fresh growth. It is bitter in taste.

Chemical constituents

Santonica possesses α-santonin (2-4%), volatile oil (2-3%), artemisin and resin. Santonin is the principal anthelmintic constituent which is a sesquiterpene lactone. Its concentration is maximum in closed flower heads and decreased quickly in mature and developed flower heads. It becomes yellow on exposure to light and is insoluble in water, but slightly soluble in alcohol, ether and chloroform. Indian plant besides santonin contains two more constituents, β-santonin with very weak anthelmintic properties and pseudo-santonin devoid of anthelmintic properties. Artemisin (8-hydroxysantonin) is responsible for the bitter taste of the drug and resin.

The drug also contains 1,8-cineole, camphor, erivanine, lumisantonin, alkhanin, hydroxy davanone, α-thujone, β-thujone and p-cymene.

Uses

Santonica is anthelmintic and santonin is more effective on roundworms than threadworms. It is used as deobstruent, stomachic, laxative and tonic. A decoction of the fresh plant is used to treat intermittent and remittent fevers.

Pharmacology

Santonin showed significant anti-inflammatory

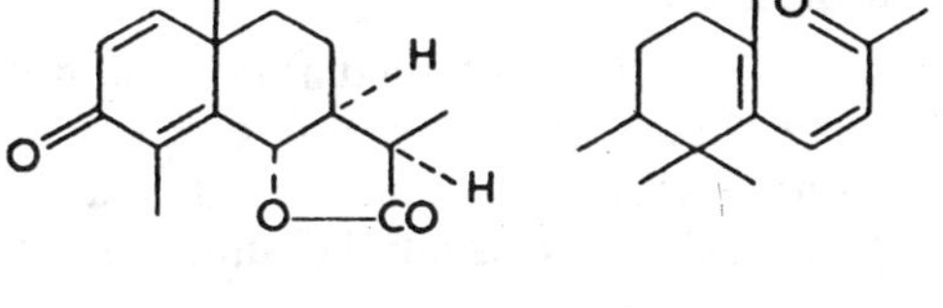

α-Santonin   β-Irone

Fig. 18.42. Chemical constituents of Santonica.

activity and inhibited granuloma formation. It exhibited antipyretic effect in mice.

SAUSSUREA

Synonyms

Kuth, Kut, Costus.

Biological Source

Saussurea is the dried roots of *Saussurea lappa* C.B. Clarke. (Family : Asteraceae).

Habitat

The plant is found in Kashmir at altitudes from 2700 m to 4300. It is cultivated in the Himalayan region of Kulu, Manali, Lahul and Garhwal.

Cultivation

Saussurea is a robust, erect, perennial herb, 1-2 meters in height, with large cordate, radical and alternate leaves. It requires a cool and humid climate. A deep rich porous soil is preferred and plants growing on such soils develop long and thick roots. It can be propagated either by root cuttings or by seeds. Seeds for propagation purposes are collected in September from the crop. The seeds retain their viability for a year or more. In nature kuth seed is shed in autumn, lies under the snow in winter and begins to sprout during April-June as the snow melts. For propagation by seed under cultivation the same time table is adopted or seed can be sown in spring also. Seeds can be sown in a nursery and the seedlings transplanted at a spacing of 8.9 m x 0.9 m when they are one year old. Direct sowing also gives successful results. The shoots die back each winter and recommence growing when the winter snow melts in the following spring. Roots are harvested during October. They are dried and cut into pieces 10 cm long and dried in the sun.

Morphology

Saussurea roots are 7-15 cm long, 1-5.5 cm wide. The roots are fusiform or conical and tapering, collapse in the centre; thin roots are cylindrical, broad, light and stout, usually contain longitudinal wrinkles with anastomose or ridges running straight or spiral; fresh roots are dirty grey to light yellow, dried ones are brown or dull-red; fracture is short and

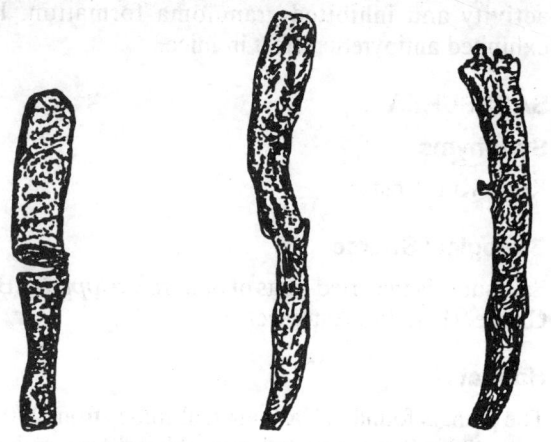

Fig. 18.43. *Saussurea lappa* root.

horny; odour is strong, sweet and aromatic and taste is bitter.

Chemical constituents

Saussurea contains volatile oil (1.5-2.5%), nitrogenous base saussarine (0.05%), inulin (15%), potassium nitrate, sugars, kushtin and bitter resin. The essential oil is the mixture of sesquiterpene lactones like costuslactone and its dihydro derivatives, costusic acid, 12-methoxy dihydrocostunolide, costol, aplotoxin, α-and β-costenes, phellandrene, camphene, and terpene alcohol. Saussurea also contains β-sitosterol, stigmasterol, betulin, aplotaxene, β-selinene, β-elemene, α- and β-ionones, α- and β-cyclocostunolides, costic, palmitic and linoleic acids, dehydro-costulactone, isoalantolactone, elema-1,3,11(13)-trien-12-ol and -12-al, selina-4,11-diene, α-*trans*-bergamotene, *trans*-bergamota-2,12-dien-14-al, arcurcumene, (–)-caryophyllene oxide, 6,10-dimethyl-9-methylideneundec-5-en-2-one, taraxasterol, its acetate, isodehydrocostus lactone, isozaluzanin C, 12-methoxy-dihydrodehydro-costuslactone, saussureal, 4β-methoxydehydro-costuslactone, 15-hydroxy-dehydrocostus lactone, amino acid-sesquiterpene adducts and saussure-amines A, B, C, D and E and (–)-massoniresinol-4"-O-β-glucoside.

The oil is a pale yellow to brownish, very viscous liquid. It has a peculiar soft but tenacious odour.

Extraction of the root with benzene or petroleum ether produces a concrete of rich and true natural odour. It is commercially called the costus resinoid. Alcoholic extract of the root contains the alkaloid saussurine.

Uses

Saussurea roots have tonic, disinfectant, stomachic, spasmolytic, carminative and stimulant properties and are used as spasmodic in asthma, cough and cholera and as alterative in chronic skin diseases and rheumatism. It is also used for preserving silk and expensive wool fabrics, as an incense in religious ceremonies and as insect repellent.

The essential oil is valued in high class perfumery and cosmetics where it is used for blending purposes. The oil is expensive, and is therefore extensively adulterated with elecampane oil.

Pharmacology

The essential oil stimulated heart in low concentration and depressed it in higher doses. Lactone fraction and delactonized oil exhibited hypotensive, spasmolytic and bronchodilatory effect. Root oil inhibited growth of Meth-A tumor cells. Costunolide and dehydrocostuslactone exhibited cholagogic and anti-ulcer effect in mice and inhibited KC1-induced contractions of aorta. An acetone extract of roots enhanced gastro-intestinal motility in mice. Saussureal exhibited plant growth regulatory activity.

The essential oil of Kuth has strong antiseptic and disinfectant properties especially against *Streptococcus* and *Staphylococcus*. It has marked carminative properties.

LEMONGRASS OIL

Synonyms

East India lemongrass, Malabar or Cochin Lemongrass.

Biological source

Lemongrass oil is obtained form *Cymbopogon flexuosus* Stapf. (syn. *Andropogon nardus* var. *flexuosus* Hack.). It contains not less than 75% of aldehydes calculated as citral (Family : Poaceae).

Habitat

Lemongrass is indigenous to India and is found in

Tinnevelli, Travancore and Cochin. Two principal varieties of Lemongrass are recognized as the red-stemmed variety, the true *C. flexuosus,* which is a source of East Indian Lemongrass oil and the white-stemmed variety which is designated as *C. flexuosus* var. *albescens.* The oil from the latter is low in aldehyde content and is slightly soluble in 70% alcohol.

Cultivation

Lemongrass grows best in well-drained sandy loam or in light sandy soil. Dark, heavy, rich soil, gives a higher yield of grass, but the oil obtained from it has a lower citral content. Warmth and sunshine favour oil development. The grass grown on lower slopes, less exposed to heavy rains, is rich in oil content.

The grass is cultivated in forest clearings or on hill slopes at an altitude of about 700 m. The ground is ploughed in March-April and seeds are sown at random. The grass come up with the first shower of the monsoon. Weeding is carried out systematically in the plantation. Protection against grazing is necessary. The grass is ready for cutting at the end of May or early in June and may be harvested every 35-40 days till November or December. The citral content of the oil is high (83%) when it is obtained from grass harvested during September-December. After cutting, the stubbles are burnt before the sporadic April monsoon shower. Fresh shoots come up from the roots with the start of regular monsoon, and the grass is ready for harvesting by the end of May. Plantations are renewed every 6-8 years.

Characters of oil

A light coloured oil, rich in citral content, is obtained by steam distillation. The yield varies form 0.25 to 0.5% per acre.

Chemical constituents

Lemongrass oil is the principal source of citral (68-85%) from which ionone is derived. The oil also contains methyl heptanone, decyl aldehyde, geraniol, linalool, limonene, dipentene, citronellal, triacontane, triacontanol, intermedeol, isointer-medeol, α- and β-pinene, car-3-ene, myrcene, ocimene, β-phellandrene, α-terpinene, p-cymene, terpinolene, methyl heptenone, geranyl acetate, β-caryophyllene, β-selinene, β-, γ- and δ-elemenes, α- and β-bisabolene, α-curcumene, γ- and δ-cadinene, methyl eugenol, elemol, β-caryophyllene oxide, eugenol, β-eudesmol, elemicin, farnesol, juniper-camphor, geraniol, anisaldehyde, terpinen-4-ol, α- and β-terpineol, borneol and p-cymene.

Uses

The oil is used in perfumery, soaps and cosmetics and as a mosquito repellent. Ionones obtained from citral are required for synthetic violet perfumes.

SANDALWOOD OIL

Synonyms

Chandan oil, Sandal oil; Yellow Sandalwood oil; Liginum.

Biological Source

Sandalwood oil is obtained by distillation of sandalwood, *Santalum album* Linn. (Family : Santalaceae).

Habitat

Sandal is a small to medium sized, evergreen semi-parasitic tree found in the dry regions of peninsular India from Vindhya Mountains south-wards, especially in Mysore and Tamil Nadu. It has also been introduced in Rajasthan, parts of U.P., M.P. and Orissa.

Cultivation

Sandal tree grows mostly on red, ferruginous loam overlying metamorphic rocks, chiefly gneiss, and tolerates shallow, rocky ground and stony or gravelly soils, avoiding saline and calcareous situations. It is not found on the black-cotton soil. The growth is luxuriant on rich and fairly moist soils, such as garden loam and on well-drained deep alluvium along the river banks, but the heartwood from these trees is deficient in oil. The trees grown on poor soils, particularly on stony or gravelly soil, produce more highly scented wood, giving a better yield of the oil.

It reproduces from seeds dispersed by birds. Germination is profuse in the forests immediately after the monsoons. For artificial regeneration, it is necessary to provide suitable climatic, and ecological conditions. For procuring seeds, the fruits are collected during January-March. Germination is up to 80%. Just after the first monsoon showers, the sandal seeds are dibbed and protected by thorny bushes. The seeds germinate in about 8-14 days. The seedlings grow rapidly, *i.e.*, up to 20-30 cm high, at the end of the first year.

Properties

Sandalwood oil is viscous, yellowish liquid having a peculiar, heavy, sweet and very lasting odour. It has sp. gr. 0.97-0.98, viscosity 1.5, and acid value 0.5-0.8.

Chemical constituents

The main odorous and medicinal constituent of Sandalwood is santalol ($C_{15}H_{24}O$). This primary sesquiterpene alcohol forms more than 90% of the oil and is present as a mixture of two isomers, α-santalol and β-santalol, the former predominating. The other constituents reported are hydrocarbons santene, nortricycloekasantalene, α- and β- santalenes, the alcohols santenol and teresantalol, the aldehyde nortricyclo-ekasantalal, isovaleraldehyde, the ketones l-santalone and the acids teresantalic acid, α and β-santalic acids, exo-norbicycloekasantalol, bicycloekasantalic and dihydro-β-santalic acid, (+)-epi-β-norekasantalic acid, β- and epi-β-ekasantalic acid, 11-keto-dihydro-α-santalic acid, bisabolenols A-E, tricyclo-ekasantolol, α- and β-santalals, *trans*-α-bergamotene, α-curcumone, muciferol, dihydro-α-norcurcumenic acid, α-bergamotenic acid and dihydro-α-santalic acid.

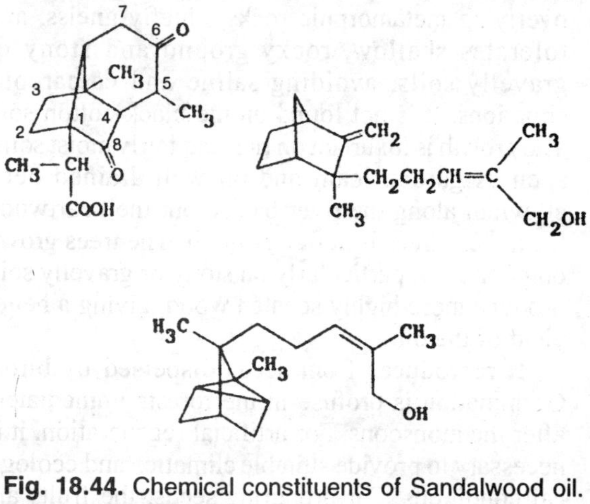

Fig. 18.44. Chemical constituents of Sandalwood oil.

Uses

Sandalwood oil is highly used in perfumery creations and finds an important place in soaps, face creams and toilet powders. A chemo-protective action on liver carcinogenesis in mice has been demonstrated.

Substitutes and adulterants

Oil from several plant sources are either used as substitutes for or as adulterants of natural sandalwood oil. Oil obtained from the Australian plant *Fusanus spicatus* (*Eucarya spicata*) is used as a substitute for genuine Sandalwood oil. Wood and oil of *Santalum yasi* have a feeble odour which is not delicate like that of Indian Sandalwood oil. East Africa markets the wood and oil derived from *Osyris tenuifolia,* the wood is similar to sandal and is used as an adulterant. An oil from Mauritius possesses most of the characteristics of the Indian oil. In West Indies an oil derived from *Amyris balsamifera* Linn. is marketed as a cheap substitute for Indian Sandalwood oil. In India, the wood of *Erythroxylum monogynum* Roxb. is used as an adulterant. The wood of *Mansonia gagei* Drum. resembles Sandalwood closely in its physical and other characteristics. Another species, which is common in southern India and used as an adultrant, is *Ximenia americana* Linn. The oil is adulterated with polyethylene glycols.

BLACK PEPPER

Synonyms

Kalimirch; Golmirch.

Biological Source

Black pepper consists of the dried, fully developed unripe fruits of *Piper nigrum* L. (Family : Piperaceae).

Habitat

Pepper is cultivated in the hills of south-western India from North Karnataka to Kanyakumari.

Cultivation

Black pepper is cultivated mostly as a mixed crop in homestead gardens. The pepper plant is a climbing vine found growing up to an altitude of 1,500

m. Supports or standards have to be provided for the plant to grow on. The standards usually preferred are quick growing trees, which not only provide support but also shade. Planting is done in April-May during the early rains so that their standards grow sufficiently to allow pepper vines to be planted in July-September. When planted as a mixed crop in coconut, arecanut, tea or coffee plantation, the main crop or the shade trees serve as standards besides providing the shade.

The Pepper vine can be propagated either vegetatively or by seeds. The planting of the pepper vine is done either in July or August. The pits for planting are made perferably on the north and north-eastern sides of the standard so that the severe western sun is avoided. Pepper is an exhausting crop and the soil needs high level of nitrogenous substances.

The wilt and *pollu* are the two important diseases of Pepper. The Pepper vine starts bearing from the third year of its growth. Usually there are two crops in a year, one in August-September and the other in March-April. The harvest season of Pepper extends from the middle of December to the middle of March in coastal areas.

Morphology

It is nearly globular in shape, about 4-5 mm in diameter with a characteristic coat with deep set wrinkles. The pericarp is thin and encloses a single seed with a hollow centre. The perisperm is horny in the outer part and floury around the central cavity.

For preparing Black Pepper, the freshly har-vested spikes are spread on mats or concrete floors and dried in sun for about a week with frequent turning over to prevent infection by mildew. During drying, the green or red fruits gradually change in colour to dark brown or almost black and their skin becomes tough and wrinkled. The fruits are detached from the stalks by beating the heaped up material with sticks or treading upon it barefood. Impurities are picked by hand.

Chemical constituents

Black Pepper contains the alkaloids piperine, chavicine, piperidine and piperetine. The characteristic aromatic odour of Pepper is due to the

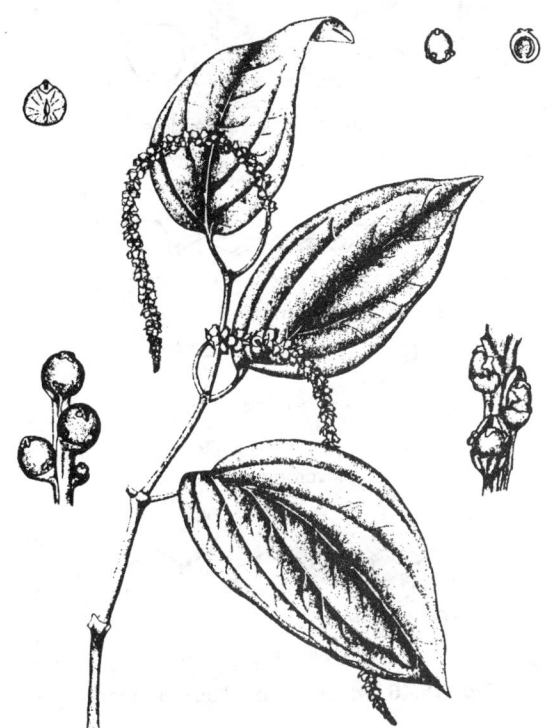

Fig. 18.45. Black pepper plant.

presence of a colourless volatile oil (1-2.6%) in the cells of pericarp which contains phellandrene, caryophyllene, piperonal, dihydrocarveol, caryophyllene oxide, cryptone, α-and β-pinenes, epoxydihydrocaryophyllene, phenylacetic acid, citronellol, α-*cis*- and β-*cis*-bergamotenes, sesquisabinene, pipercide, N-*trans*-feruloyltyramine, guineensine, pellitorine, N-*trans*-feruloyl-piperidine, feruperine, dihydroferuperine; decadienamide, tridecatrienamide and undecatrienamide derivatives, piperoleine B, β-ocimene, δ-guaiene, farnesol and guaiacol. Starch (45-63%) is the predominant constituent of pepper. It also contains thiamine, riboflavin, nicotinic acid, ascorbic acid and carotene.

Uses

Black Pepper is mostly used for its characteristic delicate penetrating aroma and pungent, biting taste. It is employed as an aromatic stimulant in cholera, weakness following fevers, vertigo and toma, as a stomachic in dyspepsia and flatulence, as an anti-

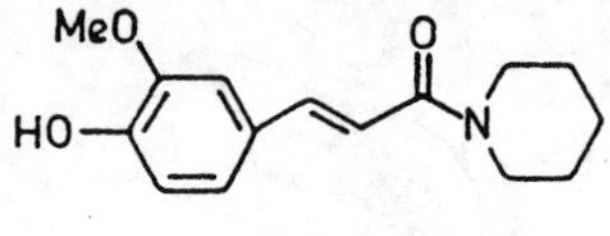

N-trans-Feruloylpiperidine

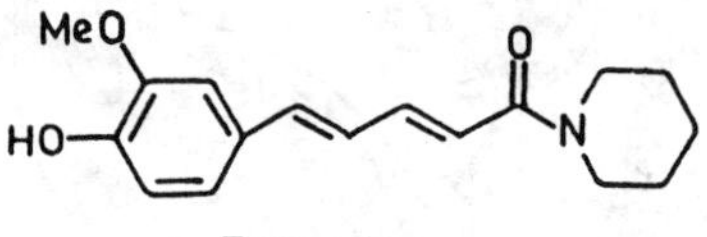

Feruperine

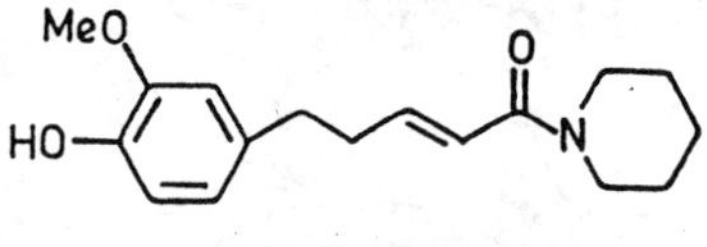

Dihydroferuperine

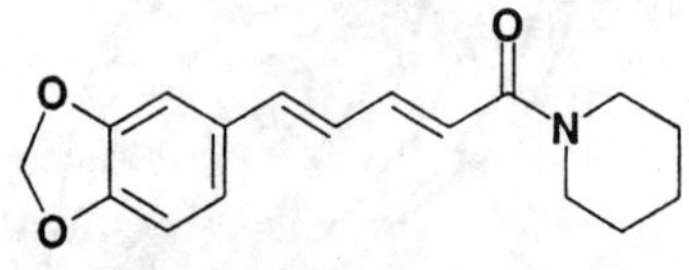

Piperine

Fig. 18.46. Alkaloids of Black pepper.

periodic in malarial fever and as an alterative in paraplegia and arthritic diseases. Externally it is valued for its rubefacient properties and as a local application for relaxed sore throat, piles and some skin diseases.

Pharmacology

Pipercide showed insecticidal activity against adzuki bean weevil. 2,4-Decadienamide; 2,4,12-tridecatrienamide and 2,4,10-undecatrienamide derivatives showed insecticidal activity. Piperonal, piperine and piperoleine B inhibited development of larva of *Drosophila*. Piperine exhibited antibacterial and antitumor activities against *Pseudomonas aeryginosa* and *Alcaligenes*. It stimulated γ-glutamyl transpeptidase activity, enhanced uptake of amino acids and increased lipid peroxidation in epithelial cells of rat jejunum.

CANTHARIDES

Synonyms

Spanish fly; Blistering fly; Blistering beetle, Russian flies; Cantharizo.

Biological source

Cantharides are the dried insects, *Cantharis vesicatoria* (Linn.) De Geer. (Family : Meloidae).

Habitat

Spain, Italy, Poland, Sicily, South Russia, and Romania.

Collection

Cantharides are found on some shrubs of the families Caprifoliaceae and Oleaceae. The mature insects have brilliant green colour with metallic luster. They appear in June-July and their presence can be detected from a distance due to strong unpleasant odour. Due to cold night, the insects become sluggish in the early morning. A large piece of cloth is spread under plants and the shrubs are shaken or beaten with a stick. The insects fall on the cloth and are collected. As the insects cause irritation on touching, the collector protects his body parts from them. The insects are killed by putting them in dilute vinegar, chloroform or ether or by exposing to the fumes of ammonia or sulphur dioxide. Then the insects are dried carefully below 40°C, stored in air tight containers and preserved from attack of other insects by adding few drops of chloroform or carbon tetrachloride.

Characters

Cantharides are 1.5-2.5 cm long, 5-8 mm broad, wings are brown, transparent and membraneous and protected by wing covers known as elytra which are copper green in colour; their body consists of three parts, *viz,* head, thorax and abdomen. A pair of antennae and two small black eyes are present on the head. Three pairs of legs are attached to the thorax. Abdomen is covered completely with wings. Dried Cantharides have strong unpleasant typical odour.

Chemical constituents

Cantharides contain the vesicating principle cantharidin (0.6-1%), fat (10-15%), resinous mass, acetic and uric acids. Cantharidin, mp 218°C, is a crystalline lactone or anhydride of cantharidic acid, sublimes at about 110°, insoluble in cold water and soluble in acetone, chloroform, ether and ethyl acetate.

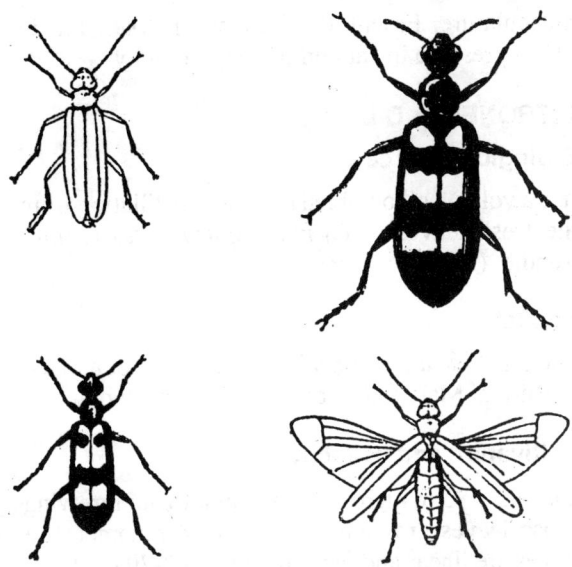

Fig. 18.47. (A) *Cantharis vesicatoria* (B) *Mylabris sidoe.*

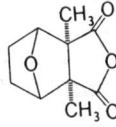

Fig. 18.48. Cantharidin.

Uses

Cantharides are vesicant, counter-irritant and rube-facient. Cantharidin is used externally in a solution form as a counter-irritant and to remove certain types of warts, in some hair tonic formulations and as an aphrodisiac.

If taken internally, it is excreted by the kidney, irritates the urinary tract, and can result in priapism. This accounts for the drug's popular reputation as an aphrodisiac. Internal administration of cantharides is potentially dangerous. Topical application of a solution of cantharidin is effective in the removal of certain types of warts; preparations containing 0.7% cantharidin in collodion are available for this purpose.

Allied drug

Mylabris (syn. Chinese Cantharides, Chinese

blistering flies) is the dried blistering beetle of *Mylabris sidoe* Fabr (Fam. Meloidae). The beetles are found in China and some parts of eastern India and used as a substitute for cantharides. These beetles are blackish brown in colour, cylindrical body, rounded above, flattish below; two black antennae with eleven segments at the globular head and abdomen containing black wings covered with black elytra with three tawny bright yellow bands and wing cases marked with a spot at point of insertion. Mylabris contains cantharidin (1-2%) and fixed oil. It is used as a substitute of cantharides.

AJOWAN

Biological source

Ajowan is the ripe dried seeds of *Trachyspermum ammi* (L.) Sprague (syn. *Carum copticum*, Benth. & Hookif) (Family : Apiaceae).

Habitat

It is a native of Egypt and grown through out India, Mediterranean region and in south-west Asian countries such as Iraq, Iran, Afghanistan and Pakistan.

Ajowan is an erect, glabrous or minutely pubescent, branched annual herb, up to 90 cm tall. The crop is grown in cold weather, both as a dry crop and under irrigation. It grows on all kinds of soil, but does well on loams or clayey loams. Seeds are sown broadcast in the moist soil from September to November. Germination takes in 5-15 days, depending upon climatic conditions. First irrigation should be light. The flowering takes place in about two months. The harvesting period is February or March. The fruits become ready for harvesting when the flower heads turn brown. The plants then pulled out by the roots and dried. The dried fruits are separated by carefully rubbing with hands or feet.

The drug occurs as entire cremocarps or separated mericarps. Cremocarps are ovoid-cordate to ovate, laterally compressed; 1.7-3.0 mm long; 1.5-2.4 mm broad, dirty yellow to yellowish brown in colour and half to two-thirds apical portion has slight purplish tinge. At the top of the cremocarp is a bifid stylopod surrounded by five minute sepals. Each mericarp shows five light-coloured ridges and is covered with light yellow protuberances. The drug has an agreeable odour and aromatic and warming taste.

Chemical constituents

Ajowan contains an essential oil (2-3.5%), protein (17.1%) and fat (21.8%). Ajowan oil is a colourless or brownish yellow liquid possessing a characteristic odour of thymol and a sharp taste. The principal constituents of the oil are phenol, mainly thymol (35-60%), carvacrol, p-cymene, γ-terpinene, α- and β-pinenes and dipentene. The fatty oil is composed of palmitic, petroselinic, oleic, linoleic and 5, 6-octadecenoic acids. The seeds also contain a phenolic glycosides, 3-galac-tosyloxy-5-hydroxytoluene, galactose, β-methyl-galactoside, 2-methyl-3-glucosyloxy-5-isopropyl phenol.

Uses

Ajowan is widely used as a spice in curries; in pickles, certain types of biscuits, confectionery, beverages and in *pan*-mixtures. It is valued for its antispasmodic, stimulant, tonic and carminative properties. It is given in flatulence, atonic dyspepsia, diarrhoea and cholera. It is used most frequently in conjunction with asafoetida, myrobalans and rocksalt. Ajowan is also effective in relaxed sore throat and in bronchitis, and often constitutes an ingredient of cough-mixture. It is taken with buttermilk for relieving difficult expectoration due to dried up phlegm. Externally, a paste of the crushed fruit is applied for relieving colic pains, and as a hot and dry fometation of the fruits on the chest in asthma. It is also used to prepare lotions and ointments and applied for checking chronic discharge. It has antibiotic activity.

Ajowan oil is used as an antiseptic, aromatic, carminative, for perfuming disinfectant soaps and as an insecticide. The action of the oil and its uses are similar to those of thymol. The oil is useful as an expectorant in emphysema, bronchial pneumonia and some other respiratory ailments.

The fatty oil is recommended as an external application in cases of rheumatism.

Pharmacology

The glycosidal fraction and essential oil contracted isolated ileum, tracheal chain and bronchial musculature. Essential oil caused marked fall in blood pressure in cat and had low toxicity.

CITRONELLA OIL

Biological source

It is a volatile oil obtained by steam distillation from the fresh leaves of *Cympopogon nardus* (Linn.) Rendle. (Family : Poaceae).

Habitat

The plant is native of Sri Lanka and now cultivated in Burma, Malaysia, Indonesia, Fiji and India.

Cultivation and collection

It is tall, 1.75 m high, perennial plant with throwing dense leaves growing from a short rhizome. The leaves are linear and tapering, up to 60-70 cm long, glabrous green and lower ribs are red in colour. It is cultivated by vegetative propagation. Regular irrigation is required during winter and summer. The crop is ready for harvesting after 8 months and it can be harvested several times with regular intervals. About 20 tonnes of grass can be harvested per hectare. It contains about 0.5% of volatile oil.

Description

The oil is pale-greenish yellow in colour. It has pungent taste. It is insoluble in fixed oils.

Chemical constituents

Citronella grass contains 0.3 to 0.9% of volatile oil. The main constituents of the oil are geraniol (40-60%) and citronellal (15-20%). Other constituents are d-camphene, limonene, dipentene, borneol, linalool, cadinene, elemicin, methyl eugenol, isocaproic acid, isovaleric, butyric and propionic acids, citral, isovaleraldehyde, pelargonaldehyde and citronellol. Java variety possesses citronellal (25-50%), geraniol (25-40%), camphene, limenene and dipentene.

Uses

The oil is used as perfume for soap, brilliantines, in mosquito-repellent ointments and sprays and as a flavouring agent for liniments, lotions and cosmetics.

TURPENTINE OIL

Synonyms

Oleum Terbinathae; Rectified oil of Turpentine.

Biological source

Turpentine oil is obtained by distillation of oleoresin of *Pinus palustris* (long leaf pine) and other species of *Pinus* such as *P. longifolia* Roxb., *P. elliottii* and *P. radiata*. (Family : Pinaceae).

Geographical source

The oil is prepared on commercial scale in India, France, Russia and U.S.A.

Cultivation and collection

In India *Pinus longifolia* and *P. gerardiana* are found naturally in Himalayas from Kashmir to Bhutan. *P. longifolia* is cultivated in Himachal Pradesh, Jammu, Punjab and Uttar Pradesh. The plant grows well at altitude 600 to 2400 m, in rainfall between 100 to 175 cm, temperature 30 to 38°C and on variety of soils like limestone, quartz and clay, stand stone and on bare rocks. It is grown by seed germination in March and April. The 20-25 year old plants are used for the collection of the Colophony (resin) and the volatile oil.

Preparation

Suitable number of blazes are made and then heavy tapping is done. The resin flows which is collected in earthenware or other suitable containers. It continues for 8 to 10 years. This type of tapping produces schizogenous ducts. The crude oleo-resin is purified by heating in a steam jacketed vessel with spiral tube. Vegetable debris, sand particles and other impurities are removed by setting or floating. The clear resin is re-distilled in a distillation plant after treatment with sodium hydroxide or lime water to remove resins, acids and phenols. It is then dried over sodium sulphate and packed in suitable containers. The oleoresin produces Turpentine oil (25%) and Colophony (70%). The Terpentine oil after treatment with alkalies is known is *rectified turpentine oil*. U.S.A. is main producer of the total world production which is about 70%.

Description

The oil is colourless or slightly yellow in colour, clear, transparent liquid. Odour is strong, characteristic and becomes much stronger on storage with less pleasantness; taste is bitter and pungent. It is insoluble in water, soluble in alcohol, chloroform, carbon disulphide, glacial acetic acid, benzene, petroleum ether and fixed oils.

Chemical constituents

About 40 monoterpenes are reported in the oil. The major components are α-pinene (20-30%), β-pinene (5-10%), camphene, β-phellandrene, δ-3-carene, *p*-cymene, longifoline, estragol and limonene. Americal oil contains α-pinene (65%) and β-pinene (30%) as the principal constituents.

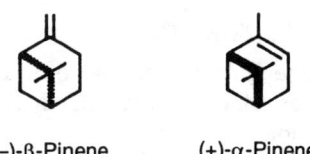

(–)-β-Pinene   (+)-α-Pinene

Fig. 18.49. Chemical consituents of Terpentine oil.

The oil also contains isopimeric acid, α-longipinene, longicyclene and car-3-ene.

Oil of turpentine is optically active, but the rotation varies not only with the species of pine from which it has been obtained, but also in samples taken from the same tree at different periods.

The varying optical rotations of differing turpentines are mainly due to the varying proportions of the (+)- and (–)-α-pinenes present; (–)-β-pinene is found in almost all *Pinus* spp. Pinene isomers have opposite absolute configurations.

Uses

Externally it is used as a counter-irritant and rubefacient. For inhalation, terebene is used which is prepared from the oil by the action of cold sulphuric acid. It is used in the treatment of chronic bronchitis. Commercially, it is used to prepare synthetic pine oil, disinfectants, denaturants and insecticides, paints, varnishes, fragrances and vitamins.

Turpentine oil is used as a counterirritant in Vicks.

Rectified turpentine oil is turpentine oil rectified by distillation from an aqueous solution of sodium hydroxide. It is dispensed when turpentine oil is required for internal use. It has been used as an expectorant.

Terpine hydrate or terpinol is formed by the action of nitric acid on rectified turpentine oil in the presence of alcohol. It is *cis-p*-menthane-1,8-diol hydrate.

Terpin hydrate is a stimulant to mucous membranes; therefore, it is used as an expectorant in the form of terpin hydrate elixir.

Adulterants

The common adulterants are resin oil, wood turpentine and petroleum jelly. The last adulterant is detected by low weight per ml of the oil and resin oil forms a stain of fatty matters on staining on a paper.

INDIAN TURPENTINE OIL

The turpentine industry has become one of the major sources of raw materials to the organic chemical complex.

The terpenes from Indian turpentine, viz., α-pinene, β-pinene, Δ-3-carene and longifolene are materials of considerable industrial importance, finding use in the manufacture of such essential commodities of everyday life as soaps and cosmetics; scents and incense; detergents; paints and varnishes; coatings and lacquers; rubber and adhesives; paper; textiles disinfectants, insecticides and pesticides; leather and a very wide range of other goods which are vital for economic and industrial development of India. The technology of terpene chemicals synthesis has advanced so fast that perfumery chemicals made from the various constituents of turpentine have virtually replaced or duplicated all "isolates" which were derived from natural essential oils.

The success in the utilization of Indian oil of turpentine has been mainly achieved by fractionation to recover its various constituents, particularly α-pinene, for use in the synthesis of camphor. The fractionation of other constituents, viz. β-pinene and particularly Δ-3-carene and longifolene in high purity has paved the way for manufacture of many new products which were earlier produced only from pinenes.

Production of turpentine oil

Oil of turpentine is obtained by distillation of oleo-

gum resin, collected from pine trees (*Pinus* spp.; Fam. *Pinaceae*) occurring in the Himalayan forest belt extending from Kashmir to Assam covering an area of approximately 8,00,000 hectares. The following five species are found in this country, of these, only the first three are being commercially exploited.

(a) *Pinus longifolia* [syn. *Pinus roxburghii* (Chir)]
(b) *Pinus khasya* (Khasi pine)
(c) *Pinus excelsa* [or *Pinus wallichiana* (Blue pine or Kail)]
(d) *Pinus merkussii*
(e) *Pinus gerardiana*

The processing of oleoresin gum in the country is undertaken by six Government Units, two Cooperative Units and three Private Units in the organized sector. There are as many as 20 units also in the small scale sector. The combined processing capacity of all the Government and Private Units in the organized sector is estimated at 70,000 tonnes of oleoresin.

Turpentine oil

Extraction : For extraction of turpentine oil, the crude oleoresin is first purified by melting in steam-jacketed containers provided with spiral mixers. Impurities such as chips and lighter particles floating to the top, and sand and silt settling at the bottom, are removed. The clarified resin is then distilled in steam or vacuum stills. The resin is heated in the jacketed-still to steam temperature and steam at low pressure is injected directly into the resin mass. The steam pressure is gradually increased as distillation proceeds. The vapours are passed through condensers and the distillate is collected in vessels with outlet pipes. Turpentine oil which collects as the top layer of the distillate is drawn off, passed through lime-water to remove rosin acids, and rectified and fractionated into light (Grade I) and heavy (Grade II) grades. The oil is then dehydrated with common salt and anhydrous sodium sulphate. The dehydrated product is stored in tanks before marketing, and any water still remaining is drained off.

The yield of turpentine oil from resin varies with locality, depending also on the time of the year when the resin is collected. On an average, 100 kg of resin yields about 20 litres of first grade turpentine oil,

2.5-3.75 litres of other grades, and 72.5-75 kg of rosin.

Properties : Turpentine oil is a clear, limpid and transparent liquid, with a pungent and bitter taste. The characteristic odour and taste of the oil become stronger and less pleasant on storage or exposure to air. The quality of the oil varies considerably depending upon the area and mode of collection, storage and processing of oleoresin. Average composition of turpentine oil from *P. roxburghii* the main Indian source for the oil, is as follows : α-pinene, 20-30; β-pinene, 5-10; Δ-3-carene, 55-65; ω-longifolene and other terpenes, 2-10%. β-Carene and longicyclene have also been reported in the oil. Indian turpentine oil is characterizaed by its comparatively low pinene and high carene contents, and is similar in some respects to the Russian product (from *P. sylvestris*). Its odour is soft and distinct. It is, however, considered inferior to American turpentine oil which is almost entirely made up of α- and β-pinenes.

Turpentine oil from the Khasi pine is a colourless mobile liquid with a characteristic odour. The Burmese oil has been reported to contain over 75% of α-pinene and 19% of β-pinene.

Turpentine oil from the blue pine has a high pinene content (88%; in one sample, 96%), and is suitable for all purposes where the American product can be used. The oil from Chilgoza pine is also of good quality (α-pinene, 70-80%), with a pale-yellow colour.

Grades and specifications : Indian standard on oil of turpentine, recognizes two grades, viz. Grade I and Grade II. Grade I turpentine oil can be used for pharmaceutical and perfumery purposes and is also preferred for the manufacture of high class paints.

Utilization

Medicine : Oil of turpentine is used in medicine and is included in the Indian Pharmacopoeia and the Indian Pharmaceutical Codex under the name Oleum Terebinthinae. It is locally irritant and is feebly antiseptic. It acts as a stimulant expectorant and is useful in chronic bronchitis and in gangrene of the lungs. It is used as a carminative in flatulent colic and typhoid and to arrest minor haemorrhages in tooth-sockets and nose. Externally, oil of turpentine is used as rubefacient in the form of liniments in rheumatic affections such as lumbago, arthritis and neuralgia. As an enema, the oil is considered useful in obstinate constipation, tympanitis and seatworm infestation. In the form of turpentine stupe, it is used as a counter-irritant in deep-seated inflammations, particularly of the abdomen.

Turpentine oil is widely used as a solvent in a paint, varnish and boot polish industries, in pharmaceuticals, perfumery, and for making synthetic camphor and pine oil, insecticides, disinfectants, and denaturants. Chlorinated turpentine (60-80% chlorine) is comparable to DDT in its insecticidal activity against mosquitoes, houseflies and cockroaches. The use of turpentine oil from the Khasi pine as a solvent for extraction of quinine from cinchona bark with low alkaloids, has been suggested.

Camphor and other terpene chemicals : Oil of turpentine is one of the most important basic raw materials for the production of camphor, and other terpene chemicals which are used in a wide range of industries, such as adhesives, lubrication additives, synthetic resins, solvents, plasticizers, paints and varnishes, soap, perfumery and cosmetics, and paper and rubber chemicals. Most of these products are based on the α- and β-pinenes which can be recovered from turpentine by fractionation. Due to low pinene content, Indian turpentine had not been used till recently in the terpene chemical industry, α-Pinene of a high purity is now being recovered from turpentine for the manufacture of synthetic camphor, and the intermediate product camphene. Camphene, in turn, can be employed for making several compounds useful in insecticides and perfumery. Synthetic resins and perfumery chemicals can be made from β-pinene. Δ-3-Carene, the principal constituent of Indian turpentine, can be used for making terpineols and synthetic oil of pine. Longifolene derivatives, oxygenated and acetylated, are now being increasingly used in perfumery. Dipentene, another fractionation product of turpentine is useful for making *p*-menthane and limonene.

One of the four stereo-isomers of a diterpenoid, 4β, 10x-dimethyl-1,2,3,4,5,10-hexa-hydrofluorine-4α, 6-dicarboxylic acid, synthesized from pine rosin, has 1300-1800 times the sweetness of sucrose.

Camphor & Allied Products Ltd., Mumbai is

manufacturing camphor from α-pinene. Both technical and pharmaceutical grades of camphor are being produced. The distilled oil of turpentine (i.e. the oil remaining after the fractionation of α-pinene from turpentine) and pine tar are the two valuable byproducts obtained in the manufacture of synthetic camphor. The distilled turpentine oil consists principally of Δ-3-carene and finds application as a solvent in several of the industries, in place of whole turpentine. Pine tar is produced by blending the terpenes available as byproducts in the production of synthetic camphor. It is used mainly as a plasticizer in rubber manufacture, and is being marketed in three grades, viz., light, medium and heavy.

Production of other chemicals from turpentine, viz. terpineol and esters, isoborneol acetate and esters, polyterpene resins and thanite insecticides has also commenced.

Synthetic pine oil : Pinenes, along with carene and longifolene present in the turpentine, are hydroxylated and etherified to yield a mixture of terpineols and terpene ethers which are the principal constituents of natural pine oil, obtainable by the steam-distillation of pine wood. The synthetic product is a straw-coloured liquid with a pleasantly mild and aromatic odour. It is as good as natural pine oil in its uses, and can be used in paints and varnishes, lacquers, distempers, soaps and detergents, and in perfumery and pharmaceuticals. Pine oil is also used in textiles, leather, insecticides, paper and rubber industries.

Prabhat General Agencies, Hoshiarpur, was the first unit in India, set up in 1960, to start manufacture of synthetic pine oil from turpentine. Subsequently two more units, Dujodwala Industries, Faridabad and Camphor & Allied Products were added.

The terpenes, α-pinene, β-pinene, camphene, limonene and to some extent Δ-3-carene and longifolene have been subjected to a variety of reactions like isomerization, oxidation, hydration, hydroboration and subsequent oxidation; hydrochlorination and hydroxylation; acetylation, Prins reaction; pyrolysis, polymerization and co-polymerization to give terpene alcohols, esters, ketones, aldehydes having remarkable odours. viz., woody, camphoraceous, citrus, minty, grassy, earthy, fruity and floral finding extensive applications is perfumery, flavours and pharmaceuticals and polymers which are valuable ingredients in the manufacture of paint, varnish, adhesive and rubber goods.

The residue left after fractionation of turpentine oil commonly referred to as "pitch" has been utilized for the manufacture of various grades of pine tars for use in Rubber Industry.

Constituents of oil of turpentine and their derivatives

The specification limits for the various constituents of oil of turpentine available after fractionation.

α-Pinene

α-Pinene is one of the best known terpenes utilized for chemical synthesis for a number of decades. In India, α-pinene is being recovered in high purity for the manufacture of synthetic camphor and the intermediate product camphene. Terpineol, produced from α-pinene, till recently was imported to meet the requirement of various industries. Camphene produces many useful items, such as isobornyl thiocyano acetate (thanite insecticide) and chlorinated camphene (toxaphene) for use in household sprays and for controlling agricultural pests. Perfumery products like isobornyl acetate, isoborneol are also manufactured from camphene. A recent development has been the synthesis of isocamphyl-cyclohexanols and cyclohexanones from camphene which are products having pronounced sandalwood odour.

β-Pinene

β-Pinene is being used in many countries for the manufacture of a wide range of products including polyterpene resins and perfumery chemicals. The β-pinene on pyrolysis gives myrcene which on hydrochlorination and subsequent treatment gives geranyl acetate, neryl acetate and linalyl acetate under different conditions and further leading to geraniol, nerol, linalool, citral, citronellol, hydroxy citronellol, α- and β-ionones. Myrcene is also used for producing dihydromyrcenol and dihydromyrcenol acetate which are one of the most valuable perfumery materials in the world market today. β-Pinene gives nopol and nopyl acetate when subjected to Prins reaction. These items have considerable export market.

Δ-3-Carene

Δ-3-Carene, on hydrochlorination and further treatment gives mixture of methadienes, terpineols and sylviterpineols, which is thus a new source of pine oils, products of great industrial value.

Production of 4-acetyl, Δ-2-carene by acetylation and 4-hydroxylmethyl and 4-acetoxy methyl, Δ-2-carene by Prins reaction is well established. All these products are excellent perfumery materials.

Under suitable conditions Δ-3-carene can be converted into Δ-2-carene which in turn has shown much greater potential leading to synthetic (–)-menthol and (+) menthol. Production of synthetic (–)-menthol and (+)-menthol from Δ-3-carene has already started in the country.

Production of a mixture of *para-* and *meta-* cymenes in high yields by pyrolysis of Δ-3-carene has paved the way for the manufacture of cresols and acetone via cymene hydroperoxide.

Of particular significance to this country is the development of terpene phenol resins from Δ-3-carene. These resins have tremendous applications in a number of industries like paints, varnishes, printing inks, rubber and adhesives. Thus many products like limonene, carvone, caranols cresols, thymol, (–)-menthol, resins and insecticides have established routes from Δ-3-carene.

Longifolene

Longifolene is a sesquiterpene in Indian turpentine oil from *P. roxburghii*. Other closely related terpenes such as longicyclene and longipinene also occur naturally. Longifolene is a rare constituent of Indian turpentine oil. On acid isomerization, longifolene gives another sesquiterpene abroad, isolongifolene, which has shown a greater industrial potential as a basic raw material for the production of perfumery derivatives.

A large number of longifolene derivatives have unusual and pleasing fragrance similar to that of isomeric compounds of cedrine because of which they are gradually finding an increased use in perfumery industry.

Thus, products like longibornane-9-o1 formate and longibornane-9-o1 are compounds having resinous sweet woody character useful in perfumery.

ω-Acetyl longifolene possesses a very pleasant and sweet woody odour of vetivert and sandalwood type.

Production of 9-oxo-isolongifolene and 8-oxo-isolongifolene by the oxidation of isolongifolene is an important development. These compounds have excellent perfumery value.

Longimusk and several other alcoholic and ketonic derivatives have also been prepared from isolongifolene.

HOPS

Hops (*Humulus*) are the dried strobiles of *Humulus lupulus* Linn. (Cannabinaceae). Only the pistillate plants are cultivated in England (particularly Kent), Germany, Belgium, France, Russia and California. The strobiles are collected, dried in kilns and pressed into bales known as 'pockets'. They are sometimes exposed to the fumes of burning sulphur, to modify the sulphur components already in the hops and to stabilize the aroma and colour.

There are numerous shining glands on the fruits and bases of the bracts. These, when separated, constitute the drug lupulin. The commercial product is very impure. It occurs as a granular, reddish-brown powder with a characteristic odour and bitter aromatic taste.

The bracts and stipules of the hop contain tannin. The odour and taste of the drug are mainly due to a complex secretion present in the lupulin glands. On distillation the fruits yield 0.30-1.0% of an essential oil composed of over 100 components

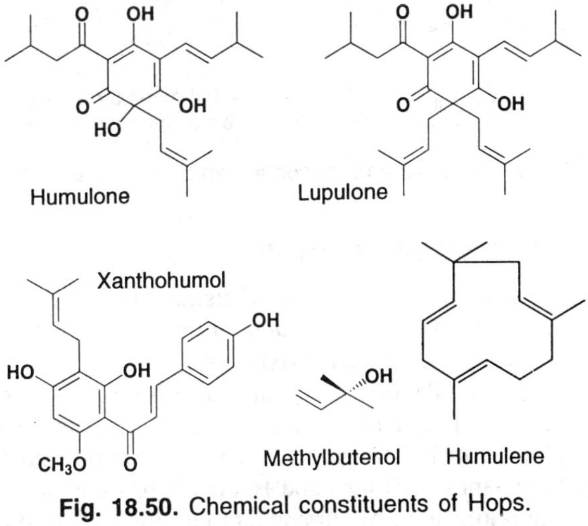

Fig. 18.50. Chemical constituents of Hops.

and containing terpenes, sesquiterpenes and esters. The bitterness is due to crystalline phloroglucinol derivatives known as α-acids (e.g., humulone), β-acids (e.g., lupulone) and about 10% of resins. 2,3,4-Trithiopentane, S-methylthio-2-methylbutanoate, S-methylthio-4-methyl-pentanoate and 4,5-epithio-caryophyllene have been isolated from the volatile oil of unsulphurated hops. The valerian-like odour is formed due to decomposition of the oil and one of the resins.

Hops are aromatic bitter and sedative due to 2-methyl-3-buten-2-ol. They are used in the preparation of beer.

CANELLA BARK (White cinnamon, Wild cinnamon)

Canella bark is the dried rossed bark of *Canella alba* (*C. winterana*) (Canellaceae), a small tree growing in the Bahamas and Florida. It occurs in quills or channelled pieces up to 5 cm long and 5 mm thick. It contains about 1% of volatile oil composed of monoterpenes, eugenol and myristicin.

It contains a novel antimicrobial sesquiterpene dialdehyde (canell) and 3-methoxy-4,5-methylene-dioxycinnamaldehyde. Canellal has insect antifeedant, antifungal and cytoxic properties.

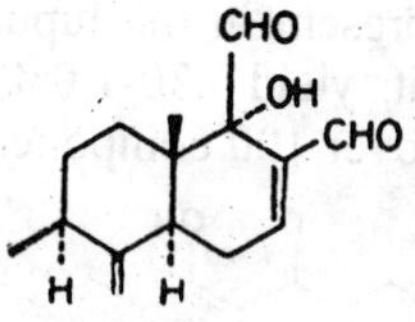

Canellal 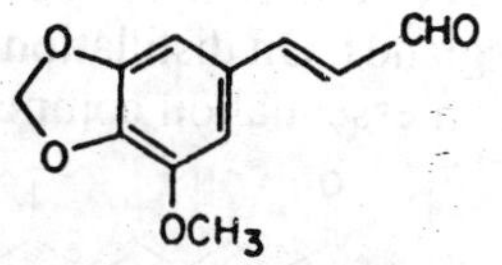   3-Methoxy-4,5-methylene-
                            dioxycinnamaldehyde

Fig. 18.51. Chemical constituents of Canella bark.

CAJUPUT OIL (Kayaputi)

Oil of Cajuput is a volatile oil distilled from the fresh leaves of *Melaleuca leucadendron* L. and other species of *Melaleuca* (Myrtaceae) and rectified by steam distillation. The plants are evergreen shrubs or trees found in the East Indies and Australia; planted in Indian gardens. The oil is produced in the islands of Bouru and Banda. It has a pleasant, camphoraceous odour and a bitter aromatic taste. It

contains about 50-60% of cineole, terpineol, its acetate and sesquiterpenes.

Medicinally, the oil is used both internally and externally as antiseptic, stimulant, rubefacient, mosquito repellent, to treat rheumatism, diarrhoea, psoriasis, pityriasis, acne and eczema.

ARNICA

The drug is derived from *Arnica montana L.* (Asteraceae), a perennial herb with a creeping rhizome and found in the meadows of the lower mountain slopes of central Europe. Volatile oil is present in both the flowers (0.5-1.0%) and rhizomes (*c*. 0.5%). The flowers contains methylated flavones and some 13 sesquiterpene lactones of the pseudoguaianolide type including some esters which involve acetic acid and various C_4 and C_5 acids. Tinctures and infusions of the dried flower-heads and rhizomes are used for the treatment of sprains and bruises. It should not be applied to broken skin and treatment should be discontinued when dermatitis develop.

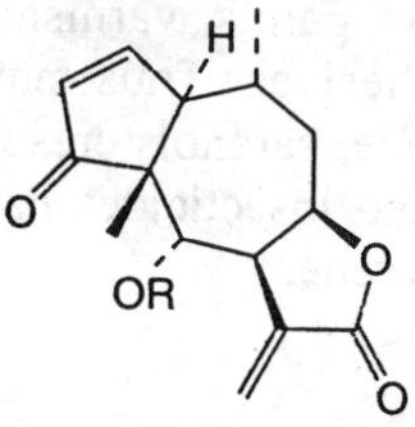

R = H (helenalin) 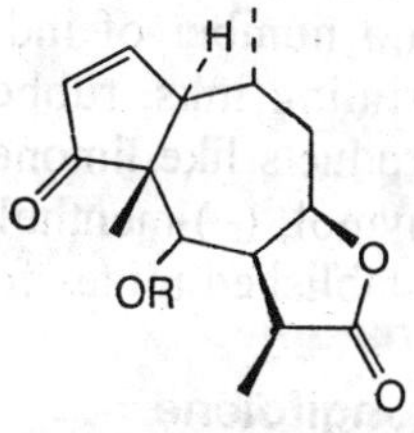   R = H (11,13-dihydrohelenalin)

Fig. 18.52. Sesquiterpenes of Arnica.

PIMENTO (Allspice)

Pimento (*Jamaica* or *Clove Pepper*) is the dried nearly ripe fruit of *Pimenta dioica* (Myrtaceae), an evergreen tree grown in the West Indies (Jamaica, Cuba and Trinidad) and Central America.

The fruits are collected before they are quite ripe, since on ripening they lose much of their aroma and become filled with a sweet pulp. They are dried artificial or in sunlight.

The pimento flower and fruit closely resemble Clove. The biocular ovary develops two seeds, whereas only one is produced in the Clove. Pimento fruits are globular and 4-7 mm in diameter. At the apex of the fruit are four small calyx teeth surrounding a short style. The pericarp is reddish-brown, rough and woody, and about 1 mm thick. Numerous oil glands are present in the pericarp. Each of the two loculi contains a single planoconvex seed. Pimento has a characteristic aromatic odour and taste.

Pimento fruits yield 3-4.5% of volatile oil having a phenol content of 65-80%. The oil also contains mainly eugenol, cineole, (–)-phellandrene and caryophyllene and some 40 other compounds.

ORRIS

Orris rhizome is obtained from three species of *Iris* (Iridaceae), namely *I. florentina. Iris germanica* and *Iris pallida*, all found in Europe.

Collection and preparation

The 3 years old plants are dug up in August and September, and the cork is easily removed. The aerial leaves and the roots are cut off and the rhizomes peeled. When fresh, the rhizomes are practically odourless and have an acrid taste. The characteristic fragrant odour is developed on slow drying. The peeled rhizomes are dried in the sun and stored for about 3 years in order to develop their full aroma.

Characters

Florentine orris occurs in dorsiventrally flattened pieces about 5-10 cm long and 2-3 cm diameter; whitish in colour, free from cork. The apex shows the remains of the flowering shoot and one or two short lateral branches terminating in cup-shaped scars. The age of the rhizome is indicated by the number of constrictions which represents the regions of winter growth. On the upper surface are lines of small vascular bundles left by the leaves and on the lower surface are numerous root scars. Odour, pleasantly aromatic; taste, bigger.

The rhizome of mogadore orris, usually inferior to the European, is smaller, darker and less fragrant. The peeling is incomplete and the drug bears patches of reddish cork and the remains of the leaves.

Chemical constituents

Orris rhizome contains volatile oil composed of irone, a substance having an odour of violets. An isomeric substance, ionone, is used as a synthetic violet perfume. Orris also contains starch, calcium oxalate, iridin (a flavone related to rutin), isoflavones, β-sitosterol and its glycosides.

Uses

Powdered orris root is used in dusting powders, while the oil is used in perfumery for its delicate odour and as a fixative for artificial violet perfumes.

FISH BERRIES

Fish berries (cocculus indicus) consists of the dried fruits of *Anamirta cocculus* (L.) W. & A. (Menispermaceae), a climbing shrub found in southeastern Asia (Malabar coast of India) and the East Indies.

The dorsal side of the fruit grows more rapidly than the ventral and the fruit becomes reniform and the base and apex both lie on the concave side. The pericarp is rough and woody and the cut-shaped seed consists of an oily endosperm surrounding the embryo, which lies with its radicle pointing towards the apex of the fruit. The two cotyledons occupy separate slit-like cavities in the endosperm. The drug has no odour; the pericarp is tasteless, but the seed is intensely bitter.

The seed contains picrotoxin (1.5%), a bitter toxic substance. This consists of picrotoxinin, $C_{15}H_{18}O_7$, and picrotin, $C_{15}H_{18}O_7$. Picrotoxinin is a highly oxygenated sesquiterpene derivative. The seeds also contain about 50% of fat.

Picrotoxin is used intravenously in poisoning by barbiturates and other narcotics. Very small quantities of the fruits are sufficient to stupefy fish.

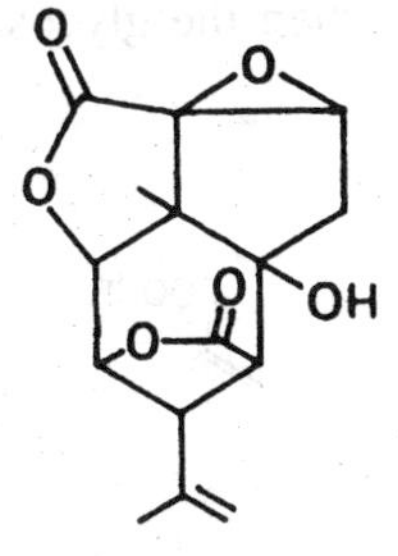

Fig. 18.53. Picrotoxinin.

GAULTHERIA OIL

Gaultheria, wintergreen, teaberry, or checkerberry consists of the dried leaves of *Gaultheria procumbens* Linn. (Fam. Ericaceae), a low shrub-like perennial with slender creeping or subterranean stems and branches that ascent from 5 to 15 cm in height. The leaves are alternate and evergreen, the flowers are white and axillary, and the fruit is a bright red, globular, aromatic berry. The plant is found in coniferous woods throughout the eastern United States and Canada. The leaves are coriaceous, the upper surface is dark green and shining, and the under surface is pale green. The odour is distinct and aromatic, and the taste is aromatic and astringent.

Methyl salicylate

In India, gaultheria oil is obtained from the fresh plant of *Gaultheria fragrantissima* and contains about 98% of esters calculated as methyl salicylate. It is produced synthetically or is obtained by maceration and subsequent distillation with steam from the leaves of *Gaultheria* species or from the bark of *Betula lenata* Linn. (Fam. Betulaceae).

The oil is obtained by distilling wintergreen plants that have been chopped into small pieces and allowed to stand in water for about 12 hours. The oil may be purified by rectification with steam. Methyl salicylate is made synthetically by dis tilling a mixture of salicylic acid and methyl alcohol.

Methyl salicylate is a colourless, yellow or red liquid that has the characteristic odour and taste of wintergreen. Synthetic oil and that obtained from *Betula* are optically inactive, but the oil obtained from *Gaultheria* is slightly levorotatory.

Methyl salicylate, the chief constituent of this oil, is formed when the glycoside, gaultherin, is

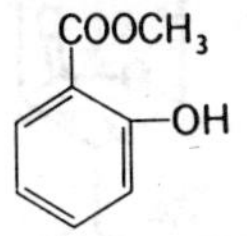

Fig. 18.54. Methyl salicylate.

hydrolyzed by the naturally occurring enzyme, gaultherase, in the presence of water.

In addition to methyl salicylate, wintergreen oil contains an ester that splits into enanthic alcohol and an acid. Enanthic alcohol and its ester possess the characteristic odour that distinguishes natural wintergreen oil from synthetic methyl salicylate.

Uses

Methyl salicylate is a pharmaceutic aid (flavor) for aromatic Cascara sagrada fluid extract. It has local irritant, antiseptic and antirheumatic pro-perties. For topical use, 10 to 25% concentrations in lotions and solutions are employed. Large doses of this drug have produced toxic symptoms. Ingestion of 10 ml by children has caused death. Symptoms of poisoning include nausea, vomiting, pulmonary edema and convulsions.

The principal adulterant of natural wintergreen oil is synthetic methyl salicylate.

Canada turpentine

Canada turpentine, or 'Canada balsam' is an oleoresin obtained from the stem of *Abies balsamea* (Pinaceae), the balsam fir. It is collected in eastern Canada and in the State of Maine in the USA. The oleoresin in the bark occurs in schizogenous ducts and large cavities. As the cavities fill with secretion, blister-like swellings develop on the trunk, and from these that the oleoresin is collected.

Canada turpentine when fresh is a pale-yellow liquid with a slight, greenish fluorescence and is of honey-like consistency. It has a pleasant, terebinthinate odour and a bitter, acrid taste. On exposure to air, Canada turpentine becomes more viscous and finally forms a glass-like varnish, a property which rendered it suitable as a microscopic mountant and as a cement for lenses. It contains volatile oil (23-24%) and a number of terpenoid acids.

Pumilio pine oil

A distillation of the fresh leaves of the pumilio pine, *Pinus muso* var. *pumilio* (Pinaceae) yields the oil. It is produced in Albania, former Yugoslavia, the former USSR, Bulgaria and Austria.

The oil has an agreeable odour and contains principally terpenes and sesquiterpenes, with up to

10% bornyl acetate. It is used as a decongestant inhalant, in the preparation of compound thymol glycerin, and as a constituent of zinc undecenoate dusting powder.

Savin tops

These are the young shoots of *Juniperus sabina* (Cupressaceae), an evergreen shrub about 2-6 m high. It grows wild in the mountains of Austria, Switzerland, Italy, France and Spain. The leaves are imbricated, sessile, adnate to the stem and usually opposite and decussate. This oil gland is oval in young leaves but more elongated in old ones. Savin contains a volatile oil (1-3%) which is a powerful irritant. It contains the terpene alcohol sabinol and its acetate. Other constituents are podophyllotoxin (0.2%), coumarins, savinin and many diterpenoids with various skeletal structures.

Oil of cade

Oil of cade is obtained by the destructive distillation of the woody portions of *Juniperus oxycedrus* (Cupressaceae) in Portugal, Spain and former Yugoslavia.

Oil of cade is a reddish-brown or blackish, oily liquid. Odour empyreumatic; taste aromatic, bitter and acrid. The chief constituents are sesquiterpenes (e.g., cadinene, and phenolic compounds (guaiacol, ethyl guaiacol and cresol).

Oil of cade is used for veterinary purposes and for skin diseases.

Juniper berries and oil

Juniper berries are the dried ripe fruits of *Juniperus communis* (Cupressaceae), an evergreen shrub or small tree found in former Yugoslavia, Italy, Hungary, Poland, Thuringia, Sweden and other countries. The berries from the more southern countries contain the most oil.

The berry-like fruit takes 2 years to ripen, developing a deep purple colour and a bluish-grey bloom. On drying, the berries become darker and shrivel slightly. They are about 3-10 mm in diameter. The apex shows a triradiate mark and depression indicating the sutures of the three fleshy scales. At the base there are usually six, small, pointed bracts arranged in two whorls.

The drug has a pleasant, somewhat terebinthinate odour, and a sweetish taste.

The main constituents are volatile oil (0.5-1.5%), invert sugar (about 33%) and resin. Oil is juniper contains over 60 compounds, of which the terpenes α-pinene and camphene, the sesquiterpene cadinene, alcohols and esters are the most prominent. The oil from the leaves contains similar compounds.

Juniper berries are used for the preparation of oil of juniper and in making certain varieties of gin. The oil has diuretic and antiseptic properties. The commercial oil vary in composition and prolonged intake of some may cause kidney damage.

ROSE OIL

Oil of rose (*Otto* or *Attar of Rose, Oleum Rosae*) is a volatile oil obtained by distillation from the fresh flowers of *Rosa damascena, R. gallica, R. alba* and *R. centifolia* (Rosaceae). The chief producing countries are Bulgaria, Turkey and Morocco.

The oil prepared is very expensive and widely adulterated.

The oil is a pale yellow semisolid. About 15-20% oil is solidified at ordinary temperatures which consists of odourless stearoptene containing principally saturated aliphatic hydrocarbons (C_{14}-C_{23} normal paraffins). The liquid portion forms a clear solution and consists of the alcohols geraniol, citronellol, nerol and 2-phenylethanol with smaller quantities of esters and other odorous principles. The odour is so modified by sulphur containing compounds. Phenylalanine acts as a precursor of the 2-phenylethanol; acetate and mevalonate are incorporated into the terpene alcohols.

From *Rosa rugosa* var. *plena* growing in central China 108 compounds have been identified in the flower oil including citronellol (60%), gera-niol (8.6%), nerol (2.8%), citronellyl acetate (2.7%) and E,E-farnesol (2.5%).

Oil of rose is of great importance in perfumery.

ROSEMARY OIL

Oil of Rosemary is distilled from the flowering tops of leafy twigs of *Rosmarinus officinalis* (Lamiaceae). The plant is native to southern Europe and the oil is produced principally in Spain and North Africa.

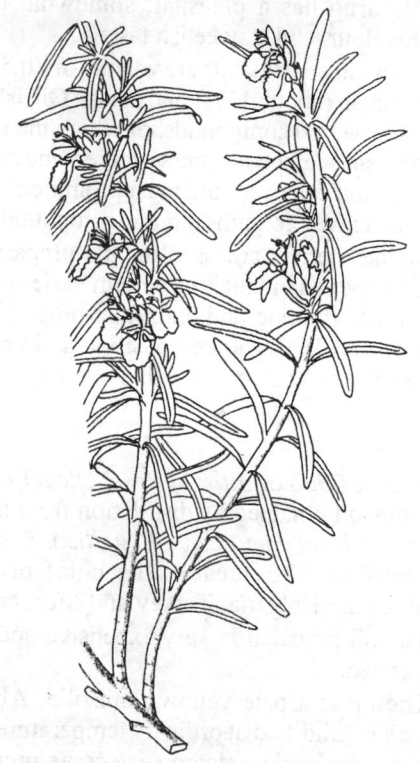

Fig. 18.55. *Rosmarinus officinalis* L.

Rosmarinic acid

Carnosol

Rosmanol
R = α–OH
Epirosmanol
R = β–OH

Isorosmanol

Rosmariquinone

Rofficerone

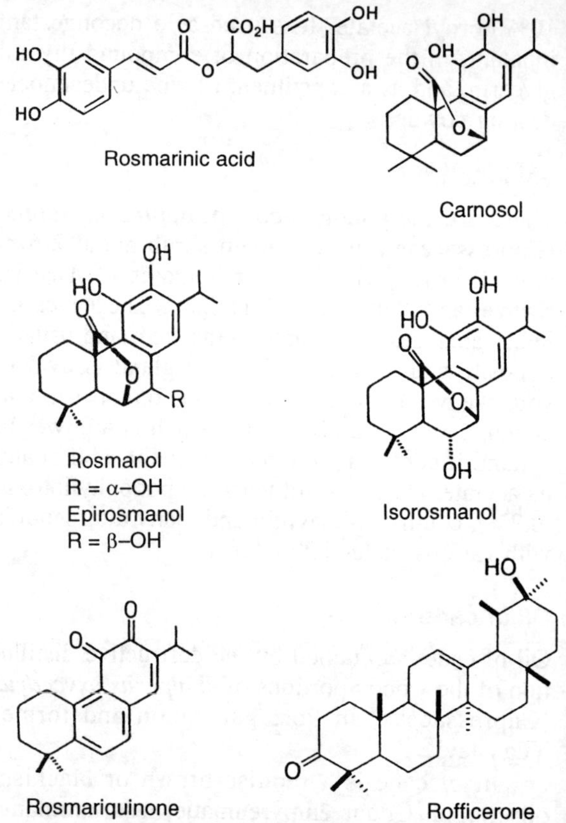

Fig. 18.56. Chemical constituents of Rosemary.

Rosemary is an evergreen shrub with rigid, opposite, sessile, persistent, linear and coriaceous leaves from about 3.5 cm long and 2-4 mm broad. Numerous branched trichomes make the lower leaf surface grey and woolly; typical labiate glandular hairs contain the volatile oil.

The fresh material yields about 1-2% of volatile oil containing 0.8-6% of esters, and 8-20% of alcohols. The principal constituents are 1,8-cincole, borneol, camphor, bornyl acetate, and monoterpene hydrocarbons. Rosemary leaves also contain the triterpene alcohols α- and β-amyrins, rosmarinic acid (a caffeic acid ester of 3,4-dihydroxyphenyl-lactic acid), rofficerone caffeic acid, chlorogenic acid, α-hydroxydihydrocaffeic acid, glycosides of luteolin and diosmetin, carnosolic acid, carnosol, rosmanol, epirosmanol, isorosmanol, rosmaridi-phenol, rosmariquinone, rosmadial, petulin and β-sitosterol together with epi-α-amyrin, which is unusual in having a *cis*-configuration at C-3.

Adulteration of the oil with Spanish eucalyptus oil, camphor oil and turpentine fractions is common.

The oil is mainly used in the perfumery industry. It is a component of soap Liniment and is frequently used in aromatherapy. The oil is also used for gastrointestinal disturbances, to enhance urinary and digestive elimination function and as a choleretic or cholagogue. Topically, it is applied to clear nasal passages, for colds, as a mouthwash and for rheumatic ailments. Rosemary extracts are used in food technology as antioxidants and preservatives.

Cornosolic acid, a diterpene isolated from *R. officinalis*, shows a strong inhibition of HIV-1-protease activity. It shows cytotoxicity at the dose which is close to effective antiviral dose.

Rosmanol and semisynthetic derivatives 7-O-methyl rosmanol, 7-O-ethyl rosmanol and 11,12-O,O-dimethyl carnasol show greater antiviral activity.

Tansy

Tansy (*Tanacetum vulgare* (L.); *Chrysanthemum vulgare* (L.) Bernh.) (Asteraceae) is used as an anthelminthic in herbal medicine but is poisonous. The herb contains about 0.2-0.6% volatile oil containing about 70% of thujone. Many sesquiterpene lactones have been isolated from the flowers and herb together with flavones.

Eriodictyon leaf

Eriodictyon or Yerba Santa consists of the dried leaf of *Eriodictyon californicum* (Hydrophyllaceae), a low evergreen shrub of the hills and mountains of California and northern Mexico.

The leaves usually occur in fragments. They are lanceolate, 5-15 cm long and 1-3 cm wide; apex acute; the base slightly tapering into a short petiole; margin is irregularly serrate or crenate-dentate; upper surface is yellowish-brown to greenish-brown and covered with a glistening resin. The lower surface is greenish-grey to yellowish grey, conspicuously reticulate, with greenish-yellow or brown veins, and minutely tomentose (cottony) between the reticulations. The leaves are thick and brittle. They have an aromatic odour and a balsamic bitter taste, which becomes sweetish and slightly acrid.

Eriodictyon contains volatile oil, resin, eriodictyol homoeriodictyol, chrysoeriodictyol, xanthoeriodictyol, eriodonol, eriodictyonic acid and ericolin.

Yerba Santa is used in the USA for the preparation of a fluid extract and Aromatic Eriodictyon syrup to mask the taste of bitter.

CHAMOMILE FLOWERS

Roman Chamomile flowers are the expanded flower-heads of *Anthemis nobilis* L. (*Chamaemelum nobile*) (Asteraceae), collected from cultivated plants and dried.

Habitat

Chamomiles are cultivated in the south of England, Belgium, France, Germany, Hungary, Poland, former Yugoslavia, Bulgaria, Egypt and Argentina. The tubular florets present in the wild plant have become ligulate, and these 'double' or 'semi-double' flower-heads form the commercial drug.

Collection

The flowers are collected in dry weather and carefully dried. The crop is often damaged by wet weather and the discoloured flowers have a much lower price than those having a good colour.

Characters

Each dried flower-head is hemispherical and about 12-20 mm in diameter. The florets are of a white to pale buff colour, the outer ones hiding the involucre of bracts. A few hermaphrodite, tubular florets are found near the apex of the solid receptacle. The ligulate florets show three teeth, the centre one being most developed. There are four principal veins. The corolla is contracted near its base into a tube from which a bifid style projects. The ovary is inferior and devoid of pappus. Each floret arises in the axil of a thin membraneous bract or palea which has a blunt apex. At the base of the receptacle is an involucre consisting of two or three rows of oblong bracts which have membraneous margins.

Chamomiles have a strong, aromatic odour and a bitter taste. The drug should contain not less than 0.7% of volatile oil and not more than 10.0% water.

Chemical constituents

Chamomiles contain 0.4-1.0% of volatile oil which is blue when freshly distilled due to the presence of azulene. Other components of the oil are *n*-butyl angelate, isoamyl angelate, 3-phenyl-propyl isobutyrate, tridecanal, pentadecanal and terpenes. Chamomiles also contain sesquiterpene lactones of the germacranolide type, hydroperoxides, dihydroxycinnamic acid, apigenin (a trihydroxy flavone), luteolin and its glucosides.

Uses

Chamomiles are used in the form of an infusion (for dyspepsia) or poultice or in shampoo. Volatile oil is obtained from the entire aerial parts.

MATRICARIA FLOWERS

Matricaria flowers (German or Hungarian chamomile flowers) are the dried flower-heads of *Matricaria chamomilla* L. (*Chamomilla recutita* (L.) Rausch.) (Asteraceae). The plant is cultivated in southern and eastern Europe.

The capitulum when spread out, is 10-17 mm in

diameter and consists of a receptacle, an involucre, 12-20 marginal ligulate florets and numerous central tabular florets. Matricaria possesses a hollow receptable which is devoid of paleae. Broken flowers are limited to 25%. The drug has a pleasant aromatic odour.

Chemical constituents

The flower-heads are required to contain not less than 0.4% of a blue volatile oil composed of the sesquiterpenes α-bisabolol, chamazulene and farnesene. Chamazulene is formed from a sesquiterpene lactone (matricin) during steam distillation.

Flavones and coumarins (e.g., herniarin) are present and the dried ligulate florets contain 7-9% of apigenin glucosides and 0.3-0.5% free apigenin. Most Turkish varieties of *M. chamomilla* yield yellow oils containing no chamazulene.

Uses

Matricaria flowers are used for their anti-inflam-

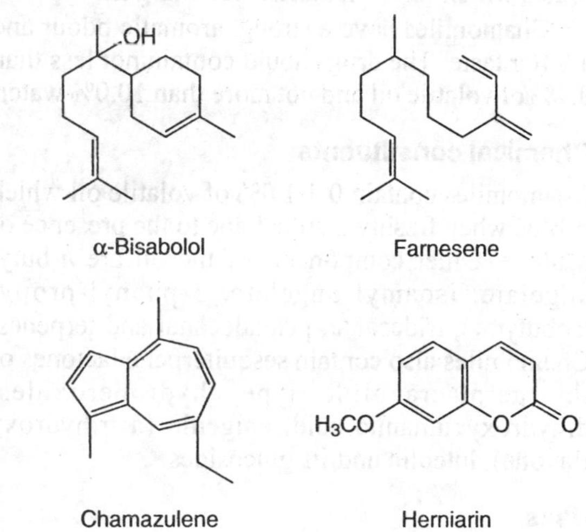

Fig. 18.57. Chemical constituents of Matricaria flowers.

matory and spasmolytic properties. The ulcer-protective properties of German chamomile have been ascribed to bisabolol-type constituents.

Allied drug

Chrysanthemum parthenium or *feverfew flowers* yields 0.07-0.4% of volatile oil. It is used as insecticide.

Kamala

Kamala consists of the trichomes and glands separated from the fruits of *Mallotus philippinensis* (Euphorbiaceae), a tree found in India, Pakistan and the East Indies. It occurs as a dull reddish-brown powder without odour or taste. It contains red resin, and radiating groups of unicellular curved trichomes. It yields the anthelminthic phloroglucinol derivatives rottlerin and isorott-lerin, resins and wax. It is used in India for the treatment of tapeworm infestation and poultry.

VANILLA

Vanilla (*Vanilla Pods*) consist of the cured fully grown but unripe fruits of *Vanilla fragrans* (Salis.) Ames (syn. *V. planifolia* Andrews) (Orchidaceae) (Mexican or Bourbon vanilla), of *V. tahitensis* (Tahiti vanilla) and *V. pompona* (West Indian vanilla).

Vanilla fragrans is grown in the woods of eastern Mexico, Reunion (or Bourbon), Mauritius, Seychelles, Madagascar, Java, Sri Lanka, Tahiti, Guadeloupe, Martinique and Indonesia. It is cultivated in tropical countries where the temperature does not fall below 18°C and where the humidity is high.

The plants are perennial, climbing, dioecious epiphytes attached to the trunks of trees by means of aerial rootlets.

Cultivation

The plant is usually propagated by means of cuttings and, after 2 or 3 years, reaches the flowering stage. The cuttings attach to trees (e.g., *Casuarina equisetifolia*) where they strike roots on the bark. It continues to bear fruit for 30 or 40 years. The flowers, approximately 30 on each plant, are hand pollinated, thus producing larger and better fruits.

The fruits are collected as they ripen to a yellow colour, 6 to 10 months after pollination, and are cured by dipping in warm water and repeated sweating between woolen blankets in the sun during the day and packing in wool-covered boxes at night. The characteristic colour and odour of the commercial drug are only developed as a result of enzyme action during the curing. Curing consists of slow drying in sheds with carefully regulated temperatures. This requires about 2 months, during which the pods lose from 70 to 80% of their original weight and take on the characteristic colour and odour of the commercial drug. The pods are then graded, tied into bundles of about 50 to 75, and sealed in tin containers for shipment.

Characters

Vanilla pods are 15-25 cm long, 8-10 mm diameter and somewhat flattened. The surface is longitudinally wrinkled, dark brown to violet-black in colour, and frequently covered with needle shaped crystals of vanillin ('frosted'). The fruits are very pliable and have a very characteristic odour and taste.

Chemical constituents

Green vanilla contains glycosides, namely glucovanillin (vanilloside) and glucovanillic alcohol. During the curing these are acted upon by an oxidizing and a hydrolysing enzyme which occur in all parts of the plant. Glucovanillic alcohol yields on hydrolysis glucose and vanillic alcohol; the latter compound is then by oxidation converted into vanillic aldehyde (vanillin). Glucovanillin yields on hydrolysis glucose and vanillin.

The vanilla species differ in their relative contents of anisyl alcohol, anisaldehyde, anisyl ethers, anisic acid esters, piperonal and *p*-hydroxybenzoic acid. These minor components, together with the two diastereoisomeric vitispiranes, add to the flavour of the pods.

Vanillin

Vanillin is 4-hydroxy-3-methoxybenzaldehyde or methylprotocatechuic aldehyde and has been synthesized in a number of ways. Large quantities of it are prepared synthetically from other sources: (1) coniferin, a glycoside present in the cambium

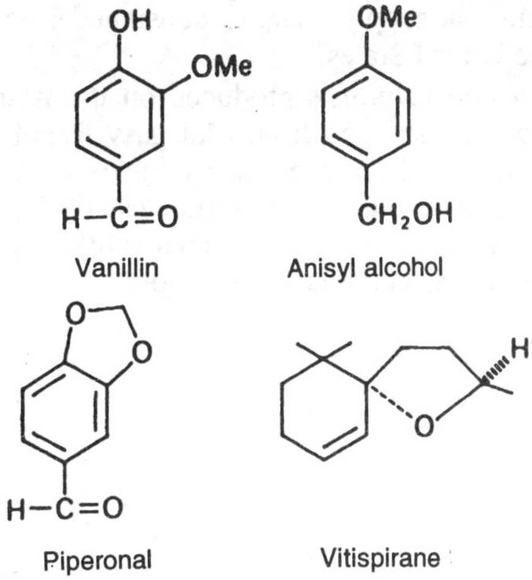

Fig. 18.58. Chemical constituents of Vanilla.

sap of pine trees; (2) eugenol, a phenol present in clove oil; (3) lignin, a byproduct of the pulp industry; and (4) guaiacol (methyl catechol). Most of the vanillin in commerce is made from lignin. In the plant glucovanillin is biosynthesized via ferulic acid. Synthesis begins when elongation of the fruit ceases, which is about 8 months after pollination, before this other phenolic glycosides predominate.

Vanillin consists of fine, white to slightly yellow, needle-like crystals that have an odour and a taste resembling vanilla. It is slightly soluble in water and glycerin and is freely soluble in alcohol, chloroform and ether. Vanillin is used as a flavouring agent.

Ethyl vanillin, a synthetic analog of vanillin, is also used as a flavouring agent.

Adulteration

Extracts of Mexican origin may be adulterated by coumarin, probably arising from the use of tonka beans.

Uses

Vanilla pods are widely used in confectionery and in perfumery.

Commercial varieties

Mexican or Vera Cruz vanilla is the best grade on the market, the pods frequently attain a length of 30 to 35 cm. The supply is largely consumed in Mexico and the United States.

Bourbon vanilla is produced on the island of Reunion and shipped from Malagasy Republic. It resembles the Mexican variety but is about two thirds as long, blacker in colour, usually covered with a sublimate or needle-shaped vanillin crystals and possesses a coumarin-like odour.

Tahiti vanilla, grown in Tahiti and Hawaii, is reddish brown in colour and about as long as the Mexican variety but sharply attenuated and twisted in the lower portion. The odour is unpleasant, and the variety is less suitable for flavouring.

Vanilla splits and cuts represent the more mature fruits in which dehiscence has taken place. They are cut into short lengths.

Resins

Resins are solid or semisolid plant exudates formed in schizogenous or schizolysigenous ducts or cavities. They are complex mixtures of compounds like resin alcohols (resinols), resin acids, resinotannols, (resin phenols), esters and resenes. Some resins (*e.g.*, Benzoin and Balsam of Tolu) are formed when the plant is injured. These resins are called as pathological resins.

The resins commonly used in pharmacy are derived from natural sources and almost are plant products - Shellac, an insect secretion, being an important exception.

Resins are classified on the basis of their occurrence in combination with another compounds as :

Balsams : Balsams are resinous substances which contain large proportions of benzoic or cinnamic acids either free or in combination or their esters. Tolu Balsam contains 35 to 50% of balsamic acids (chiefly benzoic and cinnamic acids) which are present partly in the free state and partly in combination with complex 'resin alcohols'. Benzoin, Peru Balsam and Storax are another examples of balsams.

Oleoresins : When resins occur with volatile oils, the mixture is called as oleoresins. Turpentine, Capsicum, Ginger, Male Fern, Canada Balsam and Copaiba are oleoresins.

Gum resins : When resins are found in combination with gums, then such resins are known as *gum resins*. These resins are purified by dissolving the associated gum in water. Asafoetida, Gambage and Myrrh are gum resins.

Oleo-gum resins : Oleo-gum resins are associated with gum and volatile oil both. The volatile oil is removed by steam distillation while gum is separated by dissolving in water, *e.g.*, Myrrh, Ipomoea and Asafoetida.

Glycoresins (*Glucoresins*) : Some resins are found in combination with glycosides. These resins occur in Ipomoea, Scammony, Jalap and Podophyllum. On hydrolysis they produce sugars and complex resin acids as aglycones.

Formation of resins

In many instances a resin in plants is formed in special passages or tubes called schizogenous or schizolysigenous ducts or cavities, which are usually anastomose. Thus, a single incision may drain the resin from a considerable area of the plant. The cells lining the ducts possess a layer (called the resinogenous layer) of slimy matter bonded by a fine cuticle and resin is secreted in this layer. It is excreted through the cuticle layer into the resin duct.

In some cases, *e.g.*, Copaiba, numerous resin ducts are present. Tapping is necessary to drain the ducts. Such resin is called as normal or physiologically-produced resin. In other instances, *e.g.*, turpentine, only a few resin ducts are normally present, but following injury to the cambium the new or secondary wood subsequently formed which contains very large number of ducts. The resin from these ducts is called wound, traumatic or pathologically-produced resin.

Resin may continue to flow for a considerable

period from wounding, or in some cases it may be necessary to inflict wounds at frequent intervals. Further, invasion of the wound by fungi and bacteria sometimes plays an important part in the composition of the resin exuded. For example, the simple wound resin of Styrax and Benzoin differs materially from the resin exuded after fungal invasion of the wound.

They are often preformed in the plant but the yield is usually increased by injury (*e.g.*, in the case of *Pinus*). Many products (*e.g.*, Benzoin and Balsam of Tolu) are not formed by the plant until it has been injured: that is, they are of pathological origin. The resin gums usually resemble Acacia gum in chemical nature and they are often accompanied by oxidase enzymes. The resins are also found in the heartwood of guaiacum, in the external glands of Indian hemp, in the internal glands of male fern or in the glands on the surface of the lac insect.

Characters

Purified resins are amorphous, brittle, transluscent, hard solids. On heating they are softened and then melted. They are practically insoluble in water but dissolve in organic solvents like alcohol, ether and chloroform. Varnish-like film is formed on evaporation of the solvent. They produce smoky flame on burning.

Chemical constituents

Chemically, the resins are complex mixtures of the following compounds :

1. *Resin acids* : Resin acids are the mixture of oxyacids, carboxylic acids and phenolic acids. They are present in the free state or as esters. They are soluble in aqueous alkaline solutions which form soap-like froth on shaking. Abietic acid in Rosin or Colophony, copaivic acid and oxycopaivic acid in Copaiba, guaiaconic acid in Guaiac, pimaric (pimarinic) acid in Frankincense, sandaracolic acid in Sandarac, aleuritic acid in Shellac and commiphoric acid in Myrrh are the examples of resin acids.

2. *Resin alcohols* : Resin alcohols are complex molecules with high molecular weight. They are present in the free state or as esters of simple aromatic acids, *e.g.*, benzoic acid, salicylic acid

and cinnamic acid. They are further subdivided as :

   (i) *Resinotannols* : They are tannins and form blue colour with ferric chloride, *e.g.*, aloe-resinotannol from Aloe, amoresinotannol and galbaresinotannol from Ammoniac, peruresinotannol from Balsam of Peru, siaresinotannol and sumaresinotannol from Benzoin.

   (ii) *Resinols* : Resinols do not contain tannins. Benzoresinol from Benzoin, storesinol from Storax and guaiacresinol from Guaiac resin are the examples of resinols.

3. *Resenes* : Resenes are complex neutral compounds which do not respond to any chemical reaction. They are insoluble in acids and alkalies and do not form any salts or esters, *e.g.*, alban and fluavil from Gutta percha, copalresene from Copal, dammaresene from Dammar, dracoresene from Dragon's blood and olibanoresene from Olibanum.

Resin containing drugs possess purgative (Podophyllum), cathartic (Colocynth, Gamboge, Ipomoea), hydragogue (Jalap), sedative (Cannabis), counter-irritant (Capsicum, Turpentine), anthelmintic (Asphidium), expectorant (White Pine, Copaiba, Storax, Tolu Balsam, Benzoin) and laxative (Asafoetida) properties. Externally resins are used as mild antiseptic in the form of cerates, ointments and plasters. They are employed in the preparation of emulsions.

COLOPHONY

Synonyms

Rosin, Yellow resin; Abietic anhydride; Colophony resin; Amber resin; Resin; Coloponium.

Biological source

Colophony is a solid residue left after distilling off the volatile oil from the oleoresin obtained from *Pinus palustris* (long leaf pine) and other species of *Pinus* such as *P. elliottii* (slash pine), *P. pinaster* (syn. *P. maritima*), *P. halepensis*, *P. massoniana*, *P. tabuliformis*, *P. carribacea* var. *hondurensis*, *P. oocarpa*, *P. radiata*, and *P. roxburghii* (syn. *P. longifolia*). Family : Pinaceae.

Habitat

The genus *Pinus* is widely found in many countries including USA, France, Italy, Portugal, Spain, Greece, New Zealand, China, India (Himalayan region) and Pakistan.

Colophony is chiefly produced in USA contributing about 80% of world supply. Other countries producing the resin are China, France, Spain, India, Greece, Morocco, Honduras, Poland and Russia.

Collection

The collection of the oleoresin is very laborous procedure. Although Colophony is a normal (Physiological) resin of *Pinus* species, its amount is increased by injuring the plant. For its collection a few-feet long groove or blaze is made in the bark with the help of knife or some other instrument. A metal or earthenware cup is attached below the groove by nails. The cup is adjusted accordingly when the size of groove increases. The resin is taken out at different intervals and sent for further processing.

The flow of oleoresin is increased by applying sulphuric acid (50%), plant hormones or cultures of *Fusarium* species to the grooves. By such treatment the living xylem cells produce excess amount of oleoresin which is leaked to the adjacent cells. The acid treatment has the effect of collapsing the thin-walled cells lining the ducts, thus enlarging the channels, with the production of a more rapid flow of the oleoresin. The application of paraquat to the wood causes the living xylem cells to synthesize large quantities of oleoresin which then leaks into adjacent areas until they become saturated. About 250,000 trees are required to sustain a small commercial processing plant.

Cup and gutter method

This method is used in America, European countries, India and Pakistan. The 60-100 cm long blaze or longitudinal groove is cut with a suitable instrument. It is enlarged at intervals and in about 4 years is about 4 m long. The metal or earthenware cups are attached to the trunk by nails and one or two strips of galvanized iron are placed above each to direct the flow of oleoresin. As the grooves are lengthened the cups are moved higher up the tree and new grooves are started when the old ones become exhausted or collection is difficult. The cups are emptied at intervals and the oleoresin sent to the distillery. Trees can be tapped by this method for about 40 years.

Preparation

The crude oleoresin arrives at the distillery in barrels. It is mixed with about 20% by weight of turpentine in a heated stainless steel vessel and allowed to stand to separate water and other impurities. The diluted oleoresin is then transferred to copper or stainless steel stills and the turpentine is removed by steam distillation. When distillation is complete the molten resin is run through wire strainers into barrels, in which it cools and is exported.

The resin obtained from trees during their first year of tapping is of a lighter colour than that obtained later on. The following grades of American rosin are recognized: B, FF (for wood rosin only), D, E, F, G, H, I, K, L, M, N, WG (window-glass), WW (water-white) and the extra-white X grades and American and Portuguese qualities (XA, XB, XC). A great deal of the American tall oil rosin is now paler than grade X. Grade B is almost black.

Characters

Colophony occurs as translucent, hard, shiny, sharp,

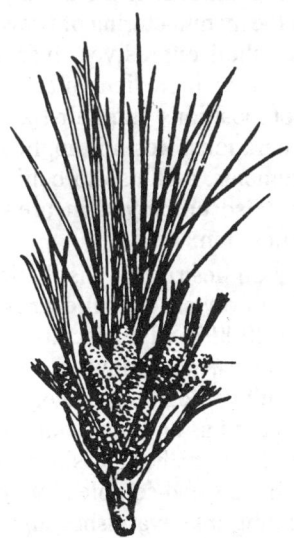

Fig. 19.1. *Pinus roxburghii.*

pale yellow to amber fragments, fracture brittle at ordinary temperature, burns with smoky flame, slight turpentine-like odour and taste, melts readily on heating, density 1.07-1.09. Acid number is not less than 150. It is insoluble in water but freely soluble in alcohol, benzene, ether, glacial acetic acid, oils, carbon disulphide and alkali solutions.

Chemical tests

1. To a solution of powdered resin (0.1 g) in acetic acid (10 ml) one drop of conc. sulphuric acid is added in a dry test tube. A purple colour, readily changing to violet, is formed.
2. To a petroleum ether solution of powdered Colophony twice its volume of dilute solution of copper acetate is shaken. The colour of the petroleum ether layer changes to emerald-green due to formation of copper salt of abietic acid.
3. To alcoholic solution of Colophony sufficient water is added. It becomes milky white due to precipitation of chemical compounds.
4. Alcoholic solution of Colophony turns blue litmus to red due to the presence of diterpenic acids.

Chemical constituents

Colophony contains resin acids (about 90%), resenes and fatty acid esters. Of the resin acids about 90% are isomeric α-, β- and γ-abietic acids (sylvic acid, $C_{20}H_{30}O_2$); the other 10% is a mixture of dihydro-abietic acid and dehydroabietic acid. Before distillation the resin contains excess amounts of (+) and (–) pimaric acids. During distillation the (–) pimaric acid is converted into abietic acid while (+) pimaric acid is stable. On heating at 300°C abietic acid is transformed into *neo*-abietic acid. The other constituents of Colophony are sipinic acid and a hydrocarbon.

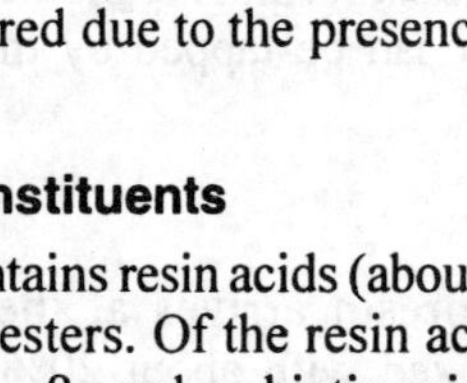

Fig. 19.2. Abietic acid.

Colophony obtained from *P. massoniana* contains pimara-8 (14), 15-diene, derivatives of 7,13-abietadien-18-oic acid, podocarpen-7,13-dien-18-oic acid, abietatrien-18-oic acid and podo-carpatrien-18-oic acid; pimaric, l-pimaric, palustric, neoabietic, dehydroabietic, 7-oxodehydroabietic and 7α-hydroxydehydroabietic acids. Pimaric, l-pimaric, palustric and neoabietic acids showed inhibition of aggregation of platelets.

Uses

Colophony is used as stiffening agent in ointments, adhesives, plasters and cerates and as a diuretic in veterinary medicine. Commercially it is used to manufacture varnishes, printing inks, cements, soap, sealing wax, wood polishes, floor coverings, paper, plastics, fireworks, tree wax, rosin oil and for water proofing cardboard.

The abietic acids show antimicrobial, antiulcer and cardiovascular; some have filmogenic, surfactant and antifeedant properties.

Much rosin is artificially modified by hydrogenation or polymerization; these products are used for paper size, adhesives, printing inks, rubber, linoleum, thermoplastic floor tiles and surface coatings.

Colophony is used in rubber industry, in casein glues, as binder in roofing cements, in dry battery insulating compositions, in soldering pastes and fluxes, and in the manufacturing of fireworks, match compositions, shell explosives, insecticides and disinfectants. It is an ingredient of core oils, certain lubricating compositions and hair-fixing and nail-polishing preparations. Rosin is applied to bows of musical instruments, and also to belting to reduce slipping. It is also employed in brewing and in mineral beneficiation.

Colophony on destructive distillation yields 3-10% of pale yellowish oil called rosin spirit or pinolime, and 80-85% of a viscous brown liquid with a green fluorescence, known as rosin oil. Rosin spirit consists of hydrocarbons and oxygenated substances, and is used as an illuminant and substitute for turpentine in varnishes. Rosin oil consists of abietic acid, phenols and complex hydrocarbons. It is used in printing inks, varnishes and antiseptics; as a binder for making micanite from mica splittings and to adulterate boiled linseed, olive, rape and sperm oil.

INDIAN PINE RESIN

Pine resin or Turpentine resin is an oleoresin tapped from several species of pine. On distillation, it yields two commercial products—an essential oil, known as Oil of Turpentine or Turpentine, and a non-volatile product termed Rosin or Colophony.

Pine resin

Four resin-yielding *Pinus* spp. occur wild in India, of which only Chir pine (*P. roxburghii* Sarg., syn. *P. longifolia* Roxb.) is of commercial significance as a source of pine resin. Several exotic pines have been introduced into India but none has attained any economic importance. The most important *Pinus* spp. exploited in the USA for pine resin are *P. palustris* and *P. caribaea*. French pine resin is obtained from *P. maritima* and Russian pine resin from *P. sylvestris*.

Chir (*P. roxburghii*) is found in the Himalayas from Kashmir to Bhutan and in the Siwalik Hills at altitudes of 450-2,400 m. Khasi pine (*P. insularis* Endl. syn. *P. khasya* Royle) occurs in the Khasi, Jaintia, Lushai, Manipur and Naga hills and in the NEFA. It is exploited for the oleoresin to a very limited extent. Chilgoza pine (*P. gerardiana* Wall.) found locally in the inner arid valleys of the north-west Himalayas at altitudes of 1,800-3,000 m and blue pine (*P. gerardiana* Wall.) found locally in the inner arid valleys of the north-west Himalayas at altitudes of 1,800-3,000 m and blue pine (*P. wallichiana* A.B. Jackson, syn. *P. excelsa* Wall. ex D. Don) found in the Himalayas from Kashmir to Bhutan at altitudes of 1,800-3,700 m and in the Balipara tract of Assam, also yield oleoresins. The resin from these two pines is of experimental interest only.

Tapping of resin from Chir commences in March and continues till November after which the flow of resin practically ceases. The average yield of pine oleoresin is about 250 kg per 100 blazes. The yield of crude is influenced by several factors such as season, locality, year of tapping, period of freshening of the blazes, etc. The yield per blaze is greater in hot, dry years and on the southern than the northern slopes. The yield is smallest in the first year reaching a maximum in the third year; there is a decline of yield in the fifth year.

Among the other pines, the yield of oleoresin from the blue pine (*P. wallichiana*) is low, being about half of that from chir pine. Chilgoza pine, on tapping, yields a good quality resin. However, its availability is limited and the tree is valued more for its edible seeds.

Production

Pine resin is produced in Jammu & Kashmir, Uttaranchal and Himachal Pradesh. The tapping and selling of the oleoresin in these States is managed almost entirely by the respective Government Forest Departments. It is not easy to obtain reliable data on the total production of the resin in the country.

Rosin constitutes the solid residue remaining in the still after distilling off the turpentine from the oleoresin. It is recovered from the still and the molten mass is strained through filtering trays, filled into wooden casks and allowed to cool for 1-2 days before marketing. The yield of rosin is about 75% on the quantity of pine resin distilled.

Commercial rosin varies in colour from pale amber to black. Rosin produced from fresh oleoresin is pale while that from aged samples is dark in colour. Rosin is classified according to its colour into three types, namely pale, medium and dark which are further graded into eight colour grades.

Manufacturing units

The manufacture of rosin and turpentine oil from pine resin is a well-established and a sizeable industry in India. There are four stateowned units engaged in the manufacture of rosin and turpentine. These are : Indian Turpentine & Rosin Co. Ltd., Clutterbuckganj (Bareilly); Himachal Govt. Rosin & Turpentine Factory, one unit at Nahan and another at Bilaspur; and Jammu Rosin & Turpentine Factory, Miransahib, Jammu. Of these, only the first named unit is in the large scale sector. Another important unit is the UP Cooperative Resin Processing Factory, at Haldwani. In addition, there are 30-35 small private units located at Hoshiarpur, Raipur, Bareilly, Haldwani and Delhi. A number of private units have been set up at Bari Brahmina and around Jammu in the state of Jammu & Kashmir.

BALSAM TOLU

Synonyms

Tolu Balsam; Thomas Balsam; Opobalsam; Resin Tolu; Balsam of Tolu; Balsamum tolutanum.

Biological source

Balsam Tolu is obtained by incision of stem of *Myroxylon balsamum* (L.) Harms. Family : Papilionaceae.

Habitat

The plant grows in Colombia (near lower Magdalena and Canca rivers), West Indies, Cuba, Venezuela and Peru. The trees are cultivated in the West Indies.

Collection

Balsam Tolu is a pathological resin and is formed in trunk tissues as a result of injuries. It is collected all the year except the period of heavy rains by making V-shaped incisions in the bark and sap wood. Calabash cups are placed to receive the flow of balsam. Many other incisions are made on higher portion on the trees. Collected balsam is transferred into larger tin containers and exported.

Characters

Tolu Balsam occurs as soft, yellowish-brown or brown, semi-solid or plastic solid, transparent in thin layers, brittle when old, dried or kept in cold, odour aromatic, and taste is aromatic, vanilla-like and slightly pungent. It is insoluble in water and petroleum ether; soluble in alcohol, benzene, chloroform, ether, glacial acetic acid and partially soluble in carbon disulphide and NaOH solution.

On keeping it turns to a brown, brittle solid. It softens on warming. Under microscopical examination shows crystals of cinnamic acid, amorphous resin and vegetable debris. Odour is aromatic and fragrant; taste, aromatic; the drug forms a plastic mass when chewed.

The alcohol solution is acidic to litmus, and gives a green colour with ferric chloride (due to the presence of resinotannol). It yields an odour of benzaldehyde when a filtered decoction is oxidized with potassium permanganate solution.

Chemical tests

1. Alcoholic solution of Balsam Tolu (1 g) gives green colour with ferric chloride due to toluresinotannols.
2. Alcoholic solution of Balsam Tolu is acidic to litmus paper.
3. To filtered solution of Balsam Tolu (1 g) in water (5 ml) aqueous potassium permanganate solution is added and heated for 5-10 minutes. Odour of benzaldehyde is produced due to oxidation of cinnamic acid.

Chemical constituents

Tolu Balsam contains resin (~80%) which is a mixture of resin alcohols combined with cinnamic and benzoic acids. The aromatic acids are also present in free state in proportions 8-15 per cent. The other constituents reported in the drug are benzyl benzoate, benzyl cinnamate, vanillin, styrene, eugenol, ferulic acid, 1,2-diphenylethane (bibenzyl), mono- and sesquiterpene hydrocarbons, alcohols and triterpenoids. Tolu Balsam contains from 35 to 50% of total balsamic acids calculated on the dry alcohol-soluble matter.

Carbreuvin (3',4',7-trimethoxyisoflavone), isoflavones afromosin, 7-hydroxy-4'-methoxyisoflavanone, 7,3'-dihydroxy-4'-methoxyisoflavanone and 2-(2',4'-dihydroxyphenyl)-5,6-dimethoxybenzofuran from the wood; 1(5),6-guaiadiene and epi-1(5), 6-guaiadiene from the resin are reported.

Uses

Balsam of Tolu is used as an expectorant, stimulant and antiseptic. It is an ingredient of cough mixtures and Compound Benzoin tincture. It is also used as a pleasant flavouring agent in medicinal syrups, confectionery, chewing gums and perfumery.

Adulteration

Commercial preparations are usually adulterated with rosin but the general sophistication is the natural balsam from which the aromatic substances have been isolated.

PERU BALSAM

Synonyms

Peruvian Balsam; Indian Balsam; China oil; Black

Balsam; Honduras Balsam; Surnam Balsam; Balsam of Peru; Balsamum peruvianum.

Biological source

Peru balsam is obtained by incision of the stem of *Myroxylon balsamum* var. *pereirae* (Royle) Klotsch at high temperature. Family : Papilionaceae

Habitat

The plant is most widely found in Colombia, Venezuela, Central America (San Salvador), in forests near Pacific coast and cultivated in West Indies, Cuba, Florida and Sri Lanka.

Collection

M. pereirae is a large tree, about 25 meters in height. Peru balsam is a pathological resin and is formed when the plant is injured. The 10 years old tree is beaten on four sides in November or December. The cracked bark is scorched with torch to separate it from the trunk. Within a week the bark is dropped from trunk and the balsam begins to flow from the exposed wood. The injured part is covered with cloths or rags in which the resin is absorbed. When the cloths are saturated with exudate, they are removed from time to time and boiled with water. On cooling the water extracted balsam is settled out which is removed, strained, packed in tin cans and exported to get *balsamo de trapo*.

The balsam produced in the bark is obtained by boiling the bark in water and is known as *tacuasonte* (prepared without fire) or *balsamo de cascara* (balsam of the bark).

By the removal of narrow strips of bark and the replacement of scorching with the use of a hot iron the tree recovers in 6 months. The drug is chiefly exported from Acajutla (San Salvador) and Belize (British Honduras) in tin container holding about 27 kg.

Characters

Fresh Peru Balsam is a soft, yellow, viscous syrupy liquid or semi-solid. On keeping it becomes dark brown, or nearly black, brittle solid. It softens on heating in which crystals of cinnamic acid may be visible under microscope. It does not stick, has an empyreumatic, aromatic, vanilla-like odour and a bitter, acrid, persistent taste. It is insoluble in water and olive oil but soluble in alcohol, chloroform, and glacial acetic acid, usually with a slight opalescense.

The solution in alcohol (90%), becomes turbid on the addition of further solvent. The relative density, 1.14-1.17, is a good indication of purity, and if abnormal indicates adulteration with fixed oils, alcohol and kerosene.

Chemical constituents

The drug contains balsamic esters (45-70%) like benzyl cinnamate (cinnamein), C_6H_5 CH=CH COOCH$_2$ C_6H_5 (50-60%), benzyl benzoate and cinnamyl cinnamate (styracin), resin (28%) consisting of peruresinotannol combined with cinnamic and benzoic acids, alcohols [nerolidol (peruviol) farnesol and benzyl alcohol] and small amounts of vanillin and free cinnamic acid.

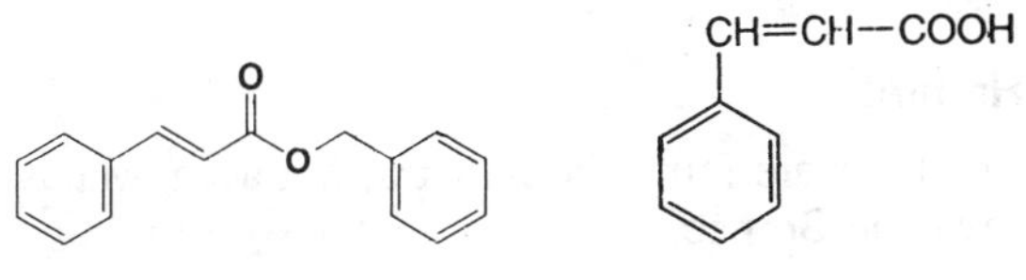

Benzyl cinnamate   Cinnamic acid

Fig. 19.3. Cinnamic acid and benzyl cinnamate.

Chemical tests

1. Its alcoholic solution gives green colour with ferric chloride.
2. TLC of its ethyl acetate shows two main spots of benzylic esters under UV light.
3. TLC sprayed with phosphomolybdic acid shows the presence of nerolidol.
4. It reacts with potassium permanganate to yield benzaldehyde.

Uses

Peru Balsam is used as miticide, to aid in healing of indolent wounds, as scabicide and parasiticide, in skin catarrh, diarrhoea, ulcer therapy, as local protectant and rubefacient. It is an antiseptic and vulnerary and as a stimulating expectorant. It is also employed in perfumery and some chocolate flavourings, also in making of odours.

Peruvian Balsam is topically used as an antiseptic to treat burns, frost-bites, cracks, erythema, pruritus, ulcers and wounds. Its suppositories are used to cure pain, pruritus, piles and other anal disorders. It is an ingredient in cosmetic and hygiene products (soups, creams, lotions, detergents) and in fixative. It can cause contact dermatitis in some people.

SUMATRA BENZOIN

Synonyms

Gum Benjamin; Benzoinum; Benzoin; Luban (Hindi).

Biological source

Sumatra Benzoin is obtained from the incised stem of *Styrax benzoin* Dryander and *Styrax paralleloneurus* Perkins. It contains about 25% of total balsamic acids, calculated as cinnamic acid. Family : Styraceae.

Habitat

The trees are found in Sumatra, Malacca, Malaya, Java and Borneo.

Collection

The plants are medium size trees. Sumatra Benzoin is a pathological resin which is formed by making incision and by attack of fungi. In Sumatra the seeds are sown in rice fields. The rice plants provide protection to benzoin plants during first year. After harvesting of the rice crop the trees are allowed to grow. When they are 7 years old, three triangular wounds are made in a vertical row. Tapping consists of making in each trunk three lines of incisions which are gradually lengthened. The first triangular wounds are made in a vertical row about 40 cm apart, the bark between the wounds being then scraped smooth. The first secretion is very sticky and is rejected. After making further cuts, each about 4 cm above the preceding ones, a harder secretion is obtained. Further incisions are made at 3-monthly intervals and the secretion becomes crystalline. About 6 weeks after each fresh tapping the product is scraped off, the outer layer (finest quality) being kept separate from the next layer (intermediate quality). About 2 weeks later the strip is scraped again, giving a lower quality darker in colour and containing fragments of bark. Fresh incisions are then made and the above process is repeated. Second exudation is milky white and is used for medicinal purpose. The stem is incised four times during one year. All types of exudations are sent to industry for further processing. A single tree yields about 10 kg of resin per year and is completely exhausted by the 19th year of its life.

The best grade contains the most 'almonds' and the worst contains a few almonds but abundant resinous matrix. The blending is done by breaking up the drug, mixing different proportions of the three qualities and softening in the sun. It is exported after stamping in plaited containers with a plastic wrapping.

Characters

Sumatra benzoin occurs in brittle masses consisting of opaque, whitish or reddish tears embedded in a translucent, reddish-brown or greyish-brown, resinous matrix. Odour, agreeable and balsamic, taste, slightly acrid. *Siamese benzoin* occurs in tears or in blocks. The tears are of variable size and flattened; they are yellowish-brown or reddish-brown externally, but milky-white and opaque internally. The block form consists of small tears embedded in a glassy, reddish-brown, resinous matrix. It has a vanilla-like odour and a balsamic taste.

When heated, benzoin evolves white fumes of cinnamic and benzoic acids which readily condense on a cool surface as a crystalline sublimate.

Chemical constituents

Sumatra Benzoin consists of free balsamic acid (cinnamic and benzoic acids) (25%) and their esters. The amount of cinnamic acid is usually double that of benzoic acid. It also contains triterpenic acids like siaresinolic acid (19-hydroxy-oleanolic acid) and sumaresinolic acid (6-hydroxy-oleanolic acid); traces of vanillin, phenylpropyl cinnamate, cinnamyl cinnamate and phenylethylene.

Uses

Sumatra Benzoin possesses expectorant, antiseptic, carminative, stimulant and diuretic properties. It is used in cosmetic lotions, perfumery and to prepare Compound Benzoin. It forms an ingredient of inhalations in the treatment of catarrh of upper respiratory tract in the form of Compound Benzoin Tincture. Benzoin is used as an external antiseptic and protective, and is one of the main ingredients of Friar's Balsam. It is also used to fix the odour of incenses, skin-soaps, perfumes and other cosmetics and for fixing the taste of certain pharmaceutical preparations. Benzoin retards rancification of fats and is used for this purpose in the official benzoinated lard, also used in food, drinks and in incense.

Allied drug

Palembang benzoin, an inferior variety produced in Sumatra is collected from isolated trees from which the resin has not been stripped for some time. It is very light in weight and breaking with an irregular porous fracture. It consists of reddish-brown resin, with only a few very small tears embedded in it. Palembang benzoin is used as a source of natural benzoic acid.

SIAM BENZOIN

Biological source

Siam Benzoin is a balsamic resin derived from stem of *Styrax tonkinensis* Craib. (Family : Styraceae).

Habitat

The trees are present in North Laos, North Vietnam, Annam and Thailand.

Collection

Siam Benzoin is also a pathological resin produced by incising the bark and by fungus attack. The stem of 6-8 years old plant is incised when balsam exudates. The resin is obtained in the form of liquid which is solidified.

Characters

Siam Benzoin occurs as tears or in blocks of variable sizes and reddish brown externally, but milky-white or opaque internally. Matrix is glassy, reddish-brown, resinous, brittle but softening on chewing and become plastic-like on chewing. It has vanilla-like odour and a balsamic taste.

Chemical constituents

The principal constituent of Siam Benzoin is coniferyl benzoate (60-80%) (3-methoxy-4-

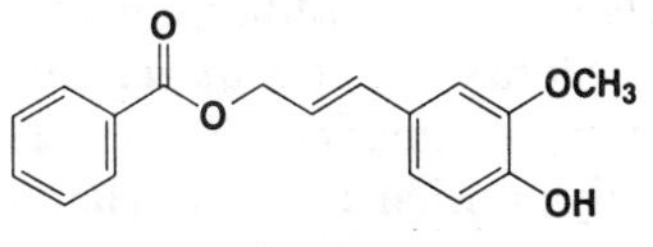

Fig. 19.4. Coniferyl benzoate.

hydroxycinnamyl alcohol). Other constituents are free benzoic acid (10%), triterpene siaresinolic acid (6%), vanillin and benzyl cinnamate.

Chemical tests

1. Heat Sumatra Benzoin (5 g) with 10% aqueous potassium permanganate solution. A bitter almond-like odour is produced due to oxidation of cinnamic acid present in Sumatra Benzoin. This test is negative in case of Siam Benzoin.

2. To a petroleum ether solution of Benzoin (0.2 g), 2-3 drops of sulphuric acid are added in a China dish. Sumatra Benzoin produces reddish-brown colour while Siam Benzoin shows purple-red colour on rotating the dish.

3. To alcoholic solution of Benzoin ferric chloride solution is added. A green colour is produced in Siam Benzoin due to the presence of phenolic compound coniferyl benzoate. This test is negative in case of Sumatra Benzoin which does not contain sufficient amount of phenolic constituents.

Uses

Siam Benzoin acts as antiseptic, vulnerary and expectorant; it is used to prepare benzoinated lard, cosmetics, fixatives and in perfumery. It is superior to the Sumatra Benzoin with respect to antioxidative effect in Lard and other fats.

STORAX

Synonyms

Styrax; Sweet oriental gum; Prepared Storax; Liquid Storax; Styrax preparatus.

Biological source

Storax is a balsam obtained from the trunk of

Liquidambar orientalis Miller, commercially known as Levant Storax, or of *Liquidambar styraciflua* Linn. known as American Storax. The balsam is subsequently purified. (Family : Hamamelidaceae).

Habitat

Levant Storax is a native to Asia Minor and southwest of Turkey. American Storax is produced chiefly in Honduras; found along the Atlantic coast from Connecticut to Central America.

Collection

Levant Storax and American Storax are medium-sized trees attaining the height of 15 m and 40 m respectively. Levant Storax is a pathological resin. In the early summer the bark of 3-4 years old tree is injured by bruising. Cambium is activated to produce new wood with balsam secreting ducts. The bark is gradually saturated with balsam which is peeled off. The pieces of bark are pressed to get the product. The bark is boiled in hot water and repressed. The crude balsam is poured into casks or cans and exported.

American Storax exudes into natural spaces present in between the bark and the wood. The presence of balsam in spaces may be detected by excresences on the outside of the bark. From these pockets the balsam is tapped with gutters into containers which is exported in tin cans.

Storax is purified by dissolving the crude balsam in alcohol, filtering and evaporating the solvent under low temperature not to lose volatile compounds. The alcohol-insoluble part consists of vegetable debris and a resin.

Characters

Levent Storax is a viscous, semiliquid, greyish, sticky, opaque mass which deposits as a dark-brown, heavier, oleoresinous product on standing. American Storax is a semisolid, sometimes solid mass softened by warming, becoming hard, opaque, and darker coloured. Storax is transparent in thin layers, has characteristic taste and odour, and is denser than water. It is insoluble in water; almost completely soluble in warm alcohol, ether, acetone and carbon disulphide. Odour is agreeable and taste is balsamic.

Chemical constituents

Storax is rich in two resin alcohol (50%), α-storesin and β-storesin and balsamic acids (30-47%). The alcohols occur partly free and partly as esters of cinnamic acid (10-20%). Storax also contains cinnamyl cinnamate or styracin (5-10%), phenyl-propyl cinnamate (10%); ethyl cinnamate, benzyl cinnamate, free cinnamic acid (5-15%), styrene, traces of vanillin and volatile oil (0.5-1%). Stream-distillation of Storax yields a pale yellow or dark brown oil (0.5-1.0%), known as oil of Storax. It has a pleasant but peculiar odour.

L. formosana resin contains liquidambronic, forucosolic, liquidambradiolic, ambronic, ambrolic and ambradiolic acids, isorugosins A, B and D, rugosins A-F, cornusiin A, captothins A and B; triterpene aldehydes liquidambronal and ambronal; bornyl *trans*-cinnamate and isorugosin E.

The presence of cinnamic acid in the drug is shown by the odour of benzaldehyde which is produced when the drug is mixed with sand and warmed with a solution of potassium permanganate. The resin also contains monoterpenes, phenylpropanes and aliphatic acids.

Allied drug

American storax obtained from *L. styraciflua*, a large tree found near the Atlantic coast from Central America to Connecticut, is also used in the USA. This balsam resembles the Levant storax in constituents. Thirty six compounds have been identified in the leaf-oil of the plant and tannins and related phenolics obtained from cell cultures.

Uses

Storax is used as a stimulant, expectorant, parasiticide, topical protectant and an antiseptic. Pharmaceutical preparations like Compound Benzoin Tincture, Friars' Balsam and Benzoin Inhalation are also prepared from the Storax.

COPAIBA

Synonyms

Balsam Copaiba; Balsam of Copaiba; Balsam Capivi; Jesuit's Balsam, Copaiva.

Biological source

Copaiba is an oleoresin obtained from trunks of South American species of *Copaifera* (*Copaiba*) like *Copaifera landsdorfii* Dest. (Family : Papilionaceae).

Habitat

Copaiba plants are found in Brazil, Venezuela and Colombia, especially the Amazon valley and banks of Orinoco.

Collection

Copaiba is a physiological resin. The tree is 18 meters in height which is tapped and the oleoresin conducted directly to containers. About 20-24 litres of the product is collected from one tree.

Characters

Copaiba is a transparent, viscid, pale yellow to brown-yellow liquid, peculiar odour; bitter acrid, nauseating taste. It is insoluble in water but soluble in benzene, chloroform, ether, oils, carbon disulphide, absolute alcohol and petroleum ether.

Chemical constituents

Copaiba contains volatile oil, resin, illuric acid ($C_{20}H_{28}O_3$), metacopaivic acid (in Maracaibo Copaiba), copaivic acid and oxycopaivic acid (in Para Copaiba). These acids are the diterpenes relating to abietic or pimaric acid. It also contains at least 24 sesquiterpene hydrocarbons and a number of diterpenes.

Uses

Copaiba has diuretic, antiseptic, expectorant and disinfectant properties and is used in leucorrhoea, gonorrhoea, in varnishes and for manufacturing photographic paper.

ASAFOETIDA

Synonyms

Devil's dung; Food of the gods; Asafoda; Asant; Hing (Hindi).

Biological source

Asafoetida is an oleo-gum-resin obtained as an exudation by incision of the decapitated rhizome and roots of *Ferula assafoetida* L., *F. foetida*, Royel, *F. rubricaulis* Boiss. and some other species of *Ferula* (Family : Apiaceae).

Habitat

The plant grows in Iran, Turkestan & Afghanistan (Karam and Chagai districts).

Collection

The plant is a perennial branching, 3 m high herb possessing large schizogeneous ducts and lysigenous cavities containing milky liquid. Upon exudation and drying of the liquid, Asafoetida is obtained. For the collection of the drug the upper part of the root is laid bare and the stem cut off close to the crown in March-April. The exposed surface is covered by a dome-shaped structure made of twigs and earth. After separating each slice, exudation of oleo-gum-resin, present as whitish gummy resinous emulsion in the schizogenous ducts of the cortex of the stem, takes place. It hardens on the cut surface which is collected, packed in tin-line cases and exported. Removal of the exudation and exposure of fresh surface proceeds until the root is exhausted. The yield is usually soft enough to agglomerate into masses when packed.

Characters

Asafoetida occurs as a soft solid mass or irregular lumps or "tears", sometimes almost semiliquid. Tears are rounded or flattened and about 5-30 mm in diameter, greyish-white or dull yellow or reddish brown in colour.

Asafoetida mass is mixed with fruits, fragments of root, sand and other impurities. Asafoetida has a strong garlic-like (alliaceous) odour and a bitter, acrid and alliaceous taste. When triturated with water, it makes a milky emulsion. It should not have more than 50% of matter insoluble in alcohol (90%) and not more than 15% of ash.

Chemical constituents

Asafoetida contains volatile oil (4-20%), resin (40-65%) and gum (~25%). The garlic-like odour of the oil is due to the presence of sulphur compounds of the formulae $C_7H_{14}S_2$, $C_{16}H_{20}S_2$, $C_8H_{16}S_2$, $C_{10}H_{18}S_2$, $C_7H_{14}S_3$ and $C_8H_{16}S_3$. The main constituent of the

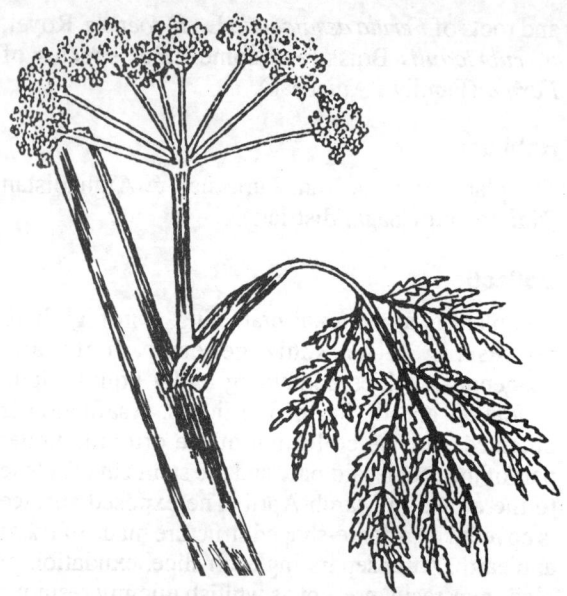

Fig. 19.5. *Ferula asafoetida.*

oil is isobutyl propanyl disulphide ($C_6H_{16}S_2$). The three sulphur compounds, viz., 1-methylpropyl-1-propenyl disulphide, 1-(methylthio)-propyl-1-propenyl disulphide and 1-methyl-propyl 3-(methylthio)-2-propenyl disulphide have also also been isolated from the resin; the latter two have pesticidal properties. The flavour is largely due to *R*-2-butyl-1-propenyl disulphide and 2-butyl-3-methylthioallyl disulphide (both as mixtures of diastereoisomers). The drug also contains a complex mixture of sesquiterpene umbelliferyl ethers mostly with a monocyclic or bicyclic terpenoid moiety. Resin consists of ester of asaresinotannol and ferulic acid, pinene, vanillin and free ferulic acid. On treatment of ferulic acid with hydrochloric acid, it is converted into umbelliferone (a coumarin) which gives blue fluorescence with ammonia.

Asafoetida also contains phellandrene, sec-butylpropenyl disulphide, geranyl acetate, bornyl acetate, α-terpineol, myristic acid, camphene, myrcene, limonene, longifolene, cadinene, β-caryophyllene, β-selinene, fenchone, eugenol, linalool, geraniol, isoborneol, borneol, guaiacol, cadinol, farnesol, E- and Z-2-butyl-1-propenyl-disulphide, dimethyl trisulphide, 2-butyl-3-methyl thioallyl disulphide, 2-butylmethyl disulphide, 2-butyl-

methyltrisulphide, di-2-butyl disulphide, di-2-butyltrisulphide, di-2-butyl tetrasulphide, chamazulene, p-menthdiols, car-3-ene, *p*-cymen-7-ol, isolongifoline, jaeskeanin, jaeskeanidin, ferutinone, ferutinianin, teferidin, ferutinin, drimatol akichenol, and jaeschkeanadiols.

The gum-resin contains coumarins assafoetidin, ferocolicin, asadisulphide, asacoumarins A and B, 5- and 8-hydroxyumbelliprenins and 8-acetoxy-5-hydroxyumbelliprenin.

Chemical tests

1. On trituration with water it produces a milky emulsion.
2. The drug (0.5 g) is boiled with hydrochloric acid (5 ml) for sometime. It is filtered and ammonia is added to the filtrate. A blue fluorescence is obtained.
3. To the fractured surface add 50% nitric acid. Green colour is produced.
4. To the fractured surface of the drug, add sulphuric acid (1 drop). A red colour is obtained which changes to violet on washing with water.

Uses

Asafoetida is used as carminative, expectorant, antispasmodic and laxative as well as externally to prevent bandage chewing by dogs; for flavouring curries, sauces and pickles; as an enema for intestinal flatulence, in hysterical and epileptic affections, in cholera, asthma, whooping cough and chronic bronchitis.

Adulteration

Asafoetida is adulterated with gum Arabic, other gum-resins, rosin, gypsum, red clay, chalk, barley or wheat flour and slices of potatoes.

Allied drugs

Galbanum and ammoniacum are oleo-gum-resins obtained, respectively, from *Ferula galbaniflua* and *Dorema ammoniacum*. Galbanum contains umbelliferone and umbelliferone ethers, up to 30% of volatile oil containing numerous mono- and sesquiterpenes, azulenes and sulphur-containing esters. Ammoniacum contains free salicylic acid but no

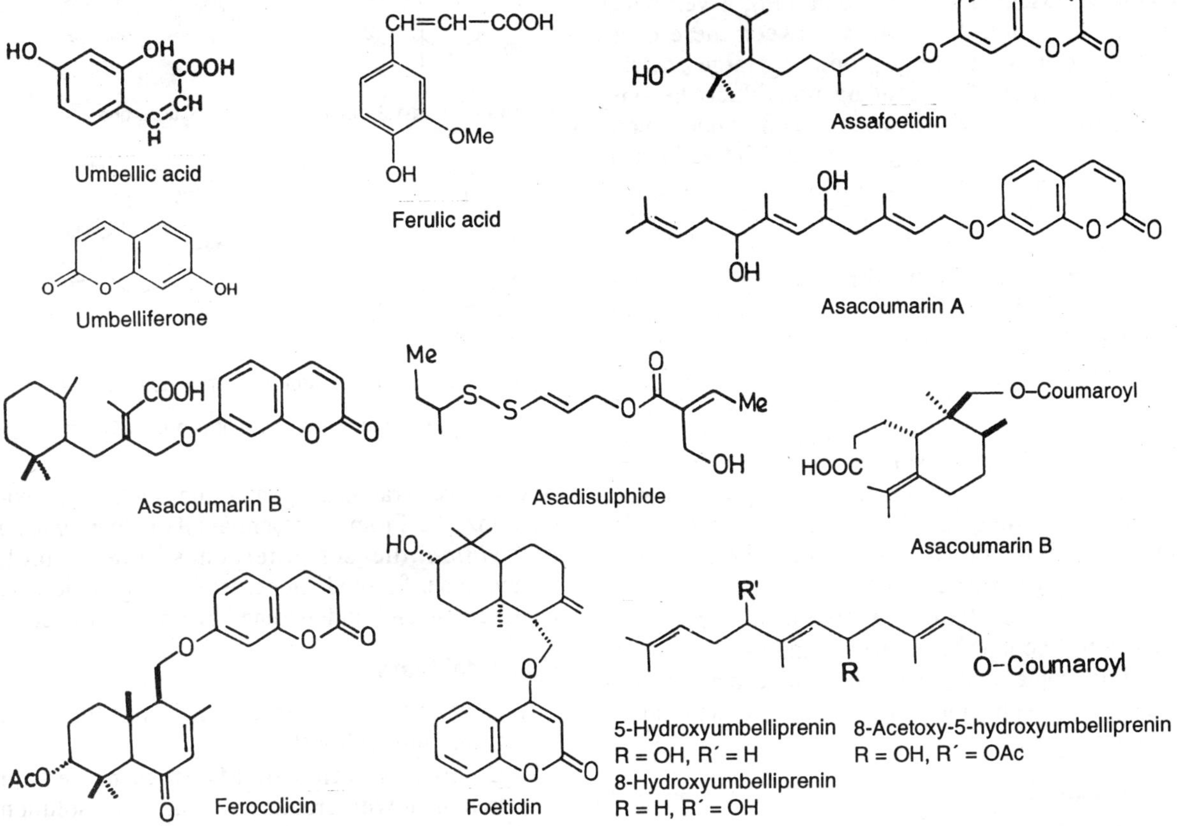

Fig. 19.6. Chemical constituents of Asafoetida.

umbelliferone. The major phenolic constituents is ammoresinol. An epimeric mixture of prenylated chromandiones termed ammodoremin is also present. The volatile oil (c. 0.5%) contains various terpenoids with ferulene as the major component.

Pharmacology

The essential oil showed significant protective action against fat induced increase in plasma fibrinogen and decrease in coagulation time and fibrinolytic activity on alimentary hyperlipaemia, serum cholesterol was also slightly lowered. Luteolin and its 7-glucoside showed anti-inflammatory activity in rats, anti-ulcer activity and anti-polio virus activity. Luteolin inhibited proliferation of human carcinoma of larynx and sarcoma 180 cells.

MYRRH

Synonyms

Gum-resin Myrrh; Gum Myrrh; Arabian or Somali Myrrh; Myrrha.

Biological source

Myrrh is an oleo gum-resin obtained from the stem of *Commiphora molmol* Eng. or *C. abyssinica* or other species of *Commiphora* (Family : Burseraceae).

Habitat

It grows in Arabian pennisula, Arabian pennisula, Ethiopia, Abyssinica, Nubia and Somaliland.

Collection

Myrrh plants are small trees up to 10 meters in

height. They have the phloem paranchyma and closely associated ducts containing a yellowish granular liquid. The tissues between these ducts often collapse, thereby producing large cavities similarly filled, i.e., schizogenous ducts become lysigenous cavities. The gum-resin exudes spontaneously or by incising the bark. The yellowish-white, viscous fluid is solidified readily to produce reddish-brown masses which are collected by the natives.

Myrrh forms a yellowish emulsion when triturated with water. When extracted with alcohol (90%), a whitish mass of gum and impurities remains. The alcohol-insoluble matter should not exceed 70%. Lump myrrh usually yields not more than 5% of ash. It may be distinguished from perfumed bdellium and similar products by allowing an ethereal extract of the drug to evaporate to dryness and passing the vapour of bromine over the resinous film produced. A violet colour is given by genuine myrrh but not by bdellium.

The crude alcohol-insoluble matter ('gum') contains about 18% of protein and 64% of carbohydrate containing galactose, arabinose and glucuronic acid. This gum is associated with an oxidase enzyme.

Characters

Myrrh occurs as irregular masses or tears weighing up to 250 g. The outer surface is powdery and reddish-brown in colour. The drug breaks and is powdered readily. Fractured surface is rich brown and oily. Odour is aromatic and taste is aromatic, bitter and acrid.

Chemical constituents

Myrrh contains resin (25-40%), gum (57-61%), and volatile oil (7-17%). Large portion of the resin is ether-soluble which contains α-, β- and γ-commiphoric acids, resenes, the esters of another resin acid and two phenolic compounds. The ether insoluble portion is a mixture of α- and β-heerabomyrrholic acids. The volatile oil is a mixture of cuminic aldehyde, eugenol, *meta*-cresol, pinene, limonene, dipentene and two sesquiterpenes. The disagreeable odour of the oil is due to mainly the disulphide, $C_{11}H_2OS_2$. The gum contains proteins (18%) and carbohydrate (64%) which is a mixture

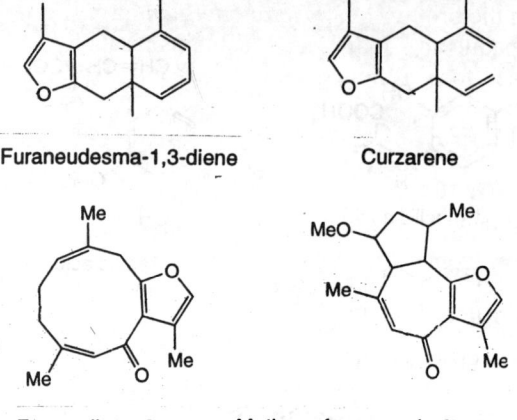

Furaneudesma-1,3-diene   Curzarene

Furanodiene-6-one   Methoxy furanoguala-9-ene-8-one

Fig. 19.7. Chemical constituents of Myrrh.

of galactose, arabinose, glucuronic acid and an oxidase enzyme. From the essential oil of *Commiphora abyssinica* the sesquiterpenes like elemol, furanodiene, furanodienone, isofuranogermacrene, curzerenone and linderstrene have been isolated.

Chemical tests

1. A yellow brown emulsion is produced on trituration with water.
2. Ethereal solution of Myrrh turns red on treatment with bromine vapours. The solution becomes purple with nitric acid.

Uses

Myrrh is used as carminative and in incense and perfumes. It has local stimulant and antiseptic properties and is utilized in tooth powder and as mouth wash. Topically it is astringent to mucous membranes.

It is used in a tincture, paint, gargle and rinse due to its disinfecting, deodourizing, and granulation-promoting actions in inflammatory conditions of the mouth and throat. Alcoholic extracts are used as fixatives in the perfumery industry.

Allied drugs

Four different varieties of 'bdellium' are present. Of these, *perfumed* or *scented bdellium* or *bissabol* is obtained from *C. erythaea* var. *glabrescens*. It resembles soft myrrh in appearance but more aromatic odour and does not give a violet colour with the bromine test. *Hotai bdellium* or *gum hotai* is opaque and odourless; it contains a saponin and is used for washing the hair.

MALE FERN

Synonyms

Aspidium, Male shield-fern, Filix mas (B.P.); Male fern rhizome; Rhizoma filicis maris.

Biological source

Male Ferm consists of the rhizome, frond bases and apical bud of *Dryopteris filix-mas* (L.) Schot, known as European Aspidium or Male Fern, or of *Dryopteris marginalis*, known as American Aspidium or Marginal Fern collected late in autumn, divested of the roots and dead portions, and carefully dried retaining its internal green colour. (Family : Polypodiaceae).

Dryopteris filix-mas aggregate is composed of a complex of three related species—*D. filix-mas* (L.) Schott, *D. borreri* Newm. and *D. abbreviata* (Lam and D.C.) Newm. Hybridization readily occurs and *D. filix-mas* itself, with 164 chromosomes, is an allotetraploid with half its chromosomes derived from *D. abbreviata* and the others from an unknown source. Twelve varieties of *D. borreri* are present.

Habitat

Dryopteris filix-mas is native of Europe, North Africa, Northern Asia, North America, Rocky Mountains and Andes of South America. *Dryopteris marginalis* occurs in eastern and central USA and India.

Collection

Male Fern is a perennial woody fern. The underground parts of the plant are collected in late autumn; roots, and dead portions are removed, dried and preserved carefully.

Macroscopical characters

The drug occurs in pieces about 7-25 mm in length, consisting of a rhizome about 2-5 cm diameter surrounded by frond bases. The frond bases are brown externally and densely covered with ramenta; internally they are green, and show in transverse section from six to nine pale yellow meristeles. The

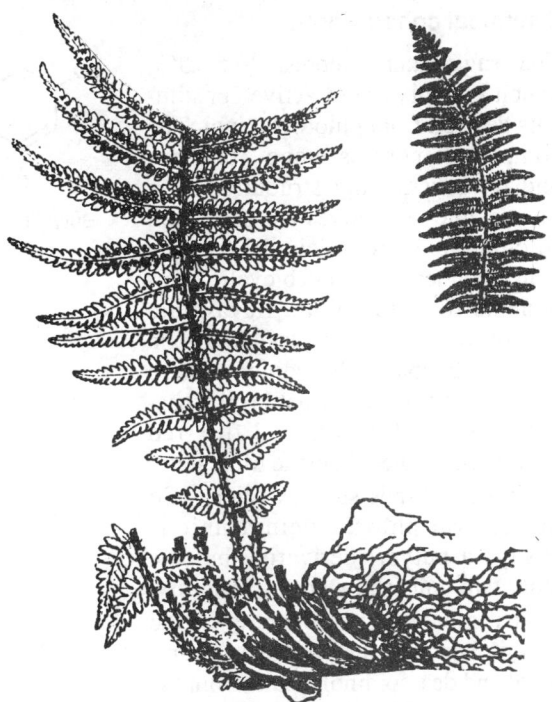

Fig. 19.8. *Dryopteris filix-mas.*

rhizome is brownish externally and yellow-green internally. On long storage the interior becomes brown, the activity decreases and the drug is no longer fit for use. Internally the rhizome shows from six to nine large meristeles arranged in a diffuse cycle and external to those the surface meristeles running from the fronds. The crude drug should contain 1.5% of filicin and 21-23% oleoresin. The odour is slight; taste is sweet in the beginning and bitter and nauseous later on.

Microscopical characters

A sections of the rhizome shows (1) a hypodermis of brownish nonlignified sclerenchymatous fibres; (2) a ground parenchyma which is rich in starch grains and which possesses shortly stalked, internal secreting glands in its intercellular spaces. These internal glandular hairs biosynthesize the anthelminthic compounds; (3) meristeles, which are largely composed of large tracheids with pointed ends and scalariform thickening. Crystals of calcium oxalate are absent. The ramenta have two-celled marginal projection.

Chemical constituents

The drug contains oleoresin (6.5-15%) which is a mixture of active constituents derived from phloroglucinol. The compounds possess mono-, bi-, tri-, and tetracyclic ring structures. The monocyclic derivatives are aspidinol, filicinic acid and filicinyl butanone which condense to yield bicyclic components like albaspidin, flavaspidic acid or tricyclic derivatives like filixic acid and dryopterin. In addition to these aromatic compounds, volatile oil asbaspidin, filicin, filmaron and filix red have been isolated from the Male Fern.

In compounds such as filicic acid the central phloroglucinol unit is always a butyryl derivative but the other two units show great variability.

The monomers do not present in the living plant, and the presence of aspidinol and desaspidinol results from the breakdown of larger molecules, particularly in the presence of alkali.

The chief active principle of the Male Fern is the complex dibasic acid, filmarone, an amorphous brownish yellow acid.

The phloroglucides of male fern are formed via the acetate pathway, with methionine acting as a donor for the methoxy and methylene bridge groups. Monomeric compounds (*e.g.*, aspidinol) injected into *D. marginalis* have been shown to be incorporated into dimeric compounds such as desaspidin.

The crude drug deteriorates rapidly in storage. The oleoresin, which is comparatively more stable, is extracted from the drug. The oleo-resin is obtained by exhausting the fresh coarsely powdered drug with ether in a perculator and evaporating the extract into a thick syrup. The official oleoresin should contain 24-26% filicin by weight.

D. marginata contains margaspidin, phloraspidinol, phloraspin, para-aspidin, trisparaaspidin, filixic acid, aspindol and flavaspidic acid.

Pharmacology

The plant extract showed antiviral activity against vesicular stomatitis virus in monkey cell culture.

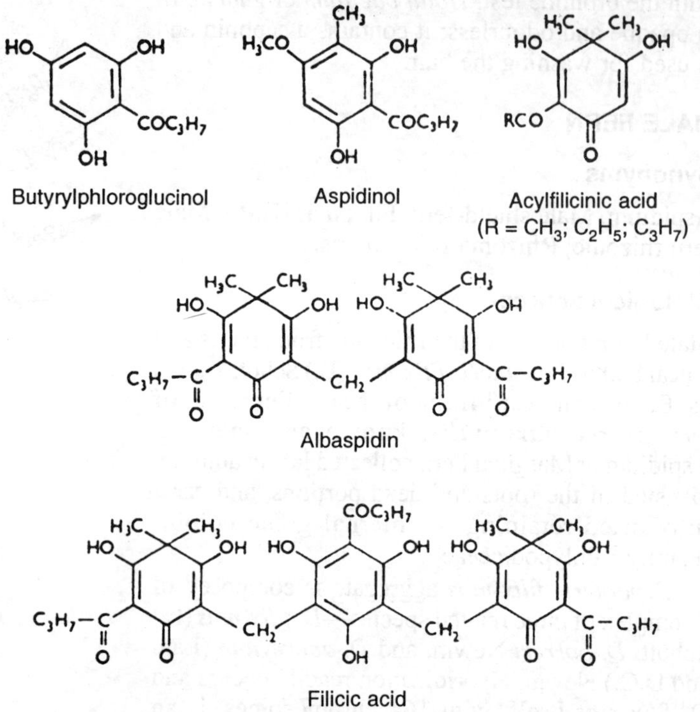

Fig. 19.9. Phloroglucinol derivatives of Male fern.

Uses

Male Fern is used as taenicide due to its anthelmintic properties. The side effects of the drug are stomach pains, colic, diarrhoea, blood in stool, albuminuria, nervous excitement, mental disturbances, defects in vision and blindness.

Filicin is an active vermifuge, especially effective for the expulsion of tapeworm. It is administered in capsules or in pills. Taenia are expelled in a few hour after administration. In combination with calomel, both vermifugal and purgative actions are ensured.

Substituents and adulterants

Many ferns yield substantial amounts of extract. Many Indian ferns contained 1.5% or more of filicin. Some European ferns, besides male fern, contain adequate amounts of filicin, as also the American *D. marginalis*.

Athyrium filix-foemina, the lady fern, is used as a substituent.

Dryopteris spinulosa, the shield fern, has small glands on the margins of the ramenta.

PODOPHYLLUM

Synonyms

May apple; Mandrake root; Indian apple; Vegetable calomel; Podophyllum rhizome, American Mandrake; Rhizoma podophylli.

Biological source

Podophyllum consists of the dried rhizome and roots of *Podophyllum peltatum* Linn. (Family : Berberidaceae).

Habitat

Podophyllum is found in eastern parts of Canada and the USA.

Collection

The plant is a perennial herb growing in marshy, shady situations. It bears a single rhizome which is a meter in length. This is dug up, cut into 10 cm long pieces and dried. The bulk of the crop is gathered in late summer and autumn, cut into 10-20 cm long pieces, dried and the rootlets are usually removed. The rhizomes contain a higher %age of active constituents in late spring and early summer, but drug collected at these times contains very little starch and abundance of water, and consequently there is considerable shrinkage upon drying.

Macroscopical characters

Podophyllum occurs in subcylindrical reddish-brown pieces, 5-20 cm long and 5-6 mm thick; outer surface smooth or wrinkled. The remains of the aerial stems are present on the upper surface as large cup-shaped scars surrounded by the remains of the cataphyllary leaves. On the lower side of each node are about 5-12 root scars or portions of roots, 2-7 cm long and about 1.5 mm diameter. The fracture is short, starchy or horny interior. The transverse section of the internode shows a starchy bark and pith and a ring of 20-30 small fibrovascular bundles. A section of the node shows branches from the ring of bundles running upwards to the cup-shaped scar of the aerial stem or downwards to the roots. Odour, slight; taste, unpleasant bitter and acrid.

Microscopical characters

A transverse section of the rhizome shows a dark

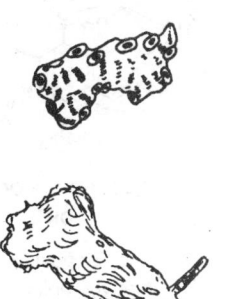
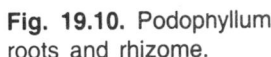
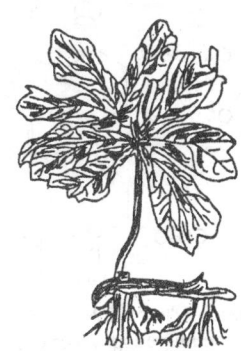

Fig. 19.10. Podophyllum roots and rhizome.   **Fig. 19.11.** *Podophyllum peltatum* entire plant.

coloured epidermis, one or two layers of cork cells, collenchymatous and parenchymatous cortex, pith and a ring of small vascular bundles with simple pores or reticulate thickening. The cells of the ground tissue contain reddish-brown masses of resin, cluster crystals of calcium oxalate and starch. The starch occurs in simple grains 3-15-25 μm in diameter and in compound grains with two to 15 components. The starch shows gelatinization.

Chemical constituents

The active principles of podophyllum occur in the resin. It is prepared by pouring an alcoholic extract of the drug into water and collecting and drying the precipitate. The resin (3.5-6%) contains active principles as lignans (C_{18} compounds). The important lignans are podophyllotoxin (~20%), β-peltatin (~10%) and α-peltatin (~5%) occurring in free state and as glucoside. In addition to these lignans, the other closely related compounds like dimethyl podophyllotoxin and the glucoside, 4'-demethylpodophylloxin, its glycoside, desoxypodophyllotoxin and podophyllotoxone are present in the drug. All these compounds possess cytotoxic or antitumour activity. Treatment of lignans with alkali produces epimerization with formation of the stable *cis*-isomers which are physiologically inactive.

Picropodophyllin and quercetin are also present in Podophyllum.

Podophyllin is an amorphous powder, light brown to greenish yellow in colour. It has a characteristic odour, a bitter taste and is irritating to eyes

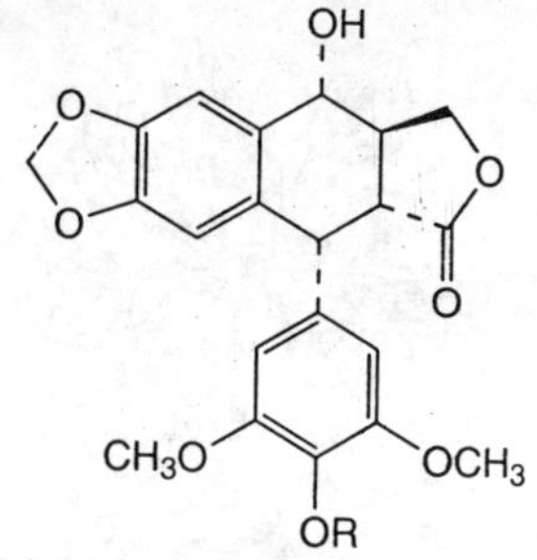

Podophyllotoxin, R = CH₃
Demethylpodophyllotoxin, R = H

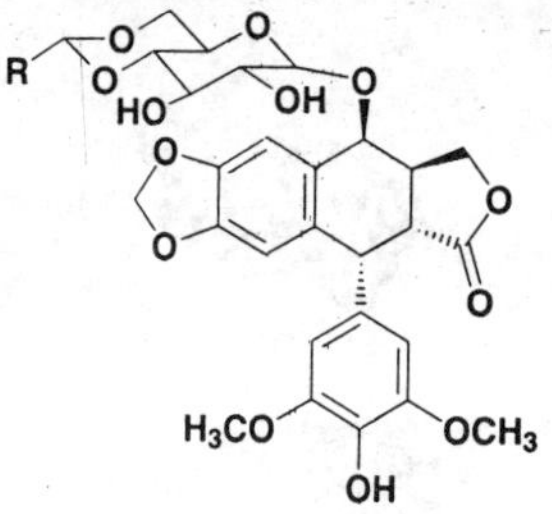

R = CH₃, Etoposide
R = thienyl, Teniposide

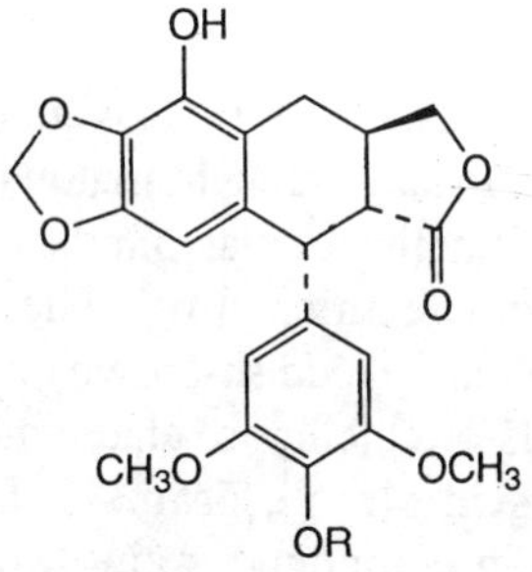

β-Peltatin, R = CH₃
α-Peltatin, R = H

Fig. 19.12. Lignans of Podophyllum.

and mucous membrane. Besides podophyllotoxin and 4'-demethylpodophyllotoxin, podophyllin has other constituents, *e.g.*, kaempferol, quercetin, podophyllotoxin-1-O-β-D-glucopyranoside, 4'-demethylpodophyllotoxin-1-O-β-D-glucopyranoside and tannins. Extraction of podophyllin with chloroform yields a residue which upon recrystallisation from benzene : methanol and hexane gives a 9:1 mixture of podophyllotoxin and 4'-demethylpodophyllotoxin (30 to 40% based upon resin). The remaining chloroform insoluble portion is called the Marc which consists of quercetin, kaempferol, tannins, podophyllotoxin-1-O-β-D-glucopyranoside and 4'-demethylpodophyllotoxin-1-O-β-D-glucopyranoside.

The introduction of anticancer drug Etoposide and Teniposide has created a demand for podophyllotoxin, the natural tetralin lignan (podophyllotoxin) is used for the semi-synthesis of these drugs. Since the total synthesis of podophyllotoxin is still uneconomic, future production of these drugs will depend upon either systematic cultivation of Podophyllum plants or the use of tissue culture techniques to obtain podophyllotoxins.

The lignans of podophyllum can be divided into: Podophyllum aglycones and Podophyllum glycosides.

Podophyllum aglycones

Podophyllotoxin, isolated in 1880 by Podwyssotzki, is the main compound of Podophyllum species. Picropodophyllotoxin is easily formed by base catalyzed rearrangement of podophyllotoxin. Desoxypodophyllotoxin, isolated from all the Podophyllum species, was known earlier also from the roots of *Anthriscus sylvestris* (Apiaceae) Kawanami and was named "anthricin".

The modern techniques of separation and purification such as column chromatography and thin layer chromatography yielded α-peltatin, β-peltatin, 4'-demethyl podophyllotoxin. The solvent partition, and paper chromatography led to the separation of desoxypodophyllotoxin and glucosides of podophyllotoxin and 4'-demethyl-podoohyllotoxin, β-peltatin and α-peltatin.

Podophyllum glycosides

Picropodophyllotoxin-1-O-β-D-glucoside is present in Indian podophyllin. Water soluble lignan glucosides are present in Podophyllum rhizomes.

Uses

Podophyllum possesses purgative, cholagogue and anti-cancer properties. It has a cytotoxic action and is used as a paint in the treatment of soft venereal

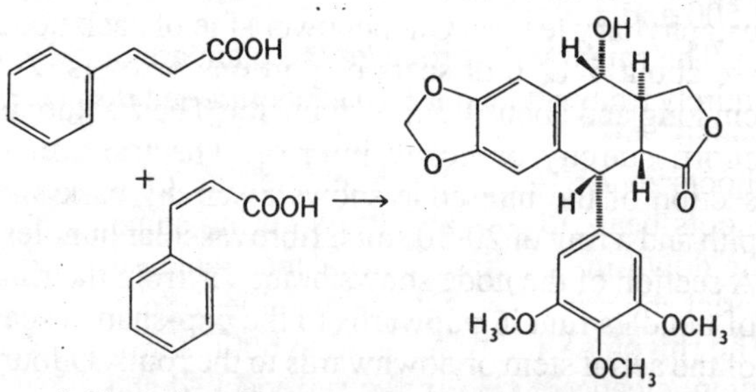

2 Cinnamic acid   Podophyllotoxin

Fig. 19.13. Biosynthetic origin of podophyllotoxin.

and other warts. Etoposide (4'-demethyl-epipodo-phyllotoxin ethylideneglucoside) is a lignan derivative obtained semisynthetically from podophyllotoxin and used in the treatment of small-cell lung cancer and testicular cancer as well as lymphomas and leukaemias. The related thenylidene derivative teniposide has similar anticancer properties. Ectoposide has value in paediatric neuroblastoma, lymphocytic leukaemia, brain tumours in children, Hodgkin's disease, pronchogenic carcinomas, placental carcinomas and breast cancer. The main side effects are granulopenia and thrombopenia.

INDIAN PODOPHYLLUM

Synonyms

Papra (Hindi); Rhizoma Podophylli indici; Indian Podophyllum rhizome.

Biological source

Indian Podophyllum consists of the dried rhizome and roots of *Podophyllum hexandrum* Royle (syn. *P. emodi* Wall. ex Hook). It contains 40-50% of podophyllotoxin (Family : Berberidaceae).

Habitat

Podophyllum is found in the interior ranges of Himalayas at 3000-4600 m from Sikkim to Hazara descending to 2,000 m in Kashmir. It is cultivated in Punjab, Uttar Pradesh and North West Frontier Provinces.

The plant flourishes well as an undergrowth in the fir forests, rich in humus and decayed organic matter. It is generally associated with species of *Rhododendron, Salix, Juniperus* and *Viburnum*, but it also met with in open alpine meadows. The plant loves moist and shady localities situated between 2,500 and 4,000 m.

The rhizome and roots of the plant are obtained entirely from wild plants. The underground rhizomes remain dormant during winter and produce aerial shoots in April or May after melting of ice. The shoots bear flowers and fruits during summer and die down in November. Rhizomes which bear 3-5 aerial shoots are considered suitable for collection. The rhizomes and roots are dug up in spring or autumn, cleaned, dried in the sun, packed and stored in gunny bags; sometimes they are cut into cylindrical pieces and carefully dried. Rhizomes collected in spring contain a higher resin content than those obtained in autumn. Freshly collected rhizomes possess more amount of active compounds which are lost on prolonged storing.

Characters

The plant is an erect, glabrous, succulent, perennial herb bearing 2-8 cm and 1-2 cm thick, subcylindrical, tortuous and irregular rhizomes. Internodes of the rhizomes are very short appearing knotty. Upper surface bears 3-4 cup-shaped or oval or circular depressed stem scars with an occasional bud or bud-scar on the lateral surface, lower surface contains numerous roots which are about 10 cm in length and 3 mm thick. The roots may be longitudinally wrinkled, nearly straight, curved or tortuous. Colour is earthy brown. Roots are broken off easily. Fracture is short and starchy. Odour is slight but distinct; taste bitter and acrid.

Microscopical characters

The general arrangement of the tissues is similar to that found in American podophyllum, but the vascular bundles are more elongated radially. The odour and taste are identical to those of the American drug. The calcium oxalate cluster crystals are fewer and smaller, 20-30-60 μm. The starch grains are simple or two to 20 compound.

Chemical constituents

Indian podophyllum contains excess amount of resin (6-12%) and the concentration of podophyllotoxin is up to 40 per cent. No peltatins are reported but the other constituents are almost the same as reported in the American Podophyllum. The drug also possesses quercetin, berberine, starch and calcium oxalate.

It also contains kaempferol, astragalin (kaempferol-3-glucoside), podophyllotoxin, podophyllotoxin glucoside, picropodophyllin, 1-O-glucopyranosyl-picropodophyllin, 4'-dimethyl podophyllotoxin, 4'-demethylpodophyllotoxin glucoside, dehydropodophyllotoxin, podophyllol, podophyllic acid, 4'-demethyl deoxypodopohyllotoxin glucoside, deoxypodophyllotoxin, podophyllotoxone, 4'-demethylpodophyllotoxone, 4'-demethylisopicropodophyllone and diphyllin.

Uses

Podophyllum resin (podophyllin) is used to treat soft venereal and other warts. The drug has been reported to possess anticancer, cholagogue, purgative, alterative, emetic and bitter tonic properties.

Indian podophyllum is used for the preparation of the resin and isolation of podophyllotoxin for drug use and semisynthesis of etoposide. Other less common species of *Podophyllum* (*e.g.*, *P. pleianthum*) and related genera (*e.g.*, *Diphylleia*) also contain podophyllotoxin and structurally related lignans.

Podophyllotoxin is used by pharmaceutical industry for structural modification producing therapeutically useful anticancer drugs like Podophyllinic acid ethylhydrazide (SP-1) and Podophyllotoxin benzylidene-5-D-glucopyranoside (SP-G). Some cyclic acetals and ketals of 4'-demethyl-epipodophyllotoxin-beta-D-glucopyra-noside show promising activity. Two of them, the ethylidene derivatives (Etoposide) and the thenylidene derivative (Teniposide) are marketed as anticancer drugs by Sandoz. In contrast to Podophyllotoxin (a classical spindle poison or antimitotic causing arrest of cells in the metaphase), Etoposide and Teniposide do not affect microtubule assembly. Instead they prevent cells from entering mitosis and arrest cells in the late S or G2 phases of the cell cycle. Epipodophyllotoxin derivatives interact with topo-isomerase II[282]. Etoposide is proved to be useful in the treatment of patients with small-cell lung cancer, testicular cancer, Kaposi's sarcoma, lymphoma and leukaemia, while Teniposide in cases of acute lymphatic leukaemia, neuroblastoma and non-Hodgkin's lymphoma and brain tumour in children.

Podophyllotoxin is extremely toxic causing gastrointestinal distress, encephalopathy and peripheral neuropathy. It induces walking difficulties and other neurological problems.

Podophyllotoxin is converted into podophyllinic acid ethylhydrazide and podophyllotoxin benzylidene-5-D-glucopyranoside which are useful anticancer drugs. The ethylidene derivative (etoposide) and the thenylidene derivative (teniposide) of 4'-demethyl-epi-podophyllotoxin-β-D-glucopyranoside are marketed as anticancer drugs by Sandoz. These derivatives do not affect microtubule assembly and they prevent cells from entering mitosis and arrest cells in the late S or G2 phases of the cell cycles. Etoposide is useful to treat patients with small cell lung cancer, testicular cancer, Kaposi's sarcoma, lymphoma and leukaemia. Teniposide is given in cases of acute lymphatic leukaemia, neuroblastoma and non-Hodgkin's lymphoma and brain tumours in children. Podophyllotoxin is a classical spindle poison or antimitotic causing arrest of cells in the metaphase.

CANNABIS

Synonyms

Indian hemp; Indian Cannabis; Marihuana; Marijuana; Bhang; Ganja; Charas; Kif; Hasach; Pot; Cannabis indica.

Biological source

Cannabis is the dried flowering tops of pistillate plants of *Cannabis sativa* Linn. (Syn. *C. indica* Linn.). It contains not more than 10% of its fruits, large foliage leaves and stems over 3 mm in diameter (Family : Cannabinaceae).

Habitat

Cannabis occurs in India, Bangladesh, Pakistan, Iran, Central America, USA, East Africa, South Africa and Asia Minor.

Cannabis products

The following products are prepared from Cannabis.

1. **Ganja :** It contains up to 10% of its fruits, large foliage leaves and stems over 3 cm. It is known as *Flat-* or *Bombay ganja* when 30 cm long pieces of the herb are made into bundles and pressed. *Round* -or *Bengal ganja* is prepared by rolling the wilted tops between the hands. Ganja is legally produced only by a few licensed growers in Bengal and southern India. The seeds are sown in rows about 1.3 m apart and male plants are discarded. The resinous tops of the unfertilized plants are cut about 5 months after sowing and pressed into cakes. The yield is nearly 120 kg per acre.

2. **Bhang or Hashish :** It consists of the larger leaves and twigs of both male and female plants. It is smoked with or without tobacco. It is unfit for medicinal use owing to deficiency of resin. It is also taken in the form of an electuary made by digestion with melted butter.

3. **Charas :** It is the crude resin obtained by rubbing the tops between the hands and beating them on a piece of cloth. This is an inferior product. It may be collected by beating the flowering tops in coarse cotton cloths spread on the ground. A greenish-brown soft mass adheres, and may be purified by pressing it through the cloths. The resin is scraped off. It is mixed with many smoking mixtures.

Morphology

Cannabis occurs in flattened, rough, dull dusky green masses. The dried resin is hard, brittle and does not stick. The flat-ganja is flattened mass of a dull green colour. The odour is very marked in the fresh drug and becomes faint alterwards; taste is slightly bitter.

The flat- or Bombay-ganja occurs in agglutinated flattened masses of a dull green or greenish-brown colour. The resin is not sticky but hard and brittle; the odour, which is very marked in the fresh drug, is faint. The drug has a slightly bitter taste.

The lower digitate leaves of the plant are not found in the drug. The thin, longitudinally furrowed stems bear simple or lobed, stipulate bracts which subtend the bracteoles, enclosing the pistillate flowers. The bracts are stipulate and the lamina may be simple or three-lobed. The bracteole enclosing each flower is simple.

Microscopical characters

The resin is secreted by numerous glandular hairs. The head is usually eight-celled and the pedicel multiseriate or unicellular. Corrigan and Lynch, a reagent consisting of vanillin in ethanolic sulphuric acid, stains the cannabis glands a deep reddish-purple. Abundant conical, curved, unicellular hairs are also found, many having cystoliths of calcium carbonate in their enlarged bases. These cystolith hairs are not confined solely to the genus *Cannabis*. Cluster crystals of calcium oxalate are abundant, particularly in the bracteoles.

Resin production

Two varieties of *Cannabis sativa* are recognized: one produces fibre and the other resin. Canabinoid production is not directly dependent on the presence of chlorophyll. The plant's ability to produce resin is governed mainly by the environment. When progeny of seeds of European fibre-producing plants are grown in Egypt they reverted to resin-producing plants in a matter of a few years and, conversely, seeds from resin-producing plants of the Middle East failed to produce abundant narcotic resin when grown in temperate Europe. Cannabis has the chemical capacity to become either fibrous or resinous, depending on the climate. It is not possible to raise resin-containing plants in temperate regions.

Δ^9-THC levels are higher for continental than for maritime and insular climates.

Plants raised in the European countries from overseas seed-stock (Morocco, Sri Lanka, Zambia) for a number of generations broadly retained the cannabinoid content typical of the source countries but tetra-hydrocannabinolic acid (THCA) predominated over THC.

Resin-producing plants exist as chemical races. The principal chemotypes contain Δ^9-THC, CBD or cannabigerol together with others having various ratios of THC/CBD. There may also be a variation in resin content between male and female plants. Wild-growing plants of cannabis collected in northern India at different altitudes and locations

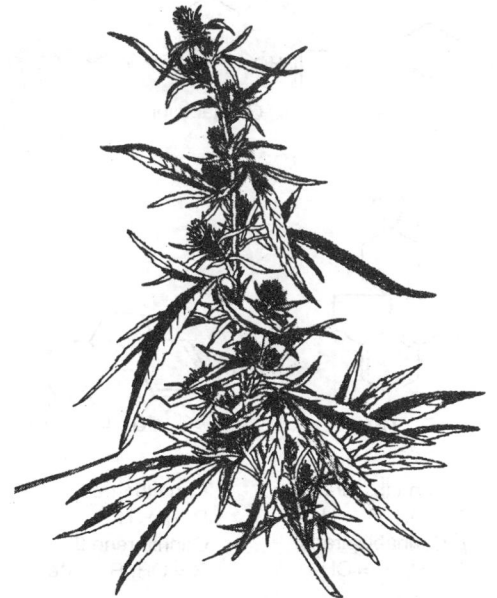

Fig. 19.14. *Cannabis sativa* branch.

showed great variations in the proportions of cannabinoids present.

There is very variable narcotic action of different samples of the drug.

Chemical constituents

Cannabis yields resin (15-20%) which is brown, amorphous, semi-solid mass, soluble in alcohol, ether and carbon disulphide. It contains more than 60 compounds (cannabinoids). Some principal active compounds are cannabinol, tetrahydrocannabinol, cannabidiol, cannabidiol -carboxylic acid, cannabigerol and cannabichromene. The tetrahydrocannabinols (Δ^8-and Δ^9-THC) possess euphoric activity. In addition to cannabinoids the plant also contains volatile oil which is a mixture of 30 compounds; the bases choline, trigonelline, spermidine and cannabisativine (alkaloid); flavo-noid O-glucosides of both vitexin and orientin, and calcium carbonate.

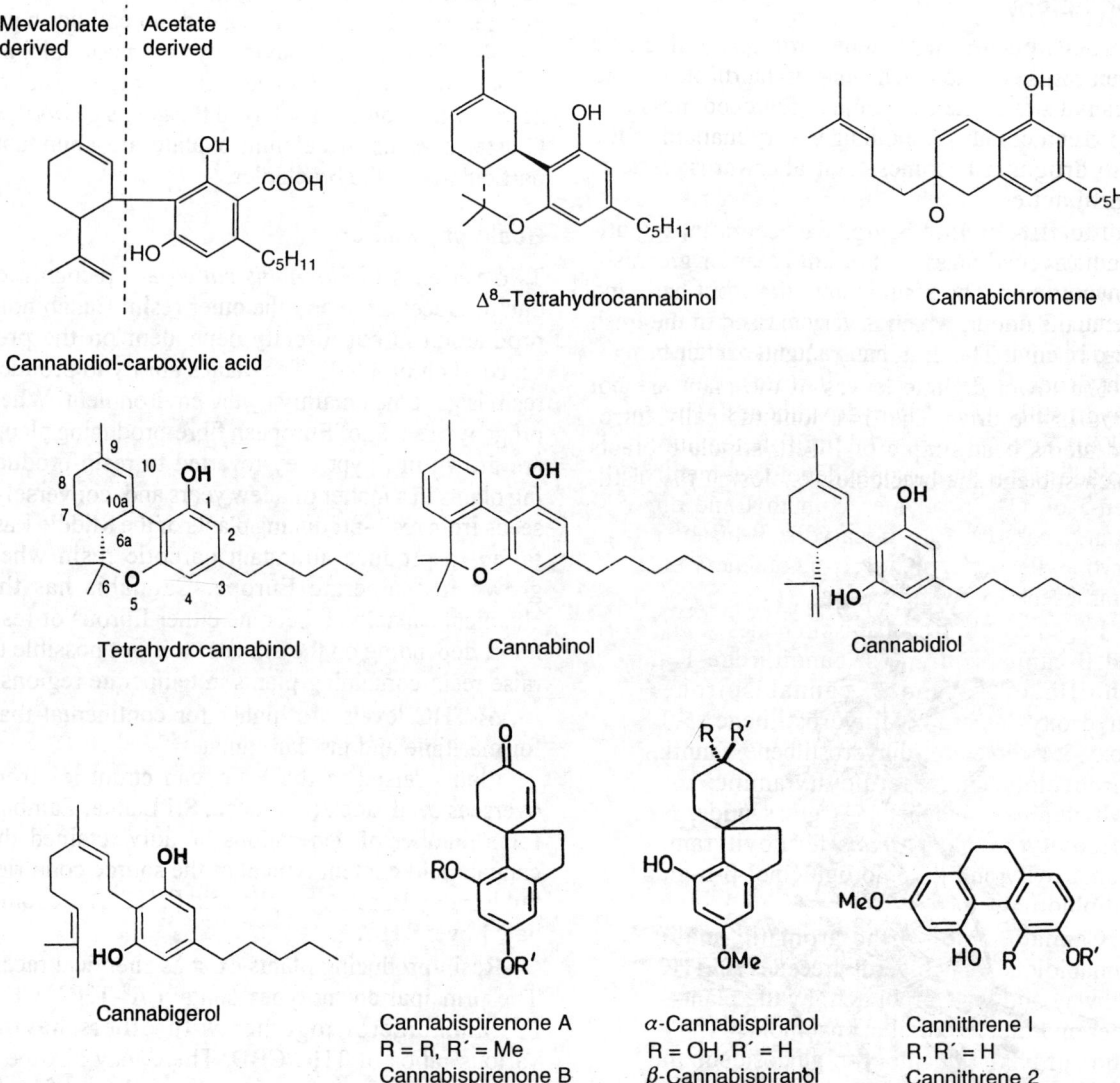

Fig. 19.15. Cannabinoids of *Cannabis sativa*.

Cannabis also contains 1-dehydrotetrahydro-cannabinol, cannabidivarin, tetrahydrocannabi-varin, 1-dehydrotetrahydrocannabinol, cannabi-varichromene, cannabidiolic and tetrahydro-cannabinolic acids, L-(+)-isoleucine-betaine, cannabicitran, cannabitriol, N-acetylglucosamine, N-acetylgalactosamine, cannabispiran, cannabitriol, 1-dehydro-3,4-*cis*-tetrahydrocannabivarinic acid, cannabidivarinic acid, cannabichromevarinic acid, cannabigerovarinic acid, C-3 cannabichromanone, C-3 cannabielsoin, C-3 cannabielsoic acid B, cannabispirol, acetylcannabispirol, cannabispirone, cannabispirenone, 8,9-dihydroxy-9a(10a)-dehydro-tetrahydrocannabinol, cannabicoumaronone, tetra-hydrocannabivarol, cannabiglendol, cannabispiran, dehydrocannabispiran, β-cannabispiranol, cannabitetrol, isocannabispiran, cannabistilbenes, canniprene, cannabispiradienone, campesterol, stigmasterol, β-sitosterol, *trans*-cinnamic acid, nonacosane, vitexin, isovitexin, orientin, apigenol acetate, 3-methyl alkenes, friedelin, epifriedelinol, 1,2-diphenylethanes, orientin and vitexin glucosides, anhydrocannabisativine (alkaloid), canniprene, dihydrostilbene and dehydrostilbenes. The essen-tial oil is composed of longifolene, humulene epoxides I and II, caryophyllenol I, *m*-mentha-1,8-dien-5-ol, C_9-C_{39} alkanes, 3-methyl and dimethyl alkanes, carvone, dihydrocarvone, β-bisabolene, β-caryophyllene, its epoxide, α-humulene, γ-elemene, α-farnesene and β-farnesene.

It also contains cannabispirenones A and B, α- and β-cannabispiranols, cannithrene-1 and -2, canniflavone 1 and 2, cannabispirone, 5,4'-dihydroxy-3-methoxydihydrostilbene, 5,3'-dihy-droxy-3,4'-dimethoxydihydrostilbene, cannflavin, 1-spirocyclohexanes, feruloyltyramine, *p*-couma-royltyramine, cannabisin A, grossamide, N-*trans*-caffeoyltyramine, N-*trans*-feruloyltyramine, N-coumaroyltyramine, phloroglucinol-β-D-glucoside and phloroglucinol.

Cannabinodiol is the aromatic analogue of cannabidiol. Cannabigerol precedes Δ^9-THC in the pathway and is incorporated, by the plant, into the latter and other neutral cannabinoids. The identifi-cation of phloroglucinol β-D-glucoside in the shoot laticifer exudate of *C. sativa*, and phloroglucinol as a prominent component, and the only phenol, in the glandular trichomes suggests that it may have an

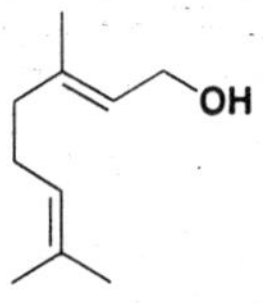

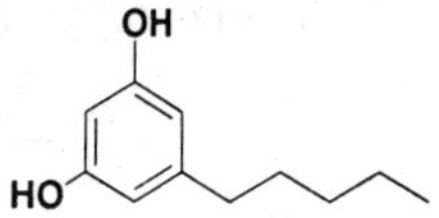

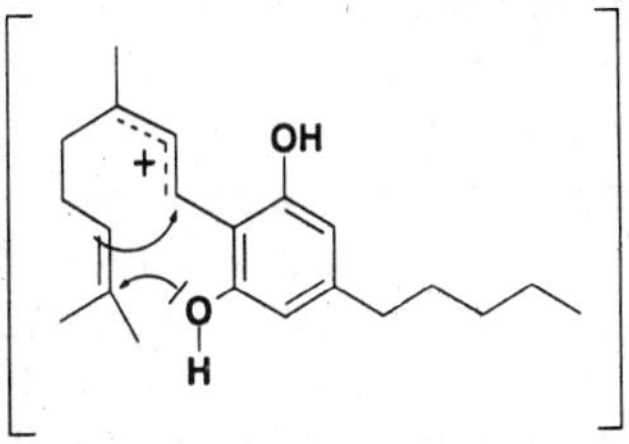

Fig. 19.16. Cannabinoid biosynthesis.

important role in the *in vivo* enzymatically regulated biosnthesis of the cannabinoids.

Cannabipinol contains a bicyclic monoterpene moiety in addition to the acetate-derived portion. Cannabidivarin is a cannabidiol homologue with a 5-propyl-resorcinol moiety.

These compounds arise from the condensation of a molecule of geranyl pyrophosphate with a phenol such as olivetol, and this may explain the formation of cannabigerol; the latter leads, by oxidation and allylic rearrangement to CBD, then THC. The occurrence of *Cannabis* forms that do not elaborate CBD suggests the existence of other pathways from cannabigerol to THC.

Uses

Cannabis is used as tonic, intoxicant, stomachic, antispasmodic, analgesic, narcotic, anticonvulsant, anti-anxiety and antitussive agent. When ingested or inhaled as smoke, it may cause euphoria, delirium, hallucinations, weakness, hyporeflexia, and drowsi-ness. It is a drug of abuse.

Cannabis evaluation

Cannabis preparations can be evaluated on their Δ^9-THC content. A relatively simple relationship is based on the combined Δ^9-THC and cannabinol (CBN) in relation to cannabidiol (CBD).

The phenotype is expressed as :

$$= \frac{\Delta^9\text{-THC} + \text{CBN}}{\text{CBD}}$$

A sample with a value greater than 1 = a drug type of cannabis; a sample with a value less than 1 = a fibre type.

A formula based on a ratio between cannabinoids, taking into account quantifiable homologues and separating the cannabinoids into their ring systems is proposed.

Addiction has been common in many parts of Asia and the problem becomes worldwide. Cannabis is not produced under optimum conditions for the production of high activity, under ordinary conditions of storage, hemp and hemp products rapidly lose activity and become almost inert after 2 years. In dried samples most of the cannabinoid content is present as CBN. Δ^9-THC still present in low concentration in all the samples.

Pharmacology

Cannabis extract produced complete arrest of spermatogenesis in mice, increased sensitivity to stimulation and reduced tolerance to pain caused prolongation of sleeping time in mice, showed reduction in body weight and in weights of seminal vesicles, ventral prostrate, epididymis and prepatial gland in male mice, produced marked degenerative changes in testes of toad, caused significant increase in blood glucose of rats and produced dose-related potentiation of analgesic action of a sub-analgesic dose of morphine. Plant resin produced hypothermia, analgesia and mixed excitation-depression effects, showed anticonvulsant activity against metrazol-induced and electro-shock seizures and antipyretic and anti-inflammatory actions and potentiated d-amphetamine toxicity in mice. Drug extract activated hypophysealadrenal axis in rats.

Cannabinol and 1-dehydro-THC exhibited depression of intestinal motility in mice. 1-Dehydro-THC had enhanced central depressant effect in mice, caused immediate and prolonged fall in blood pressure and reduction in pulse rate, produced bronchodilation in asthetic patients, showed antinoceptive effect in mice, was found to be potent stimulant of ACTH secretion, decreased blood pressure, heart rate, cardiac output and right ventricular contractile force in intact dogs, produced prolongation of ether anaesthesia up to the highest dose of 40 mg/kg, completely abolished seizures, lowered normal intraocular pressure by 15-50% in humans and caused reversible depression in luteinizing hormone levels in female monkeys. 1-Dehydro-THC was extremely allergic in guinea pigs and the immune response to it was accompanied by antibody formation. It caused complex behavioural response in rats including stereotype, catatonia and hyper-reactivity, decreased specific attack behaviour in animals, prolonged pentobarbitone sleep and inhibited phenazone metabolism.

8-Dehydro-THC failed to elicit CNS and cardiovascular effects in animals. Cannabidiol was also devoid of behavioural effects but showed marked hypotension in dogs. Flavocannabiside and flavosativaside weakly inhibited lens aldose reductase. 6-Dehydro-THC produced hypothermia in rats.

Marihuana smoking caused a specific decrease in epididymal sperm of mature rats. Cannabis extract caused testicular lesions resulting in mass atrophy of spermatogenic elements, inhibited mitochondrial monoamine oxidase of human brain, decreased uterine alkaline and acid phosphatase activities and caused inhibition of total microsomal oxidase and of aryl hydroxylase. Marihuana smoke and THC are toxic to lung and impair pulmonary antibacterial defence system. An active plant extract containing choline was effective to treat intestinal obstruction.

1-Dehydro-THC produced overall increase in avoidance performance in mice in 100 mg/kg. It produced marked hypothermia, anorexia, adipsia and depression in location, increased ATPase and cyclic AMP phosphodiesterase activities and cyclic AMP content of human spermatozoa. 1-Dehydro-THC decreased levels of lipid, phospholipid and total cholesterol in testes of rats and had no effect on testicular level of cholesterol, decreased fructolysis rate. Testosterone levels were depressed in male rats both after smoking one marihuana cigarette and after i.v. infusion of L-dehydro-THC. Large doses of 6-dehydro- and 1-dehydro-THC increased brain acetylcholine levels in rodents. THC had no effect on plasma testosterone levels but significantly increased plasma dihydrotestosterone levels. 1-Dehydro-THC did not show hypokinetic effect itself in rat. Cannabi-chromene showed anti-inflammatory properties as effective as phenylbutazone. 1-Dehydro-THC produced highly significant analgesic effect, inhibit serotonin release from platelets in plasm of migraine patients, and reduced content of brain tele-methylhistamine in rats. Cannabidiol had limited effect on heart rate but increased contractile force and coronary flow. 1-Dehydro-THC decreased levels of some uterine biochemical components and exhibited immuno-suppressive effect against autoimmune encephalomyelitis in animals.

9-Dehydro-THC markedly suppressed normal behavioural elements in rats. Cannabinoids were effective in ontagonizing TPA-induced erythema of skin. Connaflavins A and B inhibited prostaglandin E2 production by human rheumatoid synovial cells. Phenylpropane derivative inhibited plasmin, trypsin and thrombin. Cannabichromene suppressed rat paw oedema completely. Cannabidiol inhibited hepatic 6β-testosterone hydroxylase and erythromycin N-demethylase activities. 1-Dehydro-THC suppressed macrophage soluble cytolytic activity by affecting tumor necrosis factor-α.

KALADANA

Synonyms

Mirchi (Hindi), Krishnabija (Sanskrit).

Biological source

Kaladana consists of the dried ripe seeds of *Ipomoea hederacea* (L.) (syn *I. nil* Roth.). (Family: Convolvulaceae).

Habitat

It grows throughout India both cultivated and apparently wild, up to 2,000 m in the Himalayas.

Morphology

The seeds are 5-6 mm long, 3.7 mm wide, triangular, brownish black in colour. Each seed has two flat faces joining at an angle of 60° to 80°. At the base of joint there is a cordate hilum. Testa is dull black, hard, smooth and glabrous. Taste is first sweetish then acrid.

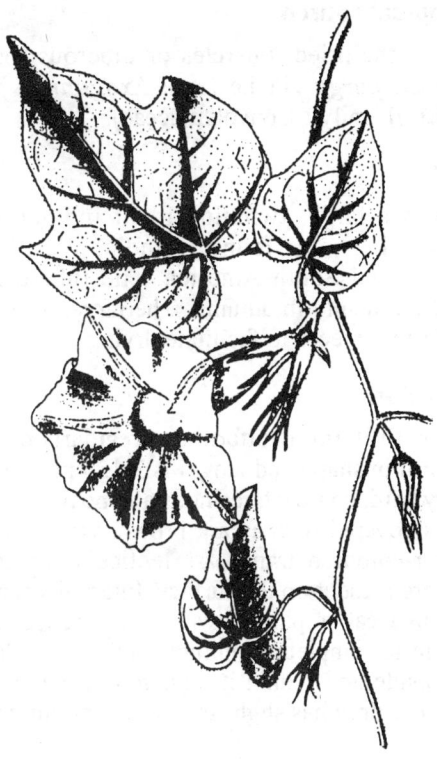

Fig. 19.17. *Ipomoea hederacea.*

Chemical constituents

Drug contains resin (about 15%), mucilage, fixed oil and saponin. Hydrolysis of the resin affords hydroxypalmitic acid and sugar. Lysergol, heder-aceterpenol, hederaceteriol, hederaterpenoside, β-sitosterol glucopyranoside and chanoclavine are also present in Kaladana.

The seed oil is composed of glycerides of palmitic, stearic (20.3%), arachidic, oleic (43.9%), linoleic (14.5%) and linolenic acids.

Uses

Kaladana is used as purgative and substituted for Jalap.

JALAP

Synonyms

Jalap root; Radix jalapae; Mexican or Vera cruz Jalap.

Biological source

Jalap is the dried tubercles or tuberous roots of *Ipomoea purga* Hayne (syn. *Exogonium purga* Benth). *(*Family : Convolvulaceae).

Habitat

Jalap is a large, twinning plant indigenous to Mexico. It is also found in India, West Indies, Jamaica and South America. The tubercles are collected mainly in autumn. The larger specimens are cut into pieces to facilitate drying.

Characters

Jalap is fusiform, napiform or irregularly ovoid or pyriform in shape and length is 3-15 cm. The drug is very hard, compact, resinous and heavy. The surface is covered with a dark brown, wrinkled cork. Lighter-coloured transverse lenticels and rootlet scars are present on the surface. Internally the drug contains weak to pale brown, with dark secondary, concentric complete cambium zones fairly close to the outside and within it numerous irregular dark lines. The drug has slight smoke-like odour, taste is

starchy and sweet in the beginning and acrid afterwards.

Chemcial constituents

Jalap contains resins (8-12%), volatile oil, starch, gum and sugar. The main constituent of Jalap resin is convolvulin which contains 8 hydroxy groups esterified with valeric, tiglic and exogonic acids. It also contains ipurganol, jalapin, β-methyl esculetin, palmitic and stearic acids and mannitol. Convolvulin on hydrolysis gives glucose, rhamnose and convolvulinic acid. Convolvulsin is composed of β-D-quinovoside of tetrahydroxy-decanoic acid.

Uses

It is a hydragogue, cathartic and drastic purgative.

$C_{45}H_{72}O_{20}(OH)_8$ $CH_3CH_2CH_2CH_2COOH$
Convolvulinic acid Valeric acid

$CH_3CH=C(CH_3)COOH$ $C_{10}H_{14}O_3$
Methylcrotonic acid Exogonic acid

$CH_3(CH_2)_4CH-(CH_2)_9-COOH$
        |
        OH
Jalapinolic acid
(11-Hydroxyhexadecanoic acid)

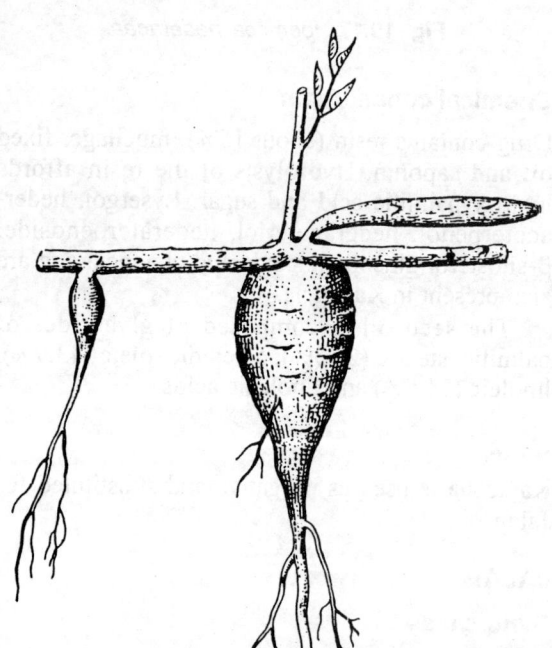

Exogonic acid

Fig. 19.19. Chemical constituents of Jalap.

INDIAN JALAP

Synonyms

Turpeth root; Nishodh (Hindi); Black Nishodh.

Biological source

Indian jalap consists of dried roots of *Ipomoea turpethum* R. Br.; syn. *Operculina turpethum (L.)* Silva Manso. (Family : Convolvulaceae).

Habitat

It is found throughout India up to 1,000 m.

Characters

Indian jalap occurs in cylindrical or spirally twisted

Fig. 19.18. *Ipomoea purga.*

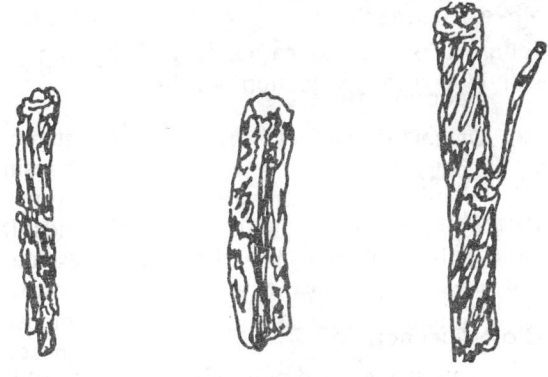

Fig. 19.20. Indian Jalap.

form, length 2-15 cm, diameter 3-5 mm. Outer surface is greyish-brown containing longitudinal wrinkles. Fracture is irregular. Roots are darker containing longitudinally furrows. Odour is slight and distinct; taste is unpleasant.

Chemical constituents

Indian jalap contains resin (7-8%) and volatile oil. Alcoholic soluble portion of the resin is a mixture of gluco-gluco-rhamnosides of turpethinic acids like 11-hydroxypalmitic acid (jalapinolic acid), 3,12-dihydroxypentadecanoic acid (operculonic acid); 4, 12-dihydroxy-pentadecanoic acid; and 4, 12-dihydroxypalmitic acid.

The resin is composed of turpethinic acids A (glycoside of 3,12-dihydroxypentadecanoic acid), B (glycoside of 4,12-dihydroxypentadecanoic acid), C (glycoside of 3,12-dihydroxyhexadecanoic acid), D (glycoside of 4,12-dihydroxyhexadecanoic acid) and E (glycoside of 11-hydroxyhexadecanoic acid).

Uses

Indian jalap is used as purgative.

Allied drug

In Indian system of medicine white Nishoth consists of roots of *Marsdenia tenacissima*. (Family:

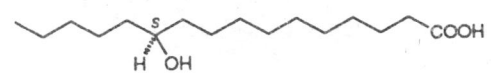

Fig. 19.21. 11S-Jalapinolic acid.

Asclepiadaceae). The plant is a large twinning shrub occurring throughout India. Roots are cylindrical, cut into pieces. Outer surface contains longitudinal furrows, ridges and irregular cracks. Colour is yellow to buff, fracture is short and starchy in the bark and splintery in the wood. Odour is musty and taste is bland first, then acrid. Its roots contain 17α- and 17β-marsdenin, cymarose, β-D-glucosyl-L-thevetose, cinnamic acid and acetic acid obtained by acid hydrolysis of pregnane esters tenasogenin A-C, isodrevogen P, drevogenin Q, cissogenin and tenasogenin. The stem yields tenacissosides A-E. The plant also contains polyoxypregnanes.

Brazillian Jalap rhizome

It is derived from *Ipomoea operculata* and constitutes a substitute for Mexican jalap. It contains 18 operculins (ether-soluble resin glycosides). These resemble the other known jalapins in that they are monomers with similar intramolecular macrocyclic ester structures in the glycosidic acid moieties. However, their component acids (*n*-decanoic and *n*-dodecanoic acids) are different from those of previously known resin glycosides (isobutyric, 2-methyl-butyric, tiglic and nilic acids). On alkaline hydrolysis a particular operculin will give a characteristic operculinic acid along with *n*-decanoic and *n*-dodecanoic acids. Operculinic acid E, is 11S-jalapinolic acid 11-*O*-α-L-rhamnopyra-nosyl-(1 → 2)-β-D-glucopyranoside.

Ipomoea batatus

This species is widely cultivated as a food. The roots contain a mixture of hexa-, hepta- and octadecylferulates; five ether-soluble resin glycosides called simonins I-V.

The roots of *Convolvulus scammonia* (*vide supra*) contain ether-soluble resin glycosides called scammonins; they possess a glycosidic acid, *e.g.*, scammonic acid A and have an intra-molecular macrocyclic ester structure involving various sugars.

Pharmacology

Polyoxypregnanes exhibited cytotoxic activity against KB cell line. Alcoholic extract of root abolished contractions induced by histamine and acetylcholine in guinea pig ileum. It also induced mild CNS depression.

$$CH_3 (CH_2)_3 \underset{OH}{CH} (CH_2)_8 \underset{OH}{CH}\text{-}CH_2 COOH$$

Operculinolic acid (3:12-Dihydroxyhexadecanoic acid)

IPOMOEA

Synonyms

Mexican Scammony (root); Orizaba Jalap root; Orizaba Jalap; Mexican Scammony root; Ipomoea radix.

Biological source

Ipomoea consists of the dried root of *Ipomoea orizabensis* (Pellet) Led. yielding not less than 15% of resin. (Family : Convolvulaceae).

Habitat

Orizaba, Mexico.

Characters

The plant is a perennial vine, the underground portion is a fusiform, 60 cm long root. Drug usually occurs as transversely cut slices of 3-12 cm in diameter and 1-5 cm thick. Outer surface is brown to grey, longitudinally wrinkled, fracture is short, irregular and resinous; texture is hard and tough, breaking with difficulty. Odour is slight; taste is acrid and resinous.

Chemical constituents

Ipomoea, when extracted with alcohol (90%), yields about 10-20% of a complex resinous mixture, of which about 65% is soluble in ether.

Ipomoea contains resin (10-20%), scopoletin (coumarin), volatile fatty acids, sugars, β-sitosterol, and calcium oxalate. The 65 per cent of the resinous mass is ether soluble. The prominent constituents of Ipomoea resin (Jalapin) are the methyl pentosides and other glycosides of jalapinolic acid and its methyl ester, phytosterol glycosides, (ipuranol), ipurolic acid and convolvullinic acid. Other compounds reported in ipomoea are 3, 4-dihydroxycinnamic acid, cetyl alcohol and gum.

Uses

Ipomoea is used as cathartic with hydragogue activity and for preparation of resin.

COLOCYNTH

Synonyms

Bitter apple; Bitter cucumber; Bitter gourd; Colocynth pulp; Indrayan (Hindi); Colocynthis; Fructus Colocynthidis.

Biological source

Colocynth is the dried pulp of the unripe but fully grown fruit of *Citrullus colocynthis* Schrad (Family : Cucurbitaceae).

Habitat

The plant occurs in Syria, Cyprus, Sudan, North Africa, Turkey, Spain and throughout India.

Collection

The plant is a perennial herbaceous vine. The collected fruits are peeled to separate the epicarp and immediately dried in the sun.

Morphology

The fruit is almost a globular berry, 4-10 cm in diameter. The peeled fruits are 4-8 cm in diameter, subspherical, nearly white, light in density and show sometimes small patches and impressions due to cuts occurred by knife. Transverse section of the fruit shows three segments, divided by the radiating placentas, with seeds attached to the internal

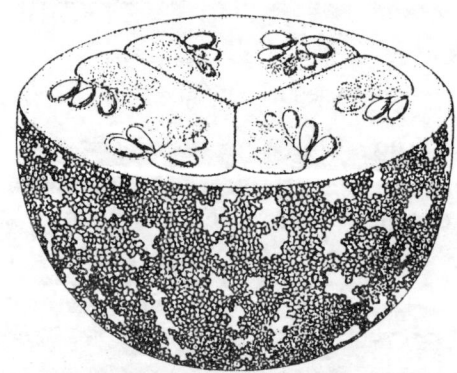

Fig. 19.22. Colocynth.

margins. Pulp is light, pithy and spongy, easily broken white or light yellow in colour.

Flat, ovoid seeds, 200-300 in each fruit, are present which are compressed, brown or orange in colour, one end somewhat pointed with rounded margin, 7 mm long and 4.5 mm wide. Fruit is odourless and taste is very bitter.

Chemical constituents

Colocynth contains an ether-chloroform soluble resin, a phytosterol glycoside, citrullol, pectin, colocynthin, colocynthetin, albuminoids and other glycosides. The glycosides on hydrolysis form cucurbitacin E (α-elaterin), and cucurbitacin L (dihydroelatericin B). Choline and two alkaloids have also been isolated from the drug.

The other compounds present in colocynth are a bitter oil 'citbittol', glucose, α-spinasterol, citrullol,

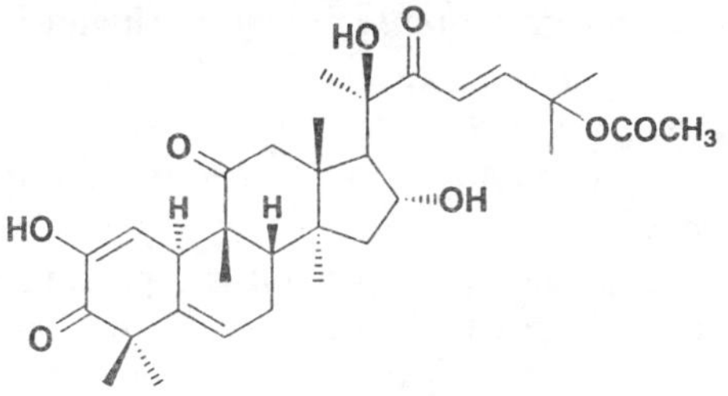

Cucurbitacin E

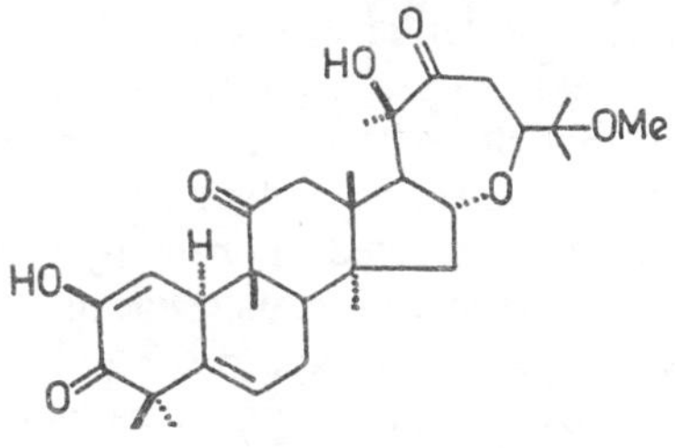

Cucurbitacin T

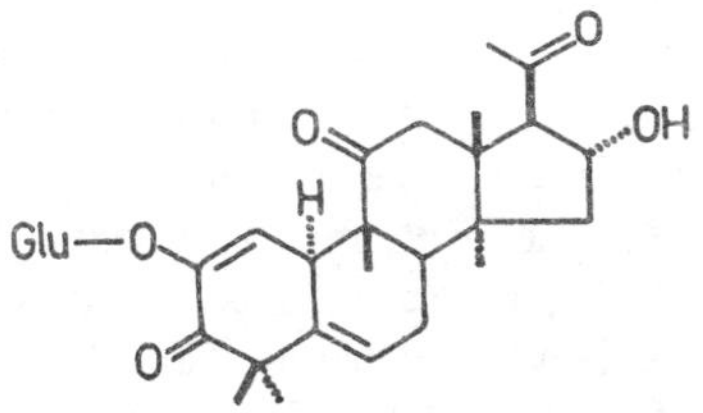

Fig. 19.23. Cucurbitacins of Colocynth.

cucurbitacins B, I, E-2, J, elateridine, hexanor-cucurbitacin I, its 16-O-acetyl derivative and 2-O-glucoside, cucurbitacin L glucoside, hentriacontane, n-octacosanol and 1,26-hexacosanediol.

The fruit peel possesses 11,14-dimethylhexadecan-14-ol-2-one, 10,14-dimethyl-hexadecan-14-ol-2-one, n-alkanes, lauric, myristic, palmitic, hexadecenoic, stearic, oleic, linoleic and arachidic acids, hexadecanol, octadecanol, eicosanol, docosanol, tetracosanol, hexacosanol, methyl heptenone, citronellol, citronellal, phenylethyl alcohol, methyleugenol, docosanyl acetate, 10,13-dimethylpenta-13-decen-1-al.

Uses

Colocynth is a very powerful cathartic. Cucurbitacin E is reported to possess anticancer activity.

GINGER

Synonyms

Zingiber, Saunth (Hindi); Rhizoma zingiberis.

Biological source

Ginger is the dried rhizome of *Zingiber officinale* Rosc, scraped to remove the darker outer skin and dried in the sun (Family : Zingiberaceae).

Habitat

It grows in southern Asia, West Indies. China, Africa and India; cultivated in all tropical countries.

A number of commercial varieties of root, oleoresin and essential oil are available, derived from *Z. officinale*. These arise from different chemical races, from differences in cultivation and harvesting techniques or from different climatic conditions. They vary in sensory characters. Australian oils are characterized by a 'lemon, citrus-like' odour. Oil from Fiji has a high citral content and a high content of 1,8-cineole similar to Japanese oil.

Nigerian Ginger closely resembles the Jamaica drug, darker colour, its smaller size and it is less deeply scraped. Nigerian ginger has a more pungent taste and less aroma than Jamaican. It yields less volatile oil (about 0.7-1%).

African Ginger is darker in colour, more pungent in taste and less flavour than *Jamaica Ginger. African Ginger* is mostly unpeeled, much of the ventral and dorsal surfaces bear patches of wrinkled cork of an earthy-brown colour. It is darker and smaller than Cochin Ginger in bulk, and appears discoloured due to lack of care during preparation. The fracture is short, odour strongly aromatic and taste pungent. The small exposed portions of cortex on the lateral sides are grey to blackish in colour. It lacks the fine aroma of the Jamaica drug, although exceeding it in pungency. *Bombay ginger* resembles the African.

The rhizomes of *Jamaican Ginger*, the best quality ginger, are unbleached, devoid of outer suberized layers and pale yellowish brown to yellowish orange. The fracture is short and uneven, fibrous and resinous. It is pleasantly pungent and aromatic. An inferior grade of Jamaican Ginger, known as *Rotoon Ginger*, is also marketed.

Indian Ginger is cultivated in southern India. It occurs in both coated and scraped forms. The coated variety bears a wrinkled reddish-grey cork which readily exfoliates. Pieces are similar in size and shape as the Jamaican and is considered only second to *Jamaican* in quality. There are two main types of Indian Ginger : (i) *Cochin Ginger*, which comes from central Kerala, is the peeled type, light brown to yellowish grey externally, more starchy, fracture short; and (ii) *Calicut Ginger*, from Malabar, is orange or reddish brown, resembling *African Ginger*, but the periderm is usually removed. It is inferior to *Cochin Ginger* in quality. Another type, *Calcutta Ginger*, is greyish brown to greyish blue externally. Indian Ginger is more strachy and is almost as pungent as *Jamaican Ginger*, but is less agreeable in odour. *Indian Ginger* has a faint lemon-like odour due to the presence of citral.

Chinese Ginger is white and is free from fibre. It is inferior in aroma to the *Jamaican Ginger* and consists of rhizomes which are not fully ripe. *Chinese ginger* is produced in large quantity and is sliced as opposed to split. The peeled drug is reported to be of Jamaican quality. It is the main variety available in the UK.

Japanese ginger is derived from *Z. mioga*. Its volatile oil differs in physical properties from that of the official species and gives the drug a bergamot-like odour. The taste is less pungent than that of *Z. officinale* and the starch grains are compound and less eccentric.

Preserved ginger consists of young undried rhizomes which are preserved by boiling in syrup. The West Indian variety is made from the official plant, but that from China is said to be obtained from the greater galangal, *Alpinia galanga* (Zingiberaceae).

Galangal rhizome is derived from the lesser galangal, *A. officinarum*.

The other Ginger is *Martinique Ginger (Z. zerumbet)*.

Cultivation : Ginger plant is a perennial herb about 1 m high with branching rhizome. The plant is propagated by rhizome cuttings each bearing a bud. The pieces of rhizome are planted in holes during March or April in a well-drained clayey loam. In December or January rhizomes are collected. When the stems wither, the rhizomes are ready for collection. For the scraped drug, after removal of soil, the rhizomes are killed by boiling water. They are then carefully peeled, thoroughly washed and then dried in the sun on mats. During drying they are turned up and down and protected during any damp weather. This first drying usually takes about 5 or 6 days. To obtain a whiter product the ginger is again moistened and dried for a further two days, when it is ready for export.

Ginger grows well at subtropical temperatures where the rainfall is at least 1.98 m per annum. As the plant is sterile, it is grown by vegetative means. Selected pieces of rhizome each bearing a bud are planted. Ginger requires a warm and humid atmosphere. A well distributed rainfall is required for its cultivation. If areas receiving less rainfall, the crop needs regular irrigation.

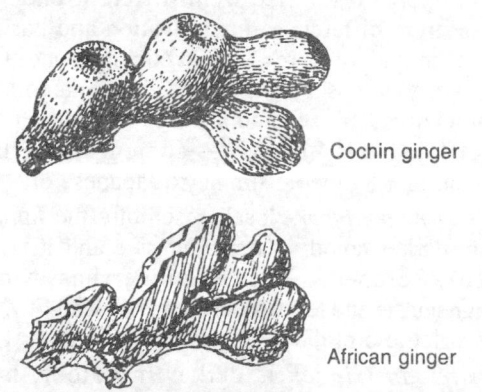

Cochin ginger

African ginger

Fig. 19.24. Ginger rhizome.

Morphology

Rhizomes are thick, horizontal, laterally compressed, often palmately branched, each having at its apex a depressed scar, showing longitudinal striations and occasional loose fibres, size 5-15 cm long, 3-4 cm wide and 1-15 cm thick: fracture-short and starchy with projecting fibres. Fractured surface shows a narrow cortex, a well marked endodermis and a wide stele; the whole showing numerous scattered greyish points. Colour is buff; odour is agreeable and aromatic; taste is pungent.

The unscraped rhizome is covered by brownish layers of cork with conspicuous ridges; the cork readily exfoliates from the lateral surfaces but persists between the branches.

Microscopy

A transverse section of unpeeled Ginger rhizome shows a zone of cork cells, cortex, endodermis and ground tissues.

Outer zone of cork tissue consists of irregularly arranged cells. The cork cambium is differentiated. Within the cork is a broad cortex with an outer zone of flattened parenchyma and an inner zone of normal parenchyma. The cortical cells contain simple, ovoid or sack-shaped starch grains with a markedly eccentric hilum. Numerous oil cells, with suberized walls enclosing yellowish-brown oleoresin, are scattered in the cortex. The inner cortical zone contains about three rings of collateral, closed vascular bundles. The larger bundles are enclosed in a sheath of septate, non-lignified fibres. Each vascular bundle contains phloem, showing well-marked sieve-tubes and a xylem composed of 1-14 vessels with annular, spiral or reticulate thickening. The inner part of the cortex is marked by a single-layered endodermis free from starch. The outermost layer of the stele is marked by a single layered pericycle. The vascular bundles of stele resemble those of the cortex and are scattered as in monocotyledonous stems.

Ground tissue contains large parenchymatous, rounded, polygonal cells containing excess of starch, oleo-resin and vascular bundles. Starch occurs as flattened, oval or subrectangular, transversely striated, simple granules, each with a hilum in a projection towards one end. Oleo-resin cells contains suberized cell walls and yellow contents. Pigment cells contain dark, reddish brown contents and occur either singly in ground tissue or in axial rows accompanying the vascular bundles. Sclereids and calcium oxalate crystals are absent.

The inner cortical zone contains about three rings of collateral, closed vascular bundles. The larger bundles are enclosed in a sheath of septate, nonlignified fibres. Each vascular bundle contains phloem, with well-marked sieve-tubes and a xylem composed of 1-14 vessels with annular, spiral or reticulate thickening. These vessels do not give lignin reaction with phloroglucinol and hydrochloric acid. Axially elongated secretion cells with dark contents may be present in the vessels. The inner limit of the cortex is marked by a single-layered endodermis free from starch. The outermost layer of the stele is marked by a single-layered pericycle. The vascular bundles of the stele resemble those of the cortex, and are, scattered as is typical of monocotyledonous stems. The ground mass of the stele is composed of parenchyma resembling the cortical parenchyma and containing much starch and numerous oil cells. Cork cells are not present in the scraped drug.

Chemical constituents

Ginger contains acrid resinous substances (5-8%), volatile oil (1-3%), starch (5%), protein (2-3%) and sugars such as sucrose, raffinose and glucose. The chemical constituents from the Ginger rhizome can be divided into two classes, the pungent and the

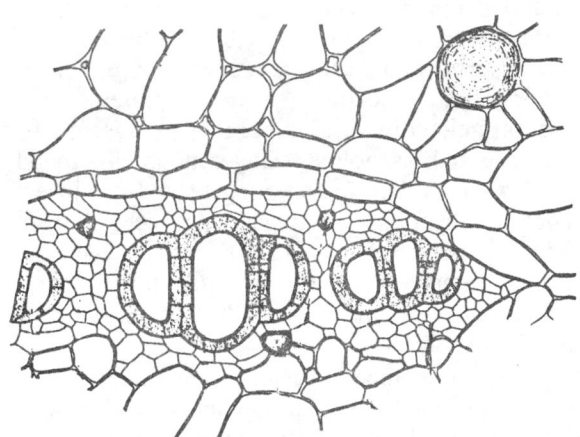

Fig. 19.25. T.S. of Ginger rhizome.

flavouring principles. The pungent substances, gingerols are 1-(4-hydroxy-3-methoxyphenyl)-5-hydroxy alkan-3-ones with an S (+)-configurations, having side chains of different lengths. On the basis of the length of side chain, gingerols are designated as [3]-, [4]-, [5]-, [6]-, [8]- and [10]- gingerols. The other gingerol analogues are zingerone or [4(4-hydroxy-3-methoxy-phenyl-butanone], [6]-shogaol, [4]-, [6]-, [8]- and [10]-gingediols, methylgingediols, their acetates, hexahydrocurcumin, dimethyl hexahydrocurcumin, dimethyl hexahydrocurcumin, gingerdiones, dehydrogingerdiones, capsaicin, dihydrogingerol, desmethylhexahydrocurcumin, diaryl heptanoids, methoxyphenyl decane derivatives and 6,4'-dichloroflavan.

Gingerols and shogaols are non-volatile phenolic compounds with different side-chains. Gingerol is formed in the plant from phenylalanine, malonate and hexanoate.

The pungency of gingerol is destroyed by boiling with 2% potassium hydroxide. Boiling with baryta water decomposes it with formation of a phenolic ketone called zingerone and aliphatic aldehydes (mainly normal heptaldehyde). Zingerone also occurs in the rhizome and its pungency is destroyed by prolonged contact with 5% sodium hydroxide. Shogaols, components of the oil, represent compounds formed by loss of water from the gingerols and do not appear to be present in the fresh rhizome.

Volatile oil is a mixture of more than 25 components of monoterpenes (β-phellandrene, camphene α-and β-pinenes, cumene, myrcene, limonene, citral, borneol, p-cymene, 1,8-cineole, linalool, neral, etc.) and sesquiterpenes (zingiberene, farnesene, γ-selinene, ar-curcumene, β-sesquiphellandrene, zingiberol, β-eudesmol, β-elemene and bisaboline). Zingerone is also found in rhizome which is also pungent and has sweet odour. Dehydration of gingerol produces shogaol which is not present in fresh rhizomes. The oxygenated monoterpenes are 2-heptanol, 2-nonanol, n-nonanal, n-decanal, methyl heptenone, borneol and bornyl acetate.

The other compound detected are *cis*- and *trans*-sesquiphellandrol, sesquithujene, sesquisabinene hydrate, zingiberenol, heptane, octane, isovaleraldehyde, nonanol, ethyl pinene, car-3-ene, α-

terpinene, α-terpineol, nerol, neral, geranyl acetate, β-sesquiphellandrene, α-copaene, undecan-2-one, citronellal, heptane-2-ol and 6-methylhept-5-en-2-one.

The roots contain zerumbone, zerumbodienone and humulene epoxides I and II. Japanese Ginger possesses galanolactone, (E)-8β, 17-epoxylabd-12-en-15,16-dial, [6]-shogaol, [6]-, [8]- and [10]-gingerols.

Uses : Ginger is used as an antiemetic, positive inotropic, spasmolytic, aromatic stimulant, carminative, condiment and flavouring agent. It is prescribed in dyspepsia, flatulent colic, vomiting spasms, as an adjunct to many tonic and stimulating remedies, for painful affections of the stomach, cold, cough and asthma. Sore throat, hoarseness and loss of voice are benefited by chewing a piece of ginger.

Ginger stimulates the flow of saliva, raises the tonus of the intestinal musculature and activates peristalsis.

Powdered ginger may be a more effective antiemetic than dimenhydrinate (dramamine). It may ameliorate the effects of motion sickness in the gastrointestinal tract itself, in contrast to antihistamines, which act centrally. Gingerols show the potent inhibitory actions against prostaglandin synthetase which correspond with the anti-inflammatory and antiplatelet aggregation properties of the drug. These compounds, together with [6]-shogaol, also produce enhanced gastrointestinal activity with effects on bile secretion. The C_{20}-dial has a cholesterol-biosynthesis inhibitory activity in animal preparations and is assumed to be a HMG-CoA reduce inhibitor. The sesquiterpene hydrocarbons possess antiulcer activity of the drug. The rhizome shows a strong antibac-terial and antifungal action.

Adulteration

Ginger may be adulterated by addition of 'wormy' drug or 'spent ginger' which has been exhausted in the extraction of resins and volatile oil. This adulteration may be detected by the official standards, for alcohol-soluble portion, water-soluble portion, total ash and water-soluble ash. Sometimes pungency of exhausted Ginger is increased by the addition of Capsicum or seeds or *Aframomum melequeta* (grains of paradise, fam. Zingiberaceae).

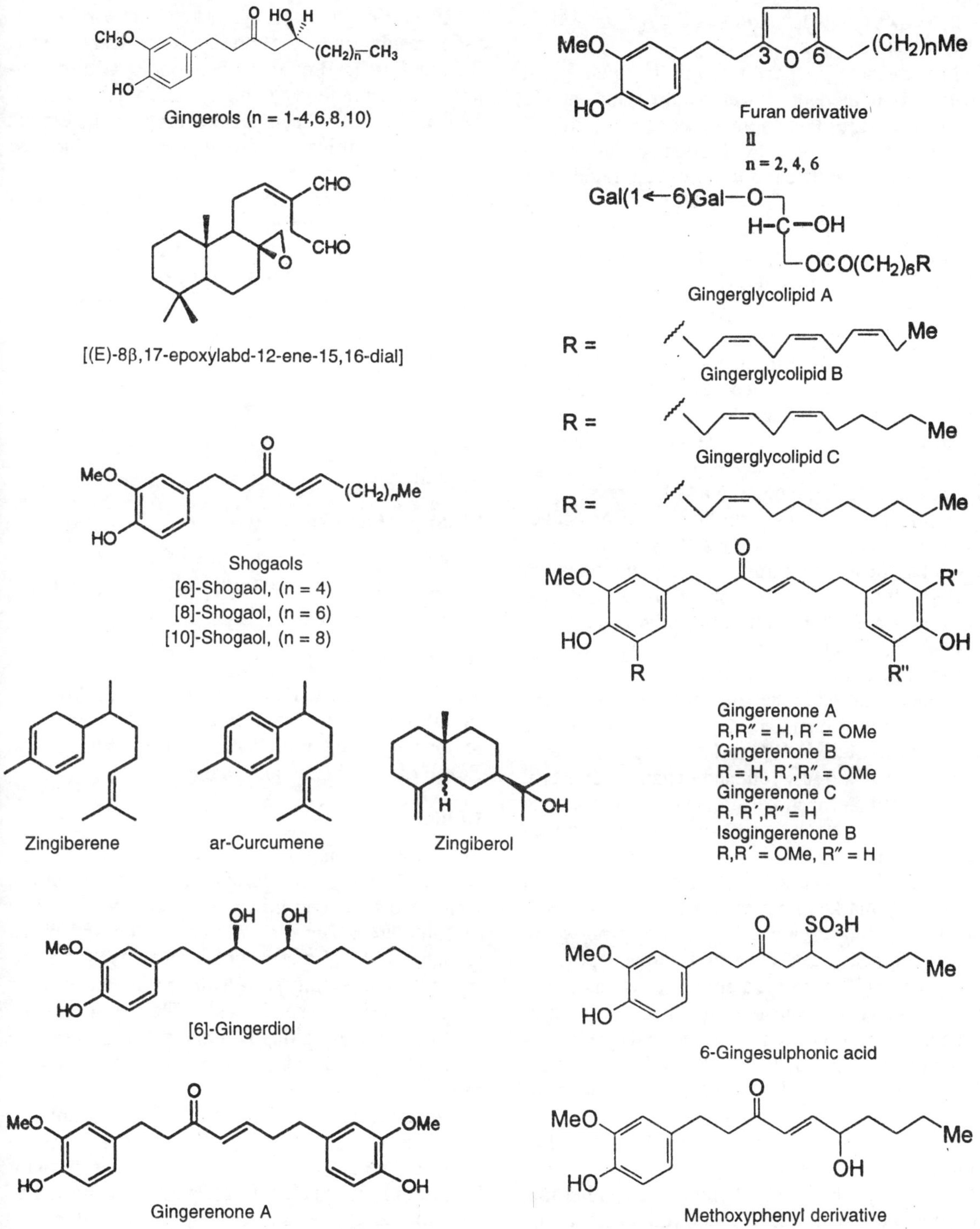

CH_3O
HO
O HO H
$(CH_2)_n$–CH_3
Gingerols (n = 1-4,6,8,10)
MeO
HO
3 O 6
$(CH_2)_nMe$
Furan derivative
II
n = 2, 4, 6
CHO
CHO
O
[(E)-8β,17-epoxylabd-12-ene-15,16-dial]
Gal(1←6)Gal—O
H–C–OH
$OCO(CH_2)_6R$
Gingerglycolipid A
R =
Me
Gingerglycolipid B
R =
Me
Gingerglycolipid C
R =
Me
MeO
HO
O
$(CH_2)_nMe$
Shogaols
[6]-Shogaol, (n = 4)
[8]-Shogaol, (n = 6)
[10]-Shogaol, (n = 8)
MeO
HO
R
O
R'
OH
R''
Zingiberene
ar-Curcumene
H
OH
Zingiberol
Gingerenone A
R,R″ = H, R′ = OMe
Gingerenone B
R = H, R′,R″ = OMe
Gingerenone C
R, R′,R″ = H
Isogingerenone B
R,R′ = OMe, R″ = H
OH OH
MeO
HO
[6]-Gingerdiol
O SO_3H
MeO
HO
Me
6-Gingesulphonic acid
O
MeO
HO
OMe
OH
Gingerenone A
O
MeO
HO
Me
OH
Methoxyphenyl derivative

Fig. 19.26. Chemical constituents of Ginger.

Such type of pungency is not destroyed by boiling with an alkali.

The extract prepared from the suspected powder, is heated on a water-bath with caustic alkali. The liquid is then evaporated, and the residue acidified with hydrochloric acid and shaken with ether. The ethereal solution evaporated on a watch glass gives a residue which is not markedly pungent to taste. This test depends on the fact that gingerol is more readily decomposed by alkalies than are capsaicin or paradol.

Pharmacology

Oral or intravenous administration of [6]-gingerol or [6]-shogaol to rats produced an inhibition of spontaneous motor activity, showed antipyretic and analgesic effects and prolonged hexabarbital-induced sleeping time. [6]-Shogaol was more effective than [6]-gingerol. Both the compounds suppressed gastric contraction. The methanolic extract of Ginger rhizome or its active ingredients, the gingerols, possess potent positive inotropic effects on guinea pig isolated left atria. [6]-Gingerol and the gingerdione derivatives are potent inhibitors of prostaglandin biosynthesis. Gingerols and shogaols exhibited significant antihepatotoxic action against cytotoxicity in primary cultured rat hepatocytes. The semi-purified powdered protease of Ginger showed a high proteolytic activity at pH 4.5-6.0. Ginger oleoresin significantly lowered serum and hepatic cholesterol and increased faecal cholesterol excretion. Rhizome extract showed a positive inotropic effect on guinea pig isolated left atria. [6]-Shogaol showed triphasic effect on blood pressure in rats, an initial fall followed by marked pressor response, bradycardia and apnea. It induced contractile response in isolated guinea pig trachea and showed positive inotropic and chronotropic activities on isolated atria in rats. Gingerols I and II from rhizomes potentiated contractions induced by prostanoids and inhibited contractions produced by PGD_2, TXA_2 and LT on isolated blood vessels of mice and rats. Gingerols acted as modulator of eicosanoid responses in vascular smooth muscles due to their prostaglandin-related chemical structures. [6]-Shogaol from active fraction inhibited 5HT-induced hypothermia. Gingerenone A exhibited moderate anticoccidium activity in cultured kidney cells of chicken and

strong antifungal effect against *Pyricularia oryzae*. 6-Gingesulphonic acid inhibited antiulcer activity. β-Sesquiphellandrene showed activity against rhinovirus. Zerumbone completely inhibited growth of mouse L 1210 leukaemia cells. An acetone extract of Ginger significantly inhibited serotonin induced hypothermia and 5HT-induced diarrhoea and showed antimicrobial activity against *Bacillus subtillis* and *Escherichia coli* k-12. Addition of dry ginger with fatty meal of male volunteers significantly inhibited platelet aggregation induced by ADP and epinephrine and enhanced platelet aggregation.

TURMERIC

Synonyms

Saffron Indian; Haldi (Hindi); Curcuma; Rhizoma curcumae.

Biological source

Turmeric is the dried rhizome of *Curcuma longa* Linn. (syn. *C. domestica* Valeton). (Family : Zingiberaceae).

Habitat

The plant is a native to southern Asia (Probably India) and is cultivated extensively in temperate regions. It is grown on a larger scale in India, China, East Indies, Pakistan and Malaya.

Cultivation

Turmeric plant is a perennial herb, 60-90 cm high with a short stem and tufted leaves; the rhizomes, which are short and thick, constitute the Turmeric of commerce. The crop requires a hot and moist climate, a liberal water supply and a well-drained soil. It thrives on any soil-loamy or alluvial, but the soil should be loose and friable. The field should be well prepared by ploughing and turning over to a depth of about 30 cm and liberally manured with farmyard and green manures. Sets or fingers of the previous crop with one or two buds are planted 7 cm deep at distance of 30-37 cm from April to August. The crop is ready for harvesting in about 9-10 months when the lower leaves turn yellow. The rhizomes are carefully dug up with hard picks, washed and dried.

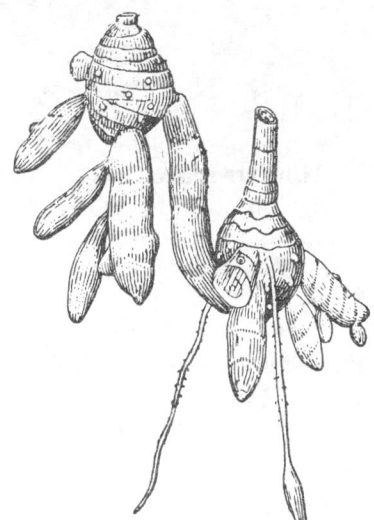

Fig. 19.27. Turmeric rhizome.

Macroscopical characters

The primary rhizomes are ovate or pear-shaped, oblong or pyriform or cylindrical and often short branched. The rhizomes are known as 'bulb' or 'round' turmeric. The secondary, more cylindrical, lateral branched, tapering on both ends, rhizomes are 4-7 cm long and 1-1.5 cm wide and called as 'fingers'. The bulbous and finger-shaped parts are separated and the long fingers are broken into convenient bits. They are freed from adhering dirt and fibrous roots and subjected to curing and polishing process. The curing consists of cooking the rhizomes along with few leaves in water until they become soft. The cooked rhizomes are cooled, dried in open air with intermittent turning over and rubbed on a rough surface. Colour is deep yellow to orange, with root scar and encircling ridge-like rings or annulations, the latter from the scar of leaf base. Fracture is horny and the cut surface is waxy and resinous in appearance. Outer surface is deep yellow to brown and longitudinally wrinkled. Taste is aromatic, pungent and bitter; odour is distinct.

Microscopical characters

The transverse section of the rhizome is characterized by the presence of mostly thin walled rounded parenchyma cells, scattered vascular bundles, definite endodermis, few layers of cork developed under the epidermis and scattered oleoresin cells with

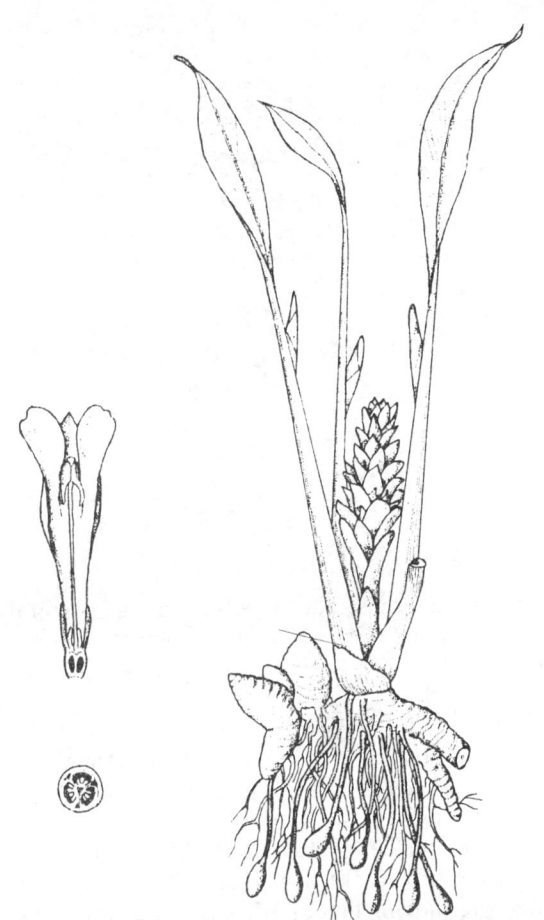

Fig. 19.28. Turmeric plant.

brownish contents. The epidermis is consisted of thick walled cells, cubical in shape, of various dimensions. The cork cambium is developed from the sub-epidermal layers and even after the development of the cork, the epidermis is retained. Cork is generally composed of 4-6 layers of thin-walled brick-shaped parenchymatous cells. The parenchyma of the pith and cortex contains grains altered to a paste, in which sometimes long lens shaped unaltered starch grains of 4-15 μm diameter are found. Oil cells have suberised walls and contain either orange-yellow globules of a volatile oil or amorphous resinous masses. Cortical vascular bundles are scattered and are of a collateral type. The vascular bundles in the pith region are mostly scattered and they form disconti-nuous ring just un-

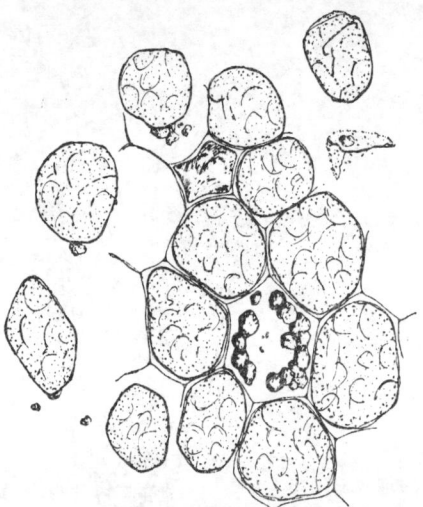

Fig. 19.29. T.S. of Turmeric rhizome.

Diphenyl heptatrien–3–one

Diphenyl pentadien–3–ones

R = OMe   R = H

Procurcumadiol

ar-Tumerone

(–)-Zingiberene

Curcumin

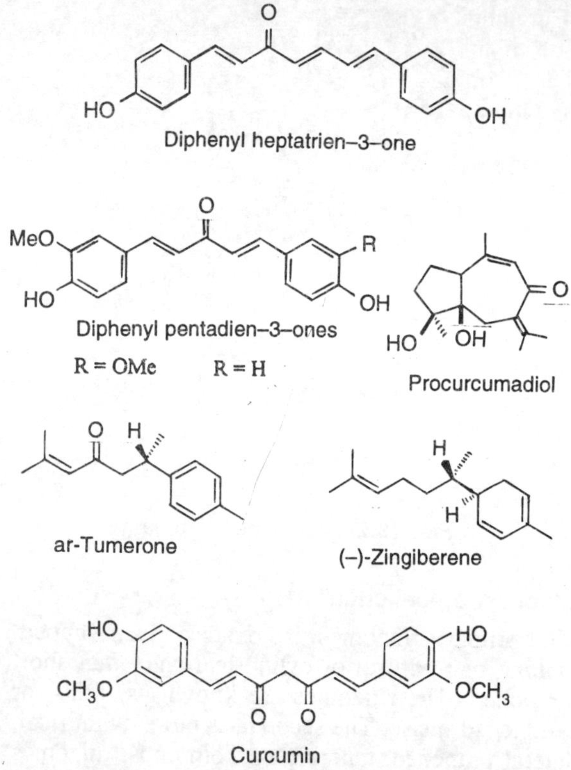

Fig. 19.30. Chemical constituents of Turmeric.

der the endodermis. The vessels have mainly spiral thickenings and only a few have reticulate and annular structure.

Chemical constituents

Turmeric contains yellow colouring matter called as curcuminoids (5%) and essential oil (~6%). The chief constituent of the colouring matter is curcumin I (diferuloylmethane) (60%) in addition with small quantities of dicaffeoylmethane (curcumin III), caffeoylferuloylmethane (curcumin II) and dihydrocurcumin. The volatile oil contains mono- and sesquiterpenes like zingiberene (25%), α-phellandrene, sabinene, turmerone, arturmerone, borneol and cineole. Choleretic action of the essential oil is attributed to p-tolylmethyl carbinol.

The volatile oil also contains α- and β-pinene, camphene, limonene, terpinene, terpinolene, caryophyllene, linalool, isoborneol, camphor, eugenol, curdione, curzerenone, curlone, ar-curcumenes, β-curcumene, γ-curcumene. α- and β-turmerones and curzerenone.

The rhizomes possess arabinose (1%), fructose (12%), glucose (28%), starch grains, p-α-dimethylbenzyl alcohol, 1-methyl-4-acetyl-1-cyclohexene, caprylic acid, campesterol, stigmasterol, β-sitosterol, cholesterol, dihydrocurcumin, monodesmethoxycurcumin, didemethoxy curcumin, 2-(hydroxymethyl) anthraquinone, sesquiterpenes I and II, sesquiterpenes germacran-13-al, procurcumadiol, bisaboladiene derivatives, dehydrocurdione, bisacumol, bisacurone, curcumenol, isoprocurcumenol, zedaronediol, procurcumenol, epiprocurcumenol, turmerin, turmerol, α-atlantone; glycans ukonans A, B, C and D, 5'-methoxycurcumin and some phenolics.

Uses

Turmeric is used as aromatic, anti-inflammatory, stomachic, uretic, anodyne for billiary calculus, stimulant, tonic, carminative, blood purifier, antiperiodic, alterative, spice, colouring agent for ointments and a common household remedy for cold and cough. Externally, it is used in the form of a cream to improve complexion. Dye-stuff acts as a cholagogue causing the contraction of the gall bladder. It is also used in menstrual pains. Curcumin has choleretic and cholagogue action and is used in liver diseases. Curcumin is a non-toxic authorized colour, heat resistant and sensitive to changes in pH.

Curcuminoids have antiphlogistic activity which is due to inhibition of leukotriene biosynthesis. ar-Turmerone has anti-snake venom activity and blocks the haemorrhagic effect of venom.

Chemical tests

1. Turmeric powder on treatment with concentrated sulphuric acid forms red colour.
2. On addition of alkali solution to Turmeric powder red to violet colour is produced.
3. With acetic anhydride and concentrated sulphuric acid Turmeric gives voilet colour. Under U.V. light this colour is seen as an intense red fluorescence.
4. A paper containing Turmeric extract produces a green colour with borax solution.
5. On addition of boric acid a reddish-brown colour is formed which, on addition of alkalies, changes to greenish-blue.
6. A piece of filter paper is impregnated with an alcohol extract, dried and then moistened with boric acid solution slightly acidified with hydrochloric acid, and re-dried. Pink or brownish-red colour is developed on the filter paper which becomes deep blue on addition of alkali.

All these tests are due to the presence of curcuminoids in the drug.

Pharmacology

The essential oil and ethenolic extract of *C. longa* and curcumin inhibit the growth of microorganisms present in cholecystitis. Curcumin and its analogues show anti-inflammatory action and inhibit contractions induced by nicotine, acetylcholine, serotinin, histamine and barium chloride on isolated guinea pig ileum. Curcumin was more potent inflammation inhibitor than ibuprofen. Curcumin caused an increase in bile flow in dogs by nearly 100% without any appreciable disturbance in blood pressure and respiration. There was an increase of total excretion of bile salts, bilirubin and cholesterol, whereas fatty acid contents remained almost constant. The plasma level was markedly stimulated by duodenal infusion of curcumin in dogs and human beings. Curcumin and its analogues possessed significant antihepatotoxic action against CCl_4-induced liver damage in mice. Curcumin inhibited the cyclo-oxygenase activity of platelets *in vitro*, inhibited the production of 5-hydroxyeicosatetraenoic acid in intact human neutrophils and showed anticoagulant activity. It inhibited ADP-, epinephrine- and collagen-induced platelet aggregation in monkey plasma. Intravenous injection of curcumin produced transient hypotension and bradycardia in dogs and cats which may be due to its myocardial depressant action. Curcumin exhibited a negative inotropic and chronotropic effect on isolated perfused rabbit heart, and an antispasmodic effect on smooth muscle of dog intestine, but no effect on the rectus abdominis muscle of frog. Turmeric or curcumin caused no adverse effects on growth, feed efficiency ratio, blood counts, or clinical blood chemistry. Turmeric oleoresin containing curcumin showed a reduction in weight gain and in feed efficiency in pigs. Turmeric extract inhibited cell growth in Chinese hamster ovary cell culture and was cytotoxic to lymphocytes and Dalton's lymphoma cells. Curcumin administered orally to rats was found to be excreted in feces to about 75%, while negligible amount was found in urine. It was poorly absorbed from the gut. The major biliary metabolites were glucuronides of tetrahydrocurcumin, hexahydrocurcumin, dihydroferulic acid and traces of ferulic acid.

An aqueous extract of turmeric completely suppressed carrageenin-induced oedema. The essential oil in rats showed significantly more marked anti-inflammatory effect that cortisone acetate. The plant definitely reduced cough and dyspnoea in a clinical trial. Diferuloylmethane, feruloyl-*p*-coumaroylmethane and di-*p*-coumaroylmethane showed cytotoxic activity.

Curcumin produced gastric ulceration in albino rats due to marked reduction in mucin content of gastric juice. Plant extract caused significant reduction in ratio of total cholesterol/phospholipids in hyperlipidaemic rats and elevated HDL-cholesterol and total cholesterol ratio. Curcumin and its derivatives exhibited anticoagulant activity. Curcumin showed cytotoxicity to lymphocytes and Dalton's lymphome cells, reduced development of animal tumors, protected mice against thrombotic challenge, inhibited cyclooxygenase activity of platelets and catalysed degradation of hyaluronic acid.

Effect of curcuminoids was inhibited by addition of a OH radical quen-cher (mannitol).

Ukonans A, B, C and D showed marked reticulo-endothelial potentiating activity. Arturmerone inhibited proliferation and natural killer activity of human lymphocytes. Curcumin exhibited inhibition of calcium/calcium ionophore-stimulated formation of leukotriene B_4, inhibited responses to phyto-haemagglutinin and mixed lymphocyte reaction, inhibited proliferation of smooth muscle cells stimulated by fetal calf blood serum, protected human red blood cells against primaquine-induced oxidative damage, increased life span of cyclo-phosphamide-treated mice and reduced leukoplemia produced by cyclophosphamide.

The peptide turmerin is an efficient antioxidant and DNA-protectant. Turmerin was not cytotoxic up to 1.0 mg concentration to human lymphocytes.

Demethoxycurcumin, bisdemethoxycurcumin and 5'-methoxycurcumin showed stronger activity than curcumin.

GALANGA

Synonyms

Galangal; Colic root; East India root; Chinese ginger; Ganlang rhizome; Rasna; Barakulanjan (Hindi); Lesser galangal; Galangal rhizome; Rhizoma galangae.

Biological source

Galanga consists of dried rhizome of *Alpinia officinarum* Hance. (Family : Zingiberaceae).

Habitat

Galanga is grown in China, Thailand, eastern Himalayas, Bengal and south-west India.

Morphology

The plant is 1-2 m long perennial herb bearing rhizomes. The drug consists of irregularly branched cylindrical rhizomes, about 2-8 cm long and 1-2 cm thick. They are marked with fine, wavy annulations of lighter colour than the general surface which is reddish or rusty brown in colour. Taste is aromatic and pungent; odour is aromatic, distinct, spicy and agreeable. Fracture is very tough and fibrous, the exposed surface is lighter orange or brown in colour.

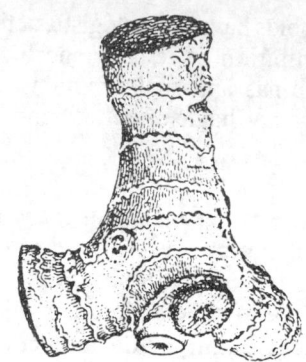

Fig. 19.31. Rhizome of *Alpinia officinarum* (Galanga).

Chemical constituents

Galanga contains volatile oil (0.5-1%), resin (20%), kaempferol, galangin, dihydroxyflavanol, galangol, phlobaphene tannins and starch in abundance. The volatile oil is a mixture of 1, 8-cineole, α-pinene, β-pinene, methyl isovalerate, camphene, limonene, *p*-cymene, camphor, β-elemene, α-bergamotene, terpinen-4-ol, δ-cadinene, γ-cadinene, methyl cinnamate and eugenol. Kaempferol, galangin and alpinin are the flavonoids.

The other compounds isolated from Galanga are quercetin, its 3-methyl ether, isorhamnetin, kaempferide, galangin-3-methyl ether, diaryl-heptonoids, *viz.*, 1,7-diphenylhept-4-en-3-one, 1,7-diphenyl-5-hydroxy-3-heptanone, 7-(4"-hydroxy-3"-methoxyphenyl)-1-phenylhept-4-en-3-one, 5-hydroxy-7-(4"-hydroxy-3"-methoxy-phenyl)-1-phe-nyl-3-heptanone, 7-(4"-hydroxy-phenyl)-1-phenyl-4-hepton-3-one, 5-methoxy-7-(4"-hydroxyphenyl)-1-phenyl-3-heptanone, 5-methoxy-1,7-diphenyl-3-heptanone and 1-(4"-hydroxyphenyl)-7-phenyl heptone-3,5-dione.

Pharmacology

Diaryl heptanoids exhibited prostaglandin biosynthesis inhibitory activity.

Uses

Galanga is used in rheumatism, fever, catarrahal affections specially in bronchial catarrah, as stomachic, stimulant, aphrodisiac, carminative and flavouring agent. It has antifungal and antibacterial properties.

Allied drugs

Alpinia galanga (Greater galanga) rhizome, a native of Java and Sumatra and cultivated in India, is substituted to the *A. officinarum*. Greater galanga is larger is size, colour deep orange brown externally and pale buff internally. The drug does not contain any flavonoid. Alcoholic extract of the drug on filter paper does not show any fluorescence under U.V. light due to absence of flavonoids.

Adulteration

The genuine drug is not available in sufficient quantities and most of it is adulterated with the rhizomes of *Acorus calamus*.

CAPSICUM

Synonyms

Chillies; Cayenne Pepper; Red Peppers; Spanish Pepper; Mirch (Hindi); Capsicum fruits; Fructus Capsici.

Biological source

Capsicum consists of the dried, ripe fruits of *Capsicum frutescens* Linn. (African Chillies) or of *Capsicum annuum* Linn. var. *conoides* (Tabasco pepper) or of *Capsicum annuum* var. *longum* (Lonusiana Long pepper), or of a hybrid between the Honka variety of Japanese Capsicum and the old Louisiana Sport Capsicum known as *Loisiana Sport Pepper* (Family : Solanaceae).

Habitat

Capsicum is native of America and cultivated in tropical regions of India, Japan, southern Europe, Mexico, Africa (Kenya, Tanzania, and Sierra Leone) and Sri Lanka.

Cultivation

Capsicum is cultivated mostly as a rainfed crop. In the gangetic area, it is a cold weather crop. The crop is raised on a variety of soils, *e.g.*, ordinary red loams, black soils and clayey loams. Good drainage is essential and water-logging is detrimental. Seedlings are first rainsed in a nursery. Seeds obtained from selected pods and mixed with ashes are sown by broadcasting. Germination occurs in about a week. The field is ploughed and manured with compost. The field is irrigated once a day until the plants are established. Flowering starts when the plants are 2.5-3.5 months old. Dew and heavy rain at flowering time are injurious. Ripe and nearly ripe fruits are picked at intervals of 5, 10 and 20 days.

Characters

Capsicum is 5-12 cm long, 2-4 cm wide, globular, ovoid or oblong in shape, pericarp is shrievelled, orange or red in colour, pedicel is prominent and bent. The calyx is toothed. The amount of calices and pedicels should not exceed beyond 3 per cent. Internally the fruits are divided into two halve parts by a membranous dissepiment to which the seeds are attached. The seeds are reniform, flattened, 3-4 mm long, with a coiled embryo and oily endosperm. Capsicum has characrteristic odour and an intense pungent taste.

Collection

The fruits are picked as they become fully ripe. The quality of the drug is in part determined by its colour. The unripe fruits fade to pale buff upon drying. The fruits are dried in sun, graded by colour; occasionally oil is rubbed on the fruits to give a glossiness to the pericarps. Most of the calices and pedicels are removed.

Chemical constituents

Capsicum contains fixed oils (4-16%), oleoresin, carotenoids, capsacutin, capsico (a volatile alkaloid), thiamine, volatile oil (1.5%) and ascorbic acid (0.2%). The resin contains an extremely pungent principle, capsaicin, (decylenic vanillyl amide) (about 0.5%). Capsaicin retains its characteristic pungency in a dilution of 1 part in 10 million parts with water. The maximum concentration of capsaicin is in the inner walls. Its pungency is uneffected by alkalies but is destroyed by oxidising agents such as potassium dichromate or permanganate. Capsanthin is the main carotenoid of red fruits. It also occurs as monoester and diester along with cryptocapsin. Other carotenoids include zeaxanthin, capsorubin, capsanthin, rubixanthin, phytofluene, capsanthin-5,6-epoxide, capsanthin-3,6-epoxide. lutein, cryptoxanthin, α- and β-carotenes, capsorubin and few xanthophylls. The carbohydrates reported in chillies are fructose, galactose, sucrose,

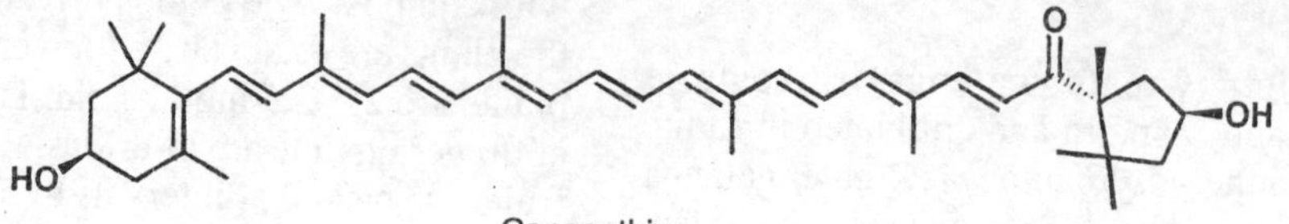

Capsanthin

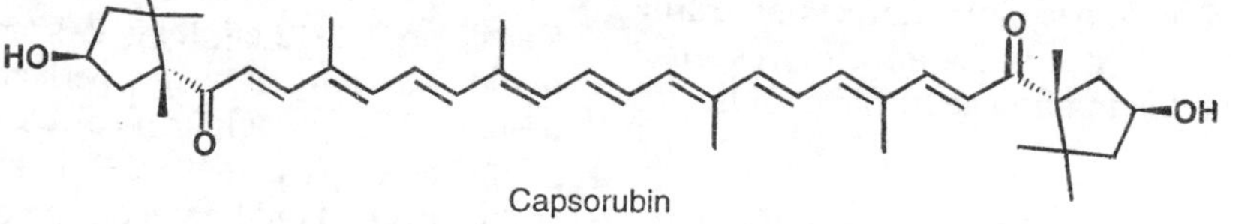

Capsorubin

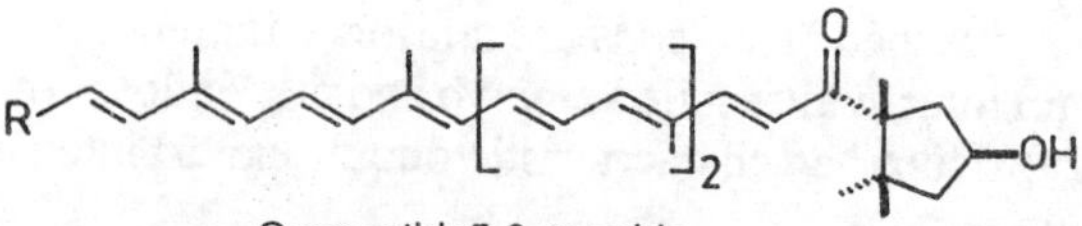

Capsanthin5,6-epoxide

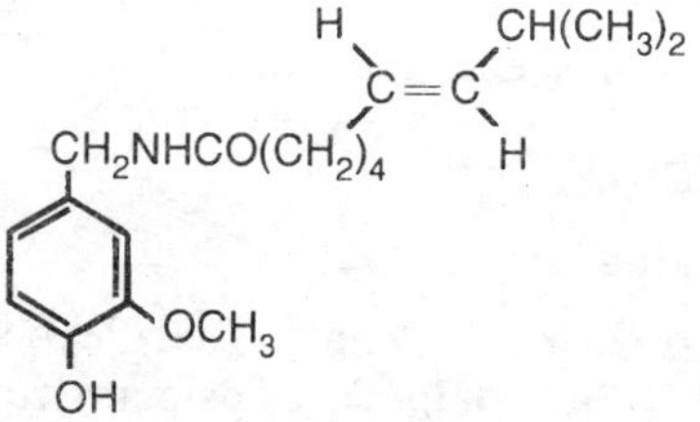

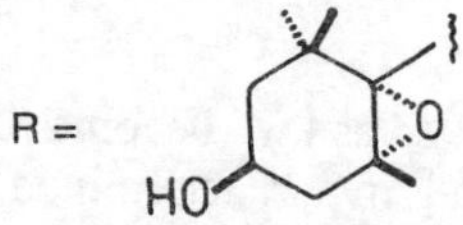

R =

Capsanthin 3,6-epoxide

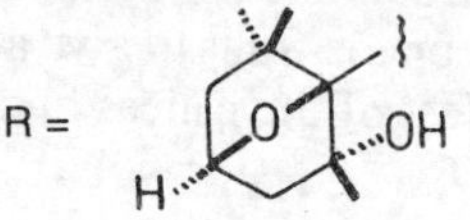

R =

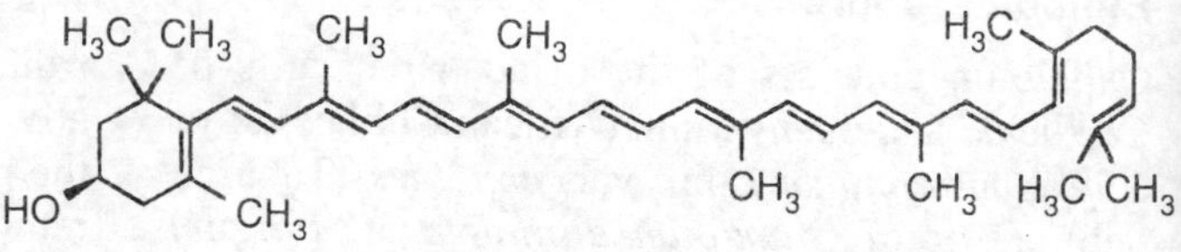

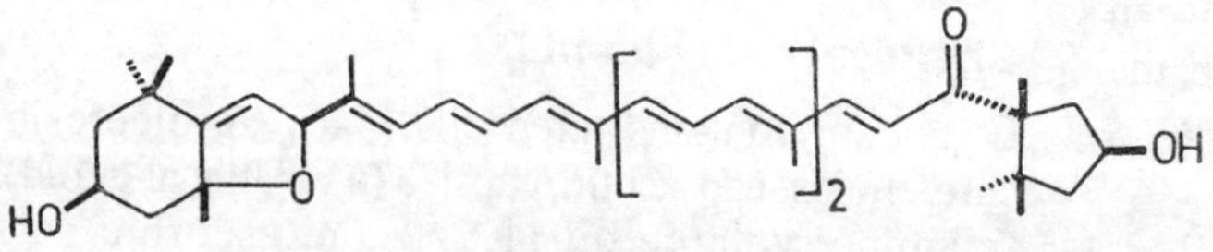

Capsaicin

Capsochrome

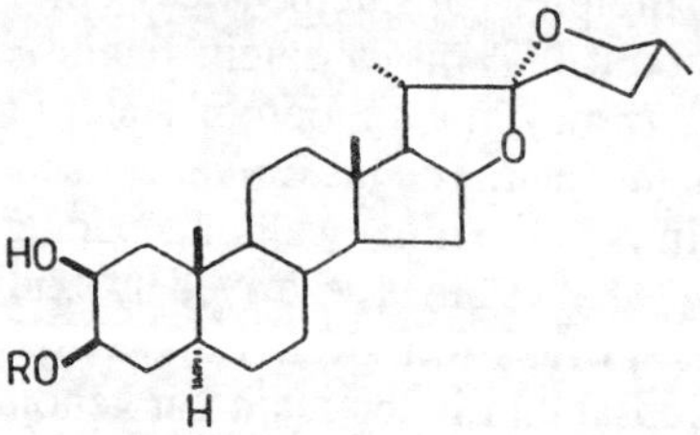

Capsicoside A1
R = Gal
Capsicoside B1
R = Gal(4→1)Glu
Capsicoside Cl
R = Gal(4→1)Glu (3→1)Xyl

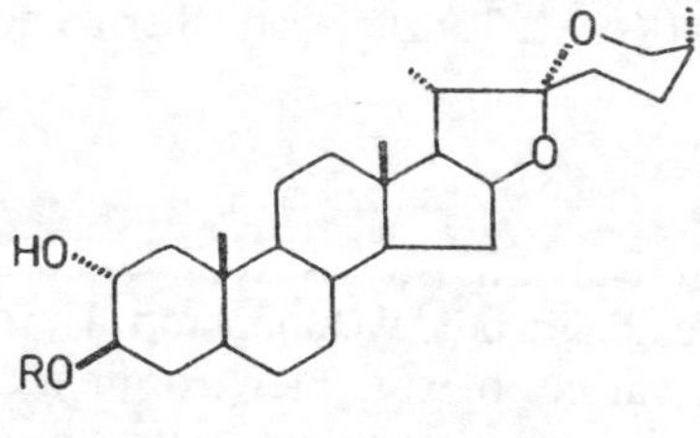

Capsicosin D1
R = Gal(4→1)Glu[(2→1)Gal](3→1)Xyl
Capsicosin E1
R = Gal(4→1)Glu(2→1)Gal(4→1)Glu(3→1)Xyl

Fig. 19.32. Chemical constituents of Capsicum.

fructosyl-sucrose, planteose and planteobiose. Tocopherol (vitamin E) is present in trace amounts (~2.4 mg/100 g).

The pungent compounds of *C. annuum* are capsaicin (69%), 6,7-dihydrocapsaicin (22%), nordihydrocapsiacin (7%), homocapsaicin (1%) and homodihydrocapsaicin (1%).

The other compounds isolated from Capsicum are saponin capsicidin, capsicoside, lanosterol, cycloartenol, cycloartanol, cholesterol, 24-methyl-cholesterol, 24-ethylcholesterol, stigmasterol, 24-methylcholesta-5,24-diol, 28-isofucosterol, 24-methylenecholesterol, 24-ethylcholesta-5,24-dienol, cholest-7-enol, 24-ethyl-cholest-22-enol, 4α-methyl-cholest-8(14)-en-3β-ol, lanost-8-en-3β-ol, 24-methylene lanost-8-en-3β-ol, 24-methylene cycloartanol, lupeol, β-amyrin, daturaolone and daturadiol (from seeds).

The seed oil contains 4α-methylsterols, 31-norlanost-9(11)-enol, 24-methyl-31-norlanost-9(11)-enol, 4α, 2n-dimethylcholesta-7,24-dienol, 4α-methyl-24-ethylcholesta-7-,24-dienol, 31-norcycloartanol, 31-norcycloartenol, cycloeuca-lenol, 31-norlanost-8-enol, obtusifoliol, 4α,14α, 24-trimethylcholesta-8,24-dienol, 4α-methyl-cholest-8-enol, lophenol, 24-methyllophenol, 24-ethyllo-phenol, gramisterol and citrostadienol.

The capsaicin content of fruits varies appreciably in a range up to 1.5% and is influenced by environmental conditions and age of the fruit. It occurs principally in the dissepiments of the fruits, *e.g.*, entire fruit 0.49, pericarp 0.10, dissepiment 1.79, seed 0.07.

The fruits yield about 20-25% of alcoholic extract (capsicin) and about 5% (official limit 8%) of ash. Hungarian capsicums or 'Paprika' are derived from a mild race of *C. annuum* and are a convenient source of ascorbic acid.

The water-soluble constituents of the fruits of three varieties of *C. annuum* contain acyclic glycosides (geranyl linalool derivatives) named capsianosides A-F (dimeric esters of acyclic diterpene glycosides) and capsianosides I-V (monomeric compounds of acrylic diterpene glycosides).

A number of colorimetric assays can be used for the quantitative determination of capsaicin, e.g., ultraviolet absorption at 248 and 296 nm for the ointment and oleoresin.

Biogenesis of capsaicin

Phenylalanine is incorporated into the C_6-C_1 vanillyl unit of capsaicin, the C-3 of phenylalanine giving the methylene group of the vanillyl-amine residues via cinnamic, *p*-coumaric, caffeic and protocat-echuic acids. Tyrosine is not a probable precursor. The C_{10} isodecanoic acid is formed from isobutyryl coenzyme A and three acetate units. The homo derivatives (C_{11} acid) are formed from leucine and isoleucine.

A prior active accumulation of *p*-coumaroyl, caffeoyl and 3,4-dimethoxycinnamoyl glycosides, 3-*O*-rhamnosylquercetin and 7-*O*-glucosylluteolin takes place the ontogenetic formation of capsai-cinoids in the fruits of *C. frutescens*. When the fruit ceases to increase in length the amount of these compounds falls. Capsaicinoid synthesis occurs together with that of the glycosides of vanillic acid and *p*-hydroxybenzaldehyde.

Cell cultures

Capsaicin production takes place as 10 times greater in immobilized cell cultures than in control suspension cultures.

Allied drugs

Japanese Chillies (*C. frutescens*) are about 3-4 cm long. They are usually free from pedicels and cali-ces and have a bright red pericarp. They possess about one-quarter of the pungency of the African Chillies.

Bombay Capsicums (*C. annuum* L.). The pericarp is thicker and tougher than in the chillies, and the pedicel is frequently bent. They are much less pungent than African chillies.

Natal Capsicums are larger than the Bombay variety, being up to 8 cm long. They have a very bright red, transparent pericarp. They are much less pungent than chillies.

Uses

Capsicum has been used externally as stimulant, counter irritant, rubefacient, in sore throat, scar-latina, hoarseness and yellow fever. Internally it is used as carminative, stomachic, atonic dyspepsia and flatulence. In the form of ointment, plaster and medicated wool it is used for the relief of rheumatism and lumbago. Capsaicin is used for the treatment of migraine and cluster headache, and for some patients with neurogenic bladder dysfunction.

Pharmacology

Capsaicin caused transient rise in blood pressure in dogs, whereas in rabbits it caused hypotension. It impaired heat-reinforced behaviour in rats, attenuated analgesic effect of morphine in rats and did not affect morphine analgesia. Capsaicin released acetylcholine from isolated myenteric plexus longitudinal muscle strips of guinea pig ileum. Capsaicin pretreatment reduced gastric acid secretion elicited by s.c. injection of histamine. It caused rapid fall in blood pressure, induced pressor response in pithed rats and induced contractile response in isolated guinea pig trachea. Capsaicin markedly inhibited responsiveness of platelets to aggregation by agonists.

DAMIANA

Damiana consists of the dried leaves of *Turnera diffusa* var. *aphrodisiaca* (Turneraceae), and other species of *Turnera*. The plant is found in Bolivia and Mexico. The leaves are yellowish-green to green in colour, broadly lanceolate, shortly petiolate, and 10-25 cm long; margin with 3-6 teeth on each side; veins pinnate and prominent on the lower surface. The drug consists of the reddish-brown, cylindrical twigs, flowers and spherical fruits. Damiana has an aromatic odour and taste. It contains 0.5-1.0% of volatile oil composed thymol, α-copaene, δ-cadinene and calamenenes; a brown amorphous substance, damianin, resins and gum.

Uses

Damiana is used in Mexico and southern USA to revive libido with subconscious causative factors. Elixir of Damiana and Saw Palmetto are used as an aphrodisiac for men.

GAMBOGE

Gamboge is a gum-resin obtained from *Garcinia hanburii* (Clusiaceae), a tree native to South-East Asia.

Spiral incisions are made in the bark and the exudate is collected in the internode of a large bamboo. It solidifies in about a month. The bamboos are then heated until they crack and the gamboge is removed.

Gambogs is a gum-resin. It forms a yellow emulsion with water. Gamboge contains 70-80% of resin (gambogic acid) and 15-20% of water-soluble gum along with an oxidase enzyme. Gamboge acts as a purgative and as a pigment.

MASTIC

Mastic is an oleoresin containing little oil, obtained from a cultivated variety of *Pistacia lentiscus* var. *chia* (Anacardiaceae) in the Greek island of Chios. The plant is an evergreen dioecious shrub.

Tapping is done from July to October. The stem and larger branches are wounded by means of a gouge-like instrument to make an incision about 2 cm long and 3 mm deep. Each plant is tapped repeatedly for about 5 to 6 weeks, making 200-300 wounds. A special tool is used for removing the tears which harden on the plant. These are graded, washed and dried before being exported in wooden boxes. Chios exports about 2,50,000 kg annually.

Mastic occurs in yellow or greenish-yellow rounded or pear-shaped tears about 3 mm diameter. The tears are brittle but become plastic when chewed. Odour, slightly balsamic; taste, mildly terebinthinate.

The resin contains tri-, tetra- and pentacyclic triterpene acids and alcohols. Over 60 compounds have been reported from mastic and up to 250 recorded in plant oils (2%). The principal components are α-pinene, β-myrcene and camphene. The acid value is about 50. East Indian or Bombay mastic has an acid value of more than 100.

Mastic is used in the preparation of Compound Mastic Paint and as a microscopical mountant.

SANDARAC

Sandarac is a resin obtained from the stem of *Tetraclinis articulata* (Cupressaceae), a tree 6-12 m high, found in North and North-West Africa and in Spain

Sandarac occurs in small tears; 0.5-1.5 cm in length; having elongated, stalactic or cylindrical shape, globular or pear-shaped tears. The surface is covered with a yellowish dust, but the interior is transparent, and contains small insects. The drug is easily powdered and when chewed remains gritty, showing no tendency to form a plastic mass. The drug has a faint, terebinthinate odour, and a bitter taste.

Sandarac resin consists of sandarocopimaric acid (inactive pimaric acid), sandaracinic acid, sandaracinolic acid, sandaracoresene a bitter pirnciple and 0.26-1.3% of volatile oil.

GRINDELIA

Grindelia or gum plant consists of the dried leaves and flowering tops of *Grindelia camporum* (*G. robusta*), *G. humilis* and *G. squarrosa* (Asteraceae), found in the south-western USA. The plants are herbs with cylindrical stems, sessile or amplexicaul leaves, and resinous flower-heads surrounded by an involucre of linear-lanceolate bracts. Odour, balsamic; taste, aromatic and bitter.

Grindelia contains about 20% of resin, which consists of labdane diterpene acids known as grindelanes and methyl esters. The plants yield about 0.2% of a volatile oil containing over 100 components; bornyl acetate and α-pinene are the major components of the monoterpenoid fraction.

The herb is used to treat bronchitis and asthma and in the form of a lotion for dermatitis produced by the poison ivy, *Rhus toxicodendron* (Anacardiaceae). Some grindelanes show antifeeding deterrent activity towards aphids.

GUAIACUM RESIN

Guaiacum resin is obtained from the heartwood of *Guaiacum officinale* and *G. sanctum* (Zygophyllaceae), small evergreen trees. *G. officinale* is found on the coast of Venezuela and Colombia and in the West Indies, while *G. sanctum* occurs in Cuba, Haiti, the Bahamas and Florida.

Guaiacum resin occurs in large blocks or rounded tears; 2-3 cm diameter. The freshly fractured surface is brown and glassy. The powder is greyish but becomes green on exposure; taste, acrid; odour aromatic. Guaiacum is soluble in alcohol, chloroform and solutions of alkalies. An alcoholic solution gives a deep blue colour (guaiac-blue) on the addition of oxidizing agents such as ferric chloride. This colour is destroyed by reducing agents. Colophony, an adulterant, is detected by the cupric acetate test.

Some of the main resinous constituents are lignans having a C_{18} structure formed from two C_6-C_3 units. Guaiaretic acid (10%) is a diaryl butane.

The flowers, fruit and bark of the tree contain triperpenoid and nortriterpenoid saponins.

An alcoholic solution of the resin is used for the detection of blood stains, cyanogenetic glycosides, oxidase and peroxidase enzymes.

Guaiacum resin is used to treat chronic rheumatic conditions. It is a permitted food additive in the USA and in Europe.

OLIBANUM

Olibanum (*Frankincense*) is an oleo-gum-resin obtained by incision from the bark of *Boswellia carterii, B. frereana* and other species of *Boswellia* (Burseraceae). These are small trees native to north-eastern Africa and Arabia. The drug is present in ovoid tears, 5-25 mm long, sometimes stuck together. The surface is dusty and of a yellowish, bluish or greenish tint. Fracture, brittle; inner surface waxy and semitranslucent. Odour is characteristic, especially when burned; taste, slightly bitter. The drug contains 3-8% of volatile oil consisting of mainly *p*-cymene and sesquiterpenes, about 60-70% of resin, and 27-35% of gum. The gum contains two polysaccharides; one composed of units of galactose and arabinose and the other of galactose and galacturonic acid. Olibanum is used in incense and fumigating preparations and as a stimulant in China for the treatment of leprosy. It shows a positive anti-inflammatory activity.

Proteins and Enzymes

Proteins are highly complex molecules which contain the elements of carbon, hydrogen, nitrogen, and usually sulphur. They are synthesized by living cells and are an essential part of the structure of the cell and its nucleus. Whole glandular products, oil-bearing plant seeds, antitoxins, serums, and globulins contain proteins in combination with other biochemical substances—all these substances possess therapeutic activity. The plant proteins are easily isolated in crystalline form. Proteins are stored in plants in the form of aleurone grains. They are required for animals as the source of nitrogen in food.

The molecular weight of most proteins can be estimated only approximately by centrifugal sedi-mentation methods for soluble proteins, which vary from few thousand to many millions. Other methods are osmotic pressure measurements, X-ray diffraction, light scattering effects, gel filtration and chemical analysis.

Soluble proteins form colloidal solutions which are generally viscous and may form gel. Many of them (*e.g.*, egg albumin) are coagulated by heat or by action of acids, alkalies or certain chemicals or by U.V. light. This process is known as 'denaturation' in which solubility of the protein is decreased.

Proteins are hydrolyzed to form simpler subs-tances and ultimately amino acids. The hydrolytic process takes place during digestion by proteolytic enzymes or in laboratory by hot acids or alkalies :

Protein → Polypeptide → Peptide → Amino acids

Proteins are built up from amino acids linked together in chains or rings. The carboxylic group of one molecule is condensed with an amino group of the adjacent molecule with the formation of the amino linkage commonly known as peptide linkage.

Natural compounds formed in this way are called as 'polypeptides' if they have molecular weight below 10,000. Molecules with molecular weight above ~ 10,000 are known as proteins. In general, proteins and polypeptides differ in chemical and physical properties. Both type of compounds often exhibit physiological activity as in case of enzymes and hormones.

Proteins may be classified as :

(i) Fibrous proteins which serve as structural materials for animals, e.g., collagen, horn, feathers, nails, fibroin (silk), and

(ii) Globular proteins which are soluble in water, dilute acids and alkalies, *e.g.*, egg albumin and serum albumin.

In another classification proteins are divided as:

(i) Simple proteins, which yield only amino acid on hydrolysis, e.g., protamines, albumin and globulins.

(ii) Conjugated proteins, which contain a non-protein group, known as prosthetic group, *e.g.*, nucleoproteins, lipoproteins, and metalloproteins, and

(iii) Derived proteins, which are the degradation products obtained by the action of acids, alkalies or enzymes on proteins. For example, denatured proteins, meta-proteins, secondary proteoses, peptones, polypeptides, simple peptides and amino acids are the derived proteins.

Since proteins are present in all living organisms, they are of great importance in biochemistry. They form an important class of food, *e.g.*, meat, fish and egg are important source of animal proteins. Cereal grains, *e.g.*, wheat and pulses are plant protein foods. Whole glandular products, oil-bearing plant seeds, antitoxins, serums, and globulins contain proteins in combination with other biochemical substances. These products possess therapeutic activity. Allergens are usually proteinaceous materials producing allergic reactions.

Certain proteins are highly poisonous. Among them are plant toxalbumins, ricin from castor beans, robin from locust bark, abrin from jequirty seeds, hemolysins from salamanders and various toxins, *e.g.*, neurotoxoids from snake venum.

Proteins act as defence chemicals, include cell wall glycoproteins (hydroxyproline-rich, proline-rich, and glycine-rich glycoproteins); inhibitory proteins (many are induced and endogenous antiviral proteins, antifungal lipid transfer proteins, antibacterial α-thionins); lectins (which are carbohydrate-binding proteins); antioomycete pathogenesis-related protein, and anti-fungal defensin proteins; extracellular hydrolases (*e.g.*, cellulases, pectinases, chitinases, ribonucleases, proteases, and lipid acyl hydrolases such as patatins); and ribosome-inactivating proteins such as trichosanthin in the Chinese cucumber plant, *Trichosanthes kiriliowii*).

Properties of proteins

Proteins are amphoteric in nature. At some definite pH, characteristic for each protein, the positive and negative charges are exactly balanced and the molecules do not migrate in an electrical field. The condition is known as 'isoelectric point' and at this pH the protein has its least solubility. All proteins are optically active and may be coagulated and precipitated from aqueous solution.

Colour reactions

Proteins exhibit a variety of colour reactions, *e.g.*:

1. *Biuret reaction* : To alkaline solution of a protein (2 ml), a dilute solution of copper sulphate is added. A red or violet colour is formed with peptides containing at least two peptide linkages. A dipeptide does not give this test.
2. *Xanthoproteic reaction* : Proteins usually form a yellow colour when warmed with concentrated nitric acid. This colour becomes orange when the solution is made alkaline. The colour is due to nitration of aromatic ring present in phenylalanine, tyrosine and tryptophan.
3. *Millon's reaction* : Millon's reagent (mercuric nitrate in nitric acid containing a trace of nitrous acid) usually yields a white precipitate on addition to a protein solution which turns red on heating. This reaction is characteristic of phenols (*e.g.*, the phenolic amino acid tyrosine).
4. *Ninhydrin test* : To an aqueous solution of a protein an alcoholic solution of ninhydrin is added and then heated. Red to violet colour is formed.
5. *Nitroprusside test* : Proteins containing sulphur group form red colour with nitroprusside solution.
6. *Lead sulphide test* : Alkaline solution of sulphur containing proteins, on addition to lead acetate, produces a black precipitate.

GELATIN

Synonyms

Gelfoam; Puragel; Gelatinum.

Biological source

Gelatin is a heterogenous mixture of water-soluble proteins of high average molecular weight obtained by treating specific animal tissues like skin, tendons, ligaments and bones with hot water. Gelatin is not found in nature but derived from collagen by hydrolytic action.

Preparation

For preparation of Geltain, the insoluble collagens are converted into soluble gelatin which is then purified and concentrated to a solid form. Commercially, gelatin is obtained from by-products of slaughtered cattle, sheep and hogs. The starting materials, *e.g.*, bones, are defatted with an organic solvent. Sometimes these are decalcified with hydrochloric acid. The material is then heated with water at 85°C to convert collagens to Gelatin. The solution is decolourized, filtered by electro-osmosis, concentrated under reduced pressure, allowed to set into gel in shallow trays and dried rapidly in drying rooms at 30°, 40°, 50° and 60°C for some weeks.

Characters

Gelatin occurs as a colourless or slightly yellow, transparent, brittle, practically odourless, tasteless sheet, flakes or course grannular powder. In water it swells and absorbs 5-10 times its weight of water to form a gel in solutions below 35-40°. It is insoluble in cold water and organic solvents, soluble in hot water, glycerol, acetic acid; and is amphoteric. In dry condition it is stable in air, but when moist or in solution, it is attacked by bacteria. The gelatinizing property of Gelatin is reduced by boiling for long time. The quality of gelatin is determined on the basis of its jelly strength (Bloom strength) with the help of a Bloom gelometer. Jelly strength is used in the preparation of suppositories and pessaries.

Commercially two types of gelatin, A and B, are available. Type A has an isoelectric point between pH 7 and 9. It is incompatible with anionic compounds such as Acacia, Agar and Tragacanth. Type B has an isoelectric point between 4.7 and 5 and it is used with anionic mixtures. Gelatin is coloured with a certified colour for manufacturing capsules or for coating of tablets. It may contain various additives.

Chemical constituents

Gelatin consists of the protein glutin which on hydrolysis gives a mixture of amino acids. The approximate amino acid contents are : glycine (25.5%), alanine (8.7%), valine (2.5%), leucine (3.2%), isoleucine (1.4%), cystine and cysteine (0.1%), methionine (1.0%), tyrosine (0.5%), aspartic acid (6.6%), glutamic acid (11.4%), arginine (8.1%), lysine (4.1%) and histidine (0.8%). Nutritionally, gelatin is an incomplete protein lacking tryptophan. The gelatinizing compound is known as chondrin and the adhesive nature of Gelatin is due to the presence of glutin.

Uses

Gelatin is used to prepare pastilles, pastes, suppositories, capsules, pill-coatings, gelatin sponge; as suspending agent, tablet binder, coating agent, as stabilizer, thickener and texturizer in food; for manufacturing rubber substitutes, adhesives, cements, lithographic and printing inks, plastic compounds, artificial silk, photographic plates and films, matches, light filters for mercury lamps; clarifying agent; in hectographic matters; sizing paper and textiles; for inhibiting crystallization in bacteriology, for preparing cultures and as a nutrient.

It forms glycerinated gelatin with glycerin which is used as vehicle and for manufacture of suppositories. Combined with zinc, it forms zinc gelatin which is employed as a topical protectant. As a nutrient, Gelatin is used as commercial food products and bacteriologic culture media.

Absorable gelatin sponge

It is a a water-insoluble gelatin based sterile sponge. It is prepared from purified, specially treated gelatin to form a light, white porous, pliable, non-antigenic matrix. It is sterilized by heat. It absorbs about 50 times its weight of water and about 45 times its weight of blood. It is a local haemostatic and used to control capillary oozing, bleeding of veins and operative wounds. The sponge is applied to the bleeding area, held for about 15 seconds and left.

Absorbable gelatin film

It is a specially prepared cellophane-type gelatin product in neurosurgery and in thoracic and ocular surgery. It consists of a thin, nonantigenic, pliable absorbable film of purified gelatin. It occurs in pieces of about 2.5 × 5 cm or 10 × 12.5 cm in size and about 0.075 mm in thickness. It is moistened by immersion in salt solution for cutting into the shape required to fit into the contours of the incision.

Chemical test

1. Biuret test is positive.
2. Xanthoproteic test is positive.
3. Millons test is positive.
4. Ninhydrin test is positive.

5. On heating Gelatin (1 g) with soda lime, smell of ammonia is produced.
6. A solution of Gelatin (0.5 g) in water (10 ml) is precipitated to white buff coloured precipitate on addition of few drops of tannic acid (10%).
7. With picric acid Gelatin forms yellow precipitate.

Microfibrillar collagen

Microfibrillar collagen is a fibrous, water-insoluble material prepared from purified bovine corium collagen. It is an absorbable, topical hemostatic agent that is used in surgical procedures when control of bleeding by ligature or other conventional means is ineffective or impractical. It is applied dry and directly onto the bleeding surface; the microfibrillar collagen attracts platelets that adhere to the fibrils and trigger the formation of thrombi.

ENZYMES

Enzymes are organic catalysts produced in the body by living organisms. They perform many complex chemical reactions that make up life processes. Enzymes are lifeless and when isolated, they still exert their characteristic catalytic effect. Their chemical composition varies and they do show several common properties. They are colloids, soluble in water and dilute alcohol but are precipitated by concentrated alcohol. Most enzymes act best at temperatures between 35 and 40°C; temperatures above 65°C, especially in the presence of moisture, destroy them, whereas their activity is negligible at 0°C. Certain heavy metals, formaldehyde, and free iodine retard the enzymes activity. Their activity is markedly affected by the pH of the medium in which they act or by the presence of other substances in this medium. They are highly selective in their action.

The enzymes are proteins having molecular weight from about 13,000 to 840,000. At present they are divided according to their action by a complex system established by the Commission on Enzymes of the International Union of Biochemistry. Six major classes are recognized; each has 4 to 13 subclasses, and each enzyme is assigned a systematic code number (E.C.) composed of 4 digits. The major classes are as follows :

1. *Oxidoreductases* : These enzymes catalyze oxidoreductions between 2 substances.
2. *Transferases* : These enzymes catalyze a transfer of a group, other than hydrogen, between a pair of substrates.
3. *Hydrolases* : These enzymes catalyze hydrolysis of ester, ether, peptide, glycosyl, acid-anhydride, C-C, C-halide, or P-N bonds.
4. *Lyases* : These enzymes catalyze removal of groups from substrates by mechanisms other than hydrolysis, leaving double bonds.
5. *Isomerases* : These enzymes catalyze interconversion of optic, geometric, or positional isomers.
6. *Ligases* : These enzymes catalyze linkage of 2 compounds coupled to the breaking of a pyrophosphate bond in ATP or a similar compound.

The well-known trivial names ordinarily used in the pharmaceutic literature are :

1. *Esterases*, including lipase, phospholipase, acetylcholinesterase and others.
2. *Carbohydrases*, including diastase, lactase, maltase, invertase, cellulase, hyaluronidase, glucuronidase, lysozyme and others.
3. *Nucleases*, including ribonuclease, desoxyribonuclease, nucleophosphatase & others.
4. *Nuclein deaminases*, including adenase, adenosine deaminase and others.
5. *Amidases*, including argniase, urease and others.
6. *Proteolytic enzymes*, including pepsin, trypsin, chymotrypsin, papain, fibrinolysin, streptokinase, urokinase and others.

Enzymes are found in combination with inorganic or organic substances that have an important part in the catalytic action. If these are nonprotein organic compounds, they are known as coenzymes. If they are *inorganic* ions, they are referred to as *activators*. Coenzymes are integral components of a large number of enzyme systems. Several vitamins (thiamine, riboflavin, nicotinic acid) have a coenzymatic function.

Enzymes are obtained from plant and animal cells and many have been purified. They are used as therapeutic agents and as controlling factors in certain chemical reactions in industry. Pepsin, pancreatin and papain are used therapeutically as digestants. Hyaluronidase facilitates the diffusion of injected fluids. Streptokinase and streptodornase dissolve clotted blood and purulent accumulations. Zymase and rennin are used in the fermentation and cheese industries; and penicillinase inactivates the various penicillins.

The names used to designate enzymes usually end in -ase or -in. The important enzymes are given hereunder.

YEAST

Synonyms

Dried yeast; Cerevisiae fermentum; Faex medicinalis.

Biological source

Yeast are unicellular organisms, consists of the cells of a suitable strain of *Saccharomyces cerevisiae* Hansen (Fam. Saccharomycetaceae) dried to preserve the vitamins present.

Collection and preparation

Yeast are commercially available as 'Brewer's yeast' which is viscid, semifluid frothy mass and consists of living cells of *S. cerevisiae* and related species. 'Compressed yeast' is the purer strain of yeast, partially dried by expression of water and admixed with a starch. 'Dried yeast' is the dried cells of *S. cerevisiae*. Dried yeast is usually obtained as a by-product from the brewing beer made from an extract of cereal grains and hops. The yeast cells are washed to free beer and dried, and may be debittered. Dried yeast may also be obtained by growing suitable strains of yeast, using media other than those required for the production of beer, and under appropriate environmental conditions. Dried yeast is obtained by heating the compressed yeast at 30°C until the moisture content is reduced to below 9%.

Brewer's yeast or torula yeast, *Candida utilis* (Henneberg) Loder and Kreger-Van Rij (Fam. Cryptococcaceae), is grown in suitable nutrient media in large fermentation tanks, and the cell mass is recovered. If the cell mass is a by-product of beer production, the cells must be washed thoroughly, usually using one or more alkaline solutions, to re-move the insoluble acidic bitter resins from the hops. The yeast cells are dried and marketed as a granular powder or compressed tablets.

Characters

Dried yeast occurs as a pale buff to weak yellowish orange flakes, granules or powder with characteristic indicative odour. Due to the presence of dead cells, dried yeast is inactive in fermentation process.

Under the microscope it shows spherical, elliptical or ovate cells up to 8 µm long, some showing budding. They are transparent and have a cell wall enclosing a granular protoplasm in which are one or two glycogen vacuoles. The nucleus exists as a small mass near the centre of the cell and cannot usually be seen without the use of a special staining procedure. Yeast should contain no starchy material.

Chemical constituents

The principal compounds of yeast are vitamins of 'B-group' such as aneurine, nicotinic acid, riboflavine, folic acid and B_{12}. In addition to these yeast contains proteins (46%), carbohydrates (36%) particularly glycogen, fats, sterols and enzymes like zymase complex, glucogenase, invertase, maltase, emulsin and diastase, nucleoproteins. It is a rich source of biologically complete protein and is used in the manufacture of nucleic acid. Torula yeast, derived from *Candida utilis* (Cryptococcaceae), contains about 45% of protein and is rich in vitamins.

In molecular genetics *S. cerevisiae* has been utilized as a suitable organism for the over-expression of active enzymes of other plants and of animals (*e.g.*, hirudin of the medicinal leech).

Uses

Yeast is used as dietary source of B vitamins and proteins, and in the treatment of furunculosis. Mostly yeast is used in baking bread, brewing; producing alcohol by fermentation of sugar, molasses and cereals.

DIASTASE (MALT EXTRACT)

Synonyms

Maltin, Diastase of malt, Maltase.

Biological source

Diastase is a mixture of amylolytic enzymes obtained from malt.

Malt is obtained by artificially germinated barley grains, *Hordeum vulgare* Linn. (Fam. Poaceae). Barley is grown throughout the world in favourable climate. For preparing malt, wet barley grains in heaps are kept in warm room for germination until the caulicle protrudes. The grain is dried quickly to kill the embryo. The enzyme diastase in the moist warm grains converts starch to maltose which stimulates the embryo for germination. Dry malt contains maltose sugar (50-70%), dextrins (2-15%), proteins (8%), diastase and peptase enzyme. It resembles barley but is more crisp with an agreeable odour and sweet taste. It is used mainly in the brewing and alcohol industries.

Malt extract is prepared by extracting the partially germinating grains of *H. vulgare*. It contains dextrin, maltose, glucose and amylolytic enzymes. Diastase converts at least 50 times of its weight of potato starch into sugars (dextrin and maltose) in 30 minutes.

Diastase is a yellowish white amorphous powder or translucent scales obtained from an infusion of malt. It loses amylolytic power on keeping, on heating its solution at 85°, or on adding excess of acid. It is soluble in water with some turbidity; almost insoluble in alcohol.

Diastase is used to manufacture starch, converting starch into sugar and to remove starch from fabrics.

Dry malt resembles barley but is more crisp, has an agreeable odour, and has a sweet taste. It contains 50 to 70% of the sugar, maltose; 2 to 15% of dextrins; 8% of proteins; diastase; and a peptase enzyme.

Malt is used extensively in the brewing and alcohol industries.

Malt extract is the product obtained by extracting malt, the partially and artificially germinated grain of one or more varieties of *Hordeum vulgare*. The malt is infused with water at 60°C, preferably under reduced pressure.

Malt extract may be mixed with 10%, by weight of glycerin. It contains dextrin, maltose, a small amount of glucose and amylolytic enzymes. It can convert not less than 5 times its weight of starch into water-soluble sugars.

Malt extract is used as an easily digested nutritive and as an aid in digesting starch. Many commercial extracts of malt do not contain diastase, which is destroyed by the heat used for their sterilization. They are used as bulk-producing laxatives.

Diastase and amylase are well-known amylolytic enzymes. Salivary diastase or *ptyalin* and pancreatic diastase or *amylopsin* are found in the digestive tract of animals; they are called "animal diastase". *Malt diastase* is most active in solutions that are approximately neutral; acidity of pH 4 destroys the enzyme.

Invertase or sucrase, found in yeast and in the intestinal juices; hydrolyzes sucrose into glucose and fructose. *Maltase*, converts maltose into glucose and is found in yeast and the intestinal juices.

Zymase is a fermenting enzyme causing the conversion of monosaccharides (glucose, fructose) into alcohol and carbon dioxide.

Emulsin, an enzyme found in almonds, causes the hydrolysis of β-glucosides; thus, amygdalin is hydrolyzed into glucose, benzaldehyde and hydrogen cyanide.

Myrosin is found in white and black mustard. It hydrolyzes sinalbin, sinigrin and other glycosides.

The esterases

Lipase is a lipolytic enzyme present in the animal and vegetable kingdoms. It is found in the pancreatic juice of animals and in oily seeds. Lipase hydrolyzes fats into glycerin and fatty acids.

Pectase splits pectin into pectic acid and methyl dietary fat.

Urease is obtained from soybeans and is used as a laboratory reagent for converting urea to ammonia.

PAPAIN

Synonyms

Papayotin; Vegetable pepsin; Arbuz; Nematolyt; Caroid; Summetrin; Tromasin; Velardon; Vermizym.

Biological source

Papain is the dried and purified latex of the green

fruits and leaves of *Carica papaya* L. (Fam. Caricaceae). The plant is cultivated in Sri Lanka, Tanzania, Hawai and Florida. The plant is 5-6 m in height bearing fruits of about 30 cm length and a weight up to 5 kg. The epicarp adheres to the orange-coloured, fleshy sarcocarp, which surrounds the central cavity. This cavity contains a mass of nearly black seeds.

Preparation

It is distributed throughout the plant, but mostly concentrated in the latex of the fruit.

The latex is obtained by making 2-4 longitudinal incisions, about 1/8 inch deep, on the surface on four sides of nearly mature but green fruits while still on the tree. The incisions are made early in the morning, at intervals of 3-7 days. The latex flows freely for a few seconds but soon coagulates. The exudate is collected in non-metallic containers. The latex is dried as soon as possible after collection. Rapid drying or exposure to sun or higher temperature above 38°C produce dark colour product with weak in proteolytic activity. The use of artificial heat yields the better grade of crude papain. The final product should be creamy white and friable. It is sealed in air-tight containers to prevent loss of activity. If 10% common salt or 1% solution of formaldehyde is added before drying, the product retains its activity for many months.

Fully grown fruits give more latex of high enzyme potency than smaller or immature fruits. The yield of Papain varies from 20 to 250 g per tree. The yield of commercial Papain from latex is about 20%.

Papain can also be obtained from the juice of stems, leaves and petioles. The enzyme has nearly the same activity as that obtained from the fruit latex.

A highly active product is purified by dissolving the commercial product in water, saturating with hydrogen sulphide, precipitating with alcohol and drying the precipitate at low temperature.

Commercial Papain is often adulterated with arrowroot starch, dried milk of cactus, gutta percha, rice flour and pepsin. Bleaching is done for improving the colour, but this lowers the enzyme activity of the product.

Papain possesses both milk clotting and protein digesting properties. The milk clotting property is lost through oxidation with hydrogen peroxide and is regained on reduction with hydrogen cyanide or hydrogen sulphide. The pepton hydrolyzing activity is lost on oxidation with hydrogen peroxide and is regained on reduc-tion. Oxidation, however, does not affect the Gelatin hydrolyzing activity.

Papain has been referred to as "vegetable pepsin" because it contains enzymes somewhat similar to pepsin; however, unlike pepsin, papain acts in acid, neutral or alkaline media.

Characters

Papain occurs as white or greyish-white, slightly hydroscope powder. It is incompletely soluble in water and glycerol. It may digest about 35 times its weight of lean meat. Best grades render digestion of 200-300 times their weight of coagulated egg albumin in alkaline media. A temperature range of 60-90° is favourable for the digestive process with 65° the optimum point. Best pH is 5.0, but it functions also in neutral or alkaline media. It is activated by reduction (HCN and H_2S) and inactivated by oxidation (H_2O_2, iodoacetate).

Chemical constituents

Papain contains several enzymes such as proteolytic enzymes peptidase I capable of converting proteins into dipeptides and polypeptides, rennin-like enzyme, clotting enzyme similar to pectase and an enzyme having a feeble activity on fats.

The enzymes, papain, papayaproteinase and chymopapain, have been isolated in crystalline form from the latex. Papain is a typical protein digesting enzyme with isoelectric point. It contains 15.5% nitrogen and 1.2% sulphur. Crystalline Papain is most stable in the pH range 5-7 and is rapidly destroyed at 30° below pH 2.5 and above pH 12. Papain is a protein of 212 amino acids and having a molecular weight of about 23,000 daltons. It is resistant to heat, inactivated by metal ions, oxidants and reagents which react with thiols, and is an endopeptidase activated by thiols and reducing moieties, e.g., cysteine, thiosulphate and glutathione.

The leaves possess dehydrocarpaines I and II, fatty acids, carpaine, pseudocarpaine and carotenoids.

The fruits yield lauric, myristoleic, palmitoleic and arachidic acids, malonated benzyl-β-D-glucosides, 2-phenyl ethyl glucoside and 4-hydroxyphenyl-2-ethyl glucoside.

Uses

Papain is used to prevent adhesions; in infected wounds; internally as protein digestant, as anthelmintic (nemotode), to relieve the symptoms of episiotomy (incision of vulva), in meat industry for tenderizing beef, for treatment of dyspepsia, intestinal and gastric disorders, and diphtheria, for dissolving diphtheria membrane; in surgery to reduce incidence of blood clots where thromboplasma is undesirable and for local treatment of buccal, pharyngeal and laryngeal disorders.

It is used in digestive mixtures, liver tonics, for reducing enlarged tonsils, in prevention of post-operative adhesions, curbuncles and eschar burns. It is an allergic agent causing severe paroxysmal cough, vasomotor rhinitis and dyspnea. It is a powerful poison when injected intra-venously. In industry it is used in the manufacture of proteolytic preparations of meat, lever and casein, with dilute alcohol and lactic acid as meat tenderizer, as a substitute for rennet in cheese manufacture, in brewing industry for making chill-proof bear, for degumming natural milk, in prepa-ration of tooth pastes and cosmetics, in tanning industry for bathing skin and hides, and as an ingredient in cleansing solutions for soft contact lenses.

Test

Papain is reacted with a gelatin solution at 80°C in the presence of an activating cysteine chloral hydrate solution for an hour. The solution is cooled to 4°C for long time. The treated solution must not regel in comparison to a blank solution under identical conditions.

For assay, an aqueous suspension of papain is titrated at pH 7 and at 25°C in the presence of cysteine chlorohydrate by maintaining the pH with addition of sodium hydroxide. It is titrated while the enzyme esterase releases acid. The hydrolysis rates of the ethyl ester of benzoylarginine of papain to be tested and of a reference latex are compared. A microbial contamination test for total viable aerobic microorganisms *Escherichia coli, Salmonella,* *Pseudomonas aeruginose* and *Staphylococcus aureus* should be in limits.

Pharmacology

Carpaine showed antitumour activity against mouse lymphoid leukaemia, lymphocytic leukaemia and Ehrlich ascites tumor cells. It decreased systolic, diastolic and mean arterial blood pressure in rats. Carpaine caused dilatation of skin blood vessels, hypotension and cardiostimulation.

CHYMOPAPAIN

Chymopapain is a nonpyrogenic proteolytic enzyme obtained from the latex of *Carica papaya* Linn. (Fam. Caricaceae). It is a sulfhydryl enzyme similar to papain with respect to substrate specificities but differing in electrophoretic mobility, stability and solubility.

It is used to treat herniated lumbar intervertebral discs. Chymopapain is injected into the nucleus pulposus to hydrolyze the noncolla-genous polypeptides or proteins that maintain the tertiary structure of the chondromucoprotein. This relieves the compressive symptoms of lower back pain by lessening osmotic activity and thereby decreasing fluid absorption and reducing intra-discal pressure.

This treatment is successful in about 75% of the patients. The unit of chymopapain activity is the nanoKatal (nKat), and 1 mg of the enzyme contains at least 0.52 nKat units.

BROMELAIN

Synonyms

Bromelin; Ananase; Extranse; Inflamen; Traumanase.

Biological source

Bromelain is a protein-digesting and milk clotting enzyme found in pineapple fruit juice and stem tissues of *Ananas comosus* (L.) Merr. (Family : Bromeliaceae).

Enzymes from fruit juice and stem tissue are distinguished as fruit Bromelain and stem Bromelain. From pineapple juice the enzyme is obtained by precipitation with acetone and also with ammonium sulphate. Stem Bromelain has molecular weight of about 33,000 and is probably the first proteolytic enzyme of plant origin to be established as a glycoprotein.

Unlike Papain, fruit Bromelain does not disappear as the fruit ripens. Fruit and stem Bromelains are acidic and basic proteins, respectively.

Bromelain is used as adjunctive therapy to reduce inflammation and edema and to accelerate tissue repair after episiotomy. Bromelain is also used to produce protein hydrolysates, in tenderizing meats, in leather industry and as chill proofing agent in beer.

It is also used as food additive and bating reagent of hides. It is useful in determining antibody substances, dissolving necrogenic tissues, treating digestive troubles; when applied as an antiphlogistic it shows less after-effects.

Pineapple volatile oil contains ethyl acetate, ethyl 3-(methylthio) propanoate and butane-2,3-diol diacetate.

Pharmacology

Juice of unripe fruits showed marked anti-implantation and abortifacient activities in rats. Bromelain inhibited growth of Lewis lung carcinoma, YC-8 lymphoma and MCA-1 ascites tumor cells. Its cytotoxic effects were abolished by heating at 100°C or by addition of aspirin.

FICIN

Synonyms

Ficus proteinase; Ficus protease; Debricin; Higheroxyl delabarre.

Biological source

Ficin is a concentrate prepared by filtering and drying the latex of *Ficus glabrata* (Fam. Moraceae). It is a proteolytic enzyme of molecular weight about 23,800-25,500 which requires a free sulphydryl group for activity and as such as a member of a group which includes Papain and Bromelain.

Ficin occurs as a buff to cream-coloured hygroscopic powder. It has acrid odour, which grows stronger with age. It is bulky, nearly 3 ml/g, not free-flowing. It appears dry, even when 15% water is present. It is not completely soluble in water; insoluble in usual solvents. It loses about 10-20%

activity when stored 1-3 years at ordinary temperature and atmospheric conditions. Aqueous solutions are inactivated at 100°, solid partially inactivated within a few hours. Solutions are relatively stable between pH 4-8.5; incompatible with iron, copper and aluminium. The most proteins are hydrolyzed with aqueous Ficin solution. Ficin has tissue - dissolving property. Therefore, it must be handled with care. Ficin is 10-20 times more active as Papain in regard to milk clotting; 4-10 times as active in general.

Ficin, a mixture of proteases, is used as protein digestant in the brewing industry, as a chill-proofing agent in beer; in cheese industry as a substitute for rennet in the coagulation of milk; in meat industry as a meat tenderizer and as an agent for removing castings from formed sausage. In leather industry it is used for the bating of leather; in the textile industry for shrink proofing wool, for removing gelatin from sized thread, and mixed with amylases and maltases as a spot remover. It is also used in the preparation of peptones, for determining protein material in spent grains and in determination of the Rh factor. It speeds 10 times the agglutination of human blood cells by the Rh factor when in contact with the anti-Rh serum. It has been used as a trichuricide.

Ficin causes irritation to skin, eyes and mucous membranes. Large doses by mouth cause purging.

Proteolytic enzymes

Pepsin is a proteolytic enzyme present in the gastric juice. It is most active at a pH of about 1.8, but in neutral or alkaline media, pepsin is entirely inactive. It converts proteins into proteoses and peptones.

Trypsin is formed by the action of the proenzyme, trypsinogen, on the enterokinase of the intestinal juices. Trypsin is a proteolytic enzyme that is considerably more active than pepsin, converting proteoses and peptones into polypeptides and amino acids. It acts best in an alkaline medium of about pH 8 and may thus be distinguished from pepsin, which acts only in acid media.

Erepsin is a proteolytic enzyme also present in the intestinal juices. It converts proteoses and peptones into amino acids.

Rennin is a coagulating enzyme which occurs

in the mucous membrane of the stomach of mammals. It curdles the soluble casein of milk.

Papain is a mixture of active proteolytic enzymes found in the unripe fruit of the papaya tree. It is a meat tenderizer.

Oxidizing enzymes

Peroxidases are present in plants. They bring about the oxidation reactions that cause the discoloration of bruised fruits.

Thrombin converts the fibrinogen of the circulating blood into the insoluble fibrin of the blood clot.

Zymase is an oxidizing enzyme because the monosaccharide is splitted by oxidation.

Lactase is an enzyme that hydrolyzes lactose to galactose and glucose. It is obtained commercially from the yeast, *Saccharomyces lactis*, and is used as a powder to help patients with lactose intolerance to digest the lactose in milk or milk products.

PEPSIN

Pepsin contains a proteolytic enzyme obtained from the glandular layer of the fresh stomach of the hog, *Sus scrofa* Linn. var. *domesticus* Gray (Fam. Suidae).

Pepsin is prepared by digesting the minced stomach linings with hydrochloric acid. This solution is clarified, partially evaporated, dialyzed, concentrated, and either poured on glass plates to dry, thus forming *scale pepsin*, or carefully evaporated in a vacuum, forming *spongy pepsin*.

Pepsin occurs as lustrous, transparent, or translucent scales, as granular or spongy masses light yellow to light brown, or as fine white or cream-coloured amorphous powder. It is free from offensive odour and has a slightly acid or saline taste.

Pepsin digests not less than 3000 and not more than 3500 times its weight of coagulated egg albumin. A pepsin of higher digestive power may be reduced to the standard by admixture with a pepsin of lower power or with lactose.

Pepsin is administered to assist gastric diges-tion. It is a proteolytic enzyme and should be given after meals and followed by a dose of hydrochloric acid. The usual dose is 500 mg. It is often combined with pancreatin in product formulations.

PANCREATIN

Pancreatin is a substance containing enzymes, prominently amylase, lipase and protease. It is obtained from the pancreas of the hog, *Sus scrofa* Linn. var. *domesticus* Gray (Fam. Suidae), or of the ox, *Bos taurus* Linn. (Fam. Bovidae). The pancreas is a gland lying inside the posterior wall of the abdomen. The fresh glands are minced and extracted by methods similar to those used in the manufacture of pepsin.

Pancreatin is a cream-coloured amorphous powder with a faint, characteristic, but not offensive, odour. Its greatest activity is in neutral or faintly alkaline solution. Traces of mineral acids or large amounts of alkali hydroxides render pancreatin inert, and an excess of alkali carbonates inhibits its action.

Pancreatin is a digestive aid and is also used in the preparation of predigested foods for invalids. Enteric-coated granules of pancreatin have been used to treat infants with celiac disease and related pancreatic deficiencies. The usual dose is 325 mg to 1 g as tablets, capsules or granules.

PANCRELIPASE

Pancrelipase is a more concentrated form of pancreatin. In each mg it contains not less than 24 USP units of lipase activity, 100 USP units of amylase activity, and 100 USP units of protease activity. Thus the lipase activity is increased 12-fold, but the activity of amylase and protease only 4-fold when compared with pancreatin.

It is used as a digestive aid to increase the intestinal absorption of fat, thus aiding in the control of steatorrhea. It is available in the form of capsules, powder packets and tablets. The usual dose range is 8000 to 24,000 USP units of lipolytic activity prior to each meal or snack.

TRYPSIN

Crystallized trypsin is a proteolytic enzyme obtained from an extract of the pancreas gland of the ox, *Bos taurus* Linn. (Fam. Bovidae). It contains not less than 2500 USP trypsin units in each mg. It occurs as a white to yellowish white, odourless, crystalline or amorphous powder.

Crystallized trypsin is a proteolytic enzyme. It is used orally, topically, or by inhalation or local injection for debridement of necrotic and pyogenic surface lesions. Trypsin is applied topical by aerosol for wound and ulcer cleansing.

CHYMOTRYPSIN

Chymotrypsin is a proteolytic enzyme crystallized from an extract of the pancreas gland of the ox, *Bos taurus* Linn. (Fam. Bovidae). It contains not less than 1000 USP chymotrypsin units in each mg. The enzyme occurs as a white to yellowish white, odourless, crystalline or amorphous powder. Chymotrypsin is available as *chymotrypsin for ophthalmic solution.*

This proteolytic enzyme is administered in solution to the posterior chamber of the eye, under the iris, to achieve zonal lysis.

HYALURONIDASE

Hyaluronidase is a sterile, dry, soluble, enzyme product prepared from mammalian testes. It is capable of hydrolyzing mucopolysaccharides of the type of hyaluronic acid. Its potency is expressed in USP hyaluronidase units. Hyaluronidase for injection contains not more than 0.25 µg of tyrosine for each USP hyaluronidase unit.

Hyaluronidase is a mucolytic enzyme which deploymerizes and catalyzes hyaluronic acid and similar hexosamine-containing polysaccharides. It is also a spreading and a diffusing factor. It occurs in human testes, in various bacterial cultures as a metabolic product, in heads of leeches, and in snake venomes. This enzyme promotes diffusion and hastens absorption of subcutaneous infusions due to its action on hyaluronic acids.

Hyaluronidase for injection is a spreading agent and the usual dose is 150 USP units.

STREPTOKINASE

Streptokinase is a purified bacterial protein elaborated by group C β-hemolytic streptococci. It is available as a lyophilized powder. The compound acts to convert plasminogen to the proteolytic enzyme plasmin. Plasmin degrades fibrin clots, fibrinogen and other plasma proteins.

Streptokinase is used to treat of pulmonary embolism, deep vein thrombosis, arterial thrombosis and embolism, arteriovenous cannula occlusion and coronary artery thrombosis. It produces a prompt recanalization of the involved vessel. The route of administration, dosage, and duration of treatment vary for each of the above conditions. Streptokinase is marketed in sterile vials containing 250,000 to 750,000 IU.

UROKINASE

Urokinase is an enzyme isolated from human urine or obtained from human kidney cells by tissue culture techniques. There are two forms with similar clinical effects, but they differ in molecular weight. It is marketed as a sterile, lyophilized white powder.

The enzyme acts on the endogenous fibrinolytic system. It converts plasminogen to the enzyme plasmin. Plasmin degrades fibrin clots, fibrinogen and other plasma proteins. Urokinase is used in the treatment of pulmonary embolism, coronary artery thrombosis, and in restoring the patency of intravenous cateters. It may produce serious allergic reactions, presumably owing to its human origin and should be used with appropriate caution.

FIBRINOLYSIN AND DESOXYRIBONUCLEASE

Fibrinolysin is present in the blood serum as a protease and in plasma as the inactive precursor, profibrinolysin (or plasminogen). It is prepared commercially by activating a human blood plasma fraction with streptokinase. In the dried form, fibrinolysin retains its proteolytic activity almost indefinitely. In solution form, it rapidly deteriorates. Its enzymatic activity is lost completely when it is exposed to room temperature for 6 to 8 hours. It can attack the protein portions of dead tissues, exudates, and blood clots found in wounds, ulcers and burns. Fibrinolysin is used to treat of blood clots within the cardiovascular system, exclusive of thrombi of the coronary and cerebral arteries.

Desoxyribonuclease (*deoxyribonuclease*) is a nucleolytic enzyme obtained from pancreatic glands of bovine origin. It is stable in dry form but rapidly loses its activity in solution form. It can catalyze cleavage of the giant molecules of desoxyribonucleic acid into numerous fragments of smaller size (polynucleotides); thus it acts against devitalized tissues in purulent states. It is available as a combination product with bovine fibrinolysin.

SUTILAINS

Sutilains is a substance containing proteolytic enzymes obtained from the bacterium *Bacillus subtilis*. It contains not less than 2.5 million USP casein units of proteolytic activity per g. This cream-coloured powder is applied topically, in ointment form, 2 to 4 times daily, for wound debridement.

COLLAGENASE

Collagenase is an enzyme preparation obtained from fermentative cultures of *Clostridium histolyticum*. It cleaves collagen and is used topically to debride dermal ulcers and severely burned areas. Burow's solutions can be used to stop the enzyme's action if the risk of bacteremia develops. Available ointments contain 250 units of collagenase activity per g.

L-ASPARAGINASE

L-Asparaginase, an enzyme obtained from cultures of certain strains of *Escherichia coli*, induces hematologic and clinical remissions of short duration in a children with acute leukemia. The antitumour is attributed to degradation by the enzyme of circulating L-asparagine, which results in the death of cells that require exogenous sources of this amino acid for survival. The drug is related to a difference in the requirement for L-asparagine between normal cells and some neoplastic cells.

Asparaginase shows serious adverse reactions such as allergic reactions and fatal anaphylaxis. It is used in combination with other chemotherapeutic agents, such as prednisone and vincristine. Administration is intravenous.

PENICILLAMINE

Penicillamine is D-3-mercaptovaline or β,β-dimethylcystine. It is a degradation product of penicillin-type antibiotics. This substance is a metal-chelating agent used in Wilson's disease (hepatolenticular degeneration) to promote urinary excretion of excess copper, in treating lead poisoning, and in cases of severe active rheumatoid arthritis. The usual

dose in Wilson's disease is 250 mg, 4 times a day; a single daily dose of up to 1.5 g is used in rheumatoid arthritis.

HEPARIN SODIUM

Heparin sodium is the sodium salt of forms of a sulphated glycosaminoglycan of mixed mucopolysaccharide nature varying in molecular weights. It is obtained from the intestinal mucosa or other suitable tissues of domestic animals used for food by humans. Heparin sodium is a mixture of active principles that prolong the clotting time of blood through formation of a complex with the plasma protein antithrombin and by inhibition of other coagulation proteases.

It is used as an anticoagulant drug.

HEPARIN CALCIUM

Heparin calcium, a salt of heparin, is superior to heparin sodium in reducing the incidence of bleeding, hematoma formation and discomfort at the site of injection.

PROTAMINE SULPHATE

Protamine sulphate is a purified mixture of simple protein principles obtained from the sperm or testes of suitable species of fish belonging to the genera *Oncorhynchus* Suckley, *Salmo* Linne, or *Trutta* Jordan et Evermann (Fam. Salmonidae). It has the property of neutralizing heparin. Each mg of protamine sulphate neutralizes not less than 80 USP units of heparin activity derived from lung tissue and not less than 100 USP units of heparin activity derived from intestinal mucosa.

Protamine sulphate is a fine, white or off-white, amorphous or crystalline powder and is sparingly soluble in water. It is an antidote to heparin and is administered intravenously.

Protamine sulphate or injection is a sterile mixture of protamine sulphate with one or more suitable dry diluents. *Protamine sulphate injection* is a sterile isotonic solution of protamine sulphate.

PROTEIN HYDROLYSATE INJECTION

Protein hydrolysate injection is a sterile solution of amino acids and short-chain peptides that represents the approximate nutritive equivalent of the casein, lactalbumin, plasma, fibrin or other suitable protein from which it is derived by acid, enzymatic, or other method of hydrolysis. It contains not less than 50% of the total nitrogen present in the form of α-amino nitrogen.

This drug is used when the patient is unable to ingest or digest food to supply the nitrogen necessary to replace that amount lost through tissue metabolism.

Protein hydrolysate injection is a parenteral nutrient.

LEVODOPA

Levodopa or 3-hydroxy-L-tyrosine is an amino acid that occurs in the seeds of *Vicia faba* Linn. (Fam. Papilionaceae), known as the horse bean, the velvet bean, or the broad bean. Isolation of the compound from protein hydrolysate is difficult due to its tendency to become oxidized; therefore, synthetic methods of production are used.

High oral doses of levodopa are used for relieving parkinsonism. Most symptoms are relieved to some degree, but akinesia and rigidity respond more readily than tremor. The major adverse effects are transitory nausea and vomiting, orthostatic faintness and transient depression of granulocytes.

The action of levodopa presumably involves the decarboxylation in the neural ganglia of the amino acid to give the amine.

21

Alkaloids

The term alkaloid is applied to naturally occurring basic compounds and is difficult to define. The term is derived from 'vegetable alkali' (*alk* = alkali; *oid* = like). They may be defined as organic nitrogenous substances of plant origin exhibiting well-defined physiological actions. A true alkaloid has a nitrogen atom as a part of heterocyclic system; it has a complex molecular structure; it manifests significant pharmacological activity and it is restricted to the plant kingdom.

Distribution

Alkaloids have been reported in various plant parts such as in whole aerial plant (Lobelia, Tylophora, Ephedra), in leaves (Dature, Belladonna, Coca), in bark (Kurchi, Cinchona), in stem (Withania), in rhizomes and roots (Ipecac, Rauwolfia, Aconite); in flowering buds (Hyoscyamus) and in seeds (Nux vomica, Physostigma, Colchicum). Several alkaloids have been found in cultures of microorganisms, *e.g.*, in bacteria, fungi (Ergot) and algae. Amphibian alkaloids such as toad venous (bufotoxin) and salamander alkaloids (salamandarine) are of animal origin. Alkaloids with complicated chemical structures (strychnine) are less widespread in nature than simple compounds (nicotine). About 100 families out of 283 possess alkaloids. Historically, the plant alkaloids were isolated as: narcotine in 1803, morphine (1806, 1816), strychnine (1817), brucine (1819), piperine (1819), caffeine (1819), quinine (1820), colchicine (1820) and conjine (1826). Conjine was the first alkaloid to have its

structure established (Schiff, 1870) and to be synthesized (Laudenburg, 1889).

True alkaloids rarely occur in lower plants. In the fungi the lysergic acid derivatives and the sulphur-containing alkaloids, *e.g.*, the gliotoxins are present. Among the pteridophytes and gymnosperms, the lycopodium, ephedra and *Taxus* contain alkaloids. The dicotyledon orders Salicales, Fagales, Cucurbitales and Oleales are devoid of alkaloids. Alkaloids are commonly found in the orders Centrospermae (Chenopodiaceae), Magnoliales (Lauraceae, Magnoliaceae), Ranunculales (Berberidaceae, Menispermaceae, Ranunculaceae), Papaverales (Papaveraceae, Fumiariaceae), Rosales (Papilionaceae), Rutales (Rutaceae), Gentiales (Apocynaceae, Loganiaceae, Rubiaceae), Tubiflorae (Boraginaceae, Convolvulaceae, Solanaceae) and Campanulales (Campanulaceae, subfamily Lobelioideae; Asteraceae, subfamily Senecioneae).

Nearly 300 alkaloids belonging to more than 24 classes occur in the skins of amphibians along with other toxins. They include the potent neurotoxic alkaloids of frogs of the genus *Phyllobates*, which are the most poisonous substances known. Alkaloids derived from mammals are of indole and isoquinoline classes along with mammalian morphine. A few are found in both plants and animals.

The names of alkaloids have been derived from the plants yielding them (atropine, tylophorine, cocaine, nicotine); from physiologic activity (emetine, morphine) and from the discoverer (pelletierine, alihirsutine). As per chemical rules the names of all alkaloids should end in "ine".

Alkaloids exhibit a variety of physical and chemical properties. All of them possess carbon, hydrogen and nitrogen and in most cases oxygen as elements. Like basic compounds they form their crystalline salts with acids like hydrochloric acid, sulphuric acid, citric acid and tartaric acid. The free alkaloids are insoluble or slightly soluble in water but their salts are freely soluble. However, they are soluble in non-polar solvents such as ether or chloroform. Therefore, alkaloids are separated from non-polar compounds by salt formation, extracting the lipid soluble portion and basifying the solution with an alkali carbonate or ammonia. Most of the alkaloids are crystalline solids with definite melting points, some of them are amorphous and few (coniine, nicotine) are liquids. They are generally colourless compounds but few are coloured substances, *e.g.*, berberine (yellow), betaine (red), tylophorine (dull yellow), and cones-sine (pale yellow). They are generally bitter in taste and optically active. On treatment with phosphotungstic acid, phosphomolybdic acid, picric acid, potassium mercuri-iodide and tannic acid, they yield insoluble precipitates (double salts). The alkaloidal substances are often administered in solution. The differences in solubility between alkaloids and their salts provide methods for the isolation of alkaloids from the plant and their separation from the nonalkaloidal substances.

The alkaloidal salts are usually soluble in water but sparingly soluble in organic solvents. For example, strychnine hydrochloride is much more soluble in water than is strychnine base. Caffeine (base) is readily extracted from tea with water.

Some alkaloidal salts are sparingly soluble, *e.g.*, quinine sulphate is only soluble to the extent of 1 part in 1000 parts of water, although 1 part quinine hydrochloride is soluble in less than 1 part of water. The following colour tests are used to detect the presence of an alkaloid :

1. *Mayer's reagent* (Potassium mercuri-iodide solution) : It gives a white or pale yellow precipitate except with alkaloids of the purine group and few others.

2. *Dragendorff's reagent* (Potassium iodide + bismuth nitrate) : Alkaloids form orange coloured precipitate with the reagent.

3. *Wagner's reagent* (Iodine solution) : It gives a brown or reddish brown precipitate with alkaloids.

4. *Hager's reagent* (A saturated solution of picric acid in cold water) : It gives characteristic crystalline precipitate with many alkaloids.

5. *Tannic acid test* : A freshly prepared aqueous solution of tannic acid (5%, w/v) gives a precipitate with most of the alkaloids which is soluble in dilute acid or ammonia solution.

6. *Ammonia reineckate test* : A saturated aqueous solution of ammonia reineckate slightly acidified with hydrochloric acid gives a pink flocculent precipitate with most of the alkaloids.

7. *Murexide test for caffeine* : Caffeine, a purine derivative, is mixed with a small amount of potassium chlorate and a drop of hydrochloric acid. The reaction mixture is evaporated to dryness and the residue is exposed to ammonia vapours. A purple colour is produced with caffeine and other purine derivatives.

8. Treatment of indole alkaloids with sulphuric acid and *p*-dimethylaminobenzaldehyde gives bluish-violet to red colour.

Functions of alkaloids in plants

In plants alkaloids act as poisonous and stimulating agents. Sparteine acts as stimulant to an aphid when feeding on *Sarothamus scoparius*. The insect changes its feeding site according to where the highest concentration of alkaloid occurs within the host plant. Tomatin, the major alkaloid of tomato, acts as repellent. Nicotine and anabasine act as powerful repellents for many insect groups and thus protects plants from insects and herbivorous. They also act as regulatory growth factors, and reserve substances for nitrogen and other elemental supply and as end products of detoxification reactions. They occur as pigments, such as pteridine and betalains, and attract animals for pollination. The increase in putrescine in barley seedlings when grown in a medium deficient in potassium is important.

Alkaloids often occur in plants in association with characteristic acids, *e.g.*, the tropane alkaloids of the Solanac and Erythroxylaceae are esters, the cinchona alkaloids occur with quinic and cinchotannic acids, opium alkaloids are associated with meconic acid. In some cases the alkaloids could provide either a means of storing or transporting in soluble form the particular acids. Tropane esters formed in the roots of solanaceous plants are translocated to the aerial parts, where hydrolysis of the alkaloid and breakdown of the liberated acid take place. The majority of alkaloids are biosynthesized from readily available units by a series of ubiquitous reactions. They are harmless to the plant.

By the use of grafts, plants storing alkaloids in the aerial parts (*e.g.*, *Nicotiana*, *Datura*) are produced free of alkaloids, indicating the non-essential nature of the alkaloid. Plants which do not normally contain alkaloids remains unaffected when administered alkaloids (colchicine is an exception).

The alkaloids participate in plant metabolism over the long term. Daily variation in alkaloid content is very common in some species. The presence of alkaloids is not vital to the plant. They do participate in metabolic sequences and are not the waste, end-products of metabolism.

The alkaloids may have a role in the defence of the plant against singlet oxygen ($^1O_2$), which is damaging to all living organisms and is produced in plant tissues in the presence of light.

Alkaloids are capable to exhibit extensive and well-marked pharmacological activities like analgesic (cocaine, morphine, codeine), anti-amoebic and emetic (emetin), anticholinergic (atropine, hyoscyamine, scopolamine), antihypertensive (reserpine, deserpine), antimalarial (quinine, cinchonine), antitumor (vinblastine, vincristine), antitussive (codeine, noscapine), cardiac depressant (quinidine), central nervous stimulant (caffeine, strychnine, brucine), diuretic (theobromine, theophylline), oxytocic (ergometrine, ergotamine), ophthalmic relaxant (tubocurarine) and smooth muscle relaxant (papaverine, theophylline).

Classification

No systematic structural classification exists for alkaloids. The most widely accepted classification system is as :

1. *True alkaloids* (Heterocyclic alkaloids): True alkaloids are toxic, show a wide range of physiological activity; contain nitrogen in a heterocyclic ring, derived from amino acids and normally occur in plants, *e.g.*, colchicine, quinine, morphine and emetine.
2. *Protoalkaloids* (Nor-heterocyclic alkaloids): Protoalkaloids are relatively simple amines in which the amino acid nitrogen is not in a heterocyclic ring, *e.g.*, mescaline and ephedrine.
3. *Pseudoalkaloids* : These alkaloids are not derived from amino acid precursors and are usually basic in nature, *e.g.*, steroidal alkaloids (conessine) and purines (caffeine).

The nitrogen of alkaloids

Alkaloids may have a nitrogen atom which is primary (mescaline), secondary (ephedrine), tertiary (atropine) or quaternary (one of the N atoms of tubocurarine), and this factor affects the derivatives of the alkaloids. In the plant alkaloids may exist in the free state, as salts or as amine or alkaloid *N*-oxides.

Alkaloid N-oxides

N-oxidation products of alkaloids, *e.g.*, the *N*-oxides of tertiary alkaloids are easily prepared from the original base.

The formation of *N*-oxides and other *N*-oxidation products of alkaloids in animal systems is well-known. Such compounds represent artefacts arising during the extraction and work-up of tertiary alkaloids. Due to the high polarity, and water-solubility of alkaloid *N*-oxides, they were discarded by the normal alkaloid extraction procedures.

Natural *N*-oxides comprises the quinolizidines of the Boraginaceae, Asteraceae and Papilionaceae and cause liver damage in animals using plants containing them as fodder. A number of *N*-oxide alkaloids of the indole series have been isolated from plant materials, *e.g.*, simple hallucinogenic indole derivatives of *Amanita* spp., reserpine, strychnine, and some *Mitragyna* alkaloids. Fresh *Atropa*, Hyoscyamus and Scopolia yield two isomeric N-oxides of hyoscyamine. Morphine and codeine N-oxides are present in opium poppy latex. Two isomeric nicotine N-oxides are isolated from *Nicotiana* species.

Alkaloids are generally arranged in order of increasing rings, *e.g.*, pyrrolidine group (hygrine, tropinone), pyridine-piperidine group (coniine, pseudopelletierine, lobelia alkaloids, lupine alkaloids, nicotine), isoquinoline group (papaverine, dauricine), tetrahydroisoquinoline group (aporphine alkaloids, berberine, crytopine, emetine), phenanthrene or morphine group (morphine, codeine, thebaine), quinoline group (Cinchona alkaloids, quinine, cusparine, dictaminine), indole group (Ergot alkaloids, harmine, physostigmine), complex indole group (brucine, strychnine), erythrina group (β-erythroidine, erysopine) and colchicine. Atropine, hyoscyamine and scopolamine are derived from tropane, a condensed product of pyrrolidine and piperidine. Pilocarpine has the imidazole ring, caffeine and theobromine are purine bases, solanine and conessine contain steroidal nucleus.

Extraction

One of the following general methods may be used for the isolation of alkaloids :

Method A

The powdered material is moistened with water and mixed with lime, which combines with acids, tannins and other phenolic substances and sets free the salts of alkaloids. Extraction is then carried out with organic solvents such as ether, chloroform or petroleum spirit. The concentrated organic liquid is then shaken with aqueous acid and allowed to separate. Alkaloid salts are now in the aqueous liquid, while many impurities remain behind in the organic fluid.

Method B

The powdered material is extracted with water or aqueous alcohol containing dilute acid. Pigments and other unwanted materials are removed by shaking with chloroform or other organic solvents. The free alkaloids are then precipitated by the addition of excess sodium bicarbonate or ammonia and separated by filtration or by extraction with organic solvents like chloroform or ethyl acetate.

The separation and final purification of a mixture of alkaloids may be done by fractional precipitation or by fractional crystallization of salts such as oxalates, tartrates or picrates. Chromatographic methods are suitable if the mixture is a complex one and if small quantities of alkaloids are present.

Supercritical fluid extraction is of increasing importance for these compounds.

Volatile liquid alkaloids, *e.g.*, nicotine and coniine are most conveniently isolated by distillation. An aqueous extract is made alkaline with caustic soda or sodium carbonate and the alkaloid distilled off in steam. Nicotine is an important insecticide. It is prepared from those parts of the tobacco plant which cannot be used for tobacco manufacture.

PYRIDINE-PIPERIDINE ALKALOIDS

Reduction of pyridine, a tertiary base, converts it into piperidine, a secondary base. This group includes alkaloids containing piperidine, α-propylpiperidine and derivatives of nicotinic acid. This group is sometimes divided into 3 subgroups: (1) derivatives of piperidine, including lobeline from lobelia; (2) derivatives of nicotinic acid, including arecoline from areca; and (3) derivatives of both pyridine and pyrrolidine, including nicotine from tobacco. The important alkaloidal drugs and their alkaloids that are classified in this group are areca, arecoline hydrobromide, lobelia, lobeline and nicotine.

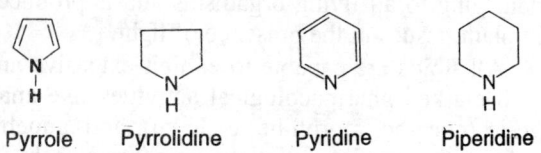

Fig. 21.1. Nitrogenous heterocyclic compounds.

Biosynthesis of alkaloids

The biosynthesis of many alkaloidal structures involve amino acids. The amino acids that most often serve as alkaloidal precursors include phenylalanine, tyrosine, tryptophan, histidine, anthranilic acid, lysine and ornithine. Some of the general reactions that are of particular importance include the decarboxylation and transamination of the amino acids to yield a corresponding amine or aldehyde. These can react to form a Schiff base which, then can react with a carbanion in a Mannich-type condensation.

Biosynthesis of ornithine-derived alkaloids

The amino acid ornithine, its decarboxylation

product, putrescine and proline constitute the basic unit of the tropane, ecgonine, nicotine (pyrrolidine ring), necine and stachydrine groups of alkaloids. Biogenetically ornithine is linked to arginine; putrescine can also be formed from arginine without the involvement of ornithine. The key intermediate is thought to be the *N*-methyl pyrrolinium ion which, through electrophilic aromatic substitution, attaches to C-3 of the pyridine ring of nicotinic acid. Nicotinic acid is formed in higher plants and certain micro-organisms via quinolinic acid by the condensation of glyceraldehyde-3-phosphate and aspartic acid.

Nicotine is formed by root metabolism, and in the leaves of plants.

PYRROLIDINE ALKALOIDS

PYRROLIZIDINE ALKALOIDS

They constitute the poisonous hepatotoxic constituents of plants of the genus *Senecio* (Asteraceae), well-known for their toxicity to livestock. Some of the alkaloids show carcinogenic and mutagenic properties. They occur in small quantities in some herbal products such as comfrey (Boraginaceae) and coltsfoot (Asteraceae). These alkaloids have an ecological role in some species of butterfly affording protection to some and converting to female flight arrestants in others. Indicine *N*-oxide has antitumour properties. Australine, present in *Castanospermum australe*, is a tetrahydroxy-pyrrolizidine alkaloid. It exhibits glycosidase inhibitory activity. The alkaloids frequently occur as esters, being linked with

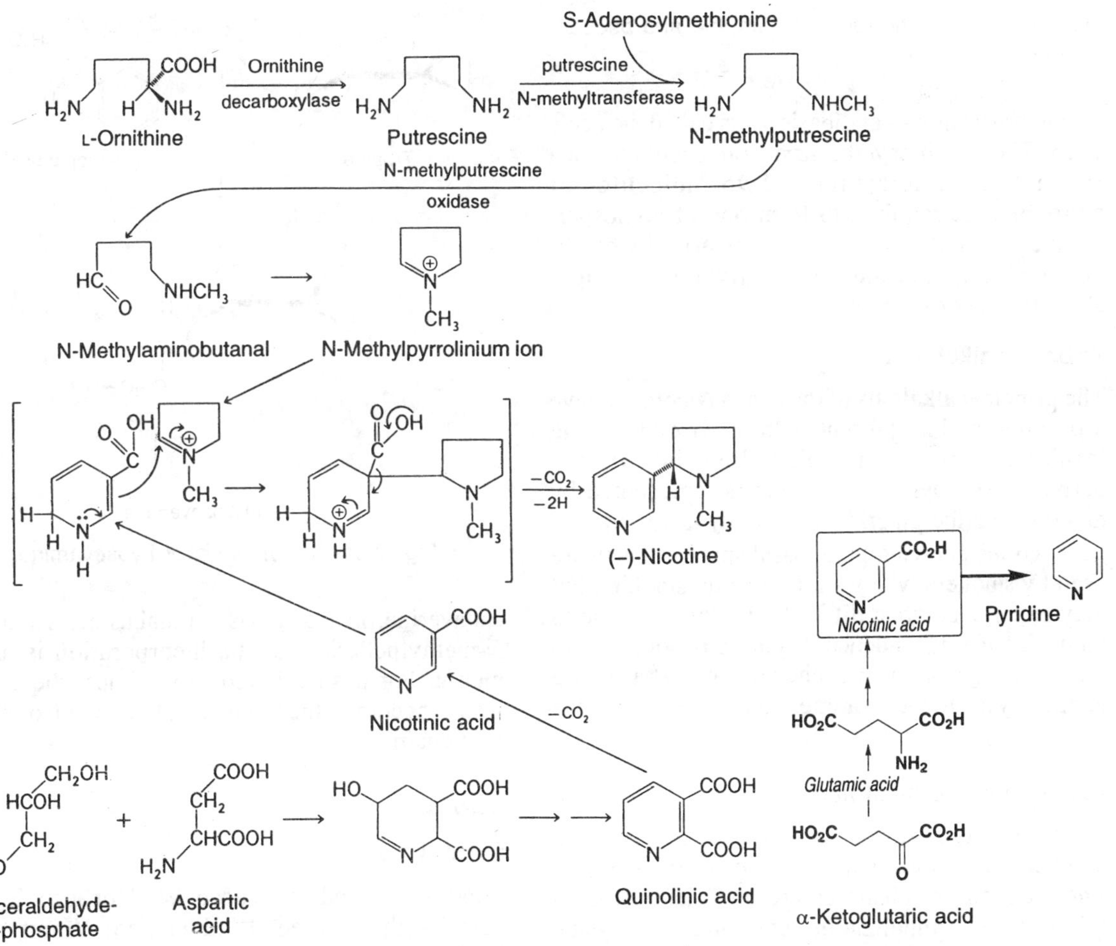

Fig. 21.2. Biosynthesis of nicotine.

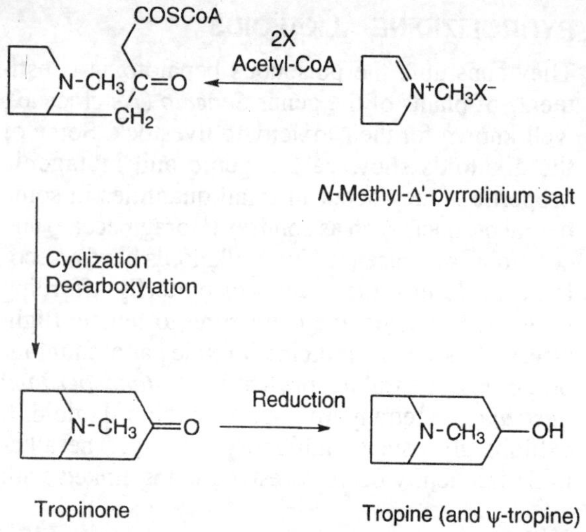

Fig. 21.3. Biogenetic routes for tropine and pseudo-tropine.

characteristic mono- or dibasic acids called the necic acids. They are biosynthesized from ornithine via a symmetrical intermediate. Two molecules of putrescine are required to form one of homospermidine. The hepatotoxic properties arise by breakdown of the alkaloids in the liver to strongly alkylating pyrrole esters.

Tobacco alkaloids

The principal alkaloids of the genus *Nicotiana* have a pyridine moiety present with a pyrrolidine ring (ornithine-derived) or a piperidine ring (lysine-derived). The pyrrolidine group is represented by nicotine and the piperidine group by anabasine.

Nicotine chewing-gum, nasal spray or patch are used by smokers who want to give up smoking but they experience great difficulty in doing so due to their nicotine dependence. Nicotine is bound to an ion exchange resin in a chewing gum base as a temporary aid to the cigarette smoker seeking to give up smoking.

Lysine-derived alkaloids

Lysine and its associated compounds give rise to a number of alkaloids, mainly of the ornithine group. The lycopodium alkaloids are also derived from lysine. In the quinolizidine lupin alkaloids, lysine is incorporated via a symmetrical precursor, *e.g.*,

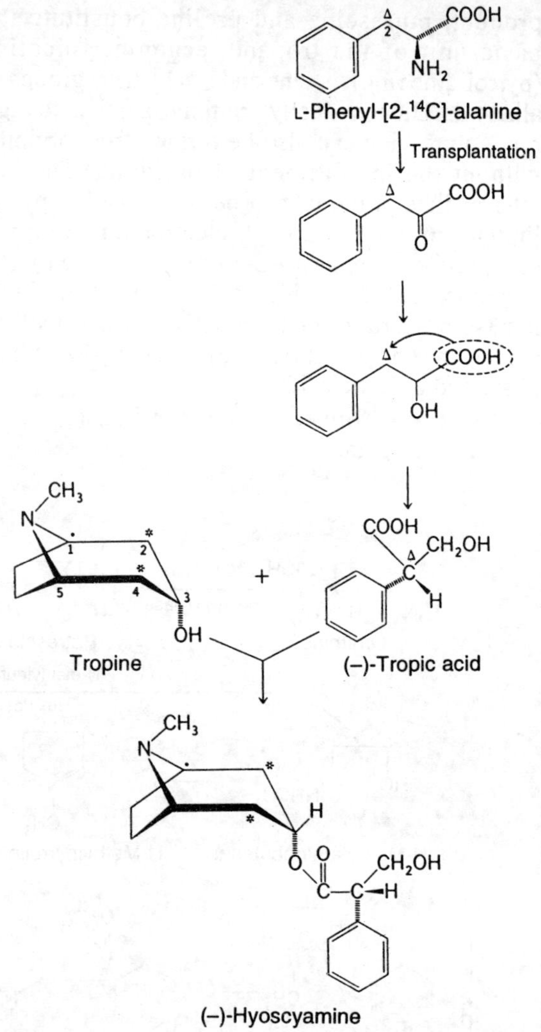

Fig. 21.4. Biosynthesis of hyoscyamine.

cadaverine, in many cases (anabasine, sedamine, *N*-methylpelletierine) the incorporation is asymmetric. For α-substituted piperidines, the C-2 of lysine becomes the point of attachment of the α side-chain.

LOBELIA

Synonyms

Lobelia herb; Indian tobacco; Wild tobacco; Emetic herb; Asthma weed; Bladder pod; Vomit wort; Herba lobeliae.

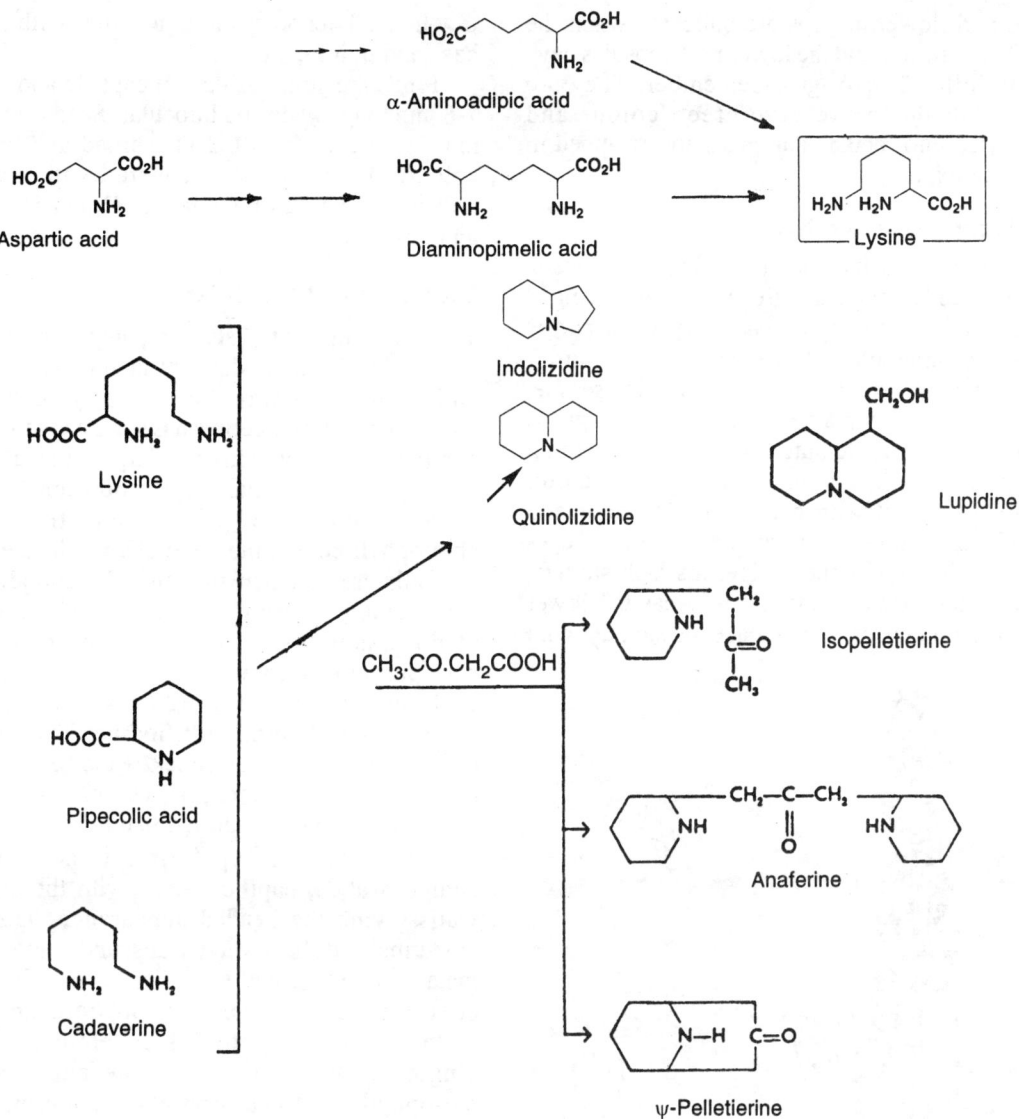

Fig. 21.5. Lysine as a precursor of alkaloids.

Official source

Lobelia consists of the dried aerial parts of *Lobelia inflata* Linn. of which 60 per cent is the stem. (Family : Lobeliaceae).

Geographical source

The plant is indigenous to the eastern USA, Canada and Holland. It is an erect annual herb, 30-90 cm high.

Cultivation and collection

Seeds of Lobelia are sown in March-April or autumn in rich, moist, loamy soil. On germination the plants are grown to produce stems of 30-50 cm in height.

The plant thrives in rich moist loam in the open or in partial shade. Seeds are sown in well prepared ground in rows 20 cm apart. Sometimes seeds are sown in beds and seedlings transplanted in the field.

Leaves and flowering tops are collected when the plants are in flower and the lowermost capsules have become inflated in August-September. They are dried in shade to preserve green colour and compressed into rectangular cakes and wrapped in pepper for export.

Macroscopical characters

Entire aerial parts include stems, leaves, flowers, fruits and seeds. Stems are greenish purple, winged and very hairy in the upper part. The lower part is rounded, channelled and less hairy. Leaves are 2 cm long, broken or entire with bristly hairs, sessile, ovate to ovate-lanceolate in shape. The margin is irregularly serrate, dentate and the teeth contain water-pores; acute and yellowish green in colour, slightly pubescent with characteristic odour and taste. Hairs are present on lamina. Base is wedge-shaped, entire. The upper epidermis lack stomata with very few or no trichomes whereas the lower one shows numerous ranunculaceous stomata with

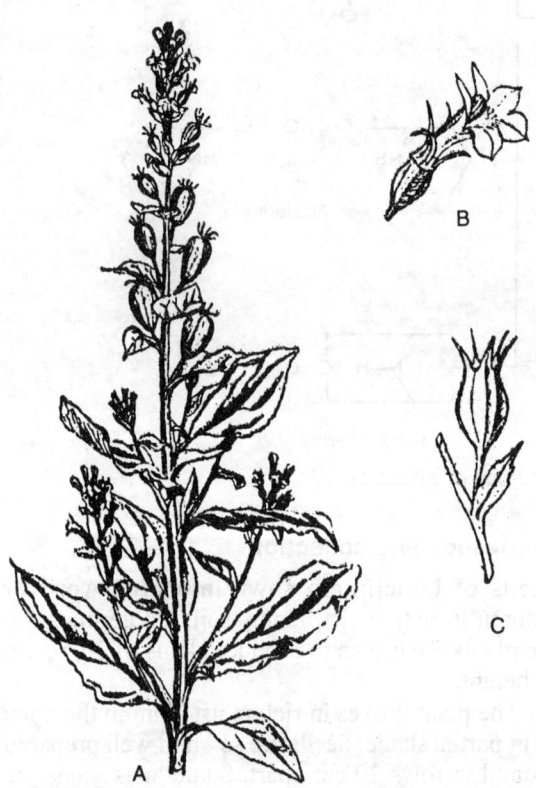

Fig. 21.6. *Lobelia inflata.*

few-hairs. Trichomes are unicellular with rounded base and pointed tips.

Fruits are yellowish green capsule and inflated, 7-8 mm long, ovate and bilocular. Seeds are 0.5-0.7 mm in length, about 0.3 mm broad and brown in colour. Outer surface is covered with elongated polygonal lignified reticulation. Odour is irritating and taste is acrid.

Microscopical characters

The epidermis of the stem is composed of rectangular cells, covered with a striated cuticle and with anticlinal pitted walls, giving a typical beaded appearance. The epidermis has stomata with the pore parallel to the stem axis and large, conical, warty-walled, unicellular hairs up to 600 μm long. The cortex is composed of rounded, thin-walled, chlorophyll containing parenchyma. In the wings, the cells are collenchymatous. The endodermis is well marked. A pericycle composed of small groups of fibres is present in the lower part of the stem. The phloem is composed of sieve-tube tissue enclosing the anastomosing latex vessels, readily visible after staining with iodine. The xylem is composed of elongated, thick-walled xylem fibres and spiral and scalariform vessels. The pith is composed of pitted lignified parenchyma.

The upper leaf epidermis is composed of straight-walled, papillose cells with the anticlinal walls giving the beaded appearance. The lower epidermal cells have wavy walls, and numerous stomata, without special subsidiary cells. Unicellular covering hairs are present on both epidermal surfaces. The mesophyll is differentiated into a single-layered palisade tissue and a spongy mesophyll. Small fat crystals are present in the mesophyll cells. The palisade tissue is present in the midrib and groups of collenchyma occur above and below the midrib bundle. The phloem contains the characteristic latex vessels. Numerous water-pores are present on the upper surface of the marginal teeth.

The surface of the seed is typically reticulate. The pollen grains are roughly spherical and show three pores.

Chemical constituents

Lobelia contains about 0.4 per cent alkaloidal

constituents of which lobeline is the important active base.

The alkaloids of Lobelia are classified into three groups :

(i) Lobeline, the most active alkaloid of the drugs is similar to nicotine in action but weaker. Lobeline group includes l-lobeline, dl-lobeline, lobelanine, *nor*lobelanine, lobelanidine and *nor*lobelanidine.

(ii) Lelobine group contains dl-lelobanidine, l-lelobanidine I and II and norlelobani-dine.

(iii) Lobinine group contains the alkaloids lobinine, isolobinine, lobinanidine and isolobinanidine.

Lobeline, (-)-lobeline, or *alpha* lobeline occurs as colourless crystals that are slightly soluble in water but readily soluble in hot alcohol.

These alkaloids possess a piperidine nucleus.

In addition to alkaloids the drug also contains a pungent volatile oil, resin, lipids, gum, sedinine, polyacetylenes, lobetyoline and lobetyol (from root culture) and β-amyrine.

Uses

Lobelia is an expectorant used to treat spasmodic asthma and chronic bronchitis. Lobeline is a respiratory stimulant, relaxant and is given in the resuscitation of newborn infants; in gas, alcohol and narcotic poisoning; in drowning in water, electric shock and collapse. Lobelia is also used to dis-

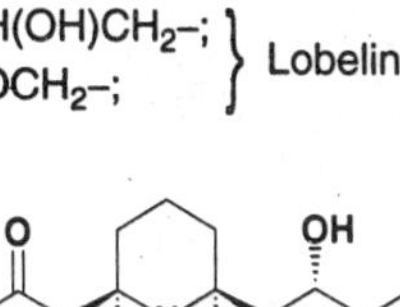

$R_1 = R_2 = C_6H_5COCH_2-$; Lobelanine
$R_1 = R_2 = C_6H_5CH(OH)CH_2-$; Lobelanidine
$R_1 = C_5H_6CH(OH)CH_2-$;
$R_2 = C_5H_6COCH_2-$; } Lobeline

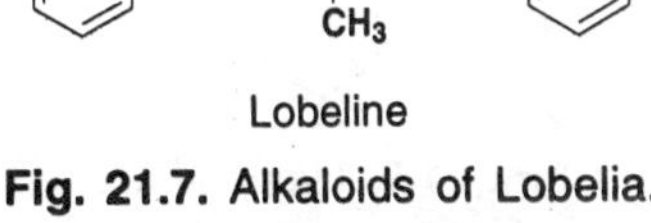

Lobeline

Fig. 21.7. Alkaloids of Lobelia.

continue smoking habit in some antismoking preparations. An injection of lobeline hydrochloride is used in the resuscitation of new-born infants. In toxic doses the drug has a paralytic effect.

INDIAN LOBELIA

Synonyms

Nala; Narasala (Hindi); Nali (Gujrati); Badanala (Bengali).

Biological source

Indian Lobelia consists of dried aerial parts of *Lobelia nicotaniaefolia* (Fam. Lobeliaceae). The drug is collected in October-November and dried in shade.

It is a large biennial or perennial herb, 1.2-3.6 m high, found in western ghats from Mumbai to Travancore at altitudes of 700-2200 m. The leaves and stems are larger in size than those of American Lobelia. The lower leaves are up to 30 cm long and 7 cm broad while the upper leaves are smaller up to 10 cm long and 2 cm wide. They are green in colour, have apex acute to acuminate, margin serrulate, venation reticulate, upper surface glabrous, lower surface glabrous to pubescent, upper epidermis has ranunculaceous stomata and few or no hairs mainly on prominent veins. Hairs and trichomes are absent in older leaves. The stomata are many on the lower epidermis. The stem is cylindrical, greenish-yellow, straight and hollow in the centre. Longitudinal striations and scars of leaf bases are present on the upper surface. Flower pedicels are up to 3 cm long, smaller in thin stems. The odour is similar to tobacco and the taste is acrid and nauseous.

The leaves of the species can be distinguished from American Lobelia on the basis of trichomes, stomata and quantitative values (palisade ratio).

Chemical constituents

Up to 0.8% total alkaloids are present in Indian lobelia. Lobelanidine, non-lobelanidine, lobeline and d-lobelanidines II and III have been isolated from the drug. The alkaloid content in *L. nicotaniaefolia* plant showed seasonal variation, being in highest concentration in October and November.

Uses

Indian lobelia is used as a respiratory stimulant and antispasmodic agent. An infusion of leaves is used as an antiseptic.

Pharmacology

Lobeline produces similar, but weaker, pharmacologic effects to those of nicotine on the peripheral circulation, neuromuscular junctions, and the central nervous system. For this reason, a 2.0 mg dose of lobeline sulfate is incorporated in tablets or lozenges that are intended to aid in breaking the tobacco habit (smoking deterrents).

(-)-Lobeline produced dose-related shortening of low intensity tail avoidance response. Its hyperalgesic potency was greater than that of morphine. β-Amyrin palmitate showed antidepressant activity. Lobeline possesses stimulant effects similar to nicotine on the peripheral circulation, neuromuscular junctions and the central nervous system. It has a placebo effect on decreasing the physical craving for cigarettes.

Biosynthesis of Lobelia alkaloids

Lobelia alkaloids are formed from a polyketo acid involving two benzoyl units and acetate. Since phenylalanine can be incorporated by the plant into lobinaline and into the related sedamine and the incorporation of lysine into the piperidine ring of lobeline, does not support this hypothesis.

LYCOPODIUM

Lycopodium consists of the spores of the club-moss, *Lycopodium clavatum* (Lycopodiaceae, Phylum Pteridophyta). The commercial drug is collected in Poland and Russia. Indian and Pakistani supplies are obtained from the Himalayas. The sporangial spikes are cut and dried and the spores are separated by shaking and then freed from vegetable debris by sieving through four sieves. The drug is exported in sacks enclosed in matting.

Lycopodium is a light yellow, highly mobile powder without odour or taste. It floats on water without being wetted. The spores are 25-40 μm diameter and have the shape of a three-sided pyramid with a convex base. The surface is covered with

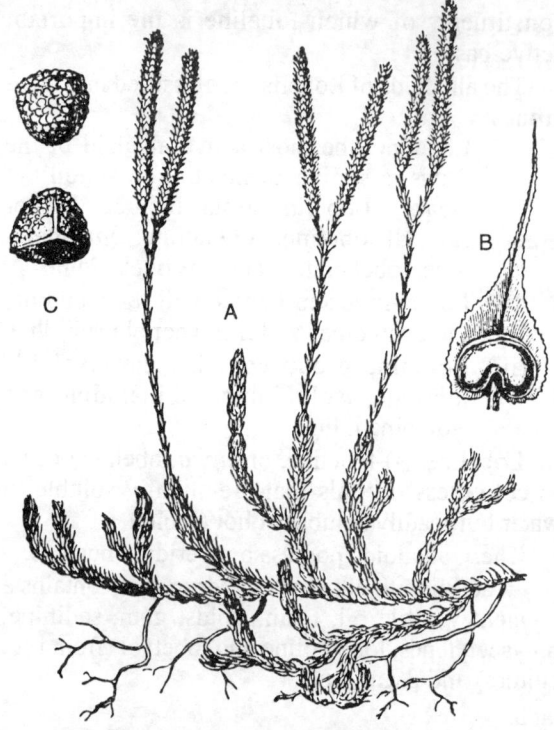

Fig. 21.8. *Lycopodium clavatum.*

polygonal-shaped reticulations which form a projecting ridge at the edge of the spore. The edges of the flat sides form a distinct, triradiate marking. On crushing, yellowish drops of oil are obtained.

Lycopodium contains about fixed oil (50%), which consists mainly of the glycerides of lycopodiumoleic acid. The drug also contains about 3% of sugars, phytosterin and alkaloids of the annotine type and traces of nicotine. The lycopodium alkaloid lycopodine is, like pelletierine, derived from lysine and acetate.

Adulteration is done with the pollen of *Pinus*

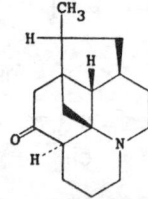

Fig. 21.9. Lycopodine.

species, *Corylus avellana* and *Typha latifolia* or with roasted and coloured starches, dextrin, sulphur or inorganic salts.

Lycopodium is used in medicated snuffs, as a dusting powder for pills and in quantitative microscopy.

ARECA NUTS

Synonyms

Betal nuts; Pinang; Semina Areacae; Supari (Hindi).

Biological source

Areca nuts are the seeds of *Areca catechu* Linn. (Family : Palmae (Palmaceae)).

Habitat

The tree is cultivated in tropical India, Sri Lanka, Malay States, South China, East Indies, Philippine Islands and parts of East Africa (including Zanzibar and Tanzania). In India it is cultivated in the coastal regions of southern Maharashtra, Tamil Nadu, Karnataka, Bengal and Assam.

Cultivation

Areca palm is mostly propagated by seeds. The palm requires a moist tropical climate for luxuriant growth; it is very sensitive to drought. It grows in areas with heavy rainfall in between temperature of 15° to 38°. It is cultivated in plains, hill-slopes and low lying valleys. The seeds are collected from 25-50 years old trees.

Collection

Areca nut is a handsome palm with a tall, slender stem crowned by large elegant leaves. Each tree contains about 100 fruits per year which are detached by means of bamboo poles, and the seeds extracted. The pericarp is fibrous and surrounds a single seed which is easily separated. The seeds are usually boiled in water with the addition of a little lime and dried.

Characters

Areca nuts are about 2.5 cm in length, bluntly rounded, conical in shape and 2-3 cm wide at the base. The testa is brown and marked with a network of small depressed lines. The ruminate endosperm is opal-white. Patches of a silvery coat, the inner layer of the pericarp, occasionally adhere to the testa. The deep-brown testa is marked with a network of depressed fissures; the colour of the testa is due to the presence of tannin. In the centre basal part of the endosperm, the small embryo is situated and an external pale area indicated its position. The seed is very hard, has a faint cheese-like odour when broken and an astringent, acrid taste.

Chemical constituents

Areca nut contains a number of alkaloids of a piperidine series such as arecoline (methyl ester of arecanine), arecaine (N-methyl guvacine), guvacine (tetrahydronicitinic acid), arecaidine, guvacoline, arecolidine, leucocyanidine, (+)-catechin, (-)-epicatechin, procyanidins A-1, B-1 and B-2; prenolic components NPF-861A, -861B, -8611A and -8611B, phthalic, lauric, myristic, palmitic and stearic acids, bis (2-ethyl hexyl) ester isoguaicine; β-sitosterol and choline. Arecoline is present in about 0.1-0.5 per cent yield and is medicinally important. In addition to alkaloids, Areca nuts contain fat (14%) and amorphous red tannin (15%) known as areca red of phlobaphene nature. The fat consists mainly of the glycerides of lauric, myristic and oleic acids.

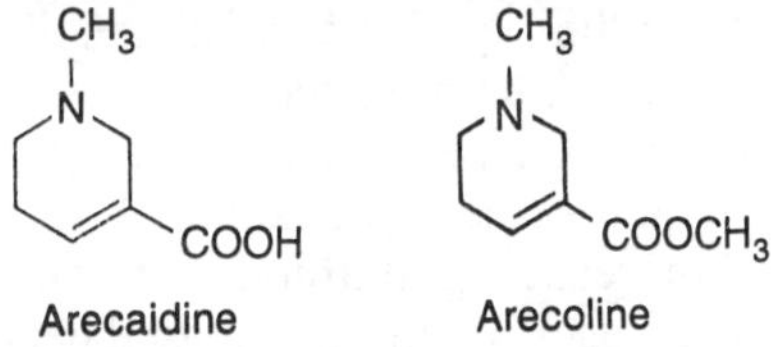

Fig. 21.10. Alkaloids of Areca nut.

Uses

Powdered Areca is used as anthelmintic, taenifuge and vermifuge for dogs. It has aphrodisiac action and useful in urinary disorders, as nervine tonic and emmenagogue. The chewing of Areca nut may cause mouth cancer.

Substituents and adulterants

Nuts from other plants, *viz. Areca caliso, A. concinna, A. ipot, A. laxa, A. nagensis, A. triandra, Caryota cumingii* and *Heterospathe elata* are used as substituents for Areca nuts. Sago palm nuts (*Metroxylon* species), dried tapioca (*Manihot esculenta*) and slices of sweet potato (*Ipomoea batatas*) form cheap adulterants that are mixed with slices of Areca nuts and prove a serious menace affecting the industry. Nuts of *Caryota urens*, cut to various shapes and sizes resembling genuine Areca nuts, and coated with concentrated Areca nut extract *kali*, form the principal adulterant. Adulteration above 10% significantly increases the fibre content of the sample, which can be used as a measure of detecting adulteration.

Pharmacology

An aqueous extract exhibited direct vasoconstriction and adrenaline potentiation in rat. Aqueous extract decreased nucleic acid and protein content in all tissues and decreased glycogen and increased sialic acid in lung and kidney tissues. Arecoline produced hypoglycaemia in rabbits. Phenolic compounds prevent dental caries and gingivitis and moderately cytotoxic activity.

Arecoline hydrobromide exerts anthelmintic action. The central effects of arecoline were mydriasis, induction of behavioural abnormalities, impairment of conditioned reactions and pseudo-analgesic properties. In mice, arecoline decreased motility and exploratory activity. It caused tremors and an increase in cerebral acetyl choline content. It stimulated the superior cervical ganglion of cats following intra-arterial injection into the ganglion. Arecoline reduced mean arterial blood pressure and cardiac output. An aqueous extract of Areca nut and arcoline increased glutathione content in liver, kidney and muscle of mice; increased hepatic DNA and RNA content and stimulated hepatic DNA and RNA synthesis.

Arecaine and guvacine inhibited uptake of GABA in brain and produced behavioural changes.

There are problems with the widespread use of khat or ghat (*Catha edulis*) and betel nut (*Areca catechu*) amongst Asians. A betel quid consists of a leaf from the plant *Piper betel* which is wrapped to form a small packet containing, tobacco, Areca nuts, Black catechu, saffron and lime. A number of ingredients are reported to be carcinogenic. The quid is placed inside the mouth between the gum and the inside cheek causing salivation and stimulation of the oral nerves. It may improve digestion. However, prolonged use causes buccal inflammation, dental decay and mouth cancer.

The betel quid may have interactions with allopathic medicines. There is a correlation between betel nut (*Areca catechu*; Palmae) and buccal carcinoma. *N*-nitroso-amines in the saliva and urine of betel chewers are derived from the nut and tobacco which is often included in the 'quid'. Chewing betel nut along with tobacco greatly increases the risk of buccal carcinoma compared with chewing betel nut alone. The betel leaf (*Piper betle*), used to wrap the 'quid', possesses anti-tumor properties.

Betel chewing does not produce broncho-constriction. However, it may affect the control and severity of asthma attacks thus contributing to the high rates of acute asthma. Betel nut is used medicinally either alone or in 'herbal' mixtures.

BROOM

The broom, the tops *Cytisus scoparius* (Papilionaceae), is a perennial shrub about 1-2 m high. The lower part is woody, branches are long green and glabrous. The upper parts of the stem bear five prominent, longitudinal ridges. The lower leaves are stalked with three obovate leaflets, the upper ones are sessile and reduced to a single leaflet.

The fruit is a black, hairy pod about 3-5 cm long. Their main constituents are quinolizidine alkaloids, *e.g.*, sparteine, a yellow isoflavone scoparin and flavonoids. The drug has diuretic and cathartic actions.

POMEGRANATE BARK

This consists of both the stem and root barks of *Punica granatum* Linn. (Punicaceae). It is present in curved or channelled pieces, 5-10 cm long, 1-3 cm wide, outer surface shows longitudinal corky furrows, a few shallow depressions and the bark apothecia of lichens. The root bark shows depres-

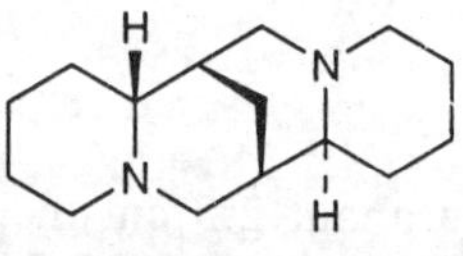

Fig. 21.11. (–)-Sparteine.

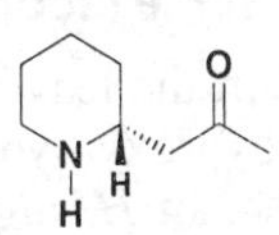

Fig. 21.12. Pelletierine.

Tropic

Apotropic acid
(atropic acid)

Angelic acid

Tiglic acid

Isovaleric acid

Tropanol
(3a-hydroxytropane)

Pseudo-tropanol
(3b-hydroxytropane)

Tropane

Tropane

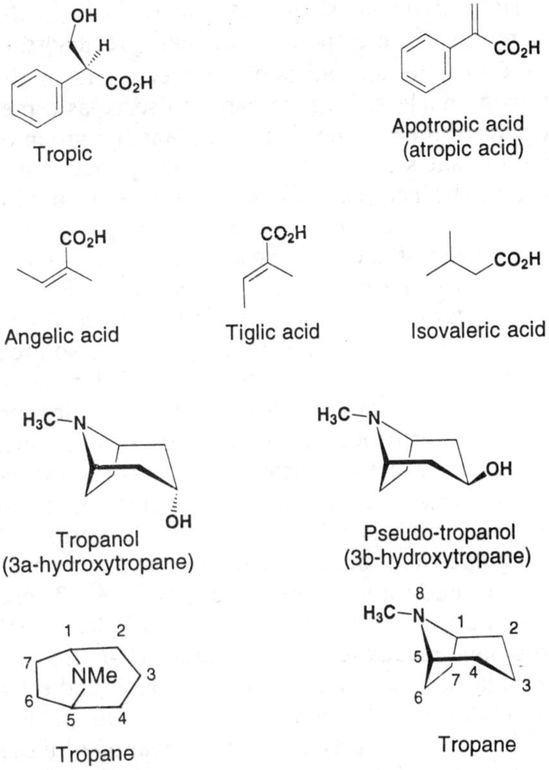

Fig. 21.13. Carboxylic acids and tropane alkaloids.

sions where the outer layers have exfoliated. The barks are smooth and yellowish on their inner surfaces and break with a short granular fracture. They contain about 0.5-0.9% of volatile liquid alkaloids, *e.g.*, pelletierine and pseudopelletierine, along with about 22% of tannin.

TROPANE ALKALOIDS

Condensation of tropane ring with piperidine constitutes the basic carbon framework of tropane nucleus. Plants of Solanaceae family are the major source of tropane alkaloids. The principal alkaloids of therapeutical interest are hyoscyamine, its more stable recemate atropine and hyoscine. The compounds occur as esters of tropic acid with tropine (tropan-3α-ol).

They are hydrolysed by heating at 60°C with baryta water. Atropine yields tropic acid and tropine; hyoscine gives tropic acid and oscine. Enzymatic hydrolysis produces scopine. The chemical treatment converts it to the more stable geometric isomer, oscine.

These alkaloids are present in Solanaceae, in which some 40 different ester bases of the tropane type have been isolated. The genera of pharmaceutical interest are *Atropa, Acnistus, Scopolia, Physochlaina, Przewalskia, Hyoscyamus, Physalis, Datura, Solandra, Duboisia* and *Anthocercis*.

Dimeric and trimeric tropanol ester alkaloids involving the dicarboxylic acids mesaconic and itaconic acids are found in *Schizanthus*. Other tropane bases occur in the Erythroxylaceae (cocaine in coca leaves), Convolvulaceae, Dioscoreaceae, Rhizophoraceae, Brassicaceae and Euphorbiaceae. The calystegines are trihydroxytropanes with a different substitution pattern. Acetic, propionic, isobutyric, isovaleric, 2-methylbutyric, tiglic, nonanoic, tropic, atropic, 2-hydroxy-3-phenylpropionic, 2,3-dihydroxy-2-phenylpropanoic, *p*-methoxy-phenylacetic and anisic acids are the esterifying acids.

Biogenesis of tropane alkaloids

The characteristic alkaloids of the group are esters of hydroxy tropanes, tropic acid and tiglic acid. There are, for each alkaloid, two distinct biogenetic moieties.

In *Datura* species, feeding studies with labelled ornithine have shown that this amino acid is incorporated stereospecifically to form the pyrrolidine ring of tropine. The remaining 3 carbon atoms are derived from acetate and thus complete the piperidine moiety. Methylation results via transmethylation from S-adenosylmethionine to complete the tropine nucleus.

Phenylalanine is the precursor of tropic acid. The side chain of the amino acid undergoes a novel type of intramolecular rearrangement during the conversion. Esterification of tropic acid with tropine produces hyoscyamine.

The formation of the tropane ring system is generally similar for all Solanaceae. There are variations between species, particularly in the stereospecific incorporation of some precursors.

Ornithine and acetate are precursors of the tropane nucleus. Hygrine can also serve as a precursor of the tropane ring. The *N*-methyl group of the tropane system can be supplied by methionine and can be incorporated at a very early stage of biosynthesis, as shown by the intact incorporation of *N*-methylornithine into hyoscine and hyoscyamine of *Datura metel* and *D. stramonium*. For *D. meteloides* the C-2 of hygrine is incorporated into the C-3 of the tropine moiety of the isolated alkaloid. Putrescine and its *N*-methyl derivative serve as precursors, which are taken in conjunction with the stereospecific incorporation of ornithine. Putrescine *N*-methyltransferase in roots of *Hyoscyamus albus* is the first committed enzyme specific to the biosynthesis of tropane. The reduction of tropinone yields both tropine (3α-hydroxytropane) and pseudotropine (3β-hydroxytropane). These reductions are brought about by two independent tropinone reductases, referred to as TR-I and TR-II. Solanaceous alkaloids with hydroxyls and ester groups are also common at C-6 and C-7 (R^2 and R^3) of the tropane ring system. Hydroxylation of these carbons probably occurs after the C-3 hydroxyl has been esterified.

Esterification

The next stage in the biosynthesis of hyoscyamine is the esterification of tropine and tropic acid. There is an involvement of two acetyl-CoA-dependent acyltransferases in the respective formation of 3α- and 3β-acetoxytropanes in *D. stramonium*-transformed root cultures.

Acid moiety

The tropic acid fragment of hyoscine and hyoscyamine is derived from phenylalanine, as is the α-hydroxy-β-phenylpropionic acid (phenyl lactic acid) of the tropane alkaloid littorine. Tropic acid is formed by an intramolecular rearrangement of phenyl lactate. Hyoscyamine is biosynthesized from littorine by a process involving the intra-molecular rearrangement of the phenyl lactate moiety of the alkaloid. Isoleucine serves as a precursor of the tigloyl and 2-methylbutanoyl moieties of various mono- and di-esters of the hydroxytropanes.

Biogenesis of hyoscine (scopolamine)

Hyoscine is formed in the leaves of *D. ferox* from hyoscyamine via 6-hydroxy-hyoscyamine and 6,7-dehydrohyoscyamine. In *H. niger* cultured roots, there is an enzyme responsible for the conversion of hyoscyamine to 6-hydroxyhyoscyamine.. When the labelled compound, [6-^{18}O]-hydroxyhyoscyamine, is fed to *Duboisia myoporoides*, hyoscyamine is converted to hyoscine and the ^{18}O is retained, thus eliminating 6,7-dehydro-hyoscyamine from the pathway. For this reaction to proceed the epoxidase enzyme requires 2-oxo-glutarate, ferrous ions and ascorbate as cofactors, together with molecular oxygen.

Ontogenesis

In belladonna and scopolia, hyoscyamine is the dominant alkaloid throughout the life cycle of the plant. In *D. stramonium* hyoscyamine is the main alkaloid at the time of flowering and after. The young plants contain principally hyoscine; in many other species of *Datura* (*e.g.*, *D. ferox*) hyoscine is the principal alkaloid of the leaves at all times. The relative proportions of hyoscine and hyoscyamine in a particular species vary with age of the plant, day length, light intensity, general climatic conditions, chemical sprays, hormones, debudding and chemical races. The root is the principal site of alkaloid synthesis; however, secondary modifications of the alkaloids may occur in the aerial parts, for example, the epoxidation of hyoscyamine to give hyoscine, and the formation of meteloidine from the corresponding 3,6-ditigloyl ester.

HYOSCYAMUS LEAF

Synonyms

Insane root; Hog's bean; Poison tobacco; Black Henbane; Henbane; Hyoscyamus herb; Khurasani-ajvayan (Hindi); Folia Hyoscyamus; Kurasani-Yomam (Tamil); Kurashanivaman (Telgu).

Biological source

Hyoscyamus leaf consists of the dried leaves and flowering tops of *Hyoscyamus niger* Linn. containing not less than 0.05% alkaloids calculated as hyoscyamine. Egyptian henbane (*H. muticus* L.) contains about 0.5% alkaloids. (Fam. Solanaceae).

Geographical source

Hyoscyamus is cultivated in England, USA, Germany, Poland, Russia and in India from Kashmir to Garhwal.

Characters

Hyoscyamus is an erect, hairy, viscid, biennial or annual herb found wild. The biennial plant has stem up to 1-5 m high, leaves sessile, ovate-oblong to triangular-ovate, stalked, up to 20 cm long, margin dentate or pinnatifid, very hairy, flowers (May-June), corolla yellowish with deep purple veins. The stem of annual species is robust up to 0.5 m in height, leaves-sessile, smaller with fewer hairs than the biennial variety with less incised margin. Flowers (July-August), corolla funnel-shaped, pale in colour with less deeply veined. Drug is collected from biennial herb.

Henbane flowers have the formula K(5), C(5), A5, G(2). The hairy, five-lobed calyx is persistent. The fruit is a small, two-celled pyxis, which contains numerous seeds.

Henbane seeds are dark grey in colour, reniform in shape and about 1.5 mm long. They have a minutely reticulated testa and an internal structure closely resembling that of stramonium seeds. Henbane seeds contain about 0.06-0.10% of alkaloids (hyoscyamine with a little hyoscine and atropine).

Cultivation

The Henbane is grown by sowing seeds in June or

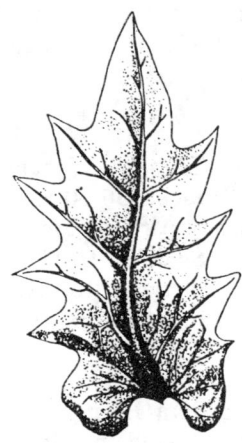

Fig. 21.14. *Hyoscyamus niger* leaf.

July. The germination of seeds is slow. It is assisted by special treatments (*e.g.*, concentrated sulphuric acid, gibberellic acid or splitting of the testa). The plant may be attacked by the potato beetle, and spraying with derris or pyrethrum may be necessary. In the first year the stem is very short, leaves are in a rosette and hairy. The leaves and flowering tops are collected and dried rapidly at 40-50°C.

The annual plant usually flowers in July or August and the biennial in May or June.

Macroscopical characters

Henbane consists of the leaves and flowering tops. The leaves are generally broken and possess greyish-green colour, very broad midrib and hairiness. The moist stems are clammy to the touch, owing to the secretion produced by the glandular hairs. The stems are less than 5 mm diameter and are also very hairy. The flowers are compressed or broken having yellowish corollas with purple veins. Henbane has a characteristic, heavy odour and a bitter, slightly acrid taste.

The leaves are broken, crumpled, sessile, oblong to ovate, colour greyish-green, very flat broad midrib with lateral veins forming acute angles, hairy. Crowded flowers, about 2 cm long, with 4 mm long pedicel. Fruits are small, 1.5 cm long, ovoid, oblong, contain numerous dark grey-coloured flat and reinform seeds. Taste of the herb is bitter.

Microscopical characters

A transverse section of a henbane leaf shows a bifacial structure. Both surfaces have a smooth cuticle, epidermal cells with wavy walls, stomata of both anisocytic and anomocytic types, and a large number of hairs, abundant on the midrib and veins. The hairs are up to 500 μm long; some are uniseriate and two to six cells long, while others have a uniseriate stalk and a large, ovoid, glandular head. Similar hairs are found on the stems. The spongy mesophyll contains calcium oxalate of single and twin prisms or clusters and micro-sphenoidal crystals. The broad midrib contains a vascular bundle, broader than that of stramonium, showing the usual bicollateral arrangement, which is also present in the stems. The mesophyll of the midrib is made up of two thin zones of collenchyma.

The calyx possesses trichomes and stomata. The

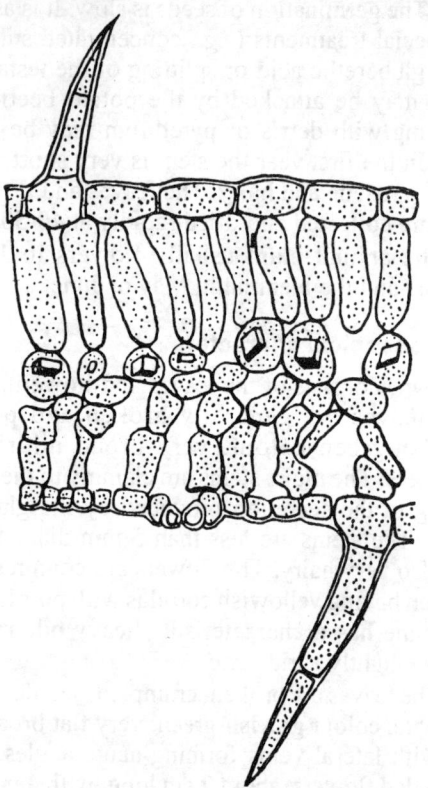

Fig. 21.15. T.S. of Hyoscyamus leaf.

Scopolamine

Apoatropine

Apoatropine

Hyoscyamine

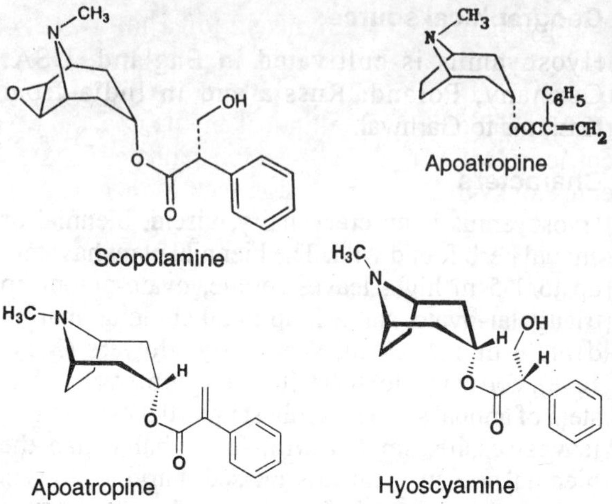

Fig. 21.16. Tropane alkaloids of Hyoscyamus leaf.

corolla is glabrous on the inner surface but exhibits trichomes on the outer surface. Bluish anthocyanins of corolla turn red with chloral hydrate solution. Numerous pollen grains are present, tricolpate with three wide pores and an irregularly, finely pitted exine. The testa of the seeds has an epidermis with lignified and wavy anticlinal walls, and sclereids are present in the pericarp.

Chemical constituents

Hyoscyamus contains tropane alkaloids (0.045-0.14%). 1-Hyoscyamine (atropine) and hyoscine (scopolamine) are the predominent alkaloids. The petioles contain more alkaloid than the lamina and stem. During isolation optical activity of hyoscyamine is lost and racemic mixture of atropine is obtained which contains a mixture of d-and 1-hyoscyamine. Hyoscipicrin and choline are also present. The alkaloid content of seeds is less than that of the leaves.

The other alkaloids isolated are hyoscyamine-N-oxide, skimmianine, apohyoscine, apoatropine, tropine, α- and β-belladonines.

Uses

Hyoscyamus is smooth muscle relaxant, sedative, narcotic, anodyne, antiseptic and mydriatic agent and used in asthma and whooping cough. Atropine has stimulant action on the central nervous system. Atropine and hyoscine are used as ophthalmintic to dilate the pupil of the eye. The parasympatholytic action of Hyoscyamus is weaker than Stramonium and Belladonna. The higher relative proportion of hyoscine in the alkaloid mixture makes the plant less likely to give rise to cerebral excitement than does belladonna. It is used to relieve spasm of the urinary tract and with strong purgatives to prevent griping.

Allied drugs

H. muticus Linn (Egyptian Henbane) is a perennial herb allied to *H. niger*, 30-60 cm high and distributed in the sandy parts of Egypt, Saudi Arabia, Iran, Baluchistan, Sind, Western Punjab and Algiers, cultivated in southern california. It differs from Hyoscyamus obtained from *H. niger* by its striated cuticle and usually branched trichomes with unicellular heads. It contains a higher percentage of total alkaloids than *H. niger*. The leaves of *H. muticus* are smoked in Africa and India for inducing intoxication.

Egyptian Henbane consists of a mixture of leaves, stem, flowers and fruits. The leaves are usually matted pubescent, pale green to yellow, rhomboidal or broadly elliptical and up to about 15 cm long. Midrib broad, venation pinnate, margin entire or with about five large teeth on each side. Petiole almost absent or up to 9 cm long. The stems are greyish-yellow, striated, slightly hairy and hollow. The flowers are shortly stalked, with large hairy bracts, a tubular five-toothed calyx and a yellowish-brown corolla. The fruit is cylindrical surrounded by a persistent calyx and contains numerous yellowish grey to brown seeds. Odour, slightly foetid; taste, bitter and acrid. Egyptian henbane contains glandular trichomes, which have a one- to four-celled stalk and unicellular heads, striated cuticle, the prisms of oxalate, twin prisms and occasional clusters and microsphenoids. *H. muticus* contains atropine, scopolamine, aliphatic constituents and β-sitosterol.

H. albus is a herb with white flowers, found in the Mediterranean region. Its properties are similar to those of official Henbane, for which it is often substituted. *H. albus* contains hyoscyamine, hyoscine, 2,3-dimethylnonacosane, hyalbidone, 6β- and 7β-hydroxyhyoscyamine, littorine, tropine, ψ-tropine, tropinone, 4'-hydroxylittorine, N-methylpyrrolidinyl cuscohygrine, 3-propionyloxytropane, 3-isobutyryloxytropane, 3β-tigloyloxynortropane, 6-hydroxy-3-phenylacetoxy-tropane. The root hairs contain 7β- and 6β-hydroxyhyoscyamine, littorine, hyoscine and hyoscyamine.

Indian henbane

It is *H. reticulatus*. This contains hyoscine and hyoscyamine and microscopically it is almost identical to *H. niger*. *H. pusillus*, a herb occurring in Ladakh, has been reported to be poisonous. This species and *H. aureus* produce hyoscine as the main alkaloid.

SOLANACEOUS ALKALOIDS

The principal alkaloids of this group are (–)-hyoscyamine; atropine, [(±)-hyoscyamine]; scopolamine (also known as hyoscine); and the anhydride of atropine (apoatropine) and its stereoisomer, belladonnine. These are tropine derivatives and esters.

Atropine is an alkaloid obtained from plant sources (from *Atropa belladonna* Linn., from species of *Datura* Linn., and from *Hyoscyamus* Linn. (Fam. Solanaceae) or produced synthetically. It is extremely poisonous. Synthetic production of atropine is more costly than extraction from natural sources and cannot compete in price. Formerly, *Hyoscyamus muticus* represented the chief natural source; however, atropine is now also obtained from species of *Duboisia*. It pre-exists in the solanaceous plants only in traces and is formed from hyoscyamine during the process of extraction.

Atropine occurs as colourless, needle-like crystals or as a white, crystalline powder; it is optically inactive but usually contains some levorotatory hyoscyamine, the limit of which produces an angular rotation not to exceed –0.70°.

Atropine sulfate occurs as colourless crystals or as a white, crystalline powder. It is extremely poisonous. It effloresces in dry air, is slowly affected by light and is an anticholinergic.

Atropine sulfate is an anticholinergic. Used in surgery as an antisialogogue to control bronchial, nasal, pharyngeal, and salivary secretions, it is usually injected intramuscularly prior to induction of anesthesia. During surgery, the drug is given intravenously when reduction in pulse range and cessation of cardiac action are attributable to increased vagal activity. It is also useful in pylorospasm and other spastic conditions of the gastrointestinal tract and for ureteral and biliary colic when administered concomitantly with morphine.

Atropine and scopolamine are competitive with acetylcholine at the postganglionic synapse (muscarinic site) of the parasympathetic nervous system. They show an antispasmodic effect and used to relieve spasms of the bowel in the treatment of spastic colitis, gastroenteritis, and peptic ulcer. Due to their antisecretory effect, they are used to reduce respiratory secretions in anesthesia (antisialogogue), gastric secretions in peptic ulcer therapy, and nasal and sinus secretions in common cold and allergy medications. Due to their mydriatic and cycloplegic effects. They are used to prevent adhesions between the iris and lens of the eye in iritis.

Atropine is an antidote for poisoning caused by cholinesterase inhibitors such as physostigmine and organophosphate insecticides.

Hyoscyamine is the tropine ester of (–)-tropic

acid and is hydrolyzed by boiling in dilute acids or alkalies to form these compounds.

The carbon atom α to the carboxyl group of tropic acid is asymmetric and forms the optical isomer. When (–)-hyoscyamine is extracted from the plants. it is racemized during the process and thus converted into the (±)-compound, which is atropine. The piperidine ring system of tropine can exist in chair and boat conformations. The chair form has the lowest energy requirement. The most active isomer has the esteratic group substituted axial at position 3, as in the case of (–)-hyoscyamine and atropine.

Hyoscyamine sulfate is extremely poisonous. Hyoscyamine sulfate occurs as white, odourless crystals or as a crystalline powder; it is deliquescent and is affected by light.

Hyoscyamine sulfate is an anticholinergic. It is used to control gastric secretion, visceral spasm, hypermotility in spastic colitis, pylorospasm and associated abdominal cramps. In parkinsonism it is used to reduce rigidity and tremors and to control associated sialorrhea and hyperhidrosis.

Scopolamine (hyoscine) occurs as an almost colourless, syrupy liquid from its chloroformic solution and as colourless crystals from its ether solution. It is levorotatory.

Scopolamine hydrobromide or hyoscine hydrobromide occurs as colourless or white crystals or as a white, granular powder that is odourless and slightly efflorescent in dry air. It is extremely poisonous and as an anticholinergic and central nervous system depressant, whereas atropine is a stimulant. For this reason, scopolamine hydrobromide is used for preanesthetic sedation and for obstetric amnesia in conjunction with analgesics and for calming delirium. It is administered subcutaneously or intramuscularly in a single dose.

Scopolamine is effective in the prevention of nausea and vomiting associated with motion sickness. It is applied as the free base in a transdermal system behind the ear at least 4 hours before the antiemetic effect is required. The scopolamine is gradually released from an adhesive matrix of mineral oil and polyisobutylene.

Scopolamine has a depressant activity on the central nervous system and is used to treat motion sickness, for preanaesthetic sedation, for obstetric amnesia in conjunction with analgesics and to calm delirium.

Toxicity symptoms occurred during the therapeutic use of atropine, scopolamine and belladonna tincture are skin rash, skin flushing, mouth dryness, difficulty in urination, eye pain, blurred vision and light sensitivity.

BELLADONNA

Synonyms

Belladonna herb; Belladonna leaf; Deadly night shade leaves; Banewort; Death's herb, Dwale; Poison black cherry; Folia belladonnae.

Biological source

Belladonna consists of dried leaves and flowering tops of *Atropa belladonna* Linn. (European Belladonna) containing about 0.35% of total alkaloids calculated as hyoscyamine. The drug may be consisted of all the aerial parts. Prepared Belladonna herb is the finely powdered drug adjusted to contain 0.28-0.32% of total alkaloids. (Fam. Solanaceae).

Geographical source

A. belladonna is cultivated in USA, Canada, UK, Germany and India.

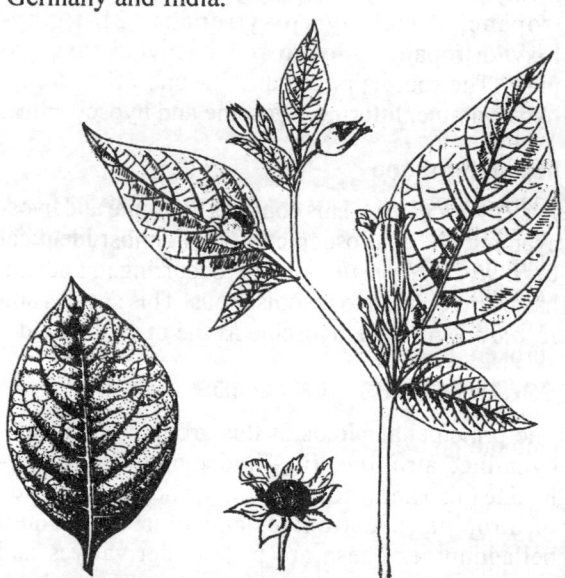

Fig. 21.17. Belladonna flowering shoot.

The plant is an erect, glandular-pubescent or glabrous, perennial herb, about 1.5 meter high. Leaves on the upper part are in pairs of two, among which one leaf is larger and the other smaller.

The leaves are richest in alkaloid at the flowering stage. A sunny position gives more active leaves than a shady one.

Cultivation and collection

Plants are cultivated by sowing seeds in nurseries and seedlings are transplanted in April to moist, calcareous and loamy soil. Weeds are removed and manure is applied for proper growth of the crop. During flowering session leaves and flowering tops are cut at least three times in a year at an interval of two months from one to three years old plants. When the plant is four years old, roots are dug out. The collected drug is dried at 40-50°C. Undried leaves deteriorate and give off ammonia. Belladonna plant infected with the fungus *Phytophthora belladonnae* should be destroyed to prevent further infection. Sometimes the leaves are damaged by flea-bettle insect and the roots by a fungus.

Morphology

The drug contains leaves, smaller stems of about 5 mm diameter, flowers and fruits. Leaves are stalked, brittle, thin, entire, long-pointed, 5-25 cm long, 2.5-12 cm wide, ovate lanceolate, slightly decurrent lamina, margine-entire, apex acuminate, colour dull-green or yellowish-green, surface glabrous, lateral veins join the mid-rib at an angle of 60°, curving upwards and are anastomose. The upper side is darker than the lower. Each has a petiole about 0.5-4 cm long and a broadly ovate, slightly decurrent lamina about 5-25 cm long and 2.5-12 cm wide. The margin is entire and the apex acuminate. A few flowers and fruits may be present. If the leaves are broken, they are characterized by the venation and roughness of the surface due to the presence of calcium oxalate in some mesophyll cells which causes minute points on the surface of the leaf on drying. The flowers blooming in June are solitary, shortly stalked, drooping and about 2.5 cm long. The corolla is campanulate, five-lobed and of a dull purplish colour. The five-lobed calyx is persistent, remaining attached to the purplish-black berry. The fruit is bilocular, contains numerous seeds and is about the size of a cherry. A yellow variety of the plant lacks the anthocyanin pigmentation.

Microscopical characters

A transverse section of the leaf of *A. belladonna* has a bifacial structure. The epidermal cells have wavy walls and a striated cuticle. Anisocytic type and some of the anomocytic type stomata are present on both surfaces but are most common on the lower. Hairs are most numerous on young leaves, uniseriate, 2-4-celled clothing hairs; or with a unicellular glandular head. Some hair have a short pedicel and a multicellular glandular head. Certain of the cells of the spongy mesophyll are filled with microsphenoidal (sandy) crystals of calcium oxalate. The midrub is convex above and shows the usual bicollateral vascular bundle. A zone of collenchyma is present in epidermis near midrib.

Chemical constituents

Belladonna contains 0.3-1.0% total alkaloids, the prominent base is 1-hyoscyamine. The other components are atropine, apoatropine, asparagine, choline, belladonnine, cuscohygrine, scopolamine, chrysatropic acid, volatile bases such as pyridine; atroscine, leucatropic acid; phytosterol, N-methylpyrroline, homatropine, hyoscyamine N-oxide, rutin, kaempferol-3-rhamnogalactoside and 7-glucoside, quercetin-7-glucoside, scopoletin (β-methylaesculetin), calcium oxalate, 14% acid soluble ash and 4% acid-insoluble ash. Addition of ammonia to the alcoholic solution of scopoletin shows blue florescence. This test is useful to detect

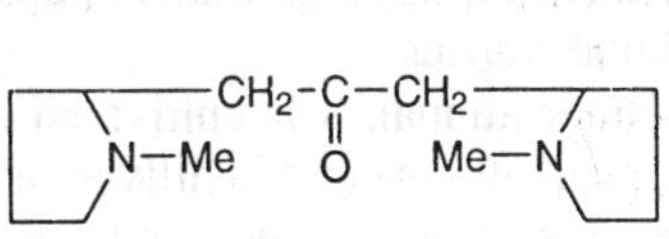

Cuscohygrine

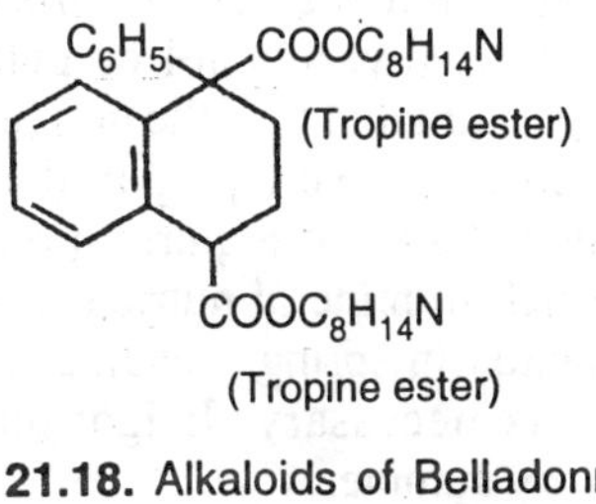

Fig. 21.18. Alkaloids of Belladonna.

Belladonna poisoning. Atropine is formed by racemization during the extraction process.

Uses

The drug is used as adjunctive therapy in the treatment of peptic ulcer; functional digestive disorders, including spastic, mucous and ulcerative colitis; diarrhoea, diverticulitis and pancreatitis. Due to anticholinergic property, it is used to control excess motor activity of the gastrointestinal tract and spasm of the urinary tract.

Belladonna is anticholinergic, narcotic, sedative, diuretic mydriatic and used as anodyne and to check secretion. Other uses are similar to Hyoscyamus. It relieves spasm of gut or respiratory tract. Consumption of Belladonna checks excessive perspiration of patients suffering from tuberculosis. Belladonna acts as a parasympathetic depressant.

INDIAN BELLADONNA

Synonyms

Sag-angur (Hindi); Yebruti (Bengali); Girbuti (Marathi), Bantanaku (Panjabi); Mait-brand (Kashmiri).

It consists of dried leaves and other aerial parts of *Atropa acuminata* Royle ex Lindley (Solanaecae). The plant is found in Kashmir, Shimla, Chamba, Kangra and Kulu.

The plant is a perennial herb, 60 cm to 3 m high, erect with dichotomous branching, leaves oblong elliptical, brownish green, 7.5-13 cm long, 4-6.5 cm wide, tapering towards apex and base, flowers are yellowish brown, drooping, funnel-shaped, solitary, fruits globular berries.

As a winter annual, it is cultivated in plains in the sub-tropical climate and in hilly areas. The plant can be propagated from seeds or from cuttings of the young shoots or from fresh root-stocks. The seeds are very small, brownish black and are obtained from berries. Seeds pre-treated with sulphuric acid, ethyl alcohol or petroleum ether give better germination than the untreated ones. The seeds are sown in well prepared nursery beds during May and July. It requires a porous, slightly acidic soil rich in mineral nutrients. The seedlings are transplanted in spring. Shading the transplants with twigs is necessary. Irrigation is required during the dry summer.

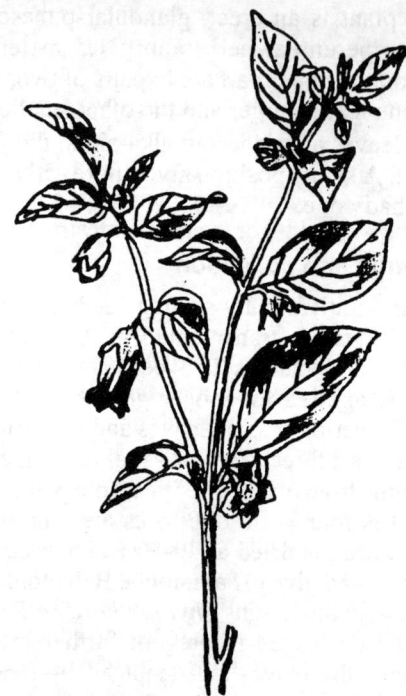

Fig. 21.19. *Atropa acuminata.*

Total alkaloidal contents in Himalayan plant are 0.5% in leaves. The constituents of Indian Belladonna leaves resemble those of the European species.

Uses

Indian Belladonna is used as sedative, anticholinergic tranquillizers, in labour, delirium tremens, toxic psychoses and maniacal states. Atropine and other Belladonna alkaloids are common constituent of proprietary medicines for the common cold and acute rhinitis. They induce bronchial dilation and give relief in bronchial asthma. They are employed in diseases of the gastro-intestinal tract, in heavy metal poisoning, Parkinsonism and in checking enurenis in children.

Belladonna preparations are reputed as local anodynes and counter irritants for external application for treating intercostal pains, rheumatism, lumbago, neuralgia and pleurisy. They are made into plasters and liniments for local application and into suppositories employed to relieve the spasm of anal fistula.

Belladonna leaves extract is used as proprietary pharmaceutical preparations to treat gastrointestinal hypermotility, hypersecretion, peptic ulcer, spastic constipation, spastic dysmenorrhoea, nocturnal enuresis, bronchial asthma, whooping cough, digestive disorders, ulcerative colitis, diarrhoea, diverticulitis and pancreatitis, to control excess motor activity of the gastrointestinal tract and spasm of the urinary tract.

Adulteration

Phytolacca decandra (Phytolaccaceae) and *Ailanthus glandulosa* (Simaroubaceae) are the most important adulterants of Belladonna. In *Phytolacca* the lamina is denser and less decurrent than in belladonna; the epidermal cells have straight walls, the stromata are of the anomocytic type and some of the mesophyll cells contain bundles of needle-shaped crystals of calcium oxalate. *Ailanthus* leaves are triangular-ovate, with straight-walled epidermal cells, a strongly striated cuticle, cluster crystals of calcium oxalate, and on both surfaces white, unicellular clothing lignified hairs with a strongly striated cuticle. The roots of *Althaea officinalis* are sometimes mixed with Belladonna roots but they can be distinguished on the basis of their fracture and absence of starch in the exposed surface. The roots contain L-arabinan, flavonoid sulphate and hypoletin-8-glucoside. *Phytolacca acinosa* grows side by side with Belladonna in nature and resembles the latter when not in flower. Its leaves are often substituted for Belladonna leaves. It can be detected in commercial samples by its ovate leaves and hollow stem. *P. acinosa* contains β-sitosterol, triterpenes phytolaccanol, epiacetyleuritolic acid, spergulagenic acid, isophytolaccinic acid A, isophytolaccagenin A, 3-O-methyl spergulagenate, phytolaccagenin A, acinosolic acids A and B, phytolaccagenic, esculentic and jaligonic acids, acinosperigenin and saponin esculentoside S. The leaves of *Solanum nigrum* and other species of *Solanum* and *Datura* are often used as adulterants.

S. nigrum contains α- and β-solamargine, solasonine, solasodine, tigogenin, solasodiene, diosgenin, chlorogenic, neochlorogenic and isochlorogenic acids, caffeoylglucose, uttronin A, uttrosides A and B, α-carotene, steroidal glycosides SN-0, SN-1, SN-2, SN-3 and SN-4 (immature fruits); totigonin, steroidal alkaloids SN-a, SN-b, SN-c, SN-d, SN-e and SN-f (immature berries); 12β-hydroxysolasadine, N-methylsolasodine, solanocapsine, tomatidenol, 23-O-acetyl-12β-hydroxy-solasodine and quercetin glycosides.

Pharmacology

Atropine inhibited cholinesterase and in small doses it potentiated toxicity of acetylcholine in mice and guinea pig ileum. Atropine showed increased tolerance to hexabarbital, inhibited learning and retention in training and memory testing experiments, exhibited strong bronchodilator effect, inhibited cholinergically, induced gastric acid secretion and gastric motility in mice, induced increased in outward movement of Na^+ in muscle and exerted central nervous system stimulant activity in rabbits. It showed tranquillizing action. Scopolamine exhibited thymoleptic effect in higher doses and antihistaminic activity. Atropine sulphate inhibited insulin release induced by oral intake of glucose in human subjects.

BELLADONNA ROOT

Synonym

Radix belladonnae.

Biological source

Belladonna root consists of the dried roots or rootstock of *Atropa belladonna* L. (Fam : Solanaceae).

Collection

Atropa belladonna produces a large branching root. The aerial stems die each year and new ones arise independently from the large crown. Roots of the first and second years are small in size and not collected although the percentage of alkaloid is high. The roots of three or four years old plant are collected in autumn. The roots are dug up, washed, cut into small pieces and dried at 40-50°.

Macroscopical characters

The drug occurs in small pieces or longitudinal slices, length 10-20 cm, diameter 3-4 cm; shape cylindrical and tapering; surface longitudinally wrinkled with scars of roots; fracture short; whitish or brownish interior after drying; cambium is

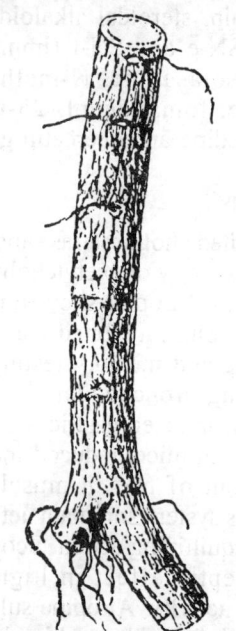

Fig. 21.20. Belladonna root.

distinct with porous xylem; odour - distinct, taste bitter.

A transverse section of the bark is nonfibrous. The wood consists of scattered groups of vessels, tracheids and fibres which are most abundant near the cambium. There is a primary xylem in the centre. The parenchyma of bark and wood contains sandy crystals of calcium oxalate and abundant simple and compound starch grains.

The structure changes when the roots is converted into rhizome. The wood becomes denser and exhibits radiate structure. The rhizome shows a distinct pith and internal phloem. The aerial stems found on the upper surface of the crown are hollow.

Chemical constituents

Belladonna root contains 0.4-1.0 per cent total alkaloids. The important alkaloids isolated are hyoscyamine, atropine and scopolamine. The other chemical components obtained are apoatropine, belladonnine, cuscohygrine, and tropine along with β-methyl aesculetin, calcium oxalate and starch. It also contains hygrine, hygroline, tropinone, pseudotropine and tropanol esters. A pseudotropine

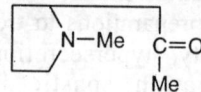

Fig. 21.21. Hygrine.

forming tropinone reductase is isolated from transformed belladonna root cultures.

Uses

Roots are narcotic, anticholinergic, sedative, diuretic, mydriatic; used as an anodyne, local anaesthetic, in cough and bronchitis and to check perspiration of tuberculosis.

Allied drugs

Indian Belladonna roots are obtained from *Atropa acuminata* which are brownish grey roots, stolons, rootstock and stem bases. The roots are cylindrical, longitudinally wrinkled, branched, and 0.5-3 cm diameter. Young roots resemble those of *A. belladonna* but older ones show concentric zonation of the secondary xylem. The rootstock is 3-9 cm diameter at the top and bears the bases of 4-12 aerial stems. The rootstock, stem bases and stolons all possess a pith which becomes hollow in the stem bases. The constituents are similar to those of European belladonna.

Adulterant

The root of *Phytolacca decandra* (Phytolaccaceae) is sliced and mixed with samples of belladonna. It shows some resemblance to belladonna root. The transverse section shows a number of concentric cambia with a ring of wood bundles. The parenchyma contains abundant acicular crystals of calcium oxalate.

STRAMONIUM
Synonyms

Thornapple leaves; Jimson or Jamestown weed; Dhatura; Stinkweed; Devil's apple; Apple of Peru; Folia stramonii.

Biological source

Stramonium consists of dried leaves and flowering tops of *Datura stramonium* Linn. or its variety

D. tatula Linn. (Family : Solanaceae). The drug is required to contain not less than 0.25% of alkaloids calculated as hyoscyamine. Prepared Stramonium is the finely powdered drug adjusted to an alkaloid content of 0.23-0.27%.

Geographical source

Stramonium is found widely in European, Asian, and American countries and in South Africa. The plant grows commonly in waste places throughout India from Kashmir to Malabar. It is cultivated in Germany, France, Hungary and South America.

Cultivation

Datura prefers a rich calcareous soil. It can be grown from seeds in spring in drills; the plants are later thinned to stand 3 m apart in raws. The plant is sensitive to frost and sheltered situations are preferred for cultivation. Entire plants are cut down when the fruits are mature. Nitrogen manuring, which favours the growth of plants, also flavours alkaloid formation. At the end of August leaves and flowering tops are collected and dried at 45-50°C.

Plant habitat and morphology

D. stramonium is a bushy annual herb, 1.5 m high, having whitish roots and numerous rootlets. The stem is herbaceous, round, smooth, green branched, glabrous and shows dichasial branching with leaf adnation. Leaves stalked, ovate, 8-25 cm long, 7-15 cm wide, coarsely and irregularly lobed and toothed. Flowers are solitary, axillary, short stalk, single, white, have sweet scent, calyx tubular, 5-toothed, 5-ribbed, corolla funnel-shaped. The ripe fruits are thorny capsule about 3-4 cm long. Seeds are numerous dark brown or blackish in colour, reinform in outline, 3 mm long. The testa is reticulated and finely pitted; smell is slightly unpleasant and taste is bitter.

Macroscopical characters

The dried leaves are greyish-green in colour, thin, brittle, twisted, broken, whole leaves 8-25 cm long and 7-15 cm wide; shortly petiolate, ovate or triangular-ovate in shape, acuminate at the apex and have a sinuate-dentate margin. The margin possesses teeth dividing the sinuses; the lateral veins run into the marginal teeth.

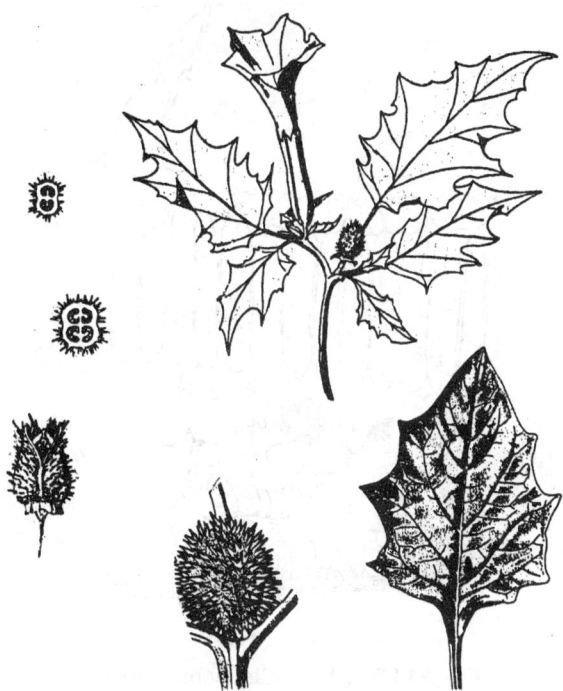

Fig. 21.22. Stramonium leaf.

Microscopical characters

A transverse section of a leaf has a bifacial structure; covered with a smooth cuticle and possess both stomata and hairs. Microsphenoidal and prismatic cluster crystals of calcium oxalate are abundant in the mesophyll. The stomata are of the anisocytic and anomocytic types. The epidermal cells have wavy walls. The uniseriate clothing hairs are three- to five-celled, slightly curved, and have thin, warty walls. Small glandular hairs with a one or two-celled pedicel and an oval head of two to seven cells are also present.

The midrib has a bicollateral structure and characteristic subepidermal masses of collenchyma on both surfaces. The xylem is a curved arc. Sclerenchyma is absent.

Stem diameter is about 5 mm. They possess epidermal hairs and perimedullary phloem. The stem parenchyma contains calcium oxalate similar to that found in the leaf.

Chemical constituents

Stramonium contains 0.2-0.6% alkaloids. The main

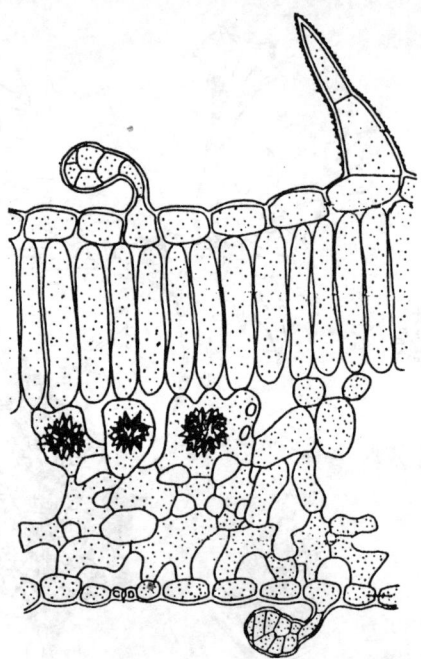

Fig. 21.23. T.S. of Stramonium leaf.

alkaloids are hyoscyamine and hyoscine (scopolamine). It also contains protein albumin and atropine.

Atropine is formed from hyoscyamine by racemization. At the time of collection these alkaloids are usually present in the proportion of about two parts of hyoscyamine to one part of hyoscine, but in young plants hyoscine is the predominant alkaloid. The larger stems contain small amount of alkaloid and the official drug should contain not more than 3% stem with a diameter exceeding 5 mm.

Ditigloyl esters of 3,6-dihydroxytropane and 3, 6, 7-trihydroxytropane have also been isolated from the roots in addition to hyoscine, hyoscyamine, tropine and pseudotropine.

D. stramonium also contains 6-hydroxyhyos cyamine, skimmianine, meteloidine, acetyl derivatives of caffeic, p-coumaric and ferulic acids, β-sitosterol, stigmasterol, campesterol, withanolide 1, vitastramonolide, daturalactone; steroidal glycosides daturataturins A and B; flavonoids chrysins, quercetin and kaempferol and their esters.

Uses

It is a narcotic, antispasmodic and anodyne drug and used to relieve the spasm of the bronchioles in asthma. The leaves are ingredient of *Pulvis stramonii compositus* and other powders used for the relief of asthma. The leaves may be made into cigarettes or smoked in a pipe to relieve asthma. They are also used in the treatment of parkinsonism, boils, sores and fish-bites. The flower juice is used to treat earache.

The fruit juice is applied to the scalp for curing dandruff and falling hair. Stramonium ointment, containing lanolin, yellow wax and petroleum, is employed to cure haemorrhoids. Stramonium is one of the chief ingredient of the Ayurvedic preparation, *Kanaka asaves*, used as demulcent, expectorant, antispasmodic and anodyne in cough, asthma and phthisis.

Atropine and hyoscine are used to dilate the pupil of the eye.

Adulterants

The leaves of *Datura innoxia* and *D. metel* are used as substitutes for Stramonium. The dried leaves are curled and twisted, but are usually somewhat browner in colour, with entire margins and with differences in venation and trichomes. The leaves contain about 0.5% of alkaloids. Over 30 alkaloids, and two novel hygrines, have been characterized from *D. innoxia*. The leaves of *Xanthium strumarium*, *Carthamus helenioides* and *Chenopodium hybridum* are used as adulterants. The leaves of *D. innoxia* contains hyoscyamine, hyoscine, meteloidine and N-methylpyrrolidinyl hygrines.

The leaves of *D. metel* yields scopolamine, hyoscine, hyoscyamine, datumetine; p-hydroxycinnamic acid of tyramine, withanolides daturametelins A-G, daturilinol, withametelin, isowithametelin, secowithametelin, 12-deoxywithastramonolide, physalindicanol A, withametelins B, C, D and E, lycium substance B, withfastuosins A and B.

X. strumarium contains sesquitorpenoids, xanthinin, xanthanol, 6,9-dihydroxy-8-epixanthatin, epixanthumin, isoxanthanol, xanthumin, carboxyatractyloside, isohexanone, chlorobutanol, stearyl alcohol, palmitic acid, strumasterol, oleic and 3,4-dihydroxycinnamic acids, β-sitosterol and its glucoside, heptacosanol, 8-epixanthatin-5β-epoxide, β-amyrin, octacosanol and stigmasterol.

Xanthumin showed CNS depressant and antibacterial activities.

Datura seeds are derived mainly from *D. metel.* Each seed is light brown in colour and ear-shaped. They are larger and more flattened than stramonium seeds but resemble the latter in internal structure. The alkaloid content, hyoscine with traces of hyoscyamine and atropine, is about 0.2%. *D. ferox,* having very large spines on its capsules, contains as its major alkaloids hyoscine and meteloidine.

The 'tree-daturas' is *D. sanguinea* indigenous to South America and cultivated as ornaments. It produces large, white or coloured trumpet-shaped flowers and pendant unarmed fruits. It contains tropane alkaloids. Some 400 tonnes of dried leaf are produced annually in Ecuador and yield about 0.8% hyoscine. One of chemical races of *D. sanguinea* produces large amounts of 6 β-acetoxy-3α-tigloyloxytropane.

Pharmacology

Scopolamine disrupted regulation of local blood flow in brain and altered basal tone of cerebral pial artery system in rats. It inhibited play fighting in prepubescent male rats and showed analgesic activity in rat. Scopolamine exaggerated response of heart rate. It increased ECGP-R variance during standing condition and caused dryness of the mouth. Scopolamine facilitated performance of avoidance task in normal animals. Scopolamine markedly increased spontaneous activity of rats and exhibited antiulcer activity against gastric ulcer. It inhibited gastric acid secretion and pepsin activity.

WITHANIA (ASHWAGANDHA)

Synonyms

Ashwagandha; Withania root.

Biological source

Withania consists of the dried roots of *Withania somnifera* Dunal. (Family : Solanaceae).

Geographical source

Withania is widely distributed from southern Europe to Africa. In India it is found widely in the drier parts ascending to 1800 m in the Himalayas and cultivated in Neemuch near Ajmer and in Manasa (MP).

Plant habitat and macroscopy

The plant is tomentose, evergreen, perennial, branched, erect shrub. The tuberous roots are cut into small pieces and used. The roots are straight, unbranched, conical and 5-12 mm thick. The outer surface is longitudinally wrinkled and buff to greyish yellow. On the crown 2-6 stem bases are present. Taste is macilaginous and bitter.

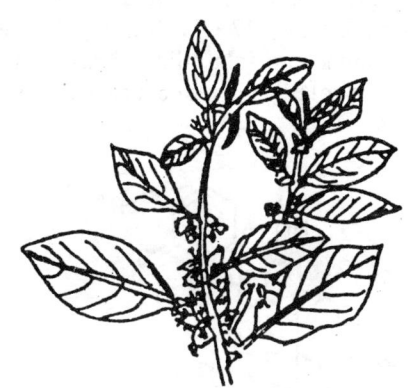

Fig. 21.24. Withania twig.

The plant is cultivated in soils that are unsuited for other crops. Seeds are sown broadcast in the nursery just before the onset of rainy season. Nitrogenous fertilizers promote heavy leaf growth. The plants flower and fruit in December. The entire plant is uprooted for roots, which are separated from the aerial parts by cutting. They are transversely cut into smaller pieces for drying. The pieces are dark brown with a creamy interior. They are straight, unbranched and conical. The main root bears fibre-like secondary roots. Their outer surface is buff to grey-yellow with longitudinal wrinkles. The stem bases are variously thickened, cylindrical and green and have longitudinal wrinkles. The roots have a short and uneven fracture, a strong odour and mucilaginous bitter and acrid taste.

Chemical constituents

Withania contains alkaloids and withanolides. The important alkaloids isolated are tropine, pseudo-tropine, hygrine (pyrrolidine derivatives), iso-pelletierine (piperidine derivative), cuscohygrine (two pyrrolidine moieties), anaferine (two piperidine moieties), anahygrine (one pyrrolidine moiety and one piperidine moiety), withasomnine (phenyl 1: 5 trimethylene pyrrazole), nicotine, somniferine, somniferinine, withaninine, witha-nine, pseudowithaninine, choline, withasomine, visamine, withaniol (mixture of two withanolides), withanolides like like withaferine A, withanolides N, O, D, S, Q, R, G, H, I, J, K, V, sitoindosides IX, VII and VII, a withanolide 5,2-O-α(R)-dihydroxy-6α-7α-epoxy-1-oxo-(15α)-witha-2,24-dienolide, withasomidienone, 27-OH-3-oxo-(22R)-witha-1,4,24-trienolide and solasodine. Besides these the drug contains volatile oil, reducing sugar, starch and amino acids.

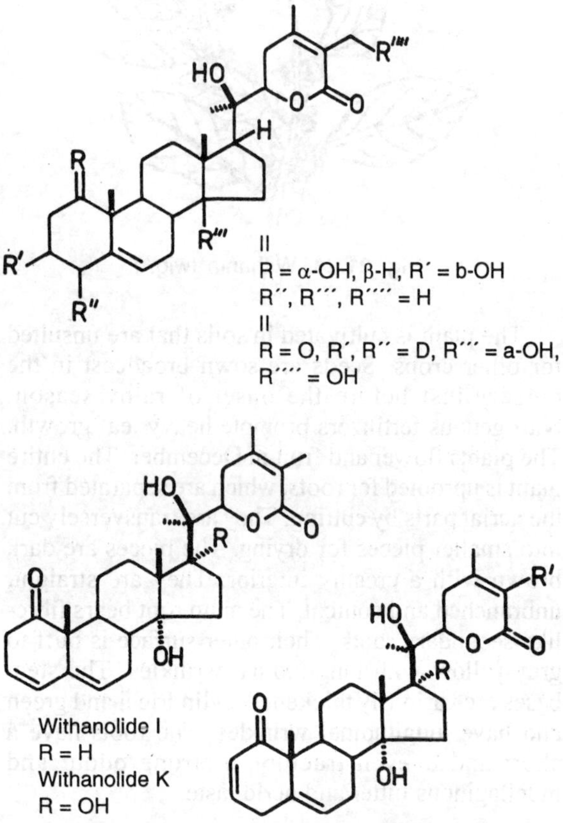

Withanolide I
R = H
Withanolide K
R = OH

II
R = α-OH, β-H, R′ = b-OH
R″, R‴, R‴″ = H
II
R = O, R′, R″ = D, R‴ = a-OH,
R‴″ = OH

Withanolide G
R = H, R′ = Me
Withanolide H
R = H, R′ = CH₂OH
Withanolide J
R = OH, R′ = Me

Fig. 21.25. Withanolides of Withania.

W. somnifera also contains compounds A₁, A₂, A₃, A₄ and A₅, 3α-trigloyloxytropane, withanolide WS-12 C, N, U, 14β-hydroxywithanone, 14,17,20-trihydroxy and 4,14,17,20-tetrahydroxy - 5,6-epoxy-withanolides, sitoindoside X, 5-dehydroxy-withanolide R, withasomniferin A, sominone, sominolide and withasomidienone.

Uses

Withania is considered as alterative, anodyne, aphrodisiac, tonic, anti-inflammatory drug, nervine tonic, sedative deobstruent, diuretic, narcotic and abortifacient. It is used in rheumatism, consumption, debility from old age, emaciation of children, asthma, bronchitis, tuberculosis, leucorrhoea, insomnia, epilepsy and hypertension. Due to its adaptogenic property the drug is much reputed.

Pharmacology

The pharmacological activity of the drug (roots and leaves) is attributed to alkaloids and withanolides.

The drug show antistress, analgesic, anti-inflammatory, antitumor, antibiotic, anticonvulsant, antihepatotoxic, psychotropic, hypotensive, antispasmodic and CNS depressant activities. The drug is highly safe, the LD₅₀ value being 1260 mg/kg. Withanolides possess immunosuppressive and immunomodulatory properties. The sitoindosides VII, VIII and withaferin A, in combination exert antistress activity. Sitoindosides IX and X exert adaptogenic and immunostimulatory activities.

Decrease in serum cholesterol was more and erythrocyte sedimentation rate much higher in treated group than in placebo group. Withanolide D exhibited significant antitumor activity against sarcoma 180 and Ehrlich ascites carcinoma and cells from human epidermoid carcinoma of nasopharynx. Withaferin A showed significantly protective effect against CCl₄-induced hepatotoxicity in rats. Root extract contains an ingredient which has GABA mimetic activity. A methanolic fraction of the plant extract showed anti-inflammatory activity. A steroidal lactone 5,20-(R)-di-hydroxy-6,7-α-epoxy-1-oxo-(5α)-witha-2,24-dienolide and solasodine isolated from the drug also exhibited adaptogenic and immuno-modulating activities.

Withanolides possess anti-inflammatory and antiarthritic activities. The antitumor activity of the drug is attributed to withaferin A and withanolide D. Withaferin A shows the activity due to the presence of unsaturated lactone ring in the side chain with allylic primary alcohol group at C-25 and highly oxygenated ring at the other ring of the molecule. The drug increases the effect of radiation on tumor regression and growth delay. Withaferin A is a potential antibiotic compound. The extract of the drug exhibits good anticonvulsant activity. It has CNS depressant effect, the total alkaloidal fraction of root extract showed prolonged hypotensive, bradycardiac and respiratory stimulant activities in dogs. Compounds A_1-A_5 were effective against aerobic bacilli. Visamine prolonged hexanal-induced sleeping time and showed hypothermic and nicotinolytic effects in mice. Withaferin A and withanolide E exhibited specific immunosuppressive effect on human B and T lymphocytes. Withanolide E showed antitumor activity and immunosuppressive pro-perties. In a clinical trial, root powder showed significant increase in haemoglobin, RBC, hair melanin and seated stature.

DUBOISIA LEAVES

Three species of *Duboisia*, e.g., *D. hopwoodii*, *D. myoporoides* and *D. leichhardtii* contain tropane alkaloids. *D. hopwoodii* contains nicotine and related alkaloids. These plants are found in Australia.

D. myoporoides occurs along the east coast of Australia, where the rainfall exceeds a monthly mean of 5 cm for 11 months of the year and where frosts rarely occur. *D. leichhardtii* occurs naturally in a limited area of south-east Queensland known locally as the South West Burnett. *D. hopwoodii* is distributed in western and central Australia.

D. myoporoides has larger and more densely leaves. For collection, the small branches are removed, tied in bundles and stood in sheds to dry; the leaves are then easily removed by beating.

Duboisia contains hyoscine and hyoscyamine as the main alkaloids alongwith norhyoscyamine, 6β-hydroxyhyoscyamine, valeroidine, tigloidine, poroidine, isoporoidine, valtropine, 3α-tigloyloxytropane, butropine, apohyoscine, 3α-non-anoyl oxytropane, two discopine esters, triterpenoids ursolic acid and betulonic acid and a number of aliphatic constituents.

A number of chemical races of *D. myoporoides*, include the 'northern' and 'southern' races which differ in their relative contents of hyoscine and hyoscyamine, and a race which contains nicotine and anabasine as principal bases.

The total alkaloid content of the leaves remains the same throughout the year but there is a decrease in hyoscine content from January to June (summer to autumn) and a gradual increase from June to September; the reverse is true for hyoscyamine. Repeated sprayings of plants with cytokinin solution in the form of a seaweed extract enhances the hyoscine yield.

SCOPOLIA

All species of *Scopolia*, e.g., *S. caucasia*, *S. lurida* and *S. tanguica*, resemble those of belladonna, although they are more lanceolate and translucent. The cuticle is striated, sandy crystals are less numerous, hairs are rare or absent, and stomata are present on the lower surface only. The fruit, which is a pyxis, is present in the drug. The rhizomes, which are black in colour and bear numerous depressed stem scars, are used similarly to belladonna root. The drug contains hyoscyamine, hyoscine, cusco-hygrine, 3α-tigloyloxytropane, pseudotropine, tropine, 6-hydroxyhyoscyamine and daturamine (anisodine) which is a 'hydroxyhyoscine'. The dried rhizomes of *S. japonica* ('Japanese Bella-donna Root') were official in the *Japanese Pharmacopoeia*, 1961 and steroidal glycosides (scopolosides) are reported from this species.

Przewalskia tangutica is a tropane alkaloid-containing plant in Tibet. The roots have a high content of hyoscyamine, 6β-hydroxyhyoscyamine and small amounts of hyoscine.

MANDRAKE

The true mandrake, *Mandragora officinarium*, is a Mediterranean species. The roots occur in fusiform or two-branched pieces. The drug, like belladonna, has long been known to contain atropine and fluorescent substance scopoletin.

COCA LEAVES

Synonyms

Coca; Huanaco coca, Truxillo coca; Java coca; Folia cocae.

Biological source

Coca or coca leaves have been described as the dried leaves of *Erythroxylum coca* Lam (Huanaco Coca) or of *Erythroxylum truxillense* Rusby (Truxillo Coca) (Family : Erythroxylaceae).

Geographical source

It is cultivated in Colombia, Java, Sri Lanka, Bolivia, Peru, Indonesia and India. It is a shrub or small tree, pyramidal in shape, up to 6 m high, with dark green, ovate leaves.

Cultivation

Coca plant is grown similarly to tea-plantation. Seeds are sown in rich, light and well drained soil at an altitude of 500-2000 meters.

It requires a humid atmosphere, rainfall not below 75-80 inch and temperature between 59-68°F. It thrives best in well drained moist loams rich in humus. The plant can be propagated by cutting, but for raising plantations, seedlings are raised in nurseries and transplanted. The first crop of leaves is gathered in 1-3 years after planting. Only the stiff ripe leaves, easily detached, are collected. The young leaves are reported to be rich in cinnamyl-cocaine and this is replaced in the old leaves by cocaine or truxilline. The cultivated plants are usually kept up to 2 m in height. Three harvests are collected annually, the first from the pruned twigs, the second in June and the third in November. The leaves are dried and packed in bags.

Morphology

1. Huanaco or Bolivian Coca leaves are entire,

3-8 cm long, 1.5-4 cm wide, shortly petiolated, apex acute, base tapering, lamina-brown and glabrous, margin entire, midrib prominent on the lower surface with a ridge on its upper surface, apex acute, surface glabrous, slightly glossy, texture thin, odour-distinct, taste bitter. The lower surface shows two, very characteristic, curved lines, one on either side of the midrib. Odour, characteristic; taste, at first bitter and slightly aromatic, the alkaloids afterwards causing numbness of the tongue and lips.

2. Truxillo or Peruvian coca are broken, pale green in colour, lamina is 1.6-6 cm long, shape elliptical, margin entire, venation is identical but ridges on lower surface are conspicuous, apex acute, base tapering, surface glabrous, not glossy, texture thin odour is distinct and taste is bitter.

3. *Javanese coca* leaves are of the Truxillo type. Large quantities are exported for the manufacture of cocaine.

Microscopical characters

A transverse section of a coca leaf show upper epidermis, palisade parenchyma with prisms of calcium oxalate, spongy parenchyma and a characte-

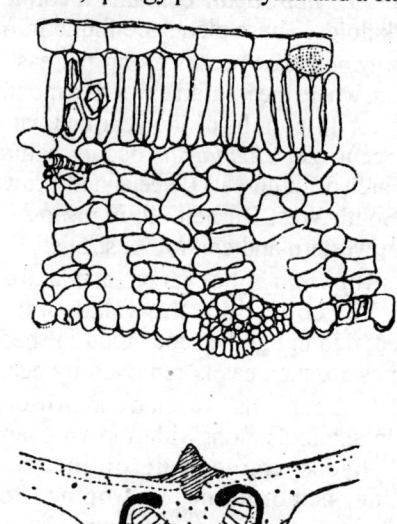

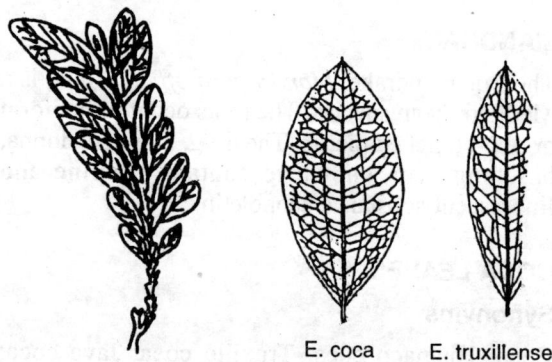

E. coca   E. truxillense

Fig. 21.26. Coca leaves.

Fig. 21.27. T.S. of Coca leaf.

ristic lower papillose epidermis with numerous stomata. The midrib is partly surrounded by an arc of pericyclic fibres. The lower epidermis shows the papillae and circles, and numerous stomata, each with four subsidiary cells. The long axes of two cells are parallel to the pore.

Chemical constituents

Coca leaves contain 0.7-1.5% of alkaloids which are of three type derivatives of :
  (i) ecgonine (cocaine, cinnamylcocaine, α-and β-truxilline)
  (ii) tropine (tropococaine, valerine) and
  (iii) hygrine (hygroline, cuscohygrine)

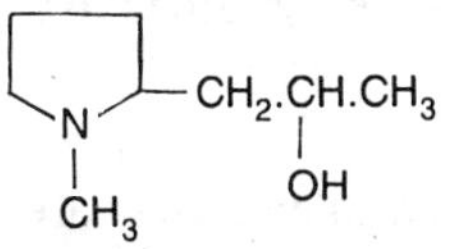

The alkaloidal composition varies according to the variety of the plant and stage of development of leaves. Cocaine, cinnamylcocaine and α-truxilline are the most important alkaloids. Javanese leaves are usually richest in total alkaloids, of which the main is cinnamylcocaine. Bolivian, Peruvian and Ceylon leaves contain less total alkaloid but a higher proportion of cocaine. 1-Hydroxytropacocaine (free hydroxyl situated at a bridgehead carbon) has been isolated as a major alkaloid of greenhouse-cultivated *E. novogranatense* var. *novogranatense*; much lower amounts were detected in var. *truxillense* and in field cultivated coca from Colombia and Bolivia.

The constituents isolated from the leaves are simple alkaloids (hygrine, dihydrocuscohygrine), tropococaine, yellow crystalline glycosides, cocatannic acid and essential oil.

Cocaine is the methyl ester of benzoylecgonine. On hydrolysis it yields ecgonine, benzoic acid and methyl alcohol. Cinnamylcocaine on hydrolysis gives ecgonine, methyl alcohol and cinnamic acid, while α-truxilline forms ecgonine, methyl alcohol and α-truxillic acid.

Besides the alkaloids, coca leaves contain an essential oil (0.06 - 0.13%), the chief constituent of which is methyl salicylate up to 13.6%, together with N-methylpyrrole (3.7%), *N,N*-dimethylbenzylamine (0.5%) and two dihydrobenzaldehydes (38.9%). The grassy odour of the leaves is due to the presence in the oil of *trans*-2-hexenal (10.4%) and *cis*-3-hexen-1-ol (16.1%); no mono- or sesquiterpenes were detected. A colouring matter, coca citrin, has been reported from the leaves.

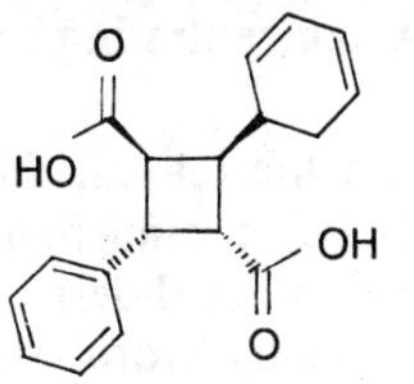

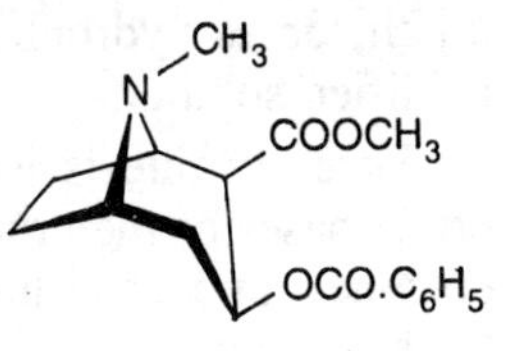

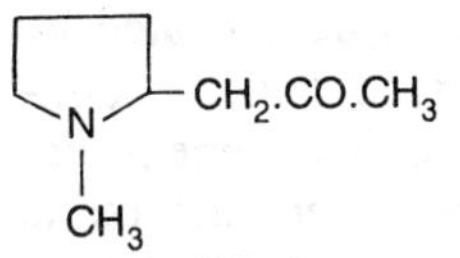

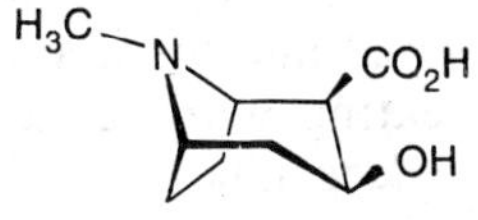

Fig. 21.28. Chemical constituents of Coca leaves.

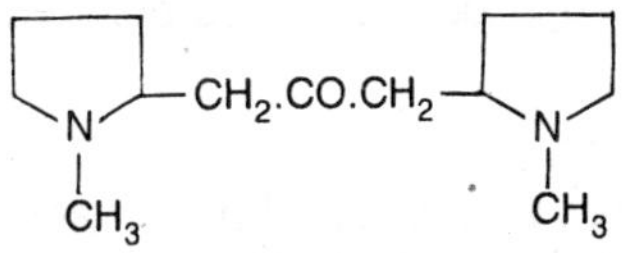

Biosynthesis of cocaine

Ecgonine, the basic moiety of the cocaines, is ornithine-derived via hygrine. Systematic degradation of the labelled cocaine indicated that, unlike hyoscyamine, the alkaloid is formed via a symmetrical precursor (*e.g.*, putrescine). A mechanism for the condensation of the intermediate N-methyl-Δ^1-pyrrolinium ion with an acetate-type compound has been proposed for *E. coca*. This involved two successive reactions with malonyl CoA as in polyketide biosynthesis.

The benzoyl moiety of cocaine is derived from phenylalanine. The incorporation of labelled 1-methyl-Δ^1-pyrrolinium chloride into cuscohygrine, indicate the alkaloid to be a mixture of its *meso* and optically active diastereomers.

Manufacture of cocaine

The crude alkaloids is extracted with dilute sulphuric acid or by treatment with lime and petroleum or other organic solvents. Non-alkaloidal matter is separated by transferring the alkaloids from one solvent to another. The crude alkaloids are obtained in solid form as free bases by precipitation with alkali, or as hydrochlorides by concentrating an acidified solution.

Pure cocaine is isolated from the leaves, the crude bases or the crude salts. Cocaine, cinnamylcocaine and α-truxilline are closely related derivatives of ecgonine, which is produced by hydrolysis with boiling dilute hydrochloric acid.

The ecgonine hydrochloride is purified and converted into the free base. This is benzoylated by treating with benzoic anhydride and the benzoylecgonine purified. The benzoylecgonine is methylated with methyl iodide and sodium methoxide in methyl alcohol solution, to give methylbenzoylecgonine or cocaine which is converted into the hydrochloride and purified by recrystallization.

Uses

Coca leaves are stimulant and astringent. They are used in masticatory. Cocaine is local anaesthetic and has stimulant action on CNS and is used in dental anaesthesia and minor local surgery of ophthalmic, ear, nose and throat.

Adulterants

Novocaine, boric acid, sodium carbonate and bicarbonate, lime, chalk and starch are among the adulterants of cocaine. Lactose and even quinine, have been used. Flowers of a species of *Inga* (Mimosoideae) are sometimes added to the leaves.

Pharmacology

Cocaine hydrochloride enhanced spontaneous locomotor activity in rats, produced an increase in fight duration in male mice and inhibited polymorphonuclear leukocyte oxidative microbicidal and natural killer cell activities.

Allied species

There are over 200 species of *Erythroxylum* found throughout the world. The majority of these plants contain a range of tropane alkaloids.

Cocaine

It is the methyl ester of benzoyl ecgonine. Cocaine is prepared by semi-synthetic method from plant-derived ecgonine. When hydrolyzed, it yields ecgo-

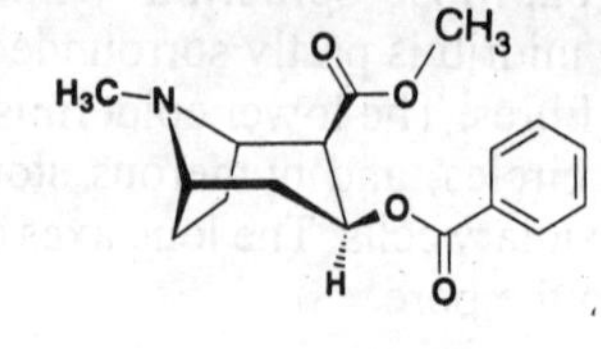

Fig. 21.29. Cocaine.

nine, benzoic acid and methyl alcohol. The total plant bases are extracted, the ester alkaloids are converted to (–)-ecgonine by acid-hydrolysis and its esterification first with methanol and than with benzoic acid yields cocaine.

Cocaine shows central and peripheral nervous system actions. It is a psychomotor stimulant with a strong abusing property. The abuse liability is through a prolongation of dopamine in the synapse by blocking the dopamine reuptake mechanism. Cocaine has the ability to dominate behaviour, reducing other behaviours such as eating and sleeping. It has reinforcing potential of any drug.

Cocaine hydrochloride is an ingredient in Bromptom's cocktail, which is used to control severe pain in terminal cancer. It counteracts the narcotic-induced sedation and respiratory depression together with the narcotic analgesic ingredient, like methadone or morphine, used in cocktail. It potentiates the analgesic effects. Cocaine is absorbed by pulmonary capillaries and moves from the lungs to the left side of the heart and then directly to the brain. The effects are perceptible in 7-10 seconds. Repeated use results in psychic dependence and tolerance. Therefore, cocaine is classified as a Schedule II drug.

Cocaine and cocaine hydrochloride are generally inhaled or sniffed and are rapidly absorbed across the pharyngeal mucosa, resulting in cerebral stimulation and euphoria. They are also injected intravenously and subcutaneously, and cocaine freebase is smoked. Inhalation of the vapours of alkaloidal cocaine is a popular practice because of the rapidity of onset and the intensity of the euphoric experience. The reason for converting cocaine hydrochloride to the free amine is that the latter substance volatilizes at about 98ºC whereas the salt volatilizes at 195ºC, a temperature at which some of the cocaine is decomposed.

QUINOLINE ALKALOIDS

Alkaloids containing quinoline as their base nucleus have been isolated from Cinchona, Acronychia and viridicatin. Cinchona alkaloids are the compounds of therapeutic importance.

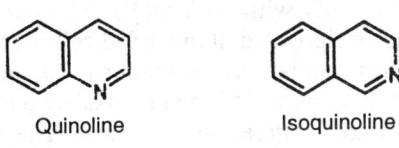

Quinoline   Isoquinoline

Fig. 21.30. Quinoline and Isoquinoline.

CINCHONA BARK

Synonyms

Peruvian bark; Cinchona; Calisaya bark; Jesuit's bark; Cortex cinchonae.

Biological source

Cinchona bark consists of dried bark of stem or of the root of *Cinchona succirubra*, *Cinchona calisaya*, *Cinchona ledgeriana* or *Cinchona officinalis* or their hybrids containing about 6.5 per cent of total alkaloids, 30-60 per cent of which are quinine-type alkaloids. (Family : Rubiaceae).

Geographical source

Cinchona is the native of Peruvian Andes, South America. Now the plant is cultivated in Indonesia, Java, Zaire, India, Guatemala and Bolivia. In India *C. calisaya* is cultivated at elevations from 500-1000 m in Sikkim and the Moyar valley in the Nilgiris. *C. officinalis* is cultivated in Ootacamund (Ooty) in the Nilgiris. *C. succirubra* is grown in the Nilgiris and Naduvattam plantation in South India, Sikkim, and in parts of Satpura range in M.P. *C. ledgeriana* is found in Bengal, on the Anamalai hills in Tinnevelly district of south India and on the Khasia and Jaintia hills.

The barks of cinchona were originally obtained from trees growing wild. The fully grown tree was cut down near the ground level and the bark removed from both stem and branches; this method is rarely used at the present time. The bark of the root of cinchona contains alkaloid in notable amount and, consequently, in plantations of cinchona, the method of uprooting has now been largely adopted. The tree at an age of from ten to fifteen years is cut down and the root is dug up; the bark is then removed from the trunk and branches and also from the root. A second method of treatment is known as coppicing. The trees are allowed to grow to an age varying from about three to eight years for tropical trees such as cinnamon and cinchona, the stems are then cut down to within a short distance from the ground and the bark is removed from the trunk and branches. The stools, *i.e.*, the stumps which remain in the ground, are allowed to send out a certain number of shoots, which are removed when they have grown to an age of from one and a half to seven years, and the bark is stripped from them. The stools then produce more shoots and the plantation will yield regularly for a long period of years.

Cultivation

For cultivation of Cinchona the seeds are sown in tropical countries. Seedings need careful treatment and propagation to avoid diseases. The temperature should be 10-30°. A rainfall from 75" to 180" per

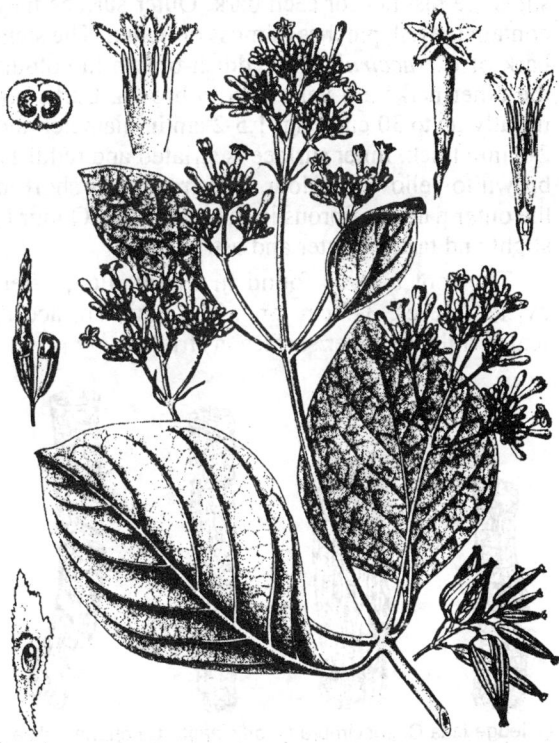

Fig. 21.31. *Cinchona succirubra*.

year is required and there should be no frost. Selected stains of seedlings are transplanted at a distance of 1 meter in rich, porous and well drained soils in slopes when the plant is two years old. The plants are protected from wind by growing banana trees in between them. The hybrids of *C. ledgeriana - C. calisaya* produce a higher amount of alkaloids. The stems grow tall, the lower branches die and drop off and the tree crown are very close. Shade favours the higher production of quinine. The minimum amount of alkaloid in bark is obtained when the trees are 6-9 years old. The bark of trunk and roots can be removed by hand from the uprooted plants. The young bark contains three more alkaloids than the old trees.

Characters

The barks of different species differ in the presence of ridges, cracks, quills and protuberances. The stem bark is curved, single or double quill. Outer rough surface contains longitudinal and transverse cracks, fissures, ridges and protuberances. Cracks and fissures are distinct for each bark. Outer surface may contain greyish patches of moss or lichen. The stem bark of *C. succirubra* is reddish-brown in colour; the other barks are yellowish to brown. Barks are usually up to 30 cm long, 1.5-2 cm in diameter and 2-8 mm thick. Inner surface is striated and reddish-brown to yellow in colour. The fracture is short in the outer part but fibrous in the inner side. Odour is slight and taste is bitter and astringent.

The root bark is found in Channelled, often twisted pieces, 3-7 cm long. The outer surface is scaly while the inner surface is striated.

Microscopical characters

In Cinchona barks, the cork has several layers of thin-walled cork cells, arranged in regular radial rows and appearing polygonal in surface view. Their cell contents are dark reddish in colour. Phelloderm of the cork cambium is composed of several layers of regular cells with dark walls. The cortex has tangentially elongated, thin-walled cells containing amorphous reddish-brown matter or small starch grains. Microcrystals of calcium oxalate and secretion cells are scattered in the cortex. The phloem

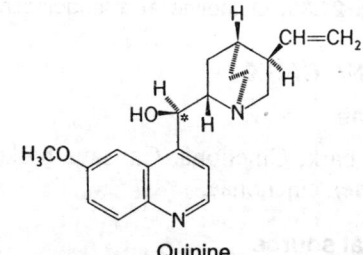

Quinine

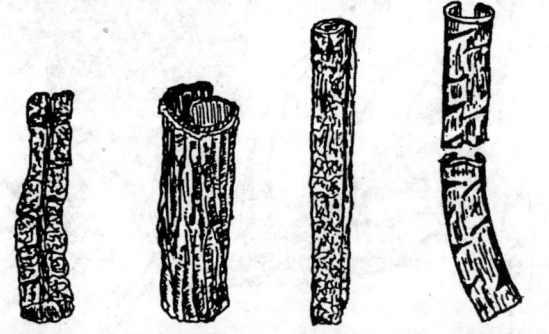

C. ledgeriana C. succirubra C. officinalis Cinchona calisaya

Fig. 21.32. Cinchona bark.

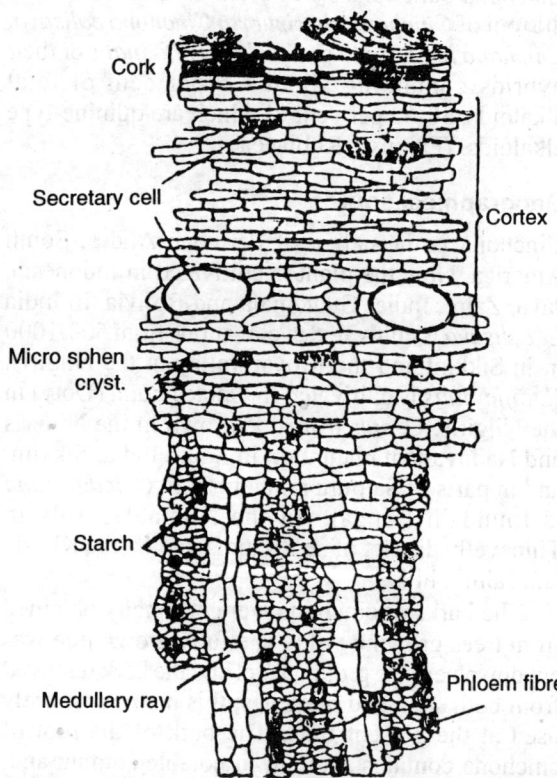

Fig. 21.33. Transverse section of Cinchona bark.

consists of narrow sieve-tubes with transverse sieve plates, phloem parenchyma resembling that of the cortex and large characteristic spindle-shaped phloem fibres with thick conspicuously striated walls traversed by funnel-shaped pits. The phloem fibres are isolated or in irregular radial rows. The distribution and size of the phloem fibres differ in the various species. The medullary rays are two or three thin-walled and radially elongated.

Chemical constituents

The Cinchona bark contains about 35 alkaloids (6.5%). The cultivated bark contains 7-10% total alkaloids. The main alkaloids are quinine (70%), quinidine, cinchonine and cinchonidine. The alkaloids are present in combination with quinic acid (5-8%), quinovic acid and cinchotannic acid. Cinchotannic acid is a pholobatannin and its major amount is decomposed to give 'Cinchona red'. Other constituents are quinovin (a glycoside), which on hydrolysis gives quinovic acid and quinovose, red colouring oxidase, calcium oxalate and starch. C.

succirubra and some other varieties contain more cinchonidine and cinchonine and sometimes quinidine than the cultivated variety. A white crystalline substance, cinchocerotin, is present in the bark of *C. calisaya*. A green colouring matter, tschirchin, different from chlorophyll, is present in the bark of *C. calisaya*.

C. ledgeriana also contains alkaloids quinoidine, epiquinine, epiquinidine, cinchophyllamine, isocinchophyllamine, quininone, quinamine, aricine, 3-epiquinamine, cinchophyllines I-V, 10-methoxycinchonamine, triterpenes cincholic acid, quinovin, reynoutrin; delphinidin; kaempferol, quercetin, norsolorimic acid and β-sitosterol.

C. succirubra contains alkaloids quinine, cinchonine, quinidine, cichonidine, cuperine, succirubin, methylsuccirubin; flavan-3-ols cinchonain Ia, Ib, Ic and Id, caffeic acid, (−)-epicatechin and proanthocyanidin dimers cinchonain IIa and IIb.

Avicularin is present in the leaves of *C. officinalis* and *C. robusta*.

The quinine series has the configuration 8S.9*R*

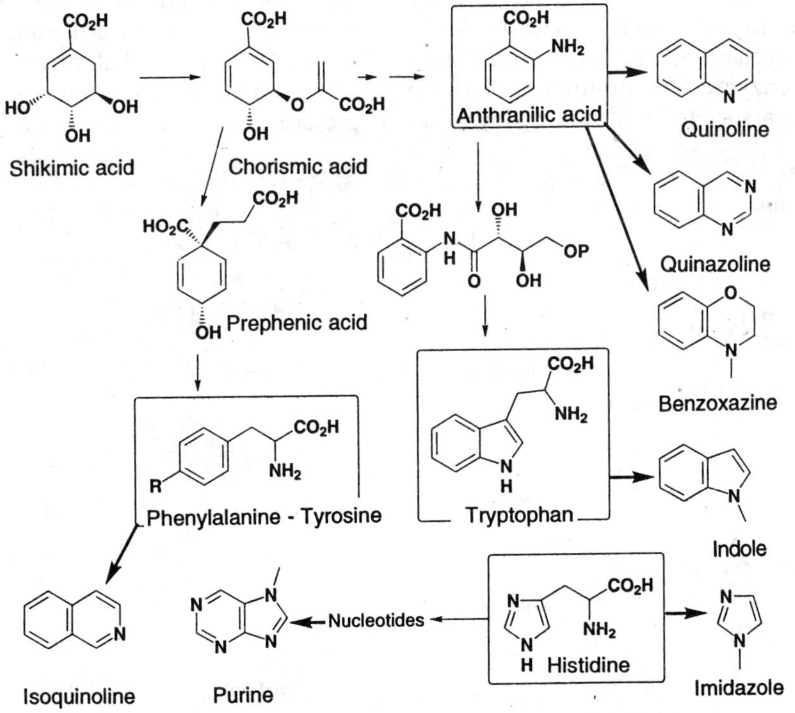

Fig. 21.34. Amino acids and origin of the chief heterocyclic rings.

and the quinidine 8R.9S. Some of these (*e.g.*, quinicine and cinchonicine) are amorphous. The amount of alkaloids present and the ratios between them vary in the different species and hybrids, also according to the environment and the age of the tree and method of collection of the bark.

The alkaloids are present in the parenchymatous tissues of the bark in combination with quinic acid and cinchotannic acid.

Biosynthesis of alkaloids

The alkaloids are formed in the aerial parts of the plant. The quinoline alkaloids have structures suggesting anthranilic acid as a biological precursor derived from indolic precursors by the specific incorporation of tryptophan (indole moiety), loganin and geraniol (terpenoid moiety) into the quinine of *Cinchona* spp. The pathway involves alkaloids of the serpentine type.

The proposed biosynthetic route has been supported and elaborated by enzyme studies. The important role of strictosidine synthase in the initial stages of the biogenesis of some tryptophan-derived alkaloids and its isolation from *C. robusta* are determined. The enzyme tryptophan decarboxylase, which provides tryptamine, is involved in these early reactions. An enzyme (cinchoninone: NADPH oxidoreductase) associated with the pathway has

been isolated from cells of a suspension culture of *Cinchona ledgeriana*; it catalyses the reduction of cinchoninone to an unequal mixture of cinchonine and cinchonidine. The enzyme was resolved (by ion exchange) into two isoenzymic forms both of which had an absolute requirement for NADPH and catalysed reversible reactions. Isoenzyme I acts specifically on cinchoninone in the forward direction of the pathway and on cinchonidine and cinchonine in the reverse direction. Isoenzyme II has a broad specificity acting on all the quinoline alkaloids of cinchona tested.

Chemical tests

1. *Thalleioquin test* : Cinchona, slightly moistened with glacial acetic acid, on heating in a test tube gives blood-red drops on the side of the tube, due to reaction for phlobatannin.
2. Cinchona bark moistened with sulphuric acid shows a blue fluorescence in U.V. light.

Uses

Cinchona bark has antimalarial, antipyretic and analgesic properties. Quinidine is used to treat prophylaxis of cardiac arrhythmias and atrial fibrillation. The barks and all preparations of Cinchona are specially valuable in intermittent fever. They are prescribed as tonic in dyspepsia, gastric catarrh, and

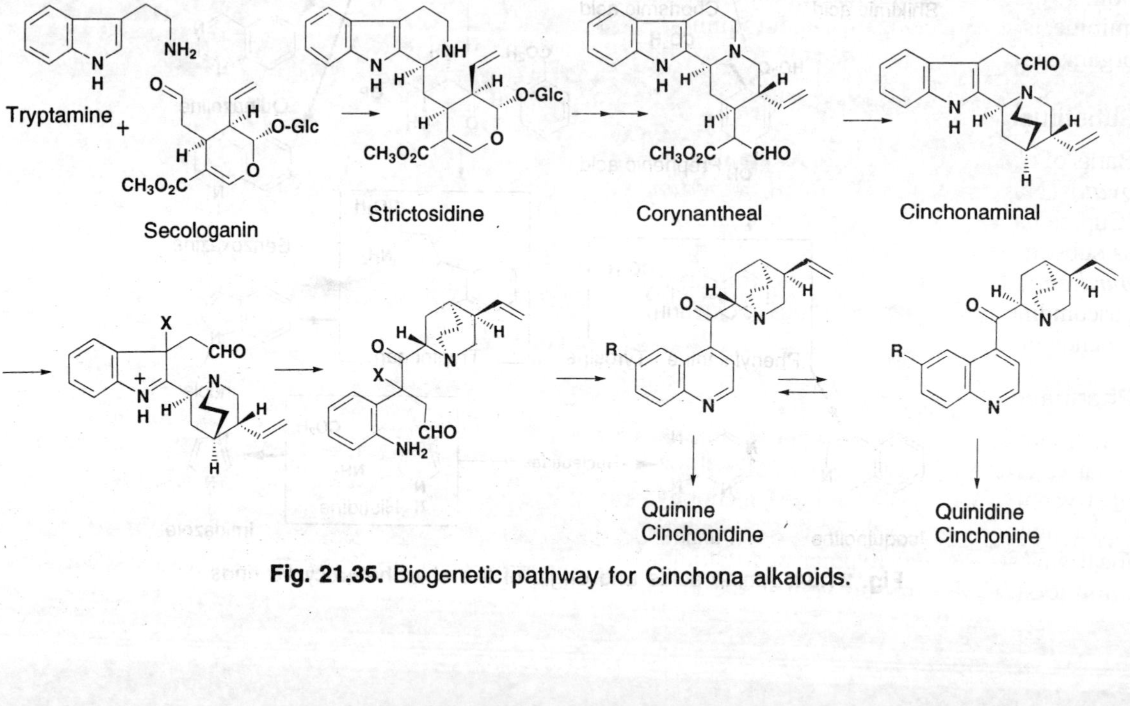

Fig. 21.35. Biogenetic pathway for Cinchona alkaloids.

convalescence from fever, and as antiperiodic; in the prophylaxis and treatment of malaria. Ten grain dose has been given in whooping cough, hay-fever, enlargement of spleen, hemicrania and other neuralgic affections. It is valued in small pox, septic fevers, pneumonia, acute rheumatism, tonsillitis, nasal catarrh and pyaemia. As an antiseptic it is recommended in abscesses, cavities, ulcers and as a wash and gargle in sore-throat. The indiscriminate use of quinine in continuous and large doses produces weakness of heart, restlessness and cachexia. It is a good ingredient in dentifrice. The Cinchona alkaloids cause disturbances of C.N.S. system, deliriant conditions, spasm, convulsion, and collapse. The most usual manifestations of cinchonism are abdominal pains, cholera, nostras, paralysis of limbs, regors, cold sweats, somnolence, icterus, albuminuria, fever, cyanosis, in chronic cinchonism, emaciation and cachexia. Quinine may cause blindness and deafness preceded by violant noises in the ears. It destroys the erythrocytes and causes quinine haemolysis.

Quinine is suitable for the treatment of *Plasmodium falciparum* infections (falciparum malaria) in many areas where the organism is now resistant to chloroquine and other antimalarials.

Quinidine is used for the prophylaxis of cardiac arrhythmias and for the treatment of atrial fibrillation; it also has antimalarial properties and like quinine is effective against chloroquine-resistant organisms.

Substituents

Barks of *Cinchona lancifolia*, (Colombian bark), *C. ovata* (Naranjada bark), *Remijia pedunculata* (Cuprea bark) and *Remijia purdiena* are often used as substitutes for Cinchona. False cuprea bark (*R. purdiena*) contains no quinine but an alkaloid cusconidine and small proportions of cinchonine and cinchonamine.

Pharmacology

Cinchophyllamine showed hypothermic and poor sedative effects in mice and decreased the toxicity of strychnine and amphetamine. Cinchophyllamine and cinchophylline are weak CNS depressants, local anaesthetic and hypotensors. Quinidine and quinine sulphates raised ventricular fibrillation threshold, reversed aconitine-induced atrial fibrillation, decreased abnormal ventricular beats and increased atrial refractory periods. Quinidine and cinchonine had higher affinities for clumping site of *Plasmodium berghei* than quinine.

Quinine's antimalarial action is believed to be the intercalation of the quinoline moiety into the DNA of the *Plasmodium* parasite, thereby reducing the effectiveness of DNA to act as a template. Intercalating agents such as quinine are rigid planar polycyclic molecules that insert between the adjacent stacked base pairs of the double helix of DNA. This results in DNA that has increased length, and because of a greater electrostatic interaction between the intercalated molecule and the two DNA strands, there is an inhibition of the strand separation that is required for replication and transcription of the genetic code. It suppresses but does not cure vivax malaria. It is used in the treatment of chloroquine-resistant falciparum malaria in combination with pyrimethamine and sulfadiazine or tetracycline. Quinine has a skeletal muscle relaxant effect, increasing the refractory period by direct action on the muscle fiber, decreasing the excitability of the motor end-plate by a curariform action, and affecting the distribution of calcium within the muscle fiber. Therefore, it is used for the prevention and treatment of nocturnal recumbency leg cramps.

Cinchona alkaloids

Quinidine, a stereoisomer of quinine, depresses myocardial excitability, conduction velocity and contractility.

Quinidine sulfate occurs as fine, needle-like, white crystals, odourless, has a bitter taste, and darkens when exposed to light. It is readily soluble in water, alcohol, methanol and chloroform.

Quinidine is used to treat various cardiac arrhythmias such as premature atrial, AV junctional and ventricular contractions; atrial and ventricular tachycardia; atrial flutter; and atrial fibrillation. When administered orally, the peak serum levels are slightly lower with the gluconate and polygalacturonate salt than with the sulfate salt. Toxic reactions occur at levels above 8 µg/ml. The patient should be instructed to notify the physician if skin rash, fever, unusual bleeding or bruising, ringing in the ears, or visual disturbance occurs.

Quinidine gluconate occurs as a white powder that is odourless and has a bitter taste. It is available in sustained release tablets.

Quinidine polygalacturonate affords controlled and uniform absorption through the intestinal mucosa and produces a lower incidence of gastro-intestinal irritation.

Quinine, a diastereoisomer of quinidine, occurs as white, odourless, bulky, bitter crystals or as a crystalline powder. It darkens when exposed to light and effloresces in dry air. It is freely soluble in alcohol, ether and chloroform but slightly soluble in water.

Quinine sulfate occurs as white, odourless, bitter, fine, needlelike crystals that are usually lusterless. It becomes brownish when exposed to light, It is insoluble in water, alcohol, chloroform and ether.

ISOQUINOLINE ALKALOIDS

Alkaloids containing the isoquinoline structure have been isolated from Ipecac, Hydrastis, Berberis, Sanguinaria, Curare and Opium.

IPECAC

Synonyms

Ipecacuanha; Brazilian or Johore Ipecac; Hippo; Ipecacuanha root; Radix ipecacuanhae.

Biological source

Ipecac consists of the dried root or rhizome of *Cephaelis ipecacuanha* (Brot.) A. Rich. (Rio or Brazilian Ipecac) or of *Cephaelis acuminata* Karst. (Cartagena, Nicaragua or Panama Ipecac). It should contain about 2% of ether soluble alkaloids calculated as emetine. (Family : Rubiaceae).

Geographical source

The plant is indigenous to Brazil and also found in Colombia, Cartagena, Nicaragua, Savantilla, Malaya, Burma, Panama and West Bengal. In India it is cultivated at Mungpoo (Darjeeling), in Nilgiris near Kollar and in Sikkim.

Collection

The plant is a low, straggling shrub containing slender rhizome with annulated wiry roots.

The roots are smooth, slender and whitish when young, develop on maturation a thick brownish bark with numerous closely placed transverse furrows.

The plant is unusually slow-growing. It thrives best in forest areas on sandy loams in humus, pot-ash, magnesia and lime. A maximum rainfall of 90 inch is required throughout the year. A temperature between 15-40°C and shaded situations are essential for successful cultivation. Temperature fluctuations should be narrow and the soil should be well drained. Propagation is by stem or root cuttings planted about a foot apart each way. Roots are harvested when the plants are about 2.5 years old and the alkaloid content exceeds 20 per cent. The plant may be dug up at any time of the year; the roots are washed and dried in shade.

In the Matto Grosso (Brazil) the drug is collected from wild plants by using a pointed stick. It levers the plant from the ground, then most of the roots are separated. The root is replaced in the ground, where it usually lives to produce further crops. The roots are dried in the sun or by fires and transported to ports from where they are exported in bales.

Morphology

The rhizome is thin, or sometimes thick and annulated. Rhio Ipecac is 5-15 cm long, 6 mm in diameter, shape is cylindrical, slightly tortuous, external surface is broadly annulated, brick red to brown in colour, the ridges are rounded and encircle the root, fracture of root is short and shows a thick, greyish bark and small dense wood. Odour is slight and taste is bitter and acrid.

Cartagena Ipecac is 4-6.5 mm in diameter greyish-brown in colour, less crowded and less projecting annulations, has transverse ridges. Half of the portion contains bark.

The Matto Grosso drug occurs in tortuous pieces, up to 15 cm long and 6 mm diameter. The colour of the outer surface varies from a deep brick-red to a very dark brown, the colour is dependent on the type of soil in which the plant has been grown. Most of the roots are annulated externally, and some have a portion of the rhizome and non-annulated roots are also found. The ridges are rounded and completely encircle the root; in some parts the bark has completely separated from the wood.

The fracture shows a thick greyish bark and a

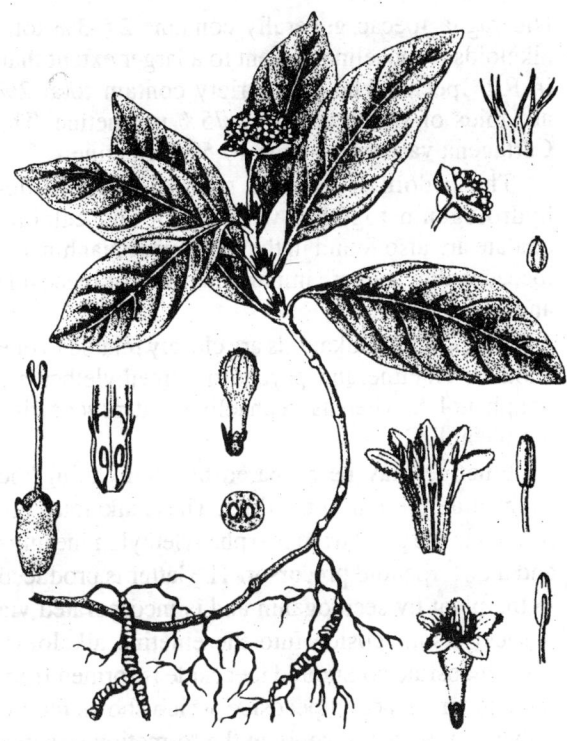

Fig. 21.36. Ipecacuanha.

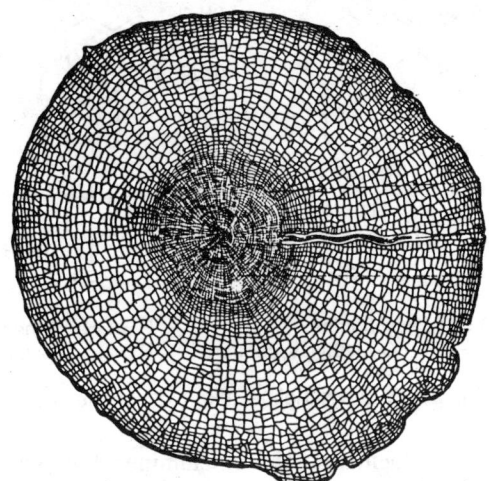

Fig. 21.37. T.S. of Ipecac.

small, dense wood, but no pith. The rhizomes have a much thinner bark and a definite pith.

Ipecacuanha stem contain the same alkaloids as the roots, but in smaller proportion. An excessive amount of stem is regarded as an adulteration.

Microscopical characters

A transverse section of the root shows a thin, brown cork, the cells of which contain brown, granular material. There is a wide secondary cortex (phelloderm), the cells of which are parenchymatous and contain starch, in compound grains with from two to eight components, or raphides of calcium oxalate. The individual starch grains are muller-shaped. The phloem is parenchymatous, containing no sclerenchymatous cells or fibres. The compact central mass of xylem is composed of small tracheidal vessels, tracheids, substitute fibres, xylem fibres and xylem parenchyma. Starch is present in the xylem parenchyma and in substitute fibres.

The transverse section of ipecacuanha rhizome shows a ring of xylem and a large pith. The

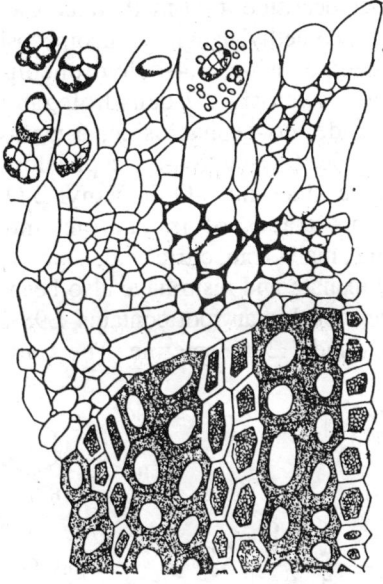

Fig. 21.38. T.S. of Ipecac.

pericycle contains characteristic sclerenchymatous cells. Spiral vessels occur in the protoxylem. The pith is composed of pitted lignified parenchyma.

Chemical constituents

Ipecac contains 2-2.5% alkaloids of which 30-75% is emetine. The other predominant alkaloids are cephaeline, psychotrine, psychotrine methyl

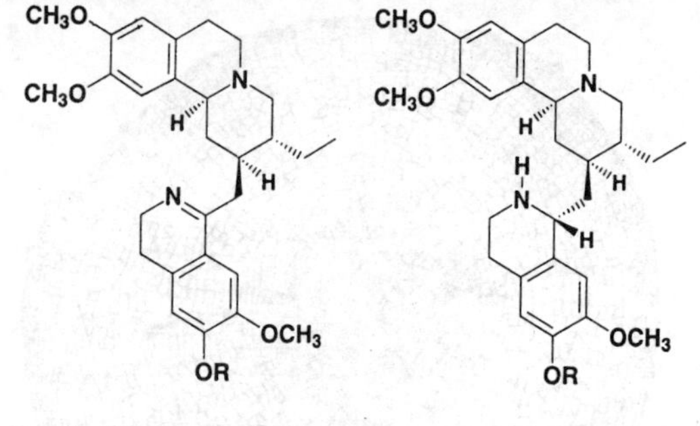

R = H : Psychotrine
R = CH₃ : O-Methylpsychotrine

R = CH₃ : Emetine
R = H : Cepheline

Fig. 21.39. Isoquinoline alkaloids of the Ipecac.

ether, protoemetine and emetamine. A crystalline glucosidal tannin, known as ipecacuanhin or ipecacuanhic acid, neutral monoterpenoid iso-quinoline glycosides (ipecoside), neoipecoside, 7-methylneoipecoside, 6-O-methylipecoside, ipecosidic acid; demethylalangiside, neoipecoside, 7-O-methylneoipecoside, 3,4-dehydroneoipecoside, alangiside, sweroside, 7-dehydrologanin, *trans*-cephaeloside, *cis*-cephaeloside, 6-methyl-*trans*-cephaeloside, 6-O-methyl-*cis*-cephaeloside, 7-O-methylipecoside and 3-O-demethyl-2-O-methyl-alangiside, traces of ipecamine and hydro-ipecamine, malic acid, citric acid, saponins, starch, calcium oxalate and resin have also been reported from the root. Indian root contains 1.98% of total alkaloids and 1.39% emetine. The Cartagena or

Nicaragua Ipecac generally contains 2.6-3% total alkaloids, cephaeline present to a larger extent than in Rio Ipecac. The Rio variety contain total 2% alkaloids of which about 60-75% is emetine. The Cartagena variety contains 40-50% emetine.

The iridoid glucosides sweroside and 7-dehydrologanin together with starch and calcium oxalate are also found in the root. Ipecacuanhin and ipecacuanhic acid are impure mixtures of ipecoside and sucrose.

The principal alkaloids are closely related to one another; emetine and psychotrine methylether are nonphenolic, whereas cephaeline and psychotrine are phenolic.

Emetine may be prepared by methylating the cephaeline present in the drug. These alkaloids are formed in the plant from two phenylethylamine units and a C₉ terpenoid precursor. The latter is produced in the plant by secologanin and is incorporated via desacetylisoipecoside into the emetine alkaloids. The glucosidic compound ipecoside is formed from the epimer desacetylipecoside which shows the involvement of secologanin in the formation of some indole alkaloids. The α-epimer, strictosodine, is formed which can serve as a precursor for alkaloids with β-configuration. The isolation of tetrahydroisoquinoline-monoterpenoid glucosides from *Alangium lamarckii* fruits, with the same stereocon-figuration as desacetylisoipecoside has supported the role of

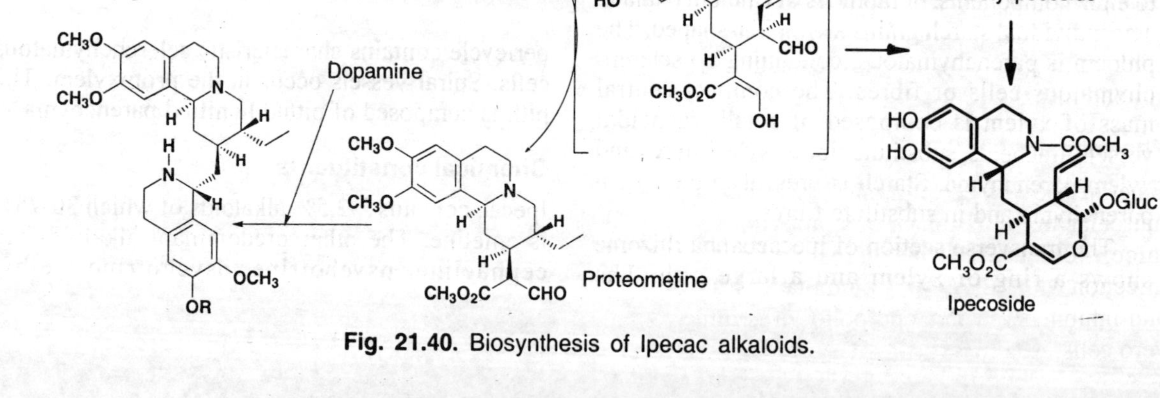

Fig. 21.40. Biosynthesis of Ipecac alkaloids.

the latter as an intermediate in the formation of emetine-type alkaloids.

In artificial culture the composition of the culture medium and the nature of the added hormones greatly influences alkaloid production. Increased growth of roots is obtained by the induction of hairy roots. Cell cultures produce more cephaeline than emetine, and immobilized cell systems give higher amounts of cephaeline compared with static cell cultures.

Test of emetine

Powdered drug (0.5 g) is mixed with HCl (20 ml) and water (5 ml), filtered and to the filtrate (2 ml) potassium chloride (0.01) is added. If emetine is present, a yellow colour develops which on standing for 1 hour gradually changes to red.

Uses

Ipecac is emetic and used as an expectorant and diaphoretic and in the treatment of amoebic dysentery. The alkaloids have local irritant action. Emetine has a more expectorant and less emetic action than cephaeline. In the treatment of amoebic dysentery emetine hydrochloride is given by injection, and emetine and bismuth iodide by mouth. Psychotrine and its *O*-methyl ether are selective inhibitors of human immuno-deficiency virus.

Adulterants

The chief adulterant of the drug is the aerial stem of the plant. It can be distinguished from the root by the longitudinal striation, presence of distinct pith composed of cells with lignified walls and by the surface scars. The drug is often substituted by stem and roots of *Richardsonia scabra*, *Cryptocoryne spiralis*, *Psychotria emetica*, *Manettia ignita*, *Hybanthus ipecacuanha*, *Asclepias curassavica*, *Anodendron paniculatum*, *Calotropis gigantea* and others. The powdered drug is often adulterated with almond meal.

Pharmacology

Emetine showed tubocurarine-like effect on neuro-muscular transmission in rats; antiviral activity in mice, 40% protection against lethality due to infection with MHV-3 or Columbia K virus in mice, and inhibited vaccinia and polio virus infection of vero cells.

Emetine hydrochloride is an antiamoebic and acts primarily in the intestinal wall and the liver. It inhibits polypeptide chain elongation, thereby blocking protein synthesis. The drug is not administered orally because it produces nausea and vomiting. Emetine hydrochloride has been used extensively as an antiprotozoan, in the treatment of amoebic dysentery, pyorrhea alveolaris and other amoebic diseases. It possesses expectorant and emetic properties.

HYDRASTIS

Synonyms

Golden seal; Yellow root; Orange root; Yellow puccoon; Indian turmeric; Hydrastis rhizome; Rhizoma hydrastis.

Biological source

Hydrastis consists of the dried rhizome and roots of *Hydrastis canadensis* Linn. containing not less than 2.5% ether soluble alkaloids (Family : Berberidaceae or Ranunculaceae).

Geographical source

Canada, eastern USA and Europe.

Characters

The plant propagates from rhizome buds. In autumn the terminal buds are replanted. The rhizomes are cylindrical, 1-5 cm long and 2-10 mm in diameter. They possess numerous, short bran-ches, which terminate in cup-shaped scars and bear encircling cataphyllary leaves. Scale leaves are present on the

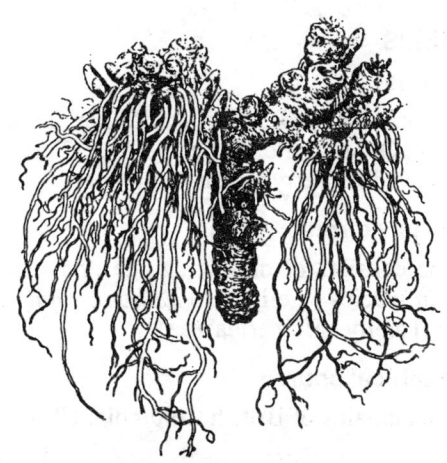

Fig. 21.41. Hydrastis.

rhizome. The outer surface of rhizome is yellowish-brown or greyish brown. The roots originate on the ventral and lateral surface, are long and wiry. The fracture of the drug is short and waxy. The odour is slight and distinct and taste is bitter.

A transverse section of the rhizome shows a thick, yellow or yellowish-brown bark; 12-20 radially elongated, bright yellow wood bundles, separated by wide medullary rays and a large pith.

Chemical constituents

Hydrastis possesses the alkaloids hydrastine (1.5-4%), berberine (0.5-6.0%) and canadine; some volatile oil and resin.

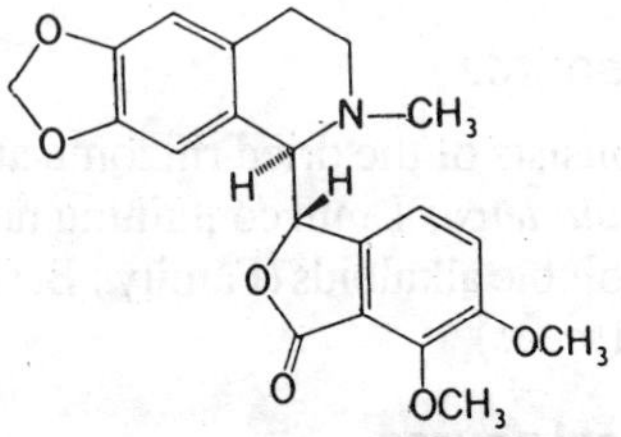

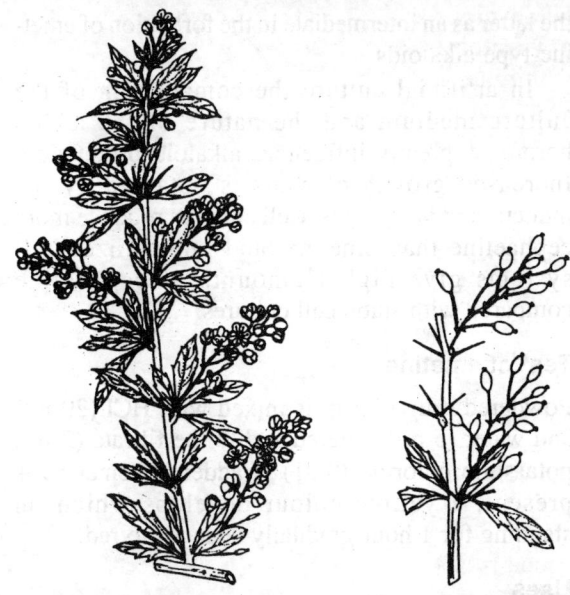

Fig. 21.43. *Berberis lycium*—flowering and fruiting branch.

Fig. 21.42. (–)-β-Hydrastine.

Uses

Hydratis is used as astringent, in inflammation of the mucous membrane, to check uterine haemorrhage, to treat of catarrhal conditions of the genitourinary tract and as a bitter stomachic. Hydrastine hydrochloride and hydrastinine hydrochloride are used in various forms to control uterine haemorrhage.

BERBERIS

Synonyms

Oregon Grape Root; Berberis aquifolium; Indian or Nepal or Ophthalmic berberry; Tree Turmeric; Holly-leaved berberry; Mountain grape.

Biological source

Berberis consists of dried rhizome and roots of *Mahonia* species chiefly from *Mahonia aquifolium* Nuttall (Family : Berberidaceae).

Geographical source

Rocky mountains of British Columbia, USA.

The plants are law trailing shrubs. The chief chemical constituents of Berberis are berberine, oxycanthine and berbamine which is an isomer of oxycanthine.

The root bark of *Berberis vulgaris* Linn. found in USA, *B. asiatica* Roxb ex. DC of Himalayan region and *B. aristata* DC of India are similarly used as *Mahonia* species. *B. asiatica* grows in dry valleys of Himalayas in Bhutan, Gharhwal, Kulu, Bihar and on the Parasnath Hill, Afghanistan. Its stem is diaphoretic and laxative and the roots are used as tonic and antiperiodic.

B. lycium Royle grows in dry hot places of western Himalayas. From the roots of *B. asiatica* berberine, palmatine, jatrorrhizine, columbamine,

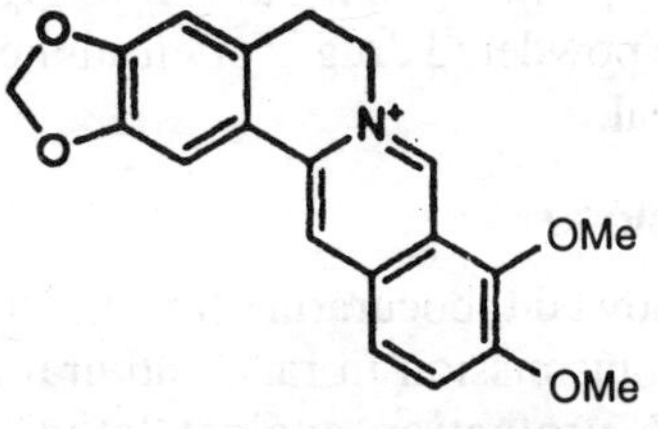

Fig. 21.44. Berberine.

tetrahydropalmatine, berbamine, oxyberberine, and oxycanthine have been isolated. Berberine and palmitine occur as chlorides. *B. lycium*, a good source of berberine, contains all these compounds in addition to berberine acetone complex.

Uses

Roots of *Berberis lycium* has antipyretic, febrifuge, carminative, aperient, anticancer and anti-protozoal properties. They are used in eye diseases, piles, diarrhoea and menorrhagia. Berberine has anti-inflammatory activity and is effective in intestinal and hepatic amoebiasis, in cholera and for controlling gastroentritis.

SANGUINARIA

Synonyms

Blood root; Red puccoon; Ped root; Puccoon root; Tetterwort; Rhizoma sanguinariae.

Biological source

Sanguinaria consists of dried rhizome of *Sanguinaria canadensis* Linn. (Fam. Papaveraceae).

The plant is found in Canada. It is a low perennial herb with horizontal branching rhizome.

Chemical constituents

Alkaloids of protopine series have been isolated

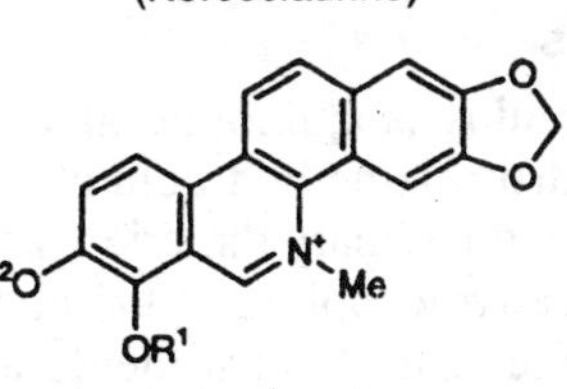

Higenamine
(Norcoclaurine)

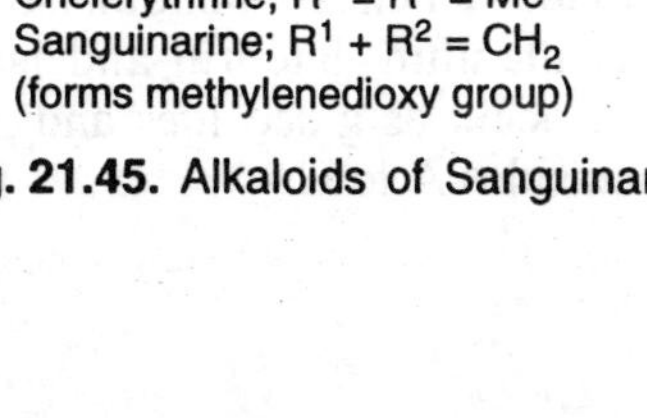

Chelerythrine; $R^1 = R^2 = Me$
Sanguinarine; $R^1 + R^2 = CH_2$
(forms methylenedioxy group)

Fig. 21.45. Alkaloids of Sanguinaria.

from Sanguinaria in addition to sanguinarine (1%), chelerythrine, allocryptopine, homochelidonine and resin.

Uses

Sanguinaria has stimulating and emetic properties. An extract of Sanguinaria is used as toothpaste base, in gingivatis and in periodical diseases.

CURARE

Synonyms

Ourari; Urari; Woorari; Woorali, South American arrow poison; Wourara.

Biological source

Curare is a crude dried extract from the bark and stems of *Strychnos castelnaei* Wedd., *S. toxifera*

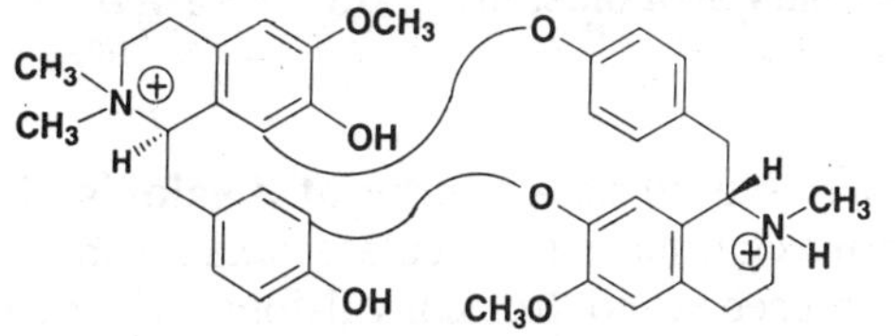

(+)-Tubocurarine

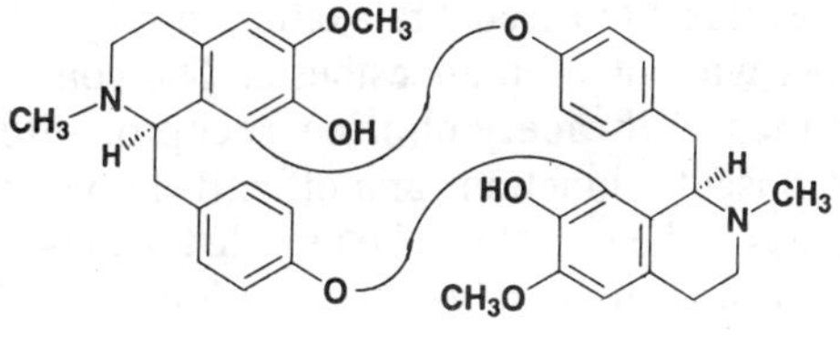

(+)-Isochondrodendrine

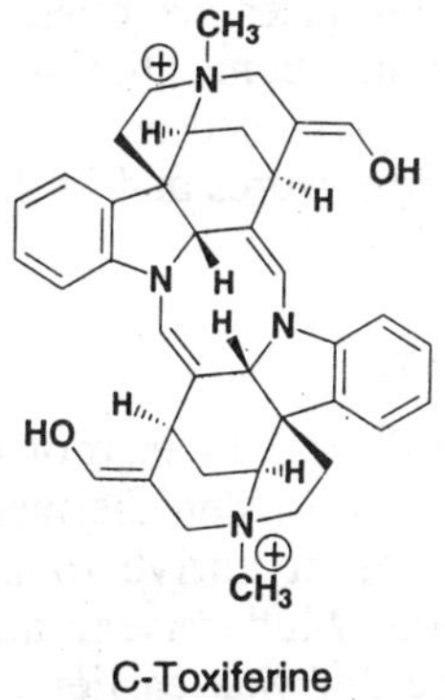

C-Toxiferine

Fig. 21.46. Curare alkaloids.

Benth., *S. crevauxii* G. Planchon, *S. jobertiana* (Family Loganiaceae) and from *Chondodendron tomentosum* Ruiz et Pavon and *C. microphyllum* (Family : Menispermaceae).

The plants generally occur in South America.

Chemical Constituents

The drug contains several alkaloids and quaternary compounds. The most important constituent is *d*-tubocurarine which is a quaternary compound of *bis*-benzylisoquinoline structure. *C. microphyllum* possesses non quaternary base (+) - bebeerine while (–) - bebeerine has been isolated from *C. tomentosum. Menispermaceous curare* has (+) - tubocurarine, (+) - isochondrodendrine, iso-chondrodendrine dimethyl ether, curine (bebeerine) and (+) - chondrocurine.

Loganiaceous curare contains 12 crystalline quaternary alkaloids, the toxiferines I-XII.

Uses

Curare is used as a source of alkaloids. Tubo-curarine chloride has muscular relaxation in surgery and is used to control convulsions of strychnine poisoning and of tetanus.

Tubocurarine chloride is also used as a skeletal muscle relaxant to secure relaxation in surgical pro-cedures without deep anaesthesia. The compound combines with acetylcholine receptor sites at neuromuscular junctions and effectively blocks all messages to the muscles. The muscle then lose their tone and become paralyzed for various periods of time.

Tubocurarine is especially useful in abdominal surgery since it produces profound surgical relax-ation with a minimal concentration of anaesthetic reagent. The drug is used as a relaxant in oral intubation, tetanic seizures and in the diagnosis of myasthenia gravis.

CALUMBA ROOT

Calumba is the dried, sliced root of *Jateorhiza palmata* (*J. columba*) (Menispermaceae), a dioe-cious climbing plant native to the forests of Mozambique and Madagascar and other east African countries. It was earlier exported from Colombo (Sri Lanka), hence the name.

Collection

The collection is done from the wild. The plant possesses a slender rhizome from which numerous large fusiform roots arise. The drug is dug up during dry weather (March). The rhizomes are rejected, the roots cut into transverse or oblique slices and dried in the shade. The imported 'natural calumba' is washed, brushed and graded, the product is known as 'washed calumba'.

Macroscopical characters

Calumba occurs in circular or oblique slices with 2-8 cm diameter and 3-12 mm thick.

Microscopical characters

The cork is thin, brown in colour and longi-tudinally wrinked. Within it lies a broad, greenish-yellow zone which extends to the cambium and contains in its outer part isolated sclerenchymatous cells within which are dark-grey, sinuous strands of sieve tissue. The greyish wood shows numerous narrow, radiating lines of yellow vessels separated by abun-dant parenchyma. The vessels are closed together in the region near the cambium and again in the extreme centre of the root, but they are less numer-ous in the intermediate zone. Some pieces show two or more concentric zones of wood. The fracture is short and starchy; odour, slight and musty; taste, bitter.

Calumba also contains some slices of *Calumba rhizome* having 2-3 cm diameter. The structure is markedly radiate.

The drug is characterized by the sclereids with thickened, yellow walls and prisms of calcium oxalate, abundant parenchymatous cells containing starch grains with an eccentric, very distinct radiate or cleft hilum, and yellow reticulate vessels.

Constituents

Calumba contains isoquinoline alkaloids (2-3%) palmatine, jatrorrhizine and columbamine. Bisja-trorrhizine is a quaternary dimeric alkaloid formed by *ortho*-oxidative coupling of the phenolic group of jatrorrhizine. Other constituents are the non-alkaloidal furanoditerpenes columbin, isocolumbin, palmarin, chasmanthin, jateorin and isojateorin. Some of these occur as glucosides and have been named palmatosides A to G.

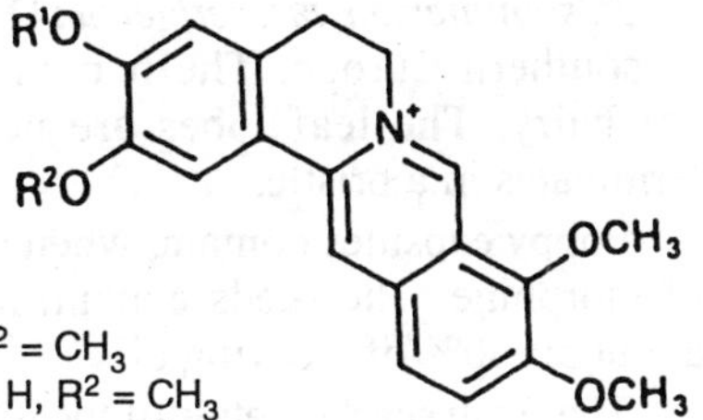

Palmatine : R^1 = R^2 = CH$_3$
Jatrorrhizine : R^1 = H, R^2 = CH$_3$
Columbamine : R^1 = CH$_3$, R^2 = H

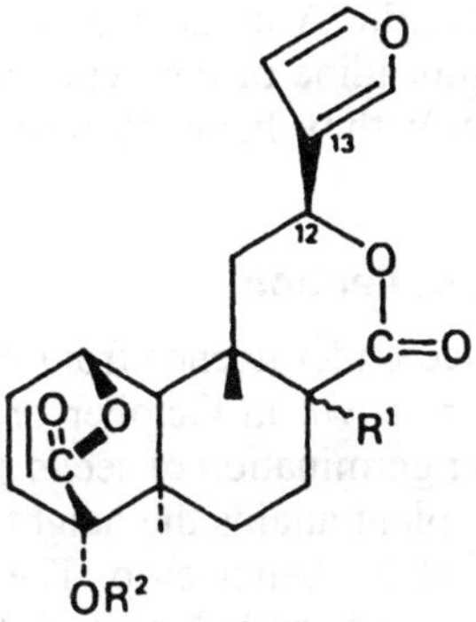

Columbin : R^1 = ◄ H, R^2 = H
Isocolumbin : R^1 = —H, R^2 = H
Columbinyl glucoside R^1 = ◄ H, R^2 = glycosyl

Fig. 21.47. Alkaloids of Columba.

Uses

Calumba is used as a bitter tonic. It may be prescribed with iron salts as it contains no tannins. It is valued for anorexia and flatulent dyspepsia.

SERPENTARY

Serpentary consists of the dried rhizome and roots of *Aristolochia reticulata* (Aristolochiaceae) known in commerce as Texan or Red River snake-root and is collected in the forests of Texas, Louisiana, Arkansas and Oklahoma.

Macroscopical characters

The fresh drug has a yellowish colour, becoming brown on keeping. It consists of small rhizomes, 1-2 cm long, 2-3 mm diameter with the remains of subaerial stems and numerous wiry roots which are about 10 cm long and 0.2-1.2 mm diameter. The drug contains up to 10% of subaerial stems. Odour, camphoraceous; taste, camphoraceous and bitter.

A transverse section of the rhizomes shows a starchy, eccentric pith, wedge-shaped, yellowish vascular bundles separated by wide medullary rays and a narrow bark.

Chemical constituents

Aristolochia species contain aristolochic acid and the tumour-inhibiting properties of this compound are of interest. Aristolochic acid is not alkaloidal. It is obtained by direct derivation from isothebaine derivatives in the plant.

Uses

Serpentary is used as an aromatic bitter. In overdoses it produces violent gastrointestinal irritation.

Allied drugs

Virginian snake-root, from *Aristolochia serpentaria*, closely resembles the Texan drug, but has smaller rhizome and more wiry roots. *Indian aristolochia* or Indian birthwort consists of the roots and rhizome of *Aristolochia indica*; it contains aristolochic acid and other phenanthrene derivatives, an *N*-glycoside and steroids. *A. clematis* (birthwort) is European and contains similar constituents to other species.

OPIUM

Synonyms

Crude Opium; Raw Opium; Gum Opium; Afim; Post.

Biological Source

Opium is the air dried milky latex obtained by incision from the unripe capsules of *Papaver somniferum* Linn. or its variety *P. album* Decand. Opium is required to contain not less than 10% of morphine and not less than 2.0% of codeine. The thebaine content is limited to 3%. It is dried partly by spontaneous evaporation and partly by artificial heat to get irregularly-shaped masses and is known in commerce as Indian opium (Fam. Papaveraceae).

Geographical source

Turkey, Russia, Yugoslavia, Tasmania, India, Pakistan, Iran, Afghanistan, China, Burma, Thailand and Laos. In India, Opium is cultivated in

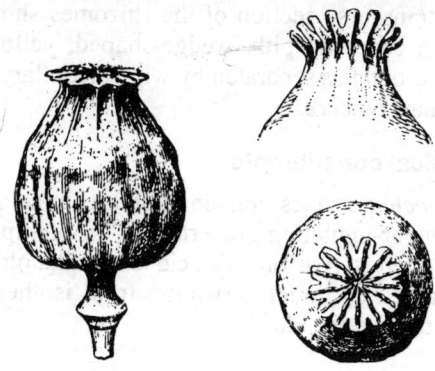

Fig. 21.48. *Papaver Somniferum* capsule.

M.P. (Neemuch) and U.P. for alkaloidal extraction and seed production.

Plant habit

The opium is an annual herb. The flowers are large, regular, terminal, solitary, white to pink in colour. It contains about eight capsules. Laticiferous vessels are found in all aerial parts which are maximum in capsule.

The opium poppy, *Papaver somniferum*, is about 50-150 cm in height. The stem and leaves are glaucous. The leaves are about 10 cm in length, entire, sessile and amplexicaul; margin is dentate. The flowers, which are borne on a slightly hairy peduncle, are solitary, nodding in the bud, and have caducous sepals. They have the floral formula K2, C2 + 2, A∝, G(∝). The unilocular ovary contains numerous ovules attached to parietal placentas. The capsule opens by means of small valves, which are equal in number to the carpels and situated below the stellate stigma.

The varieties of opium are :

P. somniferum var. *glabrum* Boiss., cultivated in Turkey; flowers purplish or white; capsule subglobular; stigmata, 10-12; seeds, white to dark violet.

P. somniferum var. *album* D.C., cultivated in India; flowers and seed white; capsules egg-shaped, 4-8 cm diameter, not pores under the stigma.

P. somniferum var. *nigrum* D.C. cultivated in Europe for the seeds, which are slate-coloured. The leaves and calyx are glabrous, the flowers violet and the capsules smaller and more globular than those of the var. *album*.

P. somniferum var. *setigerum* D.C., is found wild in southern Europe. The penduncles and leaves are hairy. The leaf lobes are pointed and each terminates in a bristle.

Poppy capsules contain, when ripe, 0.18-0.28% of morphine. The seeds contain no morphine but about 50-60% of a drying oil.

The fresh scarlet petals of the red or corn poppy, *Papaver rhoeas*, are used as a colouring matter in the form of a syrup. They contain the anthocyanidin glucoside mecocyanin. A number of alkaloids are produced (*e.g.*, rhoeadine of the benzyltetrahydro-isoquinoline type); they have no morphine like activity.

Cultivation and collection

Opium is cultivated under licence from the government. Its seeds are sown in October or March in alluvial soil. After germination of seeds snow falls. In spring the thin plant attains the height of 15 cm. Fertilizers are used for better crop. The poppy of first crop blossoms in April or May and the capsule mature in June or July. When the capsules are about 4 cm in diameter, the colour changes from green to yellow; they are incised with a knife about 1 mm deep around the circumference between midday and evening. The knife, known as a 'nushtur' bears narrow iron spikes which are drawn down the capsule to produce several longitudinal cuts. The incision must not penetrate into the interior of the capsule otherwise latex will be lost. The latex tubes open into one another. The latex, which is white in the beginning, immediately coagulates and turns brown. Next morning it is removed by scrapping with a knife and transferred to a poppy leaf. Each capsule is cut several times at intervals of 2 or 3 days. After collection the latex is placed in a tilted vessel so that the dark fluid which is not required may drain off. By exposure to air the opium acquires a suitable consistency for packing. The dried latex is kneaded into balls, wrapped in poppy leaves and dried in shade. The principal commer-cial varieties of Opium are Turkish Opium, Indian Opium, Chinese Opium, Yugoslavian Opium and Persian Opium.

Indian opium is exported in 5 kg blocks, packed 12 to a lightweight wooden case to facilitate air transport. Each block is wrapped in grease-proof paper, tied with tape and placed in a polythene bag. The drug has a soft consistency and so arrives as rounded, somewhat flattened, cakes. It contains about 9-12% of morphine. It is difficult to dry and powder due to its plastic nature.

Characters

Opium occurs in rounded or flattened mass which is 8-15 cm in diameter and weighing from 300 g to 2 kg each. The external surface is pale or chocolate-brown, texture is uniform and slightly grannular. It is plastic like when fresh and turns hard and brittle after sometime. Fragment of poppy leaves are present on the upper surface. Internal surface is coarsely granular, reddish-brown, lustrous; odour is characteristic; taste is bitter and distinct. Opium is intended only as a starting material for the manufacture of galenical preparations and is not dispensed as such.

Microscopy

Under the microscope opium shows agglomerated latex granules in irregular masses; spherical pollen grains, fragments of vessels and portions of the epicarp of the capsule. The latter showing in surface view polygonal thick-walled cells with a stellate lumen. Pointed trichomes and a few starch grains are present.

Chemical constituents

Opium contains about 35 alkaloids among which morphine (10-16%) is the most important base. The alkaloids are combined with meconic acid. The other alkaloids isolated from the drug are codeine (0.8-2.5%), narcotine, thebaine (0.5-2%). noscapine (4-8%), narceine and papaverine (0.5-2.5%). Morphine contains a phenanthrene nucleus. The different type of alkaloids isolated are :

(i) *Morphine Type* : Morphine, codeine, neopine, pseudo-or oxymorphine, thebaine and porphyroxine. Morphine consists of alkaloids which has phenanthrene nucleus whereas those of the papaverine group has benzyl-isoquinoline structure. Protopine and hydrocotarnine are of different structural types. The morphine molecule has both a phenolic and an alcoholic hydroxyl group, and acetylated form is diacetyl morphine or heroin. Codeine is an

ether of morphine (methyl-morphine). Other morphine ethers which are used medicinally are ethylmorphine and pholcodine.

(ii) *Phthalide Isoquinoline Type* : Hydrocotar-nine, narcotoline, l-narcotine, noscapine, oxynarcotine, narceine, and 5'-O-demethyl-narcotine.

(iii) *Benzyl Isoquinoline Type* : Papaverine, xanthaline, dl-laudanine, laudanidine, codamine and laudanosine.

(iv) *Cryptopine Type* : Protopine, cryptopine.

(v) *Unknown Constituents* : Aporeine, rhodeadine. meconidine, papaveramine and lanthopine.

The drug also contains sugars, sulphates, albuminous compounds, colouring matter and moisture. In addition to these anisaldehyde, vanillin, vanillic acid, *p*-hydroxystyrene, fumaric acid, lactic acid, benzyl alcohol, 2-hydroxycinchonic acid, phthalic acid, hemipinic acid, meconin and an odorous compound have also been reported.

The other compounds isolated from opium are somniferine, its methyl ether, isocorypalmine, narnotoline, 6-methylcodeine, reticuline, isoboldine, stepholidine, cotarnoline, morphine N-oxide, codeine N-oxide, narceinone, sedoheptulose, mannoheptulose, stigmasterol, β-sitosterol, nonacosanol, cyclolaudenol, cycloartenol, cycloartenone, cyclolaudenone, thebaol and aliphatic constituents.

Meconic acid, a dibasic acid, is an energy-exhausted product of the citric acid cycle whose formation controls alkaloid production. Its concentration in the latex showed considerable daily variation suggestive of active metabolism.

Chemical Tests

1. Aqueous extract of Opium with $FeCl_3$ solution gives deep reddish purple colour which persists on addition of HCl. It indicates the presence of meconic acid.

2. Morphine gives dark violet colour with conc. H_2SO_4 and HCHO.

Uses

Opium and morphine have narcotic, analgesic and sedative action and used to relieve pain, diarrhoea, dysentery and cough. Poppy capsules are astringent,

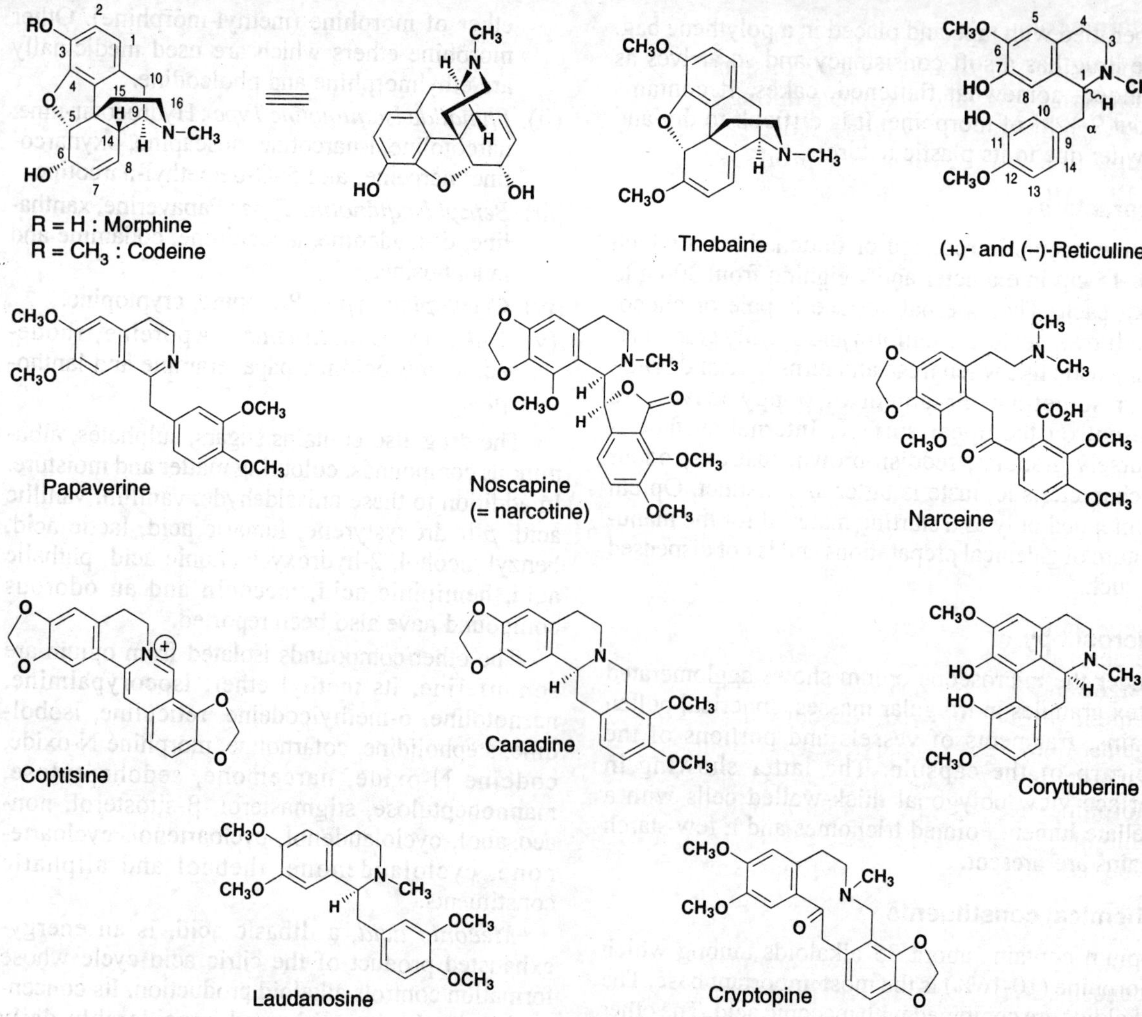

R = H : Morphine
R = CH$_3$: Codeine

Thebaine

(+)- and (–)-Reticulines

Papaverine

Noscapine
(= narcotine)

Narceine

Coptisine

Canadine

Corytuberine

Laudanosine

Cryptopine

Fig. 21.49. Alkaloids of Opium.

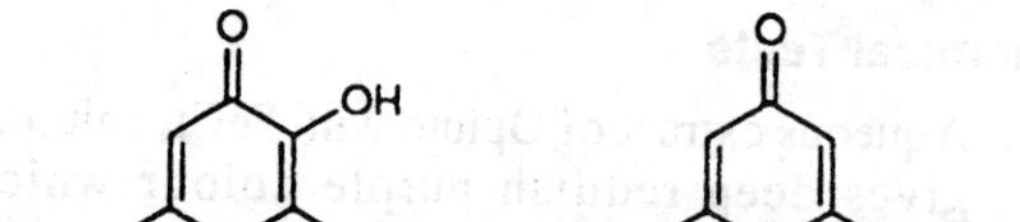

Meconic acid

Chelidonic acid

Fig. 21.50. Dibasic acids.

somniferous, soporific, sedative and narcotic and used as anodyne and emollient. As astringent, Opium checks haemorrhages, lessens bodily secretions and restrains tissue changes. Morphine is an analgesic. Codeine is mild sedative and is employed in cough mixtures. Noscapine is not narcotic and has cough suppressant action acting as a central antitussive drug. Papaverine has smooth muscle relaxant action and is used to cure muscular spasms. Opium, morphine and the diacetyl derivative heroin, cause drug addiction. Abouse leads to habituation of addiction.

Before the introduction of insulin, codeine was used to treat diabetes. Opium exerts its action more slowly and is, therefore, preferable in many cases (*e.g.*, in the treatment of diarrhoea). Opium is also used as a diaphoretic. The habitual use of codeine may, in some individuals, produce constipation.

Pharmacology

Papaverine enhanced oxygen consumption and formation of creatine phosphate during respiration in myocardial tissue of rabbits. It decreased arterial blood pressure in dogs and produced marked spasmolytic effect on corpus and isthmus of human ulcers.

Morphine decreased respiratory rate, pulse rate, blood pressure and serum pH and increased serum CO_2 level in cat; increased serum magnesium level in rats; decreased content of cytochrome p-450 and hydroxylation of progesterone and testosterone in male rats; increased brain acetyl choline in mice, elevated glucose level in blood, but did not change concentration of free fatty acids in serum of rats.

Nalorphine increased respiratory rate, decreased serum CO_2 and blood pressure.

Morphine caused decrease in vascular resistance of isolated canine gracilis muscle; caused efflux of acetylcholine into cerebral lateral ventricle from cerebral cortex; decreased body weight, thyroid weight and pituitary thyroid stimulating hormone content in rats; showed anti-convulsant activity against flurothyl and pentylene tetrazol in rats and markedly increased in locomotor activity in mice. Morphine exerted its effect on hypothalamus by inhibiting release of LH-release factor. It inhibited hypothalamic pituitary-gonadal axis; caused more side-effects than azidomorphine in humans; produced hypothermia; increased serum prolactin level of male rats; increased catecholamine-stimulated adenosine triphosphatase activities in mouse brain synapto-somes; inhibited dopamine-sensitive AT-Pase activities. Morphine produced antidiuresis in normal dogs; increased net intestinal sodium and water absorption in fed dogs; reduced arterial pressure; increased temperature of under-ear skin and tongue. Chronic morphine administration did not impair induction of humoral immune responses to bacterial or viral antigens. Morphine treatment did not alter resistance of immunized swine to PRV infection. However, cutaneous immune response to antigen was markedly suppressed. It induced potent anti-nociceptive effects in rats model of neuropathy. Acute morphine treatment altered packed cell volume, haemoglobin, serum glucose and carbomide-nitrogen levels. It produced marked attenuation of depressor and some facilitation of pressor responses and inhibited acidified ethanol-induced gastric damage in rats. Morphine sulphate suppresses hepatic phagocytosis through opiate-receptor-mediated mechanism. Morphine increases intake of preferred diet in rats. It did not block immuno-reactive neurokinin A release in dorsal spinal cord. Morphine produced pre- and post-synaphic effect on contractile activity of vas deferens. Morphine injection increased ten-fold plasma artrial natriuretic factor level.

Papaverine and eupaverine increased rate of uptake of calcium by sarcoplastic isolated vesicles of rabbit, prolonged total duration of synchronized sleep and depressed the duration of total desynchronized sleep in deprived rats; blocked Ca^{2+} uptake in depolarized smooth muscles of taenia coli of guinea pig and increased cyclic AMP and cyclic GMP in human neuroblastoma cultures. (–)-Codeine was active as analgesic while (+)-codeine had no analgesic activity. (–)-Codeine decreased heart rate. (+)-Codeine had more pronounced cardiovascular effects. Papaverine did not induce secretory action of pancreatic juice in dog; maintained compartmentation of K^+, energy metabolism and membrane fluiding of Ehrlich ascites tumor cell membranes; and enhanced cytotoxicity of nitrogen mustard in cell cultures of C1300.

Biosynthesis of Isoquinoline alkaloids (opium and related alkaloids)

These compounds result from the condensation of a phenylethylamine derivative with a phenyl-acetaldehyde derivative. Both of these moieties are derived from phenylalanine or tyrosine. Administration of tyrosine-2-^{14}C to *Papaver somniferum* resulted in the formation of papaverine labeled in corresponding positions. Norlaudanosoline is an intermediate in this reaction.

There is a structural relationship between the benzylisoquinoline alkaloids and dihydroxy-phenylalanine. Morphine could be derived from these alkaloids by rotation of the tetrahydroisoquinoline residue followed by oxidative ring closure.

Norlaudanosoline acted as a more efficient precursor for morphine than did tyrosine and yielded a labelled product. By the cultivation of poppy plants in $^4CO_2$, and by injection of labelled alkaloids into the plant, the first major alkaloid formed is thebaine;

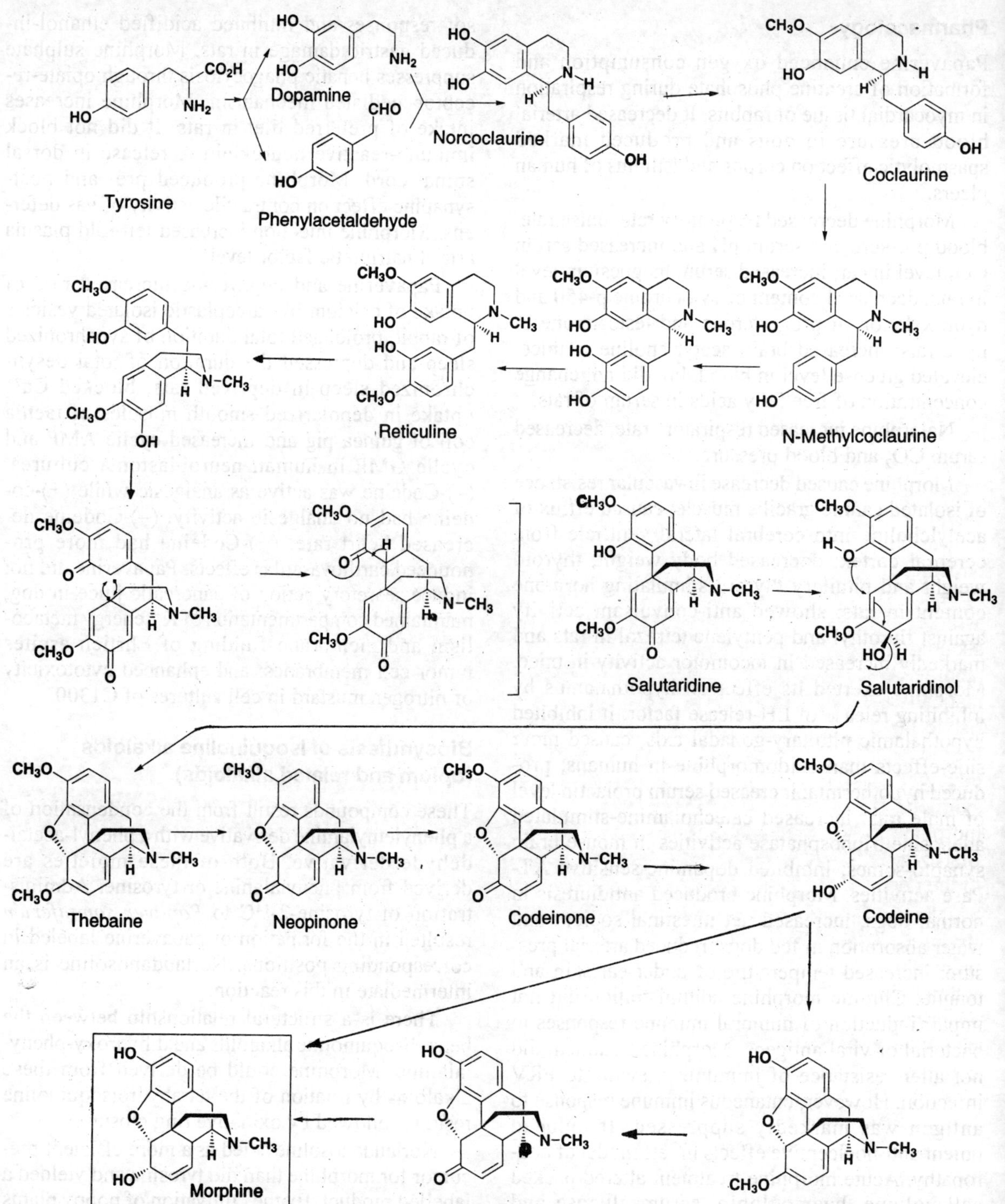

Fig. 21.51. Biosynthesis of morphine.

this is irreversibly converted to codeine and then to morphine.

In the oxidative coupling of norlaudanosoline, the hydroxyl groups are not involved in the reaction. A base of the type required, in which two of the hydroxyls were methylated, had previously been isolated from another plant (*Annona reticulata*, Annonaceae); this was reticuline. Labelled reticuline and norreticuline both proved to be very efficient precursors of morphine in the poppy, surpassing norlaudanosoline in this respect. Reticuline is a normal, minor component of *P. somniferum* is present. It is essential to some metabolic pathway but it does not accumulate.

The stages in the conversion of reticuline to thebaine and of thebaine to codeine were demonstrated by the feeding of appropriate labelled intermediates. These alkaloids are isolated as minor components of the opium alkaloid mixture.

Morphine is also formed from 2 molecules of tyrosine, and its biosynthesis is related to the biosynthesis of papaverine. Norlaudanosoline serves as a key intermediate. This medicinally important alkaloid is derived from a benzylisoquinoline metabolite. A key feature of the pathway is the enzymatically controlled methylation pattern that gives rise to (−)-reticuline, thus facilitating formation of the dienone, salutaridine, which is the first intermediate with a phenanthrene nucleus. There is a biosynthetic relationship of thebaine, codeine, and morphine; stepwise demethylation of thebaine leads first to the relatively mild analgesic codeine and then to the potent narcotic morphine.

Norcoclaurine (higenamine), a constituent of *Annona squamosa*, is a favoured trihydroxylated precursor. The (*R*)-isomer incorporates into thebaine when applied as a labelled precursor to *P. somniferum* seedlings. Dopamine and *p*-hydroxyphenylacetaldehyde (both derived from tyrosine) condense to give norcoclaurine.

A Tasmanian strain containing the alkaloid oripavine and the Indra strain converted labelled oripavine to morphine, and morphinone was also isolated with good incorporation of radioactivity. Codeine and thebaine were not radioactive, demonstrating that the demethylation of the phenolic ether of thebaine is not reversible. This alternative final stage would, therefore, appear to be thebaine→ oripavine → morphinone → morphine.

The presence of some of the other minor alkaloids of opium can be explained by various methylations and dehydrogenations of laudanosoline, reticuline and their nor-derivatives. Various oxidative couplings of reticuline account for other minor alkaloids (*e.g.*, corytuberine and isoboldine).

(+)-Reticuline also gives rise to a number of bases: narcotine (noscopine) and narceine of opium; canadine, berberine and hydrastine of *Hydrastis* (Berberidaceae); and sinomenine (the enantiomer of the opium alkaloid salutaridine of *Sinomenium acutum* (Menispermaceae). With the exception of sinomenine, these alkaloids are termed 'berberine bridged' alkaloids and they arise from norlaudanosoline and a one-carbon unit, which is derived from the *N*-methyl group group of (+)-reticuline. The methylene-dioxy group of these alkaloids is formed by oxidative cyclization of an *o*-methoxyphenol function. For berberine, 13 enzymes are involved in its biosynthesis from two molecules of tyrosine.

The cultures of *P. somniferum* do not produce morphine-type alkaloids but accumulate large amounts of sanguinarine and other alkaloids. However, some of the enzymes of the morphinan pathway are present in such cell cultures. An enzyme is characterized as 1,2-dehydroreticuline reductase, isolated from poppy seedlings.

Papaver bracteatum

Thebaine is the predominant alkaloid of this species. High yielding strains obtained from west Iran gives 3.5% thebaine in the dried capsules.

P. bracteatum produces about 27 alkaloids belonging to 10 different groups. The biogenesis of thebaine follows the same pathway as in *P. somniferum*. The plant is capable of converting codeinone to codeine. Thebaine is an end-product and yields unknown products.

Papaver orientale

This species is commonly cultivated as the ornamental poppy and a number of alkaloid chemo-types have been isolated. Generally, oripavine and mecambridine (a berberine type alkaloid) are the main alkaloids.

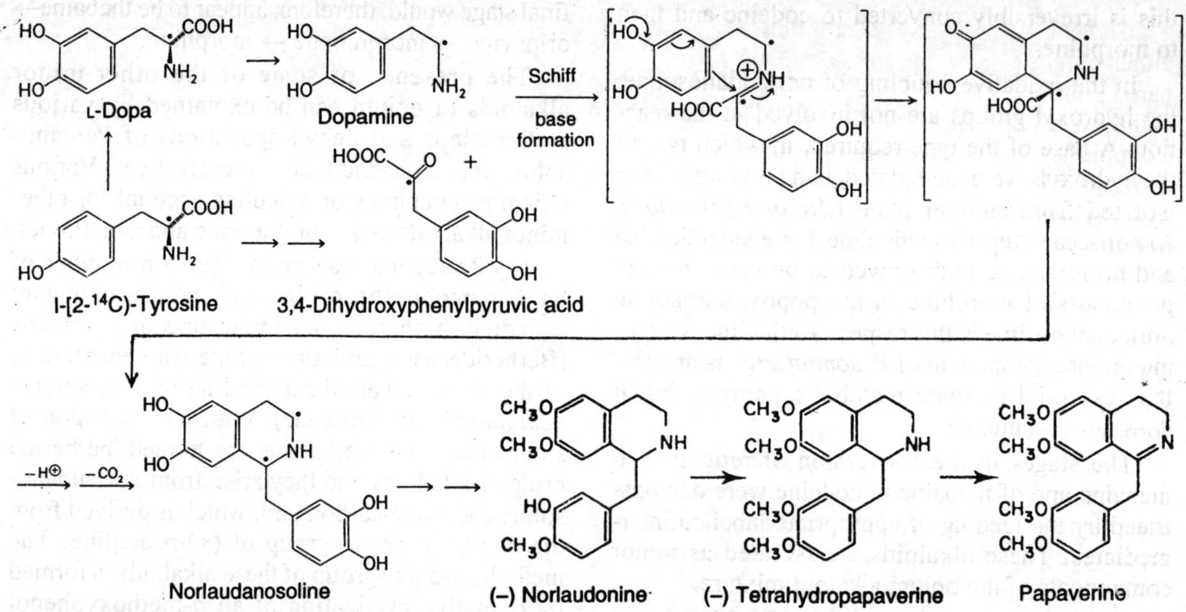

Fig. 21.52. A pathway in the biogenesis of papaverine.

Papaver pseudo-orientale

The plant ($2n = 42$) is intermediate in many of its characters of the above two species. Turkish samples contained isothebaine, mecambridine and orientalidine as major alkaloids, in addition to salutaridine and thebaine.

Poppy seed or mad seed is the dried seed of *Papaver somniferum* variety *nigrum*. The seeds are bluish black or yellowish white, reniform, from 0.1 to 1 mm in diameter, reticulate with a yellowish hilum scar, a white oily endosperm, and a curved embryo. Poppy seeds are used in baking (poppy seed rolls). They contain about 50% of a fixed oil (*poppy seed oil*), which is used in some parenteral formulations, as a drying oil, for food and salad dressings. *Poppy seed oil cake* is used as a cattle food. Poppy seed is devoid of alkaloids.

Storage

Opium is stored carefully for its morphine content. When it is dried at 100°C and stored in air-tight containers, the loss of morphine is small. A phenoloxidase enzyme, which acts on morphine, has been isolated from poppy capsules.

Adulteration

Opium is adulterated with sugary fruits, gum, powdered poppy capsules and other substances. The product is analysed and the price paid is governed by the content of morphine and other alkaloids.

Morphine is converted into other bases such as codeine, ethylmorphine and pholcodine. Kiln-drying of immature capsules at various temperatures (40-100°C) resulted in a loss of morphine content of up to about 11% without effect on codeine and thebaine.

OPIUM ALKALOIDS

Morphine

The alkaloid and its salt occur as white silky crystals. It is stable in air, odourless, and bitter-tasting.

Morphine and its salts are narcotic analgesics and strongly hypnotic. It is used to induce nausea, vomiting, constipation and habit formation.

Paregoric or camphorated opium tincture is classed as an antiperistaltic. It may be mixed before taking with a small amount of water to form a milky solution. It is used in combination with belladonna alkaloids, kaolin, pectin, and other ingredients for the treatment of diarrhoea.

Codeine is the widely used opium alkaloid. It is either obtained from opium (0.2 to 0.7%) or prepared from morphine by methylation or from thebaine by appropriate reduction and demethylation. Codeine is methylmorphine in which the methyl group replaces the hydrogen of the phenolic hydroxyl group. Codeine and its salts occur as fine needles or as white crystalline powders that effloresce in air.

Codeine and its salts are narcotic analgesics and antitussives; they are used as sedatives, in allaying coughs. The action is similar to that of morphine. Codeine is less toxic and causing less danger of habit formation.

Diacetylmorphine or heroin is formed by the acetylation of morphine; the hydrogen atoms of both the phenolic and alcoholic hydroxyl groups are replaced by acetyl groups. It has similar action but more pronounced than that of morphine. Due to its potency and the danger of habit formation, its manufacture is forbidden by law.

Apomorphine hydrochloride is formed when morphine is treated with hydrochloric acid in a sealed tube, and one molecule of water is lost. The compound decomposes readily and must be rejected if an emerald green colour is produced when it is shaken with distilled water (1 to 100).

Apomorphine is an emetic and is valuable for poisoning as it may be administered ubcutaneously.

Papaverine occurs naturally in opium to the extent of about 1%, but it may also be produced synthetically. *Papaverine hydrochloride* occurs as white crystals. It is odourless but has a slightly bitter taste.

Papaverine hydrochloride is a smooth muscle relaxant. It is used as an antitussive in combination with codeine sulfate (Copavin).

In hydromorphone hydrochloride or dihydromorphinone hydrochloride one of the hydroxyl groups of morphine is replaced by a ketone group and the adjacent double bond is removed. It is prepared by reducing morphine in hydrochloric acid solution with hydrogen in the presence of a catalyst.

The drug is a powerful narcotic analgesic and depresses the respiratory mechanism. Its dosage is smaller than that of morphine. It causes nausea and constipation less frequently and it is less habit-forming.

In hydrocodone bitartrate or dihydro-codeinone bitartrate, a ketone group replaces one of the hydroxyl groups and the adjacent double bond is saturated. It is antitussive and is used in treating a cough.

Noscapine (narcotine) exists in opium as a free base (1.3-10%). It possesses no narcotic properties and is called anarcotine. Noscapine is an antitussive. It is available in syrup and chewable tablets.

The term "*opioid*" refers to the synthetic morphine-like compounds. Many of these substances are morphine, but they are not as habit-forming. Others possess the cough-relieving activity of codeine but are not addictive.

INDOLE ALKALOIDS

The important alkaloids possessing indole as a part of their structures are strychnine and brucine (Nux vomica), lysergic acid and its derivatives (Ergot), physostigmine (Physostigma), reserpine (Rauwolfia) and vinblastine and vincristine (Catharanthus). The compounds usually contain two nitro-gens, one is present in the indole nucleus and the second is usually two carbons apart from the β-position of the indole ring.

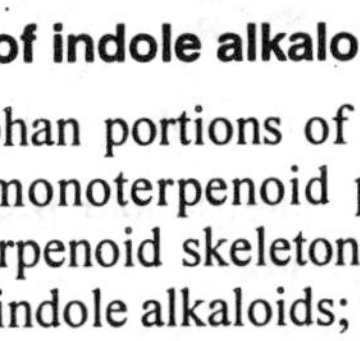

Fig. 21.53. Indole.

Biosynthesis of indole alkaloids

The nontryptophan portions of the molecules are derived from monoterpenoid precursors. These general monoterpenoid skeletons give rise to most of the complex indole alkaloids; these skeletons are designated as the *Aspidosperma, Corynanthe,* and *Iboga* types, on the basis of genera that are rich in alkaloids with the respective monoterpenoid nuclei.

The formation of the terpene involves an alde-

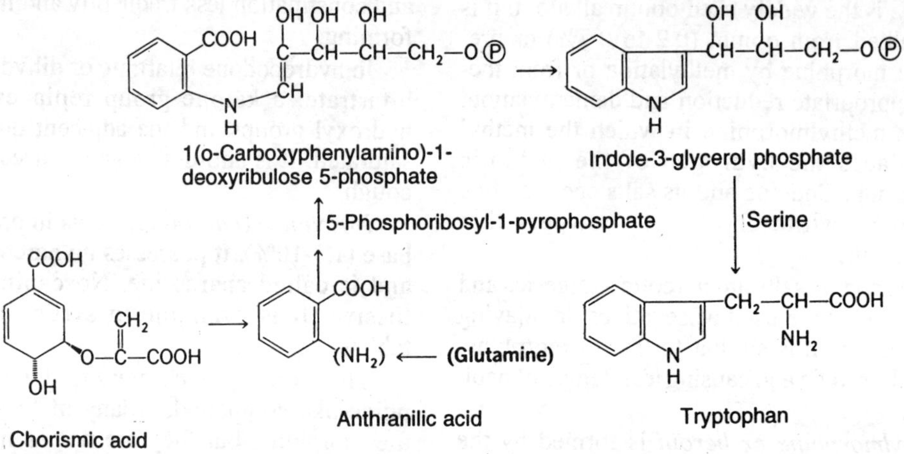

Fig. 21.54. Pathway of tryptophan biosynthesis.

hyde group, and the loss of one carbon atom during the biosynthetic process to give a C_9 unit. The *Corynanthe* type of monoterpenoid moiety is metabolically the most suitable. The glucoside, secologanin, provides the terpenoid unit and reacts initially with tryptamine to form strictosidine. The glycosidic linkage is cleaved during subsequent metabolic steps.

The *Rauwolfia* alkaloids, ajmaline, reserpine, and serpentine, are derived from a *Corynanthe*-type monoterpenoid precursor.

Aspidosperma-type   Corynanthe-type   Iboga-type

Ibogaine

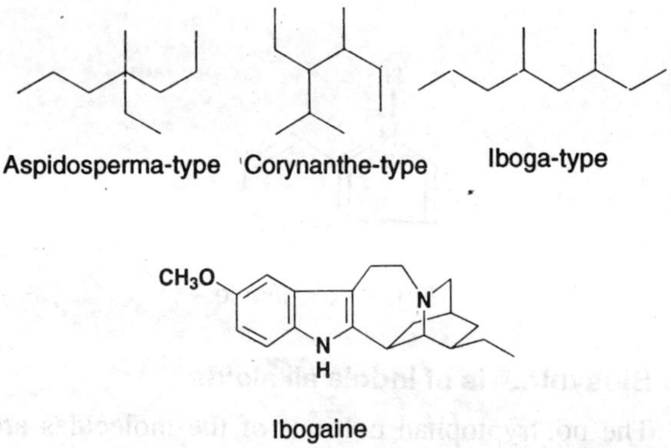

Fig. 21.55. (A) Monoterpenoid precursors of indole alkaloids, (B) Ibogaine.

NUX VOMICA

Synonyms

Nux vomica seeds; Kuchla (Hindi); Quaker buttons; Bachelor's buttons; Poison nut; Dog buttons; Vomit nut; Crow fig; Semina strychni.

Biological source

Nux vomica is the ripe, dried seed of *Strychnos nux-vomica* Linn. which should contain 1.2% of strychnine. (Family : Loganiaceae).

Geographical source

The plant is native of the East Indies and found in the forests of Sri Lanka, Malabar Coast and Northern Australia. In India it also grows in forests of Gorakhpur, Bihar, Orissa, Konkan, North Kanara, North Circars and west of Tamil Nadu up to 1300 m.

Plant habitat and morphology

The plant is a small tree up to 12 meters in height. The fruit, collected from November to February by the natives, is a berry and contains 3-5 seeds which is adhered with the white and mucilaginous bitter pulp. The epicarp is separated, seeds are obtained and washed to remove adherent pulp.

Morphology

The dried seeds are very hard, greenish-grey in colour, disc-shaped, 10-30 mm in diameter, 4-6 mm thick, flat and some concavo-convex type. The edge is acute or rounded. Numerous silky, closely appressed, radiating hairs are present on the testa.

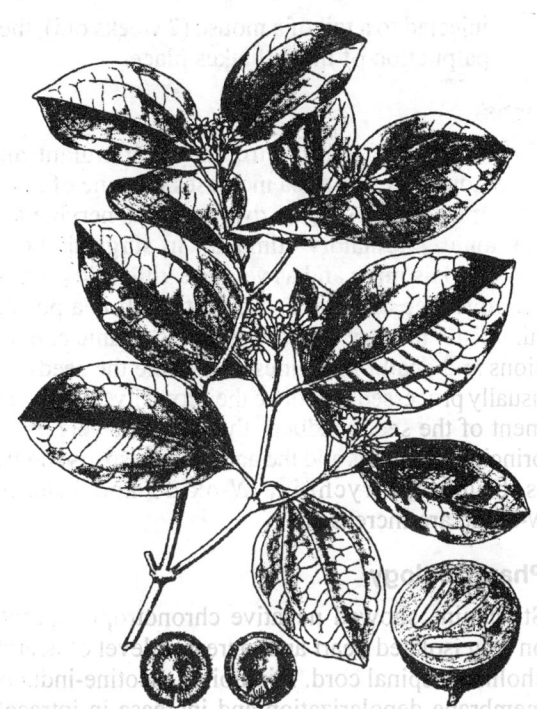

Fig. 21.56. *Strychnos nux-vomica* L.

Hilum is distinct which is present on the flattened side. From the hilum a radial ridge connects the micropyle at the circumference. A small embryo with two cordate cotyledons and a cylindrical radicle, directing towards the micropyle, is embedded in a grey, horny endosperm. A slit-like cavity is located in the centre of the seeds.

The seeds are odourless when dry; but if soaked in water and left for a day or two, they develop a very unpleasant odour. They have a very bitter taste.

Microscopical characters

A radial section shows a very thin testa consisting of collapsed parenchyma and an epidermal layer containing distinct lignified hairs. The hairs have a very large, thick-walled base with slit-like pits and they interlock with one another. The upper portions of the hairs are set a right angle to the bases and all radiate out towards the margin of the seed, giving the testa its characteristic silky appearance. On the ridge connecting hilum and micropyle, the hairs are irregularly arranged. The upper part of the wall of the hair is composed of about 10 longitudinal ridge-

like thickening united by a thin wall. The lumen is circular in the upper part, but in the base has branches corresponding with the oblique pits in the wall. Fragments of testa from a soaked seed may be disintegrated by treatment with 50% nitric acid and a little potas-sium chlorate; the hairs can then be separated.

The endosperm consists of large, non-lignified, thick walled cells, which yields galactose and mannose on hydrolysis. With iodine solution, they show well-marked protoplasmic threads (plasmodesma) passing through the walls and an oily plasma containing a few aleurone grains and the alkaloids strychnine and brucine. The presence of strychnine is detected by mounting a section in a solution of ammonium vanadate in sulphuric acid, when a violet colour is produced. The presence of brucine is determined by mounting in nitric acid, when a crimson colour is observed.

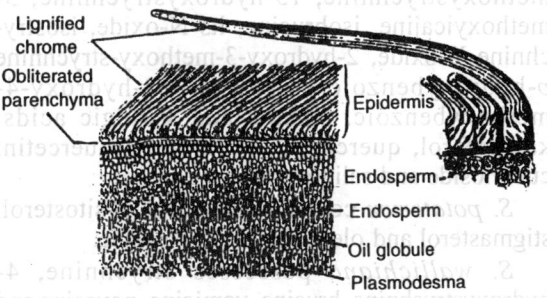

Fig. 21.57. Transverse section of Nux-vomica seed (cellular).

Chemical constituents

About 1.8–5.3% of total alkaloidal base is present in Nux vomica. The main alkaloids of therapeutic importance are strychnine (1.25%) and brucine (1.5%) which are present in large thick-walled cells of endosperm. The high concentration of strychnine is present in cells near the centre of the seeds while brucine is concentrated in the outer cells near the epidermis. The other minute alkaloids present in the drug are α-colubrine, β-colubrine, icajine, 3-methoxyicajine, protostrychnine, vomicine, novacine, N-oxystrychnine, pseudostrychnine and isostrychnine. The seeds also contain chlorogenic or igasuric or caffeotannic acid (a condensation

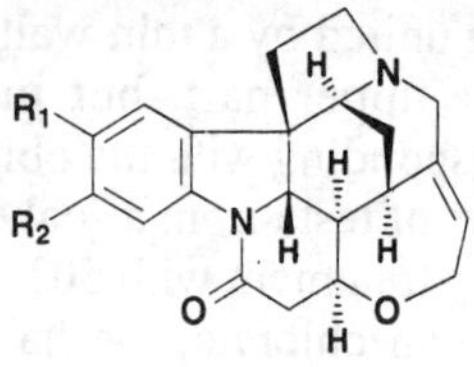

R₁ = R₂ = H : Strychnine
R₁ = R₂ = OCH₃ : Bricine

Fig. 21.58. Alkaloids of Nux vomica.

product of caffeic acid and quinic acid), loganin (a glycoside), fixed oils (3%) and proteins. Loganin is also present in the fruit pulp up to 5% along with secologanin. Hemicellulose consisting of mannan and galactan is present in the thick cell wall of endosperm. Aleurone grains are present in the endosperm of the seed.

The other compounds isolated from Nux vomica are N-methyl-*seco*-pseudo-β-colubrine, 4-hydroxy-strychnine, normacusine B, 4-hydroxy-3-methoxystrychnine, 15-hydroxystrychnine, 3-methoxyicajine, isobrucine, its N-oxide, isostrychnine N-oxide, 2-hydroxy-3-methoxy-strychnine *p*-hydroxybenzoic, vanillic, 2-hydroxy-4-methoxybenzoic, sinapic and syringic acids; kaempferol, quercetin, 3'-O-methoxyquercetin; cuchiloside and salidroside.

S. potatorum contains diaboline, β-sitosterol, stigmasterol and oleanolic acid glycoside.

S. wallichiana possesses strychnine, 4-hydroxystrychnine, brucine, vomicine, novacine and pseudostrychnine.

Chemical Tests

1. *Strychnine Test* : A mixture of ammonium vanadate and sulphuric acid on addition to strychnine or a thick section of endosperm gives purple colour.
2. *Potassium dichromate Test* : Addition of potassium dichromate and conc. H_2SO_4 with strychnine forms violet colour.
3. *Brucine Test* : Addition of conc. HNO_3 to brucine or thick section of endosperm produces yellow to orange colour.
4. *Hemicellulose Test* : When iodine and H_2SO_4 are added to a thick section, the cell walls are stained blue.
5. *Biological Test* : Strychnine (2/1000 mg) when

injected to a tail of a mouse (2 weeks old), then palpitation of the tail takes place.

Uses

Strychnine is used as circulatory stimulant and bitter tonic. Nux vomica increases the tone of intestine. It is given in atonic dyspepsia, as nervine and sex tonic, circulatory stimulant in surgical shock, alcohol poisoning and as vermine killer. Strychnine improves the appetite and digestion. It is a powerful poison in large doses, producing tetanic convulsions and death. In Chinese medicine the seeds are usually processed to reduce their toxicity. Heat-treatment of the seeds reduces the normal levels of the principal alkaloids and the amounts of isostrychnine, isobrucine, strychnine N-oxide and brucine N-oxide are increased.

Pharmacology

Strychnine showed negative chronotropic activity on frog isolated heart and increased level of acetylcholine in spinal cord. It inhibited nicotine-induced membrane depolarization and increase in intracellular Ca^{2+} concentration; also inhibited nicotine stimulation of catecholamine release from bovine culture adrenal chromaffin cells. Strychnine interacts with agonist binding site of nicotinic acetylcholine receptors.

Allied drugs

Ignatius beans are dried ripe seeds of *Strychnos ignatii* Bergius (Family-Loganiaceae). The plant is found in Philippines and Vietnam. The fruits are larger than those of Nux vomica and contain about 30 seeds. The seeds are 1.5 cm long, ovoid and dark grey. They possess irregularly arranged greyish hairs. The seeds contain 2.5-3% of total basic compounds among which strychnine is 46-62 per cent. Ignatius beans are similarly used as Nux vomica.

Strychnos tieute is found in Java and contains 1.4% of strychnine and small amount to brucine. *S. ligustrina*, *S. rheedii* and *S. aculeata* contain only brucine. The seeds of *S. triplinervia* from Mexico contain 1.8% of strychnine and brucine.

Seeds of *S. lucida* (*S. ligustrina*) from Australia contain brucine with a varying proportion of strychnine, while samples from Thailand contain

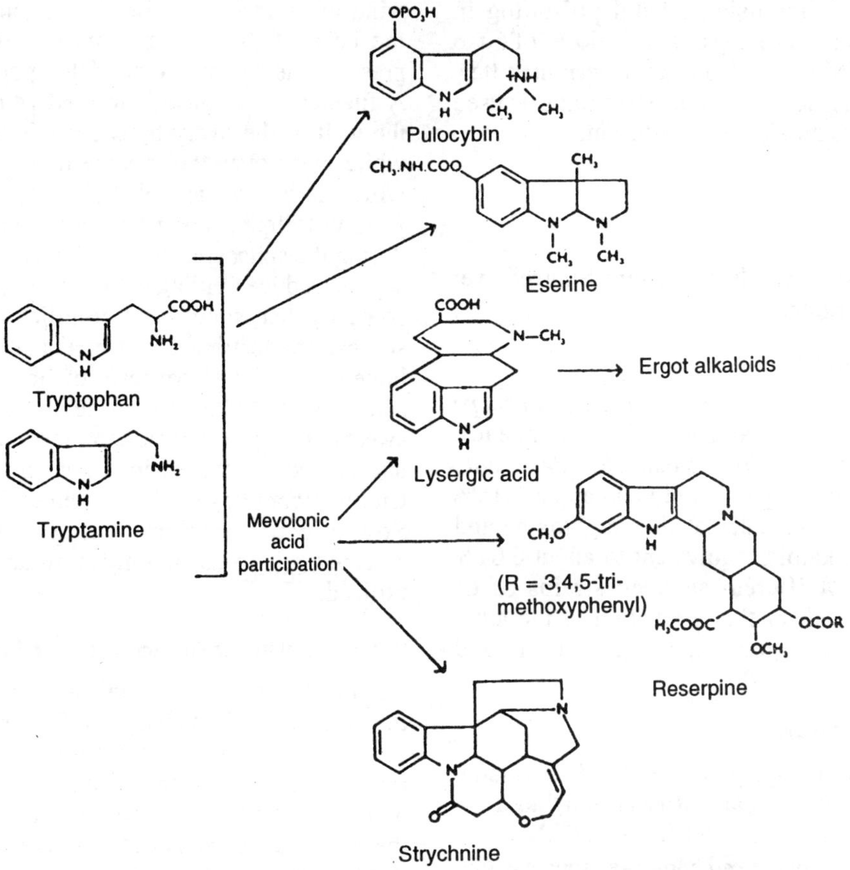

Fig. 21.59. Biosynthesis of strychnine.

only brucine. The principal alkaloid of *S. cinnamomifolia* (*S. rheedei*) seeds from southern India is 12-hydroxy-11-methoxystrychnine. *S. panamensis*, the only American species, whose seeds contain strychnine and brucine, about 0.1% of each.

In addition to the seeds, other parts of the plants of *Strychnos* spp. also contain alkaloids including strychnine.

S. potatorum, from India, and *S. nux-blanda*, from Burma, have been substituted for nux vomica; although they contain no strychnine or brucine. The seeds of *S. potatorum* contain the alkaloid diaboline and its acetyl derivative, triterpenes and sterols. They are distinguished by means of the ammonium vandate reagent. The seeds of *S. potatorum* are used for clearing water. They will also flocculate heavy metal contami-nants in water and are capable of

mopping up radioactive isotopes from nuclear waste. The protein responsible for this property has been isolated.

Strychnine and brucine (dimethoxystrychnine) are obtained from nux vomica or ignatia by extraction with dilute sulfuric acid. The solution is concentrated. The alkaloids are precipitated with lime, separated by means of solvent, and purified by recrystallization. Brucine is far more soluble in water and in alcohol than is strychnine; however, strychnine sulfate is somewhat more soluble in these 2 solvents than is brucine sulfate.

Strychnine is extremely toxic, functioning as a central stimulant. The alkaloid produces excitation of all parts of the central nervous system and blocks inhibitory spinal impulses at the postsynaptic level. This leads to an exageration in reflexes, with resulting tonic convulsions. Fatal poisoning in human beings ordinarily results from doses of 60 to 90 mg. The drug is utilized as a vermin killer. Brucine, which is less toxic than strychnine, is used commercially as an alcohol denaturant.

ERGOT

Synonyms

Ergot; Rye Ergot; Secale cornutum; Spurred rye; Ergot of rye; Ergota.

Biological source

Ergot is the dried sclerotium of a fungus, *Claviceps purpurea* Tulasne, (Family : Clavicipitaceae). developing in the ovary of rye plant, *Secale cereale* (Family Poaceae). Ergot should yield about 0.15% of the total alkaloids calculated as ergotoxine and water-soluble alkaloids equivalent to about 0.01% of ergonovine. Different selected strains of *C. purpurea* are used for the production of the alkaloids ergotamine, ergocristine, ergo-cornine and ergokryptine.

Geographical source

Czechoslovakia, Hungary , Switzerland, Germany, France, Yugoslavia, Spain, Russia and India. In India Ergot is cultivated at Kodaikanal (T.N.).

The fungus *C. purpurea* and other species such as *C. microcephala*, *C. nigricans* and *C. paspali* produce ergots on many members of the Poaceae (*e.g.*, *Triticum*, *Avena*, *Festuca*, *Poa*, *Lolium*, *Molinia* and *Nardus*) and Cryperaceae (*e.g.*, *Scirpus* and *Ampelodesma*). Many of these ergots are extremely toxic and produce typical ergotism.

Cultivation

The life cycle of the fungus, *Claviceps purpurea*, which is a parasite, passes through the following characteristic stages :
1. Sphacelia or honeydew or asexual stage
2. Sclerotium or ascigerous or sexual stage, and
3. Ascospore stage.

1. Sphacelia or Honeydew or Asexual stage

The rye plant becomes infected by the spores of the fungus in the spring session when flowers bloom for about one week. The spores are carried by the wind or by insects to the flowers and collected at the base of the young ovary where moisture is present. There germination of the spores takes place. A filamentous hyphae is formed which enters into the wall of the ovary by enzymatic action. A soft, white mass over the surface of ovary is formed, which is known as sphacelia. A sweet viscous yellowish liquid, known as honeydew, is secreted during the sphacelia stage which contains reducing sugars (reduce Fehling solution). From the ends of some hyphae small oval conidiospores (asexual spores) are abstricted which remain suspended on honeydew. The sweet taste of honeydew attracts some insects like ants and weevils. Insects suck the sweet liquid and carry the conidiospores to the plants and spread the fungal infection in the rye plants. Cultured conidiospores are used for the inoculum. Strains capable of producing about 0.35% of selected alkaloids, mainly ergotamine, are now utilized.

2. Sclerotium or Ascigerous or Sexual stage

During the sphacelia stage the hyphae enter only the outer wall of the ovary. On further development they penetrate into deeper parts, feed on the ovarian tissues and replace it by a compact, dark purple hard tissue known as pseudoparenchyma. It forms the sclerotium or resting state of the fungus. During summer the sclerotium or ergot increases in size and projects on the rye, showing sphacelial remains at its apex. It is collected at this stage by hands or machine and used as a drug. Ergot is then dried to remove moisture. About 6 weeks after inoculation, the mature sclerotia are harvested. They may be picked up by hand or collected by machine. The number and size of the ergots produced on each spike of cereal by *C. purpurea* varies, rye usually bears sclerotia, while wheat bears very few.

3. Ascospore stage

If Ergot is not collected, it falls on the ground. In the next spring session they produce stalked projections known as stromata which have globular heads. In the inner surface of the heads there are many flask-shaped pockets known as perithecia. Each of these perithecia contains many sacs (asci) which possesses eight of the thread-like ascospores. These ascospores are carried out by insects or wind

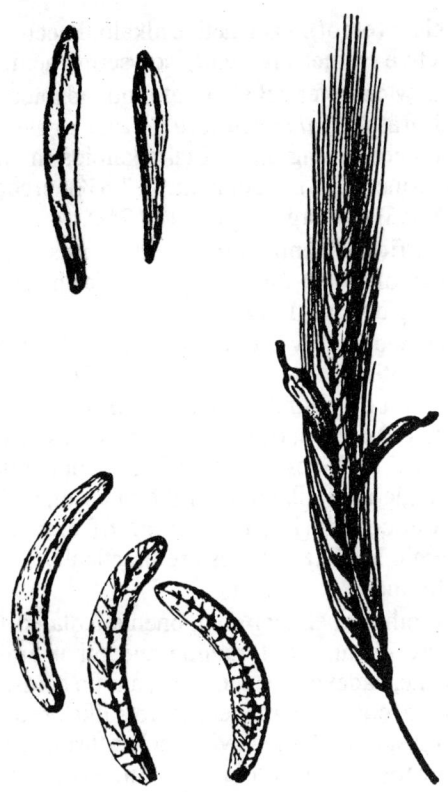

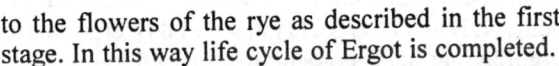

Fig. 21.60. Ergot of rye.

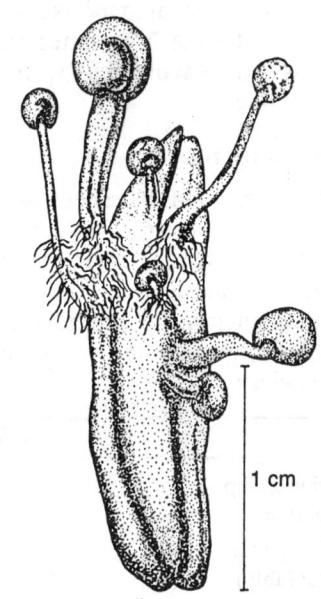

1 cm

Fig. 21.61. *Claviceps purpurea* sclerotia.

to the flowers of the rye as described in the first stage. In this way life cycle of Ergot is completed.

The ascospores may be germinated on a nutritive medium to get conidiospore-bearing cultures. The suspension of these conidiospores is usually used as a spray to infect rye plants for commercial production of Ergot.

Ergot is collected from fields of rye when the sclerotia are fully developed and projecting from the spike, or they are removed from the grain by shifting. The size of the crop varies according to weather conditions.

The vegetative phase of the fungus can, like that of other moulds, be cultivated artificially. Under such conditions the typical sclerotia do not develop.

Morphology

The size of sclerotium (Ergot) is about 1-4 cm long, 2-7 mm broad. Shape is fusiform, slightly curved, sub-cylindrical, tapering at both ends. The outer surface is dark or violet-black in colour, has longitudinal furrows and sometimes small transverse cracks. The fractured surface shows thin, dark outer layer, a whitish or pinkish-white central zone of pseudoparenchyma in which darker lines radiate from the centre. Odour is characteristic and taste is unpleasant.

Powdered ergot on treatment with sodium hydroxide solution develops a strong odour of trimethylamine. In filtered ultraviolet light it has a strong reddish colour by means of which its presence in flour may be detected.

Microscopical characters

Ergot shows an outer zone of purplish-brown, obliterated rectangular cells. The pseudoparenchyma consists of oval or rounded cells containing fixed oil and protein, and with highly refractive walls which give a reaction for chitin. Celluloe and lignin are absent.

608 Pharmacognosy and Phytochemistry

Storage

Ergot should be thoroughly dried, and the sclerotia kept entire and stored in a cool place. If the moisture content is maintained below 8 per cent, alkaloidal loss is negligible. If this figure is exceeded, deterioration is proportional to the excess moisture. The drug is liable to attack by mites and various insects, but this can be avoided by sprinkling with carbon tetrachloride.

Chemical constituents

A large number of alkaloids have been isolated from the Ergot. The most important alkaloids are ergonovine and ergotamine. On the basis of solubility in water the alkaloids are divided into two groups - water soluble ergometrine (or ergonovine) group or water-insoluble (ergotamine and ergotoxine) groups as given hereunder :

Group	Alkaloids
I. Ergometrine group (Water soluble)	Ergometrine Ergometrinine
II. Ergotamine group (Water-insoluble)	Ergotamine Ergotaminine Ergosine Ergosinine
III. Ergotoxine group (Water-insoluble)	Ergocristine Ergocristinine Ergocryptine Ergocryptinine Ergocornine Ertgocorninine

Only the first group, ergometrine group, belongs to water-soluble compounds. Alkaloids of Group II and III are polypeptides in which lysergic acid or isolysergic acid is linked to amino acids. Alkaloids obtained from lysergic acid are physiologically active compounds. In the first group, e.g., ergometrine alkaloids, lysergic acid or its isomer is linked to an amino alcohol.

The ergot alkaloids (ergolines) can also be divided into two classes (1) the clavine-type alkaloids, which are derivatives of 6,8-dimethylergoline and (2) the lysergic acid derivatives, which are peptide alkaloids and contains the pharmacologically active alkaloids that characterize the ergot

sclerotium (ergot). Each active alkaloid occurs with an inactive isomer involving isolysergic acid.

A new commercial strain of ergot adapted from a wild grass (*Anthraxan lancifolius*) to rye gave sclerotia containing 0.5% total alkaloids involving ergometrine (33%), ergotamine (17.6%), ergocornine (18.7%) and ergocryptine (22.7%).

Significant semisynthetic alkaloids include methylergonovine, dihydroergotamine, hydergine, methysergide, and LSD.

The medicinally useful alkaloids, either natural or semisynthetic, are all derivatives of (+)-lysergic acid. The compound is readily converted to its isomer, (+)-isolysergic acid, the corresponding isolysergic acid derivatives often accompany the (+)-lysergic acid alkaloids in the plant material or are produced during the course of extraction. Isolysergic acid derivatives are practically physiologically inert.

The other chemical components isolated from Ergot are histamine, tyramine and other amines, putrescine, cadaverine, agmatine, amino acids, acetylcholine, colouring matters, sterols like ergosterol and fungisterol, elymoclavine, sclerythrin, ergonovine, ergothioneine, clavicepsin, ergochrysin, ergoflavin, ergotic acid, choline, betaine, clavine, fat (15-30%), mannitol, lactic acid, succinic acid, endocrocin, clavorubin, chrysergonic acid, secaloric acids A, B and C, ergochrysins A and B, ergoflavin, ergoflavinic acid, ergochromes, hydroergotamine, dihydroergocristine, dihydroergocornine, dihydroergo-cryptine, chanoclavine, isochanoclavine, ergocerebrine, cerebrine isoergochrysin A, ergoxanthin, 6,7-*seco*-agroclavine, ergovaline, ergoptine, ergonine, N-(p-lysergly-L-valyl)-cyclo-(L-valyl-p-prolyl), N-(D-lyserglyl-L-valyl) cyclo (L-leucyl-D-propyl), costaclavine, epicostaclavine, 5'-epimer or β-ergocryptine, β-ergocryptam, β,β-ergoannam and α- and β-ergocryptines. The cell walls of Ergot are made up of chitinous layer in place of plant cellulose.

Storage

Ergot is attacked by insects, moulds and bacteria. After collection it should be thoroughly dried, kept entire, and stored in a cool, dry place. If powdered and not immediately defatted, the activity decreases, but if defatted and carefully stored in an air-tight

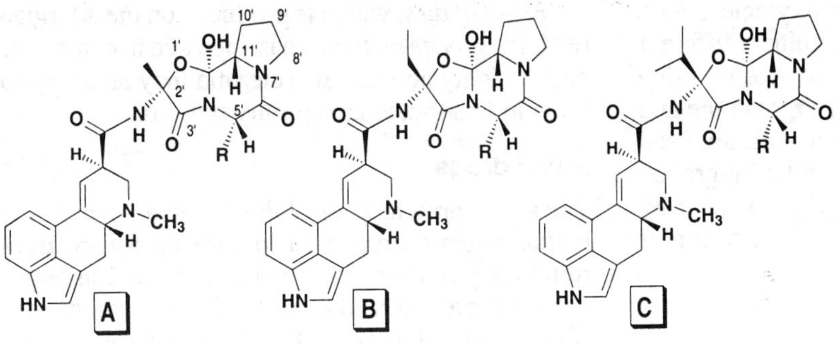

A : Ergotamines   B : Ergoxines   C : Ergotoxines

	A : Ergotamines	B : Ergoxines	C : Ergotoxines
R = CH$_2$ Ph	Ergotamine	Ergostine	Ergocristine
R = CH$_2$ CH(CH$_3$)$_2$	α-Ergosine	α-Ergoptine	α-Ergocryptine
R = CH(CH$_3$)CH$_2$CH$_3$	β-Ergosine	*	β-Ergocryptine
R = CH(CH$_3$)$_2$	Ergovaline	Ergonine	Ergocornine
R = CH$_2$CH$_3$	Ergobine	Ergobutine	Ergobutyrine

* not known

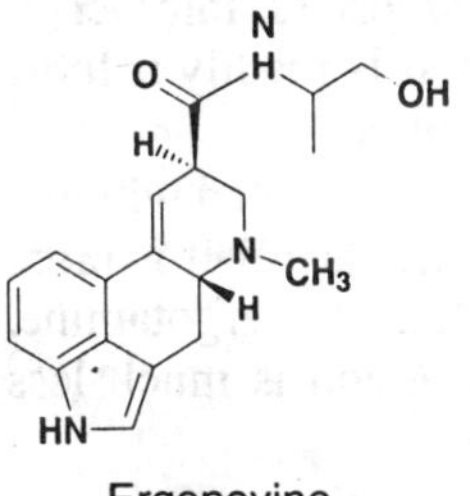

Ergonovine
(= ergometrine)

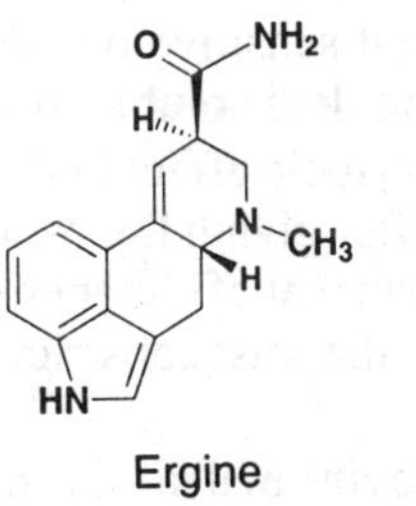

Ergine

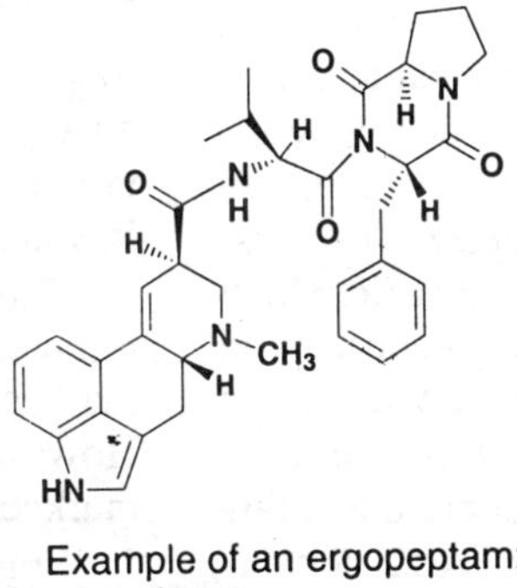

Example of an ergopeptam:
ergocristam

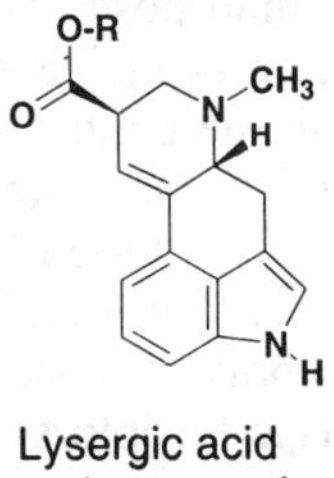

Lysergic acid
and ergopeptines

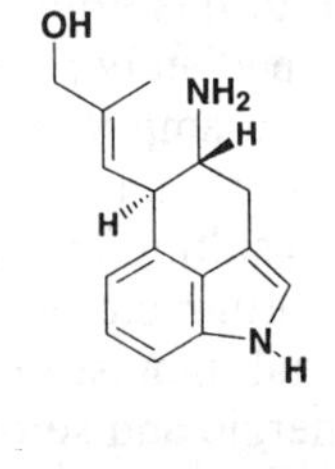

Norchanoclavine I

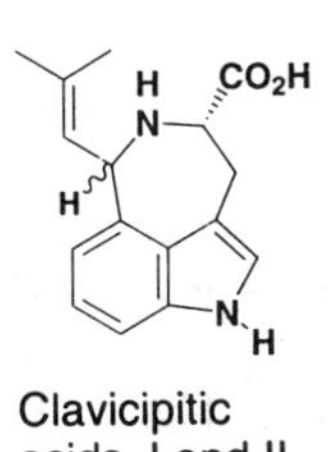

Clavicipitic
acids, I and II

Fig. 21.62. Ergot alkaloids.

container, it will remain active for a long period. Any sample of ergot which shows worm holes or a insect debris will almost certainly deteriorate further on storage.

Ergot contains not more than 8% of moisture. The use of a cartridge of a nonliquefying, inert, dehydrating agent to maintain low humidity in the container of ergot is desirable. Ergot is assayed for its alkaloid content by colorimetric procedures involving the use of *p*-dimethylamino-benzal-dehyde.

Chemical tests

1. Ergot under UV light shows a red-coloured fluorescence.
2. Ergot powder is extracted with a mixture of CHCl$_3$ and sodium carbonate. The CHCl$_3$ layer is separated and a mixture of *p*-dimethylaminobenzaldehyde (0.1g), H$_2$SO$_4$ (35%, v/v, 100 ml) and 5% ferric chloride (1.5 ml) is added. A deep blue colour is produced.

Uses

Ergot is oxytocic, vasoconstrictor and abortifacient and used to assist delivery and to reduce post-partum haemorrhage. Lysergic acid diethylamide (LSD-25), obtained by partial synthesis from lysergic acid, is a potent specific psychotomimetic. Ergometrine is oxytocic and used in delivery. It stimulates the tone of uterine muscles and prevent postpartum haemorrhage.

Only ergometrine produces an oxytocic effect, ergotoxine and ergotamine having quite a different action. Ergometrine is soluble in water or in dilute alcohol. It is known as ergonovine. Ergotamine and the semisynthetic dihydroergotamine salts are used as specific analgesics for the treatment of migraine. Lysergic acid diethylamide (LSD-25), prepared by partial synthesis from lysergic acid, is a potent specific psychotomimetic.

Pharmacology

Ergometrine caused biliary excretion of β-glucuromides of 12-hydroxy-ergometrine and 12-hydroxyergometrine; it stimulated locomotor activity in rats. Ergotamine hastened onset of esters and increased fertility rate. Ergotamine tartarate induced contractions in human veins. Ergometrine maleate stimulated gastric acid secretion in rats. Elymoclavine induced stereotype in rats and mice. It prevented development of haloperidol catalepsy in rats and decreased plasma level of prollactin.

Tissue culture of ergot

Submerged cultures did not produce the typical alkaloids associated with the sclerotium but, a series of new nonpeptide bases (clavines) which possessed no significant pharmacological action.

The commercial manufacture of simple lysergic acid derivatives is obtained by fermentative growth of a strain of *Claviceps paspali*. The alkaloids produced are converted to lysergic acid which is used for the partial-synthesis of ergometrine and related alkaloids. Other strains are now available which produce the peptide alkaloids in culture.

Ergot alkaloids have also been reported in a few other fungi—*Aspergillus fumigatus* Fres., *Penicillium chermesinum* Biourge, *Penicillium roquefortii* Thom, *Rhizopus arrhizus* Fischer and *Sphacelia typhina*. Only clavine alkaloids were detected in these latter species.

Substituents

The sclerotia *Ergot of wheat* are shorter and thicker than those of rye. Ergot on barley, rye and wheat been reported.

Ergot of oats is used medicinally in Algiers. The sclerotia are black in colour, 10-12 mm long and 3-4 mm diameter.

Ergot of diss, which is produced on the Alergian reed *Ampelodesma tenax*, has appeared in commerce and is highly active. The sclerotia may attain up to 9 cm in length and are spirally twisted.

Allied drugs

The active principles of *ololiuqui*, an ancient Aztec hallucinogenic drug used in Mexico for magico-religious purposes, have been identified as ergot alkaloids present in the seeds of *Rivea corymbosa* (Fam. Convolvulaceae) and in certain closely related *Ipomoea* species (commonly known as morning glories) & *Argyreia* species. (+)-Lysergic acid amide (ergine), the principal psychotomimetic compound in these species, is accompanied by (+)-isolysergic acid (erginine), ergonovine, (+)-lysergic acid methylcarbinolamide and certain clavine alkaloids.

Ergot alkaloids have been reported only in a few other fungi—*Aspergillus fumigatus* Fres., *Penicillium chermesinum* Biourge, *Penicillium roquefortii* Thom, *Rhizopus arrhizus* Fischer and *Sphacelia typhina*. Only clavine alkaloids were detected in these latter species.

Ergot alkaloids

Ergonovine maleate or ergometrine maleate occurs as a white or faintly yellow, odourless, microcrystalline, light sensitive powder. It is readily soluble in water but less soluble in alcohol.

The oxytocic effect of the drug is noted within 5 minutes after giving the dose and its effect is more marked than that of either ergotoxine or ergotamine. However, the vasoconstrictor action is much less marked.

Ergonovine maleate is an oxytocic and produces much faster stimulation of the uterine muscles than do other ergot alkaloids. The gravid uterus is very sensitive to this effect and small doses of alkaloid gives immediately post-partum to increase the frequency and amplitude of uterine contractions and increases the basal tone of the uterine smooth muscle, resulting in a decrease in blood loss from the postpartum uterus. It exerts its effects by acting as a partial agonist or antagonist at α-adrenergic, dopaminergic and serotonergic receptors.

Methylergonovine maleate is a semisynthetic homolog of ergonovine prepared from lysergic acid and 2-aminobutanol. It occurs as a white to pinkish tan, microcrystalline powder. It is an oxytocic reputed to be slightly more active and longer acting than ergonovine. The usual dose is the same as that for ergonovine.

Ergotamine tartarate occurs as colourless crystals or as a white, crystalline powder, sparingly soluble in water and alcohol. Ergotamine possesses oxytocic properties and is categorized as a specific analgesic in treatment of migraine. Ergotamine reduces extracranial blood flow and decreases the amplitude of pulsations in the cranial arteries that have been associated with migraine. It inhibits receptor uptake of norepinephrine at sympathetic nerve endings, increasing the vasoconstrictive action.

Ergotamine tartarate is used with caffeine for the treatment of migraine headache. Both act as cerebral vasoconstrictors; caffeine is believed to enhance the action of ergotamine.

Dihydroergotamine mesylate, a salt of a semi-synthetic alkaloid prepared from ergotamine by hydrogenation of the Δ^9 double bond in the lysergic acid nucleus, is used to treat migraine.

Ergotoxine is a variable mixture of 3 closely related alkaloids, ergocristine, ergokryptine and ergocornine. A mixture of equal parts of these component alkaloids is hydrogenated to reduce the Δ^9 double bond of the lysergic acid nucleus and to yield an equivalent mixture of dihydroergocristine, dihydroergokryptine and dihydroergocornine. The methanesulfonates of this mixture, known as *ergoloid mesylates*, are marketed for the treatment of selected symptoms in elderly patients. They produce vasorelaxation, increased cerebral blood flow, lowering of systemic blood pressure and bradycardia.

Methysergide maleate is the salt of methyler-gonovine that has an additional methyl group attached to the nitrogen at position 1 of the lysergic acid nucleus. It is prepared by semisynthesis from lysergic acid. Methysergide is a serotonin antago-nist used in the prophylaxis of vascular headache.

The patient should be advised to take medica-tion with meals. The side effects are cold, numb or painful hands, leg cramps, abdominal or chest pain, or change in skin colour occurs.

Lysergic acid diethylamide or LSD is prepared by semisynthesis. The compound has a 2-fold action, producing a predominant central sympathetic stimulation that parallels a slight depression. It is the most active and most specific psychotomimetic agent known. Due to its widespread misuse, the drug is available only to qualified scientific investigators.

Biosynthesis of ergot alkaloids

The alkaloids of ergot are derived from a com-bination of tryptophan and acetate metabolism. Initially, dimethylallyl pyrophosphate condenses at the 4-position of tryptophan. The next intermediate arises from the *N*-methylation of dimethyl-allyltryp-tophan to give N_a-methyl-dimethyl-allyltryptophan. Then decarboxylation takes place with a subsequent formation of chanoclavine-I. The number of inter-mediates and enzymatic conversions in these events is still unknown. The 2 *cis-trans* isomerizations in the isoprenoid moiety take place forming the tetracyclic ring system. If the *trans* methyl group of dimethyl-allylpyrophosphate is radioactively labelled, the *cis* methyl group of chanoclavine-I will be labelled indicating one *cis-trans* isomerization, and the *trans* methyl group of the isoprenoid moiety of agroclavine will be labelled indicating a second isomerization. Agroclavine undergoes step-wise oxidation to elymoclavine and then to lysergic acid. The carboxyl group of lysergic acid forms a peptide linkage with an amino group of a variety of amino acids or peptide residues to yield the thera-peutically useful ergot alkaloids (Fig. 21.64).

Synthesis of lysergic acid derivatives and clavine alkaloids in higher plants (*Ipomoea* species) apparently takes place from the same precursors (Fig. 21.63).

PHYSOSTIGMA

Synonyms

Calabar bean; Ordeal bean; Chop nut; Split nut; Esere nut; Semina physostigmatis.

Biological source

Physostigma is the dried ripe seeds of *Physostigma venenosum* Balfour. (Family : Papilionaceae).

It is found on the banks of streams of West Africa (near mouths of Niger and Old Calabar rivers), introduced into India and Brazil.

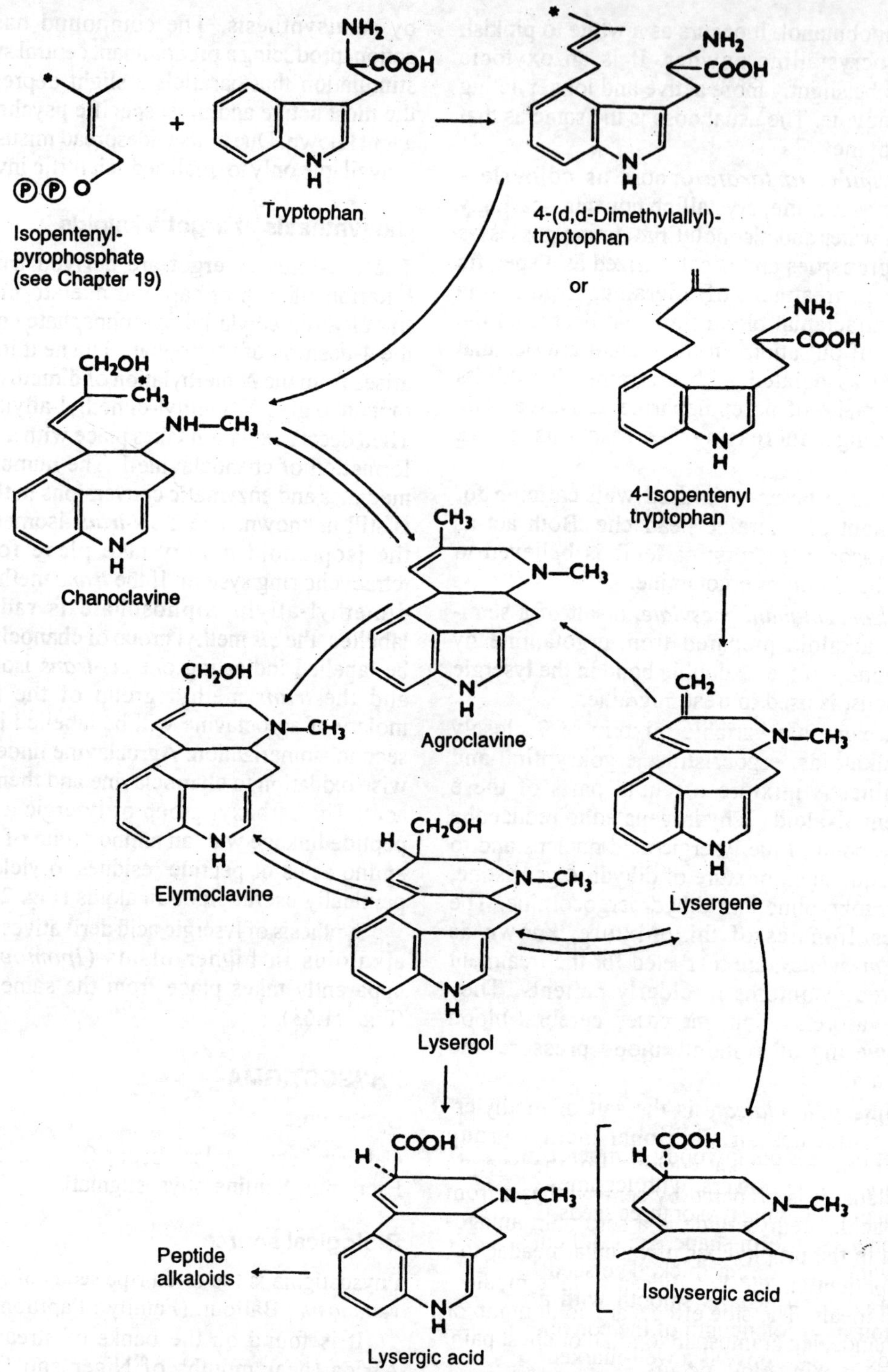

Fig. 21.63. Biogenesis of lysergic acid.

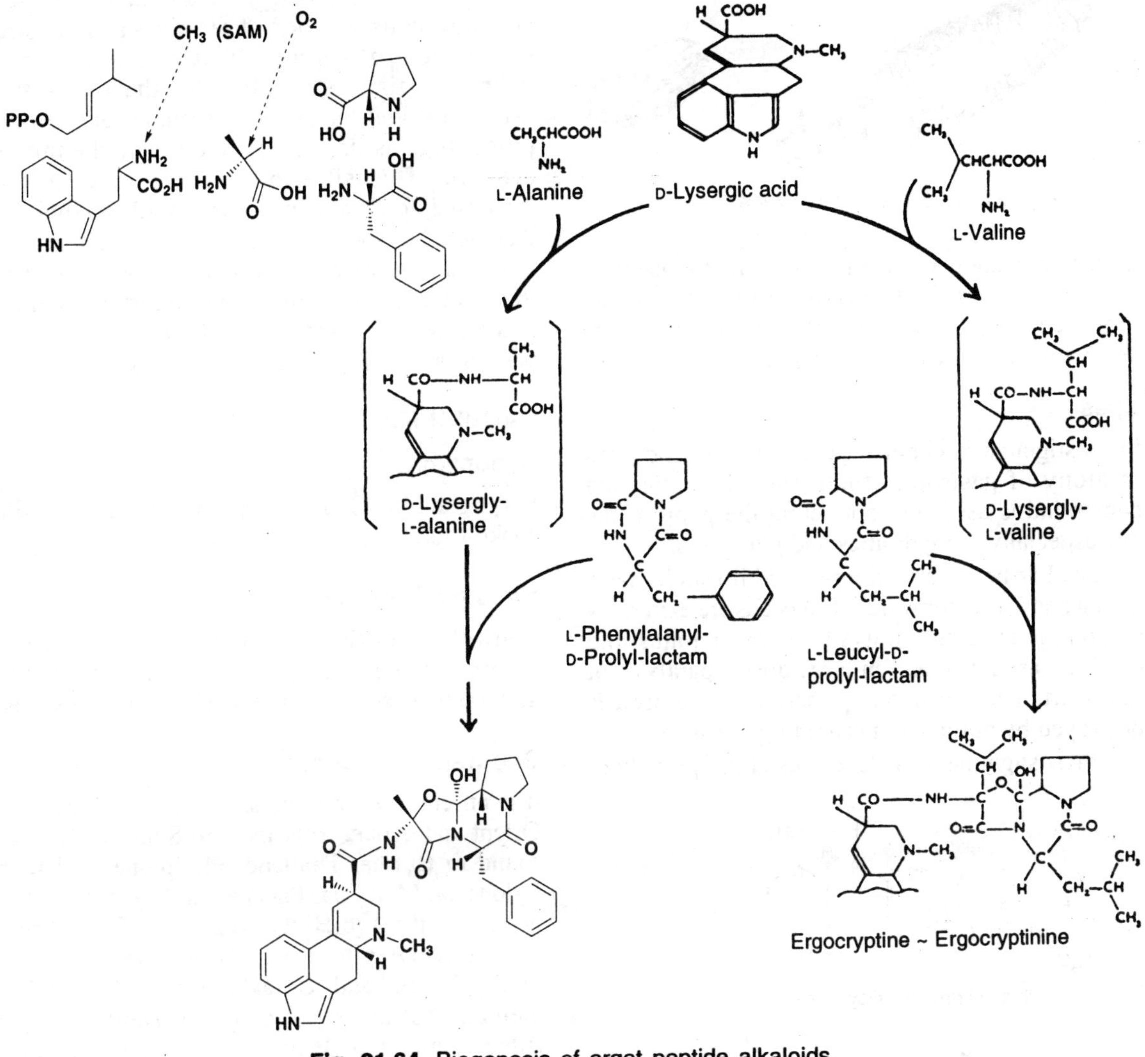

Fig. 21.64. Biogenesis of ergot peptide alkaloids.

Characters

The plant is a perennial woody climber, bears typical papilonaceous flowers, with legumes of 15 cm length, each containing two or three seeds. The beans are flattened, reniform shape, 1.5 - 3.0 cm long, 1-1.5 cm wide and 1.5 cm thick. The seeds are very hard, dark brown testa is smooth with a grooved hilum running whole length of the convex side. On either side of the groove is a well-marked ridge and in the groove itself are the greyish, papery remains of the funiculus. A transverse section shows a large central cavity and two, very hard, concavo-convex cotyledons. Physostigma is odourless with starchy taste at first and acrid afterwards.

Chemical constituents

The seeds contain 0.15-0.3% alkaloids. Physostigmine (eserine) (0.15%), eseridine, eseramine, isophysostigmine, physovenine, geneserine, N-8-norphysostigmine, calabatine and calabacine are the alkaloids isolated from the seeds. Exposure of the chief alkaloid, physostigmine, to heat, light or air

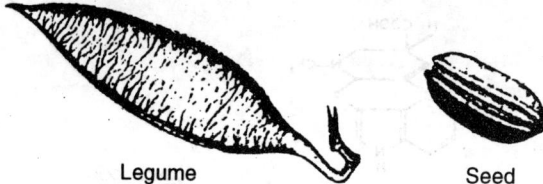

Legume   Seed

Fig. 21.65. *Physostigma venenosum.*

leads to oxidation and a red compound, rubreserine, is formed. Therefore, physostigmine should be protected from air and light. Physostigmine occurs as a white, odourless, finely crystalline powder.

Uses

Physostigmine is cholinergic and miotic and used in atony of gastrointestinal tract. Its salicylate compound is used for contracting the pupil of the eye especially in mydriatics and glaucoma.

Calabar beans are odourless with starchy taste at first and acrid afterwards. The beans are extremely poisonous causing paralysis of lower limbs and death by asphyxia, and in large doses, paralysis of the heart. The poisonous principle in the seed is destroyed by boiling and scorching the seed.

Physostigmine salicylate is used in ophthalmo-

logy to reduce intraocular tension in glaucoma, as an intravenous injection of sedatives and to correct the dilation of the pupil. It is also used in post-operative distension, atony of the intestine or urinary bladder, in tetanus, strychnine and atropine poisoning, as an antispasmodic in rheumatoid arthritis, fibrositis, bruitis and in veterinary medicine for colic in horses. With Alzheimer's disease it has shown some improvement in intellectual and cognitive performance. Physovenine has the same order of activity but that of eseramine is much lower. The seeds were formerly used by the west African tribes as an 'ordeal poison'.

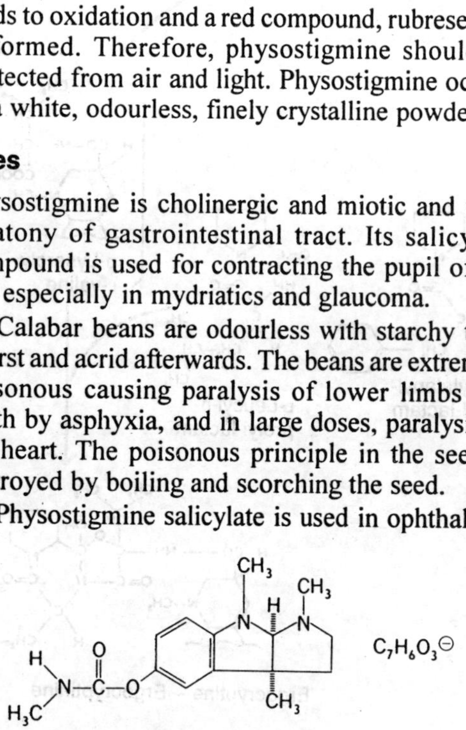

RAUWOLFIA

Synonyms

Sarpagandha, Chandrika; Chootachand; Indian snake-root.

Biological source

Rauwolfia consists of dried roots of *Rauwolfia serpentina* Benth.; sometimes pieces of rhizome and aerial stem bases are attached. (Fam. Apocynaceae).

Geographical source

It is an erect, evergreen, small shrub native to the Orient and occurs from India to Sumatra. It is also found in Burma, Thailand, Philippines, Vietnam, Indonesia, Malaysia, Pakistan and Java. In India it occurs in the sub-Himalayan tracts from Sirhind eastwards to Assam, especially in Dehradun, Siwalik range, Rohelkhand, Gorakhpur ascending to 1300 meters, east and west ghats of Tamil Nadu, in Bihar (Patna and Bhagalpur), Konkan, Karnataka and Bengal.

Cultivation

Rauwolfia grows in tropical forests at an altitude of 1200-1300 meters at temperature 10-40°. There should be enough rain or irrigation for its cultivation. The soil should be acidic (pH 4-6), clayey, and manure is applied for better crop. Propagation is done by planting seeds, root-cuttings or stem-cuttings. Better drug is obtained when the propagation is carried out with fresh seeds. The plants should be protected from nematodes, fungus and *Mosaic* virus.

Physostigmine salicylate $C_7H_6O_3^{\ominus}$

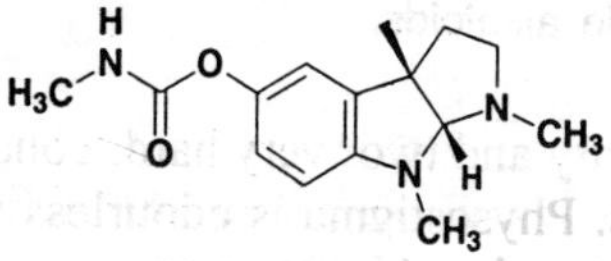

Physostigmine (eserine)

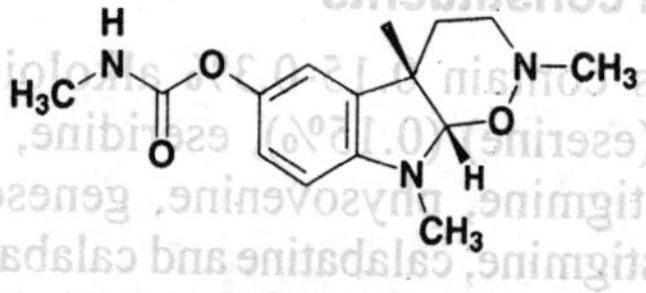

Geneserine

Fig. 21.66. Chemical constituents of Physostigma.

Collection

The drug is collected mainly from wild plants. Roots and rhizomes are dug out in October-November when the plant roots are 2-4 years old. The aerial parts and roots are separated. The roots are washed and dried in air. The roots containing moisture up to 12% should be protected from light.

Seasonal variation, genetic differences, geographic location, improper handling and drying, and other factors account for percentage differences in alkaloid amount. Certain alkaloids are hydrolyzed easily, and proper storage of the roots, the powdered drug and the compressed tablets are essential. Rauwolfia should be packaged and stored in well-closed containers in a cool, dry place that is secure against insect attack.

Morphology

The roots and rhizomes are almost identical in external characters. The drug occurs in cylindrical or slightly tapering, tortuous pieces, 2-10 cm long, 5-22 mm in diameter. The roots are rarely branched. Rootlets, 0.5- 1 mm in diameter, are rare. The outer surface is greyish-yellow, light-brown or brown. Young pieces contain slight wrinkles while old pieces have longitudinal ridges. Circular scars of rootlets are present. Bark exfoliation is present in old samples leaving behind patches of exposed wood. The fracture is short. A narrow, yellowish-brown bark and a dense pale yellow wood are present on the smooth transverse surface at both the ends. Pieces of rhizome closely resemble the root but may be identified by a small central pith. They are attached to them with small pieces of aerial stem. Slight odour is felt in recently dried drug which decreases with age; taste is bitter.

Both bark and wood contain abundant starch. Some commercial samples show mould.

Microscopical characters

The cork is stratified into two to eight zones, which consist of smaller and radially narrower suberized but unlignified cells alternating with larger radially broader cells which are lignified. In many pieces the cork is exfoliated.

Most of the cells of the secondary cortex are parenchymatous and contain starch; isolated latex

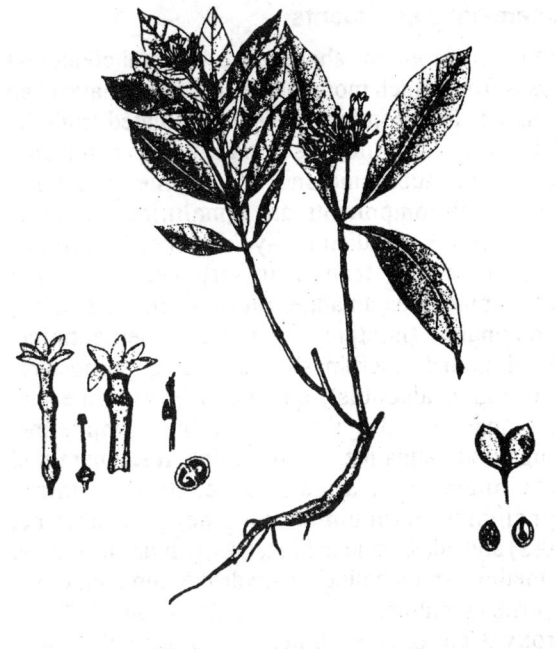

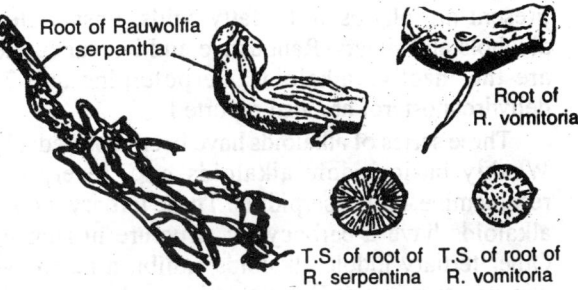

Root of Rauwolfia serpantha

Root of R. vomitoria

T.S. of root of R. serpentina   T.S. of root of R. vomitoria

Fig. 21.67. *Rauwolfia serpentina.*

cells may occur in this region. The phloem is narrow and consists mainly of parenchyma with scattered sieve tissue. Sclerenchyma is absent.

Most of the parenchymatous cells of the bark contain starch grains, and other prisms shaped crystals of calcium.

The xylem is lignified and show three to six annual rings. The medullary rays, which are one to five cells wide, contain starch and alternate with the rays of the secondary xylem, which consist of vessels, fibres and xylem parenchyma. The vessels of *R. serpentina* are small (up to 57 μm) and are less numerous than in most of the similar adulterants. The starch grains are larger in the wood than in the bark.

Chemical constituents

Rauwolfia contains about 0.7-2.4% total alkaloidal bases from which more than 80 alkaloids have been isolated. The prominent alkaloids isolated from the drug are reserpine, rescinnamine, ψ-reserpine, rescidine, raubescine and deserpidine. The other alkaloidal components are ajmalinine, ajmaline (rauwolfine), ajmalicine (δ-yohimbine), serpentine, serpentinine, tetrahydroreserpine, raubasine, reserpinine, isoajamaline, rauwolfinine, alstonine, serpajmaline (mixture of serpentine, serpentinine, ajmaline and reserpines), resajmaline (serposterol and higher alcohols), ajmalexine (reserpine and rescinnamine), 3-hydroxyserpentine, isoajmaline, raugalline, raunatine, sandwicoline, rescinnaminol, rescinnamidine, ajmalicidine, ajmalinimine, ajmalimine, in-dobinine, idobine, yohambinine, 20(S) and 20(R) raumachine, N^b-methylraumachine, 6-methoxy-raumacline, 6α-hydroxyraumacline, 12-hydroxyajmaline, 3-epi-α-yohimbine and 18β-hydroxy-3-epi-α-yohimbine. The other substances present are phytosterols, fatty acids, unsaturated alcohols and sugars. Raugustine and isoraunescine are the inactive alkaloids. Serpoterpine and 7-dehydrositosterol are also reported.

Three series of alkaloids have been reported: (1) Weakly basic indole alkaloids *e.g.*, reserpine, rescinamine, and deserpidine. These tertiary indole alkaloids have a carbocyclic structure in ring E. Other tertiary indole alkaloids exhibit a heterocyclic structure in ring E; δ-yohimbine (identical with ajmalicine, tetrahydroserpentine and raubasine) and reserpiline. (2) Indoline alkaloids of intermediate basicity, *e.g.*, ajmaline, isoajmaline, rauwolfinine, and others are listed as tertiary indoline alkaloids. These bases do not have a tranquilizing action. (3) Strongly basic adhydronium alkaloids, *e.g.*, serpentine, serpentinine and alstonine. These are not considered of practical therapeutic importance.

Pharmacology

Serpajmaline reduced systolic blood pressure of conscious dogs, pressor and chronotopic actions of adrenaline and noradrenaline. It inhibited the action of barium chloride and acetylcholine on intestine. Serpajmaline showed antihypertensive effect in dogs. It was patented in Germany as on antihypertensive and antispasmodic agent. Ajmaline showed guinidine-like action against auricular arrhythmias. It reduced hypertensive action of adrenaline and noradrenaline, but not the action of acetylcholine.

Deserpidine and its derivatives showed sedative and hypotensive effect. Rauwolfinine depressed electrical activity of brain. Rauwolscine had stimulant effect on CNS; it caused restlessness and hyper-reflexia in guinea pigs and rabbits. Raunatine lowered blood pressure in cats and reduced the pressor response to carotid occlusion. Reserpine caused increase in sugar level. Serpentine produced persistent hypoglycaemia. Reserpine decreased the toxicity of strophanthin. Reserpine, rescinnamine, raupine and yohimbine caused fall in blood pressure; yohimbine showing the maxi-mum fall. Daily administration of reserpine inhibited thyroid activity in mice; reduced oxygen consumption and body temperature.

Deserpidine showed antileukaemic activity and prolonged the survival time of mice by 50%. Reserpine, canescine and rescinnamine depleted the adrenaline store of adrenal medulla. Serpentine had quinidine-like action against auricular arrhythmias. Yohimbine resulted in increase of blood phosphorus. Rauwolscine was more potent adrenergic blocking agent than yohimbine.

Ajmalicine decreased the excitability and increased the functional refractory period of all heart tissues. Reserpinine depressed general behaviour of mice, prolonged the action of soporifics and decreased body temperature. Reserpine increased content of sodium, potassium and magnesium and decreased calcium content; increased levels of lipids of glycogen in heart and serum prolactin in dairy cows; caused decrease in weight of ovary of koel. Ajmaline increased diuresis and excretion of Na^+ in rats and dogs. Reserpine prevented increase in intraocular pressure in rabbits.

Yohimbine induced antidiuretic response in animals; stimulated vasopressin secretion and spermatogenesis; in small doses increased systolic blood pressure, heart rate and cardiac performance in dogs and in higher doses influenced cardiovascular system in opposite manner. Yohimbine caused increase in serum renin activity and heart rate in conscious rats.

Serpentine showed activity against mammary cancer MS 301 in mice. Yohimbine elevated

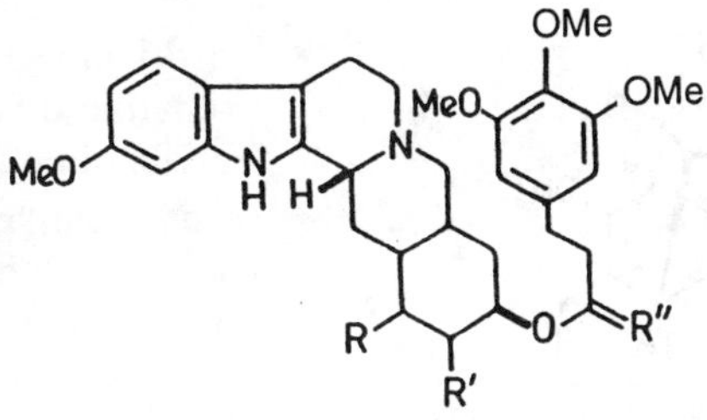

Rescinnaminol
R,R′ = H, R″ = H, OH
Rescinnamidine
R = β-COOMe, R′ = α-Ome, R″ = O

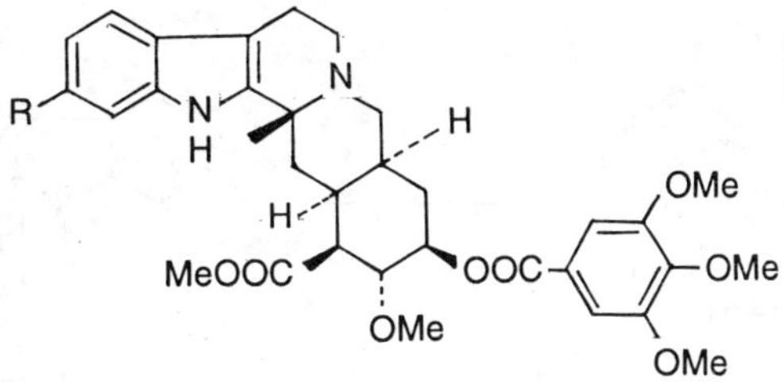

Deserpidine R = Rh
Reserpine R = OMe

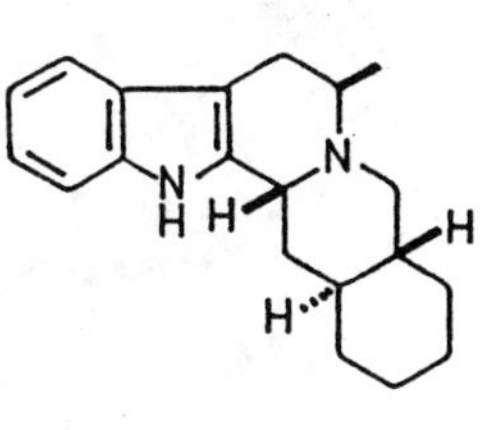

Yohambinine

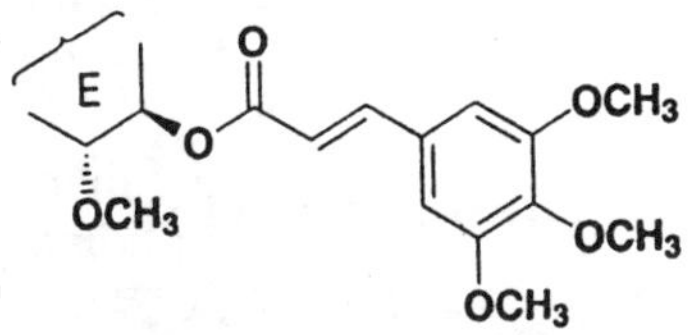

Rescinnamine

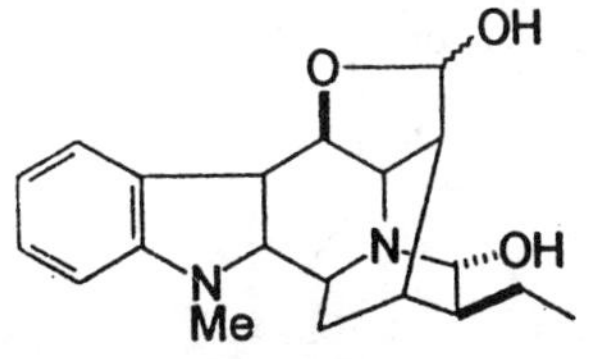

Alkaloid

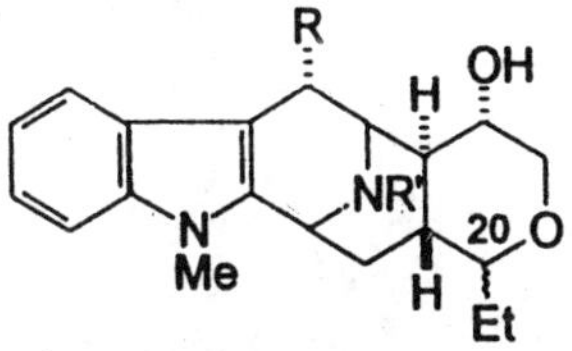

20(S)Raumacline
R,R′ = H, ~~ = β
20(R)Isoraumacline
R,R′ = H, ~~ = α
6α-Hydroxyraumacline
R = OH, R′ = H, ~~ = β
6α-Methoxyraumacline
R = OMe, R′ = H, ~~ = β
N^b = Methylraumacline
R = H, R′ = Me, ~~ = β

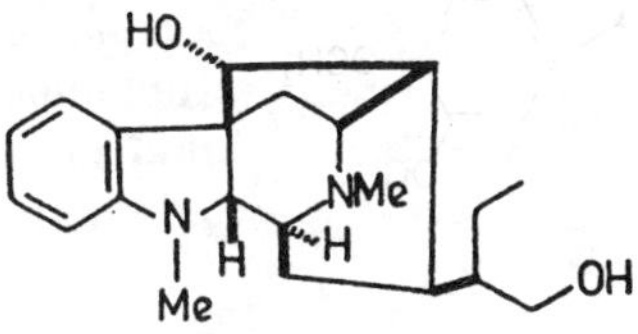

Sandwicoline

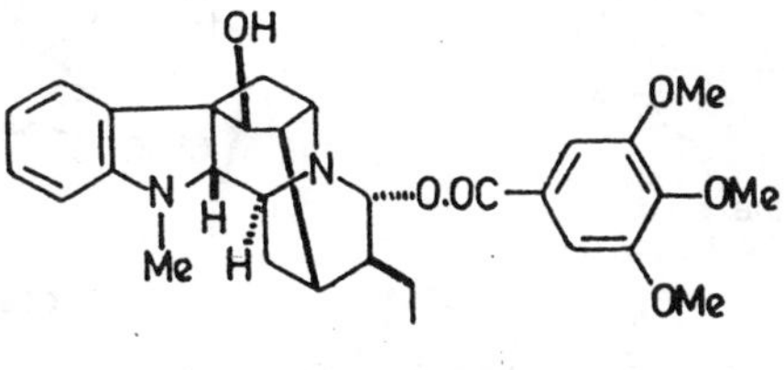

Ajmalimine

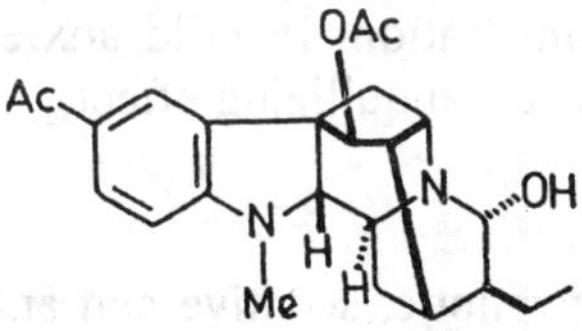

Ajmalinimine

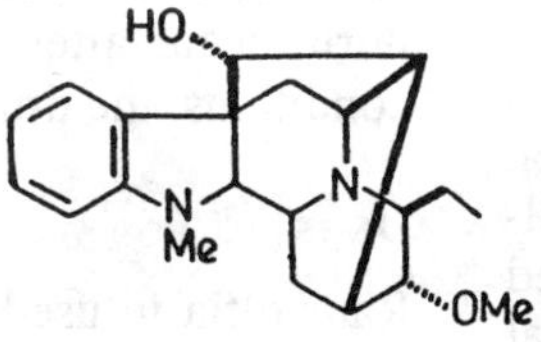

Sandwicolidine

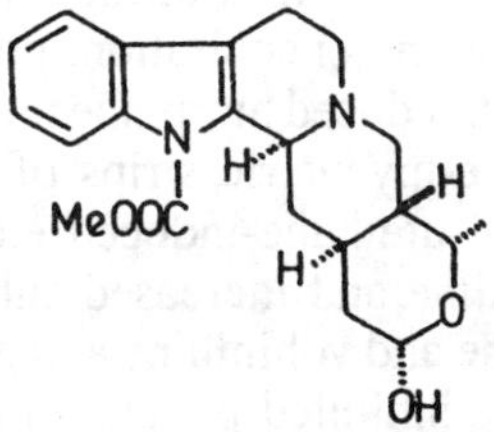

Ajmalicidine

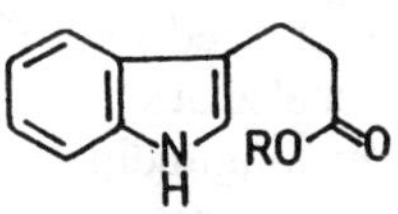

Indobine
R = Benzyl
Indobinine
R = Cyclohexyl

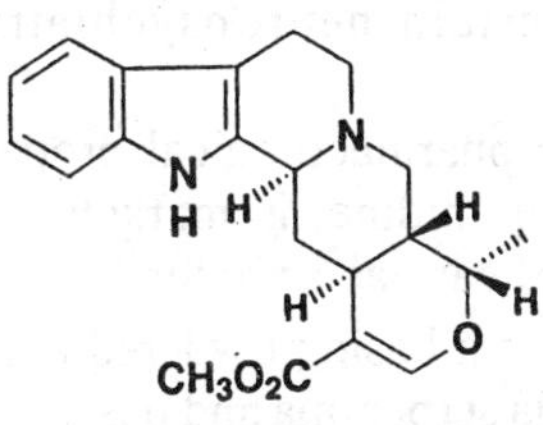

Ajmalicine (raubasine)

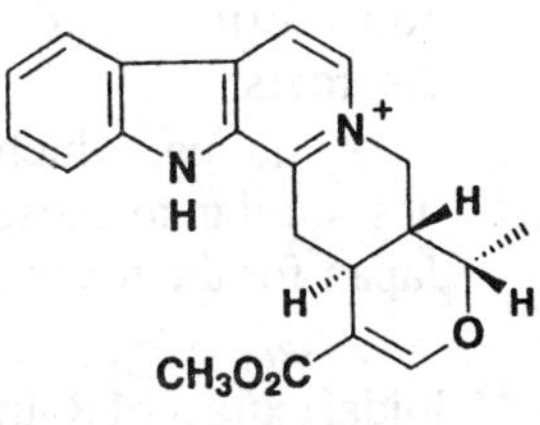

Serpentine

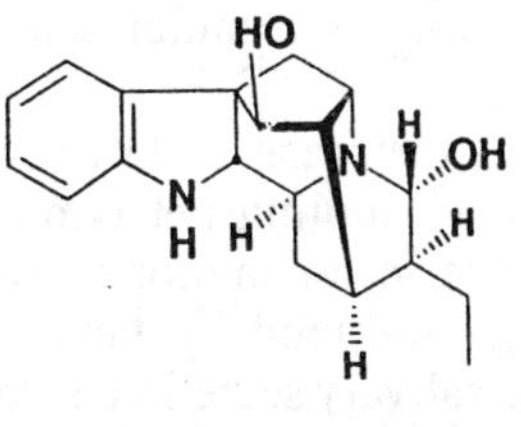

Ajmaline

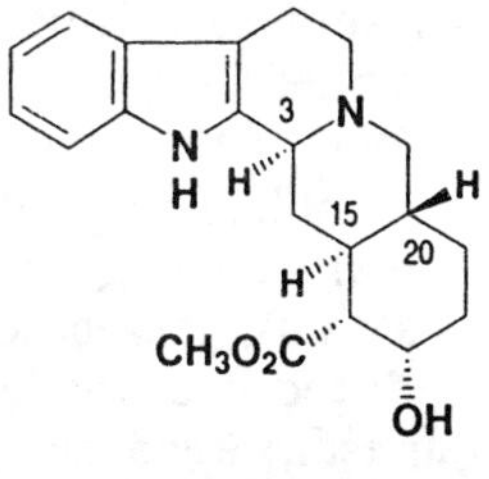

Yohimbine

Fig. 21.68. Indole alkaloids of *Rauwolfia serpentina*.

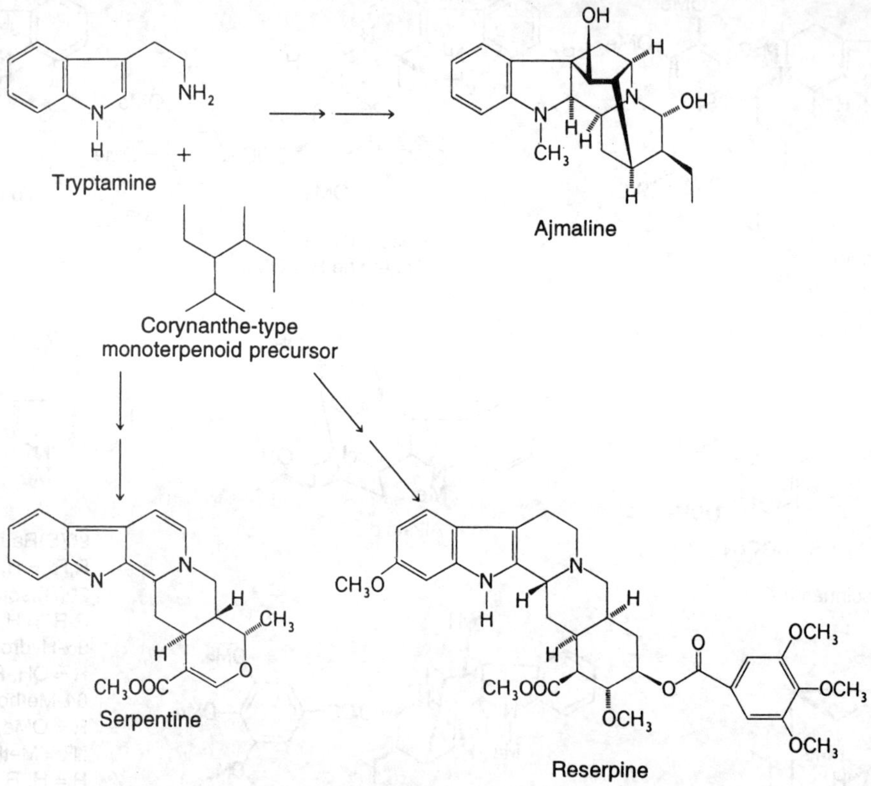

Fig. 21.69. Biosynthesis of *Rauwolfia* alkaloids.

seizure threshold in mice, anticonvulsant activity against maximal electroconvulsions in mice, increased serum prolactin concentration, produced local anaesthetic effect, reduced morphine tole-rance in longitudinal muscle-myenteric strips of guinea pig ileum, potentiated urethane-induced elevation in plasma nor-adrenaline and increased submaxillary secretion. Caffeine and yohimbine antagonized each other. Raubasine inhibited platelet biological activity in patients and reduced plasma fibrinogen. Reserpine reduced cAMP levels, potentiated degree of seizures elicited by coriaria lactone and inhibited L-type Ca^{2+} chan-nels to inhibit smooth muscle contraction.

Yohimbine produced decrease in latency to initial mounting, facilitate coupling behaviour in male rats, caused decrease in locomotor activity, reduced neuropathology induced by ketamine anaesthesia and increased salivary secretion in dogs.

The whole root exhibits a medicinal action that is different from that of reserpine. A definite lowering of blood pressure in hypertensive states, a slowing of the pulse, and a general sense of euphoria occur after administration. In mild anxiety conditions, the drug has a tranquilizing effect.

Uses

Rauwolfia in used as hypnotic, sedative and anti-hypertensive. It is specific for insanity, reduces blood pressure and cures pain due to affections of the bowels. It is given in labours to increase uterine contractions and in certain neuropsychiatric disorders.

Ajmaline, which has pharmacological proper-ties similar to those of quinidine, is marketed in Japan for the treatment of cardiac arrhythmias.

Alseroxylon fraction is a basic powdered alka-loidal extract of Rauwolfia serpentina and possesses a lack of toxicity over long-range administration.

Reserpine is a white or pale buff to slightly yellow, odourless, crystalline powder that darkens slowly when exposed to light and rapidly when in solution. Reserpine is an antihypertensive and tranquilizer.

Rescinnamine is the methyl reserpate ester of 3,4,5-trimethoxy cinnamic acid. The usual antihypertensive dose of rescinnamine is 500 μg, 2 times a day. Higher doses may cause serious mental depression.

Deserpidine (canescine, recanescine) is 11-desmethoxyreserpine. It is a wide-range tranquilizer and antihypertensive and is free from the side effects.

In more severe hypertension, Rauwolfia acts synergistically with more potent hypotensive agents.

About 3500 kg of ajmalicine is isolated annually from either *Rauwolfia* or *Catharanthus* spp. by pharmaceutical industries for the treatment of circular diseases.

Cell and root cultures

R. serpentina cell suspension cultures are an important tool in the elucidation of monoterpenoid indole alkaloid biogenesis.

By the use of cell cultures a 10-step biosynthetic pathway from strictosidine to ajmaline is established. The principal alkaloid of cell suspension cultures of *R. serpentina is* raucaffricine occurring in the nutrient medium, representing 2.3% of the dried cells. Ajmalicine, an anti-arrhythmic drug, is also produced to the extent of 0.6% together with over 30 different monoterpenoid alkaloids in trace amounts including five glucoalkaloids.

Hairy root cultures of *R. serpentina*, produced by *Agrobacterium rhizogenes* transformation, synthesized ajmaline and serpentine. *R. verticillata* hairy roots produce reserpine and ajmaline.

Allied species

There are about 86 Rauwolfia species. *R. tetraphylla (R. canescens* Linn., *R. hirsuta)* is widely distributed in tropical areas of south America, Caribbean, India and Australia. Its roots had been substituted for *R. serpentina.* It is recognized by its non-stratified cork, and sclereid groups in the phloem. The alkaloids reserpine and deserpidine are isolated on commercial scale from *R. tetraphylla.*

R. tetraphylla also contains rauwolscine, α-yohimbine, α-, β- and γ-deserpidines, raujemidine, ajmalicine, ajmaline, reserpine, sarpagine, aricine, isoreserpiline, tetrahydroalstonine and yohimbine isomer.

R. nitida is found in West India. From its root-bark 33 indole alkaloids have been isolated.

Adulterants

The roots are commonly adulterated with other parts of the plants such as the stems. Roots of other *Rauwolfia* species such as *R. beddomei, R. densiflora, R. micrantha, R. perakensis* and *R. tetraphylla* and those of *Ophiorrhiza mungos*, and white and red-flowered *Clerodendrus* species have been used as adulterants. Stems of the plant contain less quantity of alkaloids. The roots can be easily distinguished from the stems since they have a more wrinkled surface, are less flexible, thicker, more tortuous and less branched.

R. densiflora contains sarpagine (raupine), reserpine and densiflorine. Densiflorine lowered blood pressure, decreased amplitude of frog heart contraction, contracted rat ileum and increased respiration.

Ophiorrhiza mungos contains camptothecin, and 9-methoxycamptothecin.

Clerodendrum species contains steroids, their glycosides, pentacyclic triterpenoids, flavonoids hispidulin and scutellarein and their glycosides, diterpenes clerodin, uncinatone, caryoptin, 3-epicaryoptin, neolignans, cistanoside, clerodendrins, interminosides, clerodermic acid and cleroinermin.

Rauwolfia vomitoria Afz. is a bush or tree found in tropical Africa from the west coast to Mozambique. It is the most important African rauwolfia for the commercial preparation of reserpine. The tree attain a height of 10 m, the roots are larger than those of *R. serpentina.* They are cut transversely and dried. Roots are up to 5 cm or more in diameter, cylindrical or flattened pieces, up to 30 cm long. The roots taper slightly and are branched. The outer surface is greyish-brown, longitudinally furrowed or rubbed smooth. Pieces do not break easily. The fracture is short in the bark and splintery in the wood. The smoothed transverse surface shows a narrow brown bark and a buff or yellowish, finely radiate wood. Odourless; taste, bitter.

The TS of drug contains the groups of sclereids in the bark arranged in up to five discontinuous bands and by the large vessels of the wood which are up to 180 μm in diameter.

African rauwolfia contains reserpine, rescinamine, reserpoxidine, seredine, ajmaline, alstonine and yohimbine. About 42 indole alkaloids from the stem-bark are isolated. The major alkaloids were heteroyohimbines (especially reserpiline) and N^a-demethyldihydroindoles.

Other African rauwolfias containing reserpine are *R. caffra* (*R. natalensis*), *R. mombasiana, R. oreogiton, R. obscura, R. cumminsii, R. volkensii* and *R. roesa*. The roots of *R. caffra* closely resemble those of *R. vomitoria* but the cork has not the same tendency to flake off. In sections of *R. vomitoria,* there are alternating lignified and unlignified cork cells, while in *R. caffra* all the cork cells are lignified. *R. mombasiana* differs from *R. vomitoria* in the structure of the wood of the root; *R. rosea, R. volkensii* and *R. obscura* lack sclereid development.

CATHARANTHUS (VINCA)

Synonyms

Madagascar perivinkle; Shadaphul (Mar); Rattanjot (Punj.), Sadabahar.

Biological source

Catharanthus is the dried whole plant of *Catharanthus roseus* G. Don (syn. *Vinca rosea* Linn.). (Family : Apocynaceae).

Geographical source

The plant is indigenous to Madagascar but now found in tropical regions and cultivated as an ornamental plant in southern Florida, Africa, India, Thailand, Taiwan, eastern Europe and Australia.

Plant habitat

Catharanthus is an erect, everblooming pubescent herb or subshrub, 40-80 cm high, woody at the base. The leaves are oblong, with petiolate acute base, rounded apex, entire margin and oppositely arranged. The flowers are axillary, violet, rose or white with red eyes, 4-5 cm in diameter. The fruit is

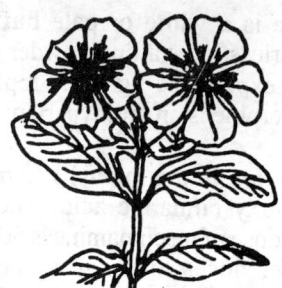

Fig. 21.70. *Catharanthus roseus* flowering part.

a divergent follicle. It has slight odour and bitter taste.

Chemical constituents

About 90 alkaloids have been reported from *C. roseus*. Vindoline and catharanthine are indole monomeric alkaloids. The alkaloids such as ajmalicine, lochnerine, reserpine, serpentine and tetrahydroalstonine are also present in other genera of Apocynaceae. About 20 dimeric alkaloids, including vindesine, vincristine and vinblastine, have been isolated from Catharanthus. These alkaloids possess antineoplastic activity. In addition to alkaloids, monoterpenes, sesquiterpene, indole and indoline glycoside have been isolated.

The other compounds isolated from catharanthus are yohimbine, vincaleukoblastine, leurosine (vinleurosine), vinolinine, vindoline, catharanthine, vindoline HCl, lochnericine, perivine, virosine, leurocristine (vinncristine), isoleurosine, lochneridine, sitsirikine, vincamicine, catharine, vindolicine, leurosidine (vinrosidine), leurosivine, rovidine, leurocristine (vincristine), alstonine, vindolinine, vincamajine, akuammidine, polyneuridine, voachalotine, macusine A, iochnerinine, carosidine, carosine, pleurosine, neoleurosidine, vincarodine, catharicine, vindolidine, neoleurocristine, vincarosine, vinosidine, lochnerivine, leurosivine, cavincine, mitraphylline, akuammicine, ammocallin, ammorosine, perosine sulphate, cavincidine sulphate, maandrosine sulphate, cathindine sulphate, pericalline, vincamicine, catharine, catharicine, perividine, catharosine, rovidine, dihydrovindolinine, coronaridine, dihydrositsirikine, isositsirikine, cleavamine, cumicine, vindorosine, deoxyvinblastin (isoleurosine), vin-

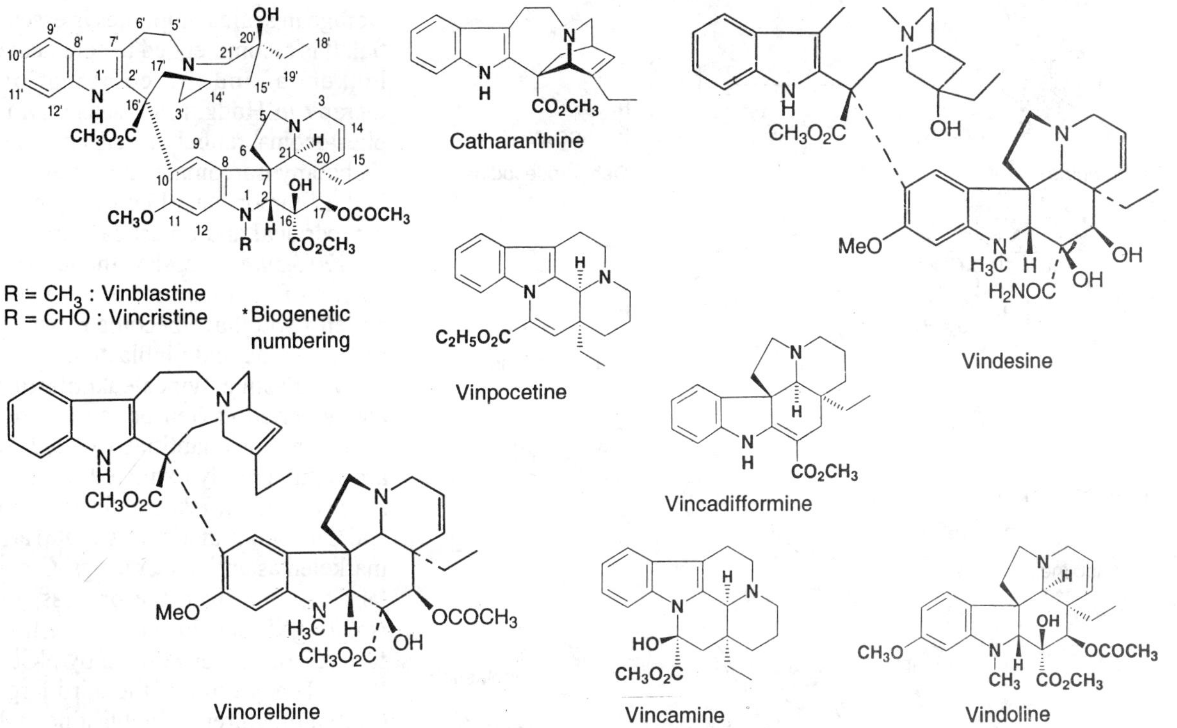

R = CH₃ : Vinblastine
R = CHO : Vincristine

*Biogenetic numbering

Fig. 21.71. Alkaloids of Catharanthus.

carodine, desacetoxy vinblastine, leurocolombine, vinamidine, pseudovinca leukoblastinediol, vincathicine, vincabine, alkaloid B, vincomajine, aquamycin, venalstonine, catharanthamine, vincapusine, pericyclivine, N-de-methylvinblastine, 17-desacetoxyleurosine, 17-desacetoxyvinblastine, rozevin, 16-epi-19S-vindolinine N-oxide, fluorocarpamine N-oxide, vindolinine N-oxide, fluorocarpamine, pleiocarpamine, roseadine, 16-epi-Z-isositsirikine, rhazimol, gomaline, 11-methoxytabersonine, mitraphylline, 16,19,20-isositsirikines, 14,15-dehydroepivineadine, 19-hydroxytabesonine, N-deformyl vincristine, rosamine, bannucine, leurosinone, 3',4'-anhydro-vinblastine, anthocyanidins petudin, malvidin, hirsutidin; deoxyloganin, loganin, sweroside, dehydrologenin, kaempferol, quercetin, ursolic acid, roseoside, oleonolic acid, its acetate and α-amyrin acetate.

Catharanthus alkaloids are generally indole and dihydroindole derivatives, some of which occur in other members of the Apocynaceae. The alkaloids with antineoplastic activity are dimeric indole-dihydroindole derivatives.

Uses

Catharanthus is used to cure diabetes and in wasp-sting. Vinblastine sulphate is an antitumor alkaloid employed to cure Hodgkin's disease and chlorio-nepithelioma. Vincristine sulphate is a cytotoxic compound and used to treat leukaemia in children. Catharanthus alkaloids are antineoplastic in nature.

The most characteristic effect of these drugs is the arrest of cell division at metaphase, in a manner resembling the effect of colchicine. Both vinblastine and vincristine bind tightly to tubulin and interfere with the functioning of the micro-tubule system, which is a component of the mitotic spindle. The alkaloids actually inhibit the polymerization of tubulin into microtubules.

Vinblastine sulfate is unstable and is available in sealed ampoules, which should be stored in a refrigerator to ensure extended stability. The alkaloid is used to treat neoplasms, Hodgkin's

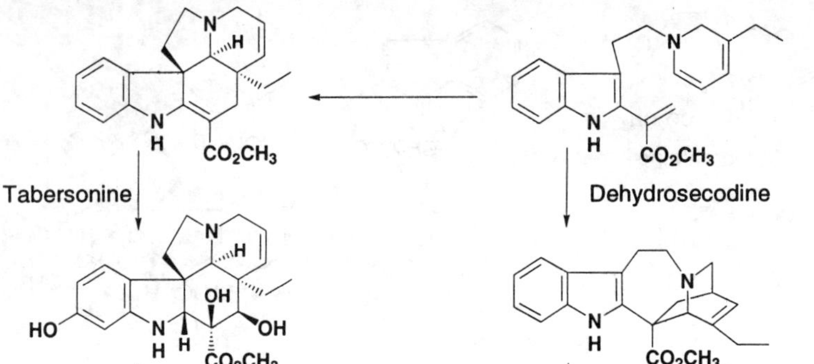

Fig. 21.72. Biosynthesis of the binary alkaloids of Catharanthus.

storage in sealed ampoules is essential. It is recommended to cure acute leukemia and in combination therapy in Hodgkin's disease, lymphosarcoma, reticulum cell sarcoma, rhabdomyosarcoma, neuroblastoma, Wilms' tumor, small cell lung cancer, cervical and breast cancers.

Vindesine, a semisynthetic derivative of vinblastine, is given to patients who have become resistant to vincristine and vinblastine.

Vinblastine (vincaleukoblastin) and vincristine (leurocristin), present in minor quantities (0.0002%) are commercially extracted from *C. roseus*. Velban (vinblastin sulfate) and Oncovin (vincristine sulfate) are marketed as anticancer drugs. Cipla labs has improved the process for isolating vinblastine and vincristine from *C. roseus* developed by NCL, Pune. Today India is the third largest manufacturer of vinblastine and vincristine in the world and is exporting these alkaloids to European countries.

These compounds are antimitotics inhibiting cell growth, at least in part, by disrupting microtubules, causing the dissolution of cell mitotic spindles and the arrest of cells at metaphase. High demand and low yield of these alkaloids in the plant, has led to starch for alternative means for their production. Nowadays, vinblastine is converted into vincristine either chemically or via microbiological N-demethylation using *Streptomyces albogriseolus*. Vinblastine is also modified structurally to yield deacetyl vinblastine amide (vindesine), introduced recently as Eldisine for use in the treatment of acute lymphoid leukaemia in children. A spirolactone (4-dioxolanone), derived from 17-deacetyl-vinblastine, exhibits antitumour activity. Biochemical coupling of alkaloids catharanthine and vindoline to get dimeric compounds is also achieved. Alpha-3',4'-anhydro-vinblastine, a precursor of vinblastine and vincristine can be enzymatically synthesized *in vitro*. A struc-

disease, lymphocytic lymphoma, histiocytic lymphoma, mycosis fungoides, advanced testicular carcinoma, Kaposi's sarcoma, and choriocarcinoma and breast cancer unresponsive to other therapies. Vinblastine is effective as a single agent but is usually administered with other antineoplastic agents in combination therapy for an enhanced therapeutic effect without additive toxicity. It is administered intravenously in doses regulated by the patient's age, body surface and white-blood-cell count.

Vincristine sulfate is identical to that of vinblastine, differing only in the substitution of an *N*-formyl group for the *N*-methyl group of vinblastine. There are differences in the antitumor spectra of the 2 compounds, and no cross-resistance has been observed. Vincristine sulfate is unstable and refrigerated tural variant 2,5'-noranhydro-vinblastine is developed as an anticancer drug and has been introduced in France. Besides these, tissue culture technique is developed for the production of these dimeric alkaloids.

Pharmacology

Vincaleukoblastine and leurocristine were effective against variety of human neoplasms. Catharanthine, leurosine, lochnerine, vindoline and tetrahydro-alstonine had hypoglycaemic activity. In brain tumors, vincristine sulphate was effective in combination with radiologic treatment. Total alkaloid and chloroform-soluble fractions exhibited hypotensive action in dogs. A plant extract was effective in stopping tumor cells in metaphase of mice. Viblastine inhibited cells in metaphase of mice and the transport of amine granules in monoamine-containing neurons, stimulated isolated frog heart and rabbit intestine, caused reduction in positive inotropic effect of noradrenergic nerve stimulation, increased platelet count in rats, produced leukopenia and agranulocytosis in rats, did not affect secretion of enzymes from rat pancreas and decreased rate of glucose uptake from medium. Vinblastine and leurosine are patented in Germany as useful cyto-static agents. Vinblastine inhibited growth of sarcoma-45 in rats and increased cell membrane fluidity of SA-1 tumor cells.

Vincristine did not decrease acetylcholine or norepinephrine in heart and salivary glands. It affected all types of spermatogenic cells except mature spermatozoa and significantly decreased fertility. Akuammidine increased blood sugar level in rats at 100 mg/kg, s.c., but decreased blood sugar at dose of 40 mg/kg; it affected motor defence reflexes and skeletal muscle tone. Yohimbine blocked hypotensive and respiratory action of clonidine in rats. It increased brain noradrena-line turnover at high dose and produced significant atony in rumen and reticulum of sheep.

Catharanthamine showed antitumor activity. Vincamine produced no useful changes in cerebral blood flow in healthy men but side effects like bradycardia; faintless and tinnitus were observed. Vinblastine sulphate inhibited intestinal sucrase and lactase of rats. Vinblastine caused reduction in output of total protein in bile. Vincristine caused reduction in sciatic nerve fibre size. It interferes with functional integrity of transport system which maintains synaptic activity. Vincristine increased urinary Mg^{2+} excretion in healthy rats. Raubasine increased regional blood flow in heart, renal cortex and medulla, spleen, liver, skeletal muscle and skin in cat. Oral administration of aqueous extract of leaves markedly lowered blood glucose level in rats. Leaf extract showed anti-inflammatory activity. Vincristine inhibited response of diaphragm to stimulation of phrenic nerve. Vincristine altered cell nucleus morphology.

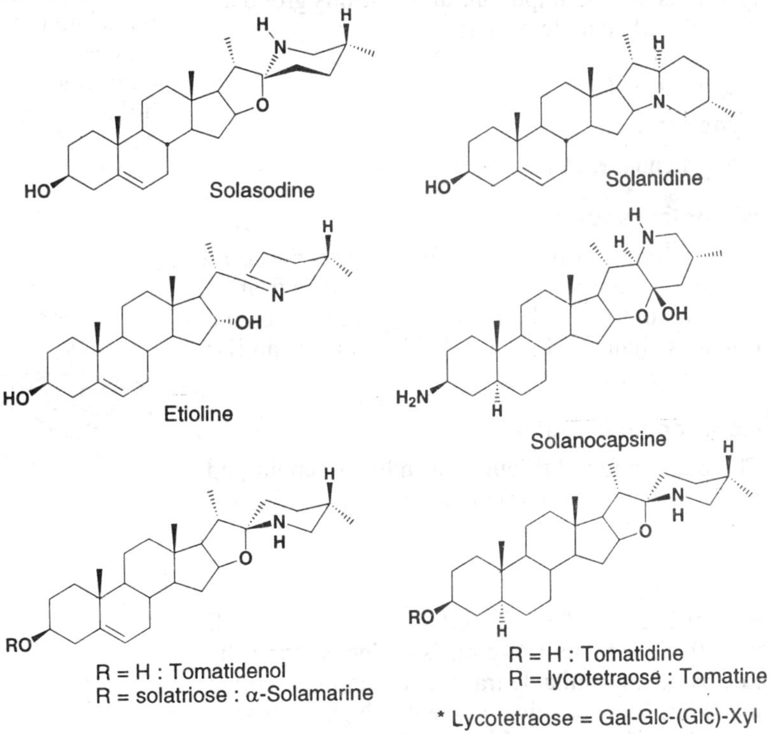

R = H : Tomatidenol
R = solatriose : α-Solamarine

R = H : Tomatidine
R = lycotetraose : Tomatine

* Lycotetraose = Gal-Glc-(Glc)-Xyl

Fig. 21.73. Steroidal alkaloids.

Leurosine and vincaleukoblastine showed anti-tumor activity against P-1534 acute lymphocytic leukaemia in mice; inhibited growth of human choriocarcinoma transplanted into hamster cheek pouch. Leurosidine and leurocristine were very active against p-1524 leukaemia in DBA/Z mice. Vindoline, dihydrovindolinine and coronaridine produced diuretic and hypoglycaemic effects.

STEROIDAL ALKALOIDS

The steroidal alkaloids possess a cyclopenteno-phenanthrene nucleus. Alkaloids with C_{27} group are known as *Solanum* alkaloids, *e.g.*, solanidine, and tomatidine. The alkaloids found in the Apocynaceae *(Holarrhena* and *Funtumia* species) and in the Buxaceae, possess 21 carbon atoms. They are produced from pregnenolone by amination at either C-3 or C-20. Conessine is a common alkamine of the group which may be used for the synthesis of some hormones (*e.g.*, aldosterone). Holaphylline is less toxic. The quaternary diamine malouetine, which is found in the same family, is a potent curare-type poison. The important drugs of this group are Kurchi bark and Veratrums.

KURCHI BARK

Synonyms

Holarrhenna; Kurchi (Hindi).

Biological source

Kurchi bark consists of dried stem bark of *Holarrhena antidysenterica* Wall. obtained from 8-12 years old tree. The bark is required to contain not less than 20% of total alkaloids. (Family: Apocynaceae).

Geographical source

The plant is found throughout India, ascending up to 1250 m in the Himalayas, especially in wet forests.

Collection

Kurchi is a deciduous laticiferous shrub or small tree, 9-10 m high. The bark is collected from the tree by making suitable transverse and longitudinal incisions. The alkaloidal content is high soon after the rains when new shoots are produced which declines during winter months.

Morphology

The pieces of Kurchi bark are small and recurved both longitudinally and transversely. The size and thickness vary from piece to piece. Outer surface is buff to reddish brown and bears numerous prominent circular or transversely elongated horizontal lenticels and longitudinal wrinkles. The thicker pieces are rugose and show numerous yellowish warts; inner surface cinnamon-brown, longitudinally striated, frequently with portions of pale yellow wood attached; fracture is brittle and splintery. The taste is acrid and bitter while the odour is not distinct.

Chemical constituents

The total alkaloidal constituents of Kurchi bark vary from 1.1 to 4.72 per cent. The main steroidal alkaloid is conessine (20-30%). The other alkaloids isolated include conarrhimine, conimine, conamine, conessimine, isoconessimine, dimethyl conkurchine, 3α- aminocon-5-ene, conkuressine, dihydroiso-conessimine, dihydroconessine, 7β- and 7α-hydroxyconessines, kurcholessine, holacine, holacimine, regholarrhenines A, B, C, D, E and F, kurchessine, holarrhimine, holarricine, kurchimine, conimine, conessidine, holarrhenine, holafrine, holarrhetine, kurchiphyllamine, kurchiphylline, holantosines A and B, N-acetylholantosines A, C and D, N-acetyl-L-holantosamine, holarosine B,

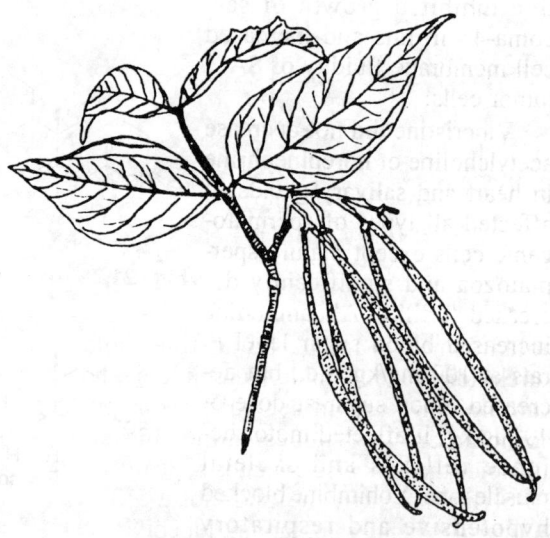

Fig. 21.74. Kurchi shoot.

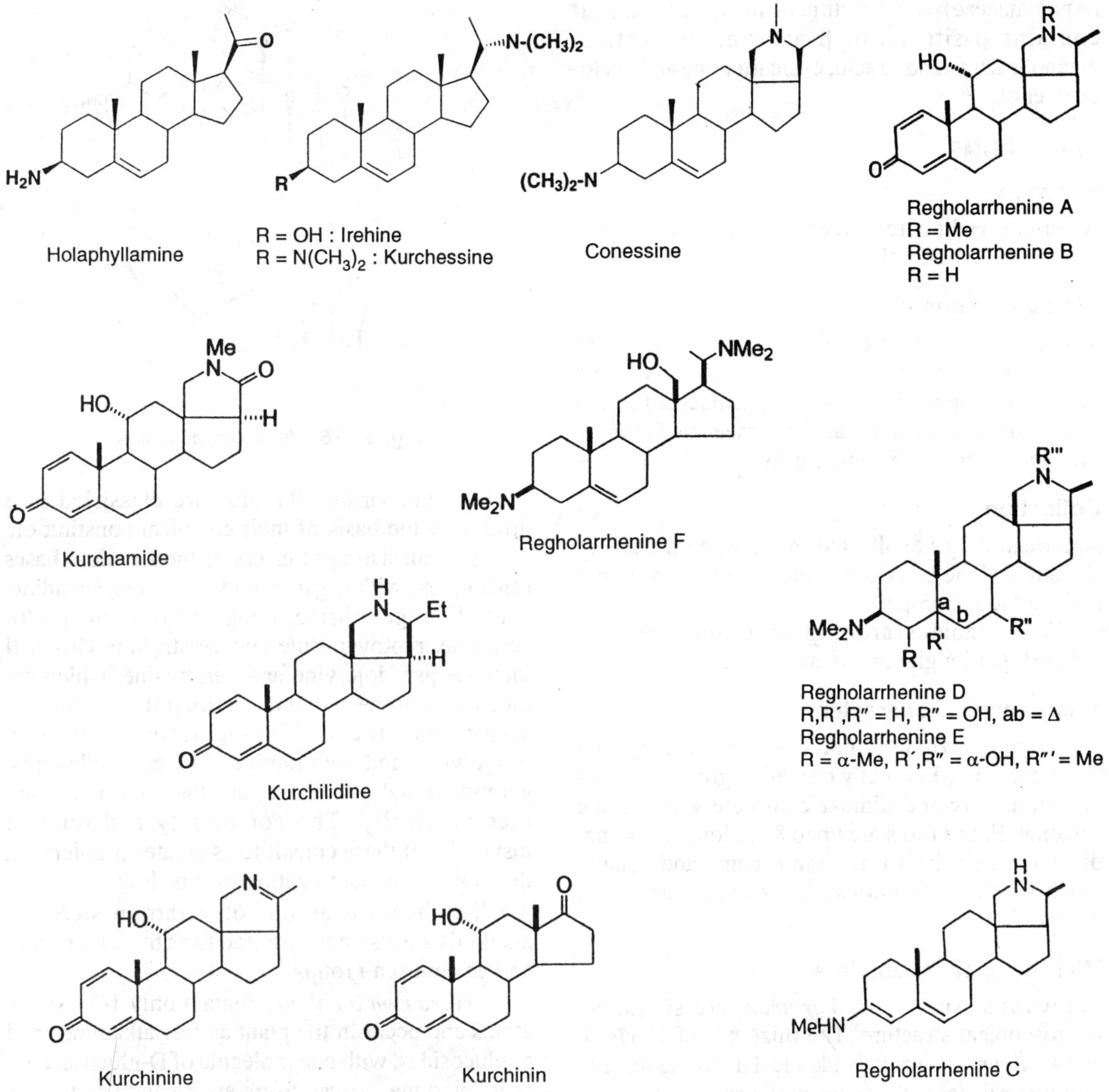

Fig. 21.75. Steroidal alkaloids of Kurchi.

holantosines E and F, holacetine, holacimine, kurchilidine, kurchamide, kurchinidine, holadiene, kurchinicin, kurchinine, holadyson, pubescine, norholadiene and pubescimine. In addition to alkaloids the bark also contains 5, 20 (29)- lupadien 3β-ol (lupenic triterpene) and sitosta-5, 23-dien-3β-ol (sterol), gum, resin, tannin, lupeol and digitenol glycoside holadysone.

Uses

The bark is considered to be stomachic, astringent, tonic, antidysenteric, febrifuge and anthelmintic. The dried bark is rubbed over the body in dropsy. Kurchi bark is used to cure amoebic dysentery and diarrhoea.

The stem bark of *Wrightia tinctoria* R.Br.

(Apocynaceae) is a substituent for kurchi bark. It contains β-sitosterol, β-amyrin, its acetate, oleanolic acid, ursolic acid, cycloartenone and cyclo-eucalenol.

VERATRUMS

Synonyms

American Hellebore; Green Hellebore; American Veratrum; Indian poke.

Biological source

Veratrum consists of dried roots and rhizomes of the perennial herbs, *Veratrum viride* Aiton and *Veratrum album* Linn. (Family : Liliaceae) found in Canada, USA, Carolina, Tennessee and Georgia. The herb is erect, rhizome fleshy.

Collection

American drug is collected in the eastern parts of Canada and the USA and white hellebore in central and southern Europe.

The rhizomes are dug in autumn season, cleaned, cut longitudinally and dried.

Macroscopical characters

The entire rhizome is conical, 3-8 cm long and 2-3.5 cm wide; externally brownish-grey. The roots are numerous and almost completely cover the rhizome. Entire roots are up to 8 cm long and 4 mm diameter, light brown to light orange, and usually much wrinkled. Odourless, but sternutatory; taste, bitter and acrid.

Microscopical characters

The various species of *Veratrum* are similar in microscopical structure. The rhizomes of *V. viride* and *V. album* are virtually identical micro-scopically but minor differences occur in the roots.

Chemical constituents

Various steroidal alkaloids have been isolated from Veratrums. The important alkaloids are jervine, pseudojervine, rubijervine, cevadine, germitrine, germidine, veratralbine, veratroidine, neogermitrine, neoprotoveratrine, protoveratrine and veratridine. Pseudojervine and veratrosine are glycosides of alkamine. Germine, jervine, rubijervine and veratramine are alkamines.

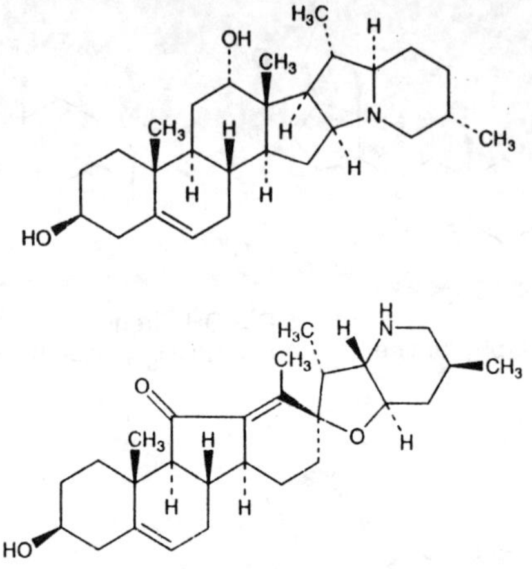

Fig. 21.76. Veratrum alkaloids.

Veratum viride alkaloids are classified in 3 groups on the basis of their chemical constitution. Group I, consisting of esters of the steroidal bases (alkamines) with organic acids, includes cevadine, germidine, germitrine, neogermitrine, neoprotoveratrine, protoveratrine and veratridine. Group II includes pseudojervine and veratrosine, which are glucosides of the alkamines. Group III contains the alkamines themselves—germine, jervine, rubijervine, and veratramine. The ester alkaloids, germidine and germitrine, are the most important therapeutically. The complexity and relative instability of these constituents creates problems in the biologic standardization of this drug.

The chemical groups of veratrum steroidal alkaloids are also now referred to as the jerveratrum and ceveratrum groups.

Jerveratrum alkaloids contain only 1-3 oxygen atoms and occur in the plant as free alkamines and as glucosides, with one molecule of D-glucose, *e.g.*, pseudojervine derived from jervine and veratrosine derived from veratramine.

Ceveratrum alkaloids are highly hyroxylated compounds with 7-9 oxygen atoms. They are present in the plant esterified with two or more various acids (acetic, α-methylbutyric, α-methyl-α-hydroxybutyric, α-methyl-α,β-dihydroxybutyric), but are also found unconjugated. These ester alkaloids are responsible for the hypotensive activity of veratrum; examples are the esters of germine, protoverine and veracevine.

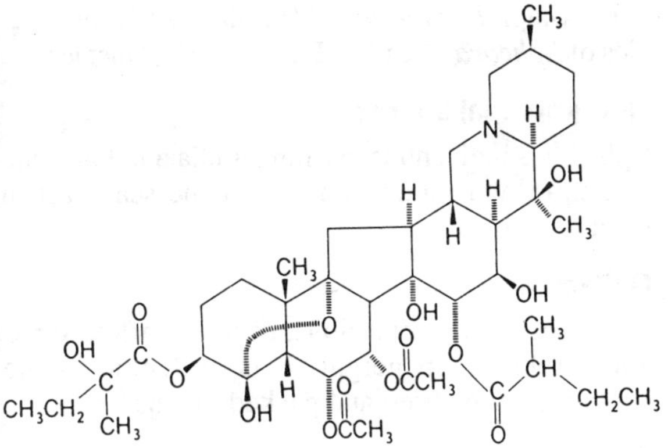

Fig. 21.77. Protoveratrine A.

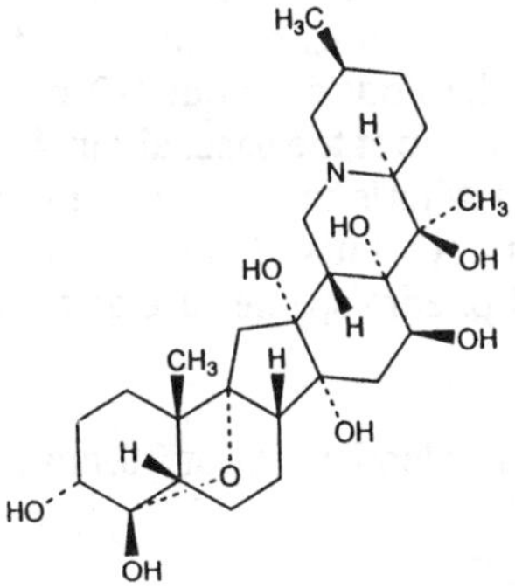

Fig. 21.78. Cevine.

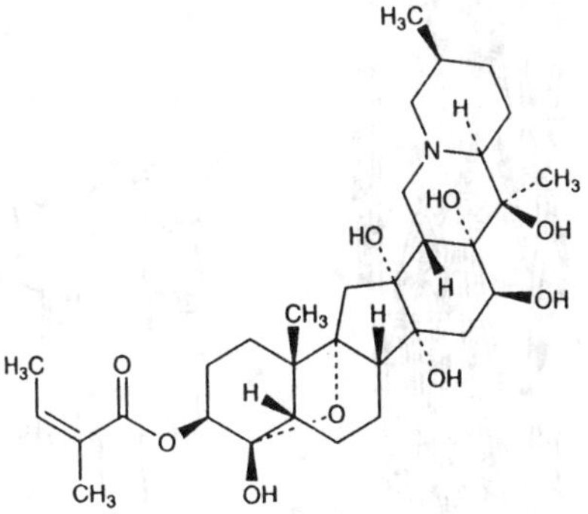

Fig. 21.79. Cevadine.

Uses

Veratrum is used as antihypertensive, cardiac depressant, sedative and insecticides. It is also used for relief in irritation of the nervous system, in convulsions, mania, neuralgia, headache, febrile and inflammatory affections of the respiratory organs and acute tonsillitis. The rhizomes are also used for insecticidal purposes in the form of sprays and in dusts. The alkaloids, especially proveratrines A and B, are effective in reducing blood pressure.

American veratrum is used for the preparation of Veriloid, a mixture of the hypotensive alkaloids. European veratrum is used for the preparation of the protoveratrines. The drugs are used as insecticides.

Allied drugs

Veratrum album, V. eschscholtzii, V. woodii, V. californicum and *V. fimbriatum* are used as allied drugs.

Over 100 steroidal alkaloids have been repor-ted from *V. album*. The drug *V. nigrum* L., var. *ussuriense* is used for the preparation of the Chinese drug 'Li-lu', together with other species. Both drugs have been used as insecticides, but their more recent importance results from those alkaloids that have hypotensive properties. Some other species, *e.g., V. californicum*, can cause serious damage to livestock grazing in locations where the plant occurs as they have teratogenic properties.

HEMLOCK FRUIT

The drug consists of the dried unripe fruits of *Conium maculatum* (Apiaceae), the spotted hemlock. It is a poisonous biennial plant indigenous to Europe.

Hemlock was the plant used by the Greeks for preparing a draught for killing criminals.

The fruit is broadly ovate, laterally compressed cremocarp, about 3 mm long with a small stylopod and the remains of the stigmas. Each mericarp has five prominent, primary ridges with a beaded appearance. The fruits does not show conspicuous vittae, although numerous very small ones are actually present. The endosperm is deeply grooved and is surrounded by well-marked, alkaloid containing layers.

When hemlock is treated with solution of potassium hydroxide, it develops a strong, mouse-like odour due to liberation of the alkaloid coniine. The alkaloid is volatile and may be steam-distilled and present up to 1-2.5% together with *N*-methyl coniine, conhydrine, pseudoconhydrine, conhydrinone and γ-coniceine.

An enzyme, mol. wt. 56200, catalyses a transamination between 5-ketooctanal and L-alanine to give γ-coniceine and pyruvic acid, has been isolated.

South African *Conium* contains a high volatile oil composition, the main component being myrcene. The alkaloids include *N*-methyl pseudoconhydrine.

Coniine is not biosynthesized in the plant directly from an amino acid, but from four molecules of acetic acid with the participation of ammonia or some other nitrogen source.

ALKALOIDAL AMINES

The alkaloids of this class do not possess nitrogen in a ring system. Most of them are simple derivatives of phenylethylamine. The important drugs of this group are Ephedra and Colchicum corm.

Phenylalanine, tyrosine- and dihydroxy-phenylalanine-derived alkaloids

These compounds and their decarboxylate products are the precursors of a large number of alkaloids which include simple protoalkaloids, the benzylisoquinolines, phthal ideisoquinolines, aporphines and proaporphines, protoberberines, protopines, naphthaphenanthridines, the *Erythrina*, Amaryllidaceae and ipecacuanha alkaloids and the morphine and rhoeadine-type alkaloids. A group of compounds is comprising of the phen-ethylisoquinoline alkaloids; it is from these that colchicine arises.

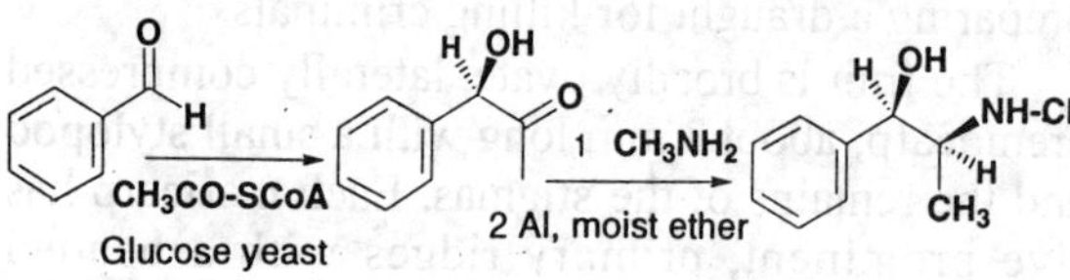

Fig. 21.80. Formation of ephedrine.

EPHEDRA

Synonyms

Ma-haung; Tsaopen Ma-huang.

Biological source

Ephedra consists of whole aerial parts of *Ephedra*

sinica Stapf, *E. equisetina* Ma Huang and other species of *Ephedra*. (Family : Ephedraceae, Gnetaceae).

Geographical source

Ephedra is indigenous to China, India and Pakistan. It is most abundantly found near the sea coast in southern China.

Collection

The plant is a low dioecious, usually leafless shrub and 60-90 cm in height. It is collected in the autumn season, dried and packed in bags.

Characters

The stems of Ephedra are slender pieces, containing numerous ridges, nodes and internodes and fine longitudinal ridges on the outer surface. The distance of internodes are nearly 3-6 cm and the diameter of the node is about 1-2 mm. The leaves are small, connate at the base, about 4 mm in length, decussate, in whorls of two, with a subulate recovered apex and a whitish lamina. The characteristic features of Ephedra species are as follows:

Ephedra sinica

The stems are slender, about 30 cm long, 4-7 mm

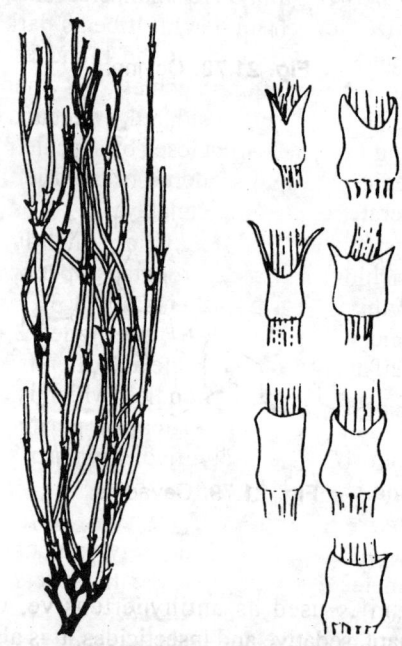

Fig. 21.81. *Ephedra sinica.*

thick, with 3-6 cm long internodes, erect, small ribbed and channeled. Branches are green, rough with longitudinal ridges. Diameter of lowest green node is 1-2 mm. Leaves are opposite, whitish, 4 mm long with subulate and recurved apex. Lamina is whitish and the base is reddish brown. Small blossoms appear in summer.

In the transverse section the young stem shows 6-10 bundles, small groups of fibres below the ridges, a few groups of fibres in the cortex and a few isolated fibres or small groups of two or three fibres in the unlignified pith.

Ephedra equisetina

The stems are more woody and branched, 25-200 cm long, yellowish green in colour, internodes are shorter, 1-2.5 cm long. The leaf apex is shorter and it is not recurved. Leaves are brownish-purple colour. Ephedra is odourless and taste is bitter.

Transverse sections show that the number of bundles in the stem is not constant (about 10). The annual rings are more pronounced than in *E. sinica*; the outer xylem has a distinct lobed outline. Cortical and pericyclic fibres are found. The pith is lignified.

Ephedra gerardiana is a small, erect shrub, variable in size, few cm in height. It bears dark green, cylindrical striated, often curved branches arising in whorls; internodes of branchlets, 1-4 cm long and 1-2 cm diameter. Fruit ovoid, red, sweet and edible, containing 1 or 2 seeds, enclosed by succulent bracts. This species is found scattered in the drier regions of temperate and alpine Himalayas.

The stems of *E. distachya* are slightly woody and branching takes place from the upper and lower parts of the main stem. Stems about 37 cm long, rough and greenish-yellow. Internodes 2.5-6 cm long. Leaf apex short but acute and often fissured at the base. The number of bundles, which is eight, is contant. There are no cortical or perimedullary fibres, but the pith is lignified. *Ephedra* has little odour and is slightly bitter taste.

Ephedra nebrodensis (syn. *E. major*) is an upright, rarely ascending, densely branched shrub, up to 2 meters high. The twigs of this species closely resemble those of *E. gerardiana*.

The plants are propagated by seeds or divisions of the rootstock. The alkaloid content increases with the age of the plant, and the best time to collect the green twigs is when the plants are 4 years old and are in blossom. Rainfall has a marked adverse effect. The alkaloidal content of the green twigs is greater than that of the woody stem. The twigs should be dried in sun. Artificial drying should be avoided. The dried drug must be stored dry. Air-dried drug stored in dry, closed containers, protected from light, retains the activity without loss for a long period. Among the Indian species, *E. major* is the richest source of ephedrine.

Chemical constituents

Ephedras contain about 0.5-2.0% total alkaloid. The chief alkaloid is ephedrine (30-90%). The other alkaloids isolated are pseudoephedrine, 1-methyl ephedrine, norephedrine and dimethylephedrine.

The minor alkaloids isolated from *Ephedra* are N-methylephedrine, N-methylpseudoephedrine, norpseudoephedrine, ephedroxane, O-benzoyl-pseudoephedrine, 2,3,5,6-tetramethylpyrazine; terpenes like α- and β-terpineol, terpine-4-ol, myrcene, dihydrocarveol, p-menth-2-en-7-ol and 1,3,4-trimethyl-3-cyclohexene-1-carboxyaldehyde.

The roots contain a number of macrocyclic alkaloids (ephedradines A, B, C and D), feruloyl-histamine which have hypotensive properties, flavonoflavanol ephedranin A and bisflavanols like mahuannins A-D.

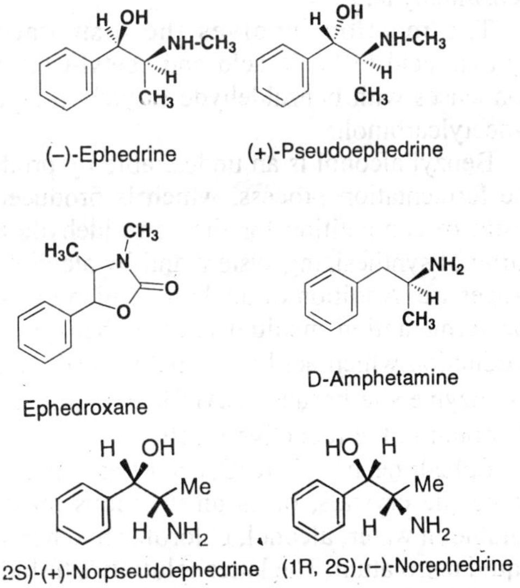

Fig. 21.82. Alkaloids of Ephedra.

Chemical Tests

To the drug (10 mg) in water (1 ml) dil. HCl (0.2 ml), copper sulphate solution (0.1 ml) and sodium hydroxide solution (2 ml) are added; the liquid turns violet. On adding solvent ether (2 ml) and shaking vigorously, the ethereal layer turns purple and the aqueous layer becomes blue.

Uses

Liquid extract of Ephedra is used for controlling asthmatic paroxysms. Tincture of Ephedra is useful as cardiac and circulatory stimulant. Decoction of stems and roots is a remedy for rheumatism and syphilis in Russia. Ephedrine is sympathomimetic, used to counteract hypotension associated with anaesthesia, as a mydriatic; in allergic reactions, as a CNS stimulant and for the relief of asthma, rhinitis, whooping cough and hay fever. Ephedrine is also a bronchodilator.

Ephedrine or (–)-erythro-α-[1-(methyl-amino) ethyl]benzyl alcohol

It is obtained either by the extraction of plant material (*Ephedra* spp.) or by a chemical procedure. A reductive condensation between L-1-phenyl-1-acetylcarbinol and methylamine yields L-ephedrine free from the D-isomer. The carbinol precursor used in the reaction is produced biosynthetically by the fermentative action of Brewer's yeast on benzaldehyde.

The reaction involves the dismutation of pyruvic acid to lactic acid and acetyl-CoA which condenses with benzaldehyde to yield L-1-phenyl-1-acetylcarbinol.

Benzyl alcohol is an undesirable by-product of the fermentation process, which is produced as a result of competition for the benzaldehyde by the carbinol synthesizing system and by alcohol dehydrogenase. Addition of analogs of nicotinamide to the fermentation medium reduces benzyl alcohol production which act by competing with NAD for its enzyme site because $NADH_2$ is required as the H^+ donor in the reductive reaction.

Ephedrine, mp 33-40°C, occurs as white, rosette or needle crystals, or as an unctuous mass. It is soluble in water, alcohol, chloroform, ether, and in liquid petrolatum. The latter solution is turbid if the ephedrine is not dry.

Ephedrine is used to treat asthma and hay fever. Its action is more prolonged than that of adrenaline and it need not be given by injection but may be administered by mouth. The ephedras are used as anti-inflammatory drugs and this action is ascribed to an oxazolidone related to ephedrine. The herb has a sudorific action. The root has antisudorific effect.

Ephedrine is a potent sympathomimetic that stimulates α, $β_1$, and $β_2$ adrenergic receptors. It excites the sympathetic nervous system, causes vasoconstriction and cardiac stimulation and produces effects similar to those of epinephrine. It produces a lasting rise in blood pressure, causes mydriasis and diminishes hyperemia.

Ephedrine sulfate occurs as fine, white, odourless crystals or as a powder and darkens when exposed to light. Ephedrine sulfate is used to combat hypotensive states and for allergic disorders, such as bronchial asthma and to treat nasal congestion.

Pharmacology

Ephedra alkaloids showed a relaxant activity on isolated guinea pig trachea. Ephedrine increased pulmonary artery blood pressure and blood resistance in cats and showed an anticholinesterase activity with acetyl-cholinesterase of human erythrocytes. Ephedrine, pseudo-ephedrine and ephedroxane showed anti-inflammatory activity in mice and inhibited arachi-donic acid release and prostaglandin production of rat peritoneal macrophages. Ephedrine and pseudoephedrine showed stimulatory activity in the CNS. However, ephedroxane exerted CNS inhibitory actions and weak antihistaminic activity. Ephedrine itself showed no mutagenic activity. In mice and rats, ephedrine was not found to be carcinogenic. After oral administration of ephedrine, about 75% of the intact ephedrine was recovered in the urine. Ephedrine decreased food intake in rats.

Feruloyl histamine, an imidazole alkaloid from *Ephedra* roots, exerted hypotensive, histidine decarboxylate inhibiting and antihepatotoxic effects in animals. Ephedradines A-D elicited hypotensive effects in rats.

Pseudoephedrine showed anti-inflammatory activity. Aerosol administration of ephedrine into nasal cavity showed mucosal ciliary transport of a test dye. Ephedrine exhibited intense CNS stimulatory activity, contracted van deferens, showed marked antihistaminic and antibarium activities, inhibited hind-paw oedema induced by histamine, serotonin, bradykinin and PGE1 in mice and decreased food intake in rats.

Biosynthesis of ephedrine and related alkaloids

These alkaloids are formed by a union of a C_6-C_1 unit and a C_2 unit. Phenylalanine is the originator of the C_6-C_1 moiety, being converted first to benzaldehyde or benzoic acid.

Benzoic acid combines with the intact CH_3CO group of pyruvic acid to form ephedrine and related alkaloids with 1-phenylpropan-1,2-dione and (*S*)-(–)-2-amino-1-phenylpropan-1-one (cathinone) serving as intermediates. 1-Phenylpropan-1,2-dione & cathinone are known constituents of *Catha edulis*.

KHAT OR ABYSSINIAN TEA

This consists of the fresh leaves of *Catha edulis* (Family : Celastraceae). The plant is cultivated in Abyssinia, in parts of east and southern Africa and in southern Arabia. Khatamine content varies between 0.1% (Yemen, Madagascar) and 0.5% (Kenya). It is widely used for chewing. Its traditional use is similar to that of coca in that the fresh leaves, when chewed, have a stimulatory effect with the alleviation of depression and of the sensations of hunger and fatigue.

The leaves contain about 1.0% of (+)-nor-pseudoephedrine and phenylpropane (–)-α-aminopropiophenone (cathinone), which is considered the principal CNS stimulant of the fresh plant. (–)-Cathinone has pharmacological properties analogous to those of (+)-amphetamine, possessing a similar potency

and the same mechanism of action. Many other components, *e.g.*, alkaloids, sesquiterpenes, triterpenes, flavonoids, numerous acids as esters and an essential oil containing about 40 components, have been characterized.

Khat-chewing is a theologically accepted and lawful custom in Arabian and African countries today.

The young, fresh leaves that come from the tips of the branches contain the optimum amount of cathinone. In older leaves, it is converted to the weakly active compounds (+)-norpseudo-ephedrine (80%) and (–)-norephedrine (20%). This conversion also occurs rapidly during the drying of young leaves.

Annona squamosa (Annonaceae)

Various parts of this plant are used for the treatment of heart disorders. The cardioactive effect are due to the alkaloid higenamine, an important precursor of other isoquinolines.

Bloodroot

Bloodroot consists of the dried rhizomes and roots of *Sanguinaria canadensis* (Papaveraceae), a perennial herb found in North America. The drug consists of dark brown cylindrical pieces of rhizome, 2-7 cm long and 5-15 mm diameter; may be branched and some show numerous wiry roots; with a short fracture and shows numerous red dots (secretion cells) distributed throughout the starch-containing parenchyma of the bark and large pith. The secretion escapes from its containing cells on drying at high temperature and the whole section assumes a deep red or brownish-red colour. A ring

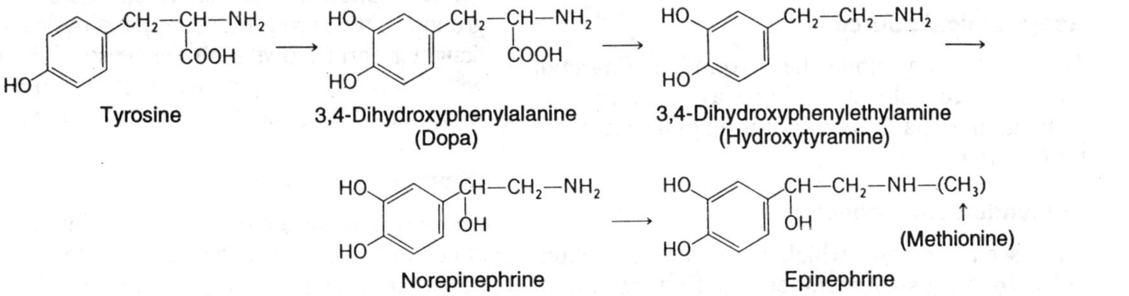

Fig. 21.83. Biogenesis of ephedrine.

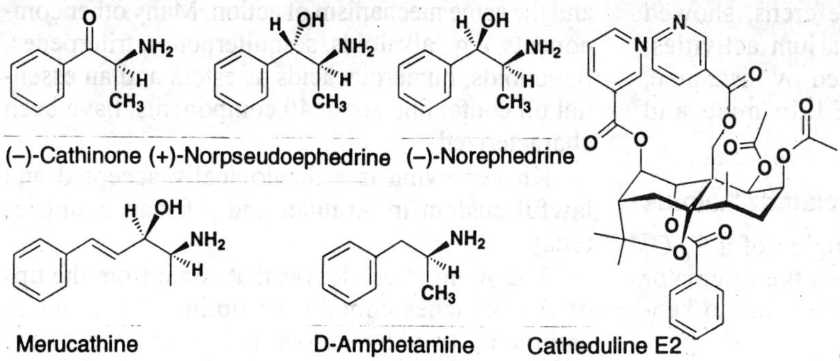

(–)-Cathinone (+)-Norpseudoephedrine (–)-Norephedrine

Merucathine   D-Amphetamine   Catheduline E2

Fig. 21.84. Chemical constituents of Khat.

of small, yellow, fibrovascular bundles lies about 1 mm from the outside. Odour, slight; taste, acrid and bitter. Bloodroot contains the benzophenanthridine alkaloids sanguinarine, chelerythrine, allocrypto-pine, protopine and dihydrosanguilutine; red resin and starch. Sanguinarine and chelerythrine form red and yellow salts, respectively.

Bloodroot is used as an ingredient of compound White Pine Syrup in USA. Sanguinarine, like colchi-cine, causes the doubling of the chromosomes in cells.

COLCHICUM CORM

Synonyms

Meadow Saffron: Autumn Crocus: Wild Saffron; Meadow Crocus; European Colchicum seed; Colchicum root.

Biological source

Colchicum seed and corm are obtained from *Colchicum autumnale* Linn. Indian drug is obtained from the species *C. luteum* Baker. (Fam. Liliaceae).

Geographical source

The plant is an annual herb found in England, Poland, Czechoslovakia, Yugoslavia, U.S.A. and Holland. In India *C. luteum* is used as a substituent for *C. autumnale*.

Cultivation and collection

Fresh seeds are sown which germinate up to about 30%. In August-September 2-6 flowers bloom which are identical to Saffron and has liliac or pale

purple colour. More than half the length of the flower is below in ground. Leaves and capsular fruit are produced in the next spring. The fruit is a three lobed, three-celled and septicidal capsule. On expansion of leaves in the spring the fruit comes out the ground. It is collected in July or August before its dehiscence and kept in muslin bags. Numerous seeds are liberated on septi-cidal dehiscence of the fruit into three valves. The matured seeds are dark in colour and surrounded by a sweet saccharine secre-tion. Before flowering corms are dug out for me-dicinal use, their outer membraneous scales are re-moved, cut in transverse or longitudinal pieces and dried up to 65°C.

The corm consists of an underground stem bearing leaves and fibrous roots. In the latter part of the summer, a new corm is developed in the axil of a scale leaf near the base of the old corm. In September the parent corm bears the remains of recently withered leaves and is larger than the daughter corm. For medicinal purposes the corm should be collected shortly after the withering of the leaves (early summer) and before the enlarge-ment of its axial bud. The corms are surrounded by a dark, membranous coat. The young corm develops fibrous roots at its base, and in August or September two to six flowers emerge from it. The flowers are 10-12 cm long. More than half the length of the flower is below ground, and the fruit lies protected throughout the winter by the surrounding corm and earth. The fruit is a three-lobed, three-celled, septicidal capsule, which is carried above ground in the spring by the expanding leaves. The daughter corm grows at the expense of the parent, which now gradually perishes. It may produce in its second spring one or more small corms.

Characters of corm

The corms, collected in July, are cut into transverse slices and dried at a temperature not exceeding 65°C. The outer membranes are rejected. The whole corms are 2-3 cm diameter. The dried drug consists of reniform, transverse slices and occasional more ovate longitudinal slices, about 2-5 mm thick. The epidermal surface is cinnamon-brown and slightly wrinkled. The interior is white and starchy and shows scattered fibrovascular bundles. The drug breaks with a short mealy fracture. The odour is marked, taste is bitter and acrid.

Fresh corm is conical in shape, 4 cm long and 3 cm wide. One side of the corm is convex and the opposite side is flat. At the apex base flowering stem is present. The outer surface is yellow to brown in colour and slightly wrinkled. A cavity having a bud is seen at the base of the flat side. New stem germinates from this bud. At the base of the corm numerous fibrous roots or their scars are present. Inner surface is fleshy and white and has fibrovascular bundles.

Microscopically there are numerous starch grains present in parenchyma, some simple but many consisting of two to seven components. The grains show a triangular or star-shaped hilum. Their shape varies from spherical or ovoid to polygonal. The vessels have a spiral or annular thickening and portions of brownish-epidermis with very occasional circular stomata.

Morphology of seeds

The seeds are collected when ripe, in July or August and dried. During drying the seeds darken in colour and become covered with a surgery exudation.

Seeds are ovoid or globular in shape and 2-3 mm in diameter. The outer surface is dark reddish brown, pitted and very hard. Endosperm is hard and oily. Small embryo is embedded at one end near the surface of the seeds at the opposite side of the hilum. A distinct strophiole is present which extends for about one quarter of the circumference from hilum. The seed is odourless and bitter in taste.

Microscopically the testa consists of thick-walled reddish-brown parenchyma; that the endosperm cells have pitted walls and contain fixed oil and aleurone grains up to 5 μm in diameter. The strophiole contains starch.

Chemical constituents

Colchicum contains the alkaloids colchicine (0.3-0.8%), colchicein, colchicoresin, demecolcine and starch. Colchicine is an amorphous, yellowish white alkaloid, readily soluble in water, alcohol or chloroform. The corm also contains a resin, fixed oils and reducing sugars.

Indian Colchicum corms contain abundant starch and alkaloid. On exposure to UV light, colchicine is changed to lumicolchicine.

C. luteum also contains luteidine, luteine, β- and γ-lumicolchicines, N-formyldesacetyl colchicine, 3-demethyl-N-desacetyl formylcolchicine, 2- and 3-demethyl colchicine, colchamine and cornigerine.

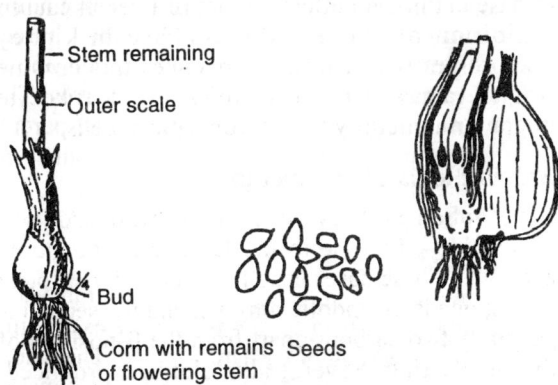

Fig. 21.85. Colchicum.

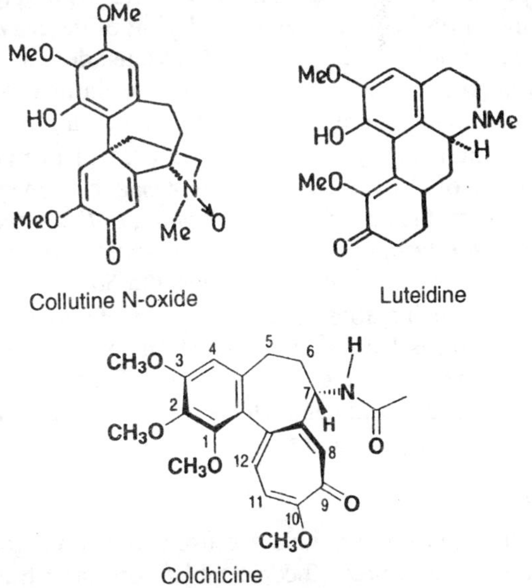

Fig. 21.86. Alkaloids of colchicum.

Chemical test

Colchicum corm with sulphuric acid (70%) or conc. HCl produces yellow colour due to the presence of colchicine.

Uses

Colchicum corm or colchicine is gout depressant and used to cure gout and rheumatism. Its higher doses colchicum causes vomiting and diarrhoea. It is also prescribed to treat myeloid leukaemia. Colchicine is also used to produce polyploidy in biological experiments. Anti-cancer activity of Colchicum has also been reported.

Colchicine

Colchicine has one amido nitrogen atom. The compound lacks pronounced basicity and does not form a well-defined series of salts as do other alkaloids. It is precipitated by many alkaloid reagents and is conventionally considered an alkaloid.

This is an amorphous pale yellow scales or powder, which darkens on exposure to light and gives a yellow colour with strong mineral acids. Colchicine is highly soluble in water, alcohol or chloroform and slightly soluble in ether or petroleum spirit. It is a weak base and extracted from either acid or alkaline solution by means of chloroform.

The richest sources of colchicine are the corms and seeds. The leaves contain only 1/5 the alkaloid content of the seeds. On slow drying of the leaves, the proportion of 2- and 3-demethylated derivatives of colchicine increases; these arise from unknown compounds as a result of enzymatic liberation.

Colchicine-type alkaloids are present in many species of *Colchicum* (*e.g.*, *C. luteum* and *C. speciosum*), and the genera *Androcymbium, Bulbocodium, Camptorrhiza, Dipidax, Gloriosa, Iphigenia, Littonia, Merendera, Ornithoglossum* and *Sandersonia*.

Colchicine does not inhibit leucocyte migration and reduces lactic acid production by leucocytes which decreases the deposition of uric acid. There is a reduction in phagocytosis which decreases the inflammatory response.

Use

Colchicum preparations are used to relieve gout. Colchicine is prescribed in tablet form and transdermal preparations containing colchicine. The alkaloid is also used in biological experiments to produce polyploidy or multiplication of the chromosomes in a cell nucleus.

The use of colchicine to double chromosomes has opened a large field in plant genetics. Any numeric change in chromosome number entails a mutation that becomes evident in a number of the characteristics of the experimental plant. New varieties of plants of economic and pharmacognostic value may be produced. The interrelationship between the action of colchicine and mitosis is being investigated in animals. Injections of colchicine can affect the dispersal of turmors. It is used in the treatment of various neoplastic diseases.

The exact mechanism of action of colchicine in the treatment of gout is not known. It reduces lactic acid production by leukocytes which results in a decreased deposition of uric acid. In addition, there is a reduction in phagocytosis which decreases the inflammatory response.

Pharmacology

Colchicine inhibited catecholamine secretion evoked by acetylcholine; suppressed development of carrageenin-induced oedema in rats; decreased polymorphonuclear leukocyte chemotaxis in human beings; did not affect liver plasma membrane-bound enzymes; inhibited phytohemagglutinin-mediated agglutination of ascitic hepatoma cells from mice; suppressed sheep red blood cell antibody titres; caused reduction in output of total protein in bile; increased alkaline phosphatase activity of liver five-fold and of kidney two-fold in rats; inhibited acid phosphatase in spleen but had no effect on liver and kidney acid phosphatase; inhibited kidney 5'-nucleotidase but had no effect on that of liver. It caused inhibition of Na^+ K^+-Mg^+-ATPase in kidney microsomes but in liver microsomes this enzyme was activated and inhibited production of leukocyte migration inhibitory factor from spleen cells.

Biosynthesis of colchicine

Tryptophan and its decarboxylation product, tryptamine, give rise to the large class of indole alkaloids. These bases usually contain two nitrogen atoms; one is the indolic nitrogen and the second is generally two carbons apart from the β-position of the indole ring. Several alkaloids are produced, depending on the type of condensation occurring

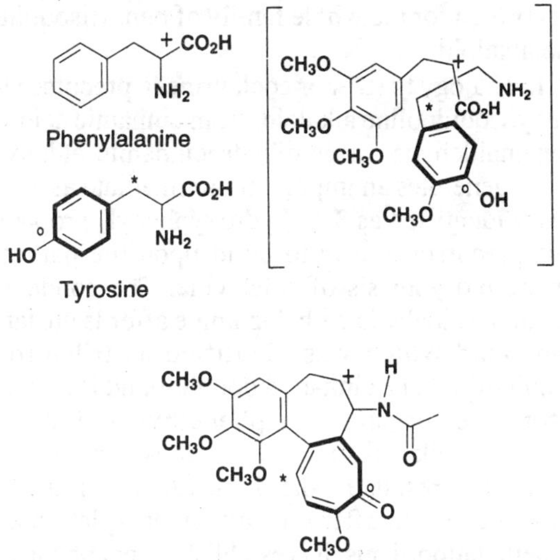

Phenylalanine

Tyrosine

Fig. 21.87. Biosynthesis of colchicine : origin of different carbon atoms.

between tryptamine and an aldehyde or ketoacid. A Mannich reaction involving the α-carbon atom of the indole nucleus affords a β-carboline derivative; reaction involving the β-position gives rise to an indolenine.

The more complex indole alkaloid contain a non-tryptophan-derived portion of the molecule and this is supplied by mevalonic acid, which in the case of the ergot alkaloids is a C_5-isopentenyl unit and with the alkaloids of the Apocynaceae, Loganiaceae, Rubiaceae etc., a C_{10}-geraniol (monoterpenoid) contribution.

Ring A and carbons 5, 6 and 7 of colchicine are derived from phenylalanine; the tropolone moiety arises from tyrosine by ring cleavage followed by closure to give a seven-membered ring. Acetate does not contribute directly to the tropo-lone ring but is effective in supplying the N-acetyl group. An intermediate formed early in the pathway due to union of two amino acids is a 1-phenylethylisoquinoline derivative. This is related to androcymbine and the

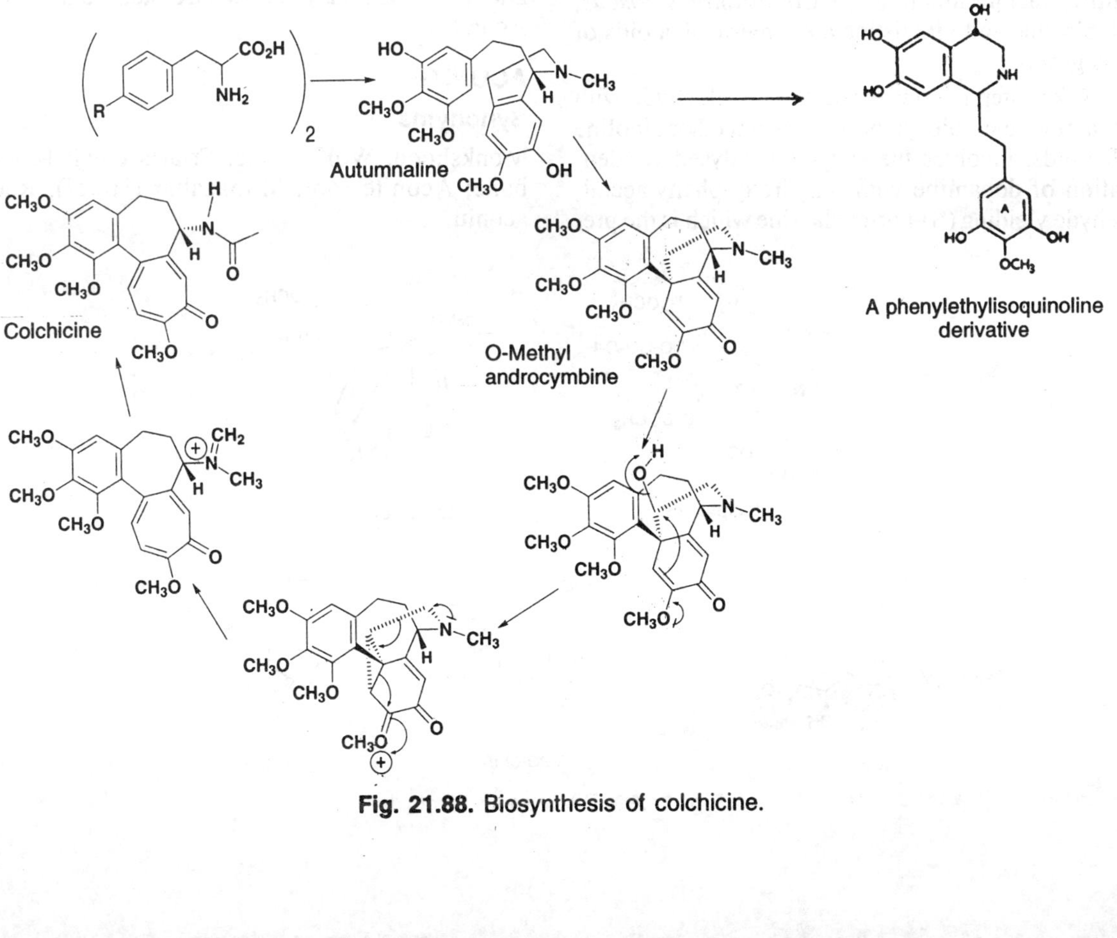

Autumnaline

A phenylethylisoquinoline derivative

Colchicine

O-Methyl androcymbine

Fig. 21.88. Biosynthesis of colchicine.

dimer melanthioidine, alkaloids of *Androcymbium melanthioides*, a close relative of colchicum. Demecolcine is an immediate precursor of colchicine.

A key intermediate in the biogenesis of the monoterpene indole alkaloids is 3α(*S*)-strictosidine formed by the enzymatic condensation by tryptamine and secologanin. The enzyme responsible for this reaction, strictosidine synthase, has been isolated and characterized from cell cultures of *Rauwolfia serpentina*, *Cinchona robusta* and *Catharanthus roseus*. The *R. serpentina* gene relating to this enzyme has been cloned and heterologously expressed in micro-organisms including *Escherichia coli* and *Saccharomyces cerevisiae* (baker's yeast), *e.g.*, the first cloning of cDNA for an enzyme of alkaloid biosynthesis. The gene is a single polypeptide M, about 34,000, possessing a 5.3% carbohydrate content. The gene is highly conserved and it is considered as an unimportant gene of secondary metabolism.

Quinine is also derived from tryptophan. The antileukaemic alkaloids of *Catharanthus roseus*, vinblastine and vincristine are dimeric alkaloids of this group.

A key step in condensation of an aldehyde with an amine, *e.g.*, biosynthesis of benzyl isoquinoline alkaloids, involves the enzyme-catalysed condensation of dopamine with 4-hydroxy-phenylacetaldehyde yielding (S)-nor-coclaurine which is the precursor then for the whole family of benzylisoquinoline alkaloid.

In analogy to (S)-nor coclaurine, a precursor for benzylisoquinoline alkaloid, from cinnamic acid via cinnamaldehyde arises dihydrocinnamic aldehyde which generates an important intermediate as a precursor identified as 3-(4-hydroxyphenyl) propanal. This precursor allows to build upon the pathway for the biosynthesis of colchicine. The condensation of the aldehyde with dopamine affords unstable compound which was identified as trihydroxy isoquinoline. The cinnamyl double-bond is reduced before the formation of phenethylisoquinoline skeleton similar to structure which was not known earlier. The results reported indicate that n-methylation may occur after aromatic hydroxylation and O-methylation. Thus, it is established that phenethyl iso-quinoline is an intact precursor for demecolcine and colchicine.

DITERPENE ALKALOIDS

Diterpene alkaloids have been isolated from the drug Aconite.

ACONITE

Synonyms

Monkshood, Wolf's-bane; Friar's cowl; Mousebane; Aconite root; Mithazahar (Hindi); Radix aconiti.

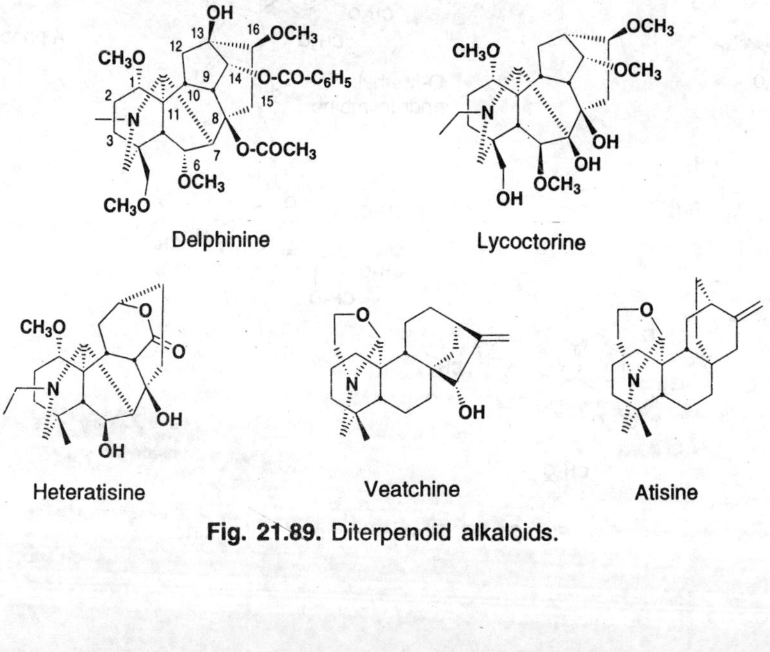

Fig. 21.89. Diterpenoid alkaloids.

Biological source

Aconite is the dried roots of *Aconitum napellus* Linn. collected from wild or cultivated plants. (Family : Ranunculaceae).

Geographical source

The plant has been originated from the mountanoeous and temperate regions of Europe. It occurs in Alps and Carpathian mountains, hills of Germany and Himalayas. The greater part of the commercial drug is derived from wild plant grown in central and southern Europe, particularly Spain.

Cultivation and plant habitat

Aconite is a perennial herb with a fusiform tuberous root. The plant is propagated from the daughter tubers. An apical bud on the apex and six lateral buds on its surface are developed. A lateral shoot bearing a thin lateral root is produced from each lateral bud. The lateral roots are called daughter roots and the main root is known as parent root. The daughter root develops gradually, becomes thick in autumn and buds are produced on its apex and surface.

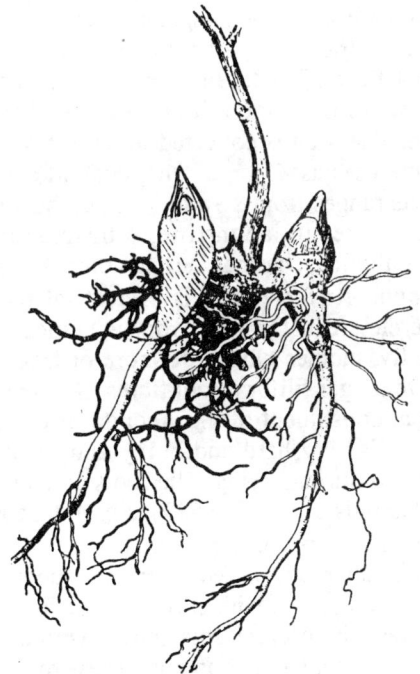

Fig. 21.90. *Aconitum napellus.*

Daughter roots are planted in soil containing leaf mould and some amount of lime. The roots are collected in autumn. Collection of Aconite from wild plants is done during flowering season. Roots are dried at 40-50°. Thus Aconite arises from one or more lateral shoots which develop into conical daughter tubers.

Morphology

Appearance of Aconite varies from season to season. Aconite collected in autumn is conical in shape and tapering below. Surface is slightly twisted bearing longitudinal ridges. Some Aconites may contain fibrous rootlets or their scars. On the top of parent root some remains of stem base are present which are more shrivelled. An apical bud is present at the apex. The colour is dark-brown. The root is 4-10 cm in length and 1-3 cm in diameter at the crown. Rootlets may be present. The fracture is short and starchy. The fractured surface is 5-8 angled, contains stellate cambium and a central pith. The odour is slight. Taste is sweet at first followed by tingling and numbness.

Transverse sections cut from the crown show a stellate cambium with five to eight angles. The amount of lignified tissues is small, the major part of the root consists of starch-containing parenchyma of the pith and secondary phloem.

Chemical constituents

Aconite contains aconitine (0.4- 0.8%), hypaconiticine, mesaconitine, aconine, napelline (isoaconitine, pseudoaconitine), neoline, ephedrine, sparteine, picraconitine, acotinic acid, itaconic acid, succinic acid, malonic acid, fat, starch, aconosine, 14-acetylneoline, hokbusine A, senbusines A and C, mesaconitine, diterpene 15α-hydroxyneoline and levulose (fructose). The aconitines are diacyl esters of polyhydric amino alcohols and are extremely poisonous. Atisines are also amino alcohols but have low toxicity. The basic skeleton of aconite alkaloid is consisted of a pentacyclic diterpene which is derived from phyllocladene. The toxicity of alkaloids is decreased on hydrolysis.

Uses

Aconite is cardiac effective. It is used externally as a local analgesic in liniments and to treat neuralgia,

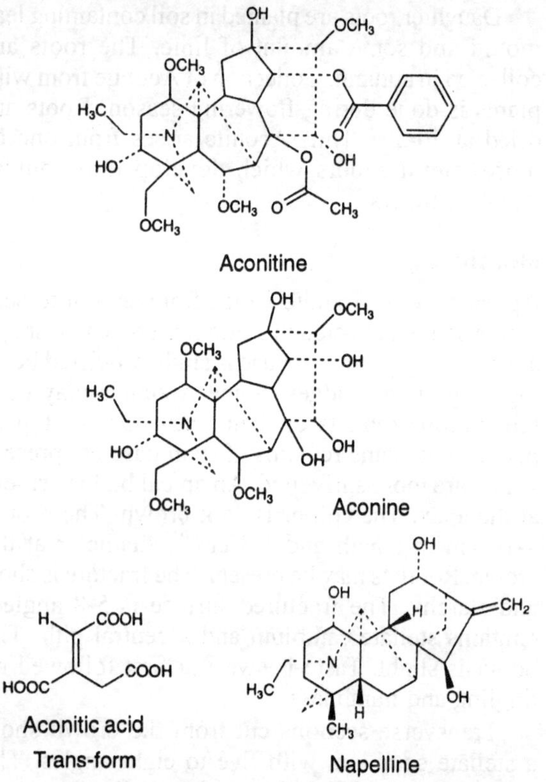

Fig. 21.91. Chemical constituents of Aconite.

rheumatism and inflammation. Tincture Aconite is antipyretic in small doses. Aconitine in amount 2-3 mg can lead respiratory failure, heart failure and in the end death. The drug is used for the preparation of an antineuralgic liniment.

INDIAN ACONITES

About 28 *Aconitum* species have been reported from India, mostly present in the alpine and sub-alpine belt of Himalayas. The roots of nine species are commonly found in the Indian markets.

Aconitum atrox (Syn. *A. balfourii*) is an erect, glabrous herb. Roots are biennial, paired; or ternate and tuberous with several attached hardened rootlets. It is a poisonous species and is one of the common constituents of *Aconitum ferox* of commerce. The roots resemble those of *A. deinorrhizum* but are somewhat shorter and thicker. They contains 1.20-2.04 % of total alkaloids, of which pseudaconitine is 0.4-0.5 per cent. The other alkaloids iso-

lated are 8-O-methyl-veratroyl pseudaconine, veratroyl-bikhaconine, balfourine, pseudoaconitine, veratroyl-pseudo-aconine, indaconitine, ludaconitine, 8-deacetyl-yunaconitine, bikhaconitine, neoline and chasma-nine.

Aconitum bisma (syn. A. palmatum) is a biennial herb. Roots are tuberous, paired, the mother root is often dry and cylindrical, the daughter root conical to long-cylindrical, external surface somewhat smooth, light brown. The roots contain five diterpene alkaloids, *viz.*, palmatisine, vakognavine, vakatisine, vakatisinine, vakatidine, 15-deacetyl-vakognavine, palmadine, palmasine, 6-acetyl heteratisine, vakognavine, heteratisine, isoatisine, vakhanatine, vakhmadine, atisine and hetisine. Benzamide is also present. The root is intensely bitter like quinine and is used in combination with long pepper for pain in the bowels, for diarrhoea, vomiting, rheumatism, sharp cuts, wounds and as a tonic.

Aconitum chasmanthum is an erect, perennial herb. Roots are biennial, paired and tuberous. This species is identical to *A. napellus*. Its roots are smaller, shorter and thicker; the mother tubers are deeply grooved and wrinkled and are black outside and brown inside. The daughter tubers are conic to conic-cylindrical with a broad base having numerous root fibres. Fracture is cartilaginous, hard and white within the cambium ring and brownish outside. The drug is collected in September. It has the same uses as *A. ferox*. The alkaloid content of the roots ranges from 2.98 to 3.11%. The alkaloids isolated are indaconitine, chasmaconitine, chasmanthinine, chasmanine and homochasmanine.

Aconitum deinorrhizum is an erect, tall plant with long terete stem. Daughter root is conical, brown externally, mother tubers are more or less similar, but have longer filiform root fibres. *A. atrox* is the principal constituent of the Aconite of commerce. The drug is very hard and horny and its starch is gelatinized during drying. The roots contains 0.9% total alkaloids of which 0.51% is pseudaconitine.

Aconitum ferox is a perennial herb. Roots are biennial, tuberous, paired, daughter tuber ovoid-oblong to ellipsoid, with filiform root fibres, dark brown, taste indifferent. It is known as Indian Aconite. The total alkaloid content varies from 0.63 to 4.7%. The alkaloids pseudaconitine, chasmaconitine, indaconitine, bikhaconitine, veratroyl pseu-daconitine, 2-(1H)-quinolinone, 3,4-dihydro-6-hy-droxy-2-(1H)-quinolinone, 14-O-acetylsenbusine A, vakognavine, chasmaconitine, crassicauline A, falconericine, bikhaconine, pseudo-aconine, neoline, senbusine A, isotalatizidine, columbianine, lipopseudaconitine, lipoyunaconitine, lipoindaconi-tine, lipobikhaconitine and diacetyl pseudaconitine are present. The roots are used after mitigation to treat neuralgia, muscular rheumatism, inflammatory joint affections, nasal catarrh, tonsilitis, sore throat, gastric disorders, debility and fever.

Aconitum heterophyllum is a tall herb. Root are biennial, tuberous, paired; daughter tuber cylindric or conic. The roots yield 0.79% of total alkaloids like atisine, heteratisine, histidine, heterophyllisine, heterophylline, heterophyllidine, atidine and hetidine. Atisine is much less toxic than aconitine and pseudaconitine. Therefore, this species is often regarded as non-poisonous. It is used as a febrifuge and bitter tonic. The roots are used to treat hysteria and throat diseases.

Aconitum spicatum is a robust and typical spe-cies. Roots are biennial, tuberous, paired and brown or blackish. The roots are used as poison. The fresh roots are soft and flexible; dried roots are hard and dark brown. The roots yield 1.75% of alkaloids which contain mainly pseudoaconitine and bikhaconitine. The other compounds isolated are IAA, zeatin, liquidambaric acid and 24-ethylcholest-5-en-3β-ol.

Aconitum falconeri is an erect herb. The bien-nial, paired roots yield two alkaloids, bishaconine and bishatisine and are used to treat disease of nervous and digestive systems and for rheumatism. *A. laciniatum* biennial roots are slightly bitter and are mixed with those *A. spicatum* and *A. ferox. A. luridum*, an erect plant, is a potent drug as *A. ferox. A. rotundifolium* contains two alkaloids in the aerial portion. *A. violaceum* is an erect plant, found mixed with the commercial varieties of Aconites. It contains 1% indaconitine, falconerine, its 8-acetate, falconericine and falconeridine.

Chinese aconites

A. carmichaeli, A. kusnezofii and *A. brachypodum* are three species used in Chinese medicine. The toxicity is reduced by soaking or boiling in water which causes some hydrolysis of the alkaloids.

Japanese aconite

The roots of Japanese aconite, formerly an article of European commerce, are shorter than the European drug, and dark grey or brownish in colour. *Aconitum japonicum* possesses cardio-tonic prop-erties and the principal alkaloid associated with this activity is higenamine [(±)-demethylcoclaurine], which is active at about the same dosage levels as the *Digitalis* glycosides. The only other cardioactive alkaloid obtained is coryneine chloride (dopamine methochloride) from *A. carmichaelii.*

Pharmacology

Three widely occurring alkaloids in aconite roots, aconitine, mesaconitine and hypaconitine, showed analgesic and anti-inflammatory activities in mice. These alkaloids induce arrhythima in rats. The arrhythmia caused by aconitine was counteracted by i.v. administration of calcium. Aconite alkaloids caused a decrease in the number of erythrocytes and in the serum levels of total protein and albumin. Aconitine caused respiratory depression in rabbits and heart fibrillation in guinea pigs. It acts directly on cardiac muscles.

Aconitine had action on CNS, CVS and respi-ratory system due to the presence of benzyl ester and hydroxy groups in the molecular structure. Acetylation of hydroxyls or saponification of benzyl ester led to sharp decrease in toxicity and arrhythmic activity.

INDOLIZIDINE AND IMIDAZOLE ALKALOIDS

Some indolizidine alkaloids are currently. known. The tetrahydroxy alkaloids castanospermine and 6-epi-castanospermine may be used as anti-AIDS drugs. Swainsonine, the toxic constituent of locoweeds and Australian *Swainsona* spp., is a powerful glycosidae inhibitor; this alkaloid is a trihydroxy-indolizidine.

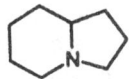

Fig. 21.92. Indolizidine

The imidazole (glyoxaline) ring is the basic

skeleton in pilocarpine isolated from pilocarpus. Pilocarpine is a monoacidic tertiary base containing a lactone group and the imidazole nucleus. This alkaloid probably is formed from histidine or a metabolic equivalent.

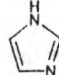

Fig. 21.93. Imidazole.

Pilocarpus and pilocarpine are the important drugs of this group.

JABORANDI LEAF AND PILOCARPINE

Jaborandi consists of the leaflets of various species of *Pilocarpus* (Rutaceae), a genus of trees and shrubs found in South America, in West Indies and Central America. Maranham jaborandi is that derived from the Brazilian plant *Pilocarpus microphyllus*. Jaborandi is now mainly used as a source of pilocarpine.

Characters

Maranham jaborandi bears imparipinnate compound leaves with about seven leaflets attached to a winged rachis which is almost glabrous (*Swartzia* is hairy). The drug consists of separated leaflets, rachis and an occasional fruit. The leaflets are 2-5 cm long, 1-3 cm broad, and emarginate at the apex. The terminal leaflets are oval, symmetrical and have a petiolule 5-15 mm long, with a winged margin which passes imperceptibly into the lamina. The remaining leaflets are obovate, asymmetrical and sessile. The veins are pinnate and anastomose near the margin. The drug is greyish-green to greenish-brown and brittle in texture. Numerous small oil cells may be seen by transmitted light. Odour, when crushed, slightly aromatic; taste, bitterish and aromatic with induction of salivation.

Pernambuco jaborandi consists of the leaflets of *Pilocarpus jaborandi*, which consists of a compound imparipinnate leaf with 1-9 leaflets.

Paraguay jaborandi, obtained from *P. pennatifolius* Lemaire. greyish-green; papery in texture; usually equal at base; veins not prominent on the upper surface and the anastomoses not marked.

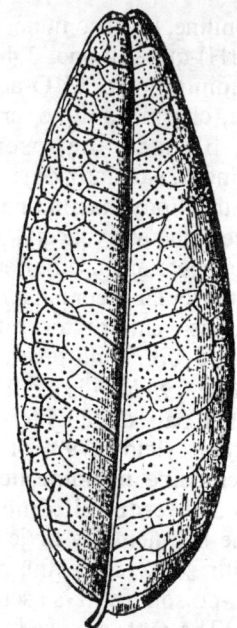

Fig. 21.94. Jaborandi leaf.

Ceara jaborandi is obtained from *P. trachylophus* Holmes and is exported from the Brazilian provinces of Ceara and Maranhao. Leaflets are smaller than those of *P. jaborandi*; oblong or elliptical; coriaceous; both surfaces bearing short curved hairs, which are particularly abundant on the lower surface.

Constituents

Maranham leaves contain about 0.7-0.8% of the alkaloids, pilocarpine, isopilocarpine, pilosine and isopilosine and about 0.5% of volatile oil. The volatile oil contains 22 components occurring throughout the samples. These included monoterpenes (*e.g.*, limonene, sabiene, α-pinene), sesquiterpenes (*e.g.*, caryophyllene) but not in *P. jaborandi*, and 2-undecanone or 2-tridecanone.

During storage, the leaves lose at least half of their alkaloidal content in 1 year through deterioration. Leaves that are 2 years old are practically useless.

Uses

Salts of pilocarpine (*e.g.*, pilocarpine hydrochloride and nitrate) are used in ophthalmic practice, as they

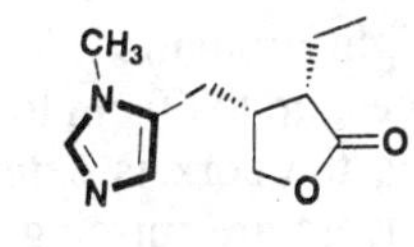

Pilocarpine

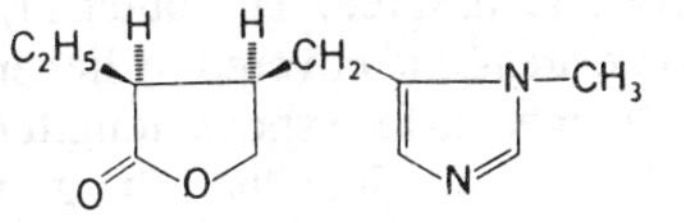

Pilocarpine

Fig. 21.95. Pilocarpine.

cause contraction of the pupil of the eye, their action being antagonistic to that of atropine. In early glaucoma treatment they serve to increase the irrigation of the eye and relieve pressure. Oral pilocarpine can possibly offer relief for patients suffering from dry mouth resulting from radiation treatment for head or neck.

Pilocarpine, the lactone of pilocarpic acid, contains a glyoxaline nucleus and with heat or alkalis is converted into its isomer isopilocarpine. Isopilocarpine occurs in small quantity in the leaf but more is formed during the extraction process. The dried leaves lose their activity on storage.

Pilocarpine is an oily, syrupy liquid, though its salts crystallize easily. It is isolated by treating the powdered leaves with sodium carbonate, extracting with benzene, and then shaking the benzene extract with dilute hydrochloric or nitric acid. The aqueous solution is then made alkaline and shaken with chloroform; the chloroform solution is then shaken with acid, and the alkaloidal salt is allowed to crystallize.

Pilocarpine stimulates the muscarinic receptors in the eye, causing constriction of the pupil and contraction of the ciliary muscle. In narrow-angle glaucoma, miosis opens the anterior chamber angle to improve the outflow of aqueous humor. In chronic open-angle glaucoma, the increase in outflow is independent of the miotic effect. Contraction of the ciliary muscle enhances the outflow of aqueous humor via indirect effects on the trabecular system.

Pilocarpine hydrochloride occurs as colourless, translucent, odourless, hygroscopic, faintly bitter crystals; pilocarpine nitrate occurs as shiny, white crystals. *Pilocarpine nitrate* is stable in air but is affected by light. Both pilocarpine hydrochloride and pilocar-pine nitrate are cholinergic (ophthalmic) drugs used to treat of glaucoma. They are applied topically to the conjunctiva, 1 to 6 times a day. The patient should be advised to wash hands immediately after application.

THEA (TEA)

Thea or *tea* consists of the prepared leaves and leaf buds of *Camellia sinensis* (Linne) O. Kuntze (Fam. Theaceae), a shrub or tree with alternate, evergreen leaves. The tea tree is indigenous to eastern Asia and is now extensively cultivated in China, Japan, India and Indonesia.

Green tea is prepared in China and Japan by rapidly drying the freshly picked leaves in copper pans over a mild artificial heat. The leaves are often rolled in the palm of the hand as they dry.

Black tea is prepared in Sri Lanka and India by heaping the fresh leaves until fermentation has begun. They are then rapidly dried artificially with heat.

Tea occurs as crumpled, bright green or blackish green masses. Its odour is agreeable and aromatic; its taste is pleasantly astringent and bitter.

Tea contains 1 to 4% of caffeine (theine) and small amounts of adenine, theobromine, theophylline, and xanthine; about 15% of gallo-tannic acid; and about 0.75% of a yellow volatile oil that is solid at ordinary temperatures and has a strongly aromatic odour and taste.

The stimulating action of tea is due to caffeine; its astringent properties are owing to the tannin con-

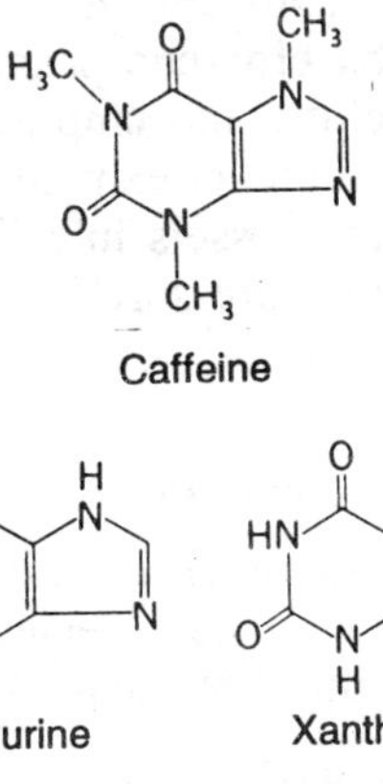

Caffeine

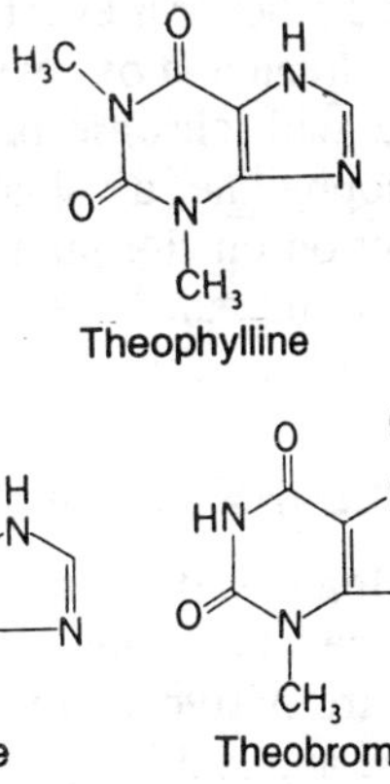

Theophylline

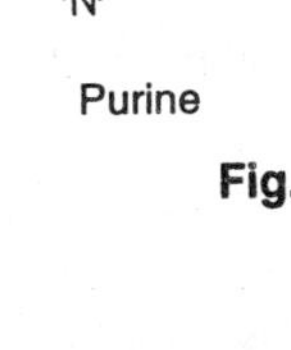

Purine

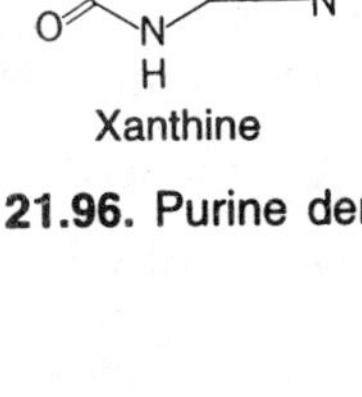

Xanthine

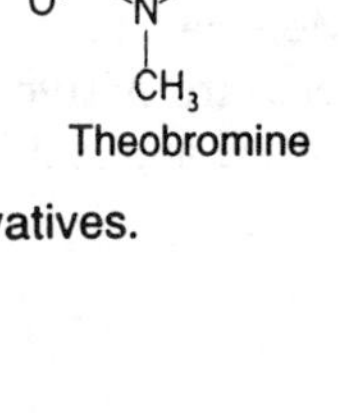

Theobromine

Fig. 21.96. Purine derivatives.

tent. Tea leaf waste and tea dust are the important sources for the extraction of caffeine.

Caffeine

Caffeine (1,3,7-*trimethylxanthine*) occurs in coffee, tea, cacao, guarana, kola and mate. It is usually prepared from tea, tea dust, or tea sweepings, or recovered from coffee roasters. Caffeine is anhydrous or contains one molecule of water of hydration.

Caffeine occurs as a white powder or as white, glistening needles matted together in fleecy masses. It has a bitter taste. Caffeine may be sublimed without decomposition when heated.

The solubility of caffeine in water is markedly increased by the presence of citric acid, benzoates, salicylates and bromides; medicinal compounds of this class are citrated caffeine and caffeine sodium benzoate. The latter is most suitable for intramuscular injection as an analeptic in the treatment of poisoning, as a stimulant in acute circulatory failure and as a diuretic.

Caffeine and its related compounds are central nervous system stimulants.

Theophylline (1,3-*dimethylxanthine*) is isomeric with theobromine. It is prepared synthetically from caffeine or by other means. Theophylline occurs as a white, odourless, bitter crystalline powder that is soluble in about 120 parts of water. It becomes more soluble when combined with basic compounds. Aminophylline or theophylline ethylenediamine, theophylline monoethanolamine, choline theophyllinate, and theophylline sodium glycinate are utilized as diuretic smooth muscle relaxants for the symptomatic relief or prevention of bronchial asthma and for the treatment of reversible bron-chospasm associated with chronic bronchitis and emphysema. Aminophylline, a valuable diuretic, exhibits dilating action on the pulmonary vessels in relieving asthma and can lower venous pressure in certain cases of heart failure.

COCILLANA (Grape bark, guapi bark)

Cocillana is the dried bark of *Guarea rusbyi* (Meliaceae) and other closely related species. The trees are native to the South American Andes, Bolivia and Haiti.

The commercial bark is slight aromatic odour, occurs in flattish or curved pieces, up to 60 cm long and 5-20 mm thick. Externally, the cork is extensive and fissured. The outer layers are missing in some areas and covered by lichen patches in others. The inner surface shows longitudinal striations and is lighter in colour than the grey-brown or orange brown outer tissues.

The bark contains 2.3% resins, 2.5% fixed oil, tannin, a small quantity of alkaloid and a glycoside.

GELSEMIUM

Gelsemium consists of the dried rhizomes and roots of the American yellow jasmine, *Gelsemium nitidum* (Loganiaceae). It is collected in the autumn in the southern USA.

The drug occurs in cylindrical pieces 3-20 cm long and 3-30 mm diameter; outer cork cells of the rhizome reddish-brown; inner ones yellowish. The roots are smaller than the rhizome have a uniform yellowish-brown cork; fracture, irregular splintery, odour slightly aromatic, taste bitter.

Gelsemium contains toxic alkaloids having a distinct carbon framework skeletal type; the main alkaloid is gelsemine. It is not as toxic as gelsemicine. Other oxindole alkaloids are sempervirine, 1-methoxy- and 21-oxogelsemine, 14-hydroxygelsemicine, gelsedine and 14-hydroxygelsedine. Blue fluorescence of the broken drug in ultraviolet light is due to scopoletin. Iridoids and glucoiri-doids are present in the aerial parts.

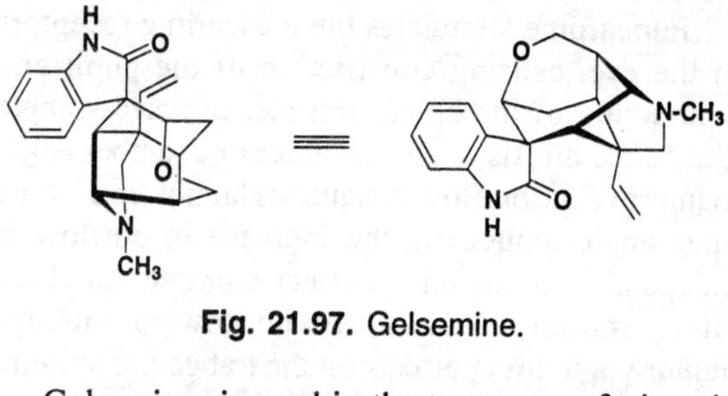

Fig. 21.97. Gelsemine.

Gelsemium is used in the treatment of trigeminal neuralgia and migraine. It has many side effects.

G. elegans is used for the same purposes as *G. nitidum*.

22

Traditional Drugs

Medicinal plants have been playing a significant role in the treatment of various ailments in India. The important traditional methods in our country are Ayurvedic, Homoeopathy, Unani and Sidha systems of medicine. Ayurveda offers traditionally a highly scientific health-care therapy as a divine gift, and as a result, the global interest of the medical profession is nucleated on the Ayurvedic and Unani systems of medicine. A traditional ingredient is fundamentally preventive, protective, nutritive and curative. Therefore, traditional medicines are safe, sure and harmless which treat the patients without any side effect.

In spite of phenomenal progress in the area of development of new drugs from synthetic sources and appearance of antibiotics as major therapeutic agents, plants continue to provide basic raw material for some of the most important drugs. An analysis of prescriptions dispensed from community pharmacies in USA showed that 41% prescriptions contained one or more products of natural origin as the therapeutic agent. Of these prescriptions, 25% were based on drugs from higher plants, some 13% represented metabolities of microbes and about 7% were of animal origin. Among 200 most frequently prescribed drugs in USA, 25% were of natural origin. The situation would appear to be similar for many other countries including India, Russia, Germany, England, Italy, China and Japan. About three hundred herbal drugs of Indian origin are used in England to treat various diseases. The *Pharmacopoeia of the Peoples Republic of China*, issued in 1978, describes 882 crude drugs of which 637 are of plant origin. *Japanese Pharmacopoeia X* released in 1981, contained 102 plant drugs.

In India there are about 700 naturally occurring drugs used in various formulations. There are about 20 large scale manufacturers of traditional drugs in addition to 1200 small manufacturers and thousands of miniature manufacturing units running by vaids and hakims.

More frequently traditional drugs are used to cure the following ailments :

Cold and cough

Senega, Ipecac, Squill, Glycyrrhiza and Ginger contain expectorant activity. The leaves of *Angelica archangelica, Pimpinella anisum* (Anise fruit), *Allium sativum* (Garlic), *Thymus vulgaris, Mentha spicata* (Mint), *Ocimum sanctum* (Tulsi), *Viola odorata* (Banafsha) and *Eucalpytus* sp. are used to treat cough, cold and bronchitis. Dried stigma of *Crocus sativus* (Saffron or Kesar) are added in cough preparations. Most of these drugs contain essential oils which are responsible for the biological activity.

Gastrointestinal disorders

Gastrointestinal disorders include colitis, constipation, diarrhoea, duodenal ulcers, dyspepsia and hyperacidity. Dried extract of *Acacia catechu* and *Geum urbanum*, leaf and bark of *Hamamelis virginiana* and root bark of *Myrica cerifera* are used to treat the inflammation of colon (colitis). Constipation is treated with seed husk of Plantago, leaves of Senna, bark of Cascara, Aloe juice, Rhubarb and Honey. Stomachic drugs include Chirata, Garlic, Kalmegh, Kapur kachari, Saffron, Nux-vomica, Picrorhiza. Agar, Aloe, Cascara, Guar gum, Isapgol, Myrobalan, Rhubarb and Senna. Carminative drugs contain volatile oils and they are Asafoetida, Black pepper, Capsicum, Caraway, Cardamom, Cinnamon, Coriander, Dill, Fennel, Garlic and Mentha oil. The herbal drugs like Ipecac, Isapgol, Kurchi and Sankhpushpi are anti-dysenteric drugs which generally contain mucilage or alkaloids. Diarrhoea is treated with Bael, Isapgol, Kurchi, Pale Catechu and Pectins.

Antiarthritic agents

Rasna (*Alpinia officinarum, Pluchea lanceolata, Vanda roxburghii,* and *Vitex negundo*) is used as a traditional remedy to cure rheumatism and arthritis. The resin obtained from *Commiphora mukul* (Gugal) and the exudate of *Boswellia serrata* (Sallai gugul) are also employed as anti-arthritic agents. *Aconitum napellus* also contains anti-rheumatic activity.

Cardiac drugs

Cardiovascular diseases are the major cause of mortality all over the world. The most popular drug is digoxin isolated from Digitalis. The cardiotonic glycoside, peruvoside, obtained from an Indian ornamental plant Kaner, *Thevetia peruviana*, (Fam. Apocynaceae) has been introduced in German under the trade name 'Encordin'. Forskolin (Coleonol) is another antihypertensive compound isolated from a fragrant herb, *Coleus forskohlii* (Fam. Lamiaceae). Asclepin, obtained from *Asclepias curassavica*, is more potent than digoxin. The popular Ayurvedic drug 'Sarpgandha' (*Rauwolfia serpentina*) shows hypotensive and tranquillizing effect. Strophanthus and Urginea are also used as cardiotonic.

Antiprotozoa! drugs

Tropical diseases include malaria where schizon-tocidal drugs are needed and drugs for multi-drug resistant blood schizonts are required. One third of the world's population may be exposed to the risk of malarial infection. Most affected areas include

Africa, India, China and East Asia. Amoebiasis caused by *Entamoeba histolytica* is the major cause of dysentery in the developing world where an estimated 42 million cases occur annually and untreated disease may progress to hepatic amoebiasis and other complications which are responsible for 75,000 deaths each year. Filaria and leishmania are two other protozoal diseases affecting our population. Many plants like *Peganum harmala, Celastrus paniculatus, Artemisia annua, Berberis aristata* and *Tiliacora triandra* show activities against various species of protozoa. For amoebicidal drugs plants like *Holarrhena antidysenterica, Berberis aristata, Allium sativum* and *Terminalia belerica* may provide potent drug. Worldwide it has been estimated that 20 million people are infected with *Leishmania* species and that 400,000 new cases occur each year. The plants which have given leads include *Plumbago zeylanica, Diospyros montana, Ricinus communis* and *Phytolacca* species.

Antiulcer drugs

Important plants for the treatment of gastrointestinal ulcers include *Prosopis glandulosa, Calendula* species, *Artocarpus heterophyllus, Mesua ferrea* (pulp) and deglycyrrhizinated *Glycyrrhiza glabra*.

Antirheumatic plants

Inflammatory diseases including different types of rheumatic diseases are very common throughout the world. Although rheumatism is one of the oldest known diseases of mankind and affects a large population of the world, no substantial progress has been so far achieved for permanent cure. Plant species of ninety six genera belonging to fifty six families have exhibited antiinflammatory activity. Most significant plants include *Aesculus hippocastanum, Azadirachta indica, Boswellia serrata, Commiphora mukul, Curcuma longa, Ochrocarpus longifolius, Pluchea lanceolata, Vitex negundo* and *Colchicum luteum*.

Antidiabetic plants

About 15.2 million people are suffering from diabetes in our country and the number is increasing every year. About 148 plants of 50 families are reported to have hypoglycaemic activity. The most important hypoglycaemic plants which need serious clinical trials include *Pterocarpus marsupium, Momordica charantia, Trigonella foenum-graecum, Salacia prinoides, Gymnema sylvestre* and *Cyamompsis tetragonoloba.*

Antiviral plants

A lyophilized infusion from flowers of *Sambucus nigra*, aerial parts of *Hypericum perforatum* and roots of *Saponaria officinalis* exhibited antiviral effect inhibiting reproduction of different strains of influenza virus type A and B and herpes simplex virus type 1.

Plant adaptogens

The resistance to disease is increased with *Withania somnifera, Ocimum sanctum, Picrorhiza kurroa, Asparagus racemosus, Pueraria tuberosa, Sida cordifolia, Desmodium gangeticum, Boerhavia diffusa* and *Cissampelos pareira.*

Hepatroprotective plants

A global estimate indicates that there are about 18,000 deaths every year because of the liver cirrhosis caused by hepatitis. Hepatocellular carcinoma is one of the ten most common tumours in the world with over 2,50,000 new cases each year. Although viruses are the main cause of liver diseases, the liver lesions arising from xenobiotics, excessive drug therapy, environmental pollution and alcoholic intoxication are not uncommon. Modern drugs have very little to offer for alleviation of hepatic ailments, whereas, potent phytoconstituents used for liver diseases include drugs like silymarin (*Silybum marianum*), catechin (*Anacardium occidentale* and others), glycyrrhizin (*Glycyrrhiza glabra*) in Japan and schizandrins (*Schizandra chinensis*) in China. In India, we have over 40 polyherbal commercial formulations reputed to have hepatoprotective action. About 160 phytoconstituents from 101 plants belonging to 52 families have antihepato-toxic activity. Kutkoside from *Picrorhiza kurroa* is a potential hepatoprotectant. *Phyllanthus amarus* is another most important plan selected for clinical trials. Antihepatotoxic activity of *Boerhavia diffusa* and *B. repanda* has been also reported. Kolaviron, a mixture of *Garcinia kola* (Guttiferae) biflavo-noids at a dose of 100 mg/kg i.p. prevented thioacetamide induced hepatotoxicity. *Withania*

fruitescens (Solanaceae) leaves exhibited protective and curative action against carbon tetrachloride induced liver toxicity.

Anti-cancer drugs

Cancer is a fatal disease affecting mankind in every country. Vinblastine was introduced in 1961 and vincristine as anticancer drugs. CIPLA has improved the process of isolating vinblastine and vincristine from *Catharanthus roseus*. Today we are the third largest manufacturer of vinblastine and vincristine in the world and we are exporting these alkaloids to European countries and the demand is steadily increasing.

Screening of plant extracts for anticancer activity started in 1961 by National Cancer Institute of the USA, and up to 1981 (20 years) about 1,14,045 plants had been screened, of which only 3.4% (representing about 3,400 different species) have been observed to be active in one or more bio-assay systems. The promising phytoconstituents include indicine N-oxide (a pyrrolizidine alkaloid) from *Heliotropium indicum*, ellipticine (a monomeric indole alkaloid) from several *Ochrosia* species, homoharringtonine (a cephalotaxine alkaloid) from *Cephalotaxus* species, taxol from *Taxus* species and camptothecine (quinoline alkaloid from *Camptotheca acuminata* a Chinese tree). The anti-cancer principles of podophyllum are contained in the resin, podophyllum resin or podophyllin. American podophyllum yields 2-8% and Indian podophyllum about 6-12% of the resin. It is not only the higher amount of the resin present in Indian podophyllum (*P. emodi* var. *hexandrum*) but there are no peltatins present in contrast to American podophyllum (*P. peltatum*) which contains α- and β-peltatins. Thus, the Indian podo-phyllum has higher amount of podophyllotoxin. In certain cases Indian podophyllum has yielded 20% resin. The higher amount is in May when the plant produces flowers. Thus the Indian podophyllum, when collected at the proper season not only contains 2½ times or even more of the resin compared to American podophyllum, but this resin has double the amount of podophyllotoxin which is the active principle used by pharmaceutical industry for structural modifications to produce anticancer drugs tenoposide and etoposide being marketed by

Sandoz. Major problem with the cultivation of this plant is that the seeds take very long time to germinate. Use of Taxol from *Taxus brevifolia* or *Taxus baccata* is the latest addition of anticancer drug especially in ovarian cancer.

Plants for urinary stones

Pashanbhed (*Rotula aquatica*) is used for uric acid calculi and Ashnibhed for biliary calculi. Decoction of Pashanbhed, Astimantaka, Satvari, Vrihati, Bhalluka, Varuna (*Crataeva nervala*), Kultha (*Dolichos biflorus*), kola and katak seeds for patients of Vataja Ashmari while Kusa, Ashmabhed, Patala, Tri-kanthaka, Sirisha, Punarnava (*Boerhavia diffusa*) and shilajit are for Pittaja Ashmari. About 4000 plants have been mentioned to be useful for dissolving stones in the urinary system. *Crataeva nervala* bark and *Tribulus terrestris* fruits have been put under clinical trials. *Cucumis trigonus* (Curcurbitaceae) has been investigated for its diuretic activity.

Plants as sedatives/tranquilizers

Indian valerian (*Valeriana wallichii*) contains 2% valepotriates and is thus four times more potent than European valerian (*V. officinalis*) which contains 0.5% valepotriates. These are triesters of poly-hydroxy cyclopentanopyran esterified with isovaleric, acetic and β-acetoxy valeric acids. Valtrates are used as tranquilizers and sedatives. Additional advantage is that these can be prescribed to alcoholic patients. Valerian also contains valernic acid having spasmolytic action. Valeranone is found in jatamansi (*Nardostachys jatamansi*) possessing sedative property.

Plant laxatives

Constipation is a common problem of Western and European countries because of protein rich diet. In the USA, 1,000 patents of vegetable origin are there which involves an annual trade of 500 million dollars. India exports 15,000 tons of plantago, 7,000 tons of senna and 1.000 tons of Rhubarb annually.

Plants for bronchial asthma

For bronchial asthma, lobeline from *Lobeliainflata* and ephedrine from Chinese plant Ma Huang (*Ephedra* species) were introduced in medicine in 1925. An infusion of the leaves of *Ammi visnaga* Lam. has been used in Egypt and neighbouring countries as a folk remedy for cough and colic. Its active principle was shown (1938) to be the furochromone - khellin, which is disodium chromoglycate marketed as an antiasthmatic drug under the trade name INTAL (Fisons) first in France (1969) and later in the USA (1973).

Antimalarial drugs

It is estimated that there are about 215 million people chronically affected by malaria and that each year there are some 150 million new cases. Most hard hit areas include Africa, India, China and the East Asia. A combination of resistance of *Plasmodium* species to antimalarial drug such as chloroquine, and the resistance of the vector mosquitoes to insecticides has resulted in malaria emerging as the world's most common tropical disease. Quinine has been used for many years as an antimalarial drug. In recent years clinicians have continued to use quinine because the resistance of *Plasmodium* strain is low when compared with other drugs.

The Chinese antimalarial drug artemisinin (Quinghausu) is a sesquiterpene lactone containing an endoperoxide moiety, which is a rare feature in natural products. Problems of low solubility in both organic and aqueous solvents have been overcome by the development of sodium dihydroartemisinin hydrogen succinate monoester. Over 2,000 malarial patients have been treated with artemisinin in China.

The Chinese use a number of other plants for the treatment of malaria, including *Dichroa febrifuga* (Saxifragaceae). Febrifugine, the active ingredient, has been used clinically against *P. vivax* and *P. ovale* and even though it causes liver damage, it is used as an antimalarial in Chinese traditional medicine.

Simaroubaceous plants are used as antimalarials in different parts of the world including Thailand (*Brucea javanica*), USA (*Castela nicholsoni*), British Honduras (*Picrasma antidesma*), Mexico (*Simaba cedron*) and India (*Ailanthus excelsa*).

The active principles are bitter substances. - quassinoids (simaroubolides). Bruceantin proved to be the most potent compound. The quassinoids without ester functions have little activity whereas those with ester functions at either C-15 or C-6 possess activity. Furthermore, activity has been demonstrated for quassinoids which possess the oxygen bridge from C-20 to C-11 (glaucarubinone) as well as for those compounds with the oxygen bridge from C-20 to C-13, e.g., bruceantin.

Plant bitters

Bitters constitute an important group of remedial agents. Quassinoids from Simaroubaceous plants, irridoid glycosides from *Swertia* and *Picrorhiza*, alkaloid quinine from Cinchona and andrographolide from *Andrographis paniculata* constitute some of the most important plant bitters having wide spectrum of biological activity.

Plant sweetners

Sucrose has a profound effect on the development of fatness, dental caries and other diseases. Since withdrawal of cyclamate, aspartmate and saccharin from the consumer's market in Japan and USA because of their toxicity, researches for new safe and economical sweetners is necessary. Leaves of *Stevia rebaudiana*, a wild herb of Paraguay, South America, has been used as a sweetening agent for tea and coffee by the natives because of the remarkable sweetness. Stevoside is the major glycoside (5-15% in the dried leaves) and is 100 times more sweet than sugar. Other glycoside - rebaudioside A-E and dulcoside A and B, reported from the leaves are also very sweet. Rebaudioside A and D are 150-200 times more than sugar, and are present in 3-4% concentration in the leaves. At present more than ten food industries in Japan are undertaking the production of *Stevia* glycosides as food additive, and the cultivation of this plant is widely carried out not only in Japan but also in the countries of South East Asia. No toxicity of *Stevia* glycosides has been reported so far. *Lippia dulcis* Trev. (Verbenaceae) yielded a volatile sweet principle - sesquiterpene hernadulcin, which is 1,000 times more sweet than sucrose. A climber *Dioscoreophyllum cuminsii* yielded from its fruit pulp a sweet protein named as Monellin which is 2,500 times more sweet than sucrose, and interestingly the seed inside the fruit contains very bitter substances like columbin and isocolumbin.

Another Nigerian plant, *Thaumatococcus danielli* (Marantaceae), has yielded from the aril of its fruit sweet proteins named as thaumatin I and II, and a patent preparation under the name of Talin which is 4,000 to 5,000 times more sweet than sucrose, and is commercially available.

Edible dyes

Annatoo plant native to tropical America and West Indies has been naturalised in India, and is found in central and southern India. It is very commonly used colour for all our dairy products like cheese and butter. We are exporting 3,000 tons of this dye to Russia every year.

As synthetic dyes are being banned in several countries slowly and slowly because of toxic effect, colouring material from plants like *Curcuma longa, Rubia cordifolia, Pterocarpus santalinus, Lawsonia inermis, Indigofera tinctoria* and *Beta vulgaris* are going to serve as basis for future development of dyes and colours. Herbal shampoos invariably incorporate saponin containing plants like *Acacia concinna* and *Sapindus mukorossi* which have not only cleansing but lice killing properties as well.

Mint/Menthol

Three decades ago we were importing menthol. Now Japanese mint, *Mentha arvensis*, is commercially cultivated, and 800 tons of menthol is being produced annually meeting not only our own requirements but meeting some export target as well.

Plants in perfumery and cosmetics

Rose oil from the flowers of *Rosa damascena* is used in cosmetics and to treat anxiety.

Demand of lavander oil in soap, perfumery and cosmetic industry is increasing. Patchouli oil is obtained from the leaves of *Pogostemon patchouli*. It is fixative in every perfume. Davana oil from the flowering plants of *Artemisia pallens* is used in food and flavour industries. About 5 tons of this oil is exported annually to USA and France.

Other disorders

Cannabis and Opium are used as analgesics and narcotics. Anthelmintic drugs include Artemisia, Chenopodium oil, Kapur kachari, Vidang, Male Fern. Ephedra, Lobella, and Sankhpushpi.

Turmeric, Punarnava, Aswagandha, Kapur kachari and Colchicum are used as anti-inflammatory drugs. Balsam Tolu, Benzoin, Camphor, Clove, Neem (*Azadirachta indica*), Eucalyptus, Myrrh, Mint, Tulsi, Turmeric and Pine oil are used as antiseptic drugs. Amla, Arjuna, Ashoka, Bahera, Black Catechu, Myrobalan and Tannic acid exhibit astringent action. Acacia, Honey, Isapgol, Aswagandha, Linseed, Sesame oil, Starch and Tragacanth have demulcent property while emollient action is exhibited by the drugs such as Arachis oil, Kokum butter, Lanolin, Linseed oil and Sesame. Ergot and Vasaka are reputed as oxytocic drugs. Coffee beans, Cocaine, Coriander, Dill, Ginger, Nux-vomica, Pipal, Rasna and Storax show stimulant action.

PUNARNAVA

Synonyms

Hog weed; Sant; Beshakapori (Hindi).

Biological source

Punarnava consists of the herb *Boerhavia diffusa* Linn. (Family : Nyctaginaceae).

Habitat

The plant is a weed found throughout India during rainy season.

Description

Stem is greenish-purple, stiff, slender, cylindrical, thickened at nodes, minutely pubescent or glabrous, prostrate or ascending, divertically branched. Leaves are opposite in unequal pairs; petiolate, ovate-oblong or suborbicular, apex is rounded or slightly pointed; base is subcordate or rounded. Lamina is green and glabrous above and whitish below, margin is entire or subundulate, turned up and pinkish in certain cases. Flowers are very small. Fruit is one-seeded nut, 6 mm long, clavate, 5-ribbed, glandular.

Chemical constituents

The active constituent is a mixture of alkaloids 'punarnavine'. Xanthine derivatives, ursolic acid, β-sitosterol, fatty acids such as stearic acid and arachidic acid, have been isolated from the drug. The plant also contains inorganic salts such as potassium nitrate, potassium sulphate and chlorides. A purine nucleoside, identified as hypoxanthine-

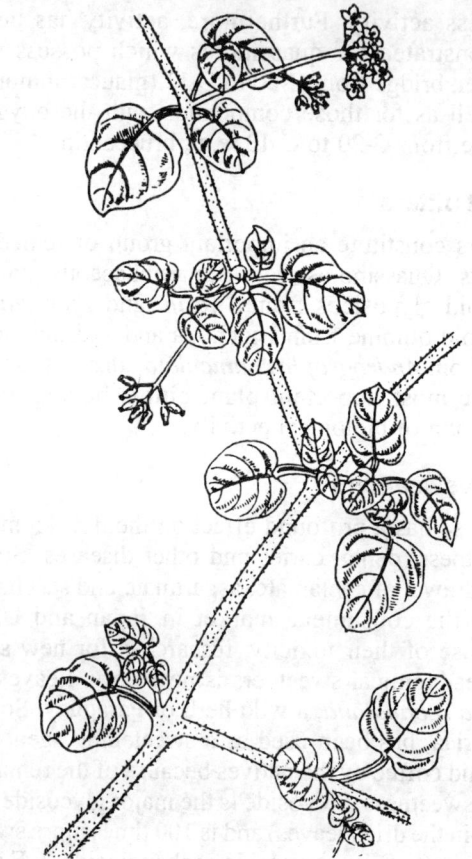

Fig. 22.1. *Boerhavia diffusa*—flowering and fruiting branch.

9-L-arabinofuranoside, a dihydroisofurano-xanthone (borhavine), C-methyl flavone, 6-O-ester of sitosteryl D-glucose, and rotenoid analogues like boeravinones A, B, C, D, E and F have been isolated from Punarnava.

The roots contain alkaloids (0.05%), triacontanol, hentriacontane, β-sitosterol, ursolic acid, 5,7-dihydroxy-3′,4′-dimethoxy-6,8-dimethyl flavone, glucose, fructose, sucrose, β-ecdysone and hypoxanthine-9-arabinoside. The roots also contain hentriacontane, β-sitosterol, ursolic acid, glycoprotein, purine nucleoside hypoxanthine-9-arabinofuranoside, punarnavoside, repenone, repenol, stigmosterol, campesterol, their glucosides, methyl esters of palmitic, heptadecylic, oleic, stearic, arachidic and behenic acids; iriodendrin, syringaresinol-β-D-glucoside, borhavine, irioden-

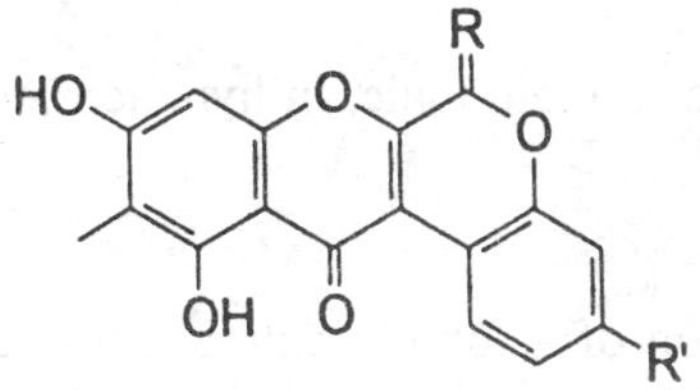

Boeravinone A
R = H, OMe, R′ = H
Boeravinone B
R = H, OH, R′ = H
Boeravinone D
R = H, OMe, R′ = OH
Boeravinone E
R = H, OH, R′ = OH
Boeravinone F
R = O, R′ = OH

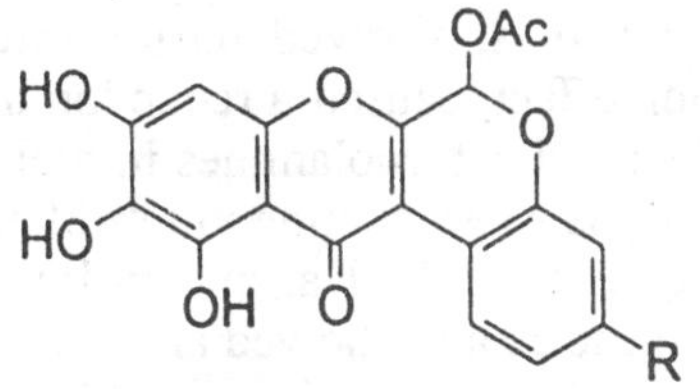

Reperone
R = H
Repenol
R = OH

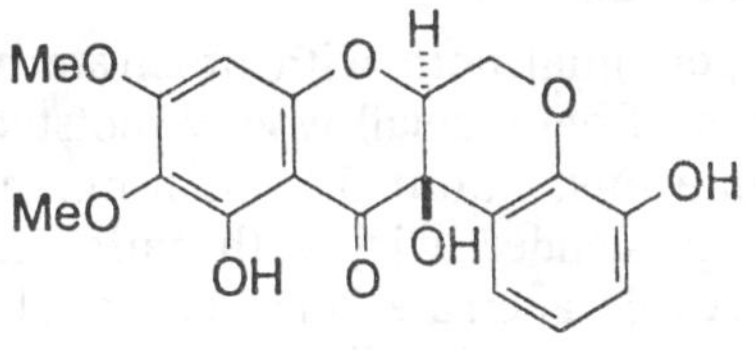

Boeravinone C

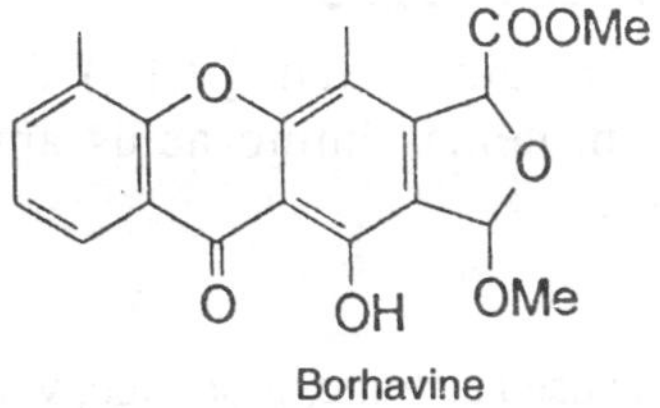

Borhavine

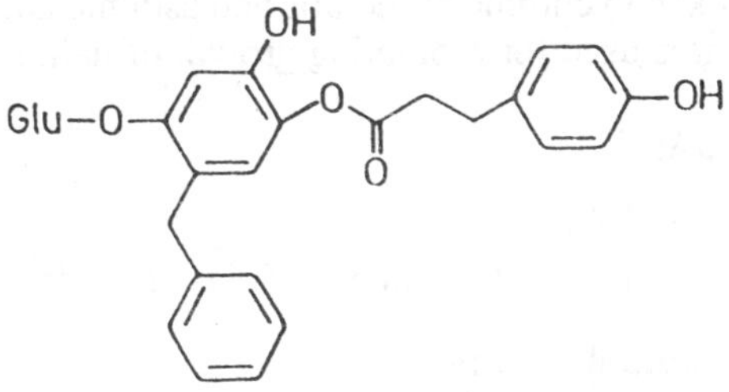

Punarnavoside

Fig. 22.2. Chemical constituents of *Boerhavia diffusa*.

drin, syringaresinol-β-D-glucoside and borhavine. The author has isolated boerhavisterol, boerha-

diffusene, boeravinone, diffusarotenoid and boerchavilanostenyl benzoate.

Uses

Punarnava is diuretic, useful in nephrotic syndrome, chronic oedema and liver diseases. The plant is used as a maintenance drug, in abdominal tumors and cancer. It also possesses anti-inflammatory, anti-bacterial and cardiotonic properties. The roots are credited with anti-convulsant, analgesic, laxative, diuretic and expectorant properties.

Adulterant

Punarnava is substituted with *Trianthema portulacastrum* (Family : Ficoidaceae), a prostrate weed, with branches up to 2 m long found in South India, Gujarat, Rajasthan and UP. Leaves are oblong, elliptic, the opposite pair somewhat unequal, flowers are dense and axillary. *T. portulacastrum* contains an alkaloid trianthemine, ecdysterone, 3, 4-dimethoxycinnamic acid and β-cyanin. The leaves are diuretic, used in oedema and dropsy and in cases of ascites especialy due to liver, peritoneal and kidney conditions.

Pharmacology

Glycoprotein was active against spherical and tubular viruses. Hypoxanthine-9-arabinofuranoside produced depressor and negative chronotropic effects in rats and cats and negative chronotropic and inotropic responses in guinea pig isolated atrial muscle. Punarnavoside stopped IUCD-associated bleeding episodes in rhesus monkey. Chloroform and methanolic extracts of roots and aerial parts exhibited hepato-protective activity in rats. Liriodendrin showed significant Ca^{2+} channel antagonistic effect in frog heart. Punarnava is effective in various eye diseases. An acetone extract of the roots showed anti-inflammatory activity. An alcoholic extract increased blood pressure in dogs and relaxant effect on rabbit ileum. Punarnava increased serum protein level and reduced urinary protein excretion in patients with nephrotic syndrome.

SHANKHPUSHPI

Biological source

Shankhpushpi consists of the whole aerial parts of *Convolvulus pluricaulis* Choisy (syn. *Convolvulus microphyllus* Sieb) and *Evolvulus alsinoides* Linn. (Family : Convolvulaceae).

Habitat

Both the plants grow widely in plains of India.

Convolvulus pluricaulis

Plant is a procumbent shrub. Stem is woody at the base, 10-30 cm long, leaves are 2.5-3 cm long, linear, oblong, villous on both sides, tapering at base, flowers are small, funnel shaped, light pink or white coloured; fruits are small, up to 2.5 mm long, glabrous, scarcely papillose.

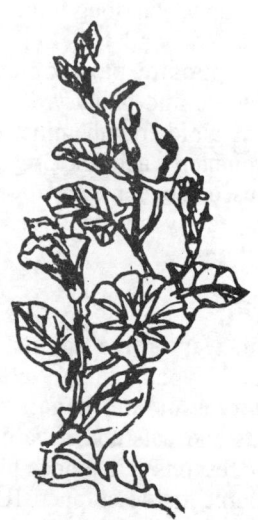

Fig. 14.3(a). Shankhpushpi : *Convolvulus pluricaulis.*

Chemical constituents

The drug contains an alkaloid known as 'shankh-pushpine', volatile oil, *n*-triacontane, higher fatty alcohols, kaempferol, its 3-D-glucoside, 2,3-dihydroxycinnamic acid, carbohydrates such as glucose, rhamnose, sucrose, starch, potassium chloride, 6-methoxy-7-hydroxycoumarin, maltose, β-sitosterol glucoside, 3,4-dihydroxycinnamic acid, *n*-octacosanol, *n*-triacontanol, β- and ε-sitosterols, convolvulusyl ester, convolvulosoic acid, octadeca-hydronaphthacenoic acid, cycloconvolvulusoic acid, convolvulusotrioic acid and cycloconvolvulusyl ester.

Uses

The drug is used as a brain tonic, in hypertension and as tranquilizer.

Pharmacology

An aqueous portion of alcoholic extract showed sedative action in rats; produced CNS mediated depression of amphibian and reduced the spontaneous motor activity of mice. The drug provided relief in anxiety neurosis, showed barbiturate hypnosis potentiation effect, caused a reduction in level of acetylcholine and catecholamines in brain tissues and provoked the sleeping time in rats after compression. Drug extract had a spasmolytic activity on smooth muscles and showed antifungal activity. It had hypotensive and cardiotonic effects.

Evolvulus alsinoides

It is a perennial herb with prostrate branching developing from a small woody rootstock. Stems are numerous, about 30 cm long, prostrate, spreading, slender, wiry with hairs. Leaves are simple, sessile, alternate, lanceolate to suborbicular. Flowers are light blue, solitary, peduncles very long, filiform and axillary. Fruit is a four angled capsule.

Chemical constituents

The herb contains betain [(CH$_3$) CH$_2$COOH⁻], evolvine, proteins, amino acids and phenolic compounds.

Uses

The plant is used as tonic, febrifuge, vermifuge and in dysentery. Cigarettes containing leaves are smoked in chronic bronchitis and asthma. Oil of the plant is used for promoting growth of hair.

VASAKA

Synonyms

Adhatoda, Vasaka folium, Adulase (Hindi).

Biological source

Vasaka consists of the fresh or dried leaves of *Adhatoda vasica* Nees. (Family : Acanthaceae).

Habitat

The plant is found throughout the plains of India, in

the sub-Himalayan tracts up to 13,00 m, Sri Lanka, Burma and Malaya.

It is an evergreen, gregarious, stiff, perennial shrub growing on waste lands. It can be raised from seeds or cuttings.

Characters

Leaves are entire when fresh and crumpled or broken when dried. Shape is lanceolate to ovate-lanceolate, margin is slightly crenate to entire; apex is acuminate, base tapering; petiole 2-8 cm long. The leaves are 10-30 cm long and 3-10 cm broad, venation is pinnate, midrib and 8-10 pairs of lateral veins, surface is glabrous or slightly pubescent, green when fresh, on drying the colour changes from brown to grey. Odour is characteristic and taste is bitter.

Chemical constituents

Vasaka leaves contains quinazoline alkaloids (0.25%) which include vasiçine, vasicinone, 6-hydroxyvascine, 1-peganine (1-vasicine), betaine, vasakin, vasicinol, 6-hydroxypeganine, vesicinine, vasicoline, adhatodine, vasicolinone, anisotine, 9-

acetamido-3,4-dihydropyrido [3,4-b]-indole, O-ethyl-α-D-galactoside, β-sitosterol-D-glucoside, galactose, deoxyvasicinone, 3'-hydroxy-4-glucosylchalcone, vasicinolone, 1,2,3,9-tetrahydro-5-methyl pyrrolo [2,1-b] quinazolin-3-ol, adhavasinone; lignins composed of guaiacyl-, syringyl- and p-hydroxyphenyl-propanes, deoxyvasicine, 37-hydroxyhexatetracont-1-en-15-one, 37-hydroxy hentetracontan-19-one, and 29-methyltriaconton-1-ol, volatile oil, fat, resin, sugar, mucilage, adhatodic acid, triacontane, β-sitosterol and vitamin C. The oil is golden yellow which contains limonene.

Uses

Vasaka is used to treat cold, cough, whooping cough, chronic bronchitis and asthma, as sedative, expectorant, antispasmodic and as anthelmintic. The drug is employed in different forms, such as fresh juice, decoction, infusion and powder; also given as alcoholic extract and liquid extract or syrup. The dried leaf is smoked as a cigarette. It is also given along with other expectorants, and forms a part of several proprietary compounds. The cough is relieved and the sputum is liquefied and is easily expelled. The leaf juice cures diarrhoea, dysentery and glandular tumor, and is given as emmenagogue.

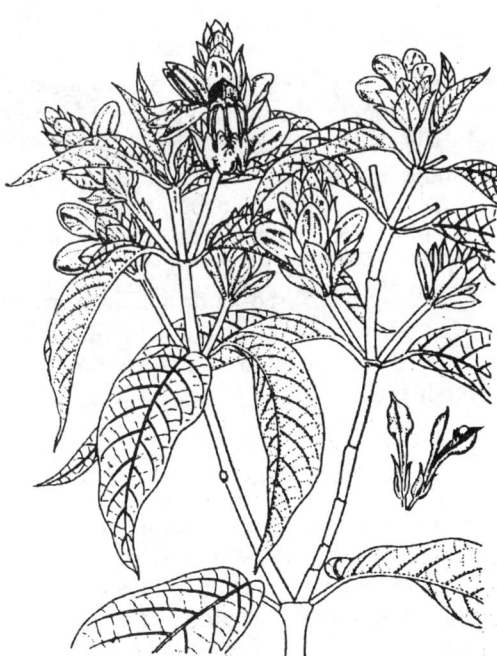

Fig. 22.3. *Adhatoda vasica*—flowering branch.

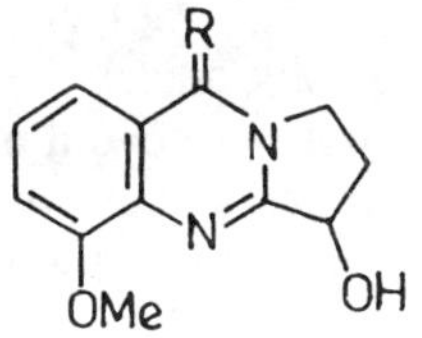

5-Methoxy-quinazoline-3-ol, R = H, H

Adhavasinone R = O

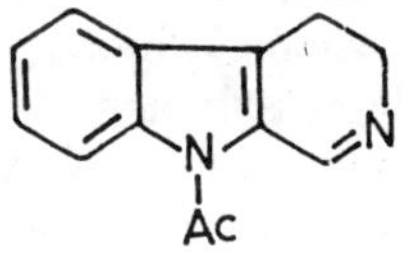

9-Acetamido-3,4-dihydro-pyrido [3,4-b]-indole

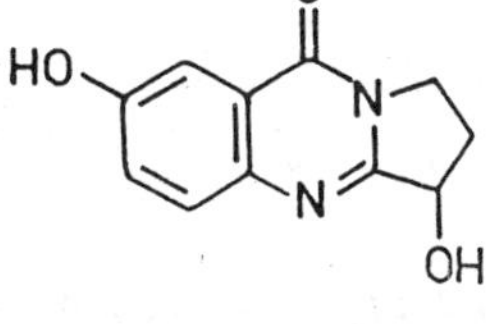

Vasicinolone

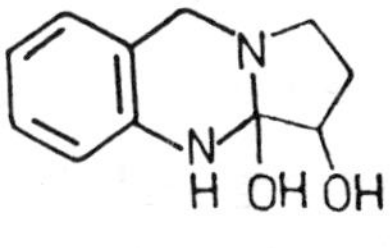

Vasicol

Fig. 22.4. Alkaloidal constituents of *Adhatoda vasica*.

The powder is used as poultice on rheumatic joints, as counter-irritant on inflammatory swellings, on fresh wounds, urticaria and in neuralgia.

The flowers and fruits are bitter and aromatic and their uses are similar to those of the leaves. The flowers are also given to improve the circulation of blood and in ophthalmia. They contain vasicine, vasicinine, β-sitosterol, an essential oil, colouring compounds luteolin, quercetin and kaempferol, α-amyrin and tritriacontane.

Pharmacology

L-Vasicine showed relaxation in a dose-dependent manner and uterotonic activity similar to that of oxytocin and methylergometrine. It exhibited bronchodilatory activity similar that of theophylline. Vasicinone showed bronchodilation *in vitro* and bronchoconstriction *in vivo*. Vasicine exhibited respiratory and uterine stimulant activity and moderate hypotensive activity. It has abortifacient effect in guinea pig.

Vasicine and Vasicinone show bronchodilatory activity comparable to that of theophylline and an individual alkaloid exerts greater activity. Vasicine and vasicinone are devoid of any anti-asthmatic activity but a minor alkaloid vasicinol (inhalative) exhibits significant activity. Brom-hexine and its derivatives also possess expectorant activity. Vasicine exhibits moderate hypotensive and cardiac depressant activities while vasicinone is devoid of these activities. Vasicine possesses strong and extremely selective uterine stimulant activity and is a promising uterotonic abortificient. It is also useful for the control of postpartum haemorrhage. The drug also shows antifungal, juvenomimetic, antifeedant, insecticidal and repellent activities. It possesses antiinflammatory properties and is effective in gingival inflammation and pyorrhoea.

PIPER LONGUM

Synonyms

Piplamul, Pippali.

Biological source

The drug consists of transversely cut pieces of roots or underground stems or of fruits of *Piper longum* Linn. (Family : Piperaceae).

Habitat

The plant is native of Phillipine and found in hotter parts of India, Sri Lanka and Malaya.

The plant is a slender aromatic climber with perennial woody roots.

Pepper is a crop of the wet tropics and is propagated from cuttings (Sarawak) or runners (India). However, it is infected to various diseases which are transmitted by vegetative propagation.

The vines are grown on poles or trees. The inflorescence is a spike of about 20-30 sessile flowers, which grows into sessile fruits. The latter are picked when the lower fruits of the spike turn red. They are then removed from the axis and dried in the open air or by artificial heat. The fire-dried spice is most esteemed.

P. longum is cultivated on a larger scale in limestone soil by layering of mature branches or by suckers planted at the beginning of the rainy season. The vines are well manured with cow dung cake and start bearing fruits 3 or 4 years after planting. The spices are harvested in January, while still green and unripe, as they are most pungent at this stage. They are dried in the sun when they turn grey. The roots and thicker parts of stem are cut and dried.

Description

Drug occurs in pieces, 0.5 to 2.5 cm long and 2-7 mm in diameter; shape is cylindrical, straight or slightly curved and some with distinct swollen internodes, showing a number of leaf rootlets and scars. Colour is light brown, odour is characteristic, taste is bitter and pungent producing numbness on the tongue.

Fruits are also used as drug. They are small, ovoid, yellowish-orange, sunk in fleshy spikes which is 2.5-3.8 cm, ovoid long, erect, blunt, blackish-green; odour is aromatic and taste is pungent.

Chemical constituents

Both roots and fruits have alkaloids like piperine, piperlonguminine, piplartine and piperlongumine. Fruits also contain volatile oil, resin, a waxy alkaloid N-isobutyl 2,4-decadienamide and sesamine.

Pepper contains 1-2.5% of volatile oil, 5-9% of the crystalline alkaloids piperine and piperettine and

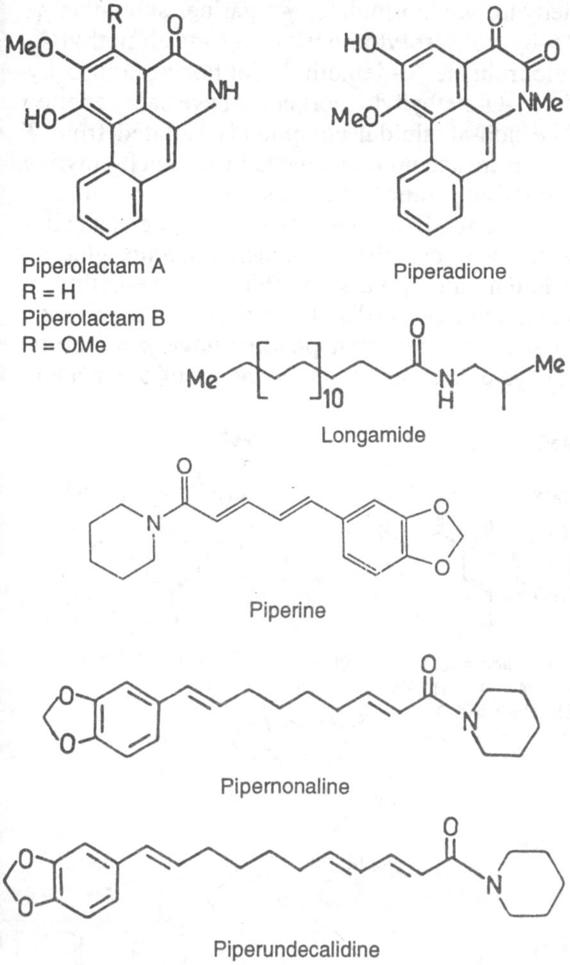

Piperolactam A
R = H
Piperolactam B
R = OMe

Piperadione

Longamide

Piperine

Pipernonaline

Piperundecalidine

Fig. 22.5. Alkaloidal constituents of *Piper longum*.

a resin. The aroma of the spice is due to the volatile oil, which consists largely of terpenes (α- and β-pinene, phellandrene, dipentene and sesquiterpenes). The pungency is due to piperine and the resin. Piperine, $C_{17}H_{19}O_3N$, is also found in the long pepper (1-2%) and in Ashanti pepper, the fruits of *Piper guineense*.

The other constituents of the drug are triacontane, dihydrostigmasterol, reducing sugars, anisotine, vasicinol, deoxyvasicine, steroidal compound vasakin, bromohexine and its derivatives like BR-227, β-sitosterol, methyl-3,4,5-trimethoxy-cinnamate, pipernonaline, piperundecalidine, piperolactams A and B, piperadione, aristolactam

A, cepharadiones A and B, cepharanone B, nor-cepharadione B, 2-hydroxy-1-methoxy-4H-di-benzo [d, g]-quinoline-4,5-(6H)-dione, longamide, guineensine, pluviatilol and methyl pluviatilol. The total alkaloidal and vasicine content is found to be highest (2.20% and 2.09%) in August and lowest (0.70 and 0.35) in February. Vasicine is bitter and gets racemized during the isolation process.

Uses

Both Piplamul and fruits are used for diseases of respiratory tract like cough, bronchitis, asthma, cold and gonorrhoea; as counter-irritant and analgesic when applied locally for muscular pain and inflammation; internally as carminative, sedative and general tonic.

Pharmacology

Piperlonguminine showed insecticidal activity against *Musca domestica*.

Allied drug

Cubebs or tailed pepper are the dried, full-grown fruits of *Piper cubeba*, a native of Indonesia, Borneo and Sumatra. The fruits are collected while green and dried in the sun. The spikes of cubebs bear more fruits than those of pepper. The upper part of the cubeb fruit is globular, 3-6 mm diameter and covered with a greyish-brown, reticulated pericarp, which is prolonged at the base into a straight stalk. Cubebs yield 10-18% of volatile oil containing monoterpenes and sesquiterpenes, (–)-cubebin, lignans, a white amorphous substance cubebic acid (1%), and amorphous resin (3%).

TYLOPHORA

Synonym

Anantmul.

Biological source

The drug consists of dried leaves of *Tylophora Indica* (Burm f.) Merr (syn. *T. asthmatica* W. et A.), (Family : Asclepiadaceae).

Habitat

The plant is a perennial branching climber with long fleshy roots. It grows widely in planes and hilly

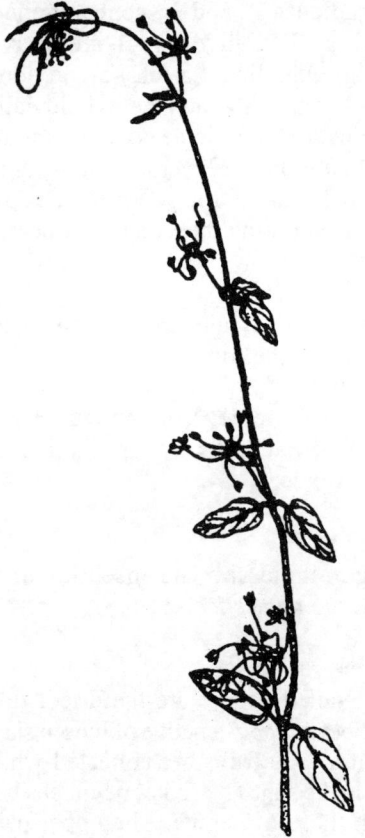

Fig. 22.6. *Tylophora indica* (Burm. f) Merr.

dehydrotylophorinidine, γ-fagarine, skimmianine, 14-hydroxyisotylocrebrine, 4,6-desdimethyliso-tylocrebrine, 6-demethyltylophorine and 5-hy-droxy-O-methyltylophorinidine have been reported. The non-alkaloidal compounds isolated from *T. indica* are kaempferol, quercetin, α- and β-amyrins, tetratriacontanol, octacosanyl octacosanoate, stigmasterol, β-sitosterol, tyloindane, cetyl alcohol, wax, resin, coutchone, pigments, tannin, glucose, calcium salts, potassium chloride, quercetin and kaempferol. Steam distillation of an alcoholic extract of the air-dried root powder gave *p*-methoxy-salicyaldehyde and a small amount of oily matter.

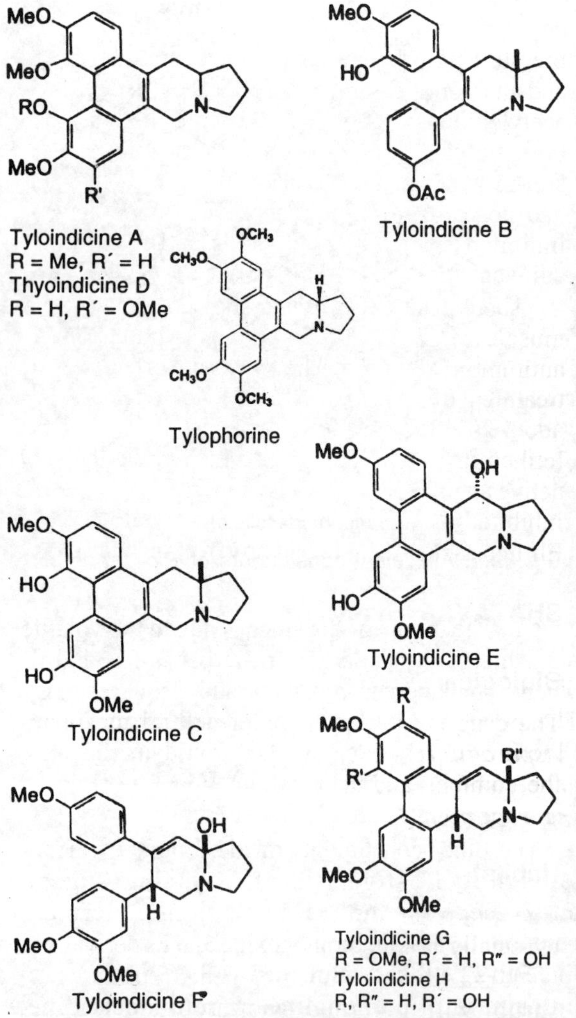

Tyloindicine A
R = Me, R′ = H
Thyoindicine D
R = H, R′ = OMe

Tyloindicine B

Tylophorine

Tyloindicine C

Tyloindicine E

Tyloindicine F

Tyloindicine G
R = OMe, R′ = H, R″ = OH
Tyloindicine H
R, R″ = H, R′ = OH

Fig. 22.7. Alkaloidal constituents of *Tylophora indica*.

places of India up to an altitude of 1,000 m in Bengal, Assam, Cachar, Orissa and southern India.

Characters

Leaves are 5-10 cm long, 2.5-5.7 cm wide, ovate or elliptic-oblong, acute or acuminate, often apiculate, glabrous, pubescent beneath, base usually cordate, petioles 6-13 mm long. The whole plant is of a pale yellow brown in colour and has no marked odour but has a sweetish and subsequent acrid taste.

Chemical constituents

The active constituents of *Tylophora indica* are phenanthroindolizidine alkaloids like tylophorine, tylophorinine, tylophorinidine and septicine. Recently some rare alkaloids, namely tyloindicines A, B, C, D, E, F, G, H, I and J, desmethyl-tylophorine, desmethyl tylophorinine, isotylocre-brine, anhydrodehydrotylophorinine, anhydro-

Uses

The dried leaves are emetic, diaphoretic and expectorant, useful in over-loaded states of the stomach, in dysentery and catarrh. The roots possess stimulant, emetic, cathartic, expectorant, stomachic and diaphoretic properties and are used in the treatment of asthma, bronchitis, whooping cough, dysentery and diarrhoea. They are recommended in rheumatic and gouty pains. They possess bacteriostatic properties and are good natural preservative for foods.

Pharmacology

Alcoholic extract and total alkaloids produced CNS depression, myocardial depression, fall of blood pressure, non-specific relaxation of smooth muscles and antagonized contractile effects of histamine and acetylcholine. Tylophorine caused CNS depression, potentiated pentobarbital sleep-ing time, showed anti-inflammatory effect in rat hind paw oedema and had no cardiovascular effects in frogs or dogs. It inhibited systemic anaphylaxis and responses of adjuvant-induced arthritis in rats.

The extract of *T. indica* showed good smooth-muscle relaxant, antihistamine, hypotensive and antitumour activities. The leaves are effective in the treatment of bronchial asthma. Tylocrebrine showed about 50% increase in life span against the L 1210 leukemia in mice. Tylophorine was marginally active against the L 1210 leukemia. These alkaloids inhibited protein synthesis in eukaryotic cells and Ehrlich ascites cell but had no effect on nucleic acid.

SHATAVAR (Shatavari)

Biological source

The drug is derived from dried tuberous roots of *Asparagus racemosus* Willd. It has been found that the commercial 'Shatawar' may not be the root of *A. racemosus* (Family : Liliaceae).

Habitat

The plant is a climber found all over India, especially in northern region.

It is a scandent, much-branched, spinous undershrub, with tuberous, short root-stock bearing numerous fusiform, succulant tuberous roots. Stem is woody, whitish grey or brown armed with strong, straight or recurved spines.

The plants can be grown successfully in black cotton soil mixed with river sand. They can be propagated from adventitious roots which are dipped in liquid cow dung for 24 hours before planting. The sprouted saplings are transferred to beds. They require hoeing and weeding during the rainy season.

Macroscopy

The roots of *A. racemosus* are borne in a compact bunch and are fleshy and spindle shaped. They are silvery white or light ash-coloured externally and white internally, smooth when fresh. The roots are peeled, dried, cylindrical, fleshy tuberous, straight or slightly curved, tapering towards the base and swollen in the middle; white to buff in colour, length 5-10 cm; diameter 1-2 cm; fracture is irregular; longitudinal furrows and minute transverse wrinkles on upper surface. Drug is hard, swells in water; taste is bitter; lack a well-marked odour.

Chemical constituents

The active constituents are steroidal saponins, *viz.*, shatavarin I-IV (0.1-0.2%). The aglycone unit is sarsapogenin. In shatavarin I three glucose and

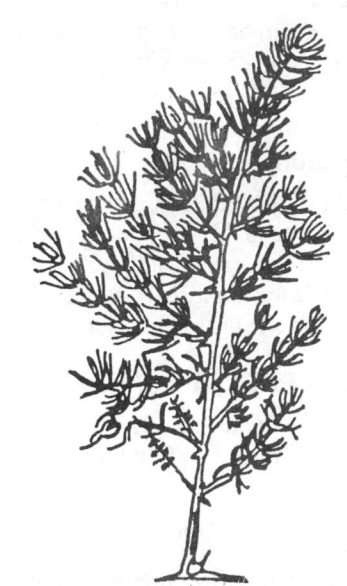

Fig. 22.8. Shatavar, *Asparagus racemosus.*

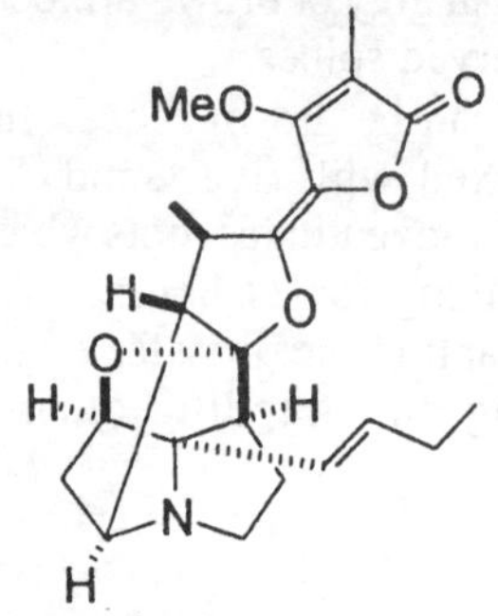

Fig. 22.9. Asparagamine A.

rhamnose molecules are attached whereas shatavarin IV possesses two glucose and one rhamnose molecules. The other compounds isolated from *A. racemosus* are β-sitosterol, stigmasterol, their glycosides, sarsasapogenin, spirostanolic acid, furostanolic saponins, 4,6-dihydroxy-2-O-(2'-hydroxyisobutyl) benzaldehyde, undecanyl cetanoate and polycyclic alkaloid asparagamine A.

Uses

Roots are refrigerant, demulcent, aphrodisiac, antiseptic, alterative, antidysenteric and galactagogue. Shatavarin I has antioxytocic property. In Ayurveda Shatavar is used to cure threatened abortion and safe delivery. Root powder relieve most of the symptoms in patients with duodenal ulcers. It did not exhibit antacid activity.

GOKHRU

Biological source

In Ayurveda two types of Gokhru are used. The smaller or Chhota Gokhru is the dried ripe seeds of *Tribulus terrestris* Linn. (Family : Zygophyllaceae). The large or Bara Gokhru consists of dried ripe fruits of *Pedalium murex* Linn. (Fam. Pedaliaceae).

TRIBULUS TERRESTRIS (Chhota gokhru)

The plant is an annual, prostrate herb with yellow flowers growing throughout India up to 3,600 m in Kashmir.

Morphology

The fruits are yellowish globose, diameter nearly 1.2 cm, containing five woody, densely hairy, spiny

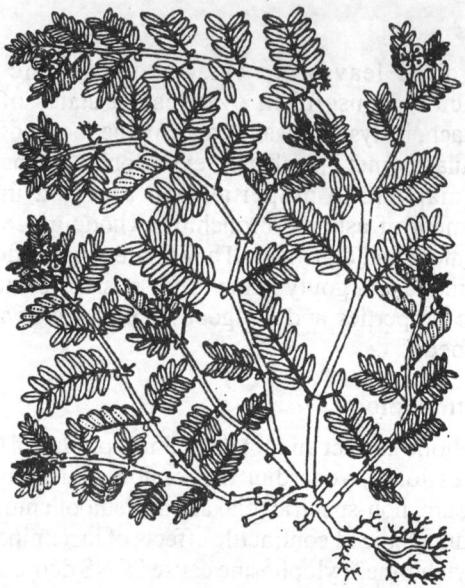

Fig. 22.10. *Tribulus terrestris.*

cocci. Each coccus possesses two large sharp, pointed spines directed towards the apex. The other two smaller shorter spines are directed downwards. Each coccus contain several seeds.

Chemical constituents

The fruits of *T. terrestris* contain saponins which produce diosgenin, ruscogenin and gitogenin on hydrolysis. The fruits also contain flavone glycosides, *viz.*, kaempferol 3-rhamnoside and kaemp-ferol 6"-p-coumaroyl 3-D-glucoside; traces

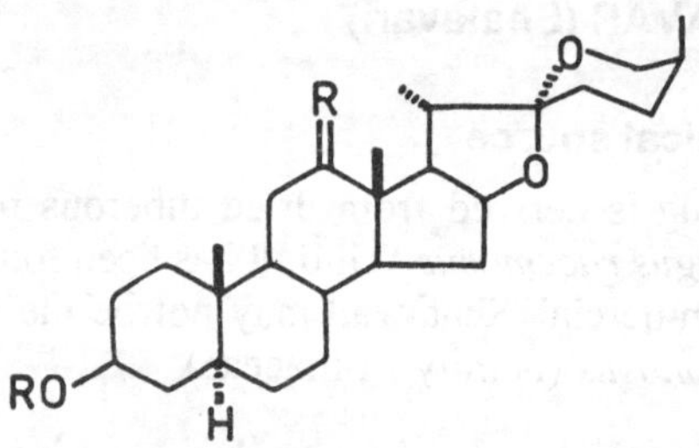

Tribulosin
R = Gal[2→1)Rha](4→1)Glu[2→1)Xyl](3→1)Xyl, R´ = H,H
Neohecogenin glucoside
R = Glu, R´ = O

Fig. 22.11. Chemical constituents of *Tribulus terrestris.*

of alkaloid, fixed oil, potassium nitrate, essential oil and resin.

The other compounds isolated from the drug are chlorogenin, kaempferol 3-rutinoside, campesterol, β-sitosterol, stigmasterol, neotigogenin, terrestroside F, saponins C and G, trillin, gracillin, dioscin, hecogenin, neohecogenin glucoside, tribulosin, quercetin glycosides, isorhamnetin glycosides, ticogenin, ruscogenin, spirosta-3,5-diene, 7-methyl hydroindanone, cinnamic amide, terrestriamide, alkaloids harmine, harmalin, tetrahydroharmine, phenanthrodode-canone, tetradecanyl ester and tribulusyl ester.

Uses

The fruit has cooling, diuretic, tonic, aphrodisiac properties and is used in painful micturition, calculus affections, urinary discharges and impotency. In the form of infusion it is useful as a diuretic in gout, kidney diseases and gravel.

Pharmacology

The plant extract showed marked CNS stimulant activity and reversed urinary oxalate excretion to normal in rats. An ethanolic extract of fruits showed activity against urolithiasis in rats. Simultaneous administration of *T. terrestris* and gentamycin to female rats decreased gentamycin induced renal damage. Leaf saponins are useful as an antisclerotic agent. Ethanolic extract showed antimicrobial activity against *Esch. coli*.

PEDALIUM MUREX (Bara Gokhru)

Pedalium murex is an annual succulent herb found near seacoasts of Kathiawar, Gujarat, Konkan, Southern Peninsula, Sri Lanka and Africa. It is also found in Rajasthan, Punjab and Delhi in autumn session.

The plant is annual, diffuse, succulent herb. The fruits are four-sided, about 2 cm long, pyramido-voidal shape and tapering at the base and apex. Each fruit has four spines and it tapers into a hollow cylindrical tube at the base.

The leaves contain pedalitin (3',4',5,6-tetra-hydroxy-7-methoxyflavone), diosmetin and dinatin.

The fruits possess amino acids, heptatriacont-4-one, hexatriacontanoic, hentriacontanoic and ursolic acids, pentatriacontane, β-sitosterol, its glucoside, vanillin, 5,7-dimethoxy-2',4',5'-tri-hydroxyflavone, triacontanyl dotriacontanoate, luteolin, rubusic acid, nonacosane, tritriacontane, triacontanoic acid and tritriacontanoic acid.

The fruits have demulcent, diuretic, antiseptic, aphrodisiac and tonic properties and given for incontinence of urine, spermatorrhoea, nocturnal emission, dysuria, gonorrhoea and impotency.

BRAHMI

Synonyms

Indian pennywort; Mandooki.

Biological source

Brahmi is the fresh or dried herb of *Centella asiatica* (L.) Urban (syn. *Hydrocotyle asiatica* Linn.) (Family : Apiaceae) and *Bacopa monnieri* (L.) Pennell (Family : Scrophulariaceae).

Habitat

The plant is found throughout India in marshy places up to 2,000 m; in Pakistan, Sri Lanka and Madagascar.

Morphology

It is herbaceous creeping herb with long prostrate reddish stem possessing long internodes and rooting at the nodes. Leaves are reniform or orbicular arising

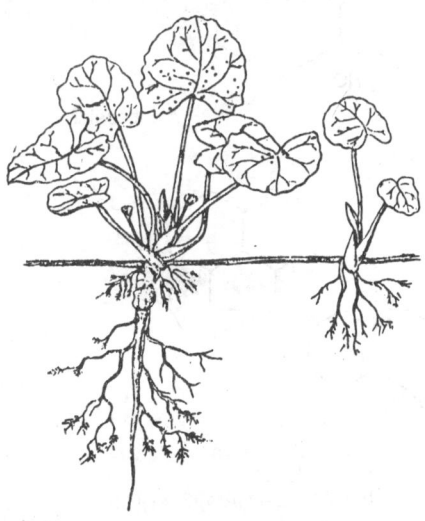

Fig. 22.12. *Centella asiatica* (Brahmi).

from each node of the stem, cupped, entire, crenate, glabrous on both sides; petioles are 7.5-15 cm long, channelled, stipules short, sheathing base. Flowers are pink, sessile, umbel consisting of 3-4 flowers.

Chemical constituents

The drug contains triterpenoid saponin glycosides called oxyasiaticoside, brahmoside, brahminoside and thankuniside. Sugar moieties are attached at carboxylic group. Hydrolysis of asiaticoside affords two molecules of glucose, one rhamnose and the aglycone asiatic acid. In addition to these the drug contains alkaloids, sterols (β-sitosterol, stigmasterol), tannins, amino acids (aspartic acid, glycine, glutamic acid, α-alanine and phenylalanine), and inorganic salts (chloride, sulphate, phosphate, iron, calcium, magnesium, sodium and potassium). Triterpenes reported in free state are brahmic acid, isobrahmic acid, betulic acid, indocentoic acid and asiatic acid. Mesoinositol and centellose have also been reported. A triterpenic acid, medasiatic acid, isolated from Brahmi, has been identified as 2α, 3β, 6β-trihydroxyurs-12-enoic acid.

C. asiatica also contains thankunic acid, asiatic acid, isothankunic acid, polyacetylenes I-V, asiacosides A and B, madecassoside, madecassic acid, isothankuniside (isothankunic acid gluco-rhamnoside), 3-glucosylquercetin, 3-glucosyl kaempferol and 7-glucosyl kaempferol.

The mono- and sesquiterpenes reported from *C. asiatica* are α-pinene, β-pinene, myrcene, γ-terpinene, bornyl acetate, α-copaene, β-elemene, β-caryophyllene, *trans*-β-farnesene, germacrene-D and bicycloelemene. Some polyacetylenes reported from the plant are pentadeca-2,9-diene-4,6-diyn-1-ol acetate, 3,8-diacetoxypentadeca-1,9-diene-4,6-diyne, 3-hydroxy-8-acetoxy-pentadeca-1,9-diene-4,6-diyne, 3-hydroxy-10-acetoxy-pentadeca-1,8-diene-4,6-diyne and pentadeca-1,8-diene-4,6-diyne-3,10-diol.

Uses

The plant has been used in diseases of skin, nerves and blood. Leaves are taken as tonic and for improving memory and useful in syphilitic skin diseases.

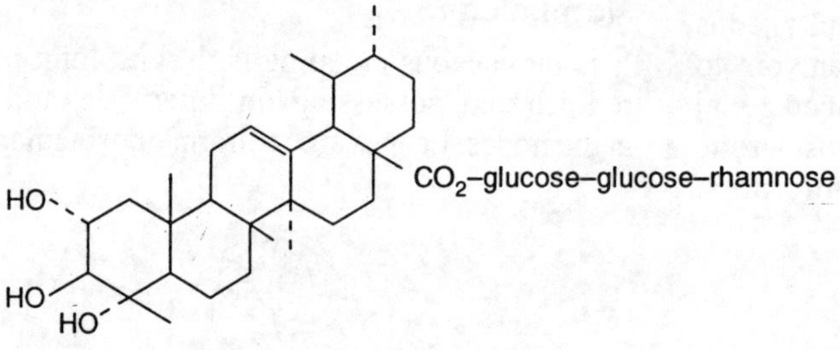

Asiaticoside

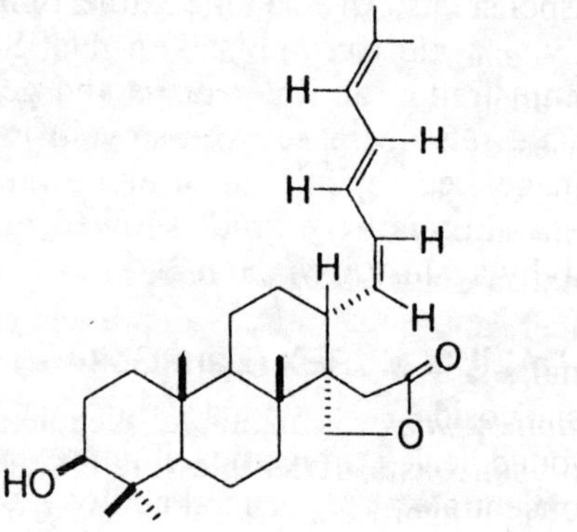

Cis-ebelin lactone

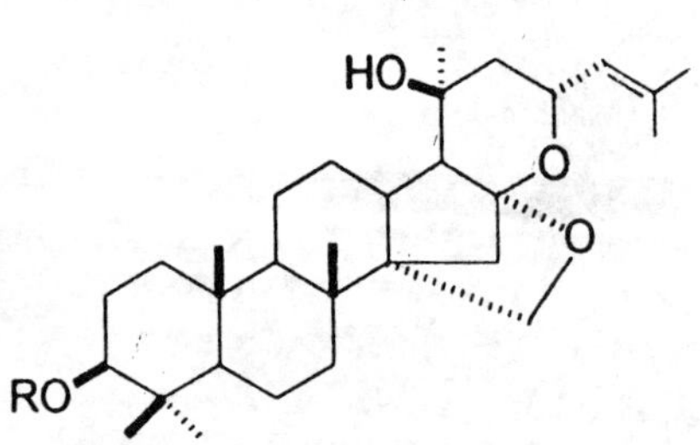

Barcoside A1
R = Ara(3→1)Ara
Bacoside A3
R = Glu[(2→1)Ara](3→1)Glu

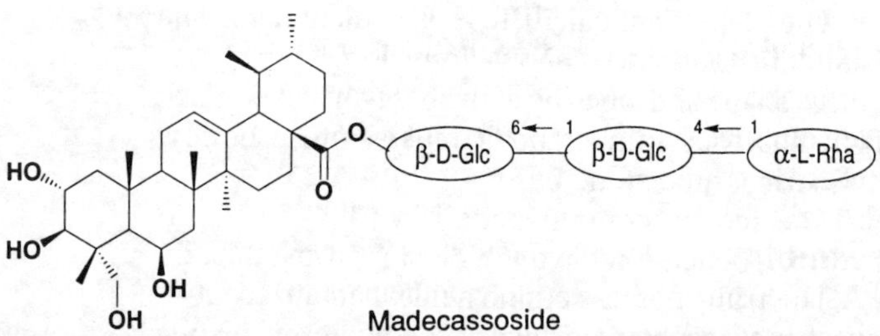

Madecassoside

Fig. 22.13. Chemical constituents of Brahmi.

Pharmacology

The plant extract showed a healing effect when applied locally to wounds or administered orally to rats. Intramuscular injection of asiaticoside into animal provoked a rapid thickening of the skin, and increases vascularization of the connective tissues, mucous secretion and hair and nail growth. Subcutaneous injection of asiaticoside to mice and rabbits increases bleeding time and haemorrhage. Addition of the total triterpene fraction of *C. asiatica* to the culture medium of human embryo fibroblasts did not influence the growth rate. It stimulated the incorporation of proline and synthesis of hyaluronic acid and chondroitin. Plant tablets showed significant increase in both general debility and behavioural pattern in mentally retarded children. Asiaticoside prevented development of cold-induced gastric ulcers in rats. Alcoholic extract produced significant changes in neurochemistry of brain and showed varying degree of sedation in mice. It reduced amphetoxicity and produces hypothermia. Total glycoside fraction of the plant produced significant plasma corticosterone levels response.

Centella asiatica is a reputed medicinal herb for its adaptogenic property and is recommended in cases of skin diseases, ulcers and for improving memory span and intelligence (brain tonic). The aqueous and alcoholic extracts of the plant show good antianxiety, antistress, antispasmodic, antiulcer, antifertility, CNS depressant and narcotic-analgesic properties. Clinically, the extract and asiaticoside possess good antiulcer, antileproitic and wound healing properties. It improves the power of concentration and general ability and behaviour of mentally retarded children. Madecassoside and madecassoic acid exert anti-inflammatory and wound healing properties while isothakunoside exhibits antifertility action. Patients treated with the drug show improvement in varicose veins and other leg circulation problems. The aqueous extract of the plant exhibits immunomodulatory activity. In Brazil, the drug is used for uterine cancer. Saponins exhibited sedative action in mice and rats. Asiaticoside prevented development of cold-induced gastric ulcers in rats and promoted wound healing. Alcoholic extract produced significant changes in neurochemistry of brain, showed anticonvulsant and sedative effects in mice, reduced amphetoxicity and produced hypothermia. Total glycosidal fraction of the plant exhibited antistress activity in rats.

BACOPA

Herb of *Bacopa monnieri* (L.) Pennell (syn. *Herpestis monniera* (L.) H.B. et K. or *Moniera cuneifolia* Michx) is also used as Brahmi. (Fam. Scrophulariaceae). The plant is found in wet, marshy and damp places throughout India and, therefore, known as Jalbrahmi or Nirbrahmi. It is a succulent, creeping herb with 10-20 cm long stem and rooting at nodes. It produces numerous branches and sessile, decussate leaves, 0.6-2.5 cm long, obovate and oblong.

The drug contains alkaloids brahmine and herpestine, D-mannitol and saponins, bacosides A and B. The saponins on hydrolysis yield the same triterpenoid aglycone bacogenin A and sugars arabinose and glucose. It also contains betulinic acid, stigmastenol, β-sitosterol, saponins monnierin, bacosides A_1 and A_3; nicotinic acid, nicotine, 3-formyl-4-hydroxy-2H-pyran, luteolin, its 7-glucoside, bacogenins A_1, A_2, A_3, A_4, apigenin-7-glucuronide and luteolin-7-glucuronide.

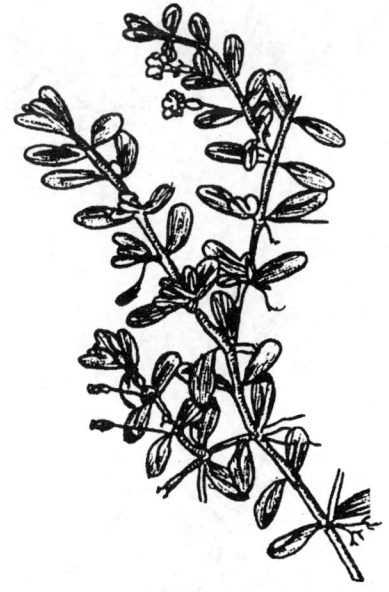

Fig. 22.14. *Bacopa monnieri.*

The plant is used as nervine tonic, diuretic and aperient and to treat asthma, epilepsy, insanity and hoarseness.

Pharmacology

Total alkaloidal fraction produced spasm of the skeletal muscle, stimulated respiration followed by depression and autonomic ganglia followed by blockade; showed tachyphylaxis and produced rigidity and convulsion in mice. It had tranquillizing property. Plant extract showed significant barbiturate hypnosis potentiation in rats. Saponins showed changes in locomotor activity and learning behaviour of normal rats. Drug-treated animals showed better acquisition, improved retention and delayed extinction. Plant extract brought about reduction of level of anxiety, adjustment, disability and leading to improved mental function.

ARJUNA BARK

Synonyms

Arjuna (Sans.); Arjun (H).

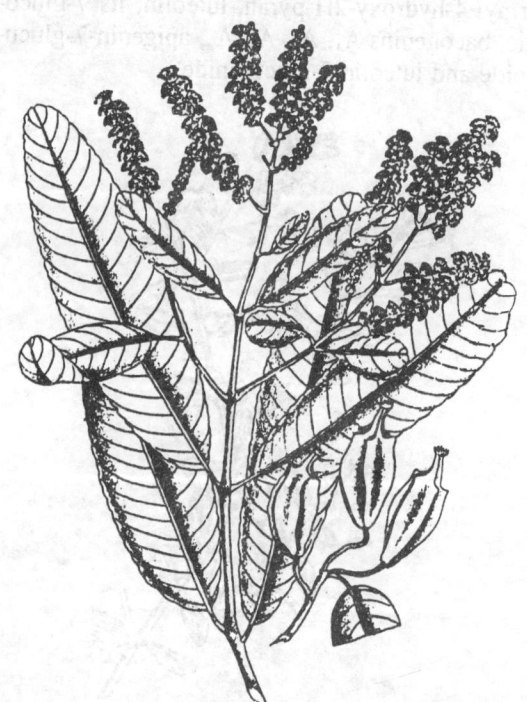

Fig. 22.15. *Terminalia arjuna* branch.

Biological source

Arjuna bark is the dried bark of *Terminalia arjuna* W. et A. (Family : Combretaceae).

Habitat

The plant is found throughout India.

Arjuna is a large deciduous evergreen tree, 20-30 meters in height. Bark is collected and dried. It occurs in flat pieces of various sizes, 3-15 cm long, 1-10 cm wide, 3 mm-1 cm thick; outer surface is smooth and grey-coloured; inner surface is striated and brown; fracture is short and fibrous; odourless, taste is astringent.

Chemical constituents

Arjuna bark contains tannins (12%), β-sitosterol, triterpenoid saponins, arjunine, arjunetin, arjunolic acid, essential oil, reducing sugars, calcium salts and traces of aluminium and magnesium salts.

The other compounds isolated from the bark are tomentosic acid, ellagic acid, (+)-leucodelphinidin, arjunic acid, arjungenin, arjunglucoside I and II, 5,7,2',4'-tetramethoxy flavone, compounds A and B, (+)-catechol, (+)-gallocatechol, epicatechol, epigallocatechol, arjunolone, baicalein, arjunglucoside III, arjunosides I, II, III and IV, terminoic acid and arjunolitin.

Uses

Arjuna bark is used as tonic, astringent, in heart diseases as a cardiac tonic, bilious affections, for sores and as an antidote to poisons. It has styptic, diuretic, febrifugal and anti-dysenteric properties. The bark gives relief in hypertension.

CHIRATA

Synonyms

Chiretta; Chirayita; Bitter stick; East Indian Balmony.

Biological source

Chirata is the entire dried plant of *Swertia chirata* Buch.-Ham. collected during formation of capsules. It should contain about 1.3 per cent bitter principles, (Family : Gentianaceae).

Habitat

The plant is found in temperate Himalayan region,

HO,,

Glu-O

COO—Glu

—OH

Arjunolitin

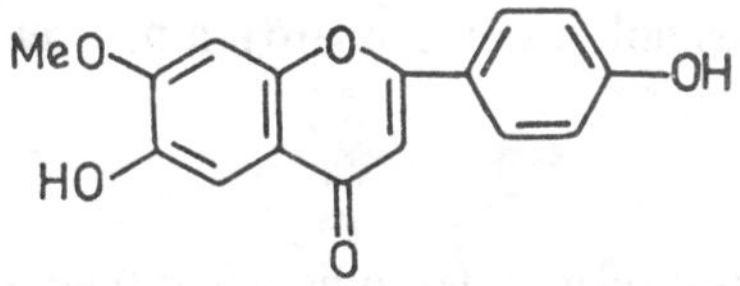

MeO

HO

O

OH

Arjunolone

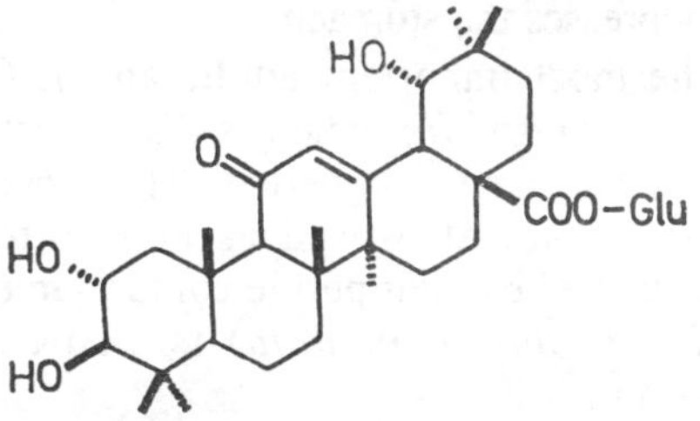

HO,,

O

HO,,

HO

COO—Glu

Arjunglucoside III

MeO

OMe

OMe O

OMe

Arjunone

HO,,

HO,,

RO

COOR'

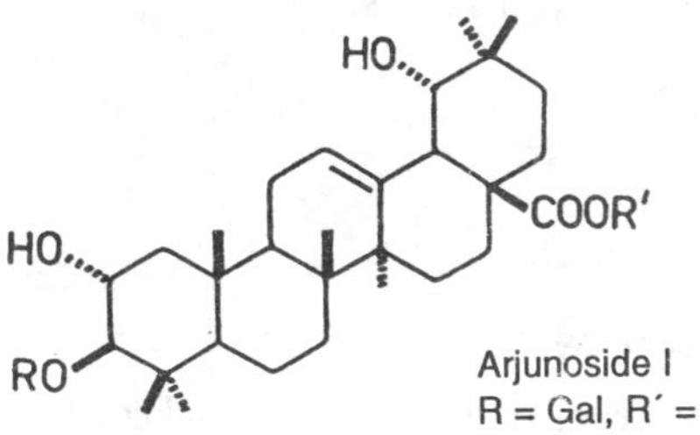

Arjunoside I
R = Gal, R´ = H
Arjunoside II
R = Glu-2-Deoxyrha, R´ = H
Arjunoside III
R = H, R´ = Gluc acid
Arjunoside IV
R = Rha, R´ = H

Fig. 22.16. Chemical constituents of Arjuna bark.

1300-3300 m from Kashmir to Bhutan and Khasia Hills.

The plant spread quickly from seeds which are shed during October-November. The herb can be cultivated in suitable localities in the temperate Himalayas. The seeds, which are very small; should be sown in a nursery and the seedlings transplanted later in the field. Flowering occurs from July to October and the plants are collected when the capsules are fully formed. The stem forms the major portion of the drug which are 1 m long, brown or purplish brown, contains a large, continuous and easily separable pith. The drug is odourless, but it has an extremely bitter taste. The whole plant is

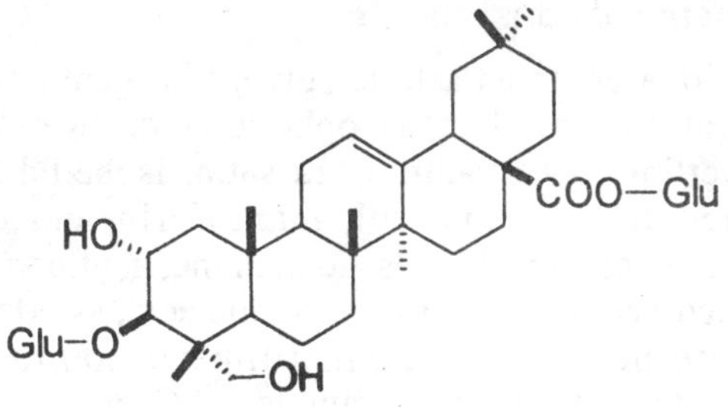

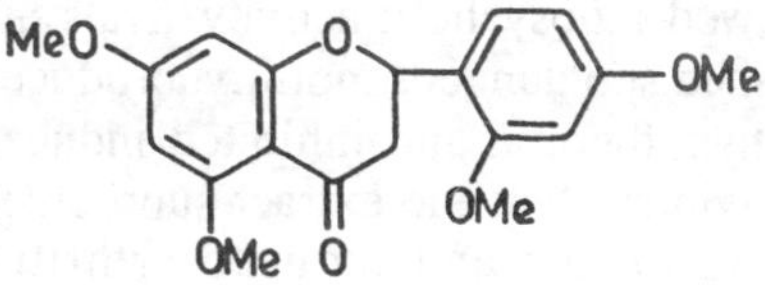

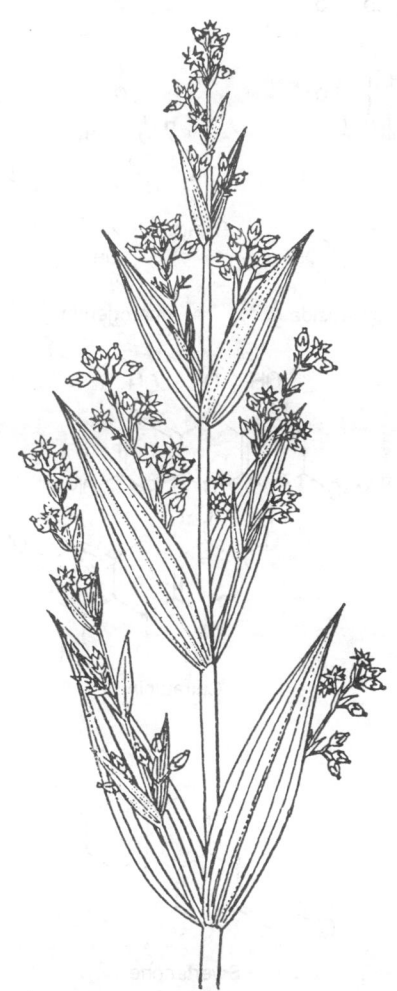

Fig. 22.17. *Swertia chirayita*—flowering branch.

medicinal but the root is the most powerful part. The root is generally small, 5-10 cm long, light brown, somewhat twisted and gradually tapering.

Characters

Chirata is a small, hairy, erect, annual herb. The stem is round, purple at the base and angular and yellowish brown at the upper side. The upper part is much branched. Leaves thin, opposite, unequal, sessile, decussate, ovate oblong with 5-7 veins. Flowers are purple, solitary, calyx and corolla are of the same size. The fruits are ovate capsules. The drug is odourless and taste is very bitter.

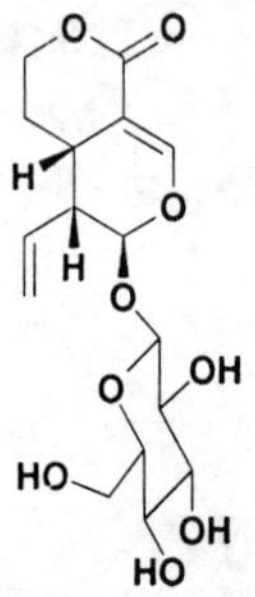

Sweroside 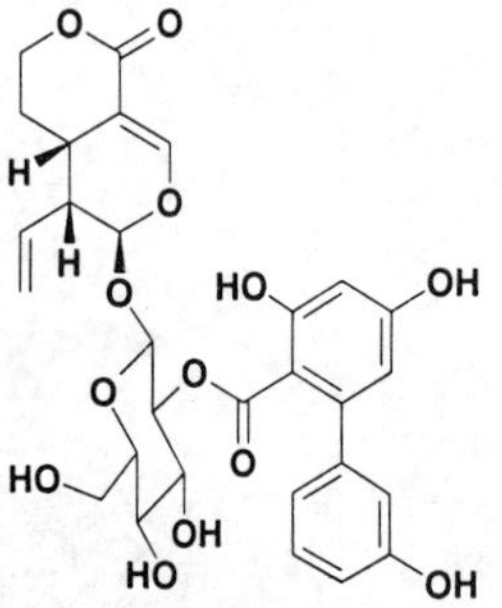   Amarogentin

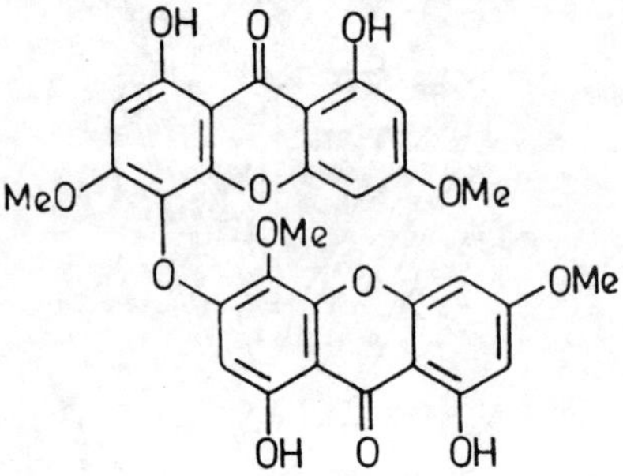

Chiratanin

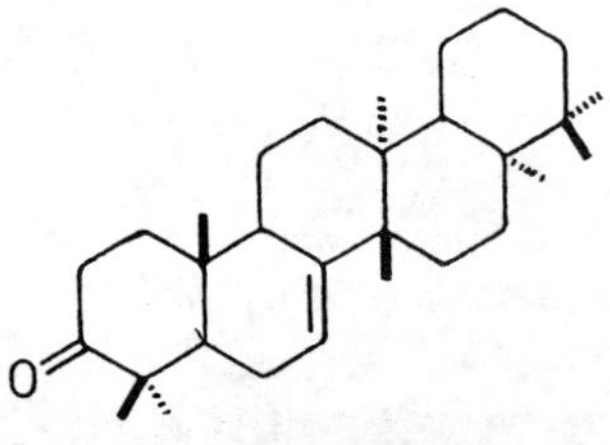

Swertanone

Fig. 22.18. Chemical constituents of *Swertia chirata.*

Chemical constituents

Chirata contains a bitter glycoside gentiopicrin; amarogentin, chiratin, ophelic acid, swerchirin, swertinin, swertianin, decussatin, isobellidifolin, friedelin, β-sitosterol, mangiferin and other xanthones, amino acids, gentiamine, gentiocrucine, enicoflavine, β-amyrin, oleanolic acid, swertanone (triterpene), chiratanin (dimeric xanthone), chiratenol (triterpene), chiratol, 7-O-methyl swertianin, swertenol, episwertenol, swerta-7,9(11)-dien-3β-ol, pichierenol, kairatenol, lignan ʳ(−)-syringaresinol, iridoids amarogenin, sweroside and amaroswerin.

Uses

Chirata is used as bitter tonic, ferbrifuge, stomachic and laxative. In excess dose it may cause nausea and oppresses the stomach.

The most important adulterant of Chirata is *Swertia angustifolia* which is distinguished by its inferior bitter tonic properties. The roots of *Rubia cordifolia* are also used as an adulterant and distinguished by their purple colour. Green Chirata (*Andrographis paniculata*) is also used as an adulterant.

Pharmacology

Gentiamine showed antipsychotic activity in rats and mice. It diminished spontaneous motility, produced catalepsy and hypothermia and inhibited induced aggressive behaviour. Benzene extract suppressed induced oedema in rats and induced arthritis. Swerchirin exhibited hypoglycaemic effect in rats. It lowered blood sugar in rats.

PICRORHIZA

Synonyms

Kathi; Kuru (Hindi); Katvee.

Biological source

It consists of dried rhizome of *Picrorhiza kurroa* Royle ex Benth., cut into small pieces and freed from attached rootlets. (Family : Scrophulariaceae).

Habitat

The plant is common on the alpine Himalayas from Kashmir to Sikkim between 3,000 to 5,000 meters.

Characters

It is a low, hairy herb with a perennial woody bitter rhizome, 15-25 cm long, covered with dry leaf-bases It occurs as pieces, 2-4 cm long and 0.3-1.0 cm in diameter. Scales at distant intervals are present; frequently small protuberances, which probably represent accessary buds, are observed both at the rhizomes and the stolones.

The drug consists of small pieces. Colour is greyish-brown, light, cylindrical, straight or slightly curved, often with remains of aerial stem which is very dark brown and wrinkled longitudinally, upper and lower surfaces bear a few small root scars, numerous scale leaves and thin scars; odour slightly unpleasant; taste very bitter.

Chemical constituents

The active constituents of Picrorhiza is picrorhizin, a glucoside which yields picrorhizetin and dextrose on hydrolysis. It also contains kutkin, a glucosidal bitter principle, picroside-I, picroside-II, picroside-III, D-mannitol, vanilic acid, kurrin, kutkiol, kutkisterol, apocynin, 6-feruloylcatalpol, vernico-side, apocynin, kutkoside, 6-feruloyl catapol, veronicoside, minecoside, picein, androsin, β-D-6-cinnamoylglucose, arvenin III, phenolic glycosides picein and androsin and seven cucurbitacin glycoside.

Uses

Picrorhiza is bitter, cathartic, stomachic, used in fever and dyspepsia and in purgative preparations. It is reputed as an anti-periodic and cholagogue, febrifuge and antimalarial. Different types of jaundice are cured with Picrorhiza. It removes kidney stone, used as emmenagogue, emetic, abortifacient, antidote for dog-bite; externally it is used in skin diseases and improves eye-sight. It is a valuable bitter tonic almost as efficacious as Gentian. It is laxative in small doses and cathartic in large doses.

It is used as an adulterant or substituted for Indian Gentian (*Gentiana kurroo*).

Pharmacology

An alcoholic extract decreased alkaline phosphatase, SGOT, SGPT and thymol turbidity. It increased body weight of rats. Root and rhizome extract exhibited hepatoprotective activity in rats. Oral administration of a plant extract to guinea pig reduced body temperature, loss in body weight, food intake and mortality induced by vaccinia virus. Plant extract suppressed inflammatory oedema. Picroliv, an alcoholic extract of the plant, showed promising anti-HBsAg-like activity, inhibited purified hepatitis B virus, provided protection against hepatic damage, increased levels of serum glutamate oxaloacetate transminase, alkaline phosphatase and liporotein-X. Kutkin, picroside I and kutkoside exhibited anti-inflammatory activity. Plant extract stimulated non-specific immune response of animals. Administration of andrographolide, andrographiside and neoandrographolide caused elevation of different enzymes of cellular antioxidant defense mechanism.

The drug possesses hepatoprotective, anti-asthmatic, immunomodulating, immuno-potentiating and bile flowing effects. The iridoid mixture from the rhizome of *P. kurroa* and picroliv exhibited hepatoprotective activity against liver damage in rats.

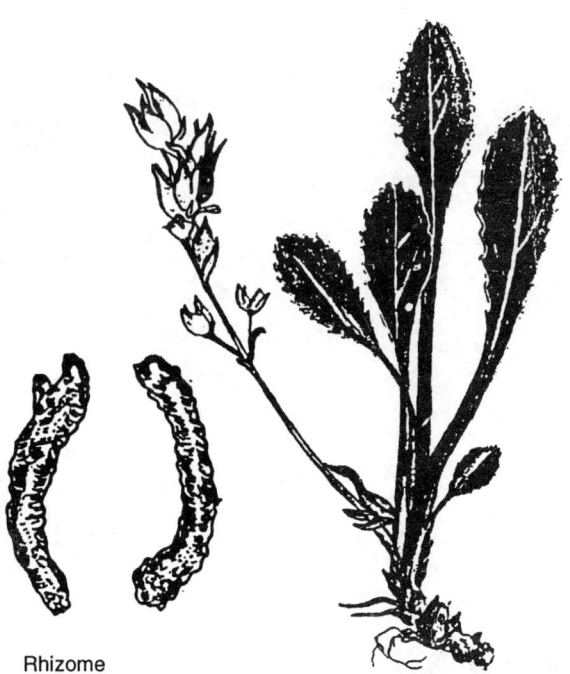

Rhizome

Fig. 22.19. *Picrorhiza kurroa.*

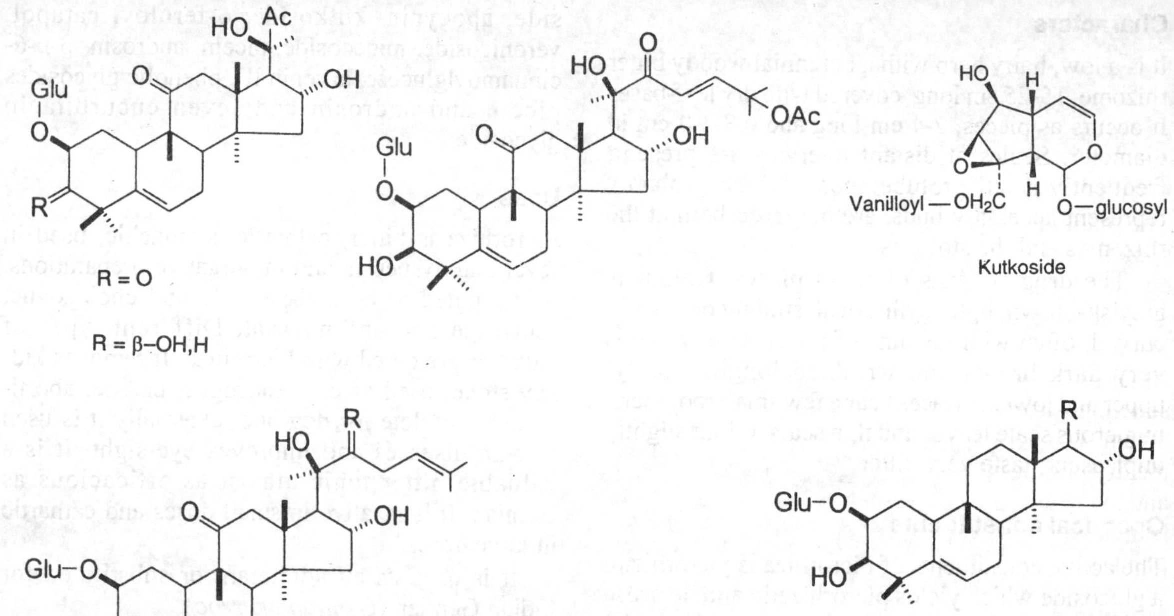

R = O

R = β–OH,H

Glu

Glu

HO

Vanilloyl — OH₂C

O—glucosyl

Kutkoside

R = O

R = OH,H

Glu–O

HO

R = H,

R = Glu(6-cinnamoyl)

Cucurbit-5-en derivatives

R =   OAc

R =   OAc

R =

R = Ac

Fig. 22.20. Chemical constituents of *Picrorhiza kurroa*.

Adulterants

The roots of *Acacia spicata, Cimicifuga foetida* and *Coptis teeta* are sold under the name '*kutki*' or '*karu*' in Mumbai. At Bengal drug shops the roots of *Gentiana Kurroo, Coscinium fenestratum* and *Swertia chirata* are available as '*Karu*'. *Lagotis cashmiriana* is an adulterant of commercial samples of *P. kurroa* in Kulu market of Himachal Pradesh. The drug samples sold in the Indian markets are mostly genuine. However, qualitywise there was lot of difference which can be attributed to collection time, age of the plant and region of collection.

KALMEGH

Synonyms

Andrographis, King of bitters, Chiretta; Bengal Chirata; Green Chirata; Kiryet (Hindi).

Biological source

Kalmegh consists of leaves or entire aerial part of *Andrographis paniculata* Nees. (Family : Acanthaceae).

Distribution

The plant occurs throughout the plains of India and sometimes cultivated. It is an annual herb, 30-100 cm in height.

The plant is gregarious and grows abundantly in moist, shady waste grounds. It prefers a sunny situation. The seeds are sown during May-June. The seedlings are transplanted at a distance of 60 cm × 30 cm. Two or three irrigations may be given during the dry period. It flowers during August-November, and the whole plant starts maturing during February-March when it is harvested for the drug. The whole plant is dried in shade and sold.

Morphology

The stem is erect, greenish brown, woody, 30-100 cm in height, and quadrangular particularly in the upper regions with four bulges arising on the four corners. The leaves are dark green, lanceolate, with a small winged petiole, 7 cm long, 2-5 cm broad, margin is entire, lamina glabrous, apex acuminate, slightly waxy and base tapering. The midrib varies in outline at different regions of the leaf. Stem branching is profuse which bears small and solitary flowers. The dried drug is odourless and taste is extremely bitter.

Chemical constituents

The plant possesses kalmeghin, a bitter crystalline diterpene lactone, *viz.* andrographolide flavonoids and phenols.

The lactones isolated from Kalmegh are andrographolide, 14-deoxy-11-oxo-andrographolide, 14-deoxy-11, 12-didehydroandrographolide, 14-deoxyandrographolide and neoandrographolide. From the leaves of Bangladesh plant homoandrographolide, andrographosterol, andrographane, andrographone, a wax and two esters have been isolated.

The roots also contain a monohydroxytrimethylflavone, andrographin, a dihydroxy-di-methoxyflavone, panicolin, neoandrographolide, 5-hydroxy-7,8,2',3'-tetramethoxyflavone, apigenin-4,7-dimethyl ester, apigenin-7,4'-di-O-methyl ether, 2',5-dihydroxy-7, 8-dimethoxyflavone, 5-hydroxy-2', 7,8-tri-methoxy flavone, 14 deoxyandrographolide, isodeoxyandrographolide, 5-hydroxy-7,8-dime-thoxyflavanone and 5-hydroxy-3,7,8,2'-tetra-methoxyflavone,. The leaves contain β-sitosterol glucoside, caffeic, chlorogenic and dicaffeoyl-quinic acids, 3,14-dideoxyandrographolide, 14-deoxyandrographiside, deoxyandrographolide-19β-D-glucoside, norandrographolide, carvacrol, eugenol, myristic acid, hentriacontane, tritriacontane, oroxylin A, wogonin, andrograpanin, 14-deoxy-12-methoxyandrographolide, andrographidines A-F and stigmasterol.

Uses

Kalmegh has febrifuge, tonic, alterative, anthelmintic, astringent, anodyne, alexipharmic and cholagogue properties. It is useful in debility, cholera, diabetes, swelling, itches, consumption, influenza, piles, gonorrhoea, bronchitis, dysentery, dyspepsia,

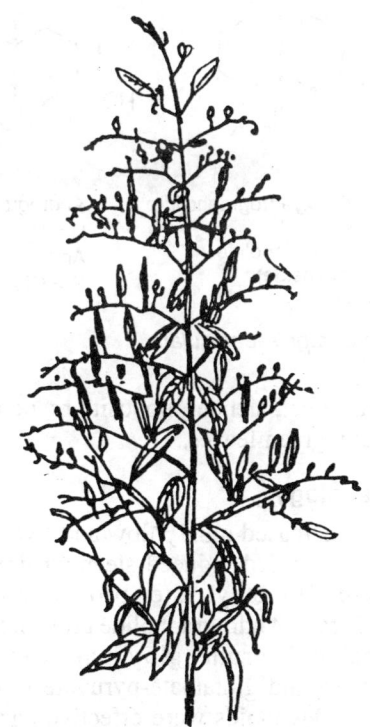

Fig. 22.21. Kalmegh (*Andrographis paniculata*).

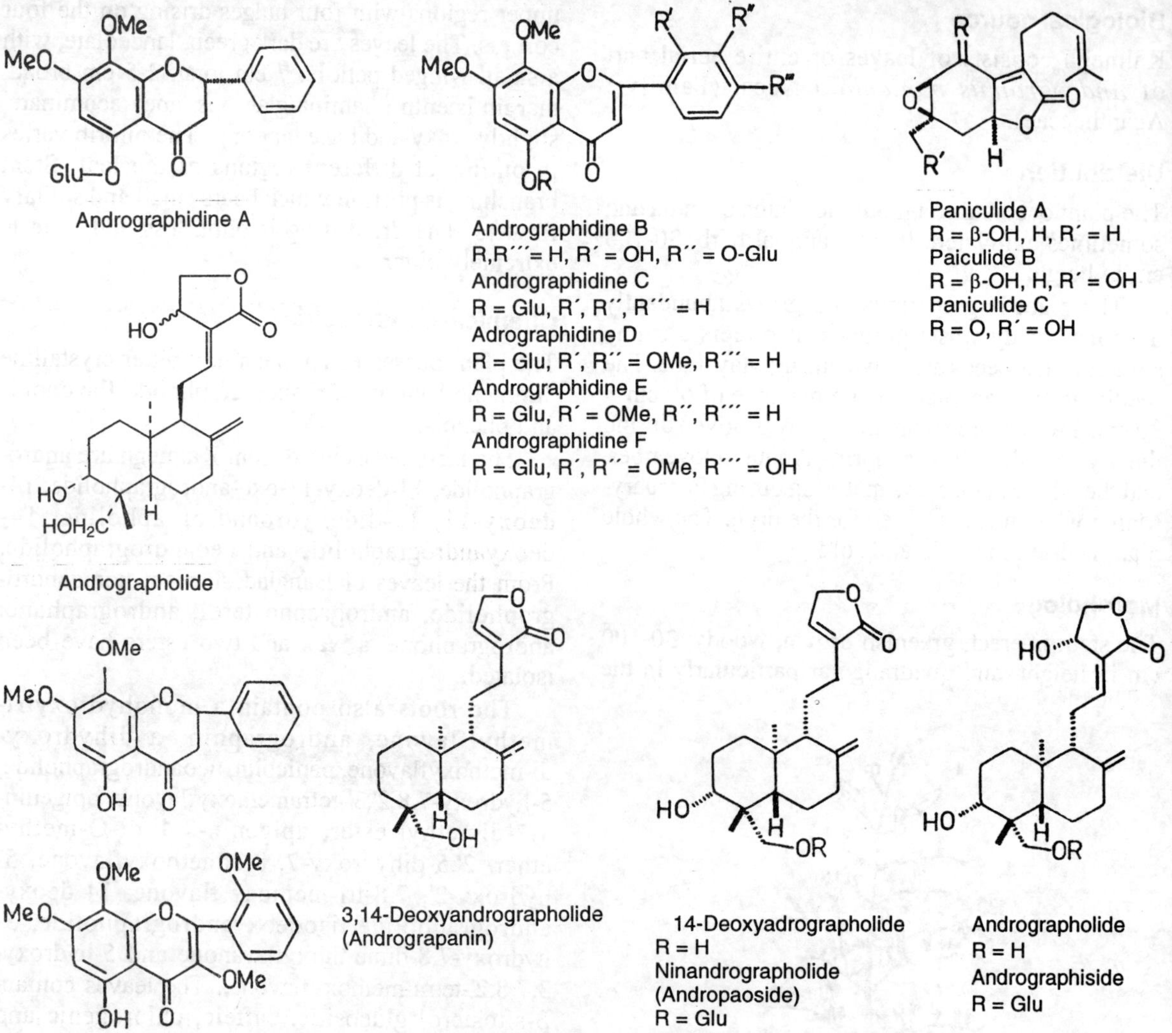

Andrographidine A

Andrographidine B
R,R‴= H, R′ = OH, R″ = O-Glu
Andrographidine C
R = Glu, R′, R″, R‴ = H
Adrographidine D
R = Glu, R′, R″ = OMe, R‴ = H
Andrographidine E
R = Glu, R′ = OMe, R″, R‴ = H
Andrographidine F
R = Glu, R′, R″ = OMe, R‴ = OH

Paniculide A
R = β-OH, H, R′ = H
Paiculide B
R = β-OH, H, R′ = OH
Paniculide C
R = O, R′ = OH

Andrographolide

3,14-Deoxyandrographolide
(Andrograpanin)

14-Deoxyadrographolide
R = H
Ninandrographolide
(Andropaoside)
R = Glu

Andrographolide
R = H
Andrographiside
R = Glu

Fig. 22.22. Chemical constituents of *Andrographis paniculata*.

fever and in weakness. A decoction of the plant is used as a blood purifier and as a cure for torphid and jaundice. It forms the major constituent of the Ayurvedic drug *SG-I Switradilepa* which is effective in treating vitiligo, a dermatological disease. The pills prepared from macerated leaves and certain spices (e.g., Cardamom, Clove and Cinnamon) are given for stomach ailments of infants.

Sometimes, the drug is mixed with the genuine Chirata (*Swertia chirata*) but can be distinguished from the latter by the green colour of its stem, numerous erect, slender, opposite branches and its lanceolate, green leaves.

Pharmacology

Kalmegh increased biliary flow and liver weight in rats and decreased induced sleeping time. Apigenin-7,4'-di-O-methyl ester produced anti-ulcer activity in rats. Andrographolide prevented induced increase of serum glutamate-oxaloacetate transminase and glutamate-pyruvate transminase. Total root flavonoids were effective against myocardial ischemic necrosis in rats. Plant alcoholic extract showed antidiarrhoeal activity. Leaf extract showed cytotoxicity against KB and P388 cells. Andrographolide and neoandrographolide showed activity similar to that of loperamide against *E. coli*. Andrographolide exhibited potent cytotoxic effect in KB and P-388 lymphocytic leukaemia; induced increase in bile flow and exhibited strong choleretic action.

BAVCHI

Synonyms

Psoralea; Bavachi fruits; Bavachi seeds; Malaya tea.

Biological source

The drug consists of the dried fruits and seeds of *Psoralea corylifolia* Linn. (Family : Papilionaceae).

Habitat

The plant grows throughout India.

Morphology

The plant is an annual herb attending a height of 60 cm to 1 m. Prominent groove of glands and white hairs are present on the stem and branches. Bluish purple flowers bloom from August to November. Fruits are minute, ovate, oblong, glabrous, rounded or mucronate and pitted; about 4 mm long, 2-3 mm

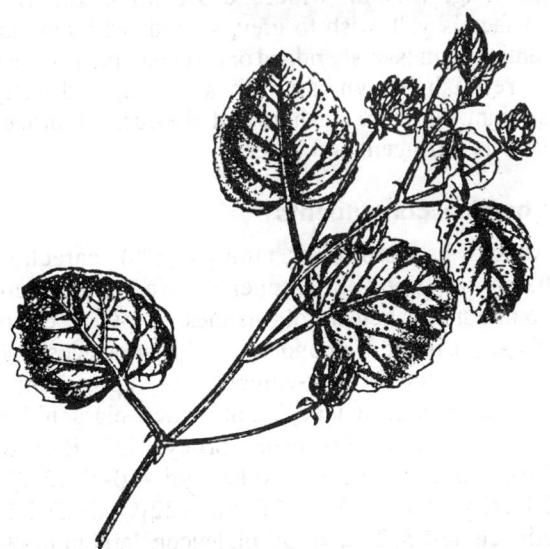

Fig. 22.23. *Psoralea corylifolia.*

broad; dark chocolate or black in colour, with pericarp attached to seeds; odourless, taste is bitter, acrid and unpleasant. Seeds are kidney shaped, 2-4 mm long, 2-3 mm broad, smooth, exalbuminous with straw coloured hard testa.

Chemical constituents

Bavchi contains fixed oil (10%), essential oil (0.2), resin and the furanocoumarins like psoralen, isopsoralen, psoralidin, isopsoralidin and corylifolean. The seeds contain flavonoids such as bavachalcone, bavachinin, isobavachalcone, bavachin and isobavachin; monoterpenoid phenol named bakuchiol. Other compounds isolated from the seeds are 4-O-methylbavachalcone, 7-O-methylbavachin, neobavaisoflavone, bavachromene, triacontane, β-sitosterol-D-glucoside and corylidine. The seed oil yielded limonene, α-elemene, limonene, γ-elemene, β-caryophyllene and its oxide, 4-terpineol, linalool, geranyl acetate, angelicin, psoralen and bakuchiol. 4'-O-nethyl-bava-chalcone, (+)-bakuchiol, neobavachalcone, corylifolin, corylifolinin, psoridin-2',3'-oxide diacetate, isoneobavachalcone, trilaurin, daidzein, coumesterol and bakuchalcone are also present in Bavchi.

Fruits of Psoralea also contain isoflavones corylin, corylinal, neobavaisoflavone, psoralenol and chalcones like 5-formyl-2, 4-dihydroxy-4'-methoxychalcone and bavachromanol.

Uses

Bavchi is used to cure leucoderma and other skin diseases. Seeds are used as stomachic, deobstruent, anthelmintic, diuretic, diaphoretic, in febrile conditions, billious affections, leprosy, psoriasis and inflammatory diseases of the skin and leucoderma. The drug is taken orally as well as locally applied in the form of a paste or ointment. Psoralen and isopsoralen possess the curative action of Psoralea in leucoderma.

Pharmacology

Seed extract possessed anthelmintic activity. Psoralen affected detoxication mechanism in rabbits. A mixture of psoralen, isopsoralen and imperatorin caused hypertrophy of liver, kidney and spleen. Seed extract showed skin photosensitising activity in guinea pigs. Corylifolinin exhibited vasodilator

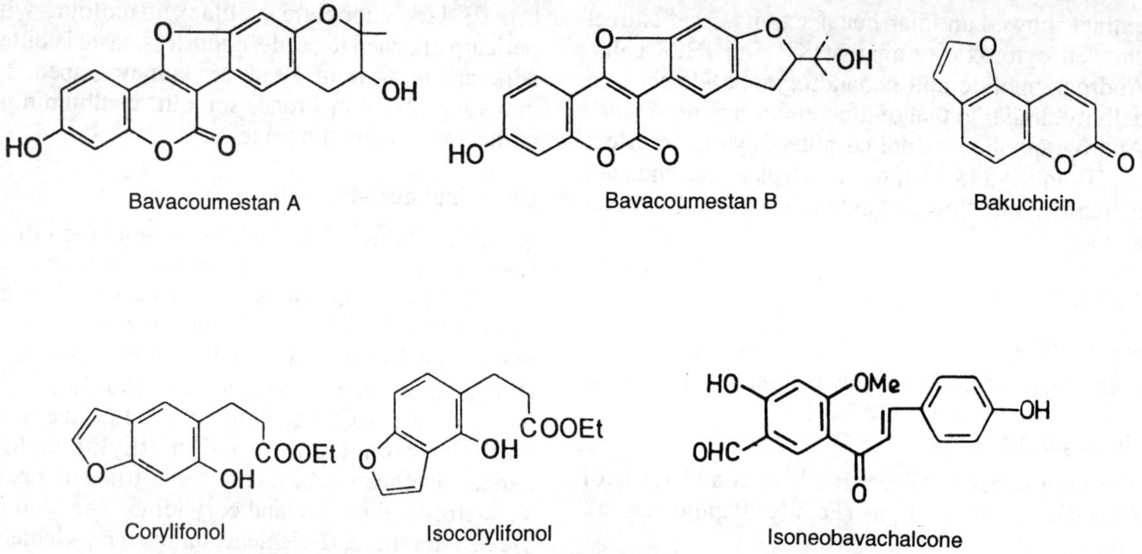

Fig. 22.24. Chemical constituents of *Psoralea corylifolia*.

activity and inhibitory effect on HeLa cells. Psoralen is used in the treatment of uterine haemorrhage in China. Bakuchiol exhibited irreversible cyto-toxicity against L929 cell culture and human cancer cell lines.

Psoralens are photosensitizing furocoumarins that occur in a number of plant families, including the (Apiaceae), where they are a common cause of phototoxicity. Methoxsalen, 8-methoxy-psoralen, or xanthotoxin, a constituent of the cremocarps of *Ammi majus* Linn. (Fam. Apiaceae), is used to facilitate repigmentation in idiopathic vitiligo (leukoderma) and for symptomatic control of psoriasis. Repigmentation therapy usually involves extended periods of time. In therapy with methox-salen, carcinogenesis, cataract development, and actinic degeneration of the skin are the side effects.

Trioxsalen, a synthetic furocoumarin, is also available for the treatment of vitiligo.

ASHOKA BARK

Synonyms

Ashoka (Hindi); Asoka (Bengali).

Biological source

Ashoka is the dried bark of stem of *Saraca indica* Linn. (Family : Papilionaceae).

Habitat

Ashoka tree is found in central and eastern Himalayas, eastern Bengal, western Peninsula, Burma, Sri Lanka and Malaya.

Morphology

Ashoka bark is available in channeled pieces, 40 cm long, 4-6 mm wide and 5-8 thick. External surface is yellowish to grey, smooth with circular lenticels, transversly ridged or cracked. Inner surface is reddish-brown, smooth and longitudinally straight. Fracture is short and fibrous; odourless; taste is astringent and bitter.

Chemical constituents

Ashoks bark contains tannins (6%), catechol, haemotoxyline, phlobaphenes, organic calcium compound, a ketosterol; alkanes (C_{20}-C_{35}), esters (C_{34}-C_{60}), primary alcohols (C_{22}-C_{30}), *n*-octacosanol, tannin, catechin, (+)-catechol, (−)-epicatechin, (−)-epicatechol, leucocyanidin, leucopelargonidin, procyanidin B_2; 11-desoxy-procyanidin B (root bark), (24ξ)-24-methylcho-lest-5-en-3β-ol, (24ξ)-24-ethylcholest-5-en-3β-ol, (22β, 24ξ)-24-ethylcholest-5, 22-dien-3β-ol, leucopelargonidin-3-O-β-D-glucoside and β-sitosterol.

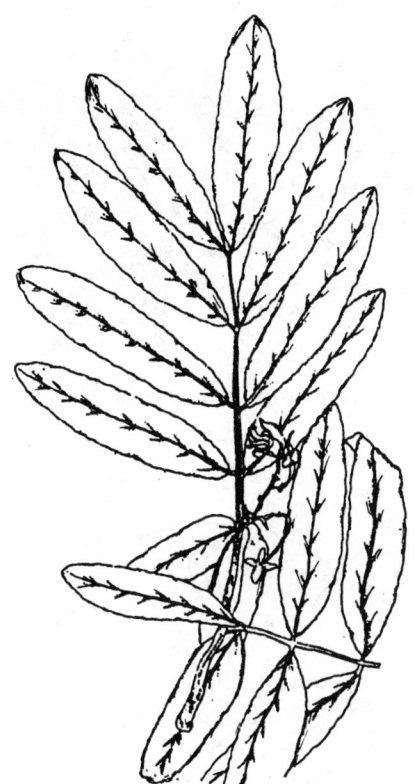

Fig. 22.25. *Saraca indica.*

Uses

Ashoka bark is astringent, used in uterine affections, biliousness, dyspepsia, dysentery, colic, piles, ulcers, pimples and in menorrhagia (excessive mensturation) and leucorrhoea.

Adulterant

The bark of *Polyalthia longifolia* (Fam. Anonaceae), known as Asopalava bark, is used in place of Ashoka bark.

AMLA

Synonyms

Embelic myrobalan; Embelica, Indian goose berry.

Biological source

Amla consists of the fresh or dried fruits of *Emblica officinalis* Gaertn. (syn. *Phyllanthus emblica* Linn) (Family : Euphorbiaceae).

Habitat

The plant is a middle-sized tree commonly found in the mixed deciduous forests of India, Sri Lanka, China and Malaya ascending to 1,500 m on the hills. It is often cultivated in gardens and homeyards.

Amla is usually propagated by seeds or by budding, cutting and inarching. The plant is sensitive to frost and drought. The tree coppices well and the coppice shoots grow vigorously. Flowers usually appear in the hot season and fruits ripen during the following winter.

Morphology

The fruit is a drupe, fleshy globose, 1.5-2.5 cm in diameter, smooth, shiny with light coloured specks. It is distinctly marked in six lobes. The fruit is green when tender but the colour changes to light yellow or brick red on maturity. A minute depression is present at one end which is left due to removal of peduncle. The taste is sour and astringent giving feeling of sweetness afterwards.

Chemical constituents

The principal chemical constituent of Amla is vitamin C (650-900 mg/100 g). The fruit juice contains about 20 times more vitamin C than orange juice. It also contains tannins (5%), glucose, pectin, and minerals like iron, phosphorus and calcium. Tannins are the mixture of gallic acid, ellagic acid and phyllembin. The presence of the tannins prevents the oxidation of the vitamin.

The other compounds isolated from Amala are

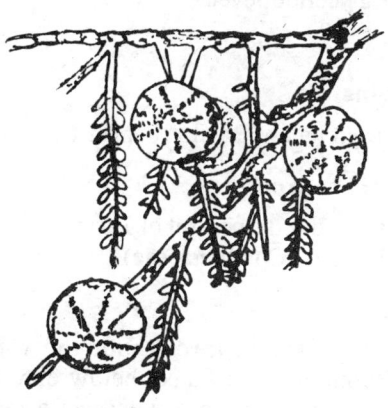

Fig. 22.26. Amla fruits.

trigalloylglucose, terchebin, corilagin, phyllembic acid, 3-O-gallated prodelphinidin and procyanidin.

The immature fruits contain indole acetic acid, auxins A_1, A_3, A_4 and A_5; growth inhibitors R_1 and R_2.

The seed fat is composed of glyceride of linoleic acid (65%).

Uses

Fruit has acrid, cooling, refrigerant, diuretic and laxative properties. Dried fruit is useful in haemorrhagic, diabetes and dysentery. In combination with iron it is used to treat anaemia, jaundice and dyspepsia. Fermented liquor prepared from the fruit is used in jaundice, dyspepsia and cough. It has antibacterial, antifungal and antiviral activities. Amla is an ingredient of the Ayurvedic formulation 'Triphala' and 'Chyavanprash'. Triphala is a laxative and used to treat headache, biliousness, dyspepsia, constipation, piles, enlarged liver and ascites. Acute bacillary dysentery is cured by drinking a sherbet of Amla with lemon juice. The exudation of the fruit is used as an external application for inflammation of the eye. The fruits are also used in the preparation of writing inks and hair dyes. The dried fruit is detergent and is used as shampoo for the head. A fixed oil extracted from the fruit is reported to promote hair growth.

Pharmacology

Fruit pulp powder reduced levels of serum, aortic and hepatic cholesterol in rabbits, but did not influence clot lysis time, platelet adhesiveness or serum triglyceride level.

BAHERA

Synonyms

Beleric Myrobalan; Bahira (Sanskrit).

Biological source

Bahera is the dried ripe fruit of *Terminalia bellirica* Roxb. (Family : Combretaceae).

Habitat

The plant is found throughout the forests of India, Burma and Sri Lanka below elevations of about 1000 m except in dry and acrid regions of Sind and Rajasthan.

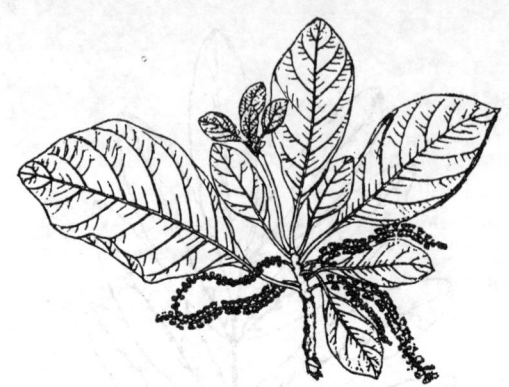

Fig. 22.27. *Terminalia bellirica*—flowering branches.

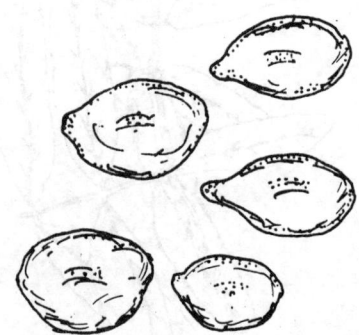

Fig. 22.28. Bahera fruits.

Bahera is a large handsome, deciduous tree, with characteristic bark, 20-35 m high and 2-3 m in girth.

The good seed crop, high germinative capacity of the healthy seeds and their quick and easy germination are favourable for the natural regeneration. The plant can be raised in fields by direct sowing. The tree is not subjected to fungal attack of any consequence.

Morphology

Fruits are globular drupes, 1.3-2.5 cm in diameter, obscurely 5-angled, ovoid, suddenly narrowing into a short stalk. Outer surface in velvety, irregularly wrinkled containing five well defined longitudinal ridges. The upper end is depressed and a prominent, sound scar of pedicel is present at one end of the fruit. The fruit is very hard and broken surface is yellow in colour. It is odourless and taste is astringent.

Chemical constituents

Bahera contains tannins (20-25%), phyllemblin, β-sitosterol, mannitol, glucose, fructose, rhamnose, fixed oil (30-40%) and hydrocarbons such as tetratriacontane, ditriacontane-2-ol, tritriacontan-9-one and *n*-tritriacontane. Tannin component is the mixture of gallic acid, ellagic acid, ethyl gallate, galloyl glucose and chebulaginic acid. A hexahydroxydiphenic acid ester has been reported which on hydrolysis yielded two moles of hexahydroxydiphenic acid. The fixed oil contains the esters of palmitic, stearic, oleic and linoleic acids.

The other compounds isolated from Bahera are bellericanin, β-sitosterol, chebulagic acid; triterpene belleric acid and its glucoside bellericoside; arjugenin, tomentosic acid (a hydrolyzed product of arjunglucoside), triterpenic acids bellerica-genins A and B and their glycosides bellericasides A and B.

Uses

The fruit has bitter, astringent, tonic, laxative, anti-pyretic activities and is used to treat piles, dropsy, dysentery, diarrhoea, leprosy, biliousness, dyspepsia and headache. It is one of the ingredient of Ayurvedic purgative medicament 'Triphala'.

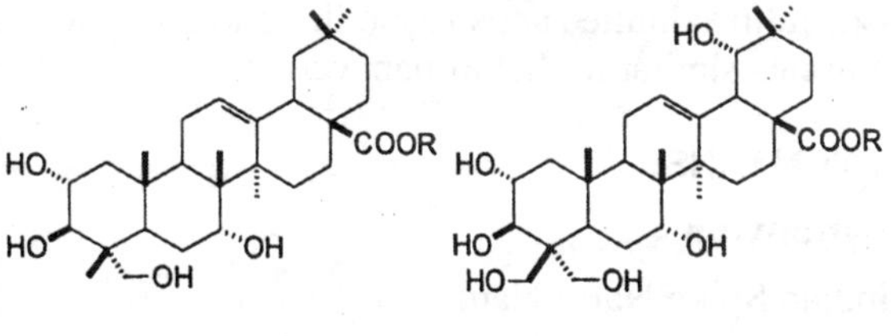

Bellericagenin A
R = H
Bellericaside A
R = Glu

Bellericagenin B
R = H
Bellericaside B
R = Glu

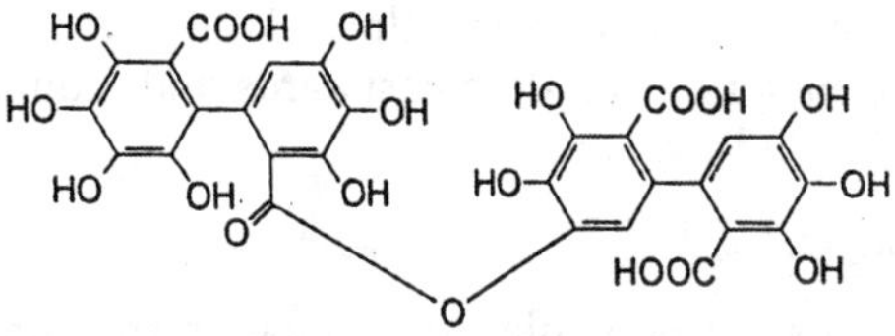

Fig. 22.29. Chemical constituents of *Terminalia bellirica*.

Pharmacology

Kernel oil showed purgative action. Fruit extract produced fall in blood pressure and increase in bile secretion.

MYROBALAN

Synonyms

Harar (Hindi), Haritaki (Bengali and Sanskrit), Hirdo (Gujarati); Hirda (Marathi).

Biological source

Myrobalan consists of dried mature fruits, known as Harde, or small fruits, known as Himaj, of the tree *Terminalia chebula* Retz. (Fam. Combretaceae).

Habitat

The plant is found abundantly in north India from Kangra and Kumaon to Bengal and southern region in Madhya Pradesh, Maharashtra, Gujarat and Travancore.

The fruits ripen from November to March,

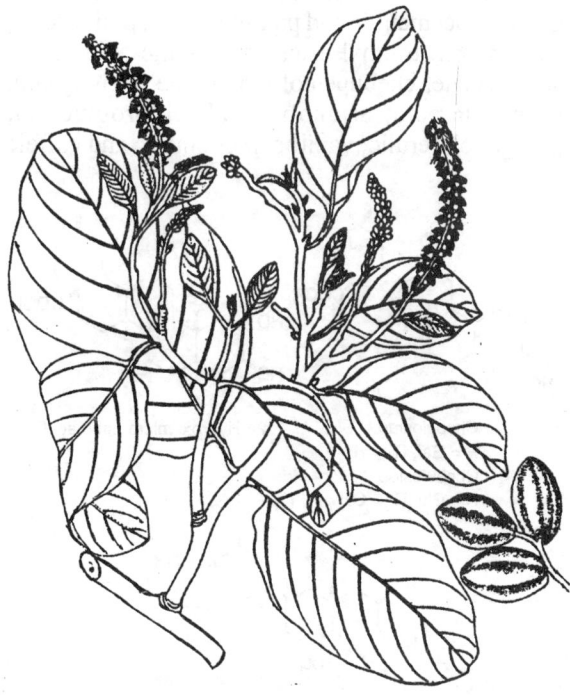

Fig. 22.30. *Terminalia chebula*–flowering branches and fruits.

depending upon the locality, and fall soon after ripening. They are dried and the seeds stored for one year. The germination capacity of the seeds is low due to the presence of hard cover and the seeds require pre-treatment.

Characters

The fruit is a drupe, ellipsoidal, ovoid; yellow to orange brown in colour; 2-3.5 cm long, 1.3-2.5 cm wide, longitudinally wrinkled; carpel, 5-6 ribbed longitudinally; hard and strong; seeds are light yellow, 1.5-2.5 cm long and rough. Odour is slight and taste is astringent and bitter.

Chemical constituents

Myrobalan contains hydrolysable tannins (30-40%), purgative compounds like anthraquinones, fixed oil containing esters of palmitic, oleic and linoleic acids, astringent compound chebulinic acid; ellagic acid, gallic acid, resin, β-sitosterol, chebulin, terchebin, terchebulin, punicalin, terfla-vins A, B, C and D; punicalagin and punicalin, maslinic and 2α-hydroxyursolic acids (from leaves); shikimic, gallic, triacontanoic and palmitic acids, β-sitosterol, daucosterol, triethyl ester of chebulic acid, gallic acid acetate, chebupentol (triterpene), arjungenin, terminoic acid, arjunolic acid, phloroglucinol, pyrogallol, ferulic, vanillic, *p*-coumaric and caffeic

Chebuloside I
R = Gal, R′ = H
Chebuloside II
R = Glu, R′ = OH

2a-Hydroxymicromeric acid

Chebupentol

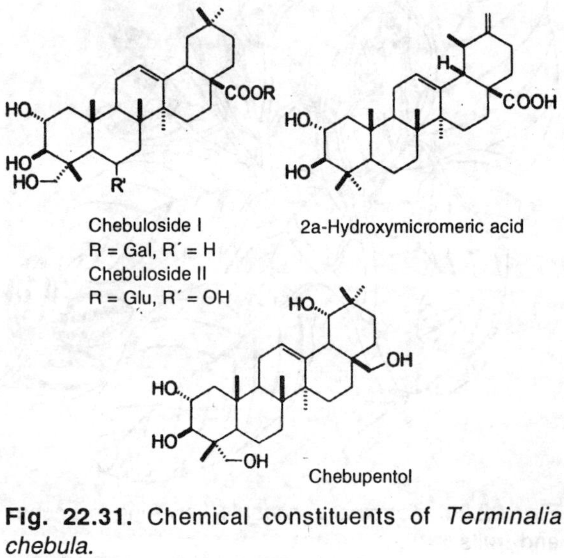

Fig. 22.31. Chemical constituents of *Terminalia chebula.*

acids. Fruit kernels yield palmitic, stearic, oleic, linoleic, arachidic and behenic acids.

The tannins in Myrobalan belong to the pyrogallol type. They are very complex. The hydrolysable tannins, chebulagic acid, chebulinic acid, and corilagin are the major tannin constituents. On hydrolysis they form chebulic acid, 3, 6-di-galloyl-glucose, ellagic acid, gallic acid, and β-glucogallin. The carbohydrates present in Myrobalan are : glucose, sorbitol, fructose, sucrose and gentiobiose. Eighteen typical amino acids are also present in addition to phosphoric, succinic, quinic, shikimic, dihydroshikimic and dehydroshikimic acids. During maturation of the fruits, the amount of tannins decreases whereas the acidity increases.

Uses

Myrobalan is astringent, laxative and alterative; used externally as a local application to chronic ulcers and wounds and as a gargle in stomatitis. Finely powdered drug is used as a dentifrice and considered useful in carious teeth, bleeding and ulcerations of the gums. Myrobalan in combination with Amla (*Emblica officinalis*) and Bahera (*T. belerica*) forms the well known Ayurvedic preparation 'Triphala', which is used as laxative and stomach disorders.

Pharmacology

Chebulin exhibited antispasmodic action on smooth muscles similar to that of papaverine.

JATAMANSI

Synonyms

Indian Spike Nard; Nard.

Biological source

Jatamansi consists of the dried rhizome of *Nardostachys jatamansi* DC. (Fam. Valerianaceae).

Geological source

The plant is found in the alpine Himalayas, 4,000-5,000 meters, extending eastwards and Kumaon to Sikkim and Bhutan.

Characters

Jatamansi is a perennial herb containing a cylindrical rhizome covered with brown to deep greyish

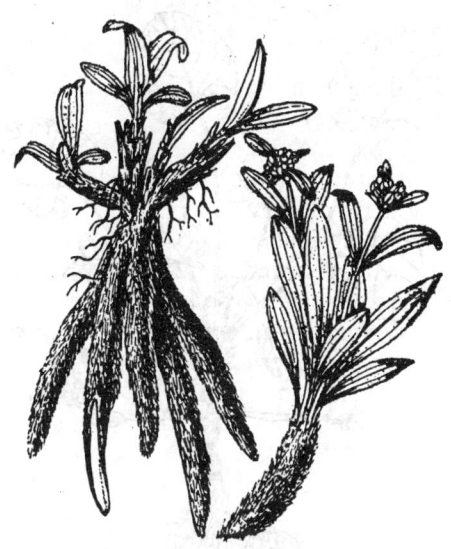

Fig. 22.32. *Nardostachys jatamansi*—with rootstocks.

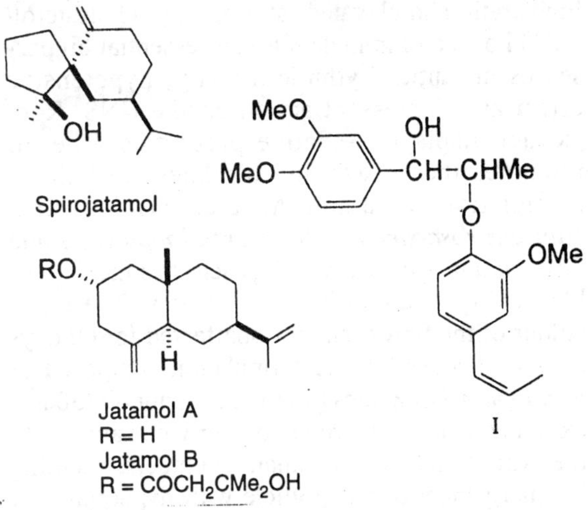

Fig. 22.33. Chemical constituents of Jatamansi.

fibres, length is 2.5-7 cm, diameter 0.5-3 cm. Fibres are produced by an accumulation of skeletons of the leaf bases. Removal of the leaf bases, aerial parts and adventitious roots shows the presence of rough surface with transverse rings. The rings indicate the scars of nodes, leaf bases and the adventitious roots. Internal colour is reddish brown. Fracture is easy and splintery. Adventitious roots are thin, branched and red to brown in colour. Odour is slight and aromatic and taste is acrid, slightly bitter and aromatic.

Chemical constituents

Volatile oil of Jatamansi possesses an alcohol and its isovaleric ester, a saturated bicyclic sesquiterpene ketone, named jatamansone, jatamansic acid, β-maaliene, calarene, jatamansin, oroselol, α-pinene, β-pinene, 3-carene, β-eudesmol, elemol, nardol, nardostachone, seychellene, seychelane, norseychelanone, patchouli alcohol, α- and β-pat-choulenes, nardostachnol, 9-dehydroaristolene, 1(10)-dehydroaristolene, 1,2,9,10-tetrahydroaris-tolene, 9-aristolen-1α-ol and (10)-aristolen-2-one.

The volatile oil of *N. jatamansi* rhizomes, collected from Garh-wal of northern Himalayas, was composed of 72 components including 41 sesquiterpenes (83.2%), 8 monoterpenes and 8 non-terpenic constituents. The important constituents of

the oil were nerolidol, ledol, jatamansic acid, nardol, calamenene, α-humulene, valencene, α-gurjunene, formic acid and propionic acid.

β-Sitosterol, angelicin, actinidine, spirojatamol, lignans virolin, (+)-pinoresinol, (+)-1-hydroxy-pinoresinol, eudesmanes jatamols A and B, nardostachyl decenoate, nardostachyl heptanoate, *n*-hexacosanyl propionate, nardostachyl cyclohexanyl ester, nonacosan-7-ol, *n*-heneitria-contane, nordostachysol, nardostachyl docosanoate, nardostachyl pentanoate and heptacosanyl pentanoate are also isolated from the rhizomes.

Uses

Jatamansi has aromatic, bitter, tonic, stimulant, spasmolytic and antiseptic properties. It is used for the treatment of epilepsy, hysteria, convulsive affections, in intestinal colic, palpitation of the heart, high blood pressure, cardiac arrhythmias and substituted for Valerian.

Adulterant

It is adulterated with rhizome of *Selinum vaginatum* (Apiaceae) which contains a volatile oil.

Pharmacology

Jatamansone showed marked tranquillizing effect in mice, anti-emetic activity in dogs and reduced aggressiveness in monkeys. Tuber extract caused significant reduction of total cholesterol/phospholipids ratio and elevated ratio of HDL-cholesterol/ total cholesterol in male rats. The essential oil possesses an antiarrhythmic activity, hypotensive effect and depressant action on the CNS. Root extract displayed sedative properties. The oil promotes the growth and blackness of hair. A formulation containing *N. jatamansi* rhizome, *Hibiscus rosa-sinensis, Saussurea lappa* roots and *Lawsonia inermis* leaves (5 g each) has the highest blackening of colourless wool fibres. The black colour of the fibres remains unaffected for 60 days at room temperature. A formulation composed of *N. jatamansi* rhizomes (50 g) in coconut oil (50 ml) exhibited maximum growth of hair when applied to the skin of rabbits and human volunteers, resulting in enlargement of hair follicle with hyperplasia of cellular constituents.

BANAFSHA

Biological source

Banafsha consists of dried flowers or aerial parts with or without flowers of *Viola odorata* Linn. (Family : Violaceae).

Geographical distribution

The plant is a herb, 30 cm in height found in Kashmir up to 1,700-2,000 meters height. It is planted in many hill stations.

It arises from a rootstock. The plant is very variable, and several single and double-flowered types are grown for ornament. It can easily be cultivated in the hilly areas of North India; in the plains, the plants do not flower freely and are grown only in winter. The plant grows well in a cool and moist climate, but exposure to heavy rain is fatal to blooming. Propagation is done by division, cuttings or seeds. The plants are repotted once or twice a year. The old plants are removed once in 4-5 years.

The drug, Banafshah, is available in commerce in three forms : (i) the dried aerial parts of the herb, *viz.*, the stems, leaves and flowers (*Kashmiri Banafshah*), (ii) only the dried flowers (*Gul-i-Banafshah*) and (iii) the aerial parts without flowers (*Berg-Banafshah*).

Morphology

Herb is glabrous or pubescent; leaves tufted, broadly

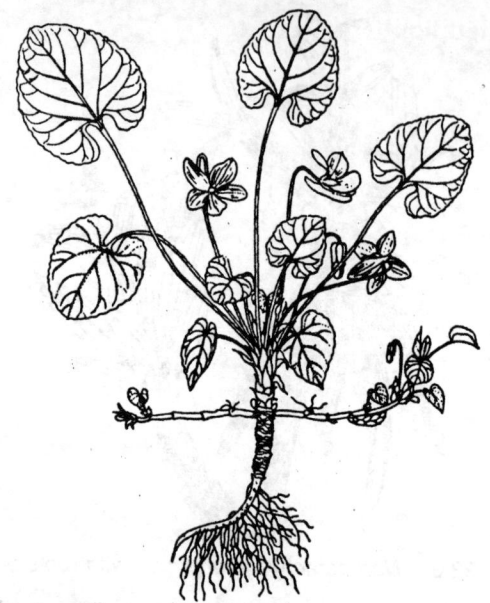

Fig. 22.34. *Viola odorata*—flowering plant.

ovate-cordate, crenate, stalked, stipulses persistent. Flowers irregular, 2-sexual, noding, on axillary stalk, usually solitary, deep violet with a white base, sweet scented. Capsules ovoid, opening horizontally by 3 boat-shaped valves, often purple.

Chemical constituents

Flowers contain a volatile oil, rutin, cyanin, glycoside of methyl salicylate and an emetic principle, called violin, which is acrid and bitter. The main components of the essential oil are α- and β-irones and α- and β-ionones. The ketones are responsible for the typical odour of the flower. Leaves possess a delightful volatile oil, an alkaloid, colouring matter, friedelin, β-sitosterol and a straight chain alcohol.

The presence of methyl salicylate, alkaloid violine, a glycoside violaquercitrin and a saponin has been reported in the roots.

The stem-volatile oil (4-12%) consists of 2, 6-nonadien-1-al as the major component (30-50%), 2, 6-nonadien-1-ol, *n*-hexanol, *n*-hexenol, *n*-heptenol, *n*-octenol, eugenol, benzyl alcohol, acids like propionic, enanthic (heptanoic), palmitic, salicylic, octanoic and octenoic acids.

Adulteration

Banafsha is adulterated with other *Viola* species, viz. *V. biflora, V. canescens, V. cinerea, V. pilosa* and *V. sylvestris*.

Uses

Banafsha is valued as an expectorant, diaphoretic, febrifuge, antipyretic and diuretic and as a laxative in bilious affections. The flowers are credited with emollient and demulcent properties and are used to treat coughs, sore throat, hoarseness and ailments of infants. Petals are made into a syrup and used as a remedy for infantile disorders. The herb is used in homoeopathy to treat diseases of skin and eyes and for relief from pain in the ear. In folk medicine, it is used as a blood-purifier.

TULSI

Biological source

Tulsi is the dried leaves of *Ocimum sanctum* Linn. (Family : Lamiaceae).

Geographical distribution

The plant is cultivated throughout India especially in houses and temples for worship.

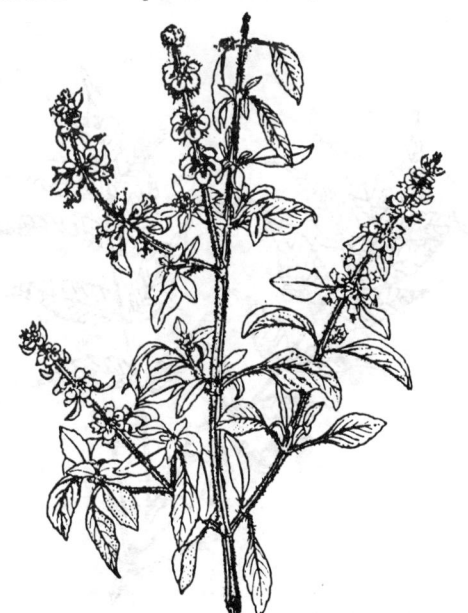

Fig. 22.35. Tulsi : *Ocimum sanctum.*

Macroscopy

Tulsi is an annual herb, 30-60 cm high, with much branched stems. The branches are generally purplish, sub-quadrangular and covered with soft hairs.

Leaves are simple, elliptical, oblong obtuse or acute, 2-5 cm long, 1.5-3.2 cm wide, margin entire or serrate, base obtuse or acute; petiole slender, 1.3-2.5 cm long, hairy surface, pubscent on both sides. Flowers are verticillate, in racemes, 15-20 cm long in close whorls. Odour and taste are aromatic and sharp.

Chemical constituents

Leaves contain 0.7% of volatile oil. The prominent constituents of the essential oil are eugenol (71%), methyl eugenol (20%), carvacrol (3%), and caryophyllene (2-32%). The oil of species grown in Phillipines contains methyl chavicol, cineole and linalool.

The other components isolated from the volatile oil are nerol, decylaldehyde, γ-selinene, β-pinene, comphene, α-pinene, cadinene, 1,8-cineole, limonene, methylchavicol and bornyl acetate.

The leaves also contain β-carotene, ursolic acid, 4-allyl-1-glucosyl-2-hydroxybenzene, 4-allyl-1-glucosyl-2-methoxybenzene, vicenin 2, apigenin-6,8-C-diglucoside, luteolin-5-O-glucoside, rosmarinic acid, cirsilineol, gallic acid, its methyl and ethyl esters; protocatechuic, vanillic, caffeic, chlorogenic and 4-hydroxybenzoic acids, vanillin, 4-hydroxybenzaldehyde and juvocimenes.

Uses

Leaves have expectorant, diaphoretic, anti-periodic, anticatarrhal, antiseptic and spasmolytic properties and are used in catarrh, bronchitis, cold, cough,

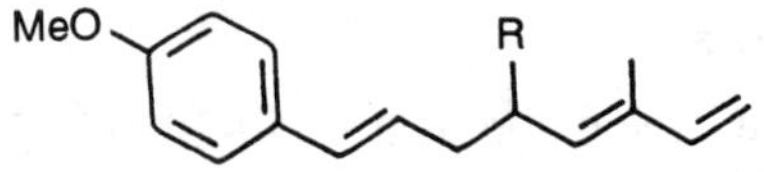

Juvocimene I
R = CH = CMe$_2$
Juvocimene II
R = 3,3-Dimethyl-2-oxiranyl

Fig. 22.36. Chemical constituents of Tulsi.

fever and gastric disorders. The leaves have been employed as aromatic, carminative, stimulant and flavouring agent. Infusion of the leaves is used as stomachic in gastric disorders of children and in hepatic affections. Dried powdered leaves are taken as snuff in ozena. Seeds are demulcent and given in disorders of the genito-urinary system. The plant is also used for snake-bite and scorpion-sting.

Pharmacology

Leaf extract modulated humoral immune responses, showed clinical and biochemical clearance of viral hepatitis in 14 days of treatment, caused decrease in uric acid level in serum and corresponding increase in urine, decreased in sexual behaviour in male rats, reduced elevated enzyme levels and, thus, protected rats against hepatic cell damage, decreased incidence of induced neoplasia in Swiss mice and induced hepatomas in rats and reduced ulcer index and acidity indicating antiulcerogenic property of the extract. Ursolic acid has antiallergic potential.

NEEM

Synonyms

Nim; Nimba (Sans.); Limba (Marathi, Gujarati); Vepa (Telgu).

Botanical source

Neem is the fresh or dried leaves and seed oil of *Azadirachta indica* J. Juss. (syn. *Melia indica* Bran. or *M. azadirachta* Linn) (Family : Meliaceae).

Habitat

Neem tree is habitated in south-eastern Asia, India, Andamans, Pakistan, Sri Lanka, Burma, Malaya, Indonesia, Japan, tropical regions of Australia and Africa.

Characters

Neem is a large glabrous tree, 10-20 m high with a straight trunk and long spreading branches. Leaves are imparipinnate, alternate, 3-6 cm long on long slender petioles; leaflets 7-17; alternate or opposite, very shortly stalked, 1-1.5 cm long, ovate-lanceolate, attenuate at the apex, unequal at the base, the upper half much longer than the lower and the leaflet

falcate, coarsely and bluntly serrate, smooth and dark green. Odour is typical and taste is bitter.

The fruit is an ovoid, bluntly pointed, smooth drupe, green when young and unripe, yellow to brown when mature and ripe, with a very scanty pulp and a hard bony endocarp. The seed is solitary with a thick testa and embryo with foliaceous cotyledons in the axis of scanty endosperm.

The seeds contain fixed acrid bitter oil (23-31%), deep greenish-yellow to brown in colour, extracted from the seeds by pressure; sp. gr. 0.91; soluble in ether, chloroform; practically insoluble in alcohol and water, odour of garlic, bitter taste.

Chemical constituents

The leaves contain nimbin, nimbinene, 6-des-acetylnimbinene, nimbandiol, nimbolide, quercetin, β-sitosterol, ascorbic acid, *n*-hexacosanol, nonacosane, amino acids, isonimbocinolide, margosinolide, isomargosinolide, isoazadirolide, nimbocinone, nimbocinolide, nimbaflavone, iso-rhamnetin, cyclic tri- and tetra-sulphides, kaemp-ferol-3-O-rutinoside and 3-O-D-glucoside, myri-cetin-3-O-rutinoside, 6-deacetylnimbinal, 28-deoxonimbolide, isoprenylated flavanone, β-sito-sterol-D-glucoside, n-hexacosanol, β-carotene,

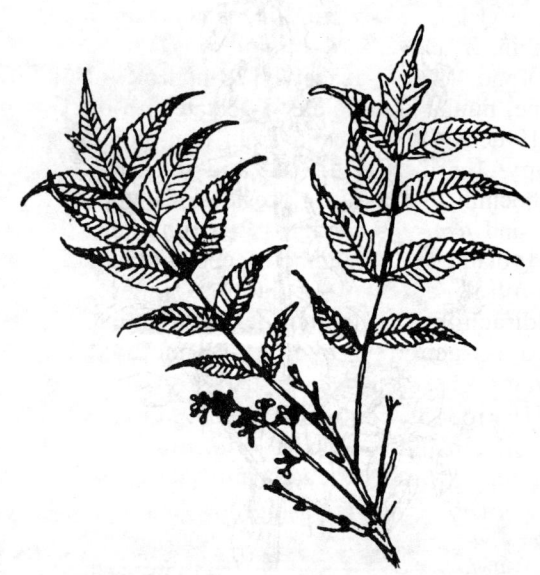

Fig. 22.37. *Azadirachta indica.*

quercetin-3-O-rhamnoside, quercetin-3-O-rutinoside, hyperoside, rutin, meldenindiol, meldenin, isomeldenin, 4α, 6α-dihydroxy-A homoazadirone, solannolide, nimocinol (6α-hydroxyazadirone), deacetylazadirachtinol, 2',3'-dehydrosalannol and azadirachtanin.

The fruits contain gedunin, 7-deacetoxy-7α-hydroxygedunin, azadiradione, azadirone, 17β-hydroxyazadiradione, 17-epiazadiradione, nimbiol, nimolinone, isonimolicinolide, nimolicinoic acid, nimbochalcin, nimbocetin, 5-hydroxymethyl furfural dipropyl disulphide, 1-cinnamoyl melianolone, 1-cinnamoyl-3,11-dihydroxymeliacarpin, naheedin, azadirachtol, eicosane, docosane, 2-methyltricosane, docosene, androsta-1,14-dien-3,16-diones, azadirachtin, epoxyazadiradione, azadirachtin, salannin, 21, 23 : 24, 25-diepoxy-tirucall-7-en-21-ol, 17-epiazadiradione, 17β-hydroxyazadiradione, nimolicinol, azadirachtol, 6-O-acetyl nimbandiol, 3-desacetylsalannin, nimbocinol, desacetylnimbinolide, desacetyl isonimbinolide.

The seeds contain six tetranortriterpenoids, viz., 1-methoxy-1, 2-dihydroepoxyazadirone, 1, 2-diepoxyazadiradione, 7-acetylneotrichilenone, 7-desacetyl-7-benzoylazadiradione, 7-desacetyl-7-benzoyl-epoxyazadiradione and 7-desacetyl-7-benzoylgedunin. They also contain azadirachtin, deacetyl nimbin, nimbidin, epoxyazadiradione, nimbin, β-sitosterol, 4-epinimbin, salannolactam-(21) and -(23), 7-deacetyl-17β-hydroxy-azadiradione, nimbanal, salannol-3-acetate, 1,3-diacetyl-11,19-deoxa-11-oxomeliacarpin, di-n-propyl and n-propyl-1-propenyl di, tri- and tetrasulphides, limbocinin, limbocidin, glycosides of stigmas-terol, cis- and trans-3,5-diethyl-1,2,4-trithiolanes from seed volatile fraction, limbonin, epoxy-azadiradione, nimbinol, azadirol, kulactone (seed coat), azadirachtin K, ohchinolide B, salamin and 1-tigloyl-3-acetyl-11-hydroxy-4β-methyl-meliacarpin.

The root bark provided nimbidiol, nimbolicin, nimbilicin, nimbocidin, gedunin, nimbilin, nimolinin, margocin, margocinin and margocilin.

Kernels yield a greenish yellow to brown, acrid, bitter fixed oil (23.5%) having a strong, disagreeable odour resembling garlic. The fatty acid composition of the oil is as : myristic (0.2%), palmitic (16.2), stearic (14.6), arachidic (3.4), oleic (56.6) and linoleic (9%). The component glycerides are : palmitodistearin, oleopalmito-stearin, oleodistearin, palmito-oleolinolein, palmitodiolein and linoleodiolein. The oil also contains 2% bitter principles which include nimbidin, nimbidinin, nimbin, nimbinin, nimbidol, nimbiol, sugiol, epoxyazadiradione, azadiradione, azadirone, meliantriol, meldenin, vipinin, tiglic acid, nimbene, 6-deacetylnimbinene, nimbandiol, 6-acetylnimbandiol and 17-epinimbocinol.

The flowers yield melicitrin, quercetin-3-galactoside and kaempferol-3-glucoside.

The roots contain 24-methylene cycloartanone, cycloeucalenone, 24-methylene cycloartanol, 4-stigmasten-3-one, 4-campesten-3-one, triacontanol, vanillic aldehyde, trans-cinnamic acid, vanillic acid and azadirinin. Neem gum is composed of a glycopeptide.

The plant also contains scopoletin, 6-hydroxy-7-methoxycoumarin, aesculetin, cinnamic acid, β-sitosterol, compesterol, isonimbolide, isolimbolide and 28-deoxonimbolide.

The stem bark contains methylnimbiol, sugiol, margolone, margolonone, isomargolonone, nimbonone, nimbonolone, polysaccharides GIII DQ$_2$ Ia, GIII DQ$_2$IIa, N9GI, CPS-I, CPS-II, CPS-III, CSSP-I, II and III, margosinone, margosinolone, nimbosterol, nimbidic acid, deacetyl nimbin, kulinone, kulactone, kulolactone, methyl kulnate, 6β-hydroxy-4-stigmasten-3-one, 6β-hydroxy-4-campesten-3-one, vilasinin, glycoprotein, arabinofucoglucans Gla and Glb, isonimbinolide, nimbionone, nimbione, nimbinone, nimosone, nimbosone, methyl nimbionone, nimbosodione, nimbisonol, demethylnimbionol, margosone and mergosolone.

Trunk wood possesses nimbolins A and B, β-sitosterol, its glucoside, 24-methylenecyclo-artanol, melianins A and B, cycloeucalenone, fraxinellone, azedaric acid, nimbolin A, gedunin, 7-deace-tyl-7-oxogedunin, 4,14α-dimethyl-5α-ergosta-8,24(28)-dien-3β-ol and 24-methyleneleuphenol.

Uses

Neem oil (margosa oil) is stimulant, antiseptic, alternative and used in rheumatism and skin diseases. Anti-inflammatory, anti-bacterial, antipyretic

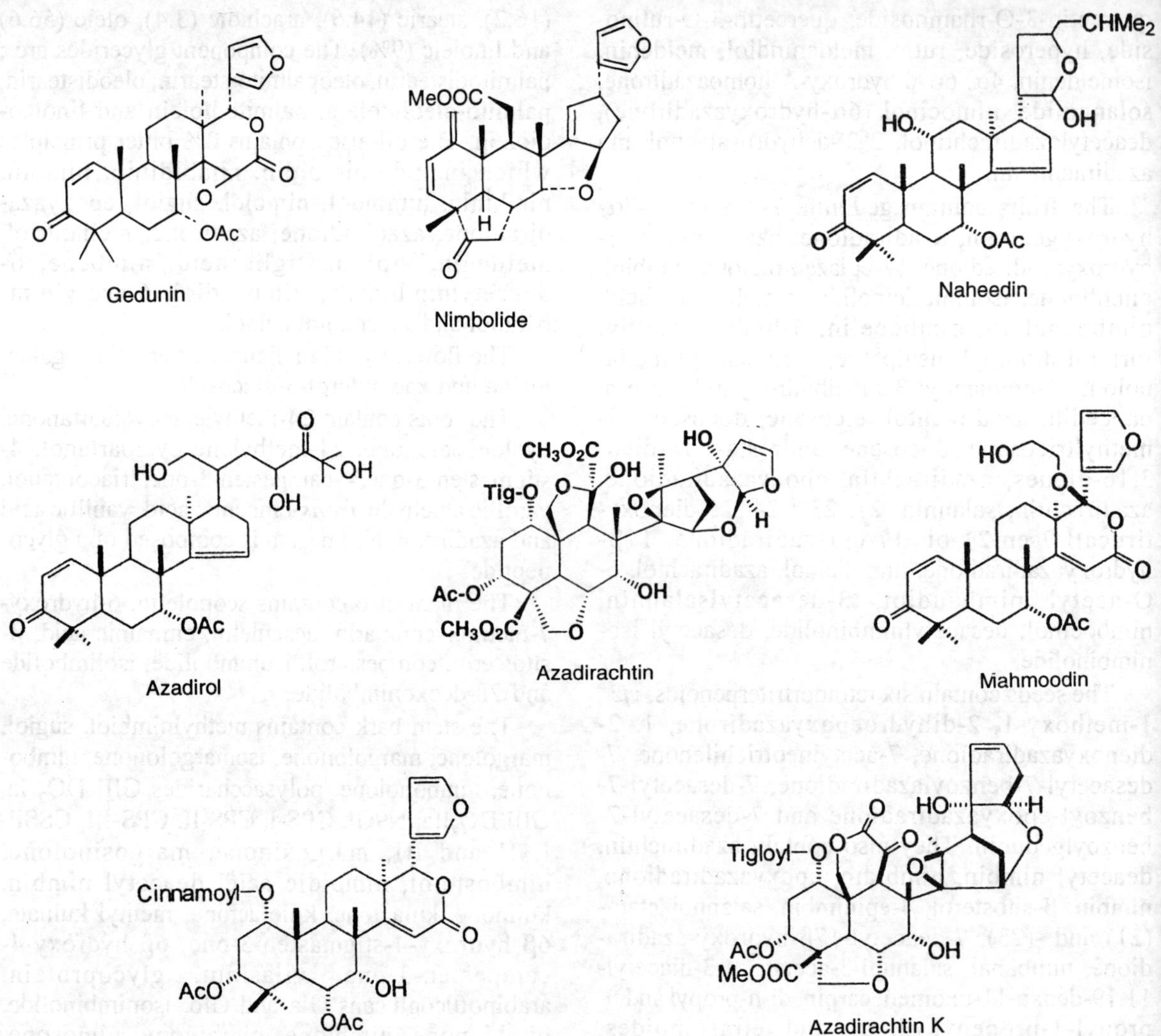

Fig. 22.38. Chemical constituents of *Azadirachta indica*.

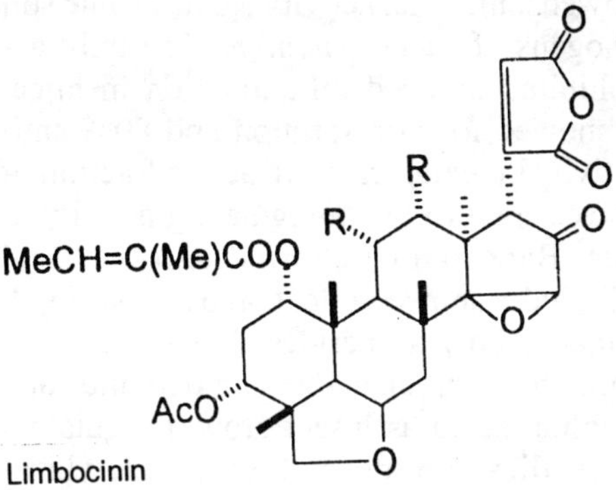

Limbocinin
R = H
Limbocidin
R = OH

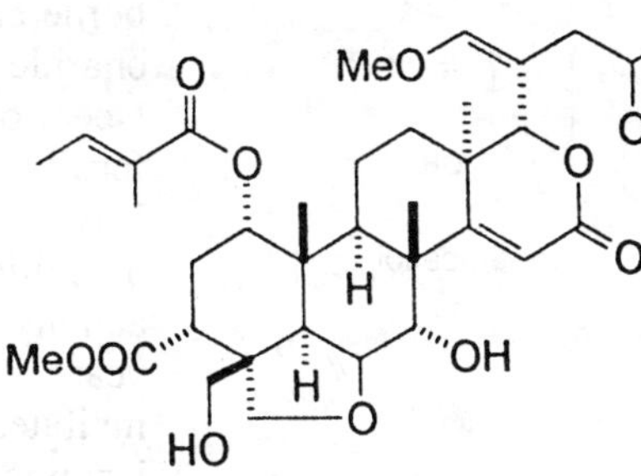

MeCH=C(Me)COO

AcO''''

R''''

R

Limbonin

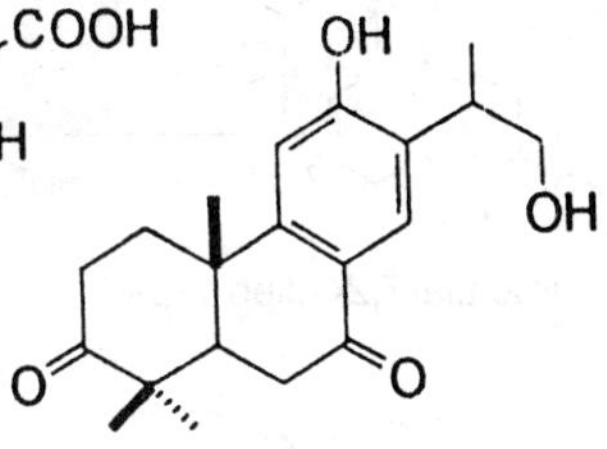

MeO

COOH

OH

MeOOC''''

HO

H

H

OH

O

Margocinin

OH

OH

O

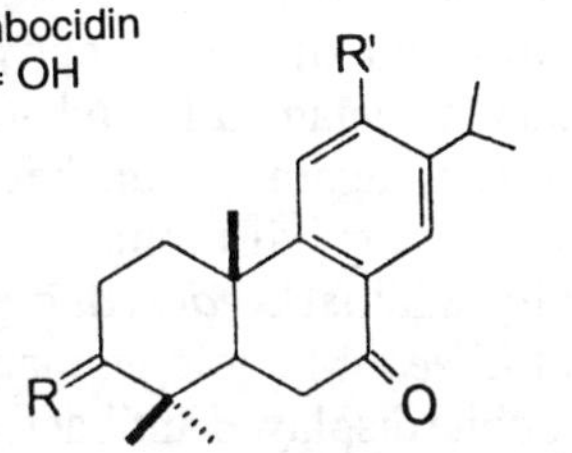

Margocilin
R = OH, H, R' = OH
Margocin
R = O, R' = H

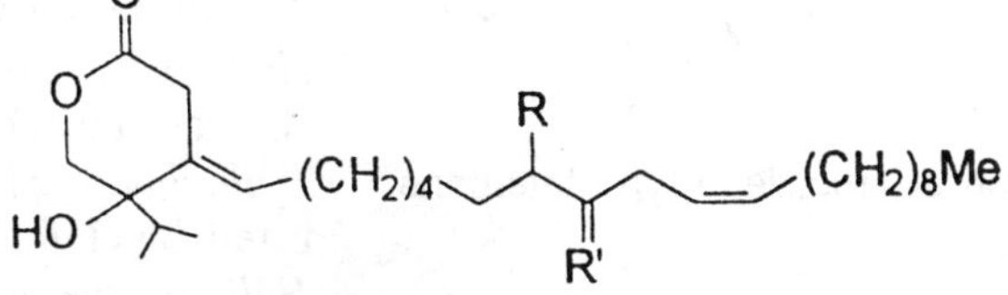

R'

R

O

Margosinone
R = H, R' = O
Margosinolone
R = OH, R' = CH₃

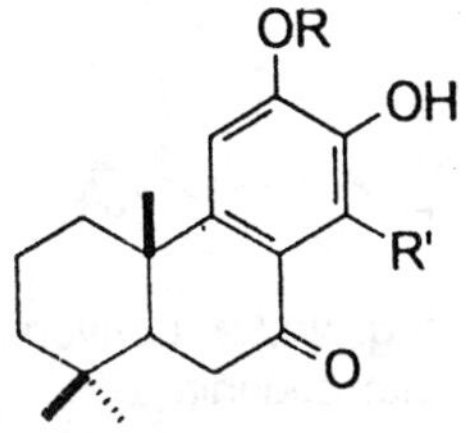

HO

R

R'

(CH₂)₄

(CH₂)₈Me

Margosone
R = H, R' = CHMe₂
Margosolone
R = Me, R' = H

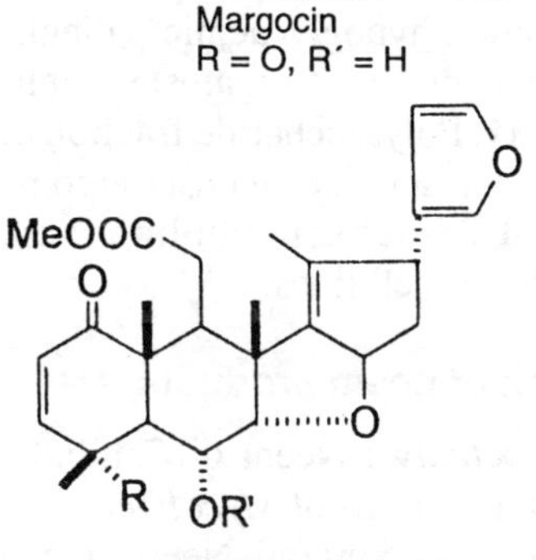

OR

OH

R'

O

Nimbinol
R = CH₂OH, R'= Ac
6-Deacetylnimbinal
R = CHO, R' = H

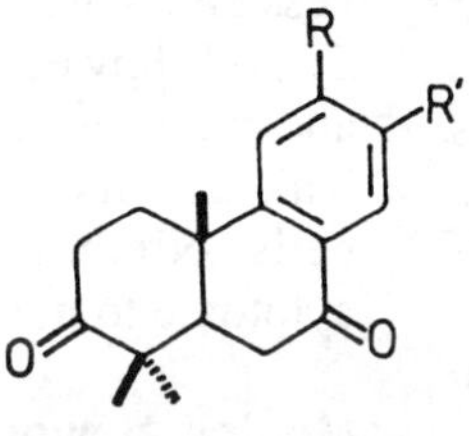

MeOOC

O

R

OR'

Nimbione,
R = Me, R' = OH
Nimbinone
R = OH, R' = Me

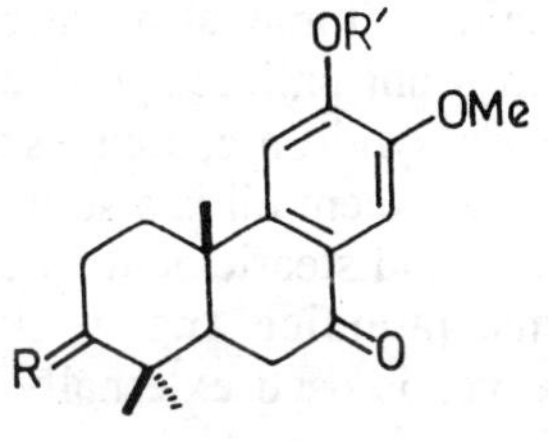

R

R'

O

Nimbionone
R = Q, R' = H
Methyl nimbionone
R = O, R' = Me
Nimbionol
R = b-OH, H, R' = H

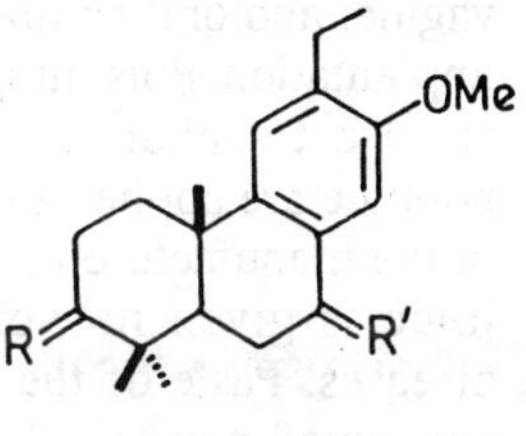

OR'

OMe

R

O

Nimbonone
R = H, H, R' = O
Nimbonolone
R = O, R' = N, H

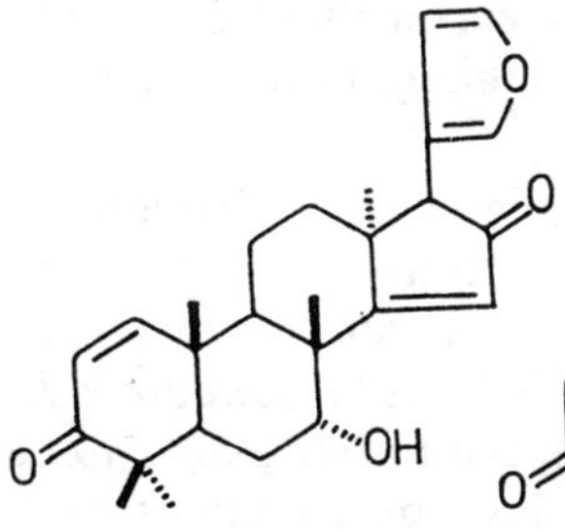

OMe

R

R'

Nimbocinol

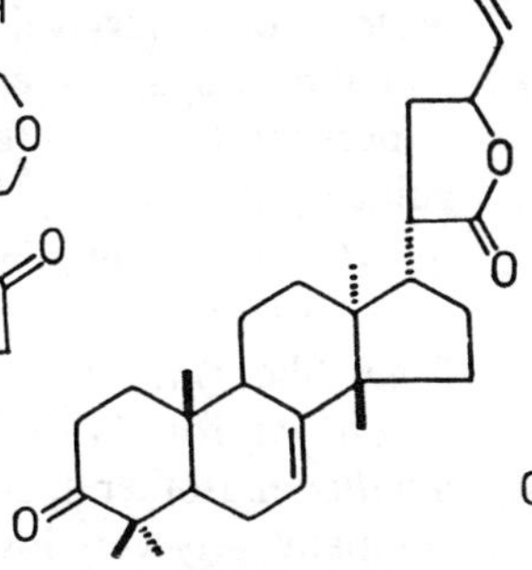

O

OH

Nimolinone

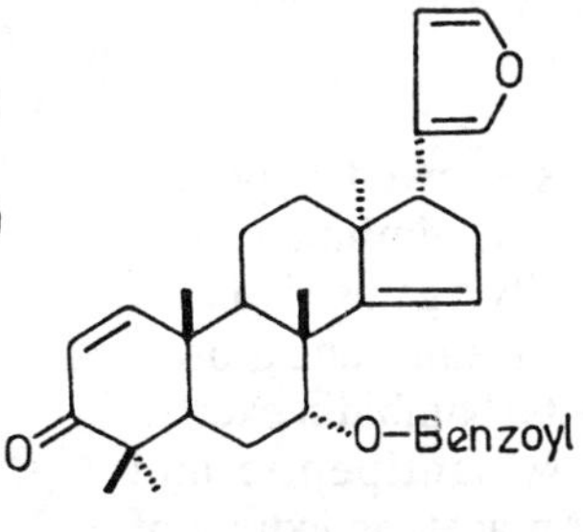

O

O

Nimocin

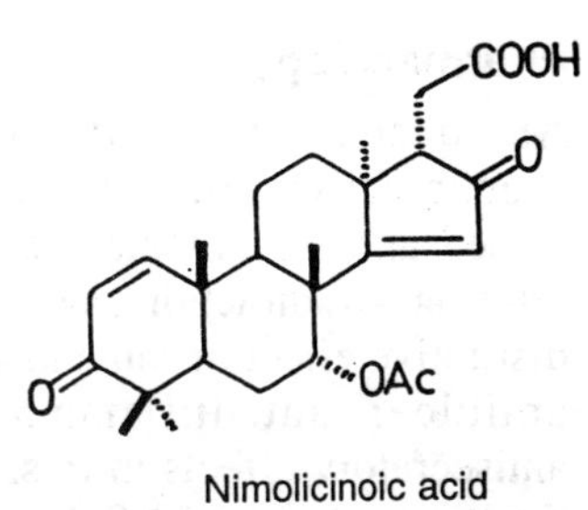

O

O–Benzoyl

Nimolicinoic acid

COOH

O

OAc

Fig. 22.38. Chemical constituents of *Azadirachta indica. (Contd.)*

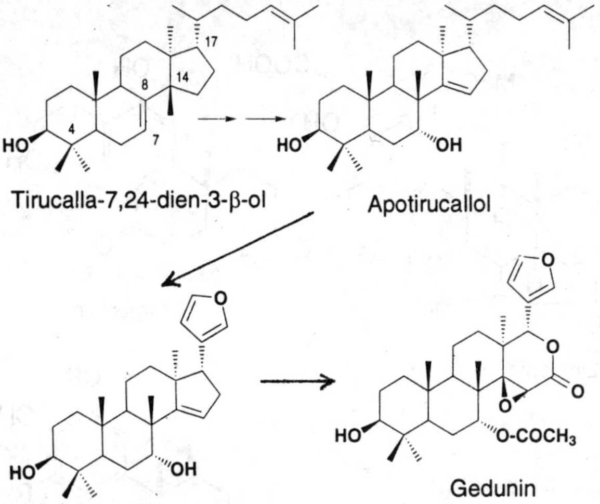

Tirucalla-7,24-dien-3-β-ol   Apotirucallol

Gedunin

Fig. 22.39. Conversion of tirucallene type triterpene into gedunin.

and hypoglycaemic activities have been noted in neem oil. As an antifertility agent, it appears to have potential, both in including male infertility and as a vaginal and oral contraceptive; it may also prevent implantation. Poisoning in young children produces an effect similar to Reye's syndrome. Leaves as poultice are applied to boils. Neem oil is also used in the manufacture of oleic and stearic acids. Leaf juice is given in worms, jaundice and in skin diseases. Paste of the leaves is used externally to cure small-pox.

The tender leaves along with *Piper nigrum* are used in intestinal helminthiasis. The paste of leaves is useful in ulceration of cow-pox. Fresh, mature leaves along with the seeds of *Psoralea corylifolia* and *Cicer arietinum* are used to prepare an effective medicine for leueoderma. The leaves are used as an insect repellent, antiviral and antifungal.

Pharmacology

An aqueous extract of leaves showed hypoglycaemic activity in dogs. Sodium nimbinate possessed anti-inflammatory activity against induced arthritis. Azadirachtin exhibited feeding and growth disruptive effect in some insects. Nimbidin exerted antiulcer, anti-inflammatory, antipeptic and antisecretory effects in rats. An acetone extract of the leaves showed CNS depressant, positive inotropic and blood pressure lowering effects. Plant

extract showed antifungal activity against some soil borne pathogens of *Cicer arietinum*. The polysaccharide inhibited induced inflammation in mice. Neem oil showed foetal resorption and 80% antifertility activity in female rats. An acidic fraction of leaves showed insect growth-regulating activity in mosquitoes. Bark extract showed anti-bacterial activity. Nimbidin showed effect on psoriasis in 60 years old males. Polysaccharides CPS-I and N9GI inhibited growth of sarcoma-180. Nimocinolide and isonimocinolide acted as insect growth regulators against houseflies and mosquitoes. Deacetylazadirachtinol and 7-deacetyl-17β-hydroxyazadiradione showed inhibition of insect ecdysis *Heliothis virescens*. Salannolactam-(21) and -(23) showed antifeedant activity against bean beetle, *Epilachna varivestis*. Di-*n*-propyldisulphide exhibited larvicidal activity against *Aedes aegypti*, *Heliothis virescens* and *H. zea*. Margolone, margolonone and isomer-golonone displayed antibacterial activity. Neem oil is effective in secondary diabetes and provided relief in itching, dyspepsia, tiredness and muscular pain in hypoglycaemic patients. The oil showed antifeedant activity against nymphs and adults of strawberry. Polysaccharide fraction of bark exhibited antitumor activity against sarcoma cells. Nimbolide and 28-deoxonimbolide were cytotoxic to human tumor cell lines.

Medicinal evaluation of neem products

1. *Anti-tubercular activity* : Neem oil inhibited the growth of all the strains of *Mycobacterium* in a concentration of 12.5 mg/ml. Neem oil and nimbidol in higher concentrations exhibited partial inhibitory influence whereas nimbidin prolonged the survival period of mice affected with tuberculosis. Neem oil also depressed the hypersensitivity to tuberculinin sensitized guinea pigs.

2. *Anti-fungal* : Nimbidin, nimbin, nimbidol and neem oil are very effective against various fungi like *Tinea rubrum* ring worm fungus, *Trichophyton interdigitale*, *Coccidiodes immitis* and other species of *Trichophyton* at comparatively very low concentrations.
   Neem oil also possessed good anti-fungal activity against *Microsporum gypsum*,

Aspergillus fumigatus, Penicillium litacinum and *Fusarium nivale.*

3. *Anti-protozoal* : Nimbidin and sodium nimbidinate killed *Paramaecium candatum* in 1/500 dilution in 1 minute. The action of sodium nimbidinate was found to be more potent than nimbidin. Nimbidol, however, proved more potent than nimbidin at a dose of 25 mg/100 g of body wt given orally, in suppressing the infection of *Plasmodium gellinaecum* in chicks.

4. *Anti-allergic* : Nimbin inhibited the stimulation produced by histamine in guinea pig ileum in a dose of 1 mg/ml. In doses of 2 mg/ml nimbidin blocked the stimulant action of acetylcholine in frog rectus abdominus muscles. Nimbidin is reported to be effective against eosinophilia with marked symptomatic relief.

5. *Dermatological diseases* : Nimbidin is also effective against various skin diseases such as furunculosis, arsenical dermitis, eczema, scabies and seborrhoeic dermatitis.

6. *Dental diseases* : Nimbidin gargle and dentifrices have been found to be effective in bleeding gums and pyorrhoea. '*Silvose T*' and '*Silvo TRS*' which are patented extracts of the bark of Neem are intended as an active ingredient in toothpastes and other oral hygiene preparations. Neem extract when added to a toothpaste produced remarkable results, in preventing and healing the inflammation of the gum and paradontosis.

7. *Other minor activities* : Various neem products show antibacterial, antiviral, spermicidal, anti-inflammatory, anti-ulcer, anti-pyretic and cardiovascular activities.

The major problem in using neem oil in soap manufacture is its objectionable odour. In toilet soap manufacture, the dark colour, high unsaponificable matter and other undesirables such as sulphur compounds and resinous materials are objectionable.

Neem cake

Neem cake is the major byproduct of the neem oilseed crushing industry. Neem cake contains more sulphur (1.07 to 1.36%) than any other cake. The nitrogen content varies from 2 to 3% of the cake. It is bulky and can be used as an organic manure.

The cake exerts an inhibitory or retarding effect on nitrification capacity of the soil due to the presence of oil. Urea coated with neem extract increased the protein content of rice due to high availability of nitrogen even after flowering. Coating of the fertilizer's (urea) granules with neem cake is more effective than any other form of blending. The berries (fruit) as such or its aqueous alcoholic extracts are toxic to pigs, rabbits, cow and buffalo calves.

TOBACCO

Synonyms

Leaf Tobacco : Tamaku (Hindi).

Biological source

Tobacco consists of the cured and dried leaves of *Nicotiana tabacum* Linn. (Family : Solanaceae).

Habitat

Tobacco is a tall annual herb indigenous to tropical

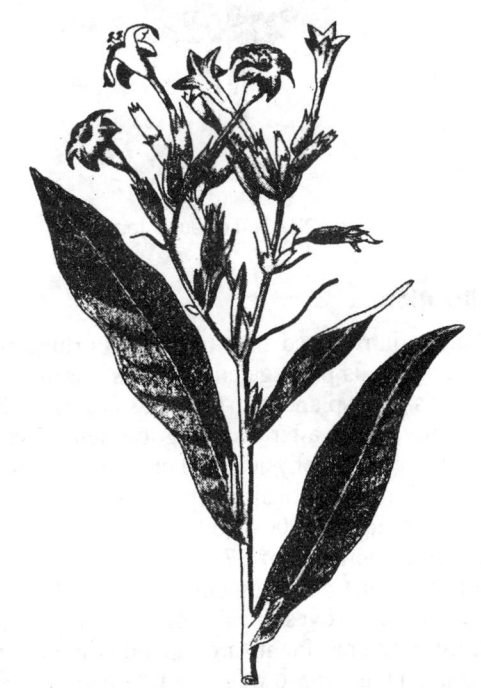

Fig. 22.40. *Nicotiana tabacum* flowering branches.

America. It is cultivated in tropical countries especially in Brazil, Sri Lanka and India.

Characters

The stem is simple, giving rise to large, pubescent, ovate, entire, simple, decurrent leaves; the veins are prominent and hairy. The flowers are long tubular, pink or reddish, sepals (5), united, persistent, funnel or cup-shaped, lobes valvate or twisted, occur in terminal spreading cymes. The leaves are hung in barns, slowly cured and dried. They are ovate, elliptic or lanceolate, up to 10 cm or more in length, usually sessile, sometimes petiolate.

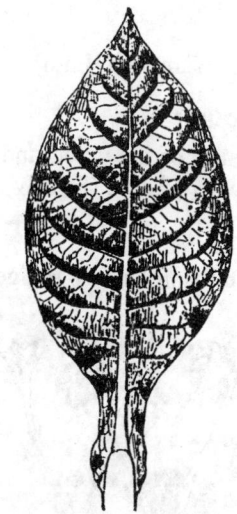

Fig. 22.41. Tobacco leaf.

Cultivation

Tobacco, introduced into India by Portuguese in 17th century, is propagated by seeds raised in nursery beds. Transplanting to the fields is done by hand on a rainy day or after irrigating the field. Tobacco is sensitive to the physical and chemical properties of the soil. The best soil is open, well drained and aerated. It requires 100-120 frost free days with an average temperature of 27° to mature. Nitrogen is required for the development of leaves. Phosphate application improves the size of leaf and promotes uniform ripening. Plants are topped when they are 90-100 cm high or 5-6 weeks old. Tobacco is cured in the sun.

Chemical composition

Tobacco contains several pyridine alkaloids (4-6%) of which nicotine (0.6-9%) is the most important. The other basic components are nicotyrine, nicotimine, *l*-nornicotine, *d*-nornico-tine, piperidine, pyrrolidine, anabasine and anatabine. Tobacco contains 25-50% carbohydrates, mainly sucrose, starch, pectins, cellulose, and lignin. Dextrin maltose, stachyose, raffinose, rhamnose, ribose, inositol and sorbitol have been identified. Tobacco contains a high percentage of organic acids (~20%), mainly malic, citric and oxalic acids. Other acids identified are maleic, fumaric, lactic, malonic, terephthalic, succinic, acetic, methylvaleric, glyceric, crotonic, propionic, methyl ethyl acetic, benzoic and 2-furoic acids. Palmitic, oleic, linoleic and linolenic acids are also reported. Polyphenolic compounds like rutin, chlorogenic acid, quinic acid, shikimic acid, quercitrin, isoquercitrin and its 7-glucoside, sco-polin, aesculetin and its 7-glucoside, and kaempferol glycosides are present. The phenolic compounds reported are caffeic acid, melilotic acid, phenol, guaiacol, eugenol, isoeugenol, *p*-allyl-catechol, *m*-cresol and *o*-hydroxyacetophenone. Nearly sixty phenolic compounds have been distinguished in the extract of flue cured leaf. Tobacco also contains resins, paraffins, amino acids, enzymes, mineral contents, vitamins, sterols, gibberellins nicotiana α, β and γ, gibberellins A and A$_3$, anatalline, 1'-hexanoyl-nornicotine, 1-octanoylnornicotine, 1'-(6-hydro-xyoctanoyl) nornicotine, 1'-(7-hydroxyoctanoyl) nornicotine, pyridine alkaloids 5-methyl-2,3'-bipyridine, N-formylnornicotine, N-acetylnornicotine; solanofuran, spiroxabovolide, 2-methyl-5-(2-methyl-5-isopropenyl-tetrahydro-2-furyl)-furans, driman-8-ol, driman-8,11-diol, caffeoyl putrescine, caffeoyl spermidine, dicaffeoyl spermidine, 3-hydroxy-β-ionone, bombiprenone, cycloartanol, cycloartenol, 24-methylene cyclo-artanol, lanost-8-en-3β-ol, β-amyrin, solavetivone, cholesterol, cholest-7-enol, 24-methylene-cholesterol, campesterol, stigmasterol, sitosterol, 28-isofucosterol, lanosterol, 31-norlanosterol, lanost-8-enol, obtusifoliol, 31-norcyclo-artenol, cycloeucalenol, gramisterol, citrostadienol, β-amyrin, lupeol, cycloartanol, 24-methylene cyclo-artanol, hentriacontane, dotriacontane, solanascone, sphingolipids, 31-nor-lanost-9(11)-enol, 24-methyl-

31-norlanost-9(11)-enol, 4,24-dimethylcholesta-7, 24-dienol, cyclo-eucalenol, 31-norlanost-8-enol, 4-methyl-cholesta-8-enol, lophenol, 24-methyllophenol, 24-ethyllophenol, gramisterol, citrostadienol, megastigma-5,8-dien-4-one, dehydrololiolide, N'-formylanabasine, N'-formylanatabine; labdanic dilerpenes, C-13 norcarotenoids, loliolide, isololiolide, phytuberin, phytuberol, galactose, galacturonic acid, rhamnose, arabinose, solanesol, 8,9-dehydrothea-spirone, 8,11-epoxy-2,6-cembradien-4,12-diol and other cembranoids, capsidiol, solavetivone, 3-hydroxysolavetivone, 3-hydroxy lubimin, rishitin, epirishitin, glutinosone, oxyglutinosone, 7,8-epoxy-4-basman-6-one, cembratrienetriols, 3-oxo-α-ionol-β-glucoside, blumenol C-β-glucoside, rishitin-1,2-diglucoside, 3β-hydroxysolanascone-3-O-sophoroside, 3β-hydroxy-solavetivone-3-O-glucoside, rishitin glycoside, megastigmene-5,6,9-triol, 18-oxo-3-virgene; 9β- and 10β-hydroxysolanascone-β-glucosides, 1β-hydroxydebneyol-12-O-β-glucoside, glutamine synthetase polypeptides and penten-4/5-olides.

Uses

Tobacco is sedative, narcotic, emetic, antiseptic, used in rheumatic swelling, skin diseases and for insect poisoning. It is widely used for smoking and as agricultural insecticide. Tobacco snuff is useful in nasal polypi, nasal catarrh, headache, chronic giddiness and fainting. Its excessive use produces dispepsia, chronic inflammation of bronchial mucous membrane, nervous depression, diseases of liver, sleeplessness, general anaemia, loss of vision or blindness, weakness, cancer, throat troubles, mental fatigue and cardiac diseases.

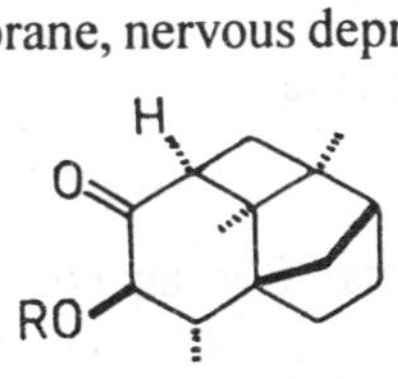

Pharmacology

Nicotine inhibited gastric and duodenal contractile activity in dogs; increased heart rate, myocardial oxygen consumption and coronary blood flow; showed self-stimulation in rats; influenced force of contraction in depolarized cat ventricular muscle; blocked contractile effect of muscarine on isolated rabbit ileum; and increased sexual receptivity in estrogen-treated female rats. (+)-Nicotine had both agonistic and antagonistic action similar to (−)-nicotine in CNS. Nicotine caused significant pressor response and increase in jejunal blood flow in dogs. Oxygen consumption was significantly reduced during first 5 minute of micotine infusion, then return to control level and then rose above control level post-infusion. Nicotine caused hyperglycaemia. Nicotine treatment did not affect apomorphine-induced locomotor activity in rats. Nicotine produced a transient contraction of isolated iris sphincter muscle of rabbit and transient contraction of isolated strips of guinea pig urinary bladder. Cembranoic diterpene inhibited action of MIAA by 50%. Aliphatic diones exhibited anti-oxidative activity. Nicotine inactivates nicotinic cholinergic receptors in brain by allosteric mechanism. Nicotine activates capsaicin-sensitive sensory nerves via nicotinic receptors. Cigarette smoking or low dose of nicotine improved mental functioning. A low dose of nicotine directly affects attention or stimulus-processing components of information processing.

3β-Hydroxysolanascone-3-O-sophoroside
R = Glu(2→1)Glu

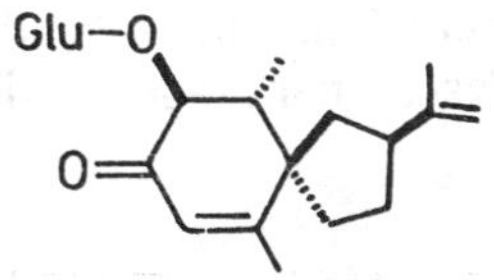

3β-Hydroxysolavetivone-3-O-glucoside

Fig. 22.42. Chemical constituents of Tobacco.

GUGGAL

Synonyms

Indian bdellium, Salai-gogil.

Biological source

Guggal is a gum-resin obtained by incision of the bark of *Commiphora mukul* (H. & S.) Engl. (syn. *Balsamodendron mukul* Hook. ex Stocks) (Family: Burseraceae).

Geographical source

The tree grows in Sind, Rajasthan, Bengal, South India, Maysore and Baluchistan.

Collection

Guggal tree is small, 1.2-1.8 m high, branches slightly ascending. It is sometimes planted in hedges. The ash coloured bark comes off in rough flakes exposing the underbark. Each plant yields about one kilogram of the product which is collected in cold season.

Characters

Guggal occurs as yellowish viscid, brown tears; or in fragment pieces, mixed with hairy stem, pieces of bark; colour brownish dark to golden yellow. It hardens very slowly. With water it forms a milky emulsion with terebinthinate odour, but fainter. Taste is bitter aromatic.

Chemical constituents

Oleo-gum resin of guggal contains gum (32%), essential oil (1.45%), sterols (guggulsterols I to VI, β-sitosterol, cholesterol, E- and Z-guggul-sterols pregnen-3-ones, guggulsterone), sugars (sucrose, fructose), amino acids, α-camphorene, cembrene, allylcembrol, flavonoids (viz., quercetrin and its glycosides), ellagic acid, myricyl alcohol, mukulol (allylcembrol), aliphatic tetrols, quercetin and its glycosides.

Uses

The gum resin is astringent, antirheumatic, antiseptic, expectorant, aphrodisiac, blood purifier, demulcent, aperient, and emmenagogue. It is used in the form of a lotion for indolent ulcers and as a gargle in caries of the teeth, weak and spongy gums, pyorrhoea alveolaris, chronic tonsiltis and pharyngitis and ulcerated throat, as a stomachic and intestinal disinfectant in chronic catarrh of the diarrhoea. It is believed to stimulate the appetite, improves the general condition, reduces fever and secretion from diseased surfaces. It is a valuable aphrodisiac and has marked antisuppurative properties. Like other oleoresins it causes an increase of leucocytes in the blood and stimulates phagocytosis. It acts as a diaphoretic, expectorant, diuretic and a uterine stimulant.

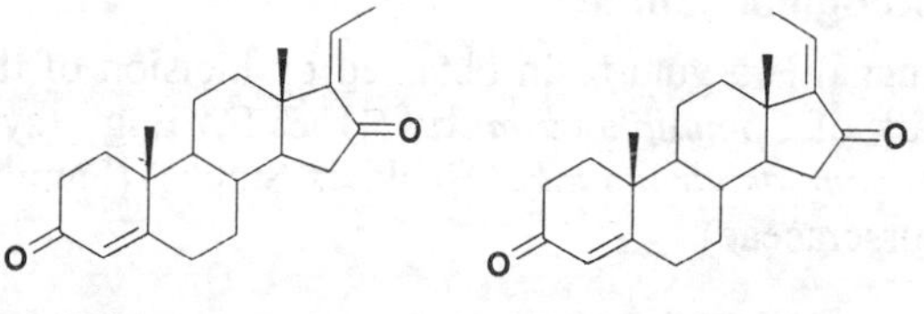

Pharmacology

Guggul containing drugs exhibit antiarthritic, anticholesteraemic, antilipidaemic, antiobesity, anti-inflammatory and anti-acne properties. Platelet aggregation inhibitory action and fibrinolytic action are also reported and the drug is prescribed to patients with heart diseases. It also possesses immunomodulatory activity. Z-Guggulsterone shows good thyroid stimulating activity in rats which leads to reduction of serum cholesterol and serum lipids. Volatile oil of the resin shows good anthelmintic activity against tapeworms and hookworms and it is better than piperazine phosphate and hexylresorcinol, respectively. Guggulip, an antihyperlipidaemic formulation, is marketed by Cipla in India and is used to treat piles. A purified guggulin steroid mixture completely inhibited ADP-adrenaline-induced platelet aggregation. Guggulipid is completely safe and devoid of any effect on liver function, blood sugar and blood urea levels. It decreased serum cholesterol and serum triglyceride levels.

PTEROCARPUS

Synonyms

Malabar kino tree; Bijasar.

Biological source

Pterocarpus consists of an aqueous extract of the wood and other parts of *Pterocarpus marsupium* Roxb. (Family : Papilionaceae).

Habitat

The tree is found commonly in hilly regions throughout the southern India and extending to Gujarat, Madhya Pradesh, Uttar Pradesh, Bihar and Orissa.

Characters

It is a moderate-sized to large deciduous tree, up to 30 m high and a girth of 2.5 m with a straight clean

Z-Guggulsterone   E-Guggulsterone

Fig. 22.43. Steroids of *Commiphora mukul.*

bole. Bark grey, rough, longitudinally fissured and scaly; blaze pink and whitish markings, older tree exuding a blood red gum-resin; leaves imparipinnate, leaflets usually 5-7, oblong; flowers in large panicles, yellow, fragrant; pods orbicular, flat, winged, up to 5 cm in diameter; seeds 1-2, convex and bony.

The tree is found in deciduous forests both on undulating and flat ground and grows on a variety of formations, provided the drainage is good. It prefers a soil with a fair proportion of sand, though it is often found on red loam with a certain amount of clay. The normal rainfall in its natural habitat ranges from 75 to 200 cm. It produces root suckers. It is planted as a shade tree in coffee estates in South India.

Natural reproduction is through seeds. The early development of seedlings is favoured by shelter from the sun and a loose soil clear of weeds. Seedlings may show little stem develop-ment or may die back annually for several years but ultimately shoot up after they have developed a long stout tap root. Whole pods are sown and germination can be hastened by cutting across their ends and then soaking

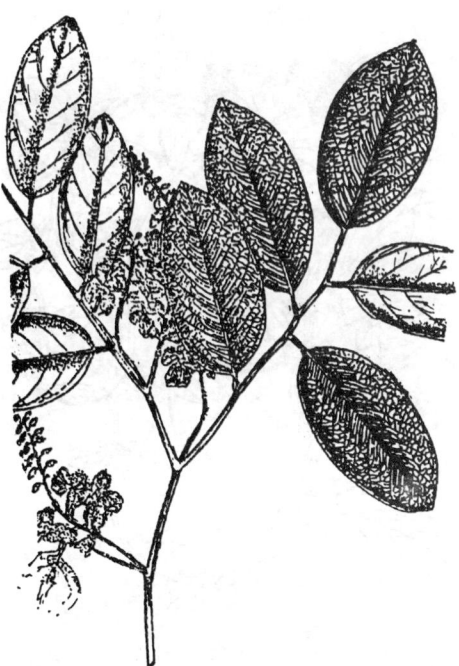

Fig. 22.44. *Pterocarpus marsupium.*

them in water for a few days prior to sowing. Stump planting of one year old plants raised in nursery gives good results. Seedlings may also be raised in bamboo baskets for planting out. The tree is attacked by a number of insects, mostly defoliators, and some fungi which cause rooting of the wood.

The tree yields a gum kino which exudes when an incision is made through the bark up to the cambium. The exudate is collected and dried in the sun or shade to give 340 g dried gum per tree. Kino occurs in small (3-5 mm), angular, glistering, brittle fragments, appearing almost black in colour. The edges looked ruby-red and transparent when viewed by transmitted light. It is odourless and bitter with astringent taste and colours saliva pink when masticated.

Chemical constituents

The bark contains 1-epicatechin and a reddish brown colouring matter. The heartwood yields liquirigenin, isoliquiritigenin, a neutral unidentified compound (mp 160), alkaloid (0.017%), resin (0.9%), a yellow colouring matter, an essential oil and a semi-drying fixed oil (0.52%). Kino contains a non-glucosidal tannin kinotannic acid (25-80%), kinoin and kino-red in addition to small quantities of catechol (pyrocatechin), protocatechuic acid, resin, pectin and gallic acid. Kino-red is the anhydride of kinoin, which is a phlobaphene produced from kinotannic acid by the action of an oxidase enzyme present in the kino.

The other compounds isolated from *P. marsupium* are marsupol (hydrobenzoin), 5, 4'-di-methoxy-8-methylisoflavone-7-rhamnoside, ses-quiterpenes selin-4(15)-en-1β, 11-diol, β-eudes-mol, erythrodiol 3-monoacetate, pterostilbene; marsupsin; pterosupin, pseudobaptigenin, liquiri-tigenin, isoliquiritigenin, garbenzol, 5-deoxy-kaempferol, *p*-hydroxybenzaldehyde (from roots); retusin-7-O-β-D-glucoside, irisolidone-7-O-α-L-rhamnoside, 5,7-dihydroxy-6-methoxy-7-O-α-L-rhamnoside, 7-hydroxy-5,4'-dimethoxy-8-methy-lisoflavone-7-rhamnoside, pterostilbene, 7-hy-droxyflavanone, 7,4'-dihydroxyflavone, pterosupin, *p*-hydroxybenzaldehyde, 3(*p*-hydroxyphenyl) lactic acid, propterol, oleanolic acid, 4,2', 4'-trihydroxychalcone, 8-C-β-D-glucosyl-3,7,4'-trihy-droxy- and 3,7,3',4'-tetrahydroxy flavones, 3'-C-β-

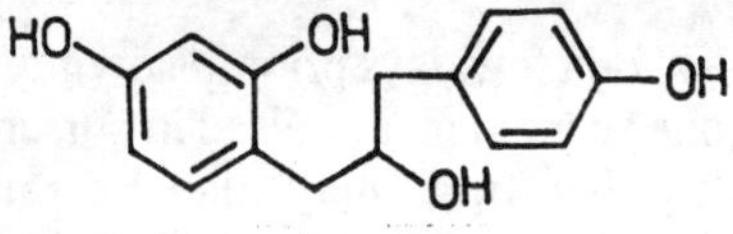

Propterol B

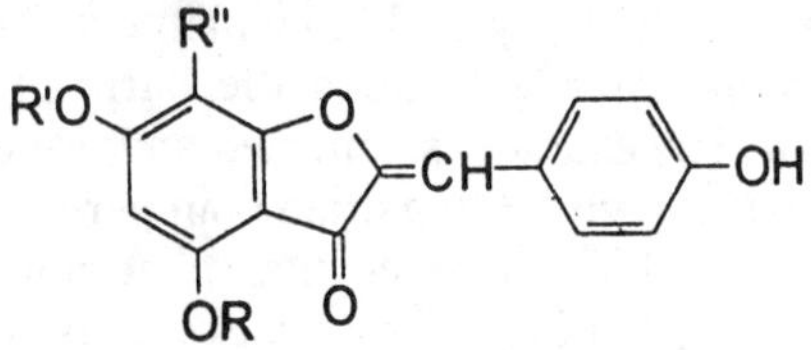

R, R″ = H, R′ = Rha
R = Rha, R′ = H, R″ = Me

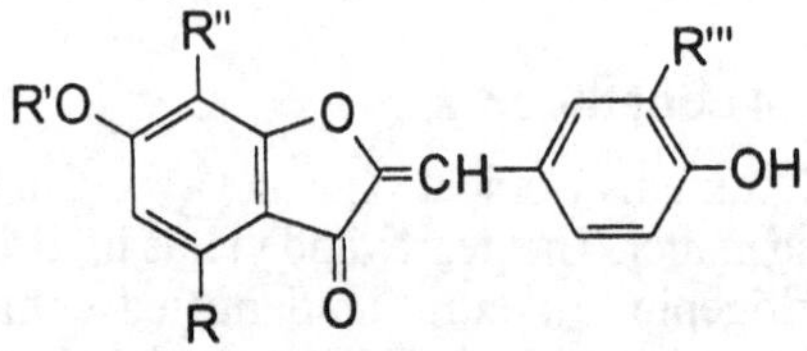

R, R‴ = H, R′ = Rha, R″ = Me
R, R‴ = OH, R′ = Rha, R″ = H

Fig. 22.45. Chemical constituents of *Pterocarpus marsupium*.

D-glucosyl-α-hydroxydichalcones, retusin-8-O-α-L-arabinoside, lupeol, naringenin, aurones 6,4'-dihydroxy-7-methylaurone-6-O-rhamnoside and 4,6,3',4'-tetrahydroxy aurone-6-O-rhamnoside.

Uses

An aqueous infusion of the wood is used in diabetes. The bark is used as an astringent and in toothache. The flowers are antipyretic. The leaves are employed as an external application for boils, sores and skin diseases. Kino is a powerful astringent and used in the treatment of diarrhoea and dysentery. It is locally applied in leucorrhoea, in passive haemorrhage and in toothache. Kino finds application in dyeing, tanning and printing and is of potential use for the paper industry.

Pharmacology

Heartwood extract showed hypoglycaemic action in fasting rabbits. (–)-Epicatechin, when given before or within 24 hours after alloxan, reversed hyperglycaemia in diabetic rats. It showed positive chronotropic and inotropic effects on isolated frog heart which was blocked by propranol. In higher doses, (–)-epicatechin caused hyperglycaemia in rats and this effect was also blocked by propranol. Ethyl acetate produced significant reduction in levels of serum triglycerides and total cholesterol. Liquiritigenin and pterosupin lowered serum cholesterol, LDL-cholesterol and atherogenic index in rats. Pterosupin lowered serum triglycerides.

GYMNEMA SYLVESTRE

Synonym

Gur-mar (Hindi).

Biological source

The drug consists of leaves of *Gymnema sylvestre* R.Br. (Fam. Asclepidaceae).

It is a large, pubescent, woody climber found in southern India, occasionally cultivated as a medicinal plant. The leaves are opposite, usually elliptic

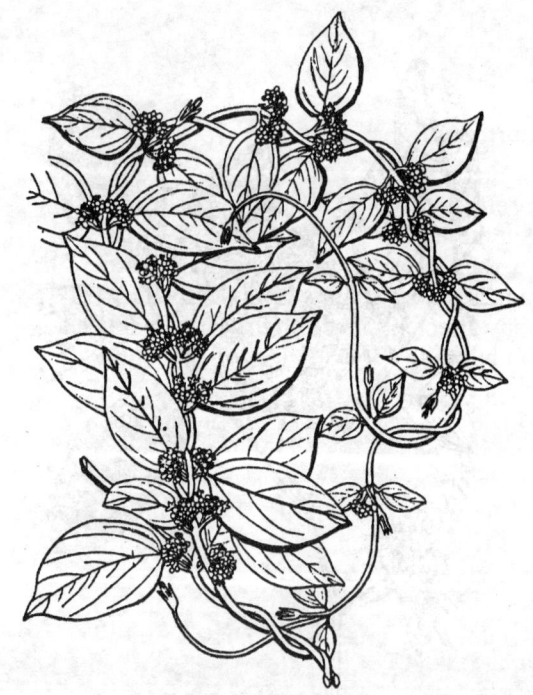

Fig. 22.46. *Gymnema sylvestre*—flowering branch.

or ovate; flowers small, yellow, in umbellate cymes; follicles terete, lanceolate, up to 8 cm in length.

Chemical constituents

The leaves contain albumin, organic acids, pararabin, hentriacontane, pentatriacontane, α- and β-chlorophylls, phytin, resins, tartaric acid, formic acid, butyric acid, anthraquinone derivatives, inositol, *d*-quercitol and gymnemic acid which is an impure complex mixture. The leaves give positive tests for alkaloids.

The other compounds isolated from the plant are nonacosane, triacontane, gymnesterogenin (hexahydroxyolean-12-ene), gymnamine, gymnemagenin, gymnemic acids I-VII, gypenosides II, V, XLIII, XLVII and LXXIV, gynosaponin TN-2, gymnemic acids III, IV, V, VIII, IX, X, XII, XV, XVI, XVII and XVIII, conduritol A, gymnemasaponins I, II, III, IV and V; gymnemasides XXVIII, XXXVII, LV, LXII and LXIII.

Uses

The plant is stomachic, stimulant, laxative and diuretic. It is used in cough, biliousness and sore eyes. The leaves are used as a remedy for diabetes. The drug is used as an errhine and for parageusia and furunculosis.

Pharmacology

The alcoholic extract or leaf powder does not show any effect on the concentration of sugar in the blood or in the urine of patients suffering from diabetes. But they cause hypoglycaemia in experimental animals when administered. This effect is not due to any direct influence on the carbohydrate metabolism but to indirect stimulation of insulin secretion by pancreas.

The leaf powder is tasteless with faint pleasant aromatic odour. It stimulates the heart and the circulatory system, increases the secretion of urine and activates the uterus. The laxative property is attributed to the presence of anthraquinone derivatives.

Gymnemic acids inhibited glucan formation of *Streptococcus mutans*, markedly inhibited the activity of glucosyl transferase from the bacterial coat and prevented the formation of dental plaque and caries. Leaf extract inhibited glucose absorption in small intenstine of rats. Gymnemic acid had

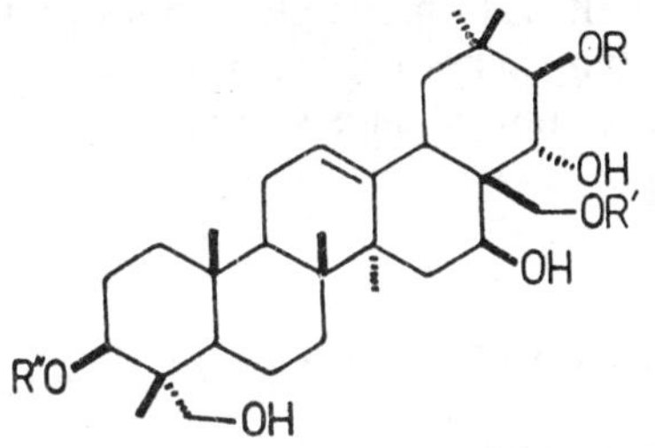

Gymnemic acid I
R = Tigloyl, R′ = Acetyl, R″ = Gluc. acid
Gymnemic acid II
R = 2-Methylbutyryl, R′ = Acetyl, R″ = Gluc. acid
Gymnemic acid III
R = 2-Methylbutyryl, R′ = H, R″ = Gluc. acid
Gymnemic acid IV
R = Tigloyl, R′ = H, R″ = Gluc. acid

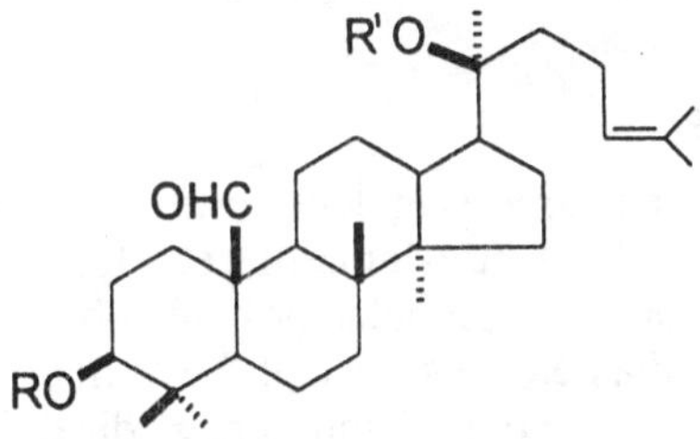

Gymnemaside I
R,R′ = Glu
Gymnemaside II
R = Glu(2→1)Glu, R′ = Glu
Gymnemaside III
R = Ara(2→1)Glu, R′ = Glu
Gymnemaside IV
R = Glu, R′ = Glu(6→1)Xyl
Gymnemaside V
R = Glu(2→1)Glu, R′ = Glu(6→1)Xyl

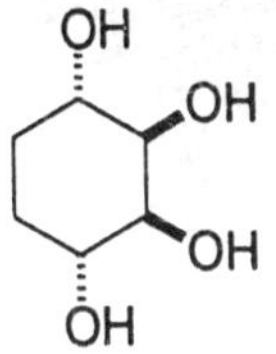

Conduritol A

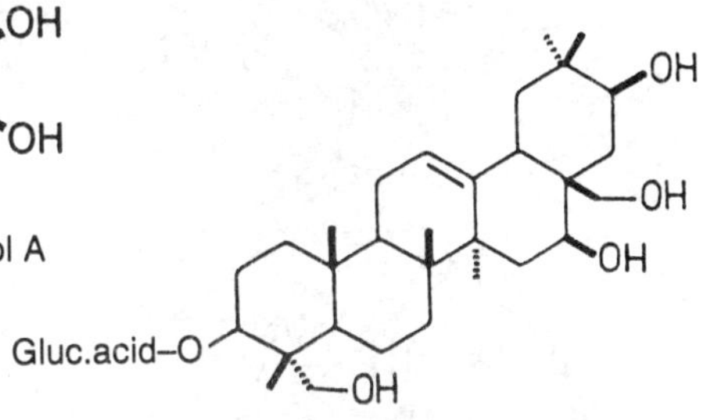

Gymnemic acid VII

Fig. 22.47. Chemical constituents of *Gymnema sylvestre*.

suppressed effect in blood glucose level after oral sucrose feeding in normal rats. Gymnema saponins III, IV and V showed antisweet activity.

VIDANG

Synonyms

Embeia; Black Vidang; Baberang (Hindi).

Biological source

Vidang consists of dried ripe fruits of *Embelia ribes* Burm. f. containing 2 per cent of embelin (Family : Myrsinaceae).

Geographical distribution

Vidang is common in the mixed deciduous forests of India ascending to 1500 m in Sri Lanka, Burma and South China. It is often cultivated in gardens and homeyards.

Characters

The plant is a large scandent shrub with slender branches and elliptic-lanceolate, gland-dotted leaves. Vidang is a globular brownish-black fruit, 2-4 mm in diameter, warty with beak like projection at the apex, about 1.2 mm long pedicel may be present in some fruits. A persistent calyx with 3-5 sepals is present. When pedicel absent, a single seed

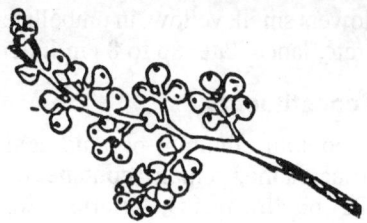

Fig. 22.49. Vidang.

covered with thin membrane. The seed is covered with a small yellow spots of crystalline embelin. Vidang contains an aromatic odour and hot astringent taste.

Chemical constituents

Vidang contains 2-3% hydroquinone embelin (2, 5-dihydroxy-3-lauryl-*p*-benzoquinone), a dimer of embelin known as vilangin, an alkaloid christembine, tannins, quercitol and minute amount of volatile oil. Embelin occurs in golden yellow needles, is insoluble in water but soluble in alcohol, chloroform and benzene. Fatty ingredients are also present in the fruits.

Tests for identification

1. A mixture of ethereal extract of Vidang powder and aqueous sodium hydroxide gives deep violet colour in aqueous layer. With dilute ammonia solution a bluish violet precipitate is formed (Test for embelin).
2. Alcoholic extract (10 ml) of powdered drug (2 g) with lead acetate solution produces green precipitate.
3. Alcoholic extract of the drug gives reddish brown precipitate with ferric chloride.

Uses

Vidang is anthelmintic especially against tapeworm. The fruit has astringent, carminative, stimulant, alternative and tonic properties. It is used to cure fevers, coughs and diarrhoea. Children suffering from tapeworms are treated by giving milk boiled with the drug. It has no activity against roundworms or threadworms.

Pharmacology

Berry extract showed antifertility and anti-oestrogenic activities in rats.

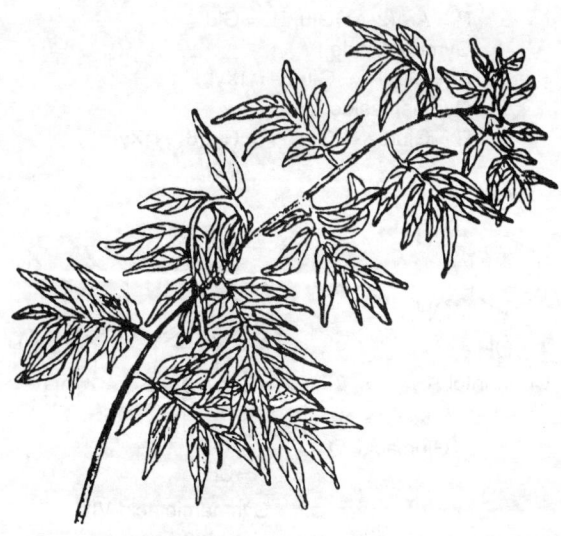

Fig. 22.48. *Embelia ribes.*

Substituent - Red Vidang

In commercial supply of Vidang sometimes Red Vidang is mixed which is dried ripe fruits of *Embelia robusta* Roxb. (syn. *E. tsjeriam-cottam* DC) (Fam. Myrsinaceae). The plant occurs on the Malabar coasts of India, Sri Lanka and Sylhet. The fruits are relatively larger in size (4-5 mm in diameter) and possess distinctly reddish wrinkled surface. The persistent calyx is more prominent with 5 distinct sepals. It contains embelin (1.5%) and minute amount of volatile oil.

ACHYRANTHES

Biological source

Achyranthes consists of the entire plant of *Achyranthes aspera* Linn. (Fam. Amaranthaceae).

Description

The plant is an erect or procumbent, annual or perennial herb, 1-2 m in height, often with a woody base, commonly found as a weed of way-sides and waste places throughout India up to an altitude of 2,100 m. Stems are angular, ribbed, simple or branched from the base, often tinged with reddish purple colour, leaves thick, ovate-elliptic or obovate-rounded, but variable in shape and size; flowers greenish white, numerous in axillary or terminal spikes, up to 75 cm long; seeds sub-cylindric, turncate at the apex, rounded at the base, reddish brown.

The plant is very variable, thrives best in the community of *Cassia tora* and is commonly found in shady places as a weed. It also grows in dried situations but does not tolerate waterlogging.

Chemical constituents

The seeds contain saponins, pentatriacontane, 6-pentatriacontanone; hexatriacontane, triacontane, hentriacontane and ecdysterone. The whole plant contains the alkaloids, achyranthine and betain. Achyranthine, a water-soluble alkaloid, dilates the blood vessels, lowers the blood-pressure, depresses the heart, and increases the rate and ampitude of respiration. Ecdysterone is also present in stem and leaves.

Plant also contains, ecdysterone (polypodine A) and ecdysone (from roots), oleanolic acid saponins

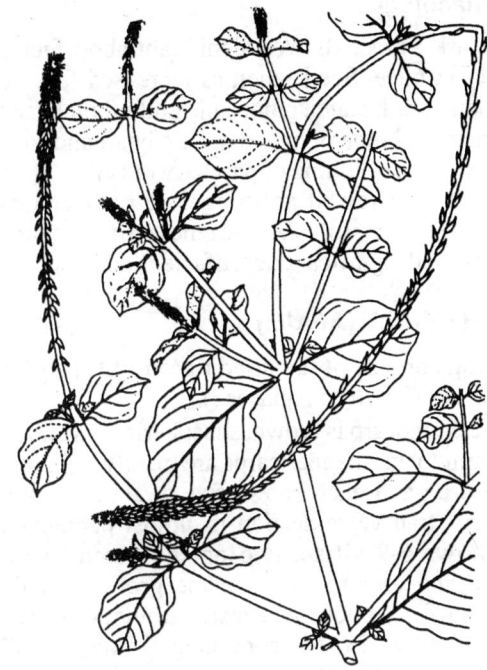

Fig. 22.50. *Achyranthes aspera*—flowering portion.

C and D; 36, 47-dihydroxyhenpenta-contan-4-one, 17-pentatriacontanol, 27-cyclohexyl heptacosan-7-ol and 16-hydroxy-26-methyl heptacosan-2-one.

The seed oil is composed of the glycerides of linoleic (50%), oleic (23%), palmitic (19%), stearic, behenic, arachidic, myristic and lauric acids.

Uses

The plant is pungent, astringent, pectoral and diuretic. It is used as an emmenagogue and to cure piles and skin eruptions. A decoction of the plant is useful in pneumonia and renal dropsy. The juice of the plant is used in ophthalmia, toothache and dysentery.

The leaves are used as a cure for gonorrhoea and excessive perspiration. Their extracts showed antibiotic action. The roots are astringent; their paste is applied to clear opacity of cornea and to wounds as an haemostatic. A decoction of the roots is used for stomach troubles and an aqueous extract for stones in bladder. The flowers are used for menorrhagia and to treat rabies. Seeds are emetic and given for biliousness. A medicated oil prepared from the plant is dropped into the ear in deafness.

Pharmacology

Stem bark extract showed significant abortifacient activity in mice. Seed saponins increased force of contraction of isolated guinea pig and rabbit hearts, also increased tone of hypodynamic heart and force of contraction of failing of papillary muscles. Shoot essential oil showed antifungal activity against *Aspergillus carneus*. The benzene extract of stem bark showed significant abortifacient activity.

CELERY FRUIT (APIUM)

The drug consists of the dried ripe fruits of *Apium graveolens* (Family : Apiaceae).

The cremocarp is brown, subspherical and about 1-1.5 mm long. The mericarps are mostly separated in the drug and each shows five straight primary ridges. A transverse section is almost pentagonal and shows 6-9 vittae, two on the commissural surface and four to seven in the grooves of the dorsal surface; odour and taste, aromatic. Celery fruits contain 2-3% of oil consisting of terpenes with smaller quantities of the anhydride of sedanonic acid, the lactone of sedanolic acid, phenols, coumarins, furanocoumarins and coumarin glycosides.

Celery fruits are used in the treatment of rheumatic diseases.

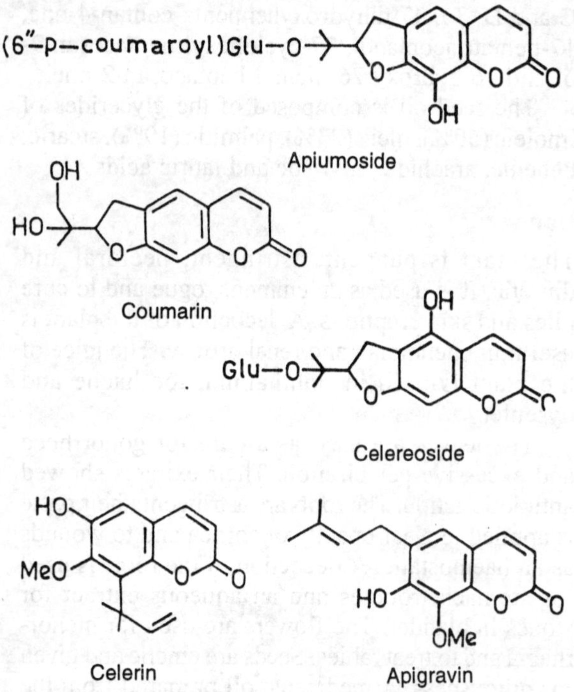

TAMARIND

The drug consists of the fruit of the tree *Tamarindus indica* (Papilionaceae) deprived of the brittle, outer part of the pericarp and preserved with sugar. The fruits are about 5-15 cm long with a brittle epicarp, a pulpy mesocarp containing five to nine branched fibres, and a leathery endocarp. The endocarp contains four to twelve chambers, in each of which is a single seed.

The epicarps are removed, the fruits are packed in layers in barrels, and boiling syrup is poured over them.

Tamarind pulp occurs as a reddish-brown, moist, sticky mass, in which the yellowish-brown fibres are readily seen. Odour, pleasant with powdered sugar.

The seeds are found, each enclosed in a leathery endocarp to which it is attached by a short funicle.

(6″-p-coumaroyl)Glu—O→

Apiumoside

HO→

Coumarin

Glu—O→

Celereoside

Celerin

Apigravin

Fig. 22.51. Chemical constituents of *Apium graveolens*.

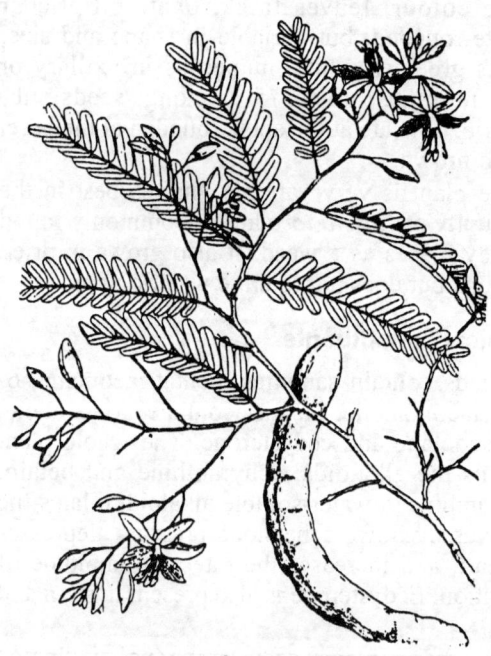

Fig. 22.52. *Tamarindus indica*.

The seeds are four-sided or ovate and about 15 mm long. They have a brown testa marked with a large patch. Within the testa, which is very thick and hard, lies the embryo. The large cotyledons are composed of hemicellulose, which stains blue with iodine.

The pulp contains free organic acids (about 10% of tartaric, citric and malic acids), their salts (about 8% of potassium hydrogen tartrate), nicotinic acid and about 30-40% of invert sugar. The tartaric acid is synthesized in the actively metabolizing leaves of the plant and then translocated to the fruits as they develop. Sugar is added as a preservative.

Flavonoid *C*-glycosides (vitexin, isovitexin, orientin and iso-orientin) occur in the leaves. The fixed oil of the seeds contains a mixture of glycerides of saturated and unsaturated (oleic, linoleic) acids.

Tamarind pulp is a mild laxative. The leaves are commercial source of tartaric acid.

ALLIUM CEPA (onion)

Allium cepa (Liliaceae) is a bulbous biennial, cultivated throughout Indian subcontinent. Bulb is used for culinary, vegetable and medicinal purposes. It is used as rubifacient, poultice for boils and abscesses, tonic, diuretic, stomachic, stimulant and expectorant. It contains amino acids (alliin and allicin), proteins, carbohydrates, vitamin C, volatile oil (0.005%), phenolic acids, flavonoids, anthocyanins, oleanolic acid, diphe-nylamine, steroidal glycosides, alliospiroside A, alliospiroside B, alliofuroside, phytoalexins, thiosulfinates, dithietanes and alpha sufinyl disulfides (capaenes). The oil and its individual constituents possess hypoglycaemic (diphenylamine), aphrodisiac, hypocholestraemic, platelet aggregation inhibitor (1-methyl-(sulfinyl)-propyl- methyl-disulphide), antiasthmatic (α- and β-unsaturated thiosulfinates (capaenes), antifungal, antimicrobial (steroidal glycosides), abortive, juvenoid, antiartheroscle-rotic and immunosuppressive, properties.

GINGKO BILOBA

Gingko biloba (Gingkoaceae) is a large perennial tree indigenous to China. It is the only surviving species of Gingkoales (Gymnosperm) which evolved about 240 million years ago and is considered as a "Living fossil" by Darwin. It is cultivated in China, Japan, Europe and occasionally in hilly

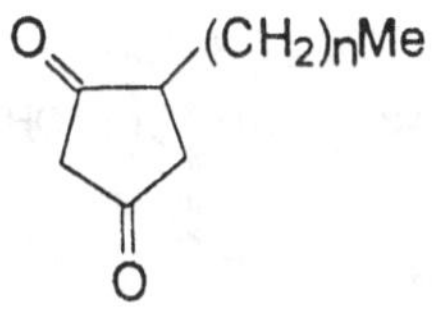

Tsibulin 1
n = 7
Tsibulin 2
n = 5

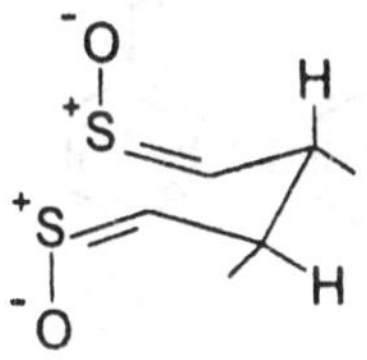

2,3-Dimethyl-1,4-butanedithial-1,4-dioxide

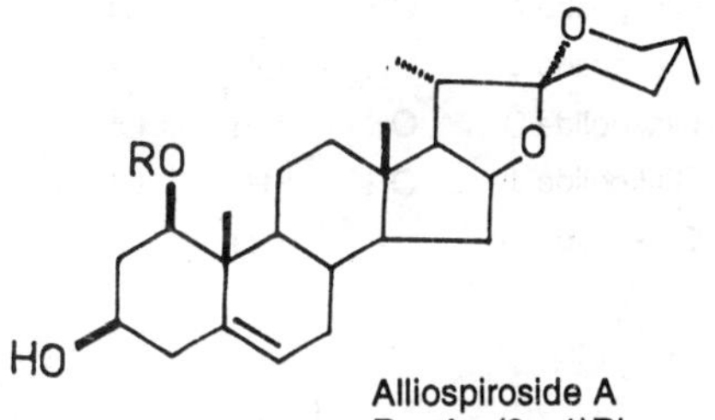

Alliospiroside A
R = Ara(2→1)Rha
Alliospiroside B
R = Gal(2→1)Rha

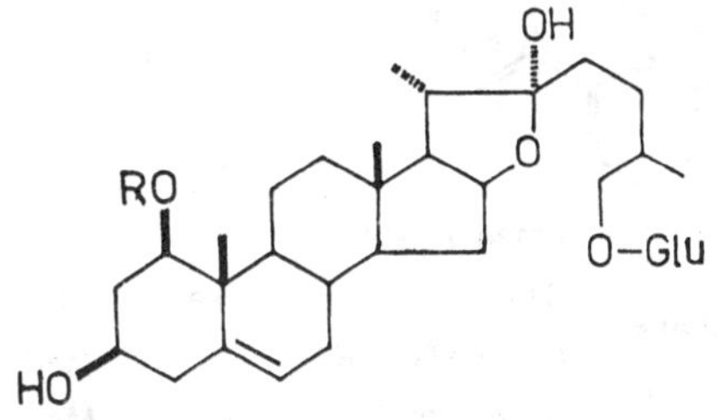

Alliofuroside A
R = Ara(2→1)Rha

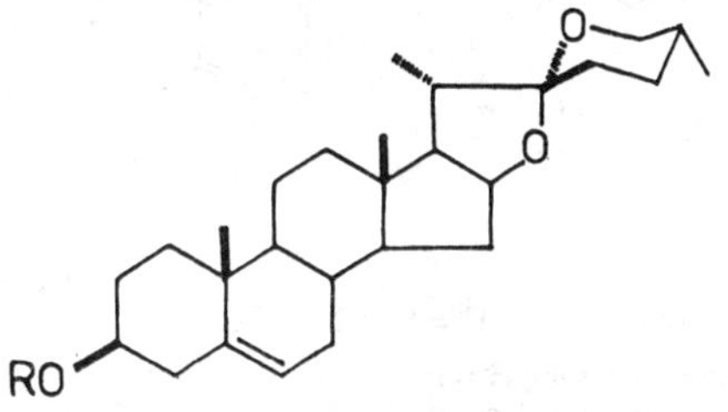

Ceposide D
R = Ara(2→1)Rha(4→1)Gal(2→1)Glu](3→1)Glu

Fig. 22.53. Chemical constituents of *Allium cepa*.

regions of India. It is used for various diseases appearing with old age, like reduced mental and physical efficiency, loss of concentration, memory impulsion, vertigo and vigilance. It enhances memory by increasing blood flow, metabolism efficiency, regulating neurotransmitters and boosting oxygen levels in the brain, and hence, it is gaining recognition as a brain tonic drug. It is also valued for its cosmetic use.

Gingko leaves contain long chain hydrocarbons and derivatives like polyprenyl acetate; anacardic acid, carbohydrates, flavonoids, isoprenoids (sterols, terpenoids), various compounds like (Z, Z')-4,4'-(1-4-pentadiene-1,5-diyl)-diphenol, catechins, proanthocyanidins, cytokinins, betalectins and carotenoids. The flavonoids kaempferol, quercetin, their mono-, di- and triglycosides like astragalin, rutin, isorhammetin, myricetin, 3'-methylmyricetin, apigenin and luteolin. The leaves contain flavonoid glycoside esters with courmaric acid. Non-glycoside biflavonoids isolated from the leaves include amentoflavone, ginkgetin, isoginkgetin, bilobetin, sciadopitysin and 5'-methoxybilobetin. The triterpenoids isolated from the leaves (0.266%) are highest in autumn.

The activity of the drug is due to ginkgolides and bilobalide. It is used in peripheral circulatory insufficiency, due to degenerative antiopathy and

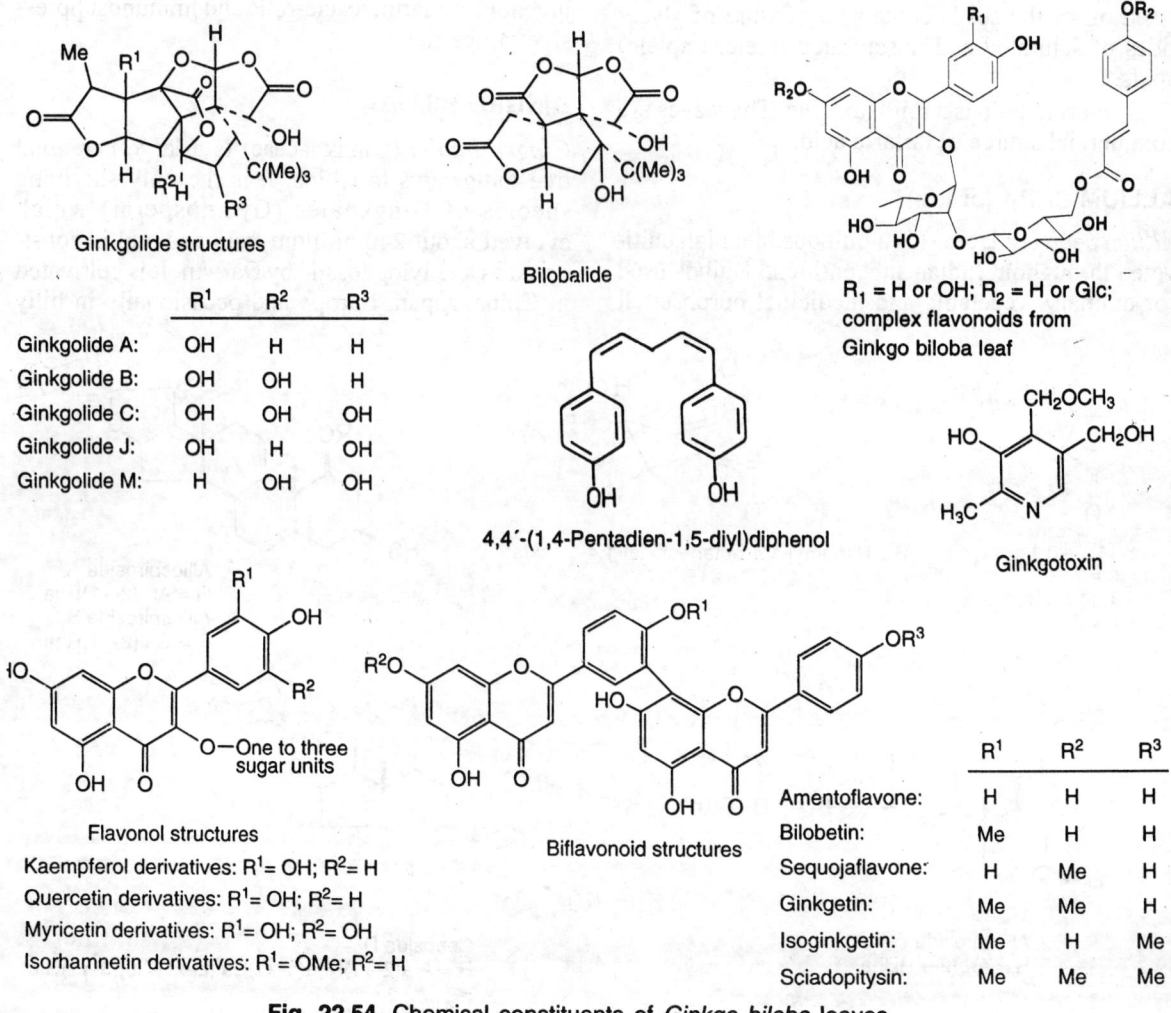

Ginkgolide structures

	R^1	R^2	R^3
Ginkgolide A:	OH	H	H
Ginkgolide B:	OH	OH	H
Ginkgolide C:	OH	OH	OH
Ginkgolide J:	OH	H	OH
Ginkgolide M:	H	OH	OH

Bilobalide

4,4′-(1,4-Pentadien-1,5-diyl)diphenol

R$_1$ = H or OH; R$_2$ = H or Glc; complex flavonoids from Ginkgo biloba leaf

Ginkgotoxin

Flavonol structures

Kaempferol derivatives: R^1= OH; R^2= H
Quercetin derivatives: R^1= OH; R^2= H
Myricetin derivatives: R^1= OH; R^2= OH
Isorhamnetin derivatives: R^1= OMe; R^2= H

O—One to three sugar units

Biflavonoid structures

	R^1	R^2	R^3
Amentoflavone:	H	H	H
Bilobetin:	Me	H	H
Sequojaflavone:	H	Me	H
Ginkgetin:	Me	Me	H
Isoginkgetin:	Me	H	Me
Sciadopitysin:	Me	Me	Me

Fig. 22.54. Chemical constituents of *Ginkgo biloba* leaves.

cerebrovascular insufficiency with symptoms of vertigo, tinnitus, headache, dementia, vigilance, mood disturbances, hearing loss and in geriatric conditions. The extract antagonises platelet aggregation induced by platelet activating factor and the four compounds responsible for this are gingkolides A, B, C and J but the activity is limited by poor bioavailability. Gingkolide B(BN-52063) acts as potent platelet activating factor antagonist. It also inhibits thrombus formation *in vivo* and produces thrombolysis. In various models of cerebral ischaemia, gingkolides exhibit hypoxia protective activity and reduction in post-ischaemic lesions. The extract inhibits immuno-complexes induced pancreatic oedema. The gingkolides subdue allergic inflammation, anaphylatic shock and asthma. Both gingkolides and bilobalides increase blood flow in patients with cerebro-vascular diseases. Bilobalide causes regeneration of motor nerves. Biflavonoids are active in peripheral vasodilation and also exhibit anti-bradykinin activity. In Europe Gingko phytoformulations based on these extracts are well known and marketed under the names of "Tebonin", "Rokan", "Tanakan" and "Gingkobil". Gincosan (PHL 00701), a combination product of standardised extract of *G. biloba* (GK501) and *P. ginseng* extract (G115), shows improved retention of learned behaviour.

SILYBUM MARIANUM

Silybium marianum (syn. *Cardus marianum*) (Asteraceae), commonly known as "Milk Thistle", is an annual or biennial plant growing as a weed in Kashmir, Punjab and other northwest parts of India, USA and Australia. The herb is also cultivated and traditionally used as a bitter digestive, liver tonic and poison antidote. Fruits contain flavonolignans such as silymarin, silybin, silydianin, silychristin, silybinin, silymonin, 3-deoxysilychristin and silandrin; flavonoids like naringenin, eridictyol, apigenin, chrysoeriol, apigenin-7-O-β-

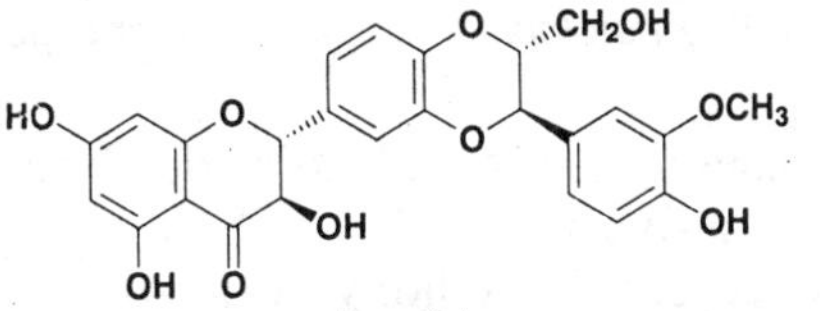

Silybin

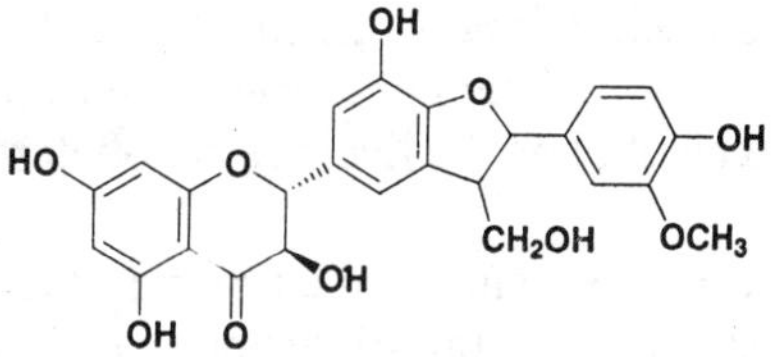

Silychristin

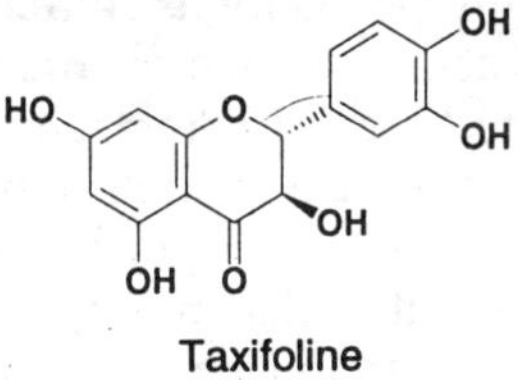

Taxifoline

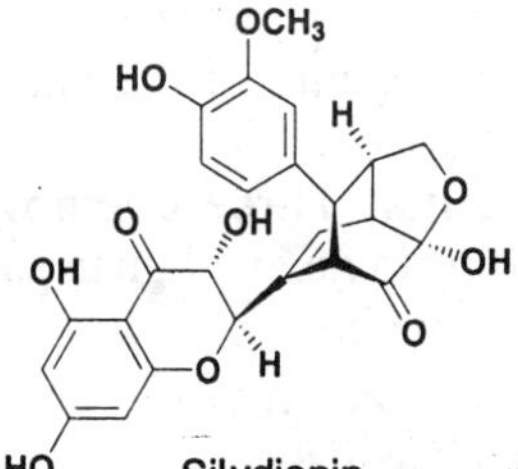

Silydianin

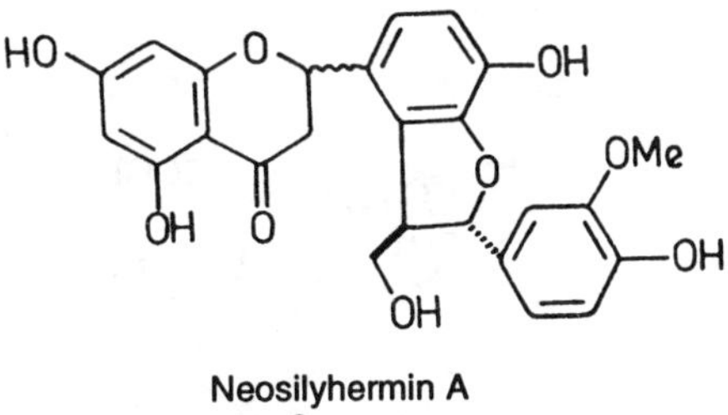

Neosilyhermin A
~~ = β
Neosilyhermin B
~~ = α

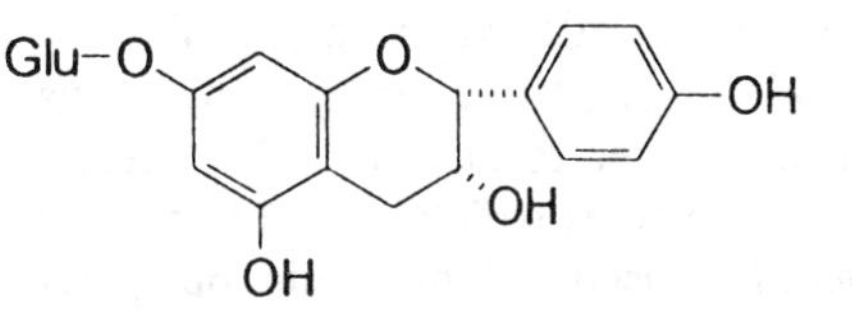

Symposide

Fig. 22.55. Chemical constituents of *Silybum marianum*.

glucuronide, 6'-ethylester, apigenin-7-O-β-galacto-side, kaempferol, taxifolin; alkaloids, saponins, phytosterols, tannins and fixed oils. The remarkable hepatoprotective activity of the drug is due to flavonolignans especially silymarin and silybin; the former is located in the thick-walled cells of the seed epidermis. Silybin is a potent hepatoprotective agent and is used as standard for evaluating herbal hepatoprotective drugs. Silybin when injected to human patients up to 48 hrs after they accidently ingested deathcap mushroom (*Amanita phalloides*) which contains most potent liver toxins known, it prevented the normally anticipated fatalities. Many commercial preparations are manufactured in Germany from the fruits. Silipide, a complex of silybin with phosphatidylcholine shows higher lipid solubility and, hence, is more active than silybin in liver damage. Silybindihemisuccinate, a soluble isomer of silymarin obtained from the drug, acts as an antidote against acetaminophenone hepatotoxicity. Symptoms of acute hepatitis, especially digestive problems and appetite, are improved within two weeks after taking Milk thistle. The detrimental effects of jaundice, drugs, environmental toxins and alcohol on the liver are encountered with the drug.

Silymarin also shows membrane stabilizing, usefulness in vascular disorders, antioxidant, cytoprotective and potassium sparing diuretic activities. Silymarin-phospholipid combination (silymarin-phytosome) possesses antiwrinkle activity controlling ageing of the skin. Silicynar, obtained from the drug, is effective in patients with chronic pancreatitis. Three chemotypes of *S. marianum* according to flavonolignan patterns in the fruits have been reported.

ARISTOLOCHIA INDICA

Aristolochia indica (Aristolochiaceae) is a perennial climber growing all over India. Roots and rhizomes of the plant are reputed for its gastric stimulant and bitter tonic drug. *A. bracteata* is another Indian species which is used as a substitute of *A. indica*. It is used as bitter tonic, purgative and anthelmintic.

Roots of *A indica* contain aristolochic acids, aristolactams, aristolochine, sesquiterpenes, steroids

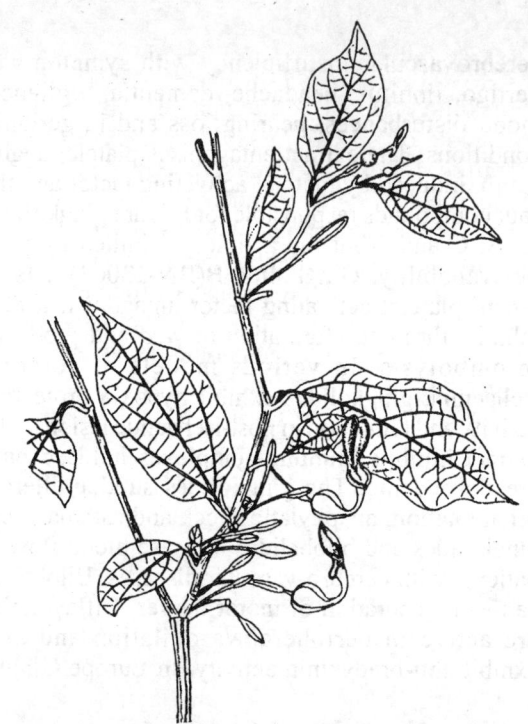

Fig. 22.56. *Aristolochia indica*—flowering portion.

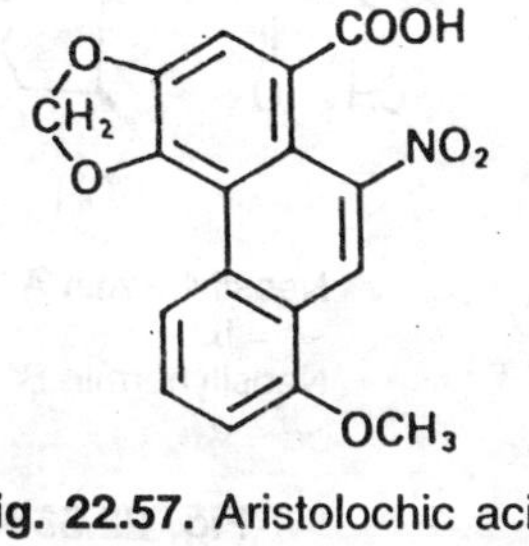

and *p*-coumaric acid. An alkaloid aristolochic acid, the chief active principle of the drug, is 3, 4 methylenedioxy-8-methoxy-10-nitro-1-phenanthrene carboxylic acid. It is intensely bitter substance and is highly valued for its antifertility, anti-implantation and abortifacient properties. Aristolochic acid is found to be good contraceptive for both males and females. It also exhibits antitubercular, antiviral, antifeedant, phagocytosis, stimulating, antineoplastic and anti-inflammatory activities. It has been proved to be carcinogenic and mutagenic.

Fig. 22.57. Aristolochic acid.

Forskolin

Forskolin, colenol, a diterpenoid is isolated from the roots of *Coleus forskohlii (Lamiaceae)*. It is reputed for its hypotensive and cardioactive properties. It stimulates adenylate cyclase, leading to an increase in cellular cAMP and thereby shows positive ionotropic effect on heart, lowers blood and intra-ocular pressure, reduces inflammation and inhibits platelet aggregation. It exerts inhibitory effect on number of membrane transport proteins and channel proteins. It has a potential as anti-metastatic agent.

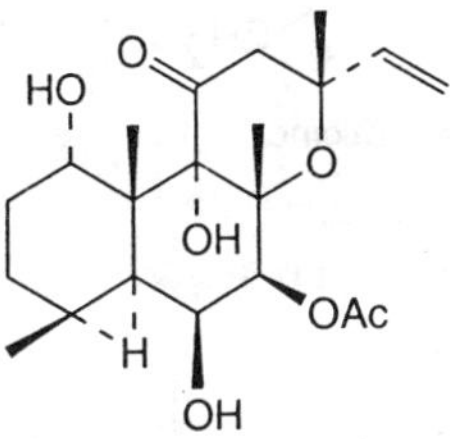

Fig. 22.58. Forskolin.

ARTEMISIA ANNUA

Huang hua hao, Chenoi, Sweet Annie, Qinghao.

Biological source

It is aerial parts of *Artemisia annua* Linn. (Family Asteraceae).

The plant is a native to China, now grows in many countries such as Australia, Argentina, Bulgaria, France, Hungary, Italy, Spain and the United States. It is cultivated in India in Delhi, Lucknow and Himalayan gardens.

Description

It is an annual, glabrous herb, 50-150 cm high. Leaves are radial, long petiolate, triangular ovate, dentate, floral leaves sessile, flower heads small, globose and pedicellate.

Chemical constituents

The herb contains artemisinin (a sesquiterpene lactose), arteannuins A and B (qinghaosu I and II), artemisitene, artemisia ketone, benzyl isovalerate, borneol acetate, cadinine, camphene, camphor, β-caryophyllene, β-pinene, scopoline, stigmasterol, 5,4'-dihydroxy-3,6,7,3'-tetramethoxy-flavone, artemitin, dihydro-epideoxy artemisinin B, artemisinic acid (artemisic acid), qinghao acid, deoxy-artemisinin (qinghaosu III), qinghaosu IV, arteannuin E (quinghaosu V), artemisilactone (arteannuin F), artemisinol, artemisic acid methyl ester, artemisitene, arteannuin C and epoxyartemisic acid.

The volatile oil of the herb cultivated in Delhi is composed of 1,8-cineole (12.8%), α-thujene (3.3%), α- and β-pinenes, *trans*-sabinene hydrate (7.1%), *p*-cymene, 4-methyl-2,3-dihydrofuran, terpinen-4-ol, myrcene, caryophyllene oxide, γ-cadinene, aromadendrene epoxide, 1,4-dihydro-acenaphthene, and artemissine. Camphor, bornyl acetate, *p*-cymol, β-myrcene, benzyl isovalerate, β-farnesene and artemisia alcohol are also reported from the volatile oil of herb at the inflorescences stage.

A. annua also contains coumarins scopoletin, esculetin; flavones 3,5-dihydroxy-6,7,3',4'-tetramethoxyflavone, 5,4'-dihydroxy-3,6,7,3'-tetramethoxyflavone and artemetin.

Camphor, 1,8-cineole, artemisia ketone, germacrene D and β-farnesene are present in the essential oil of Vietnamese plant. The other compounds isolated from the plant are nonacosanol, 2-methyltriacosa-8-one-23-ol, hentriacontanyl triacontanoate, 2,29-dimethyltriacontane (leaves and stems), axillarin, chrysoplenetin, chryso-splenol D, casticin, quercetin, its 3-rutinoside, luteolin, its 7-O-glycoside, kaempferol, its 6-methoxy derivative, 3-O-glycosides of kaempferol and quercetin, patuletin, its 3-glucoside; stigmasterol, β-sitosterol, plant growth inhibitors ABA, Me-ABA and bis (1-hydroxy-2-methyl-propyl) phthalate; artemisinin G (leaves), polyacetylene annuadiepoxide, ponticaepoxide, 5-monodecylresorcinol-3-O-methyl ether, dihydro-epideoxyarteannuin B, annulide, arteannuic acid, epideoxyarteannuin and morannuic acid.

Artemisinin is an unusual sesquiterpene lactone possessing an endoperoxide moiety and is used as a Chinese antimalarial drug Qinghaso. It is successful in treating cases of chloroquine-resistant *Plasmodium falciparum* and particularly cerebral malaria.

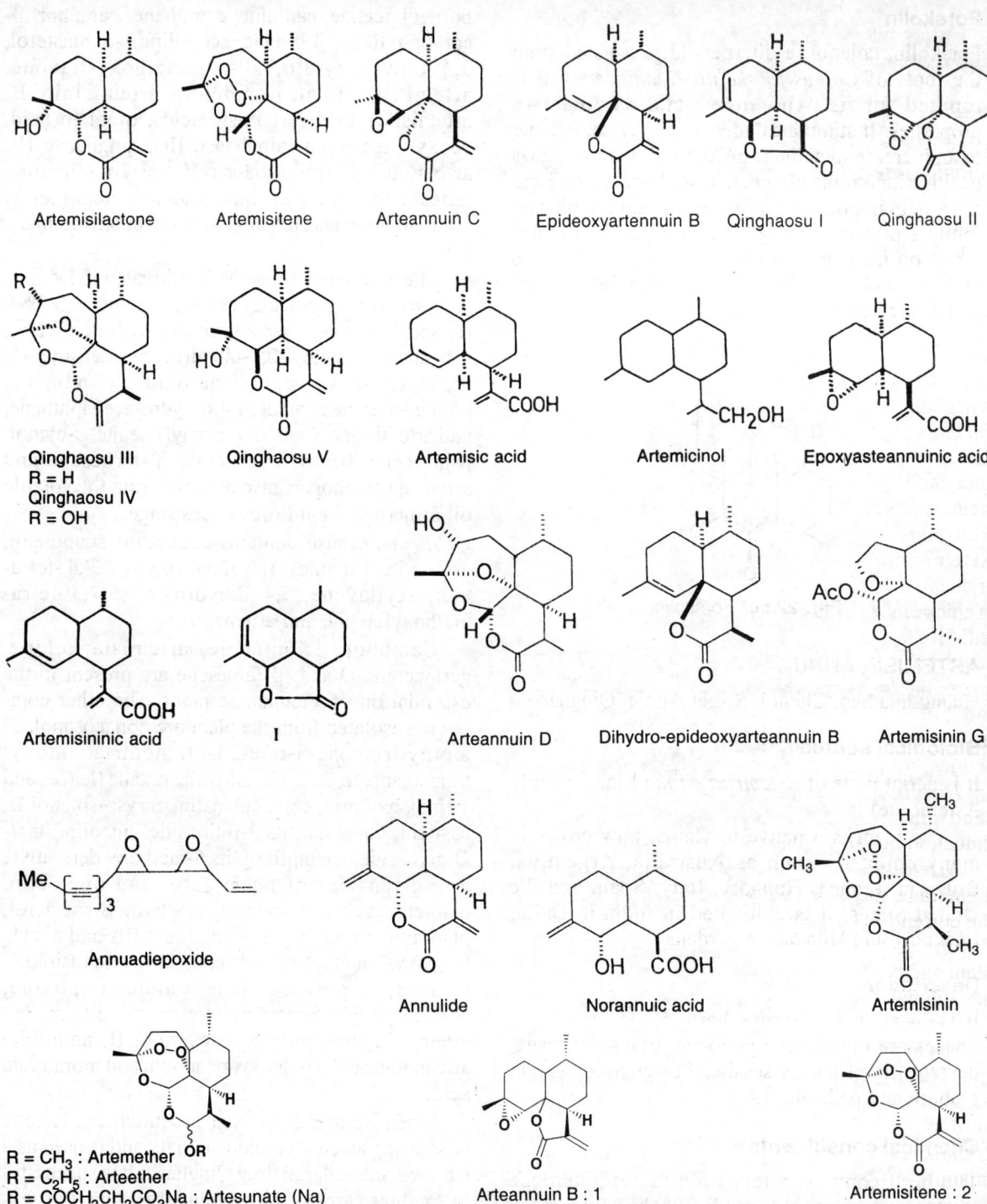

Artemisilactone   Artemisitene   Arteannuin C   Epideoxyartennuin B   Qinghaosu I   Qinghaosu II

Qinghaosu III
R = H
Qinghaosu IV
R = OH

Qinghaosu V   Artemisic acid   Artemicinol   Epoxyasteannuinic acid

Artemisininic acid   I   Arteannuin D   Dihydro-epideoxyarteannuin B   Artemisinin G

Annuadiepoxide   Annulide   Norannuic acid   Artemisinin

R = CH₃ : Artemether
R = C₂H₅ : Arteether
R = COCH₂CH₂CO₂Na : Artesunate (Na)

Arteannuin B : 1   Artemisitene : 2

Fig. 22.59. Chemical constituents of *Artemisia annua*.

Callus cultures of *Artemisia annua* produce scopoletin and a triglyceride but no artemisinin.

Uses

Artemisia is used as an antimalarial drug. It has diuretic, insecticidal, anthelmintic, antimicrobial, insecticidal and stomachic properties and is given in jaundice, diabetes and skin diseases. It is effective against chloroquine resistant strains of *Plasmodium vivax*, *P. falciparum* and against cerebral malaria.

Pharmacology

Artemisinin and two of its derivatives, artemether and artesunate are effective in both chloroquine sensitive and chloroquine resistant *Plasmodium falciparum* infection. Artemisinin and its derivatives are active against primary amoebic meningo encephalitis caused by *Naegleria fowleri*. Artemether markedly reduced worm load of *Schistosoma mansonni* and *S. japonicum* in mice and dogs. Artemisinin is active against systemic lupus erythematous and is virustatic against influenza virus in chick embryo. Artemisinin related trioxanes have anti-HIV activity. The plant exhibits anti-oxidative activity and causes cytotoxicity on P 388 and L 1210 leukemia cell lines. Plant extract exhibited high inhibition of tobacco viruses, showed anti-inflammatory, antibacterial and antinoceptive actions.

Artemisinin shows herbicidal activity. It inhibits seed germination, seedling growth and root induction in plants.

Artemisin affects the integrity of parasite's membrane, the mode of action being different from the currently synthetic antimalarials. Methoxylated flavonoids like casticin, chryolentin found in the plant and artemesin found in cell cultures, enhance the antimalarial activity of artemisinin.

Artemisinin enhanced macrophage phagocytosis in mice. It is the drug with low acute toxicity. The liver is the most important organ for metabolism of artemisinin. Sodium salt of artesunic acid is about five times more effective than artemisinin. However, it is more toxic than artemisinin but less toxic than chloroquine or artemether. A plant extract exhibited high inhibition of tobacco viruses. Various extracts of the plant showed marked antipyretic and anti-inflammatory activities and some antinocieptive and anti-bacterial activities. Artemisic acid was identified as anti-bacterial and scopoletin as anti-inflammatory agents. Bis-(1-hydroxy-2-methylpropyl) phthalate inhibited germination of wheat coleoptile and mustard seed. Artemisinin and quercetagetin-6,7,3',4'-tetramethyl ether exhibited significant cytotoxicity against P-388, A-549, HT-29, MCF-7 and KB tumor cells.

Methanolic extract obtained from callus of *A. annua* not containing artemisinin exhibits anti-plasmodial activity indicating presence of few unknown compounds. Arteannuin B and artemisinic acid can be converted to artemisinin using cell free extracts.

Synthetic derivatives like artemether, arteether, sodium artesunate, artenilic acid and beta-arteether possessing more potent activity have been developed from dihydroartemisinin. Sodium artesunate acts rapidly in restoring the consciousness of comatose patients with cerebral malaria.

Isolation of artemisinin from the plant

Air-dried leaves of *A. annua* were extracted with petroleum ether (bp 40-60ºC), which was subsequently removed *in vacuo*. The residue was redissolved in chloroform to which acetonitrile was added to precipitate inert plant components such as sugars and waxes. The concentrated extract was then chromatographed on a column of silica gel. Fractions with a high artemisinin content crystallized readily, with recrystallization being effected with cyclohexane or 50% ethanol.

Artemisinin is a poorly water-soluble, crystalline compound whose melting point is 156-157ºC, and $[\alpha]_D^{25}$ +66.3º (c 1.64 CHCl$_3$).

BHILWA

Marking nut tree, oriental cashew.

Biological source

It is the tree of *Semecarpus anacardium* Linn. f. (Family : Anacardiaceae).

It is a moderate-sized deciduous tree, 12-15 m high, found in the outer Himalayas from Sutlej to Sikkim, Assam and in hotter parts of India.

The bark is dark brown, rough, leaves large, simple, obovate-oblong; flowers small, greenish-yellow, in terminal panicles, drupes ovoid, smooth, shining, black when ripe.

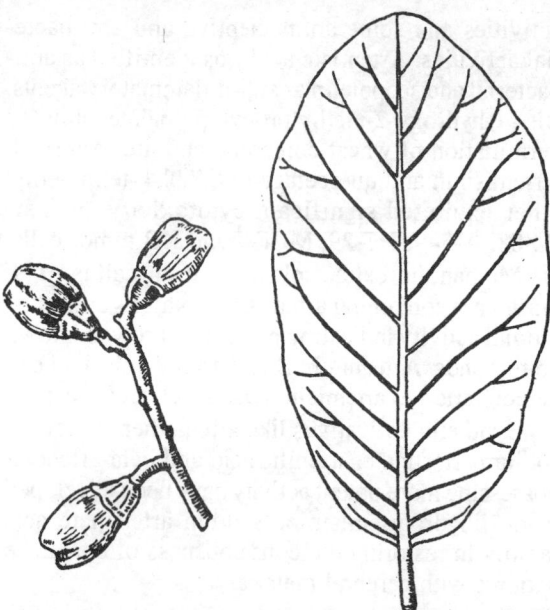

Fig. 22.60. *Semecarpus anacardium*—fruiting branch and leaf.

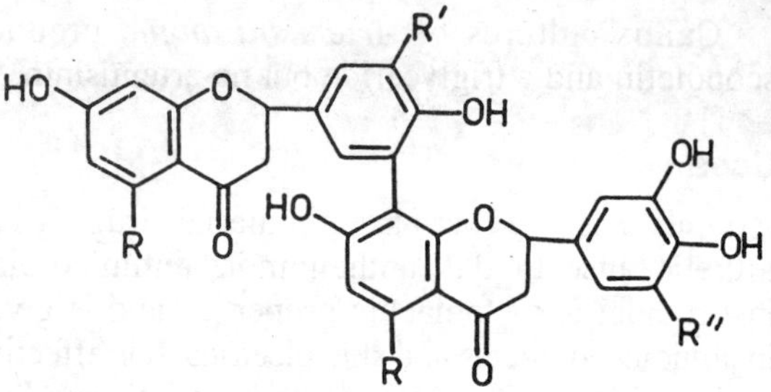

Galluflavanone
R = H, R′,R″ = OH
Jeediflavanone
R = OH, R′,R″ = H
Semecarpuflavanone
R,R′ = H, R″ = OH

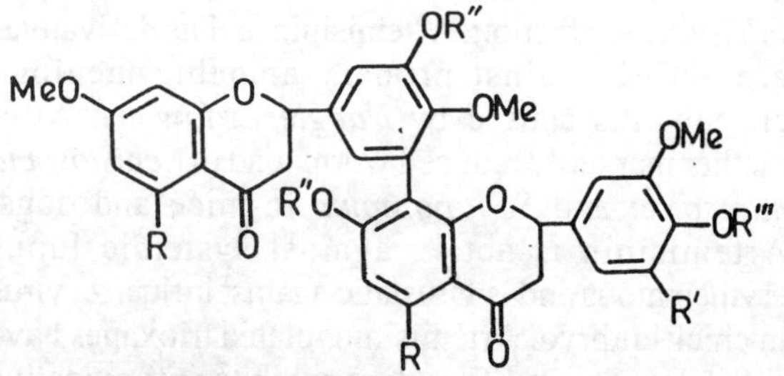

Nallaflavanone
R = OH, R′ = OMe, R″ = Me, R‴ = H
Semecarpetin
R,R′,R″= H, R‴ = Me

Fig. 22.61. Chemical constituents of *Semecarpus anacardium*.

The pericarp is abundant in a black, oily, bitter and highly vesicant juice used for marking linen, in varnish, paints and plastics. The juice, known in the trade as Bhilwan shell liquid, is a rich source of phenols. It is obtained from the nuts by extraction with petroleum ether or other solvent, by hot expression in a hydraulic press, or by roasting in a specially designed retort, or by subjecting the nuts to superheated steam at 180-230° in a close retort with an inlet for steam and an outlet for the expelled liquid.

Chemical constituents

The juice is a dark brown oily liquid or a semi-solid depending on the method of extraction. The major constituent is bhilawanol, $C_{21}H_{32}O_2$ (46%), b.p. 225-226°/3 mm. It is an O-dihydroxy compound with a catechol nucleus and an unsaturated C_{15}-side chain. It is a mixture of *cis*- and *trans*- isomers of urushenol [3-(pentadecenyl-8')-catechol]. A small quantity of a monohydroxy phenol, semicarpol, is also present. The dark tarry residue left after distillation contains high boiling phenols and hydrocarbons. Thermal degradation of the shell liquid at 400° gives catechol and a mixture of phenols and hydrocarbons.

The fruits contain nicotinic acid, riboflavin, thiamine and essential amino acids. The nuts yield anacardic acid, aromatic amines, bhilawanol, 1-pentadeca-7,10-dienyl-2,3-dihydroxy benzene, biflavanoids A, B and C, (3',8-binaringenin and 3',8-biliquiritigenin), tetrahydrobustaflavone, tetrahydro-amentoflavone and nallaflavone. The nut shell contains galluflavanone and jeediflavanone. The seed oil is composed of glycerides of linoleic, myristic, oleic, palmitic and stearic acids. Anacardu-flavanone is present in nut shells. Amentoflavone is present in the leaves. The plant also contains biflavanones A_1 and A_2.

Uses

The tree is a host plant of the lac insect. The bark is astringent. The tree exudes a gum or gum-resin, which is used in leprous affections and nervous debility, also in scrofulous and venereal affections. The fruits are used in asthma, ascites, epilepsy, neuralgia, tumors, warts, psoriasis and rheumatism; as abortifacient, anthelminitic and vermifuge. A decoction of the fruits mixed with milk and butter fat is useful in asthma, gout, hemiplegia, neuritis, piles, rheumatism and syphilitic complaints. The kernel is anthelmintic, cardiotonic, carminative and digestive. The seed oil is used externally in gout, leprosy and leucoderma. The root cooked in sour rice water causes sterility in women when eaten. The juice of the pericarp and tree trunk is a powerful counter-irritant and vesicant. It causes painful blisters. The juice is used for tattooing and for chobing elephant feet. The pericarp juice has anti-bacterial properties.

Pharmacology

Plant extract showed direct depressant effect on isolated frog heart and rabbit intestine and antagonized spasmogenic effect of carbachol, histamine, barium chloride and pitocin. It produced delayed hypotension in dogs. Nut chloroform extract increased life-span in ascites tumour systems and solid tumor systems. The fruit extract is effective against human epidermoid carcinoma of the nasopharynx.

BUCKWHEAT

Doron, Kotu, Phaphra.

It is the leaves and flowers of *Fagopyrum esculentum* Moench (Family : Polygonaceae).

It is a native to Central Asia and is cultivated in various countries as a food or fodder crop. In India, it is grown as a minor grain crop in higher altitudes (700-4000 m) of Himalayas from Kashmir to Sikkim, Khasi hills, Manipur and in Nilgiris.

It is an annual herb; 100-150 cm high, with alternate, hastate, acute leaves; flowers in axillary or terminal cymes, pinkish-white, aromatic, dimorphic and highly self-sterile; fruit a 3-cornered achene, with keeled edges, silvery grey to brown or black.

Buckwheat is a quick growing crop and prefers a moist cool climate and a well-drained sandy soil. In northern India, it is grown as a rainy season crop, sown in July and harvested in October. In Nilgiris, it is generally sown in April and harvested in August.

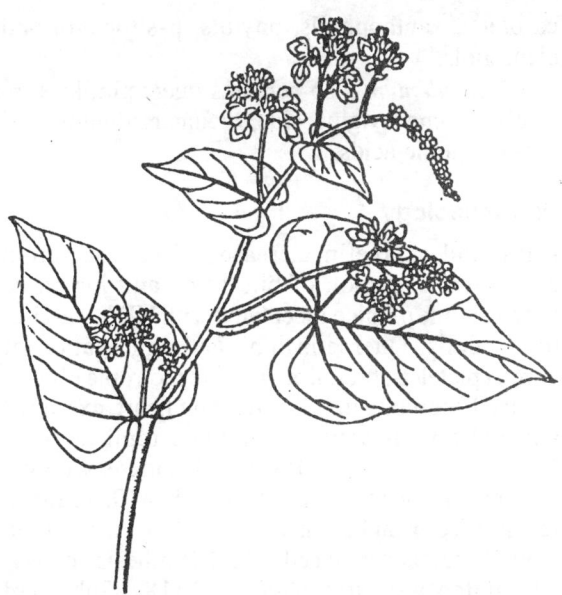

Fig. 22.62. *Fagopyrum esculentum.*

A yield up to 250 kg of grains per acre is reported from Nilgiris.

Buckwheat is used mostly in the form of flour or making bread, pancakes and porridge. The leaves of young shoots are boiled and eaten as spinach. In USA and Russia, the grains are used as stock and poultry feed.

Buckwheat plant is a promising commercial source of rutin (3-5%). Rutin is obtained from the leaves and flowers. Rutin is used to treat increased capillary fragility with associated hypertension; a condition which sometimes results in the bursting of blood vessels in the brain, leading to apoplexy or retinal haemorrhage and causing blindness. Rutin is also used for purpura, bleeding from kidney, hereditory haemorrhagic telangiectasia and haemophilia. Rutin protects against harmful effects of x-rays, as a prophylactic against gangrene due to frost bite, with other miotics in glaucoma, in combination with dicumarol, in the treatment of retinitis. It prevents weakening of capillaries due to salicylates, arsenicals, thiocyanate, sulphadiazine and gold salts.

A fatty matter of Buckwheat is composed of lecithin (2%), linolenic, oleic, linoleic and palmitic acids. The unsaponifiable fraction is composed of carotene, xanthophylls, phytols, β-sitosterol and eicosenols.

F. esculentum also contains quercetin, kaempferol-3-rhamnosylglucoside, *p*-cumaroylquinic and feruloylquinic acids.

Pharmacology

Rutin and quercetin increased biliary secretion and faecal excretion of bile acids and increased survival time of mice inoculated with NK/Ly ascites tumor cells. Quercetin inhibited aggregation of human platelets, produced positive inotropic effects, reduced heart rate in isolated rabbit heart, exhibited anti-polio virus activity, inhibited replication of herpes simplex virus in RK-13 cells, increased liver weight and hepatic cytochrome P 450, reduced levels of prostaglandin E_2 and leukotriene B_4 in pleural exudate, reduced LTB4 synthesis in cells stimulated with ionophore A-23187; inhibited growth of human gastric cancer cells, reduced intraluminal accumulation of fluid and diarrhoea induced by castor oil and decreased activities of Na^+ K^+ exchanging ATPase of rat brain plasma membrane.

CASSIA TORA

Chakunda, Panevar, Wild Senna, Foetid Senna.

Biological source

It consists of the leaves and seeds of *Cassia tora* Linn.; syn. *C. obtusifolia* L. (Fam. Caesalpiniaceae).

It is distributed throughout the tropical parts of India as a weed up to an altitude of 1,550 m in the Himalayas.

Description

A foetid, annual herb or undershrub; up to 1-2 m in height, leaves peripinnate; leaflets 3 pairs, membranous, ovate-oblong, with glands in the last two pairs; flowers small, yellow, in pairs, on short axillary peduncles; pods stout, slender, sub-4-angled; seeds green, many, flat.

Chemical constituents

The seeds contain fatty acids, physcion, rubrofusarin, its 6β-gentiobioside, aloe-emodin, chrysophanol, norrubrofusarin, 8-hydroxy-3-methyl anthraquinone-1β-gentiobioside, emodin, rhein, β-sitosterol, amino acids, chrysophanic acid, its 9-anthrone, obtusin, aurantio-obtusin, toralactone, torachrysone, questin, glucose, galactose, xylose, raffinose, castasterone, typhasterol, teasterone, 28-nor-castasterone, monopalmitin, monoolein, alaternin-1-O-β-D-glucoside, chrysoobtusin-2-O-β-D-glucoside, physcion-8-O-β-D-glucoside, obtusifolin, stigmasterol, histidine, chryso-obtusin, cystine, γ-hydroxyarginine, aspartic acid, helminthosporin, O-methyl chrysophanol, betulinic acid, 2,5-dimethoxy-benzoquinone, torosachry-sone, palmitic and linoleic acids, C16-C31 alkanes, cholesterol, β-sitosterol, 1,3-dihydroxy-8-methylanthraquinone, naphthopyrone glycosides, cassialactone, brassinolide, d-mannitol, isotoralactone and cassia lactone. The fatty acid composition of the oil is palmitic (23.5%), lignoceric, oleic (28.1%) and linoleic (45%) acids.

The protein bound amino acids are lysine, histidine, theonine, phenylalanine, valine, methionine, tryptophan, leucine, isoleucine, serine, glycine, tyrosine, aspartic acid, alanine and proline.

The leaves also contain myricyl alcohol, glucose, tigonelline, 1-stachydine, choline, tria-contanol, stigmasterol, β-sitosterol glucoside, friedelin, palmitic, stearic, succinic and d-tartaric acids, uridine, myoinositol, d-ononitol, kaempferol, quercetin, juglanin, astragalin, quercitrin, isoquercitrin and emodin. Seed volatile oil contains dihydro-actinidiolide, *m*-cresol, 3-hydroxy-4-methoxyacetophenone, methyl palmitate and methyl oleate.

Uses

The leaves possess anthelmintic and purgative properties. They are externally used for ringworm and other skin diseases. The pounded leaves are applied to cuts and wounds. They are given in cough and impetigo. A leaf-paste with egg albumin is applied as a plaster for fractured bones. A decoction of the leaves is given to children during teething and used for eye troubles.

A paste made of equal parts of the leaves and seeds is given in jaundice. The pounded leaf stupefies fish.

A leaf extract showed antifungal activity against *Curvularia verruculosa* and *Microsporon nanum*.

A tea is prepared from the leaves in Kumaun. A compound Ayurvedic oil of the plant, *Chakramardha thailamis*, is beneficial for eczema, ringworm and other skin diseases.

The seeds are official in Japanese Pharmacopoea. They are used as a stomachic and tonic. A paste of the seeds with lime juice is used for ringworm and other skin diseases. The seeds are used in eye diseases, liver complaints, and earache. A decoction of the seeds is taken as a blood-purifier and for the inflammation of the skin. The extract of the seeds showed marked contraction of the uterus of guinea pig. The pods are used in dysentery.

Chrysophanic acid-9-anthrone showed antifungal activities against *Trichophyton rubrum, T. mentagrophytes, T. granulosum, Microsporon canis, M. gypseum* and *Geotrichum candidum*.

The seeds yield a gum (7.6%) which is the most efficient suspending agent for calomel, kaolin and talk. It is used as a binding agent for tablets. The seeds contain yellow, blue and red-coloured dyes used in dyeing and tanning.

The roots possess bitter, tonic, purgative and anthelmintic properties. They are used like leaves and seeds in skin diseases. A paste of the root with lime-juice is a specific remedy for ringworm.

Pharmacology

Chrysophanic acid-9-anthrone showed fungicidal activity. Questin showed antibacterial activity against *Staphylococcus aureus*. Aloe-emodin, questin, isotoralactone, toralactone and torosachrysone showed antimicrobial activity. Cassiaside, rubrofusarin-6β-gentiobioside and naphthopyrone glycoside showed hepatoprotective activity. Emodin showed purgative action in mice and it was more effective than calcium sennosides A and B. Emodin exhibited vasorelaxant effect on isolated vascular rings of human internal mammary artery and saphenous vein, rabbit thoracic aorta, abdominal aorta and mesentric artery. Emodin may be useful immuno-suppressive agents with vasorelaxant action.

CHITRAKA

Chita, Sittragam, White Leadwort.

Biological source

It consists of the root and root bark of *Plumbago zeylanica* Linn. (Family : Plumbaginaceae).

It is found wild in peninsular India and West Bengal and cultivated in gardens throughout India.

It is a perennial, sub-scandent shrub; branches diffuse; leaves alternate, ovate, narrowed into the petiole, glabrous; flowers white, in elongated spikes; capsules oblong, pointed, enclosed by persistent viscid calyx.

The dried root occurs as cylindrical pieces of varying length, about 1-25 cm thick, reddish brown with thickly shrivelled, smooth or irregularly fissured, brittle bark with small projections. The roots have a short fracture, an acrid and biting taste and disagreeable taste.

Chemical constituents

The roots contain plumbagin, 3,3-bisplumbagin, 3-chloroplumbagin, citranone (binaphthoquinone), droserone, elliptinone, isozeylinone, isozeylanone, zeylanone, zeylinone, maritone, methylene-3,3'-diplumbagin, 2-methyl-naphthazarin, plumbazeyl-

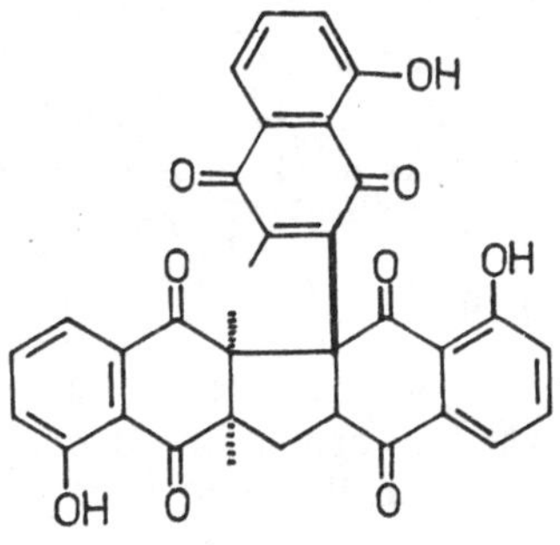

Plumbazeylanone

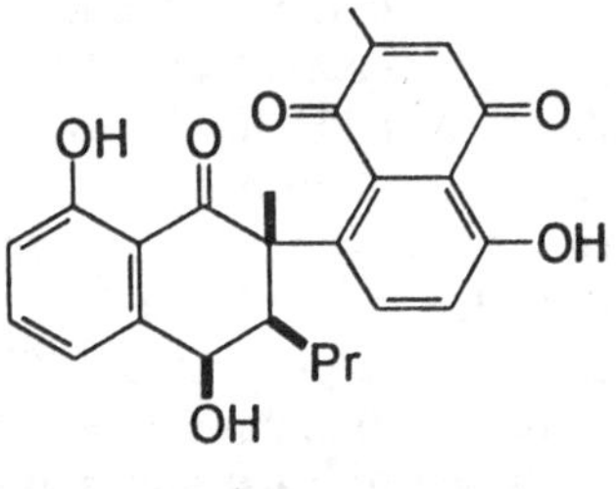

Chitanone

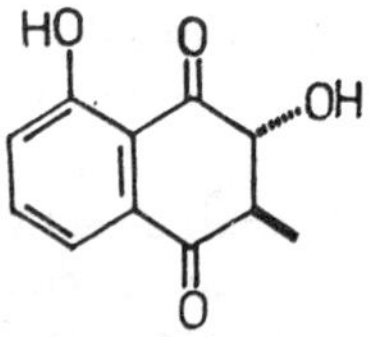

Dihydroserone

Fig. 22.63. Chemical constituents of *Plumbago zeylanica.*

anone, plumbagin trimer, catechol tannin and dihydroserone.

The root bark furnishes plumbagin, fructose, glucose, invertase and protease.

The plant also contains volatile oil (leaves and stem), α- and β-amyrins, lupeol, taraxasterol, ψ-taraxasterol, plumbagic acid, vanillic acid, 1,2(3)-tetrahydro-3,3'-bisplumbagin, isoshinanolone, dihydrosterone, β-sitosterol, aspartic acid, trypto-phan, tyrosine, threonine, alanine, histidine, glycine, methionine and hydroxyproline in aerial parts.

Uses

The root possesses abortifacient, vesicant, anti-diarrhoeal, antidyspeptic, appetizing, digestive and sudorific properties. It is used in anasarca, piles, intermittent fevers and skin diseases. A paste of the roots is applied to open abscesses. In combination with other ingredients, it is recommended in dyspepsia, epilepsy, hysteria, piles, nervous and rheumatic affections, obesity, prurigo, scabies and indolent ulcers. A paste prepared with milk, vinegar or salt and water is externally applied in leprosy and other skin disease. In Malaya, the drug is used as abortifacient. In Africa, a cold infusion of the root is used for influenza and black water fever. A tincture of the root bark is used as an antiperiodic and sudorific; milky juice is applied to scabies and ulcers.

Pharmacology

Alcoholic and aqueous extracts of the roots showed antibacterial activity against *Micrococcus pyogenes* var. *aureus, Salmonella typhi* and *Mycobacterium phlei*. An alcoholic extract acts as a powerful aphicide.

Plumbagin administered to hyperlipidaemic rabbits reduced serum cholesterol and LDL-cholesterol and elevated decreased HDL-cholesterol significantly. It prevented accumulation of cholesterol and triglycerides in liver and aorata and regressed atheromatous plaques of thoracic and abdominal aorata. Plant extract prevented 100% ovulation and implantation in female rats. Plumbagin decreased tumor growth in rats; was active against P388 lymphocytic leukaemia, showed antibacterial and antifungal activity against a wide variety of bacteria and fungi.

CIVET

Bagdas, Khatas, large Indian Civet.

Civet is the odorous secretion obtained from civet cats or civets belonging to the order *Carnivora*, family *Viverridae*, widely found in Africa, India, Malaysia, Indochina and Indonesia. The true civets are represented by the genera *Viverra, Moschothera* and *Viverricula* from Asia and *Civethictis* from Africa.

Civets have a long body, short limbs, an elongated head and pointed muzzle in comparison to cats. Civets have smooth tongue and long conspicuous moustaches. Civets are mostly nocturnal and terrestrial in habit. They feed on fowl, eggs, snakes, frogs, insects, fruits and roots. They live in woods under bushes, in thick grass or in furrows. Their hair is usually coarse and harsh; claws are partially retractile and their backs naned.

Civet which yields most of the secretion of the scent glands is the African civet, *Civettictis civetta* or *Viverra civetta*.

Viverra zibetha Linn. is found in Nepal, Sikkim, Bhutan, West Bengal, Assam, Burma, southern China, Thailand and Malay Peninsula. It contains large scent glands. Malabar civet, *Viverra civettina* Slyth; syn. *Moschothera civettina*, is found in western ghats and coasted regions of southern India.

Small Indian civet or kasturi, *Viverricula indica*, is a tawny grey brown animal found in Himalayan foothills, Punjab, from Gujarat to Tamil Nadu, Sri Lanka, Myanmar, southern China and Malaysia.

The structure of the scent glands differs in different civets. The scent gland is situated in the perineal areas, can be seen externally as a fairly large pouch with hairy swollen lips which close and open it. The secretion of the gland is discharged into a fold of skin and not into a pouch.

The function of civet secretion is not definitely known, although it is probably that the repellent odour is a means of protection, or possibly sexual attraction. For collection of civet, the cat is caged up something like a rabbit hutch to prevent the animal from turning round and biting those collecting the secreted substance. It is kept in a room, having a large fire constantly burning, so as to resemble their native climate. It is, in this state, fed with boiled sheep's head, rice and milk sweetened with honey. Once a month, sometimes even twice a week, there is a sufficiently civet secrete for gathering. When it rubs its tail against the wooden grate of its cage the keeper knows that it wants to be civeted, being in pain to get rid of the secreted substance. The civet collects in a notch or a deep cleft, between the fundament and the testicles of the male cat, from which it is scooped, or taken out by means of a liver instrument, about half a metre long, in the same manner as marrow is scooped out from bone. The secretion is greater if the animals are teased or irritated. The yield from each animal is about 30 g a week. The animals of both sexes secrete civet, the male cat produces the best. The female cat dribbles her urine into the civet reservoir which renders it very foul.

The crude civet is 500-1200 g of creamy yellow paste which turns darker and more solid on ageing. It is semi-solid when fresh, becoming darker and thicker on exposure to air. It has a strong obnoxious odour which becomes pleasant when highly diluted. It contains a large proportion of fatty material. Genuine civet has loss on drying 25%, mineral matter 2%, acetone extractive 65-80%, alcohol extractive 45-65%, ether extractive 11-24% and chloroform extractive up to 6%. The acetone resinoid has m.p. 19-25°.

The principal constituent of civet is civetone $C_{17}H_{30}O$, m.p. 31%, other compounds are (+)-(S,S)-cis-(6-methyltetrahydropyran-2-yl) acetic acid, civetol, scatole, indole, ethylamine and propylamine. Civetol is odourless and is converted into civetone by chromic acid oxidation.

The commercial product is adulterated with petroleum jelly, lanolin; mixture of scatole, indole, phenyl acetic acid and tetrahydro-paramethyl quinoline. The lack the distinct 'softness' of the odour of the natural substance on dilution is observed.

Civet is used as a fixative in perfumary trade. It increases the life of the perfume into which it is incorporated. It is mainly added in lotions. Civet extract or tincture is added in delicate floral bases. It is used for as a perfume in the manufacture of incense sticks and for flavouring tobacco. The civet, in doses of 100-800 mg/kg p.o. produced significant potentiation of pentobarbitone induced hypnosis, mild analgesia and anti-convulsant activities. Civet, when applied externally, removes localized pains and itching sensations and is useful in scabies, pimples and other skin infections. Internally, it is useful in mental retardation, insanity, fainting, convulsions, colic pains, asthma, cough and other respiratory troubles. It removes palpitation of the heart and is recommended in cardiac weakness.

GADUCHI (GILOE, TINOSPORA)

Guluchi, Amrita, Gulancha.

Habitat

It is the dried stem of *Tinospora cordifolia* Miers (Family : Menispermaceae).

It is a large, glabrous, deciduous climbing shrub; found throughout tropical India.

The stems are succulent, with long fleshy aerial roots from the branches; bark warty, creamy-white. The leaves are membranous, cordate; flowers small, yellow; drupes ovoid, red, pea-size; seed curved; wood soft, perforated.

The plant is cultivated ornamentally and is propagated by cuttings. The dry stem, with bark intake, constitute the drug.

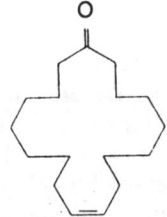

Fig. 22.64. Civetone.

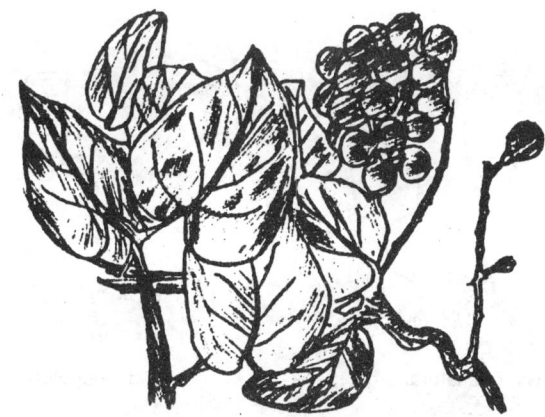

Fig. 22.65. *Tinospora cordifolia.*

Chemical constituents

The stem contains berberine, giloin (bitter glycoside), giloinin, gilosterol, tinosporon, tinosporic acid, tinosporol, magnoflorine, furanolactone diterpenoid, nonacosane-15-one, octacosanol, β-sitosterol, clerodone type diterpenes, C-6, C-12 epimer of 6-hydroxy-areangelicin, 18-norclerodane glycoside (tinosporaside), tinosporidine; cordifol, heptacosanol, octacosanol (in leaves), tinosporide,

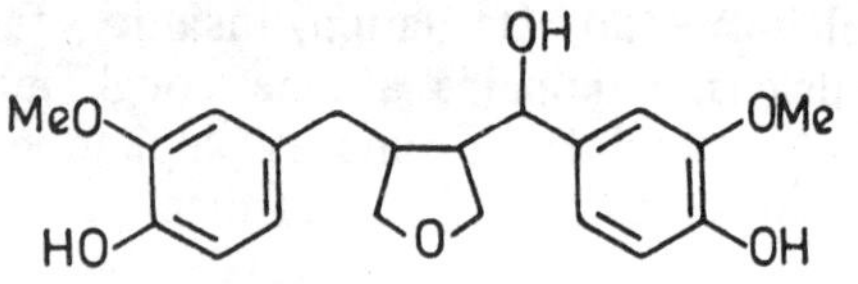

Tetrahydrofuran derivative

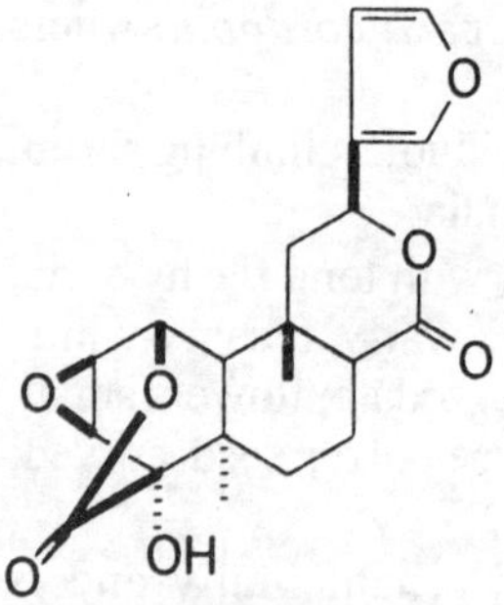

Tinosporide

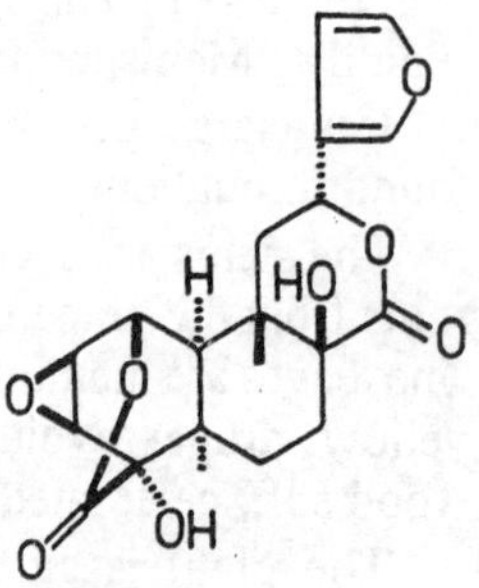

Furano-lactone

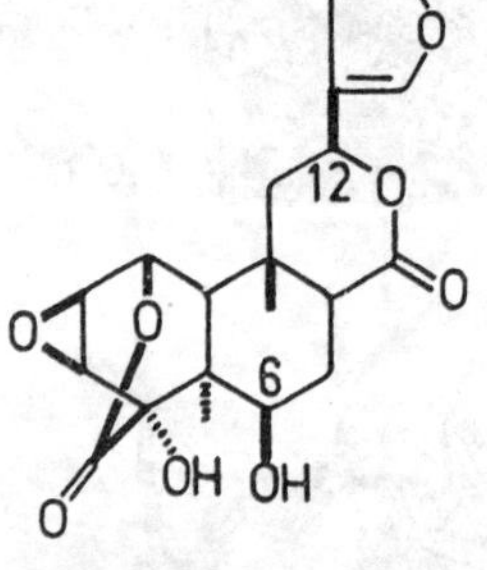

Clerodanefurano-diterpene

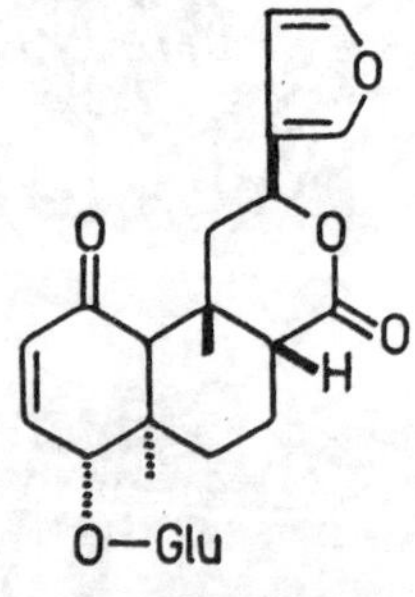

Tinosporaside

Fig. 22.66. Chemical constituents of *Tinospora cordifolia*.

tinosporin, columbin, chasmanthin, palmarin, giloinisin and substituted pyrrolidine.

Uses

It is well known for its adaptogenic and immunomodulatory, antiarthritic, antimalarial, antidiabetic, antiallergic, aphrodisiac anti-inflammatory and tonic properties. It is also useful in skin diseases, anaemia, piles and chronic fever. "Guduchi satwa" (an aqueous extract containing starch) is a nutrient and is used in chronic diarrhoea and dysentery. Juice prepared from fresh plant is used as a diuretic. The roots are used for its antistress, antileprotic and anti-malarial activities.

A decoction of the leaves is prescribed to treat gout. Young leaves, bruised in milk, are used as a liniment in erysipelas. The leaves crushed with honey are applied to ulcers. Dried and powdered fruit, mixed with honey or ghee, is used as a tonic and to treat jaundice and rheumatism. The root is a powerful emetic and given in visceral obstruction. An aqueous extract of the root is taken in leprosy.

The stem juice is valued in high fever and jaundice. A decoction of the stem mixed with *piper longum* is used in rheumatic fever, vomiting due to excessive bile secretion, and slow fever with cough. A stem paste is given with ginger in urticaria. The stem paste with the stem of *Piper nigrum* and honey is useful in heart palpitation due to flatulency. Stem juice is beneficial in elephantiasis. A stem starch, called 'palo', prepared from the aqueous extract of dried stem, acts as an antacid, antidiarrhoeal and antidysenteric agent and is used as a tonic in debility. Starch is mainly composed of 1,4-linked glucan with occasional branching. The leaves are rich in protein, calcium and phosphorus and prescribed in fever.

Pharmacology

Plant extract reduced fasting blood sugar in rabbits and rats and increased glucose tolerance in rats. An aqueous extract of the stem showed anti-inflammatory, analgesic and antipyretic action in rats and immunosuppressive effect in rabbits. It significantly inhibited antibody formation by typhoid H-antigen. It also potentiated morphine analgesia. Stem extract significantly decreased broncho-spasm induced by 5% histamine in guinea pig and reduced the number of disrupted mast cells in rats. 1,2-Substituted pyrrolidine showed CNS depressant and hypoglycaemic activities. The alcoholic extract of the stem showed anti-microbial activity against *Escherichia coli*.

The drug has analgesic effect and its aqueous extract has a high phagocytic index. The action of the drug is due to its favourable effect on the endogenous insulin secretion, glucose uptake and inhibition of peripheral glucose release.

The activity of the drug appears to be due to alkaloids. The drug shows immunomodulatory activity; It produces significant leucocytosis and predominant neutrophilia in animal models. Clinical experiments for its antistress and tonic properties subdue its use in cases of mentally retarded children. The aqueous or alcoholic extract of plant and leaf exhibits hypoglycaemic and antihyperglycaemic activities in different experimental models. A pyrrolidine derivative isolated from ethyl acetate exhibits hypoglycaemic activity in animal models. The aqueous extract exerted a significant anti-inflammatory effect which is comparable with indomethacin and the mechanism of action appears to resemble non-steroidal antiinflammatory agents. The drug possesses significant hepatoprotective, antibacterial (*M. tuberculosis*), antipyretic, hypotensive and diuretic properties. Herbal formulations Rumalaya and Septillin containing *T. cordifolia* are effective in rheumatoid arthritis and in children suffering from respiratory tract infections, respectively. Septillin showed immunostimulatory effect when tested in animals bearing tumours.

KALI-JIRI

Somraj, Purple fleabane.

Biological source

It is a whole herb of *Vernonia anthelmintica* (Willd.) Kuntze (syn. *Centratherum anthelminticum* (L.) Kuntze) (Family: Asteraceae).

It is an erect, annual herb, 15-75 cm high; stem stiff, cylindrical, striate, pubescent, slightly branched, leaves variable in size, lanceolate or elliptic, flowers pink and purple, in minute heads; achenes oblong, terete, narrow at the base.

Chemical constituents

The herb contains β-amyrin, lupeol, their acetates, β-sitosterol, stigmasterol, α-spinasterol, phenolic resins and β-amyrin.

The seed oil is composed of myristic, palmitic (23%), stearic, arachidic, behenic, oleic, linoleic (22%) and oxygenated oleic (28%) acids. The seeds contain 7, 24(28)-stigmastadienol, stigmasterol, 5-stigmasten-3β-ol, 7,22-stigmastadienol, 8,14, 24(28)-stigmastatrienol acetate and elemanolide vernodalol.

The root yields 24-hydroxytaraxer-14-ene, compesterol, α-spinasterol, lupeol acetate and 3β-acetoxyurs-19-ene.

Uses

The plant is astringent, cold, stomachic, tonic, useful in asthma, bronchitis and consumption. An infusion of the plant is used in fever. The expressed juice is given in piles, to children with incontinence of urine, and to cattle with swollen throat and suffering from indigestion. The plant possesses strong diaphoretic properties and is given to produce perspiration in fever. In combination with quinine, the plant is useful in malarial fever. In Sri Lanka, the plant is used for sores and wounds.

A poultice of the leaves is used against humid herpes, eczema and ringworm and for the extraction of guinea worms. Leaf juice is boiled with an oil and used to treat elephantiasis. In eastern India, the whole plant is given in spasm of the bladder and strangury. Fresh leaves are rubbed on scorpion bites to relieve pain and inflammation.

The seeds are commonly used as an anthelmintic and alexipharmic, effective in roundworm and threadworm infections and prescribed in cough, flatulence, intestinal colic, dysuria, leucoderma, psoriasis and other chronic skin diseases. A seed paste with lime juice is used to destroy pediculi.

The flowers are used for conjunctivitis, fever and rheumatism. The root is given in dropsy.

An ethanolic extract of the herb showed activity against *Ranikhet virus* disease and anticancer activity against Sarcoma 180 in mice. An alcoholic extract showed anthelmintic activity on earthworm and tapeworm. It caused relaxation of smooth muscles in isolated guinea pig ileum and had mild laxative action in rats.

KALI-JIRA

Kalonji, Small fennel, Black cumin.

Biological source

It consists of the seeds of *Nigella sativa* Linn. (Family : Ranunculaceae).

It is a small herb, about 45 cm high; cultivated in Punjab, Himachal Pradesh, Bihar and Assam. The leaves are 2-3 pinnatisect, alternate, cut into linear-lanceolate segments; flowers pale blue, on solitary long peduncles; seeds black, trigonous.

Chemical constituents

The seeds contain a volatile oil composed of carvone, *d*-limonene, *p*-cymene, citronellyl acetate, (+)-citronellol, nigellone, aliphatic alcohols, and α,β-unsaturated hydroxyketone.

The fixed oil of the seeds is composed of myristic, palmitic, stearic, oleic (45%) and linoleic

(36%) acids. The component glycerides of the oil are trilinolein, oleodilinolein, dioleolinolein and palmito-oleolinolein. The glycerides of some volatile acids are also present in the oil in small amounts.

Black cumin seed also contain nigellin, tannins, resins, proteins, glucose, saponins, arabic acids; free amino acids cystine, lysine, aspartic acid, glutamic acid, alanine, tryphtophan, valine and leucine; phenol glucoside, melanthin; cholesterol, campesterol, stigmasterol, β-sitosterol and α-spinasterol; isoquinoline alkaloids, nigellimine, its N-oxide, nigellicine; avenasterol-5-ene, avenasterol-7-ene, citrostadienol, cycloeucalenol, 24-ethyllophenol, gramisterol, lophenol, 24-methyl-lophenol, obtusifoliol, stigmasterol-7-ene, β-amyrine, butyrospermol, cycloartenol, 24-methylene cycloartenol, taraxerol, tirucallol, 3-O-[β-D-xylopyranosyl (1→3)-α-L-rhamnosyl (1→2)-α-L-arbinosyl-7-28-O-[α-L-rhamnosyl (1→4)-β-D-glucosyl (1→6)-β-D-glucosyl (–)-hederagenin and esters of dehydrostearic and linoleic acids.

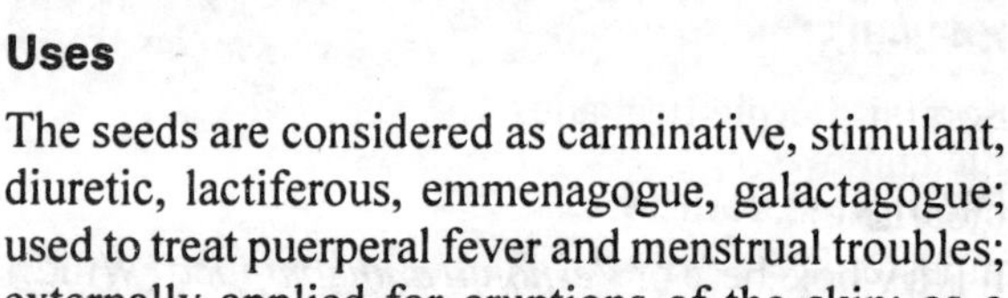

Nigellicine

Nigellimine N-oxide

Fig. 22.68. Chemical constituents of *Nigella sativa*.

Uses

The seeds are considered as carminative, stimulant, diuretic, lactiferous, emmenagogue, galactagogue; used to treat puerperal fever and menstrual troubles; externally applied for eruptions of the skin; as a stabilizing agent for edible oils and as preservative of clothes against insect attack. Powdered seeds mixed with sesame oil are externally applied to boils and scorpion sting. Essential oil of the seeds is used in common cold and cough.

The seeds are soaked in rose oil and then used as eye drops. The seeds are eaten to relieve congestion, difficult breathing, flatulence, constipation and piles.

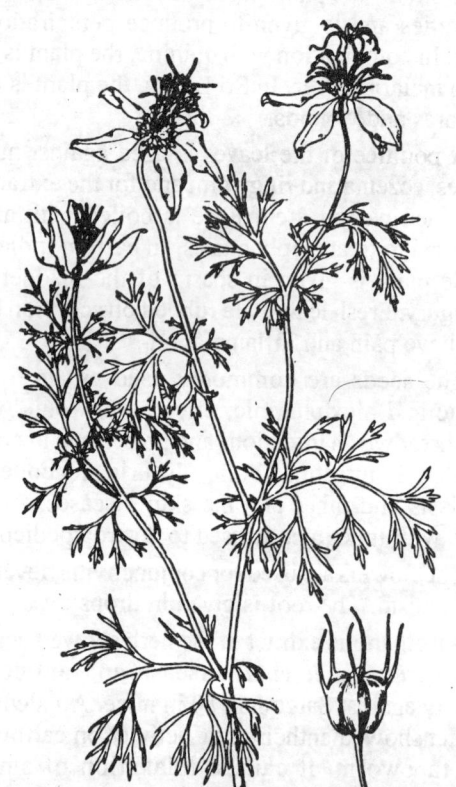

Fig. 22.67. *Nigella sativa*—flowering branch and fruit.

Pharmacology

An ether extract of the seeds when injected into lactating rats on a balanced diet showed more powerful galactagogue action than estrogen. Essential oil and nigellone protected guinea pig against histamine-induced bronchospasms. Ether extract showed more powerful galacta-gogue action than estrogen in lactating rats. Nigellone protects guinea pig against histamine induced bronchospasm.

The essential oil of the seeds was active against *Escherichia coli*, *Salmonella paratyphi*, *Staphylococcus aureus*, *Aspergillus flavus* and *Fusarium tenuis.*

An unidentified α,β-unsaturated hydroketone of the seeds exhibited antifeedant activity.

A seed extract containing certain fatty acid showed cytotoxicity against Ehrlich ascites carcinoma, Dalton's lymphoma ascites and sarcoma-180. A single injection of the seed extract significantly increased lifespan of mice bearing EAC.

KANTAKARI

Kateli, Yellow-berried nightshade.

Biological source

It consists of the whole plant of *Solanum surattense* Burm. f. (syn. *S. xanthocarpum* Schrad and Wendl.) (Family : Solanaceae).

It is very spiny diffuse herb, up to 1.2 m high, found all over India. The leaves are ovate or elliptic, flowers blue and berries globose, glabrous green.

Chemical constituents

The berries contain caffeic, chlorogenic, isochlorogenic and neochlorogenic acids; esculin, esculetin, cycloartanol, cycloartenol, cholesterol, diosgenin, campesterol, cholesterol derivatives, solasodine, solamargine, β-solamargine, solasonine, solasurine,, β-sitosterol and stigmasteryl glucoside. The fruit oil is composed of glycerides of arachidic, linoleic, oleic, palmitic and stearic acids and solanocarpine. The flowers yield diosgenin, apigenin and quercetin glycoside.

Uses

The root is reputed as antiasthmatic, antiemetic, diuretic and expectorant, used to prepare an Ayurvedic medicine, *Dasamula*. It is given in asthma, cough and pain in the chest. A decoction of the root in combination with *Tinospora cordifolia* is useful in cough and fever.

The leaves are anodyne. Leaf-juice is given with black pepper in rheumatism. The stem, flowers and fruits are bitter and carminative; useful in burning sensation of the feet accompanied by vesicular watery eruptions. The leaves are applied to relieve pain and leaf juice with black peppers is given in rheumatism. The juice of berries is used in sore throat. The seeds are given as an expectorant in asthma and cough and to relieve toothache. A powder of the berries is mixed with honey and given to children in cough.

The plant has alternative, antiasthmatic, aperient, diuretic, digestive and febrifuge properties and is used to cure bronchitis, cough, constipation and dropsy. The plant is a part of an Ayurvedic formulation *Arkadhi* which is prescribed in bronchitis, dengue fever and chest affections. A decoction of the plant is used in gonorrhoea and to promote conception.

Pharmacology

Crude plant extract caused hypotension which has been attributed to release of histamine by some constituents. Plant powder is antitussive. It is beneficial for patients of bronchial asthma and non-specific cough due to depletion of histamine from lung. Its expectorant action is due to inorganic nitrate content.

The aqueous and alcoholic extracts of the plant possess hypotensive effect and showed antiviral activity against *Ranikhet disease* virus and against *Sarcoma* 180 in mice. Extracts of shoots and fruit show antibacterial activity against *Staphylococcus aureus* and *Escherichia coli.*

LETTUCE

Kahu, Salad, Garden Lettuce.

Biological source

It consists of *Lactuca sativa* Linn.; syn. *L. scariola* Linn. var. *sativa* C.B. Clarke (Family : Asteraceae).

It grows in warmer temperate parts of western Asia, including eastern Mediterranean. It is grown mostly as a cold weather crop in the plains of India. It can be planted anytime during spring or early summer in the hills.

Description

It is an erect, glabrous, annual herb, 50-120 cm high; leaves radical, thin, nearly orbicular, oblong, obovate or lingulate, plane, bullate or curved, flower heads of yellow rays, borne on panicles, achenes lenticular oblong, dark brown, with slender beak and white pappus.

Lettuce seeds may be sown directly in the field or seedlings may be raised in nursery beds and transplanted in the fields. Seeds are very small and should be sown shallow properly. The seeds (about 85%) germinate in 4-5 days after sowing. Since lettuce is shallow rooted, it requires frequent irrigation once every 4-5 days if the weather is dry. Yellow mosaic affects the leaves turning them pale yellow and mottled and later get distorted, thickened and leathery. The causative virus is seed-borne and is spread by insects. Pythium leaf rot, caused by *Pythium aphanidermatum*, affects the lower leaves touching the ground. The incidence of the disease decreases with decrease in moisture.

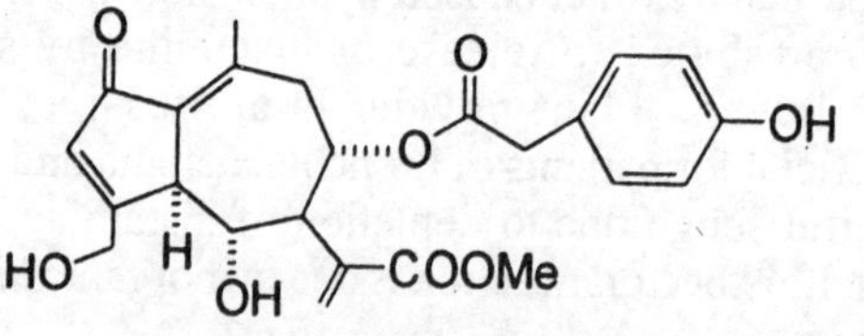

Sesquiterpene ester

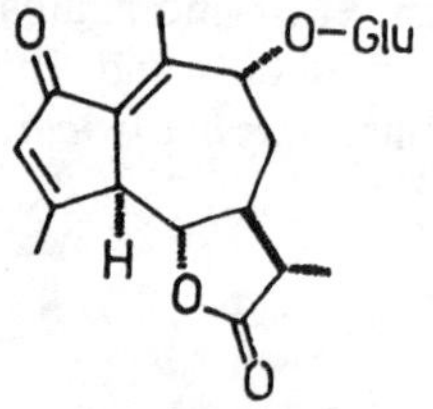

Lactuside C

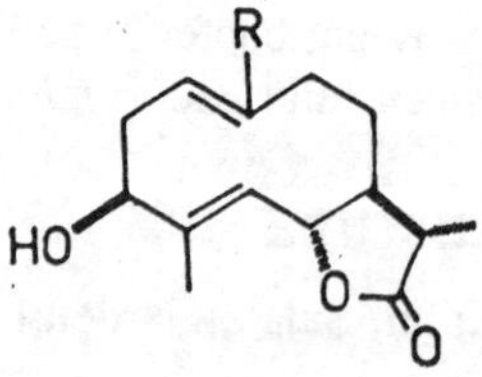

3β-Hydroxy-11β,13-dihydroacanthospermolide
R = CHO
3β,14-Dihydroxy-11β,13-dihydrocostunolide
R = CH_2OH

Fig. 22.69. Chemical constituents of *Lactuca sativa*.

Leaf lettuce may be harvested at any time after the plants are large enough for use, but before the leaves become tough and bitter. Lettuce is a popular salad crop in western countries. It is valued mainly for its vitamins and mineral contents.

Chemical constituents

Lettuce contains vitamins A, B, C, E, G and K, nicotinic acid, riboflavin, folic acid, choline, Na, K, Ca, Mg, Fe, Cu, P, S, Cl, traces of As, Ba, Mn, Ti, Zn, Al, F and I; pectic substances, organic acids (oxalic, malic and citric acids), sesquiterpenoids ceryl alcohol, amyrin and ergosterol. The latex from the stem and roots contains caoutchouc.

Uses

Garden lettuce yields lactucarium used as hypnotic in bronchitis and asthma. Lettuce is used as poutices for burns and painful ulcers.

LODH

Biological source

It consists of the stem bark of *Symplocos racemosa* Roxb. (Family : Symplocaceae).

It is an evergreen tree or shrub, 6-9 m high, abundant in the plains and lower hills throughout northern and eastern India, in Himalayas up to 1,400 m, and southwards up to Chota Nagpur. The leaves are dark green above, orbicular, oblong. The flowers are white or yellow, aromatic. The fruits are drupes, purple-black, subcylindrical, smooth; seeds 1-3.

Chemical constituents

The bark contains oxalic acid, 3-monoglucoside of 7-O-methyl leucopelargonidin, pelargonidin-3-O-glucoside; betulinic, acetyloleanolic, oleanolic and ellagic acids; flavan glycoside symposide; β-sitosterol, 28-hydroxy-20α-urs-12,18(19)-dien-3β-yl acetate, 3-oxo-20α-urs-12,18(19)-dien-28-oic, 24-hydroxyolean-12-en-3-one and butelin.

Uses

A yellow dye is extracted from the leaves and the bark. Mainly the bark is used as a mordant with other drugs. For dyeing silk yellow, it is used in combination with turmeric and *Plecospermum spinosum*. It is one of the ingredients of *abir*, a red powder used during the festival of Holi.

The astringent bark is used to treat diarrhoea, dysentery, dropsy, conjunctivitis, ophthalmial and liver complaints. A decoction of the bark is prescribed to stop bleeding of the gums. The bark is recommended with sugar to cure menorrhagia and other uterine disorders.

Pharmacology

A crystalline fraction from the bark inhibited the growth of *Micrococcus pyrogens* var. *aureus*, *Escherichia coli* and enteric and dysenteric groups of organisms.

Symposide and (–)-epiafzelechin showed anti-fibrinolytic activity.

MALKANGNI

Black-oil plant, Intellect tree.

Biological source

It consists of the seeds of *Celastrus paniculatus* Willd. (Family : Celastraceae).

It is a large, woody, climbing shrub, up to 10 m in height, distributed all over India up to an altitude of 1,800 m.

The seeds are bitter and have an unpleasant odour.

Chemical constituents

The seeds contain a fixed oil (52%), known as *Celestrus oil* or *Malkanguni oil* which is composed of the glycerides of palmitic (31%), stearic, oleic (22%), linoleic (15%) and linolenic acids. The nonglyceride portion of the oil is consisted of sesquiterpene alkaloids celapagine, celapanigine and celapanine and polyalcohol esters, *e.g.*, malkagunin (an acetate benzoate of malkaguniol), esters of poly-alcohols A, B (celaphanol), C and D, which are esterified with one or more acetic, benzoic, β-furanoic and β-nicotinic acids. The seeds also contain celastrine, paniculatadiol, β-amyrin, β-sito-sterol, a bitter resin, sesquiterpe-noids 1β, 6α-diacetoxy-9β-benzoyloxy-8β-cinnamoyloxy-β-dihydroagarofuran, 1β, 6α, 8β-triacetoxy-9α-(β-furancerbonyloxy)-β-dihydro-agarofuran, β-dihydro agarofurans VI, VII, VIII and IX; 4,4-dimethyl-1,3-dioxan-5-ol.

The root bark contains pristimerin, zeylasterone, zeylasterol, celastrol, *n*-triacontanol, β-dihydro-

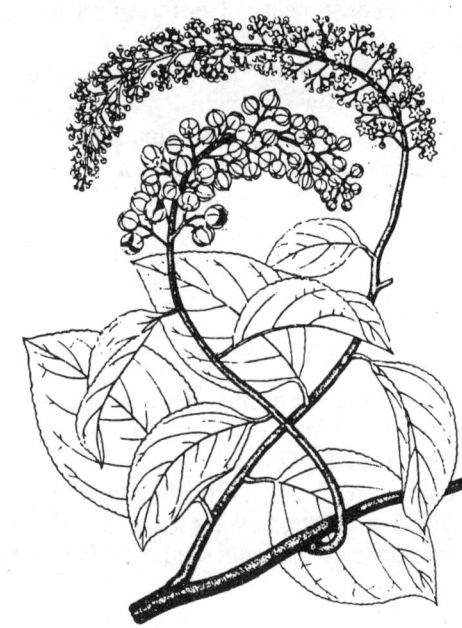

Fig. 22.70. *Celastrus paniculatus*—flowering and fruiting branch.

agarofurans, benzoic acid and a yellow oil. The bark is considered as abortifacient and its dry powder is applied on cuts for healing. The leaves are emmenagogue and anti-dysenteric. The leaf juice is given as an antidote in opium poisoning.

Uses

The seeds possess emetic, diaphoretic, febrifugal and narvine properties and are used for sharpening the memory, to cure sores, ulcers, rheumatism and gout. The seeds are taken as a tonic with sugar and ghee.

The seed oil has a powerful stimulant action. It is used in scabies and rheumatic pains, wounds, eczema, beriberi and paralysis. The oil showed a good results in treating mental depression and hysteria without any side reaction. It has tranqui-lizing effect and hastens the process of learning and memory in experimental animals. It produces fall in blood pressure in dogs. The alcoholic emulsion (96%) of the oil showed anti-bacterial activity. The oil repels mosquitoes.

The plant shows sedative, anti-inflammatory, antipyretic, anti-emetic and anti-ulcerogenic effects.

It is one of the constituent of 'Geriforte' used in senile pruritus.

The root powder is used in pneumonia, the root bark is applied on swollen veins.

A chloroform extract of root bark showed significant antimalarial activity against *Plasmodium falciparum* in vitro.

METHI

Fenugreek.

Biological source

It consists of the herb and seeds of *Trigonella foenum-graceum* Linn. (Family : Papilionaceae).

It is an aromatic, annual, 30-60 cm tall herb, widely cultivated in many parts of India. The leaves are pinnate, 3-foliolate; flowers white or yellowish-white, pods up to 15 cm long; seeds 10-20, greenish brown, oblong.

Chemical constituents

The endosperm of the seeds is rich in galactomannan (15%). The mature seeds yield amino acids, *e.g.,* 4-hydroxyisoleucine and fatty acids on hydrolysis, carotene, vitamins, saponins, *viz.,* graecunins H-N (glycosides of diosgenin), fenugrin B, sapogenins, *e.g.,* diosgenin, gitogenin, neogitogenin, homoorientin, vitexin, saponaretin, its tetrosidés B and C; trigonelloside C, 3,26-

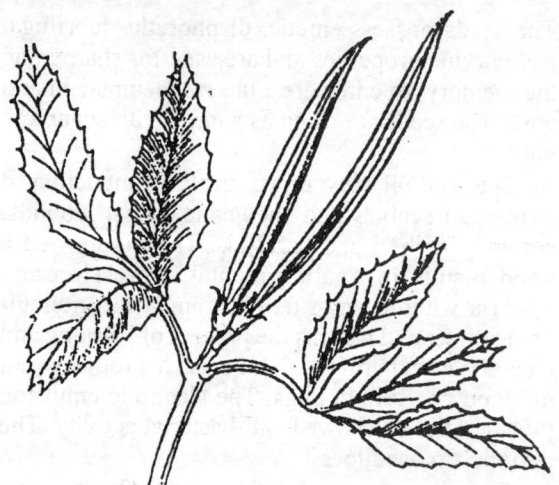

Fig. 22.71. *Trigonella foenum-graceum.*

bisglycoside, flavone C-glycoside-vitexin-2"-O-*p*-coumarate, vicenin-1 and vicenin-2.

The alkaloids, trigonelline, choline, 7-acetoxy-4-methyl coumarin, furastanol glycoside, kaempferol, luteolin and quercetin are also present

The leaves give saponins, *viz.,* diosgenin, its glycoside (graecunin B), graecunins A-G, gitogenin, tigogenin, kaempferol, quercetin and β-sitosterol. The plant also contains trigocoumarin, trigoforin, 4-methyl-7-acetoxycoumarin, *p*-coumaric acid, luteolin and quercetin. The seed oil is composed of linoleic (50.5%), palmitic, stearic, oleic (59%), linoleic (~50%) and linolenic acids.

Uses

The seeds are mucilaginous, demulcent, diuretic, carminative, aromatic, tonic, galactagogue, emmenagogue, astringent, emollient and aphrodisiac; useful in colic, flatulence, dysentery, diarrhoea, anorexia, cough, dropsy, enlargement of the livers and spleen, rheumatism, lymphatism, rickets, anaemia and diabetes. In Switzerland, they are used for flavouring cheese. Roasted seeds are used as a substitute for coffee in Africa. The seeds are used externally as poultice for abscesses, boils and ulcers, and internally as emollient for inflammation of the intestinal tract. The seeds are boiled with dried figs and dates in water and the mixture is taken in bronchitis and for soothing cough.

Powdered seeds are mixed with mustard and salt and applied for ankle sprains. The seeds are boiled in water, mixed the egg and given to the new mother for 7 days as a tonic after the baby is born. An enema made from the seeds, *Terminalia catapha*, animal fat and warm water is given to new mother to strengthen her back.

The leaves are cooling, mild aperient, externally applied to swellings and burns.

The plant possesses insect repellent properties. The dried plant is mixed with stored grains to protect them from the ravages of insects during rainy season. The entire plant is used to treat abdominal colic, bronchitis, cough and sprains.

Exports

Annually, a total of 1000-1890 tonnes of fenugreek valued at Rs. 15-27 lacs are exported from India to more than 40 countries. The main markets are Japan,

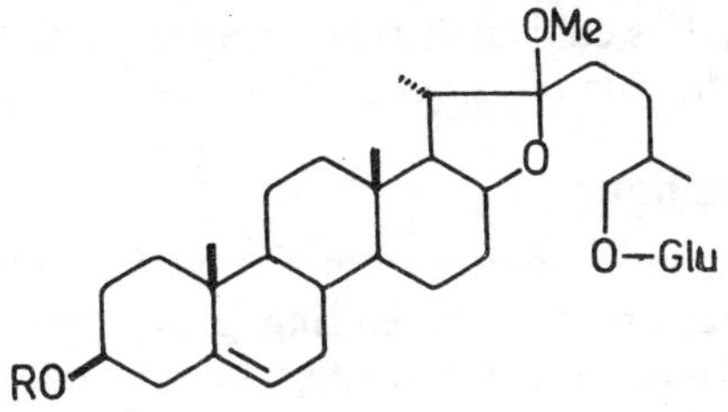

Trigofoenoside A-1
R = Glu(2→1)Rha
Trigofoenoside D-1
R = Glu[(2→1)Rha](3→1)Glu
Trigofoenoside F-1
R = Glu(6→1)Glu(2→1)Rha
Trigofoenoside G-1
R = Glu(6→1)Glu[(2→1)Rha](4→1)Xyl

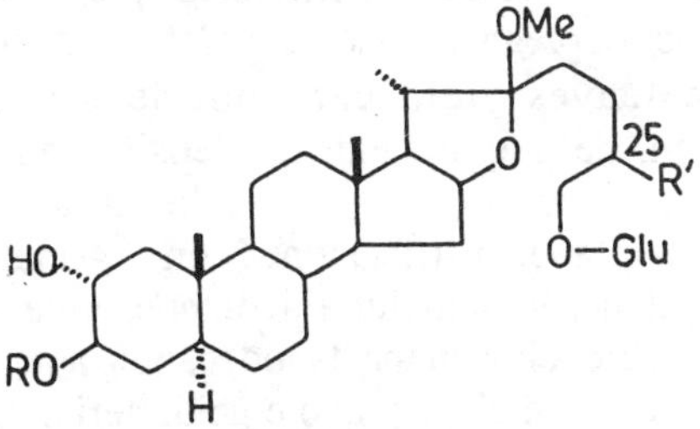

Trigofoenoside B-1
R = Glu(4→1)Rha R′ = α-Me
Trigofoenoside C-1
R = Glu[(2→1)Rha](4→1)Rha, R′ = β-Me

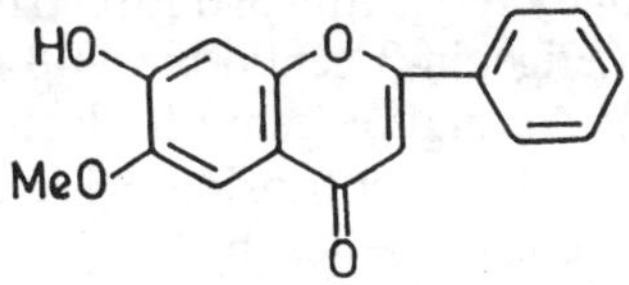

Trigraecum

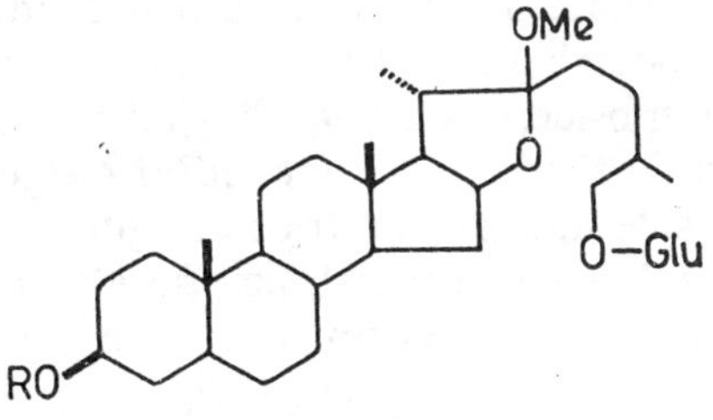

Trigofoenoside E-1
R = Glu[(2→1)Rha](4→1)Xyl

Fig. 22.72. Chemical constituents of *Trigonella foenum-graceum*.

Singapore, Sri Lanka, Saudi Arabia, Nepal, UK, USA, Canada and Kenya.

Pharmacology

Administration of a seed extract to rats enhanced food consumption and motivation to cat and induced hyperinsulinemia and hypocholesterolaemia. Seed extract exhibited mild anti-implantation activity in female rats and showed antibiotic activity against *Micrococcus pyogens* var. *aureus*.

NAGAR-MOTHA

Barik moth, Motha, Nutgrass.

Biological source

It consists of the tubers of *Cyperus rotundus* Linn (Family : Cyperaceae).

It is distributed throughout India, Pakistan and other Asian countries in warmed region as a weed.

It is a perennial herb, up to 60 cm high, bearing hard, ovoid, tunicate, black, fragrant tubers. Leaves arising from the base, longer than the stem, linear, flat, 1-nerved. Flowers in 5-7 unequal rays, each ray with 4-8 spikelets, reddish-brown.

Chemical constituents

The tubers contain saponin oleanolic acid 3-O-neohesperidoside, rotundone, 4α,5α-oxidoeudesm-11-en-3α-ol, β-selinene, cyperenone, α-cyperone, N-isobutyldeca-2,4-dienamide and securinine. A mixture of auto-oxidation products of β-selinene is most active anti-malarial substance present in the drug. The tubers also contain cuperene-1 (a tricyclic sesquiterpene), cyperene-2 (a bicyclic sesquiterpene), patchoule-none, mustakone, cyperenone, cyperolone, sugetriol triacetate and rhamnetin-3-O-rhamnosyl (1 → 4)-rhamnopyranoside.

The essential oil of the tubers is composed of copadiene, epoxyguaiene, rotundone, cyperolone, sugeonol, cyperol, isocyperol, α-rotunol, β-rotunol, kobusone and isokobusone. Caryophyllene was the major constituent of the volatile oil of tubers from a Nigerian plant.

Uses

The tubers are reputed as an aphrodisiac, astringent, cooling, galactagogue, insecticide, stimulant, useful in burning sensations, eye diseases, leprosy and

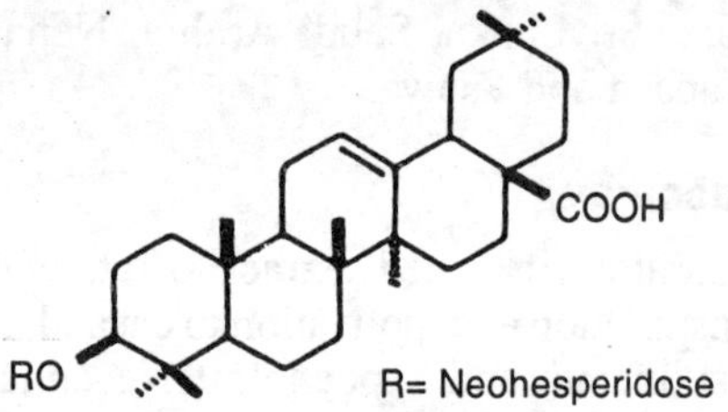

Fig. 22.73. Oleanolic acid-3-O-neohesperidoside.

indigestion. They are given to regulate menstruation. An ointment prepared from the tubers is applied to bee stings and bites and to breasts as galactagogue. In Yemen, rhizome powder is used to perfume clothes and hair. The rhizomes are also useful in uterine disorders, ulcers and to prevent tooth decay. In eastern Africa, tubers are used to treat malaria.

The seeds are used as a diuretic, to treat earache, teeth and gum problems.

The leaves are applied topically for headache.

Pharmacology

The root extract possessed tranquilizing activity. It had smooth muscle relaxant activity on rabbit ileum. The extract also showed significant anti-pyretic and anti-inflammatory activities. α-Cyperone inhibited prostaglandin biosynthesis and showed competitive type inhibition with respect to substrate.

Daily drops of root extract into the eyes of conjunctivitis cases decreased redness and reduced pain and ocular discharge in five days. The volatile oil had a marked CNS depressant effects. It potentiated hypnotic action of pentobarbital in mice and anaesthetic action of scopolamine in rabbits. It also inhibited contraction of the isolated ileum of rabbits.

NERIUM

Lal kaner, Karabi, Indian oleander.

Biological source

It consists of the bark and other parts of *Nerium indicum* Mill., syn. *N. odorum* Soland (Family : Apocynaceae).

It is a large evergreen shrub with milky juice found in Himalayas from Kashmir to Nepal, Gangetic plain, northern and central India, Afghanistan, Pakistan, Japan and Mediterranean region. It is cultivated as an ornamental plant along roadsides and in gardens.

Description

N. indicum is an evergreen shrub with a stout, 1-2 m long, erect or ascending grey stem; leaves coriaceous, linear-lanceolate, with stout midrib, dark green above, pale beneath; flowers fragrant, pink, red or white; follicles erect, striate, cylindrical; seeds villous with brown hair.

Chemical constituents

The stem bark contains odorosides A, B, D, F, G, H, K, L and M, odorobioside K, flavones quercetin 3-rhamnoglucoside, kaempferol-3-rhamno-glucoside, neriodorein, neriodorin, pregnenolone, glycosides of pregnenolone, scopoletin and scopolin.

The leaves yield cardenolide glycosides oleanolin, deacetyloleandrin, oleoside, adynerin, neriodin, neriodorin, 12-methyl-*n*-hexatriacon-tane, *n*-tritriacontane, *n*-tritriacont-3-ene, 4-methyl-*n*-tritriacontane, 9-methyldotriacontane, *n*-hentritria-contane, 12-cyclopentane-1-dodecanoic acid 10-(α-decahydronaphthyl)-heptanoic acid; nerium D, 16-anhydrodigitoxigenin (nerium F), β-D-digitaloside, nerioside, rutin, oleandrigenin-β-D-glycoside, digitoxigenin-α-L-oleandroside, neriumol and nerifol. Other cardenolide triolides and biosides from the leaves are adynerigenin-β-odorotrioside, 16-dehydroadynerigenin-β-odoro-trioside, 16-dehydroadynerigenin-β-gentio-biosyl-β-D-glucosyl-β-D-sarmetoside, digitoxigenin-β-oleatrioside, 16-dehydroneragenin-β-neritrioside, 8β-hydroxy-digi-toxigenin-β-neritrioside, 8β-hydroxydigitoxigenin-β-neritrioside, 8β-hydroxydigitoxigenin-β-neritrioside, 8β-hydroxy-16-dehydrodigitoxigenin-β-neritrioside, 8β-hydroxy-16-dehydrodigitoxi-genin-β-odorobioside, oleandrigenin-α-oleatrioside, -β-odorotrioside, -α-oleabioside, -β-neribioside and -β-D-glucoside; 16-dehydrodigitoxigenin-β-neritrioside and β-odorotrioside, gitoxigenin-α-oleatrioside, digitoxigenin-β-neritrioside, odoroside G, neriagenin-β-neritrioside, adynerigenin-β-neritrioside, 16-dehydro-adynerigenin-β-neritrio-side, -β-neribio-side and -β-odorobioside. The leaves also contain two pregnane glycosides 3-O-β-gentiobiosyl-3β, 14β-dihydroxy-5α-pregnan-20-

one and 21-O-β-D-glucosyl-14β, 21-dihydroxy-pregn-4-en-3,20-dione.

The flowers afford odoroside A, kaempferol-3-glycoside, oleanolic acid, ursolic acid, β-sitosterol and its glucoside. The seeds contain docosanoic, eicosanoic, tri-, penta-, hepta- and nonadecanoic, lauric, palmitic, myristic and stearic acids, paraffins (C_{17}-C_{27}), benzyl and β-phenylethyl alcohols, their acetates, campesterol and stigmasterol.

The roots possess neriodorein, neriodorin, neriumosides A-1, A-2, B-1, B-2 and C-1, pregnenolone glycosides, α-amyrin and plumericin. The roots also contain digitoxigenin-β-gentiotriosyl-β-D-digitaloside, uzarigenin-β-gentiobisyl-β-D-digitaloside, 5α-oleandrigenin, its β-D-digitaloside, β-D-glucosyl-β-D-diginoside and β-D-glucosyl-β-D-digitaloside; and two pregnanolone glycosides 5α-pregnanolone-O-β-D-glucosyl-glucosyl-glucoside and pregnenolone-β-D-apiosyl-β-D-glucoside. The root bark yields odoroside B, uzarizerin glycosides, kaempferol, 4-hydroxy- acetophenone, 2,4-dihydroxyacetophenone, α-amyrin, β-sitosterol, neridienones A and B, and pregnene-3,20-dione derivatives.

Uses

The roots possess abortifacient aphrodisiac, febrifuge, stomachic and diuretic properties. A root paste is applied to ulcers, piles and leprosy. A medicated oil prepared from the root bark is prescribed for skin diseases of scaly nature and leprosy. The roots are used in cardiac asthma, renal calculi and ringworm infection.

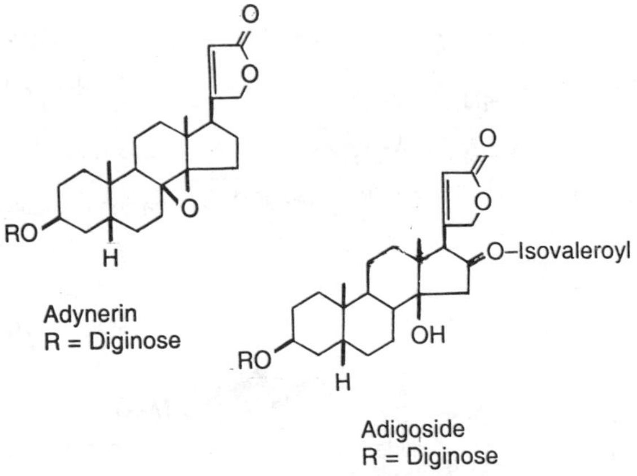

The leaves are used as an anthelmintic, antipyretic, antiseptic, to treat cardiac asthma, circulatory disorders, fever, leprosy, respiratory and skin diseases. A decoction of the leaves is given to reduce swelling. The leaves are powerful repellent and recommended in arthralgia, stomachalgia, leprosy, ulcers, scabies and piles. The juice of tender leaves is used in ophthalmia with copious lacrimation; applied to ulcers. A paste of the leaves is applied to ringworm and other skin diseases.

Pharmacology

The alcoholic extract of the bark showed molluscidal activity against *Zymmaea acumenate* snails. The nerium glycosides acted as a powerful cardiac poison and exhibited action on the heart in a lesser manner than digitoxin.

Odorin causes paralysis of experimental animals. Oleandrin and oleandrigenin-β-D-glycoside showed cardiokinetic and diuretic activities.

A glycoside containing extract showed stimulant or depressant activity on frog heart at low and high doses, respectively. It has an oxytocic activity on rat uterus and induced abortions in mice. Oleandrin increased aortic systolic, aortic means and left ventricular peak pressure in dogs. Oleandrin showed digitalis-like action on isolated animal hearts, emetic action in pigeons, cardio-kinetic and diuretic activities.

PALAS

Dhak, Bastard teak, Bengal kino tree, Flame of the forest.

Biological source

It is the whole plant of *Butea monosperma* (Lam.) Tomb; syn. *B. frondosa* Koenig ex Roxb. (Family: Papilionaceae).

It is commoly found throughout India, except in the arid regions; in Burma, outer Himalayas up to 1,008 m and Sri Lanka.

Description

The plant is a deciduous tree with crooked trunk, up to 15 m in height; bark bluish grey or light brown; branches irregular; leaves long-petioled, 3-foliolate,

Adynerin
R = Diginose

Adigoside
R = Diginose

O–Isovaleroyl

Fig. 22.74. Chemical constituents of *Nerium indicum*.

leaflets coriaceous, obovate, from a cuneate base, glabrescent above, densely finely silky below; flower buds dark brown, flowers bright orange-red, sometimes yellow, in 15 cm long racemes on bare branches; pods pendulous, silky tomentose, containing one seed at the apex, reticulately veined; seeds flat, reniform.

A red juice exudes from natural cracks and from artificial incisions in the bark. Fresh juice is ruby-red and transparent. It dries to form a gum known a *Butea gum* or *Bengal kino*. It occurs as small elongated tears or irregular, elongated masses, smaller than grains of barley, black and opaque, very brittle and can readily be pulverized into a reddish powder, and are water-soluble. On keeping, the gum becomes dull, nearly black, opaque or tough.

Chemical constituents

Butea gum contains leucocyanidin, its tetramer, procyanidin, gallic acid, riboflavin and thiamine.

The flowers contain flavonoid glycosides, butin, butein, butrin, isobutrin, palasitrin, coreopsin, isocoreopsin (butin-7-glucoside), isomonospermoside, sulfurein, palasitrin, chalcone, aurones; β-sitosterol, 4-carbomethoxy-3,6-dioxo-5-hydro-1,2,4-triazine, fructose and amino acids. The aqueous extract of the flowers contains mainly chalcone and isobutrin. The unsaponifiable matter consists mainly of myricyl alcohol and β-sitosterol. The fatty acids isolated from the wax are palmitic, stearic, arachidic, behenic, lignoceric and cerotic acids.

The roots yield glycine, monospermin, δ-lactone of *n*-heneicosanoic acid, (–)-palasonin, its methyl ester, glucose, jalaric esters I and II and laccijalaric esters III and IV.

Palasimide is present in pods. The seeds contain lipolytic and proteolytic enzymes. The proteolytic enzyme is a mixture of plant proteinase and polypeptidase and behaves like "yeast trypsin". The seeds yield alkaloid monospermin (1-N-acetyl-2-oxo-4-methoxy-3H, 5H-imidazole), a δ-lactone of *n*-heneicosanoic acid phytolectin; 15-hydroxy-pentacosanoic acid and 1-carbomethoxy-2-carbamyl hydrazine (from seed coat).

Palasonin is the anthelmintic principle present in the seeds. The anthelmintic effect of palasonin is more pronounced than either piperazine or santonin

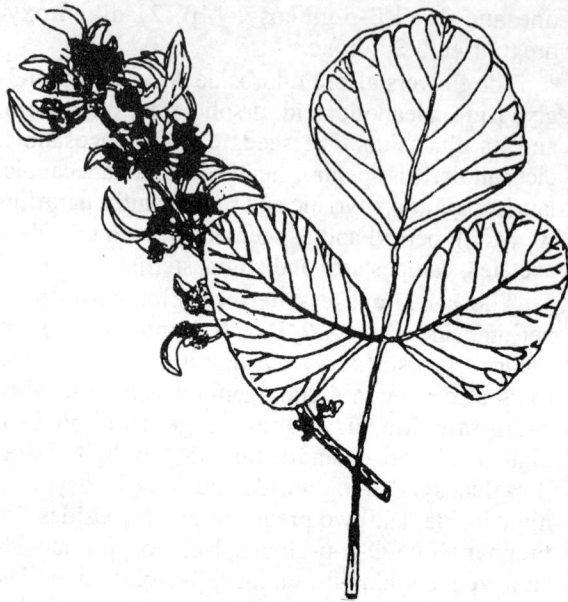

Fig. 22.75. *Butea monosperma.*

against roundworm (*Ascaris lumbricoides*) in humans. It potentiates the stimulant action on different smooth muscles.

The seed oil is composed of the glycerides of myristic, palmitic (19%), stearic, arachidic, behenic (14%), lignoceric, oleic (22%), linoleic (28%) and linolenic acid. The unsaponifiable portion of the oil contains β-sitosterol, its β-D-glucoside & α-amyrin.

The outer seed coat contains a derivative of allophanic acid and characterized as 2-hydroxy-10-methylallophanic acid.

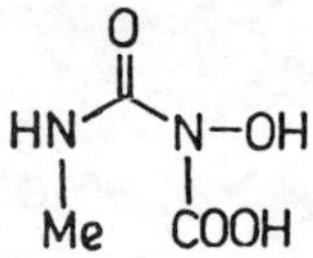

2-Hydroxy-ω-methylallophanic acid

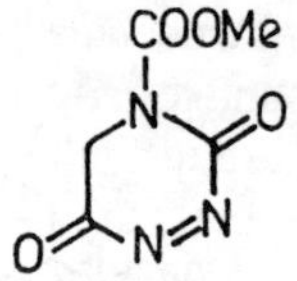

Triazine derivative

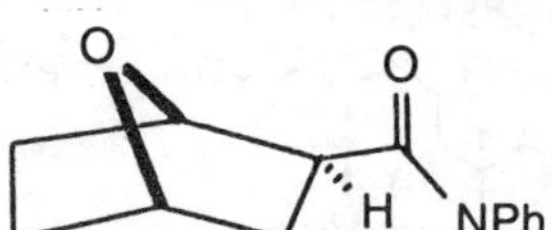

Palasimide

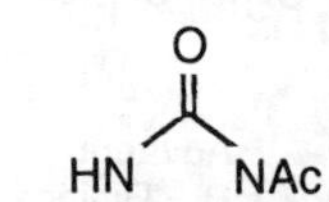

Monospermin

Fig. 22.76. Chemical constituents of *Butea monosperma.*

Uses

The fresh juice is applied to ulcers and in relaxed, congested and septic sore throat. The gum is a powerful astringent, it is given internally in diarrhoea and dysentery, phthisis, and hemorrhage from the bladder and stomach. Its infusion is applied locally in leucorrhoea. A solution of the gum is applied to bruises and erysipelatous inflammations and ringworm. The gum is substituted for or as an adulterant of genuine gum kino of commerce obtained from *Pterocarpus marsupium*.

The bark possesses astringent, bitter, pungent, alterative, aphrodisiac and anthelmintic properties. It is useful in tumors, bleeding piles and ulcers. A decoction of the bark is prescribed in cold, cough, fever, haemorrhages, in menstrual disorders and in the preparation of tonics and elixirs.

The root is useful in elephantiasis, night blindness and other defects of the eyes. It causes temporary sterility in women.

The root bark is used as an aphrodisiac, analgesic and anthelmintic. It is applied to cure sprue, piles, ulcers, tumors and dropsy.

The green leaves are commonly mixed with fodder and given to cattle to increase milk. The leaves are credited with astringent, tonic, diuretic and aphrodisiae properties. They are applied to cure boils, pimples and tumorous piles and given internally in flatulent colic, worms and piles. The shoot apex is used by the 'kani' tribal women of Kerala to prevent conception.

The flowers possess astringent, diuretic, depurative, aphrodisiac, and tonic properties. They are used as an emmenagogue, as poultice in orchitis and to reduce swellings, for bruises and strains. They are effective in leprosy, leucorrhoea and gout. The petals are given to sheep for haematuria.

The flowers yield a brilliant, but very fugitive, yellow dye. Addition of alum, lime and an alkali deepens the colour to orange and makes it less fugitive.

The seeds are slightly acrid, bitter, aperient and rubefacient, sometimes are substituted for santonin. The seeds are used as an anthelmintic, but they may produce nephrotoxicity. The seeds are used as vermifuge in veterinary medicine. The seeds kill maggots. A paste of the seeds with lemon-juice is applied to cure herpes and ring-worm. A decoction of the seeds is given in gravel.

Pharmacology

The hot alcoholic extract of the seeds showed significant anti-implantation and anti-ovulatory activity in rats and rabbits, respectively. The alcoholic extract of the seeds inhibits the growth of *Escherichia coli* and *Micrococcus pyogenes* var. *aureus*. A crude, saline extract (0.9%) of the seeds agglutinates the erythrocytes in experimental animals.

The glycosides palasitrin and butrin reduced the number of implants in the mated rats. The seed oil showed a marked and prolonged fall in the blood pressure in animals.

The seeds given orally are effective in roundworm and threadworm infections but ineffective in case of tapeworm. The side effects observed as nausea, vomiting, dizziness, general weakness and in pain in the abdomen. The extracts of the seeds and seed coat administered daily from day one post-coitum for ten days prevented pregnancy in female rats.

The fruits possess anthelmintic and aperient properties. They are used in abdominal problems, eye diseases, inflammation, piles, skin diseases, tumors and urinary discharges.

The ether, alcoholic and aqueous extracts of flowers showed anti-estrogenic activity in mice. A fraction containing sodium salt of phenolic constituents, isolated from the bark, is a potent anti-asthmatic agent.

They are active against the fungus *Helminthosporium sativum*. An alcoholic solution of the petals showed anti-estrogenic activity in mice. A decoction of the flowers is given in diarrhoea and to puerperal women. The aqueous extract of the flowers shows significant anti-implantation activity in rats. Flower extract exhibited anti-hepatotoxic activity.

RASANA

A. PLUCHEA LANCEOLATA

Biological source

It consists of the whole plant of *Pluchea lanceolata* (DC) Clarke (Family : Asteraceae).

Habitat

It is found in the saline or sandy soil of Punjab, Rajasthan and Gangetic plain and in Delhi as a weed.

Description

It is an erect undershrub, 30-60 cm tall; stem and branches terete, gray-pubescent. Leaves sessile, coriaceous, oblanceolate, obtuse, narrowed at the base, entire. Flower heads in compound corymbs, white, yellow lilac, or purple.

Chemical constituents

The leaves of *P. lanceolata* contain quercetin, moretenol, its acetate, neolupenol, isorhamnetin and quercitrin.

The flowers yield pluchine, sorghumol acetate, moretenol, its acetate, stigmasterol, neolupenol, cycloart-23-en-3β,25-diol, β-sitosterol-D-glucoside, nonacosane, heptacosane, hentriacontane and octacosane. The whole plant is a source of 23-methyl dotriaconta-3-one, 22-methyl hentriacontane-3,19-dione, pluchoic acid (2-methoxy-4-hydroxybenzoic acid), pleuchioside (urs-3α-19α-20β-triol), stigmasta-(5,11(12)-dien-3β-ol, 9,10-seco-24S-ethyl-cholest-5-en-3β-D-glucoside, plucheachro-menone, plucheasterolide, monoterpene ester [4-isopropylcyclohex-1-en-7-(2'-oxy-2'-methyl butyl) oate], plucheaursenyl acetate, pluchealactone, lanceolatoic acid, plucheasesterterpenyl ester and plucheasesquiterpenyl hexadecanoate. The roots afforded sorghumol, its acetate and boehmeryl acetate.

Uses

The herb possesses analgesic, antipyretic, laxative and nervine tonic properties. A decoction of the plant is used in bronchitis and inflammation. In Tibet, the drug is used to treat asthma, cough, hiccough, poisoning and diseases caused by *vayu*. The leaves are substituted for senna leaves.

Pharmacology

The alcoholic extract of the plant showed acetyl choline-like action and a spasmolytic action on smooth muscles. The plant has relaxation action on the isolated ileum of rat and rabbit and isolated rat uterus. The extract potentiated pentabarbital induced hypnosis in rats. A decoction of the whole plant was effective against formalin-induced arthritis. The alcoholic extract of the stems showed significant anti-inflammatory activity, decreased the adrenal gland weight and increased the adrenal ascorbic acid and cholesterol contents. A 50% ethanolic extract was devoid of antibacterial, antiprotozoal, antiviral and diuretic activities and effects on CVS, CNS and isolated tissues. The anti-inflammatory activity of boehmerol acetate was found to be highly significant. Petroleum ether and chloroform extracts of roots exhibited marked anti-inflammatory activity. The extracts from stem and leaves also showed anti-inflam-matory activity.

B. VANDA ROXBURGHII

Biological source

It is the whole plant of *Vanda roxburghii* R.Br. (syn. *V. tessellata* Hook ex. G. Don) (Fam. Orchidaceae).

It is an epiphytic orchid, 30-60 cm high, found almost all over India. The leaves are thickly coriaceous, recurved, complicate, flowers yellow with brown lines, in 6-10 flowered racemes; capsules up to 9 cm long, clavate-oblong with a short pedicel.

Chemical constituents

The plant contains tannins, resin, saponin, β- and γ-sitosterol, fatty oil, heptacosane, nonacosane and octacosanol.

The root yields tetracosyl ferulate and β-sitosterol glucoside.

Uses

Leaf paste is applied to the body to bring down fever. The leaf juice is dropped into the ear to treat otitis and other inflammation of the ear.

The roots are used in bronchitis, dyspepsia, rheumatism and fever. A medicated oil prepared by boiling the roots in mustard oil is applied externally in rheumatism and nervous troubles. The roots possess antibacterial and antitubercular properties. In Ayurveda, the root is used as a bitter, alexiteric, antipyretic, dyspepsia, bronchitis, rheumatic pains, abdomen diseases, hiccough, tremors and diseases of the nervous system.

Root extracts showed anti-inflammatory activity in rats.

RICE BRAN OIL

Biological source

It is the fixed oil obtained from rice bran (*Oryza sativa* Linn., family Poaceae), a most important bi-product of the rice milling industry. The bran comprises the germ, the pericarp and aleurone layer and is often found mixed with varying quantities of husk. The bran contains fixed oil (25%), sucrose, reducing sugars, thiamine, nicotinic acid, mineral contents calcium, phosphorus, potassium, sodium, magnesium, silica, iron, aluminium, copper, manganese, tin and chloride. The bran has a high nutritive value and is mainly used as a feed for cattle.

The oil is extracted from the bran mainly in Japan and the USA. In India, the oil is extracted in Andhra Pradesh, Maharashtra, Mysore, Uttar Pradesh and West Bengal. About 150,000 tonnes of oil is prepared in India.

The bran from shellers is best suited for the extraction of the oil. The bran from hullers contains a high proportion of husk which is difficult to remove. It can be upgraded by pneumatic separation or sieving. The bran should be extracted soon after it is milled; otherwise it deteriorates quickly. An extremely active lipase begins to act as soon as the bran is removed from rice and causes free fatty acid in the oil to increase rapidly, at the rate of 1% per hour during the first few hours of storage of the bran. The free fatty acid in the oil increased from 3% in the fresh bran to 62.5% after 100 days. Heating of the bran immediately after it is milled, at about 100° for 2 hours inactivates the lipolytic enzyme system and increase the storage life of the bran considerably. Oils with high acidity are difficult to refine and bleach to edible grades.

Preparation

The oil is obtained from the bran by expression in a hydraulic press or extraction with solvents. Hydraulic presses recover only 50% of the oil in the bran. Solven extraction is the most promising method, and hexane is the solvent commonly used. The yield of oil varies according to the source and quality of bran, the solvent used and the temperature of extraction. The average oil yield from the Indian rice bran is 12-14%.

Physical characters

The crude oil is green in colour due to the presence of chlorophyll (up to 20 p.p.m.). On standing or wintering at 20°-25°, the oil wax present in the oil (43%) settles out and can be separated by centrifuging or filtering. The oil can be completely dewaxed by mixing oil, refined by treating with 10% alkali and by bleaching with acid clay. The refining losses about 15% of the oil containing 3% free fatty acids. Prior treatment of the crude oils with additives such as sodium pyrophosphate, sodium silicate, jaggery and sugarcane molasses reduces refining losses considerably.

In an another procedure of extraction, hot alcohol extracts oil from the bran and the extract is cooled to obtain a high grade oil. The yield of refined oil is 76-79% of the oil originally present in the bran. This process is more economical than the hexane extraction process because refining loss of the oil is reduced and more by-products are recovered. The by-products include wax, fatty acids, sugar syrup rich in B-vitamins originally present in the meal and soap stock.

The refined oil is pale green in colour and possesses a good flavour. It has sp. gr. 0.91-0.92, iodine value 99-108, saponification value 181-189 and acid value 4-120. The composition of fatty acids is as : oleic (40-50%), linoleic (29-42%), linolenic (1%), stearic (1-3%), palmitic (13-18%), myristic (13-18%), arachidic, lignoceric and behenic acids. The refractive index of the oil is higher than that of most other oils having about the same iodine and saponification values; this is probably due to the unsaponifiable matter which has a high refractive index and contains squalene (202-490 mg/100 g oil). A substance similar to calciferol is also present in the oil.

Antitumor substance RBF-P, RBF-PM, RBF-X and RBF-H are isolated from rice bran. RBF-PM was a protein and RBF-X was a mixture of fatty acids and hexane-insoluble RBF-H.

Rice bran oil is a good edible oil as refined groundnut and cottonseed oils and has better keeping qualities, due to the presence of antioxidants (α- and γ-tocopherols). It is suitable for use as a salad and cooking oil, and for making soaps, oleins and stearins. The oil may be polymerized and sul-phonated for industrial uses such as textiles and leather treatment. The oil boiled for 3 hours at 200°-300° can be modified with maleic anhydride to give a varnish composition producing flexible films. Single boiled rice bran oil on treatment with oil soluble phenolic resin and with CNSL resin, yields quick-drying surface coating compositions which may be formulated into enamels.

Rice bran oil prevents cancer in the liver of rats. Tocopherol may be separated from the oil by high vacuum distillation.

RUTA GRAVEOLENS

Garden Rue, Sadab.

Biological source

It consists of a strong scented erect, glabrous herb *Ruta graveolens* Linn. (Family : Rutaceae).

It is a native of the Mediterranean region, cultivated in Indian gardens.

The plant is 30-90 cm high; leaves 2-3 pinnate, segments oblong to spathulate, strongly aromatic, flowers small, yellow, in corymbs; capsule small, lobed or rounded.

Chemical constituents

R. graveolens aerial parts contain rutin (2%), imperatorin, isoimperatorin, xanthotoxin, bergapten, psoralen; dictamnine, γ-fagarine, skimmianine, graveoline, naphthoherniarin, rutarin, rutaretin,

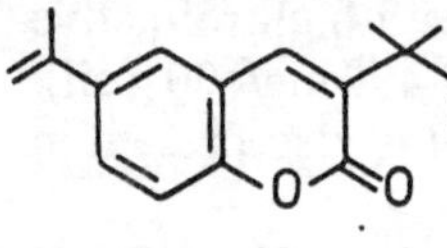

Exodehydrochalepin

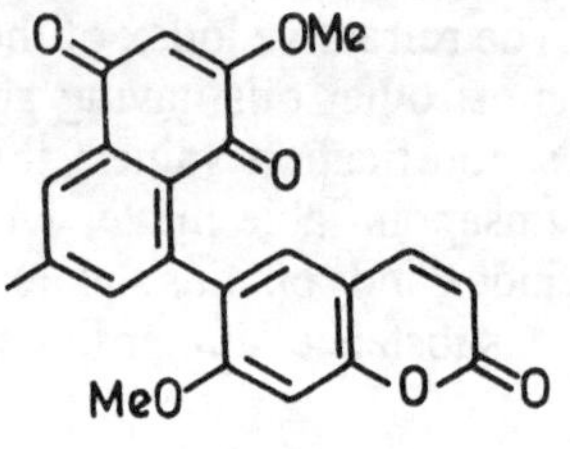

Naphthoherniarin

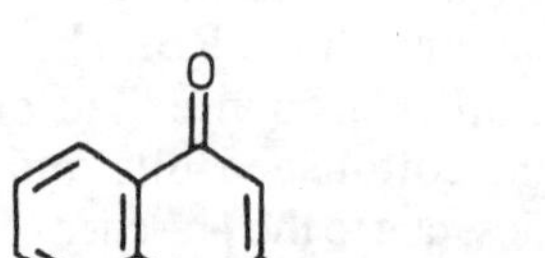

1-Methyl-2-nonyl-4-quinolone

Fig. 22.77. Chemical constituents of *Ruta graveolens.*

daphnoretin and its methyl ester, graveolinine, 2,3-dihydrokokusaginine, 2-[4-(3,4-methylenedioxy-phenyl) butyl]-4-quinolone, alkaloids ribalinium, rutalinium, N-methyl-platydesmin, kokusaginine, 1-methyl-2-*n*-nonyl-4-quinolone, rutacridone, its epoxide, gravacridonol, furacridone, 1-hydroxy-3-methoxy-N-methyl-acridone, hydroxyrutacridone epoxide, aborinine, 1-hydroxy-N-methoxy acridone, gravacridone chloride, hallacridone, dictammine, rutamine, ribalinium chloride and isopropyl dihydroxyfuro-quinoline.

The essential oil is composed of methyl nonyl ketone (80-90%), methyl heptyl ketone, α-pinene, limonene, cineole, methyl-*n*-heptyl carbinol, methyl-*n*-nonyl carbinol, ethyl valerate, methyl salicylate, methyl anthranilate, tridecan-2,4-dione, heptadecan-2,4-dione, sabinene, myrcene, caryophyllene, *trans*-α-bergamotiene, β-elemene, β-cyclocitral, β-phenylethyl butanoate, *cis*- and *trans*-cinnamyl isovalerate, 2-undecanone, 2-nonanyl acetate, 2-nonanone, 2-decanyl acetate, linalool, camphor, pregeijerene, 2-nonanol, 2-undecanol.

The seeds possess oil composed of pamitic (21%), stearic, oleic (22%) and linoleic (44%) acids; ceryl alcohol, β-sitosterol and coumarin.

The roots contain 3-(1,1-dimethylallyl) daphnetin dimethyl ether, 8-methoxy-gravelliferon, 3(1,1-dimethyl)-8-(3,3-dimethylallyl) xanthyletin, 1-(4,4-dimethyl-hexen-5-yl)-3,4-methylene dioxybenzene, suberenone, gravacridon-chloride, gravacridonol chloride, gravacridonediol, its monomethyl ether, rutacultin, rutamarin, marmesin, marmesinin, daphnorin, scopoletin, isoimperatorin, pangelin, kokusaginine, rutamine, rutamarin, isorutin, gravacridone diol, gravacridonetriol, isogravacridone, exodehydrochalepine, chalepensin gravelliferon methyl ether, 3-(1,1-dimethyl (allyl) herniarin, gravacridonediol, rutacridone, rutacridone epoxide, gravacri-donetriol, gravacridonediol and 1-hydroxy-10-methyl-acridin-9(10H)-one.

A pale yellow or greenish volatile oil, *Rue oil*, often with a fluorescence, is obtained (0.06%) on steam distillation of the fresh plant material. The oil also occurs in smaller quantities in leaves and roots and in greater amounts in seeds. Collection of flowering plant presents a problem as the pollen causes skin blisters. Rue oil has a strong odour and bitter pungent taste, and becomes brown on ageing. The oil is adulterated with turpentine and petroleum.

Uses

Rue oil is used as anthelmintic, antispasmodic, antiepileptic, rubefacient and emmenagogue, usually in veterinary medicine. In large dose, the oil acts as acronarcotic poison, causing vomiting, prostration, slow pulse, coldness of the extremities, gastroenteritis, swelling of the tongue and salivation. The oil is used as a flavouring agent and in perfumes and soap scents. Oils rich in methyl-*n*-nonyl ketone are used for the preparation of methyl-*n*-nonyl acetaldehyde, widely used as a synthetic perfume. Rutin is called as vitamin P or permeability factor. It is used to treat capillary bleeding and to increase capillary fragility.

The herb is considered resolvent, diuretic, emmenagogue, stimulant and antispasmodic. It is useful in hysteria and amenorrhoea. The juice of the herb relieves earache and toothache. The herb is useful to treat croup in poultry. In large doses it acts as a narcotic poison and abortifacient. It is applied locally to treat rheumatism of joints, feet and loins.

The spasmodic activity of the herb is attributed to the presence of coumarins in large amounts. Leaves of the herb are used as condiment and garnish, for flavouring foods and beverages. An infusion of the leaves is considered hypnotic. The leaves cause dermatitis.

Pharmacology

An alcoholic extract of the herb shows antibacterial activity against *Microcoecus pyogenes* var. *aureus* and *Escherichia coli*. Bergapten and psoralen showed marked spasmolytic effects on isolated rabbit ileum. Rutamarin and arborinine showed antispasmogenic effect on isolated smooth muscles. Rutin increased survival time of mice subjected to whole body acute lethal radiation. Daphnorctin suppressed Ehrlich ascites carcinoma growth in mice by blocking protein synthesis. Addition of rutin to tissue slices did not influence oxygen consumption. Catechol complex promoted oxygen uptake and diminished phosphate uptake by liver. Ribalinium showed ganglion-blocking and curare-like activity. Arborinine, dictamnine, γ-fagarine, skimmianine,

kokusaginine and graveolinine showed spasmolytic activity in experimental animals.

INDIAN SARPARILLA

Sariva, Anantamul, Kapuri.

Biological source

It consists of the roots of *Hemidesmus indicus* (Linn.) R.Br. (Family : Asclepiadaceae). The plant is found throughout India and Sri Lanka.

Description

The plant is a twinning undershrub with many slender wiry laticiferous branches, roots woody, aromatic, stem numerous, slender, terete, thickened at the nodes, leaves simple, opposite or whorled, linear, lanceolate to elliptic oblong, entire, shiny, dark green above, paler beneath; flowers greenish yellow or greenish-purple; follicles slender, terete, gradually narrowed divaricate; seeds oblong, flattened, black, numerous.

The roots were official in Indian Pharmacopoeia, 1966. They are cylindrical, tortuous, brownish or purple in colour, unbranched, with a short fracture

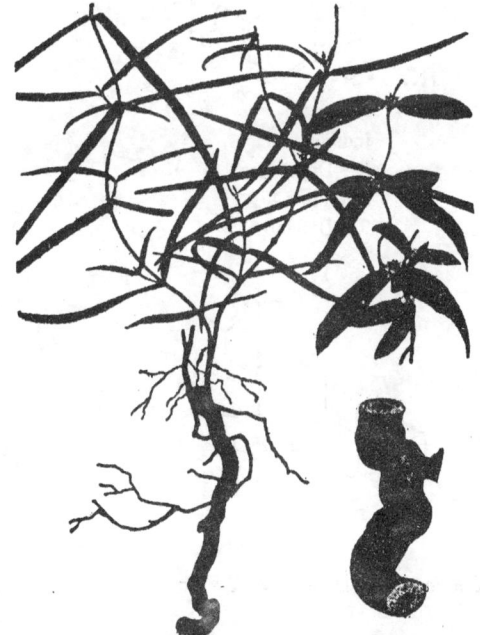

Fig. 22.78. *Hemidesmus indicus*—flowering and fruiting branches and roots.

at the periphery and fibrous at the centre, surface smooth in young roots and transversely cracked and longitudinally fissured in older roots. It should contain not more than 2% foreign organic matter, 4% ash, 15% alcohol-soluble extractive and 13.5% water-soluble extractive.

Chemical constituents

The roots contain an essential oil (0.22%) which is composed of *p*-methoxysalicylic aldehyde as a major constituent (*ca.* 80%). The root yields β-sitosterol, α- and β-amyrins, lupeol, tetracyclic triterpenes, resin acids, fatty acids, tannins, saponins, β-amyrin acetate, hexatriacontane, lupeol octaco-sanoate, coumarinolignoids hemidesminine, hemidesmins 1 and 2; hemidescine and emidine.

Uses

The drug is used as an alterative, appetizer, demulcent, diaphoretic, diuretic, blood purifier, tonic; recommended in hemicrania, nutritional disorders, syphilis, chronic rheumatism, leucoderma, asthma, bronchitis, leucorrhoea, gravel, urinary diseases and skin diseases. A syrup prepared from roots is used as a flavouring agent and in syrups.

The milky latex of the plant is used for inflamed eyes. The leaves are good for vomiting, colds, wounds and leucoderma. The stem is beneficial in disease of the brain, liver and kidney, syphilis, uterine complaints, leucoderma, paralysis, cough, asthma and as a gargle in toothache. The roots of *Ichnocarpus frutescens* R. Br. are often mixed with and substituted for Indian Sarsaparilla.

An ether extract of the roots exerts some inhibitory effect on the growth of *Escherichia coli.*

SHILAJIT

It is a bacteria-altered product of accumulated plant

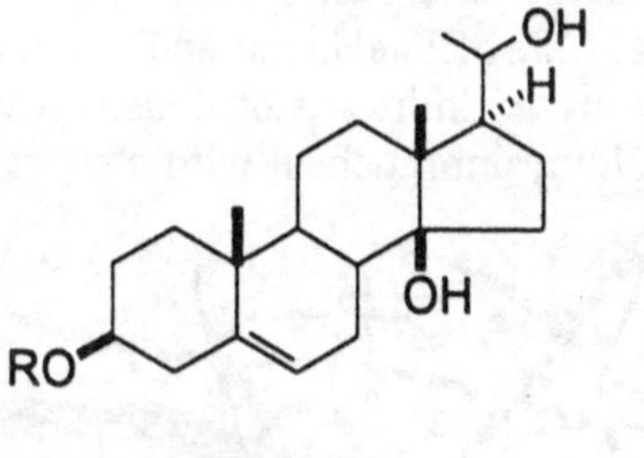

Indicine
R = Digitoxose
Hemidine
R = Boivinose

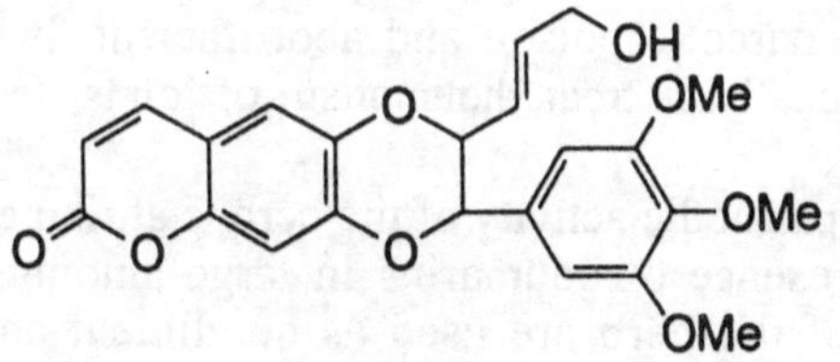

Hemidesminine

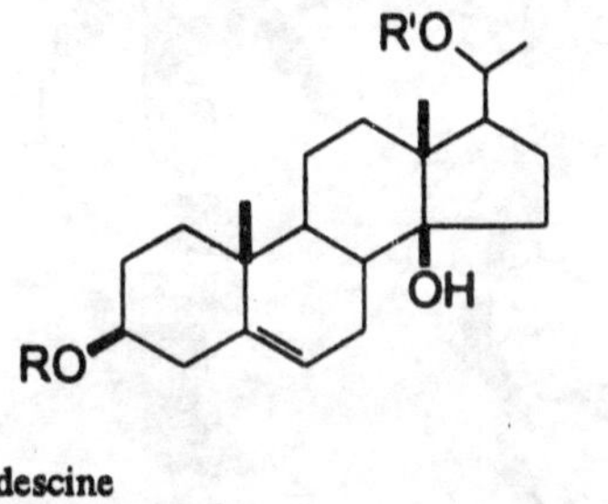

Hemidescine
R = Oleandrose(4→1)Digitoxose, R' = Ac
Emidine
R = Digitoxose(4→1)Digitoxose(4→1)Digitoxose,
R' = H

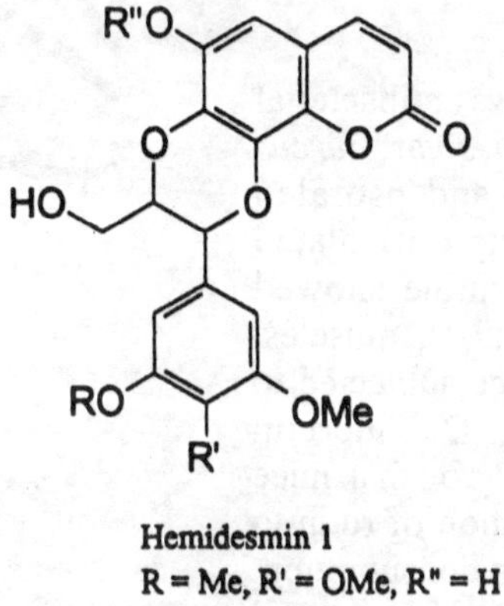

Hemidesmin 1
R = Me, R' = OMe, R" = H
Hemidesmin 2
R,R' = H, R" = Me

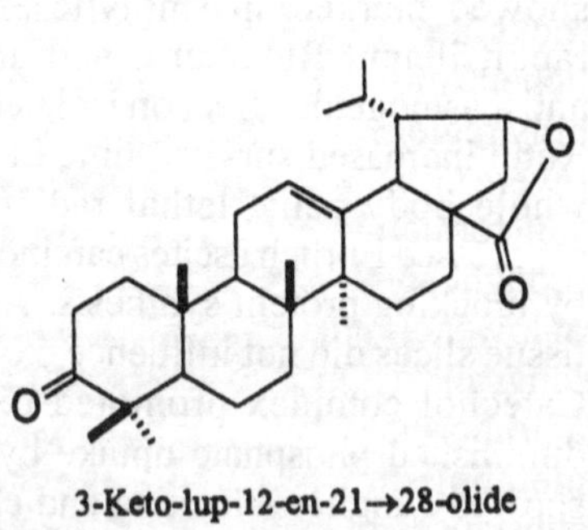

3-Keto-lup-12-en-21→28-olide

Fig. 22.79. Chemical constituents of *Hemidesmus indicus.*

material. Possibly it develops at most of the coniferous forests of northern India, Nepal, Norway, Afghanistan, Australia, Bhutan, China, Egypt, Mongolia, Russia and Pakistan. It comes out as seepages only under favourable conditions of rock and topography. In a hard and fractured or well-jointed but non-porous rock like biotite granite, it starts moving downward along fracture/joint planes due to gravity and comes out at the surface as a seepage on encountering some opening natural cutting. Sometimes the Shilajit fluid is either completely absorbed by the underlying rock or is trapped down in porous sedimentary rocks or unfractured and inconspicuously jointed non-porous sedimentary and igneous rocks. Then it is localized at or near the site of its origin thus disallowing any Shilajit seepage to occur. It is fact that Shilajit seepage mostly occur below or adjacent to the coniferous forests of Gilgil and other Himalayan regions. Apparently, there is a close link of Shilajit with these forests.

The slow moving thick acidic Shilajit fluid, along with the still undigested plant material in the form of the fibrous woody pallets and with its group of bacteria, apparently attacks the biotite and orthoclase felspar of the biotite granite and partly dissolved and carries the same on its way downwards and laterally.

The weight of a natural Shilajit body may vary from a few kilograms to 1,000 kilograms and even more. After a Shilajit body is completely removed or taken away from the site, it takes 5-7 years for the redevelopment of a workable amount there.

Current status

Humification and the concomitant weathering of rocks are caused by lithophilic vegetation, *e.g.*, lichen, mosses, algae and microorganisms in the hilly regions and in other sedimentary rocks. Under severe climatic conditions of the Antarctic, primary soil formation (humification) and wea-thering are brought about by the interactions of various groups of lower organisms, *e.g.*, blue green and green algae, fungi and actinomycetes. Humification is, therefore, a primordial biological process. The formation and metabolism of Shilajit, as also of other humic substances of origin, are currently understood as a complex series of biochemical and geochemical

reactions. The latter sequence takes place beneath the soil surface, under graded temperature and pressure. By the geochemical sequence, the organic molecules of humus are gradually transformed into petroleum intermediates and then final products. Buried Shilajit, unlike that occurs as a film on the rock outer surface, is subjected to geochemical changes resulting in diagenesis and kerogen formation.

Physical characters

Shilajit occurs in dark coloured crystalline rocks of igneous/metamorphic origin which are generally well jointed and fractured. The odour of Shilajit is that of urine of cow or simply urinous or like decaying pine wood or typical odour. It is completely soluble in water giving brown or brownish black solution. It has sandy stuff (particles of quartz, felspar and biotite), woody balls or pallets of the size 3-7 mm. Shilajit has low melting point, starts flowing at room temperature in summer days. It could ooze out through fissures and cracks of the hard igneous rocks.

The woody pallets associated with Shilajit constitute up to 80% of the raw material. The pallets burn with a flame leaving behind a black charcoal-like stuff.

Chemical constituents

Shilajit contains a number of organic compounds like sterols, triterpenes, ellagic acid, benzoic acid, phosphatidylinositol, *m*-hydroxybenzoic acid, glycine, betaine, C16–C20 fatty acids, lipids, phospholipids, benzocoumarins and 18 free amino acids. An analysis of the latex of *Euphorbia roylena* collected in summer month from the plant growing in the vicinity of Shilajit exuding rocks of the Himalayas showed the presence of identical organic compounds suggesting that the chemical constituents of Shilajit are primarily derived from the latex of *E. royleana*. Generally Shilajit contains water (15%), organic matter (55%) and minerals (30%). The organic matter is composed of gum, albuminoids, benzoic acid, hippuric acid, fatty acids, resin, wax and vegetable matter. The minerals are present as lime in the form of calcium oxide, sodium chloride, phosphorus pentaoxide, stentium oxide (tin oxide) and copper oxide.

The petroleum ether extract of Shilajit contains euphol, taraxerol, β-sitosterol, some partially identified triterpenes and sterols.

The chloroform extract of Shilajit is a mixture of benzoic acid, *m*-hydroxybenzoic acid, 3,4-benzocoumarins, *e.g.*, 7-hydroxy-3,4-benzocoumarin, its methyl ether and 2,7-dihydroxy-3,4-benzocoumarin.

The methanol extract of Shilajit yielded ellagic acid. The major amino acids of Shilajit were glycine, aspartic acid, methionine, asparagine, glutamic acid, tyrosine and phenylalanine.

Trace elements present in water-soluble fraction of Shilajit are Fe (0.6-8%), Ca (1-7%), Al (2-5%), Mg, Zn, Cu, Mn, Mo, phosphate and no Au or Ag. The pH range of these samples was quite broad (3.8-8.2).

Uses

Shilajit possesses appetite, diuretic, laxative, general tonic and tranquilizer properties. It improves digestion and general health, soothes nerves, increases mental and physical stamina, checks gaseous problems markedly and useful for sexual debility mainly through strengthening the muscles. It checks night emissions and thickens the semen. It relieves the painful joints and the frozen foot ends due to cold in winter of the ageing people. It reverses some ageing processes of the mind and body which results in the change of approach to handle the things.

The dark coloured Shilajit is more effective than the coffee brown or red variety. It must always be taken with a cup of milk 10-15 minutes after a light dinner. It is advisable to take one or more orange if suited during Shilajit intake.

The side effects of Shilajit are drowsiness or tranquillizing effect soon after the intake of the drug. Prolonged use of Shilajit causes undesirable effects. It should not be used beyond one month period.

An aqueous solution of Shilajit is used to treat asthma, chronic bronchitis, dropsy, genito-urinary infections, hypertension and nervous disorders.

THYME

Common Thyme, Garden Thyme.

Biological source

It consists of the dried leaves and floral tops of *Thymus vulgaris* Linn (Family : Lamiaceae). It should contain not more than 3% of stems over 1 mm in diameter and 2% of other foreign organic matter.

It is cultivated extensively in Germany, France, England and Greece; introduced in the Nilgiris and in the western temperate Himalayas from Kashmir to Kumaon between 1500-4000 m.

Description

It is a low, perennial undershrub, 20-80 cm height; leaves oblong-lanceolate, with orange-brown, glandular dots; coriaceous, flowers small, purple or blue or white, in pubescent verticillasters; nutlets brown.

The plant grows best in the hills. The seeds are sown in rows, about 90 cm apart and the seedlings may thinned out to 30-45 cm apart. Mulching in the winter prevents damage by frost. The crop requires inter-culturing and weeding. The leaves and flowers are ready for harvesting in about 5 months after sowing. They are plucked, dried in shade and stored in air-tight containers to prevent the loss of flavour. The yield of the dry herb is 1100-2200 per hectare in India; the yield of the volatile oil is 22 kg per hectare.

Chemical constituents

Thyme contains triterpenoid saponins, flavones, ursolic acid, caffeic acid, tannins, biphenyls, resin and a volatile oil (oil of Thyme) (0.7-2.6%). The oil is a colourless, yellow or red liquid, with a distinct, pleasant odour, and a pungent, persistent taste. It is composed of thymol (42-59%), amyl alcohol. β,γ-hexanol, β-pinene, camphene, *p*-cymene, γ-terpinene, linalool, l-borneol, geraniol, caryophyllene, 4-terpineol, *trans*-4-thujanol and a sesquiterpenic alcohol. Thymol occasionally separates as crystals from the oil.

The seeds yield a drying oil (37%) which is composed of linolenic, linoleic, oleic acids and α-hydroxylinolenic acid.

Uses

Thyme possesses aggreeable odour and an aromatic and warming taste. Due to the presence of thymol,

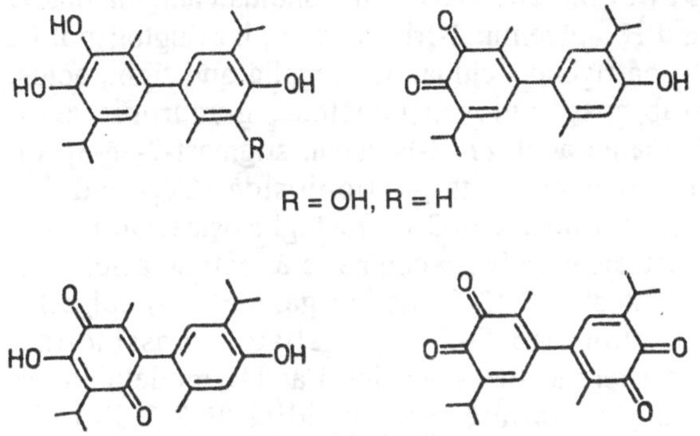

R = OH, R = H

Biphenyl derivatives

Fig. 22.80. Chemical constituents of *Thymus vulgaris*.

it shows germicidal properties and is effective against pathogenic bacteria. The leaves and flowers are used for flavouring and seasoning various foods, like preparations of meat and fish, and for garnishing. The dried Thyme is spread in clothes to repel insects. The leaves and flowers are used as incense.

The herb has a pungent taste. It possesses antiseptic, anthelmintic, expectorant, carminative, diuretic, emmenagogue and sedative properties due to the presence of a volatile oil. A liniment prepared from the shoot is applied in rheumatism and skin troubles. A decoction of the herb is useful in whooping cough.

The oil has antiseptic, antispasmodic and carminative properties. It is used as gargles and mouthwashes, to treat bronchitis and whooping cough. The oil acts as a mental stimulant and is given as a diffusable stimulant in collapse. Externally, it is used in conjugation with olive oil as a rubefacient and counterirritant. The oil is used in soap-perfumes and for flavouring the food products, such as meat, sausages, sauces and canned food. The oil is adulterated with terpenes or with 'Thymene' which is a biproduct in the manufacture of thymol from ajowain oil.

Thymol possess powerful germicidal, anti-fungal, antiseptic and anthelmintic properties. It is used as an intestinal antiseptic in treating hook-worms. It is applied for fungal infections of the skin. It has preservative properties, and is an ingredient of deodorants, mouthwashes, dentifrices and gargles. It acts as a poison in large doses and

produces a burning sensation in the stomach, nausea, vomiting, diarrhoea, tinnitus, headache, giddiness, collapse and death from respiratory failure. It may cause abortion in women and may colour urine green.

TEA

Chai, Chaha.

Biological source

It consists of the processed leaves of *Camellia sinensis* (Linn.) Kuntze (Family : Theaceae).

It is a variable evergreen shrub or a small tree, found in Assam and other hilly regions. It is cultivated in hilly areas for its leaves which furnish the tea of commerce.

The typical 'China' bush is named as *C. sinensis* var. *sinensis*, syn. *Thea sinensis* Linn.; *C. thea* Link and the 'Assam' type as *C. sinensis* var. *assamica* (Mast.) Kitamura, syn. *C. thiefera* Griff.

China Tea, is a hardy, multi-stemmed, slow-growing shrub or a small tree, 1-6 m in height. Young branches are stout, hirsute to glabrous. Leaves 4-10 cm long, erect, shortly stalked, elliptic, generally narrower with obtuse apex, base cuneate, bluntly serrulate to sinuate-serrulate, the teeth incurved and black tipped, leathery, dark glossy green above and light green and appressed villose below; flowers pedicellate, usually 1-2 in the axils of leaves of young shoots, sometimes more than 2; capsules tri- or bi-coccate, coccus one or two-seeded; seeds suborbicular or hemispherical 10-14 mm long, dull brown to reddish brown, smooth.

It flowers freely and seeds in the second year. The variety has an economic life of about 100 years; however, pruning and continued plucking reduces the life span. It is able to withstand severe winters and hot droughts of northern India. It yields less than the Assam types. It is grown at an altitude above 1,050 m in areas where there is growth pause in winter, as at Darjeeling, or a seasonal slowing down of growth as in Sri Lanka. It is highly valued for flavour.

Assam Tea is a quick-growing tender plant of more southern distribution, and is apparently indigenous to Assam, Myanmar, Thailand, Vietnam and South China. It grows into a single-stemmed tree about 17 m in height if allowed to grow unimpeded, and has an economic life of *ca* 40 years and differs from var. *sinensis* in having larger (15-20 cm long), usually thinner drooping leaves more or less acuminate at the apex. Lamina narrowly elliptic, ellipticoblong to elliptic obovate, usually spreading, thinly coriaceous, supple, light green, glossy, puberulous, chiefly along the midrib below, denticulate to undulately serrate or serrulate. In flowers and fruits the variety resembles var. *sinensis*. The teas made from China plants have a definite character and flavour, but lack strength and quality which are marked in Assam teas when grown in certain areas. Assam plants are used in North-East India, South India, Sri Lanka, Indonesia, Africa and South America.

Chemical constituents

The leaves contain proanthrocyanidin gallate, epigallocatechin (4β→8)-3-O-galloylepicatechin, diphenylamine, procyanidins B-2, B-4 and C-1, vitexin, apigenin-6,8-di-C-glucoside, kaempferol-3- and quercetin-3-rhamnodiglucoside, epitheaflagallin, epitheaflagallin-3-O-gallate, theaflagallin,

growth inhibitor ABA, flavonoids camellianins A and B, apigenin; 1-triacontanol, barringtogenol C, A_1-barrigenol, cinnamic, angelic and tiglic acids, arabinose, xylose, galactose, glucuronic acid, linolenic acid, *cis*-3-hexenal, stigmast-7-en-3β-ol, α-spinasterol, its gentiobioside, C_{30}- and C_{32} alcohols, quercetin-3-O-fructoglucoside, naringenin fructoside; gallic, *p*-coumaric & caffeic acids, (–)-epicatechin-3-(3-O-methyl gallate), (–)-epigallo-catechin-3-(3-O-methyl gallate), brassinolide, castasterone, theasinensins A and B, prodelphinidin B-2,3'-O-gallate, procyanidins B-2-3,3'-di-O-gallate, B-2 3'-O-gallate, B-4 3'-gallate; (–)-epigallocatechin 3-O-*p*-coumaroate, (–)-epigallo-catechin-3,3'-di-O-gallate, (–)-epigallocatechin, (–)-epicatechin-3-O-gallate, (–)-epigallocatechin-3-O-gallate, (+)-catechin, typhasterol, teasterone, 2-O-β-L-arabinosyl-myoinositol, polysaccharide TSA, benzyl-β-D-glucoside, camelliasides A, B, and C, schaftoside, isoschaftoside, orientin, isoorientin, isovitexin and vicenin 2. The essential oil contains linalool epoxide and theaspirone.

Uses

Tea is today the most widely used and popular nonalcoholic beverage. About half the world's population drinks tea regularly. Even in coffee consuming countries, an appreciable quantity of tea is consumed as it is one of the least expensive beverages.

When an infusion is made with hot water, the alkaloid and the volatile oil readily dissolve out and the resulting beverage has a characteristic taste and aroma. If the leaves are steeped for a longer period, the tannin dissolves and the liquid becomes bitter and loses its beneficial qualities. Drinkers of black tea have acquired a liking for the taste of the brew and for the briskness, strength and body imparted to the liquor by the condensed polyphenols. The world tea trade consists almost entirely of black tea, and green tea is required only in certain markets like North Africa.

Tea is a stimulating drink; it relieves muscular and mental fatigue and is taken for fever. The stimulating action is attributed to the purine base alkaloid, caffeine. An average consumption of 5-6 cups per day represents a caffeine intake of about 0.3 g, which is less than half the daily 'tolerable limit'

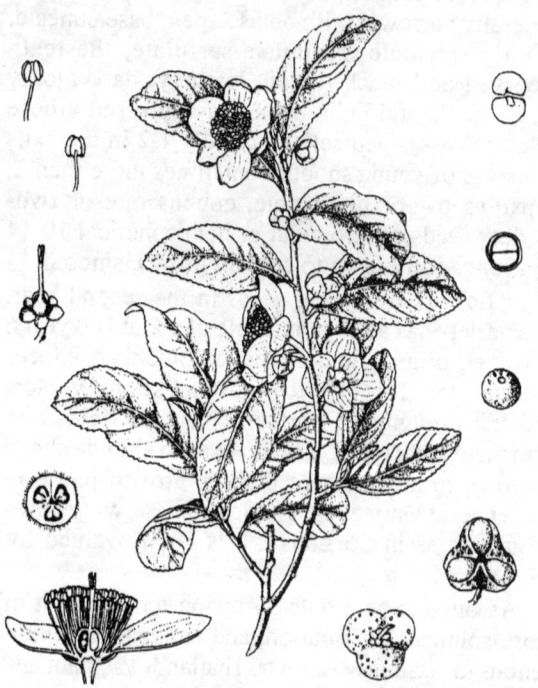

Fig. 22.81. *Camellia sinensis.*

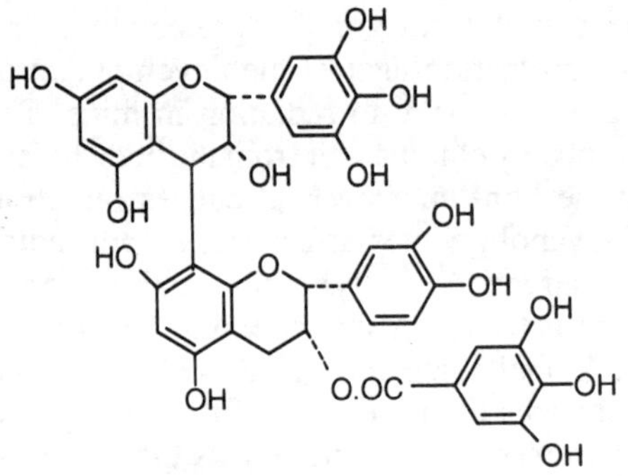

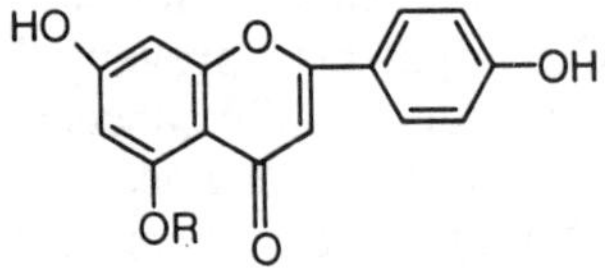

Camellianin A
R = Glu(6″-Ac)
(4→1) Rha
Camellianin B
R = Glu(4→1)Rha

Theaflagallin
R = OH, R′ = H
Epitheaflagallin
R = H, R′ = OH
Epitheaflagallin-3-O-gallate
R = H, R′ = O-Galloyl

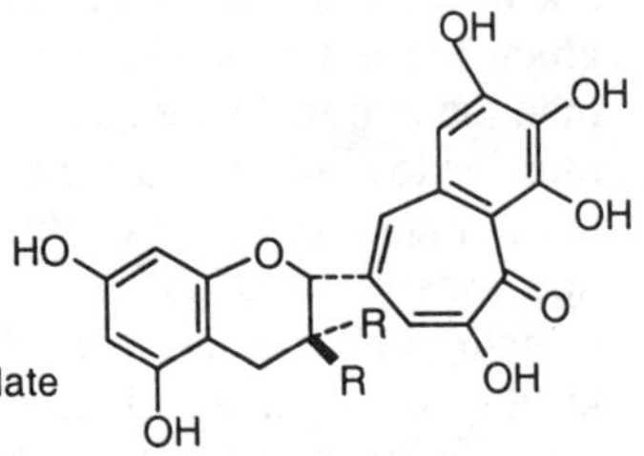

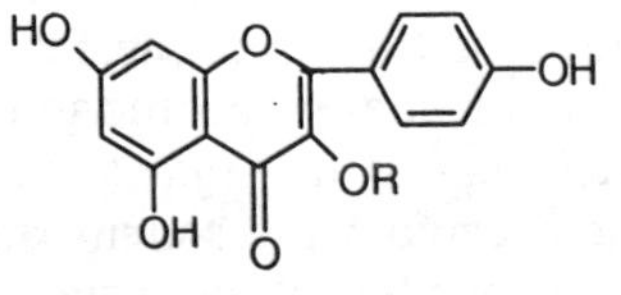

Camelliaside A
R = Glu[(2→1)
Gal](6→1)Rha
Camelliaside B
R = Glu[(2→1)Xyl]
(6→1)Rha
Camelliaside C
R = Glu(2→1)Gal

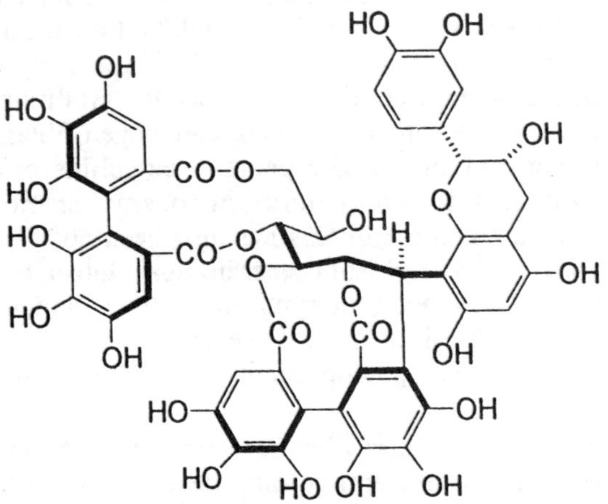

Camelliatannin A

Fig. 22.82. Chemical constituents of *Camellia sinensis*.

of 0.65 g for the medical administration of pure caffeine. The stimulation effect of tea does not have subsequent depression or hangover. Caffeine has a diuretic effect on the kidneys and stimulates gastric secretion. Hence, tea is thought to aid digestion and relieve post-prandial distress. Excessive doses of caffeine, however, can lead to anxiety and unpleasant gastric sensation. Tea may be of value in treatment of gout and restoration of fluid balance following vomiting and diarrhoea.

Pharmacology

Plant decoction showed prolonged hypertensive effect in rabbits. (–)-Gallocatechin galate reduced blood pressure in rabbits. Chinese green tea extract inhibited induced peroxidation in rat liver microsomes and mutagenicity of benzo [a] pyrene and aflatoxin B_1 and suppressed benzo [a] pyrene hydroxylase activity. The green tea polyphenol inhibited *Streptococcus mutans*. Green tea infu-sion markedly inhibited NDEA-induced tumorigenesis. It decreased lung tumor incidence and stomach tumor multiplicity. Oral administration of decaffei-nated green and black tea extracts inhibited induced lung tumorigenesis in mice by 65% due to the presence of polyphenol, (–)-epi-gallocatechin gallate. Tea flavanols reduced incidence of ischemia reperfusion arrhythmias in rat heart by about 70%.

Diphenylamine reduced blood sugar in rabbits. Catechins, gallates and all theaflavin inhibited growth of both spores and vegetable cells of *Clostridium botulinum*. Crude polyphenolic fraction of tea inhibited attachment of *Streptococcus mutans* strain formation of water-soluble glucan from sucrose by bacterial glucosyl-transferase and dental caries. (–)-Epicatechin gallate and (–)-epi-gallocatechin gallate showed marked inhibition of glucosyltransferase activity.

The diuretic property of tea is useful in therapy of cardiac oedema. It seems to reduce serum lipid, induce synthesis and secretion of catecholamines and to prevent artherosclerosis. Tea polyphenols may inhibit the absorption of dietary cholesterol and prevent the degradation of catecholamines. Successive administration of tea could stimulate the degeneration of triglycerides in the adipose tissue, thereby reducing the weight. Dimeric compounds particularly thea-flavins produced oxidatively, in the manufacture of black tea, inhibit angiotension I converting enzyme. Tea flavonoids possess anticoagulant activity and inhibit platelet aggregation in rabbits. Tea may be used in relieving bronchial asthma and difficulty in breathing due to the smooth muscle relaxant effect of caffeine. Caffeine at 40 or 80 mg per kg per day administered to male rats does not produce adverse reproductive effects. A spray prepared from tannins of tea cures allergies caused due to some mites in air.

Tea polyphenols strengthen the walls of blood vessels and regulate their permeability, an activity associated with o-dihydroxybenzene group collectively termed vitamin P or biflavonoids. Tea infusion shows anti-inflammatory activity. The constituents responsible for the anti-inflammatory and capillary strengthening properties of tea are the flavanols, (–)-epicatechin and (–)-epicatechin gallate. The efficacy of tea extracts decreases as the oxidised polyphenol content increases at the expense of flavanols and hence the Indian black teas fail to produce an effect comparable to unprocessed tea leaf or green tea.

Tea polyphenols protect ascorbic acid from oxidation in rat tissue homogenates because of their antioxidant properties. Tea extracts increase the accumulation of ascorbic acid in rat and guinea-pig tissues and reduce the level of ascorbic acid through urinary excretion. It indicates an important role of green tea in human nutrition in preventing symptoms of ascorbic acid deficiency. Black tea does not promote the accumulation of ascorbic acid as strongly as unprocessed or green tea, presumably because it has lower content of unoxidised flavanols.

Green tea polyphenols have been found to normalise thyroid hyperfunction which induces thyrotoxicosis; this has been attributed to flavanols, especially gallocatechins. Flavonol glycosides exhibit a similar action. Tea was used extensively in combating plaque in Japan. Polyphenols aid the synthesis of folic acid in rats by the intestinal microflora. Green tea infusion shows anti-bacterial activity against a number of bacteria and is an effective cure against dysentery. Without milk and sugar the tea liquor is beneficial in diarrhoea but with milk and sugar it acts as a laxative. Tea infusion shows antiviral activity on several species of enteroviruses in cell culture.

Green tea inhibits the growth of cancer tumours. Tea affords protection against the development of leukemia after exposure to radiation in mice. Tea flavanols probably eliminate Sr from the body before it reaches the bone marrow and causes radiation damage. Flavanol gallates afford significant radioprotection. Green tea polyphenols exhibit antitumourgenic activity on induced skin cancers by teleocidin. Epigallocatechin gallate (EGCG) from green tea changes the properties of the receptor on the surface of mouse cells and blocks the action of tumour promoter and thus prevents the formation of tumour cells. EGCG might also prevent the growth of tumours in human especially cancers of oesophagus, stomach and intestines. The death rate from cancer of all sites and stomach cancer in the midwest areas of Shizuoka prefecture (Japan) where green tea is the staple beverage was much lower than the national average, in both sexes. Low death rate due to stomach cancer was observed in habitual tea drinkers and high death rate in people who do not consume tea. Green tea extracts inhibit the growth of mouse sarcoma 180 at a dose of 400 mg/kg/day on oral administration. The green tea polyphenols play a role in the prevention of cancer formation probably by (i) inhibition of ultimate carcinogen formation, (ii) modulation of the metabolism of the initiating agent, (iii) direct interaction of the electrophillic ultimate carcinogenic metabolite, (iv) scavenging and free radicals, (v) inhibition of ornithine decarboxylase activity and (vi) inhibition of covalent bonding of carcinogen to DNA. Black tea is not likely to inhibit tumours as it contains only tiny amounts of EGCG. Consumption of 5 g of tea every day can reduce the synthesis of nitrosamine, which is a major carcinogen. Vitamin C and polyphenols, especially catechins block synthesis of endogenous nitrosamines. High selenium content in teas has also been correlated with low incidence of cancer in Japan. Green tea is best in preventing the synthesis of the carcinogen, followed by black and jasmine teas. Oolong tea also reduced the lung neoplasia induced by urethane in animals.

Green tea extract has been reported to be more effective in preventing tooth decay than fluoride compounds. An extract of Japanese green tea inhibited the growth of *Streptococcus mutans*

Clarke, the cariogenic bacterium responsible for causing dental caries. The main anti-bacterial substances are the polyphenolic compounds, especially (+)-gallocatechin, (–)-epigallocatechin and (–)-epigallocatechin gallate. Gallocatechin was the most active component and its minimum inhibitory concentration against the bacterium was 250 µg/ml. The green tea extract strongly inhibits the formation of dextran and levan from sucrose by the cariogenic bacteria. This also supports the role of polyphenols in inhibiting the growth of *S. mutans* and preventing the cause of caries.

Tea is considered a cure for cold and removes phlegm. It prevents the formation of stones in bladder, liver and kidney. Tea can be used as a base for the extraction of catechin, the preparations of which are useful in treating nephritis and chronic hepatitis. The bitter leaf juice is taken for abortion. Dried leaves are chewed to remove foul smell. The leaf juice is also applied to cuts and injuries as haemostatic. Tea has also been successfully used in treating severe abdominal, intestinal and cerebral haemorrhages. Green tea tannin or its active constituents may be used in treating toxic goitre. Tea can be used effectively as a vehicle for lysine fortification.

The extract of Japanese green tea shows anti-hepatotoxic effects. Tea has been found to aid liver, lessen tissue waste, promote celebration, aid mental and physical work, preserve mental equilibrium, induce tranquility and promote slender-ness.

Tea inhibits absorption of iron and leads to iron deficiency. Polyphenolic compounds in tea which form strong complexes with iron are believed to be partly responsible. Tannase, a polyphenol degrading enzyme, and lemon juice solubilize iron and also calcium in some teas might reduce the detrimental effect of tea on mineral availability.

BOSWELLIA (Salai guggal)

Kundur, Luabn, Indian frankinecense tree.

Biological source

It is the oleo-gum-resin of *Boswellia serrata* Roxb. ex Colebr (syn. *B. glabra* Roxb.), (Family : Burseraceae).

It is a medium to large-sized, deciduous,

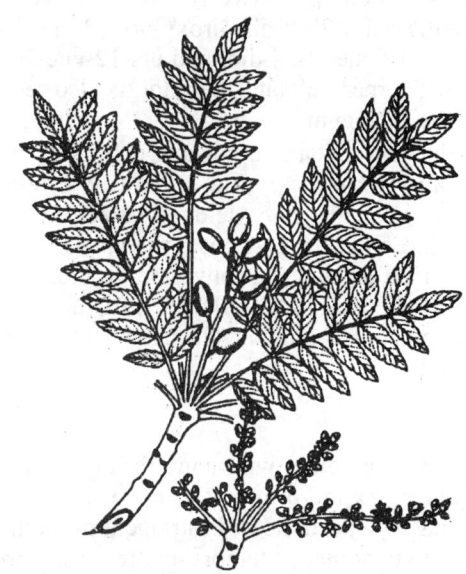

Fig. 22.83. *Boswellia serrata*—flowering and fruiting portions.

balsamiferous tree, up to 18 m in height. It is found in the dry forests from Punjab to West Bengal and in central and southern India. The tree on injury exudes an oleo-gum-resin known as Indian olibanum, Indian frankincense or *Salai guggul*. The resin is transparent and golden-yellow and solidifies to brownish yellow tears. It burns readily with an agreeable odour and is used as incense.

Chemical constituents

The oleo-gum-resin is composed of water (10%), volatile oil (10-16%), colophony (50%), gum (30%) and insoluble matter. The volatile oil contains α-thujene (50%), α- and β-pinenes, *d*-limonene, *p*-cymene, linalool, terpinolene, α-terpineol, terpinyl acetate, methyl chavicol, bornyl acetate, α-phelandrene, methyl chavicol, cadinene, geraniol and elemol. The acidic components present in the oil are phenols, α-campholenic acid, α-campholytic acid and acetic acid. Campholytic acid resembles turpentine oil. The non-volatile fraction is composed of triterpenes, *viz.*, α-anyrin, β-amyrin, methyl-chavicol, 3α-acetoxy-tirucall-8.24-dien-21-oic acid, 3-α- and 3-β-hydroxytirucall-8,24-dien-21-oic acids, β-boswellic acid, acetyl-β-boswellic acid, acetyl-11-keto-β-boswellic acid, 11-keto-β-boswellic acid, 2′-3′-dihydroxy-urs-12-ene-24-oic acid, urs-12-ene-3′-24-diol and urs-12-ene-3α, 24-diol. A diterpene alcohol, serratol, is also reported from the salai gum.

Salai gum contains uronic acid anhydride, uronic acid and oxidizing and diastatic enzymes. Hydrolysis of the gum yields D-galactose (46%), D-arabinose (12%), D-xylose, rhamnose, glucose, D-mannose, uronic acid anhydride, fructose, idose, glucuronic acid and galacturonic acid. 4-O-Methylglucurono-arabinogalactan is also present in the resin.

Uses

The gum is credited with antiarthritic, astringent, stimulant, expectorant, diaphoretic, diuretic, emmenagogue, ecbolic and astringent properties. It is used to treat ulcers, tumors, goitre, cystic breast, diarrhoea, dysentery, piles and skin diseases. An ointment of the gum is applied to sores and syphilis. Non-phenolic fraction of the oleogum-resin possesses antitumour, sedative and analgesic activities.

Pharmacology

The gum possesses excellent adhesive properties. The non-phenolic fraction of the drug possessed anti-tumour, sedative and analgesic activity and showed a marked hypotensive effect. Acid fraction significantly inhibited the migration of leucocytes into pleural cavity. It displayed no action on haemolysing activity, local irritations or cytotoxic effect. The fraction inhibited the arthritis evaluated level of connective tissue metabolites in urinary excretion hydroxyproline hexosamine and urimic acid. The acid fraction did not change in architecture of different tissue cells indicating the safety of the fraction in very high doses on prolong treatment.

The essential oil from the olibanum showed antibacterial activity. The defatted extract of the gum exudate exhibited marked anti-inflammatory and anti-arthritic activity and cholesterol and triglyceride lowering activity.

Pharmaceutical Aids and Technical Products

A number of natural products find use in various fields in addition to medicine and pharmacy. These products are called as technical products which are used in beverages, condiments, coating flavouring agents, spices, paints, varnishes, confectionaries, textiles and cosmetics.

Pharmaceutical aids

For the production of drugs various techniques such as purification, filtration, adsorption, solubilization, absorption, suspension and emulsification are employed. A number of natural products are used in these techniques. Flavouring, colouring, coating and perfuming agents are used in drug industries. These agents possess little or no therapeutic value, but they are used in the preparation of many pharmaceutical products. These agents are called as pharmaceutical aids which may be of plant, animal, mineral or synthetic origin.

In pharmaceutical industry Starch and Guar gum are used as a disintegrating agent. Sodium alginate acts as stabilizing, thickening, emulsifying, deflocculating, gelling and filming agent. Glucose and sucrose are sweetening and coating products. Agar is used as emulsifying agent and for cultural media. Acacia and Tragacanth are credited as binding, suspending and emulsifying agents. Mucilages like Ispaghol and Linseed act as demulcent and soothing agents.Quillaia contains saponins and is used in coal tar emulsion. Most of the volatile oils are flavouring products. Fixed oils like Olive, Sesame, Cottonseed, Almond and Castor oils act as emollients and vehicles for drugs. Beeswax, Spermaceti, Wool fat, Lanolin and Lard are the ointment bases. Chlorophyll, Cochineal and Saffron are the natural dyes used as colouring agents. Gelatin is a suspending agent and used for making capsules. Pyrethrum, Derris, Lonchocarpus, Cevadilla seed and Ryania are the natural insecticides. Absorbent Cotton, Jute, Hemp, Flax, Wool, Silk, Viscose and Alginate are used to prepare fibres for filtering and surgical dressings. Shellac is used for coating confections and medicinal tablets. Kaolin is employed externally as dusting powder, filtering and cleaning agent.

Technical products

In perfumery the natural substances Lavender, Sandalwood, Citronella, Balsam of Peru, Balsam of Tolu and Storax are used as technical products. Soaps are prepared from fatty acids of Castor oil, Cottonseed oil and Peanut oil. Myrrh and Quillaia are used in incense and shampoos, respectively. Wool fat, Spermaceti and White wax are the ingredients of creams. Coconut oil, Castor oil and Henna find use in hair dressings. Benzoin is added in lotions.

In food industry Acacia, Agar, Alginates, Starches and Sterculia gum are used in confection and bakery products. Citrus fruits and Ginger are added in soft drinks (beverages). The vegetable oils used as food are Coconut, Sesame, Cottonseed, Peanut and Mustard. The fruits and other parts of Capsicum, Nutmeg, Cardamom, Clove, Coriander,

Caraway and Dill are used as spices and condiments.

In Tobacco industry Glycyrrhiza and Vanilla are used in cigarettes, cigars, snuffs and other products. Hops, Yeast and Malt find use in the manufacture of bear. From Linseed oil, Castor oil, Copaiba and Colophony, paints and varnishes are manufactured. Black Catechu is applied on chewing betel leaf. In textile industry Acacia, Agar, Alginates, Catechu, Cotton, Gambir, Rosin, Starch and Sterculia gum are employed.

SPERMACETI

Synonyms

Cetaceum; Spermwax.

Biological source

Spermaceti is a solid waxy substance obtained from the oil derived from the head and blubber of the sperm whale, *Physeter macrocephalus* (Fam.: Physeteridae).

Geographical distribution

The whales are found in the Pacific, Indian and Atlantic oceans. They attend a length of 20 meters and up to 6-9 meters in circumference.

Collection and preparation

The whales are killed with torpedo harpoons upon striking the animal. In front of the cranium there is a large cavity which contains an oily fluid. The cranial cavity is opened and the oily liquid removed with buckets or by pumping. A single whale yields 10-12 barrels of oil. On cooling about 11% Spermaceti separates out. The crude material is pressed, melted, strained, and treated with boiling aqueous caustic soda to remove free acids in the form of soap. The purified Spermaceti is cooled to form cakes.

Characters

Spermaceti is white, somewhat transparent slightly unctuous masses with crystalline fracture and pearly luster. It is almost odourless and tasteless but becomes yellow and rancid on long exposure to air; density 0.93-0.94; m.p. 42-50°; viscosity 1.433, saponification number 120-136, iodine number 3-4.4. It is insoluble in water and cold alcohol; soluble in chloroform, ether, carbon disulphide, oils and boiling alcohol; slightly soluble in petroleum ether.

Chemical constituents

Spermaceti consists of chiefly cetyl palmitate ($C_{15}H_{31}OCOC_{16}H_{33}$), cetyl myristate ($C_{15}H_{31}OCOC_{13}H_{27}$), cetyl laurate, acetyl laurate and cetyl stearate; the total ester constituents are about 85%. Free cetyl alcohol is present in appreciable amounts. The esters of higher alcohols are also present. On saponification of esters with alcoholic potassium hydroxide, cetyl alcohol, ($C_{16}H_{33}OH$), m.p. 49.5°, is formed.

Uses

Spermaceti is used as a pharmaceutical aid for cold creams and as a base for ointments, cerates and an emulsion with egg yolk or expressed almond oil. It is also used in manufacture of candles, soaps, cosmetics, laundry wax; finishing and lustering linens. It possesses emollient properties.

KAOLINS

Synonyms

Bolus alba; China clay; Porcelain clay; White bole; Argilla.

Kaolins or China clays (white or high-cream burning) are derived from pegmatites or from hydrothermal alterations along fractures. They may also occur as blanket deposits in extensive areas of igneous of metamorphic rocks, bedded deposits derived from feelspathic, sandstones or as pockets in limestones.

Distribution

Kaolins are found in the Garo hills of Assam, banks of Dora river in Lakhimpur district, Makkiari near Raniganj, Birbhum district, Rajmahal hills in Bhagalpur (Bihar); Begaum, Ratnagiri, Kanera, Thana districts of Maharashtra and in some parts of M.P., Delhi, Madras, Kerala and other states.

Chemical constituents

Clays are made up of mineral grains, some of which may be of very small size. Kaolin group contains kaolinite, nacrite, dickite, annauxite and hallosysite, all $Al_2O_3 2SiO_2.2H_2O$ and allophane, $Al_2O_3.nSiO_2.$ H_2O. It contains traces of magnesium, calcium and iron.

Preparation

Kaolin is prepared when the rock in mined, excavated and the impurities are washed with water and then powdered. The rock is elutriated with water and large-sized particles are separated. On allowing the turbid liquid to settle, heavy Kaolin containing particles of large size and colloidal Kaolin containing particles of small size are separated and then dried.

Description

Kaolin, $Al_2O_3.2SiO_2.2H_2O$ (Al_2O_3 39.3%, SiO_2 46.8%, H_2O, 13.9%, sp.gr. 2.6), is an important member of the family of clay material. It is slightly plastic like and is normally white but is often tinged grey, yellow brown, blue or red due to impurities. Its softness is very characteristic. It is unctuous and soapy to touch. On rubbing with a piece of bone, it takes a high polish. It is highly refractory. Its fusion point is in between 1700-1800°. When heated in a closed tube, it gives out water. On heating with cobalt nitrate, it gives a blue mass due to the alumina present. It is not affected with dilute hydrochloric or nitric acid, but is decomposed by prolonged boiling or treatment with concentrated sulphuric acid. It becomes more resistant to acids if it is first heated to white heat.

The particles of heavy Kaolin are 20 μm in diameter, flat and irregularly arranged. With water plastic-like form is obtained which is less sticky. When the aqueous suspension is kept for sometime, the whole Kaolin settles below leaving a clear supernatant liquid. Heavy Kaolin polarizes light brightly.

The particles of fine or colloidal Kaolin are small, less than 2 μ in diameter and have various shapes and sizes. They do not polarize light. A sticky mass is obtained with water. Its aqueous suspension remains turbid permanently and only a small fraction is deposited.

Uses

Heavy Kaolin is used externally as a dusting powder, poultice, carrier of heat, filtering and cleaning agent.

Fine Kaolin is used internally as an absorbent and to coat irritated intestinal mucosa in case of diarrhoea, dysentery and intestinal fermentation. They are also used to manufacture porcelain, pottery, bricks, portland cement, ultra-marine, colour lakes, refractory mortar, plaster material, filler for paper, electric and heat insulators; clarifying liquids, drying and emollient agents.

COCHINEAL

Biological source

It consists of the dried female insects *Coccus cacti* (*Dactylopius coccus*) containing eggs and larvae. Order : Hemiptera.

Habitat

Cochineal insects are indigenous to Central America. Commercially they are grown in Peru, Mexico, Canary Islands, Algiers, Honduras, East and West Indies, Spain, Florida and California.

Eggs from the previous crop are hatched on the Cacti or Nopal tree (*Nopalea cochenillifer*, Family Cactaceae). Both male and female insects emerge. The males are about 1 mm long and possess wings, while the females are about 2 mm long and without wings. After a time fecundation takes place and the females attach themselves to the Nopal tree by means of their probosces. The males then die. The female insects grow faster and becomes to about twice their original size. The larvae mature in about 14 days and escape from the dead body of the parent. Only a small proportion of the larvae develop into males. For the next 15 days the young females crawl about the plant and the males fly. The sequence of life cycle is then repeated. It takes about 6 weeks and three to five generations of the insects may be produced in a season.

Collection and preparation

The insects are separated from the tree, killed with hot water, stove heat or by exposure to the fumes of burning sulphur or charcoal. If heat is used, the colour of insects becomes purplish-black and they are called as '*black grain*'. The fume-killed purplish-grey insects are known as '*silver grain*'. Small immature insects and larvae are separated by sieves and known as '*granilla*'. About 70,000 insects produce 450 g (1 lbs) of the Cochineal drug.

Characters

Cochineal insects are about 4 mm long and oval in shape. The convex dorsal surface shows from 9 to 11 segments without constrictions between head, thorax and abdomen. The insect has a pair of antennae with 7-joints and three pairs of very incospicuous legs. The surface contains tubular glands which secrete wax.

Chemical constituents

Cochineal contains a water soluble glycosidic colouring matter known as carminic acid or carmine red (10%) which is a C-glycoside of anthraquinone. The insect also contains fat (10%) and a wax known as coccerin (2%). Carmine is an alkaline preparation of Cochineal containing about 50 per cent of carminic acid.

The drug should be free from *Salmonellae* and *Escherichia coli*. A colour value test in which the extinction of a diluted extract of pH 8.0 is measured at 530 nm is taken as a standard parameter for the drug.

Adulteration

The weight of cochineal is increased by an inorganic matter, the colour of which is matched with the insect. No insoluble water should separate when the insects are placed in water and the ash should not exceed 7% in case of genuine drug.

Uses

Cochineal is used as a colouring agent for food products, drugs and toilet preparations. Carmine and carminic acid are used for manufacture of red and pink inks and lakes. Several grades of cochineal are available such as Silver grain, Black grain, Grannilla, Rosy-black and Red foxy.

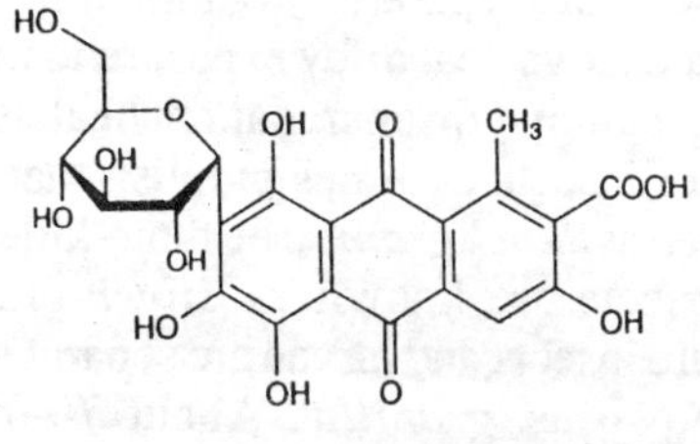

Fig. 23.1. Carminic acid.

SHELLAC

Synonyms

Lacca; Lac.

Biological source

Shellac is a resinous substance prepared from the excretion of scale insects, *Lucifer lacca*, syn. *Karria lacca* (Family Coccidae).

Habitat

Shellac is produced in Burma, Assam and India. Most Shellac is produced in Madhya Pradesh, Uttar Pradesh, Bihar and Orissa states of India.

Preparation

The insects live on the juices of various trees such as *Acacia* species, *Butea frondosa* (Papilionaceae), *Aleurites laccifera* (Euphorbiaceae), *Ficus* species (Moraceae), *Cajanus indicus*, *Shorea talura* (Dipterocarpaceae), *Schleichera trijuga* (Sapindaceae) and *Zizyphus jujuba* (Rhamnaceae).

The insects suck the juice of the tree and excrete "sticklac" almost continuously. Whitest Shellac is produced when the Kusum tree (*Schleichera trijuga*) is the host. The structure and life history of the scale insect are identical to those of Cochineal.

Collection

Shellac is found most abundantly on the smaller branches and twigs. These are broken off and the excretion is scraped from the twigs with the help of curved knives. It is ground and the colouring matter extracted with water or dilute alkali solution. The exhausted Shellac in dried form is known as *Seed lac*. The alkaline extract on dryness gives *Lac dye*. The *Seed lac* is melted in a long sausage-shaped bag suspended over a charcoal fire and the lac is squeezed out. It is cooled and then stretched into a large sheet. It is broken up to give flake Shellac of commerce. Sometimes the Shellac is poured into circular moulds and, on cooling, stamped with the maker's name. This form of Shellac is known as *Button lac*. When the Shellac is dissolved in hot alkaline solution, bleached with chlorine or sulphurous acid, precipitated with acid, collected by filtration and pulled under water into sticks, it is known as *Bleached Shellac*. When the Shellac is kept under water, it is soluble in alcohol, but the solubility decreases on exposure.

Characters

Shellac occurs in thin, very brittle, yellowish, translucent sheets or powder; m.p. 115-120, saponification no. 185-210°, iodine no. 10-18. It is soluble in alcohol, ether, benzene and petroleum ether; sparingly soluble in oil of terpentine and insoluble in water.

It is soluble in aqueous solutions of ethanolamines, alkalies and borax with slightly purple colour.

Various grades and colours are used for particular purposes. Shellac containing brownish-yellow colour is known as *orange Shellac* and the reddish-brown varieties are called *ruby* or *garnet Shellac.*

Chemical constituents

Shellac contains wax (6%), red colouring matter (6.5%), laccaic acid, resin (70-85%), few insect remains and vegetable debris. Hydrolysis of the resin gives a complex mixture of aliphatic and alicyclic hydroxy acids and their polyesters. The composition of the hydrolysate depends on the Shellac source and the time of collection. The major component of the aliphatic fraction is aleuritic acid. The resin, composed of two parts, a hard and a soft fraction, is formed from hydroxy fatty acids and sesquiterpenes. An example of the former is aleuritic acid (9,10,16-trihydroxy-palmitic acid) and of the latter, a cedrene-type sesquiterpene acid; a water-insoluble yellow pigment is erythrolaccin, a tetrahydroxy-4-methyl-anthraquinone.

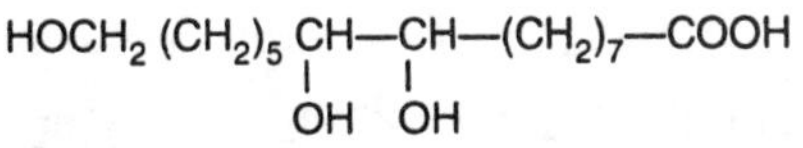

HOCH$_2$ (CH$_2$)$_5$ CH—CH—(CH$_2$)$_7$—COOH
OH   OH
Aleuritic acid

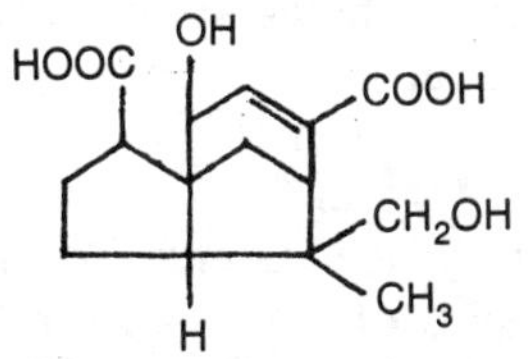

Fig. 23.2. Chemical constituents of Shellac.

Uses

Shellac is used for coating confections and medicinal tablets; finishing leather, in lacquers and varnishes, to manufacture buttons, grinding wheels, sealing wax, cements, inks, phonographs, records, paper; for stiffening hats; in electrical machines; and in polishes.

LARD

Biological source

Lard is the purified internal fat obtained from the abdomen of the hog, *Sus scrofa*, var. *domesticus* (Family Suidae).

The abdominal fat, known as *flare*, is obtained by treatment with hot water at a temperature not exceeding 57°C.

Characters

Lard is a soft, white fat, m.p. 34-41°, iodine value 52-66, saponification value 192-198. It has non-rancid odour. It is insoluble in water, very slightly soluble in alcohol and freely soluble in benzene, chloroform, solvent and petroleum ethers and in carbon disulphide. It should be free from moisture, alkalies and chlorides. It is adulterated with beef fat, Sesame oil and Cottonseed oil.

Lard oil is colourless, pale yellow liquid, density 0.90-0.91, viscosity 1.47. It solidifies in between 2 to +4°C.

Chemical constituents

Lard contains solid glycerides (40%) such as myristin, stearin and palmitin; and mixed liquid glycerides (60%) such as olein. The fractions are separated by pressure at 0°C into solid fat 'stearin' and liquid 'lard oil'. Hydrolysis of Lard yields oleic acid (48%), palmitic acid (28%), octadecadienic acid (11%), stearic acid (9%) and myristic acid (3%).

Uses

Lard is an emollient and used as a base for ointments and cerates. It has a tendency to become rancid; this can be retarded by combining lard with 1% Siam Benzoin or Sumatra Benzoin to prepare Benzoinated Lard. Lard oil is used as an antifoaming agent in the fermentations and as a tablet lubricant, illuminant, oiling wool and to manufacture soap.

WOOL FAT

Wool fat (*Anhydrous lanolin*) is a purified fat-like substance prepared from the wool of the sheep, *Ovis aries* (Bovidae).

Raw wool contains a good amount of 'wool grease' or crude lanolin, the potassium salts of fatty acids and earthy matter. Raw lanolin is separated by 'cracking' with sulphuric acid from the washings of the scouring process and purified to fit it for medicinal use. It is purified by centri-fuging with water and by bleaching.

Wool fat is a pale yellow, tenacious substance with a faint and characteristic odour. It is insoluble in water and a high proportion of water may be incorporated with it by melting (m.p. 36-42°C) and stirring; soluble in ether and chloroform. Like other waxes, it is not readily saponified by aqueous alkali, but an alcoholic solution of alkali causes saponi-fication. Saponification value 90-105; iodine value 18-32; acid value not more than 1. Hydrous wool fat or lanolin contains 25% water.

The main constituents of wool fat are choles-terol and isocholesterol, unsaturated monohydride alcohols of the formula $C_{27}H_{45}OH$, both free and combined with lanoceric, lanopalmitic, carnaubic and other fatty acids. Wool fat also contains aliphatic alcohols such as cetyl, ceryl and caranaubyl alcohols. Butylated hydroxytoluene, up to 200 p.p.m. may be added as an antioxidant. Wool alcohols are prepared by the saponification of crude lanolin and the separation of the alcohol fraction. The product consists of sterols and triterpene alcohols, including cholesterol (not less than 30%) and isocholesterol.

Chemical test

Dissolve cholesterol (0.5 g) in 5 ml of chloroform, add 1 ml acetic anhydride and two drops of sulphuric acid; a deep-green colour is formed.

. Wool fat is used as an emollient base for creams and ointments.

DIATOMITE (KIESELGHUR)

It occurs as large deposits in California, Germany, North Africa and Virginia.

The material is dried, powdered, ignited to remove organic matter, boiled with dilute hydro-chloric acid to remove iron and other impurities, washed with water and dried. Purified form occurs as a fine, white, odourless powder. It is insoluble in all acids except hydrofluoric acid. After fusion with alkalies, it is soluble in acids. It is shifted or 'air-blown' to get the finest grades.

The crude product contains silica (68-87%), or-ganic matter, clay, iron oxide and water (5-15%). The silica is amorphous. It is present in the siliceous walls of minute, unicellular plants belonging to a number of families of the Bacillariophyceae, in the walls of spicules of siliceous sponges and, in a crystalline form, as sand. Depending on the geographical origin of the diatomite, the diatoms may be either freshwater or marine forms.

Characters

Purified kieselghur is a fine, white or pale-buff odourless powder. In the olive oil mount the amorphous silica of the diatoms becomes almost invisible, while the crystalline particles of sand remain clear. Only small amounts of sand should be present.

The diatoms consist of two halves or *valves* which fit together like a pill-box. The valves show considerable variation in shape. Some samples of kieselguhr show many discoid types resembling that of the *Arachnoidiscus* found in agar. The other samples consist largely of pennate forms. A mix-ture of both types is usually most suitable for filtra-tion. In many diatoms a median cleft is found in the valves, known as the *raphe*. The valves also show dots and lines, which vary in the different species and are due to minute cavities in the wall.

Uses

It is used for the filtration of oils, fats, syrups and in the form of the Berkefeld filter for sterilization. Highly purified material is used as an inactive support in column, gas and thin layer chromato-graphy. The powder holds up to its own weight of water and still retain its powdery consistency. Diatomite is also used in face powders, pills, polishing powders and soaps, and to absorb nitroglycerin in the manufacture of dynamite.

Extract species of diatoms form an important components of plankton. They are involved in the food chains of seas and rivers.

PREPARED CHALK

Chalk is a whitish or greyish rock found in north-western Europe. It consists mainly of the shells of unicellular animals known as the Foraminifera. Chalk contains about 97 or 98% of calcium carbonate and siliceous matter, therefore, insoluble in acids. The impure chalk is finely ground with water and freed from most of the heavier siliceous impurities by elutriation. The coarser product is sold as 'whiting' and the finer elutriated product is allowed to settle. The pasty material is poured into a funnel-shaped trochiscator. The latter is tapped on a porous chalk slab and ejects the chalk to form 'cones', which are allowed to dry giving Prepared Chalk. These cones ('crab's eyes') may be powdered.

Characters

Chalk is mounted in cresol, warmed and examined microscopically. Most of the foraminiferous shells have been broken. The whole shells may be concentrated in a small bulk by removing the broken ones by elutriation. The following structures are seen:

Globigerina : The shell is consisted of calcite and perforated by large canals. Each cell has a few lobular chambers arranged in a plane or helicoid spiral. The size varies from 35 to 80 μm.

Textularia : In these the shell is composed of grains of sand cemented together by calcareous matter. They are conical or cuneiform in shape and are composed of numerous chambers in two alternating parallel series. The size varies from 50 to 180 μm.

Remains of fossil algae : Small rings or discs about 4-9 μm in diameter are termed coccoliths or morpholites.

Prepared chalk is assayed by acid-alkali back-titration.

Precipitated chalk

Precipitated chalk is prepared by the interaction of a soluble calcium salt and a soluble carbonate. The precipitate varies with the method of preparation. When precipitated at about 0°C, the product is very light and amorphous; at about 30°C a denser precipitate of minute rhombohedra is formed, and if boiling solutions are used, the precipitate consists of prismatic rhombohedra with a higher specific gravity than either of the previous forms. The assay involves a complexometric titration of calcium.

Uses

Chalk is used as an absorbent and antacid.

AMBERGRIS

It is a very expensive aromatic substance. It is a pathological product found in the intestines of sperm whales or cast by them into the sea. It occurs in streaky grey or brown waxy masses up to weight 45 kg. It has the breaks of squids on which the whales feed. Ambergris contains about 25% of ambrein. It has a fragrant musk-like odour. It gives tenacity or persistence of odour in perfumes.

MUSK

Musk is the dried secretion from the preputial follicles of the musk deer, *Moschus moschiferus*. This small deer is found in China and the Himalayas. The musk-containing sacs are brown as 'pods' which are about 5-7 cm diameter, weight up to 30 g and contain about half their weight of musk. When distilled, musk yields about 1.4% of dark brown volatile oil, the chief odorous constituent of the oil is muskone. This is a cyclic ketone having a closed chain of 15 carbon atoms. Other constituents of musk are steroidal hormones, muscopyridine and other alkaloids and peptides. A synthetic compound, which differs from muskone only in the absence of a methyl group, is cyclopentadecanone. Musk acts as a fixative and is an important ingredient of many high-class perfumes.

ROYAL JELLY, QUEEN BEE JELLY

This hive product consists of the milky fluid produced by the salivary glands of worker bees and used as essential nourishment for the development of the queen bee larvae. It contains amino acids, vitamin B complex, vitamin C, lipids, fatty acids, carbohydrates and minerals. The fresh material is unstable. It is freeze-dried or filled in capsules containing royal jelly stabilized by the addition of honey. Royal jelly is an expensive dietary supplement recommended for counteracting the effects of ageing and for the treatment of myalgic encephalomyelitis, depression, dermatitis and other conditions.

LEECH

The medicinal leech, *Hirudo medicinalis*, is about 6-10 cm long. The sucker at the anterior end has three radiating jaws containing 'teeth'. In contact with the skin, the animal produces a triradiate cut and can draw about 4-8 ml of blood. The salivary glands secrete hirudin, an acidic polypeptide of molecular weight about 7,000. It retards coagulation of blood and allows bleeding to continue after the leech has been removed. Preparations containing hirudin for the treatment of bruises are manufactured commercially. Other enzymes isolated from the leech include hementin, an antithrombin agent and orgelase, which degrades hyaluronic acid.

About 12000 kg of leeches are used annually in Europe and exported from France, Italy, Portugal and Central Europe. Some supplies of leech products are met by commercial farms and by genetically engineered organisms. The cloning and expression of a recombinant gene for hirudin in yeast and bacteria has been reported.

Leeches are often the least painful way to reduce inflammation. They have also staged a medical revival by their use in skin grafting for the removal of coagulated blood from beneath the new skin. The leech is host to *Aeromanas hydrophila*, an organism on which it depends to digest the blood consumed. This is a potential source of infection of wounds and, three types of infection, including diarrhoea, have been reported in patients receiving leech treatment which can be cured by the use of suitable anti-biotics.

RUBBER

Rubber is produced from a number of species of the families Euphorbiaceae, Apocynaceae, Moraceae, Asclepiadaceae and others.

In Malaysia, *Hevea brasiliensis* (Euphorbiaceae) is tapped in the early morning when the internal latex pressure is highest. Trees are tapped by making an overlapping spiral groove, initially 1.5 m above the ground, with a knife called a *jebong*. The exuded latex is collected in cups placed at the lower end of the groove. After about 11 years the spiral has reached ground level. The latex in vats, coagulated and bleached is cleaned with formic acid and a bleaching agent. The latex emerges as blocks which are then passed through a mill 30 times to give thin layers ready for further processing.

Rubber consists of linear chains of about 1500 to 60000 C_5-isoprenoid units linked by *cis* double bonds.

GUTTA-PERCHA

Gutta-percha is purified, coagulated latex obtained from trees of the genera *Palaquium* and *Payena* (Sapotaceae), which are found in Malaysia and Indonesia. It is collected similar to rubber but the latex flows less readily. Gutta-percha differs from rubber in being almost incapable of vulcanization, and in that it becomes plastic when heated to about 45-60°C. Gutta-percha contains a white, polymerized hydrocarbon gutta, composed of C_5-units linked by *trans* double bonds, it has less units than rubber.

Gutta-percha is applied in the form of chloroformic solution to the skin, and in the manufacture of surgical instruments. It should be preserved under water in well-closed containers protected from light.

CHICLE

Chicle is a polyisoprenoid consisting of a mixture of *cis*- and *trans*-C_5 isoprenoids obtained from *Manilkara zapota* (Sapotaceae), the sapodilla plum. It is used as a base for chewing gum.

FULLER'S EARTH

Multani mitti

It consists of certain adsorbent clays possessing the property of decolourizing and clarifying oils of animal, vegetable and mineral origins and some other liquids. Fuller's earth is distinguished from bentonite which possesses small adsorptive power unless activated by acid treatment.

Fuller's earth has high water content, foliated structure and the absence of plasticity. Dehydrated samples show a tendency to adhere strongly to the tongue. The dominant constituent is montmorillonite [(Mg, Ca) $O.Al_2O_3.5SiO_2.n H_2O$].

Beidellite [$Al_2O_3, 3SiO_2.H_2O$] is the dominant clay mineral in some of them. The ratio of silica to aluminium varies from 4 to 6 in earths of good quality.

Indian fuller's earth consists of well-bedded, non-arenaceous, unctuous clay or shale, cream to yellow, yellowish brown, buff, greenish grey or light grey in colour. It is a hydrated aluminium silicate with lime, magnesia and iron oxide as impurities. It contains up to 30% of water. It is soft when freshly excavated, but hardens on exposure to the atmosphere. It disintegrates in contact with water, it is no-plastic and does not swell. On drying at room temperature, the bleaching power of the earth is slightly altered.

Distribution

Fuller's earth occurs in Bihar, Baroda and Kolhapur districts, Hyderabad, Central India, Tamil Nadu, Karnataka and Rajasthan.

Fuller's earth is dried in rotary kilns, ground to size and screened. The final product should contain 8-10% of moisture on drying. Inactive earths are activated by treatment with hydrochloric or sulphuric acid in lead-lined tanks. The earth is dried, ground and treated with hydrochloric acid at 105° for 3-4 hours or with dilute sulphuric acid (20%) at 150° for 2 hours. The acid layer is run off and the earth washed to remove all traces of acid. The mineral is then dried and ground.

Fuller's earth is available in granular and pulverized forms. The former is suitable for use in percolators, for decolourizing an oil or material which is passed through a bed of granular earth packed in long cylindrical vessels. The pulverized form is more convenient for contact bleaching. The earth is mixed with the oil or other material to be decolourized and vigorously agitated.

Fuller's earth is tested for bleaching power, rapidity of filtration, degree of oil retention, and possibility of revivification. Earth required for refining oil should possess high decolourizing and low oil retention values. It should not impart any odour or taste to the oil.

Uses

Fuller's earth is used in refining oils, greases, lard, liquid fractions of petroleum including crude naphtha, crude kerosene and shale oil. It is employed as a carrier for pigments, size for textiles, poultice for skin eruptions, substitute for talcum powder, filler for paper and soap, and conditioner for foundry sands. Selected soft grades are mixed with graphite in pencil manufacture. In laboratory, it is used to detect colouring matter added to butter and whisky. More than 90% of fuller's earth produced in USA is used for de-colourizing mineral oil. About 6% of the earth is used for refining vegetable and animal oils.

In India, it is used as a substitute for soap in washing clothes and hair and in refining vegetable oils.

ASBESTOS

Sangresha; Shankha palita; Kalnar; Ratinara.

Asbestos is the commercial name given to various silicate minerals which can be easily split into flexible fibres, capable of being felted or spun together. The fibres are light, fire-resistant, heat, sound and electrical insulators, and non-corrosive. These properties make asbestos technically a very valuable material. Asbestos is used mainly in the manufacture of asbestos cement products and textile products and also in many other industries.

Habitat

Deposits of asbestos are widely distributed over the world. Among the largest producers of asbestos are Canada (chrysotile), Russia (chrysotile), the Republic of South Africa (amosite, blue crocidolite and chrysotile), Southern Rhodesia (chrysotile), USA (mainly chrysotile) and China (chrysotile). Italy (chrysotile and tremolite), Swaziland (chrysotile), Australia (crocidolite and some chrysotile), and some other countries are also important producers. For spinning purposes, Canadian chrysotile is considered the best in the world.

In India, Asbestos occurs in various parts of the country. Important deposits of asbestos are found in Andhra Pradesh, Bihar, Karnataka and Rajasthan. The deposits are mostly of amphibole variety; however, chrysotile variety also occurs in Andhra Pradesh and Bihar and to some extent in Rajasthan.

It occurs in various types of rocks and is formed by metamorphism. Asbestos is usually derived from basic to ultrabasic igneous rocks such as peridotite, dunite and pyroxenite, or their meta-morphosed derivatives such as states, schists and banded iron stones. Most asbestos minerals are found in veinlets, but some make up the whole mass of a rock; the length of the asbestos veins ranges from 2.5 cm to 21 m and the width from about a centimetre to a metre. There are three modes of occurrence of asbestos minerals : (1) *cross-fibre*, with fibres at right angles to the walls of the veins; (2) *slip-fibre*, with long fibres parallel or oblique to the walls of the veins, but of poor quality; (3) *mass-fibre*, with interlaced, unoriented, aggregate of fibres, sometimes radially arranged. The commercial varieties of Asbestos are:

Chrysotile or *fibrous serpentine* ($3MgO.2SiO_2.2H_2O$; sp gr, 2.4-2.6; H, 2.5-4.0) is a hydrated silicate of magnesium, usually containing small percentages of iron oxide and alumina. It has a greenish colour when in mass but separate fibres are white. It is characterized by fineness, flexibility, silkiness and strength of its fibres, these properties rendering it very suitable for spinning and weaving. It stands a fair degree of heat and is attacked easily by weak acids. It is the most valuable variety of asbestos. A brownish green, lamellar variety of serpentine is called *antigorite*.

Amosite [$Fe_5Mg_2Si_8O_{22}(OH)_2$] is a long-fibre variety of iron-rich anthophyllite; the length of the fibre is normally 10-30 cm. It is resistant to acids. The superior grade fibres are used for spinning purposes.

Crocidolite or *blue asbestos* [$Na_2O.Fe_2O_3.3FeO.8SiO_2.H_2O$] is a sodium iron silicate, usually containing a small percentage of magnesia and a little lime. It has a characteristic blue colour both in mass and when fiberized. Crocidolite usually occurs in cross-fibre seams interbedded in banded sedimentary iron stones. Crocidolite is harsher than chrysotile but usually possesses greater tensile strength and has the advantage of being much more resistant to acids and some other chemicals. It is mainly used as an insulator and in asbestos cement products. When infiltrated with silica, the variety is sold as Cat's Eye or Tiger's Eye for ornamental use.

Tremolite [$Ca_2Mg_5Si_8O_{22}(OH)_2$; sp gr. 2.9-3.2; H, 5-6] is a silicate of magnesium and calcium. It is a white to dark grey mineral. It may be soft and powdery, and when fibrous, the fibres may be long or short, strong or weak, and flexible or brittle. Its value as a fibrous, material is limited mainly because the deposits are small and uneconomical. It is used for the manufacture of boiler lagging (insulation material) and for filtration purposes.

Actinolite [$Ca_2(MgFe)_5Si_8O_{22}(OH)_2$; sp gr., 2.9-3.2; H, 5-6) is a silicate of magnesium and calcium with iron. It is a green coloured mineral of little commercial importance.

Tremolite and actinolite occur in metamorphic rocks of diverse kinds; tremolite occur in metamorphic rocks of diverse kinds; tremolite occurs in impure crystalline limestones and in calc-silicate hornfelses and also in metamorphosed ultrabasic and basic rocks, such as serpentines and green stones. Actinolite is a common metamorphic mineral occurring in derivatives of basic and ultrabasic igneous rocks such as actinolite schists and greenstones. These minerals occur in veins as slip-fibre.

Anthophyllite [$(MgFe)_7Si_8O_{22}(OH)_2$; sp gr, 3.0-3.2; H, 5.5-6.0] is a magnesium iron silicate. It is of white to grey colour, sometimes yellowish-brown, with a vitreous lustre. Anthophyllite commonly occurs as a mass-fibre and occasionally as slip-fibre; the fibres are generally harsh, short and weak. It is brittle and possesses low tensile strength. The value of this asbestos depends on its outstanding quality of being infusible and highly resistant to acids and alkalies. It is chiefly used in boiler coverings and fire-proof paints. Anthophyllite occurs as a constituent of certain metamorphic rocks (schists and gneisses), usually derived from basic or ultrabasic igneous rocks.

Preparation

The mineral as obtained from the mines by blasting and quarrying, may be dressed and sold either as "crude" or in the form of various grades of fibre which have been produced by milling. The content of fibre in the rock mined may range between 3 and 10 per cent.

"Crude" asbestos consists of hand-picked cross-fibre asbestos in its natural condition, freed from adhering rock by hand-cobbing and small pieces of short-fibred material. Crude asbestos, as marketed, may still contain from 5 to 20 per cent of rock, dust or short fibre which has to be removed by the asbestos spinner in the operation of opening up the fibre. The second method of preparing asbestos for the market consists in milling the raw material, so as to free the asbestos from the adhering rock and to liberate the fibre. The fibre is graded by sieving on rotary screens.

Grading

There is no standard classification of asbestos in India, and the grades marketed by various mine owners do not conform to the standard Canadian classification, commonly known as Quebec Asbestos Mining Association Classification or more commonly as Quebec Grading. Although the Canadian classification is universally accepted in trade, some of the other producing countries have adopted their own classifications.

The simplest way of classification of asbestos is to divide it into two types : (1) spinning type; (2) non-spinning type. In many countries the classification is based on local practice for hand-cobbing and different degrees of milling. According to standard Canadian classification, asbestos is graded into nine major groups and each group is subdivided into further sub-grades as per performance in the Quebec-Screen Test. Groups 1 and 2 are for hand-processed crudes and the remaining for milled asbestos.

Properties

Commercial utility of asbestos depends mostly on its physical properties, like spinnability, resistance to heat, acid and alkalies, filtration property, tensile strength and power to absorb cement. They play an important part in selecting a particular type asbestos for particular use. The chemical analysis of asbestos does not give any indication of its utility, and also does not help in grading. In amphibole asbestos, except tremolite, all varieties contain iron combined chemically as an essential constituent of the mineral. For some purposes, such as the manufacture of insulators for electrical appliances, it is necessary to use iron-free asbestos or treat it with acid to remove conductive constituents like iron.

Uses

Asbestos finds several uses in industry. Asbestos fabrics and asbestos-cement products are the largest uses of the mineral.

The asbestos fibres which can be spun are largely made into textile products such as cloth, tape, break-linings, clutch facings, rope cord, wick, packing-gaskets and cable coverings. Asbestos cloth is used for making protective clothing, blankets for fire fighting, filter aids, conveyors for carrying hot material, and oven and furnace insulations. It is usually a mixture of asbestos and cotton, the latter being in a proportion of 20 per cent. It has not been possible to make asbestos cloth as fine as cotton textile because of the low mechanical strength of asbestos fibre. As such, the clothes and tapes produced from it are bulky.

Asbestos cloth treated with rubber is made into gaskets for use between the abutting or flange ends of pipes, or between adjoining surfaces, such as manhole and handhole plates, to make the joints tight enough to prevent passage of air, steam or oil.

The non-spinning type of asbestos is used for compressed packing material consisting of felted mass of fibre bound with rubber and other binders such as gum, resin, lac or rubber dissolved in benzene. Certain types of compressed materials are prepared by mixing clean, well-opened fibres with fillers like clay, graphite, barytes or cellulose and then bound with some binding agents. They are of various forms known as compressed sheets, coil and spiral used for high pressure packing.

Asbestos is one of the most important fire-proofing and heat-insulating materials known. The best known and commonest of the insulating products is 85 per cent magnesia compound which is composed essentially of a mixture of 15 per cent amosite asbestos and 85 per cent magnesia. The ingredients are mixed well in water and filter-pressed into cakes and then dried in steam-heated kilns. The dry blocks are cut and bored to form cylinders of different diameters to cover pipes of various sizes, or made into different forms for insulating purposes.

The principal use of shorter fibre asbestos, having good tensile strength is in boiler coverings, mill-board and allied products in asbestos paper manufacture, and in the manufacture of asbestos-cement sheets, pipes, tiles, panelling, roofing slate and partition wall. Asbestos-cement products industry is the major consumer of chrysotile asbestos.

Chrysotile asbestos having soft, flexible and very strong fibres is especially suitable for many products for insulation like thermal insulating material, turbine jacket and blankets, mill-board, wall and ceiling sheets.

Indian Railway is the largest consumer of crocidolite for limpet spraying of coaches for heat insulation.

Recently, asbestos fibres have been employed in missile work, satellites, special packings in atomic energy equipment, in reinforcing plastics and in asphalt paving.

Consumption pattern

Asbestos-cement, asbestos products, paint, rubber, paper, foundry, chemical and refractory industries are the important consumers of asbestos in India. Asbestos-cement and asbestos products industries are the major consumers accounting for about 99 per cent of the total consumption.

Imports

Large quantities of asbestos are imported into India to meet the increasing demands. Japan, Canada, Russia, USA, Botswana, France, and Australia are the important suppliers of asbestos to India. Small quantities of asbestos are also exported.

BENTONITE

Bentonite is a naturally occurring clay, extremely fine-grained and highly absorbent, possessing bleaching characteristics. The so-called 'bleaching clays' are either activated bentonites or fuller's earths. When placed in contact with water, bentonite swells considerably forming a slippery gelatinous mass resembling soft soap; hence it is also called 'mineral soap' or 'soap clay', and is sometimes used as a substitute for soap. Bentonite finds wide and varied applications in industries like foundry, oil-well drilling, chemical (pharmaceutical), civil construction, ceramics, refractories, pelletization and various others.

Habitat

Deposits of bentonite are found to occur in various countries of the world, and commercially produced in some. The world's chief supply of bentonite comes from the United States, which produces more than half of the total world production of bentonite. Other important producers include Japan, Greece, Italy, Mexico, Rumania, Brazil and Poland.

Occurrences of bentonite are known from the various states of India. The commercially important deposits occur in Bihar, Gujarat, Jammu and Kashmir and Rajasthan.

Bentonite (sp gr, 2.4-2.8) is composed (75% or more) of crystalline clay-like minerals namely *Montmorillonite* [(Mg, Ca) O. $Al_2O_3.5SiO_2.nH_2O$] with n equal to about 8 and *beidellite* ($Al_2O_3.3SiO_2.4H_2O_2$), with small amounts of igneous rock minerals. It also contains about 5 to 10 per cent of alkaline earths and alkalies and 3 per cent of ferric iron. Bentonite has thus a variable chemical composition. It may be white, cream, yellowish green, olive green, grey or brown in colour. On exposure to moisture almost all bentonites assume a slightly darker shade. The mineral shows a conchoidal or sub-conchoidal fracture and can be easily cut with a knife into thin shavings. Freshly cut surfaces show waxy lustre and are generally soapy to touch.

Commercial bentonites can be broadly divided into two groups : (i) *Swelling type* : These absorb a large percentage of water with considerable swelling; they are sodium-based bentonites or sodium-bentonites; (ii) *Non-swelling type* : These do not swell noticeably when wetted and are calcium-based bentonites. Between these two groups, are types with intermediate properties. The non-swelling or calcium-based bentonite is identical with fuller's earth.

Bentonite nearly always occurs in well-defined beds from a few cm up to 3 to 4 m thick, but occasionally in irregular pockets. It occurs intercalated with lake and marine shales and sand-stones in beds which are remarkably uniform in thickness and extent. Most of the deposits of bentonite are regarded as being alteration products of volcanic ash, the alteration having taken place during or shortly after the deposition in water of wind-blown ash. A few deposits seem to have been formed by the alteration of glassy lava flows and still fewer from acid igneous rocks such as rhyolite.

Activation of bentonites

Many bentonites can be activated by acid and heat treatment which renders them more suitable for use in refining petroleum products or vegetable oils. The exact mode of treatment varies with the particular bentonite to be activated. In general, the process consists in crushing the dried (at 110°) mineral and heating it with sulphuric acid; the concentration of sulphuric acid and the duration of the digestion depends upon the type of bentonite. The treated mineral is washed, dried and bagged after crushing. This treatment removes some of the alumina and all the combined water thereby destroying the colloidal condition of the bentonite.

Bentonite is known and marketed under various synonyms such as soap clay, mineral soap, wilkinite, staylite, vol-clay, aquagel, ardmorite, refinite; most of these being trade names for prepared bentonites.

Properties

Since bentonites include materials of variable chemical composition, their physical and chemical properties also vary. The commercial importance of bentonites depends on such physico-chemical properties as swelling index, base-exchange capacity, setting time and gel volume.

Some bentonites are highly absorbent, absorbing up to 5 times their weight or 15 times their volume of water, with a consequent increase in volume. The swelling type (sodium-based bentonite) has single water layer particles containing Na^+ as exchangeable ion. The non-swelling type (calcium-based bentonite) has double water layer particles with Ca^{++} as exchangeable ion. A third type of montmorillonite has been identified with zero water layer particles and is probably, neutral.

Bentonites with low iron content have been found to be good catalytic agents in petroleum refining. Those having Ca and/or Mg as exchangeable ions are good decolourizers. The absorption of water in sodium-based bentonite proceeds with a considerable increase in volume, creating an excellent gel and a viscous material which is invaluable for the preparation of drilling muds. Sodium bentonite has excellent thixotropic property, i.e. the gel becoming fluid on shaking and resolidifying on standing. The swelling type bentonite when dispersed in water, separates into suspended flakes which are all finer than 0.5 μ. Calcium bentonite yields about 35 per cent flakes finer than 0.5 μ. The difference in bentonite and other clays lies in lattice structure. The sheet of atoms in bentonite is much thinner and more easily separable in water. That is why bentonite occupies more surface area than other clays.

Uses

The mineral enters into cosmetic and pharma-

ceutical preparations, such as tooth pastes, creams, lipsticks and ointments; as an emulsifying agent for asphaltic and resinous substances, in soaps, paints, pharmaceutical products, and as an adhesive agent in horticultural sprays and insecticides. Small quantities of bentonite are also used in ceramic and refractory industry; it is sometimes incorporated in white-ware ceramic bodies to increase plasticity and modulus of rupture, both before and after firing, and also as suspending agent in glaze mixtures. Bentonite is used in asbestos products, in de-inking of old newspaper, as a thixotropic agent to prevent settling of mixed paints, in bleaching crude sulphur and as an addition to Portland cements and pozzolanas. It is also used in rubber, steel, electrical, and electrode industries. Bentonite has been used in the refining of sugar. A comparatively recent use has been its development as a bonding agent in pelletizing iron ore fines.

Considerable quantities of bentonite are used in refining petroleum products, vegetable oils and greases. Petroleum products are treated with bentonite to remove tarry complexes and dissolved colouring matter, the last named by selective adsorption. For this purpose, both swelling and non-swelling type of bentonites are employed, the latter often after activation. Bentonite is a valuable constituent of drilling muds because of its thickening and suspending properties and its ability to act as a thin seal. Bentorite used for this purpose is generally of sodium or swelling type and of lower grade than that used for oil refining.

Bentonite finds extensive application in foundry practice, where the mineral is employed as a bonding agent and conditioner in moulding sand used for casting ferrous and nonferrous metals. It helps in retaining the shape of the mould by making the surface impermeable. Strength and fusion point are the two important properties desired for selecting bentonite. Generally the swelling type of bentonite is used, though other types have also been used. For use in foundry sands, it is usually sold in powder form, 90-95 per cent of which will pass a 200-mesh sieve. Bentonite of Kashmir origin is reported to be most suitable for this purpose.

Bentonite has the property of reducing considerably the permeability of the soil to water and is therefore often employed in civil construction works to make a porous medium water-tight. It can be used alone or with some other grouting material. In India, the use of bentonite has been made in sealing water tanks especially in Rajasthan. The seepage through the bottom of a tank, lagoon or lake can be effectively checked or reduced by use of bentonite.

STEATITE AND TALC

Steatite is a purer variety of talc which is the softest and the most common hydrated magnesium silicate mineral; a slightly impure variety of talc is termed soapstone. Commercially, the terms steatite, talc and soapstone are used for the same mineral, commonly referred to as talc. Pyrophyllite, a hydrated silicate of aluminium, being very similar to talc in its various physical properties and uses, is also often included amongst these minerals.

Distribution

Deposits of steatite, talc and soapstone are widely distributed in India, forming large masses in Archaean and Dharwar rocks of the Peninsula. However, many of the occurrences are small and consist merely of poststone, derived from the alteration of basic and ultrabasic rocks. Some of the deposits are of really good material, such as those found in Rajasthan, Madhya Pradesh and Andhra Pradesh. Important deposits of the mineral are also found in Bihar, Gujarat, Karnataka, Uttar Pradesh and various other States. Pyrophyllite is found in Rajasthan, Uttar Pradesh and Madhya Pradesh.

Talc is an important industrial mineral. The use of talc for carvings, ornaments and utensils is known since ancient times. It finds many applications in modern industries, viz. paint, paper, insecticides, cosmetics, ceramics, rubber and textiles. Pyrophyllite also finds similar uses.

Talc [$H_2Mg_3(SiO_3)_4$; MgO, 31.70%, SiO_2, 63.50%; H_2O, 4.80%; sp gr., 2.6-2.8 is an apple-green to white or silvery-white, or greenish-grey or dark-green mineral, crystallizing in orthorhombic or monoclinic system. It usually occurs in foliated massive aggregates; sometimes in globular and stellated groups; also granular, massive, coarse or fine; fibrous (pseudomorphous); compact and cryptocrystalline. It has a greasy lustre and a characteristic soapy feel.

There are several varieties of talc. *Steatite* is a

massive and high-grade variety of talc. *Soapstone* is a massive and impure talcose-rock, having smooth and uniform texture and soapy feel. It is also known as *potstone*, from its being carved into plates, bowls and pots. *French Chalk*, is a milky-white, soft and compact talc with a pearly lustre; it marks cloth easily.

Pyrophyllite [$H_2Al_2(SiO_3)_4$; Al_2O_3, 28.3%; SiO_2, 66.7%; H_2O, 5.0%; sp gr., 2.8-2.9; is an aluminium analog of talc. It is a white, apple-green, yellowish, silvery-grey, pinkish, brownish and also mottled mineral, crystallizing in orthorhombic system. Pyrophyllite usually occurs in compact or foliated masses, and also in radial, fibrous aggregates, sometimes granular. It resembles talc in many of its properties and uses, and can be distinguished only by optical or chemical methods. Deposits of pyrophyllite are formed by the hydrothermal replacements of silicic volcanics.

Talc (including steatite and pyrophyllite) is produced in various countries of the world. The USA and Japan are the largest talc-producing countries, followed by Russia, France, India and China.

Grades and classification

Talc is classified according to its colour and softness. Whiter varieties are preferred to dull and other tinted varieties. There is no standard basis for classifying the material. However, in Rajasthan, it is classified into four different grades: Grade I : talc of pure-white appearance and smooth feel and free from grit; Grade II: tinted variety which may be blue or green, having smooth feel, and free from grit; Grade III: off-colour variety, having smooth feel and free from grit; Grade IV or the DDT variety : white or off-colour with grit.

Properties

Talc, when pure, is a white to silvery-white or greenish mineral, which grinds to a powder of varying degrees of white. Pure talc is characterized by extreme softness, hydrophobic surface-properties and slippery feel. It is taken as the standard for softness on the Moh's scale. Some commercial talcs exhibit harder properties because of the presence of impurities and associated minerals such as tremolite, serpentine, chlorite, dolomite, and calcite. The structure of pure talc consists of a brucite-sheet sandwiched between two silica-sheets, forming layers of talc which are indefinitely superimposed. Each layer is electrically neutral; adjacent layers are held by weak van der Walls forces. The characteristic slippery property of talc results from these layers sliding over one another.

Talc has a good lustre or sheen, high 'slip' or lubricating power, good hiding-power, and ability to absorb specific types of oil and grease. It is inert in most chemical reagents, although it exhibits a marked alkaline pH (typically 9.0-9.5). It is, however, soluble in hot and concentrated phosphoric acid. It can withstand temperatures up to 1,300°, and is not affected by rapid changes of temperatures. It has a low electrical and thermal conductivity. In addition, it can easily be powdered, cut and sawn into any desired shape and size. This combination of various properties makes the talc a valuable commercial material, useful for a wide range of purposes. Pyrophyllite has a very similar crystal structure and somewhat similar physical and chemical properties, as those of talc; it is, therefore, used for similar purposes as talc in some industries.

Uses and specifications

Talc of very good quality finds use in many cosmetic and pharmaceutical preparations, such as soaps, creams, salves, rouges, toilet powders, tablets, pills and other products. The total tonnage required for this purpose is relatively small, but the material for such use must necessarily be of excellent purity and colour and good 'slip', and possess very small particle size.

Steatite and soapstone/potstone, have been used for carving small idols, model-figurines, culinary utensils, ornaments and other objects of art, and also in the construction and ornamentation of temples and palaces. Massive talc is also used in the manufacture of pencils or crayons, used for marking cloth or in steelworks and foundries. Massive slabs of steatite are cut into switch-boards, panels, table-tops, sinks, tubs and tanks, as well as into linings for furnaces and stoves. The hard-baked form of massive talc is used for the tips of gas-burners. Recently, lava-grade talc is gaining importance in the manufacture of low-loss ceramic materials which are required for high-frequency insulations in radio, radar, television and related equipment.

Pulverized talc is used in such industries as paper, ceramics, cosmetics insecticides, paint, rubber and textile.

Large quantities of talc are used in the manufacture of paper to impart opacity. Its relative cheapness, as compared with china-clay, and its high retention in the finished paper, make talc suitable for use in this industry. Generally, the material having low content of calcium carbonate is utilized. For the best-quality papers, only pure-white and fine-grained talcs, fairly free from mica, calcium carbonate, and iron oxide (limit, 1-2%), are acceptable; but the off-colour material is largely used for roofing papers.

Ground steatite or talc is increasingly being employed in ceramics, and is now a standard ingredient in many floor- and wall tiles, and is also used for electrical porcelains, enamels and refractories. Talc, as an ingredient of saggers employed to protect ware during firing, is stated to increase resistance to thermal shock. Spark-plugs, which contain a large proportion of talc, are superior to those made from ordinary porcelain mixtures because of their greater mechanical strength and electrical resistance at high temperature. Electrical porcelains include cordierite bodies which are essentially fired mixtures of clay and talc. Cordierite has a very low thermal expansion—a useful property in compounding of refractory bodies. For highly absorptive bodies, such as plates in electric heaters, almost lime-free talc is generally desirable.

Talc is largely used in paints. High-grade foliated talc is used as an inert-extender and as a pigment, whereas the fibrous variety, known under various trade-names, such as *Ashastine, Tremoline* and *Loomite* is used as a suspending agent to prevent the settling out of ready-mixed paints. Talc is chiefly used for outward application or where abrasion is likely to occur. In general, talc has a flattening effect on paint-film and is, therefore, not suitable for high-gloss paints. Colour or brightness, shape and size of particles, packing-index and oil-absorption are considered in the specifications of paint-grade talcs. A relatively fine particle size of 98.5-99.95 per cent through a 325-mesh screen is commonly desired for paints.

Talc is widely used as a filler and for dusting, especially in rubber- and insecticidal industries, where the lower grades of off-colour talc and ground soapstone are used. For insecticidal powders, such as those containing DDT, talc is said to be very suitable due to its good flowing properties and non-abrasive characters.

Talc is also used as a filler in putty, wallplasters, composition floorings, linoleum, oil-cloth, rope, string, cordage, textiles, plastics, asbestos products and polishes. It is a dusting agent in the manufacture of wirenails, linoleum, oil-cloth, felt-paper, leather, corks, glass, candy and chewing-gum. Talc also finds important use as a lubricant in many industries, as a coating for foundry-facings, glass and rubber moulds and as a scourer for some cereals, such as rice and barley.

Pyrophyllite is used in the manufacture of various refractory and ceramic products, and as a filler in rubber, paint, cosmetics, soap and other industries. Pyrophyllite has particularly proved suitably as a carrier for insecticides and fungicides. It is considered to be the best mineral medium for this purpose, as it freely flows and does not obscure the action of the insecticide or fungicide.

COLOURING AND FLAVOURING AGENTS

A formulation contains a mixture of pharmacological active constituents and other ethical or technical required material such as colouring matters, flavourings, stabilizers, emulsifiers, thickeners, preservatives, antioxidants, tablet disintegrants and coatings. In the food industry these are termed as additives and for the EEC there is a list of permitted substances that may be used in some of the above categories. Under EEC rules, for appropriate foods, such additives must be included in the labelling.

For medicinal purposes these additives are controlled by the Drug and Cosmetic Act. If a patient requires a medicament free of gluten or tartrazine it may be necessary for the pharmacist to make enquiries of the manufacturer. In recent years there is an increasing demand for materials of natural origin and, particularly regarding colouring agents, the toxic nature of many of the synthetic dyes is becoming widely recognized. The additives used in standard medical practice are covered, and used in herbal preparations, may be included in the EEC list. In some cases, e.g., Raspberry Syrup and Cherry Syrup, the preparation may have the dual role of colourant and flavouring. The oils of clove and peppermint are used as flavours but the former has antibacterial, and the latter, carminative properties. Natural gums, which are widely used as thickening, emulsifying and suspending agents have, in larger doses, a therapeutic action.

Table 23.1. Natural colourants

Colourant	Source	Shade
Cochineal	*Dactylopius coccus*	Red
Beetroot powder (betanin)	*Beta vulgaris*	Red
Carmine powder	*Dactylopius coccuus*	Purplish-red
Paprika oleo-resin (capsanthin, capsorubin)	*Capsicum annuum*	Orange-red
Saffron (crocin)	*Crocus sativus*	Yellow-orange
Carotenes	Various sources, e.g., carrot root	Orange
Annatto (bixin)	*Bixa orellana*	Yellow-orange
Curcumin	*Curcuma longa*	Yellow
Chlorophyll and complexes		Green, olive-green

Colouring agents

The essential requirements of a medicinal colou-rant are nontoxicity and stability. The effect of pH on colour, solubility in water and oils, and stability to light, heat and sugars are to be considered.

ANNATTO

Annatto seeds are obtained from *Bixa orellana* (Bixaceae). They contain on their surface an edible carotenoid pigment.

The plant is a shrub or small tree, found in northern South America and widely cultivated for the seeds or as an ornamental. There are white- and pink-flowered varieties which are propagated by seeds or cuttings. The estimated world annual production of seed is 4000 tonnes; Ecuador, India, Kenya and Peru are the principal producers. Solubility of the dye in fixed oil, e.g., castor oil makes it ideally suitable for use in the dairy industry.

The castor-oil extract of the seeds contains a small amount of essential oil composed of mainly sesquiterpene hydrocarbon ishwarane.

Production of annatto colour

Bixin is accompanied by small amount of orellin, a water soluble yellow substance, fat and resinoid of bitter stuff. The proportion of bixin in annatto varies between 10-12%. But special grades containing 15-30% are also known. The dye from the surface of the seeds is extracted by counter-current method using water during simultaneous mechanical friction of the surface of the seeds. The suspension was evaporated *in vacuo* with subsequent drying and grinding to a powder, which can be used for colouring various food articles, e.g., candies.

The colour has also been extracted by treating the seeds with a vegetable oil, with or without heating the mixture, or by treating the seeds after swelling them in water or in steam. Butter colour is manufactured in India by first heating the seeds under pressure and then extracting with a vegetable oil, preferably castor oil at 120°. The extract is then suitably diluted to specifications.

Bixin has also been extracted by boiling with ethyl acetate, acetone, alcohol or chloroform. According to one Japanese patent stabilized bixin preparation was obtained by holding bixin in alcoholic solution at pH 4.5 for one hour before spray-drying.

The commercial cheese colour is an alkaline solution that apparently contains norbixin instead of bixin. Usually it is extracted by means of dilute sodium or potassium hydroxide.

Annatto food colour is stabilized by adding curcumin, vanillin, eugenol or vitamin E.

Chemical constituents

Bixin, a C_{24}-apocarotenoid, is the principal component of the dye present in about 2.5% (dry wt) in the seeds. It belongs to crocetin (Saffron) and abscisic acid. Removal of the methyl ester group of bixin yields the dicarboxylic acid norbixin which forms the basis of the water-soluble annatto dyes. Various semisynthetic derivatives of bixin also find use as food colourants.

The seeds contain a small amount of fatty oil. The seed coat possesses a wax-like substance (3%) which is toxic and paralyzes intestinal parasites. The seeds also contain farnesyl acetate, geranyl-geranyl octadecanoate, geranyl geranyl formate, δ-tocotrienol, apocarotenoids, β-carotene, cryptoxanthin, lutein, zeaxanthin, vitamin A and iso-cutellarein. Annatto volatile oil is composed of ishwarane (30.7%), α-pinene (9.3%), β-pinene, α-elemene, valencene and amorphene.

Natural bixin has a Z-configuration between C-6 and C-7. It crystallizes as violet prisms and melts at 198°C. Ethyl bixin is used for colouring foods such as margarine. Bixin is converted to a yellow colouring material by heating with acetic acid in the presence of acetic anhydride, for colouring margarine.

The petroleum ether soluble portion of the annatto seed coat consists mostly of carotenoid dyes (about 2%) and an essential oil. The carotenoid dyes have been separated into six fractions by chromatography. A pungent smelling essential oil was obtained by steam distillation of the seeds in an yield of about 0.08%, which gets polymerized quickly.

The carbon skeleton of bixin is identical with the middle section β-carotene molecule but the chromophore is terminated by conjugated carboxyl groups. It is assumed that bixin is a product of the bio-oxidative cleavage of primarily formed C_{40}-carotenoids.

Bixin

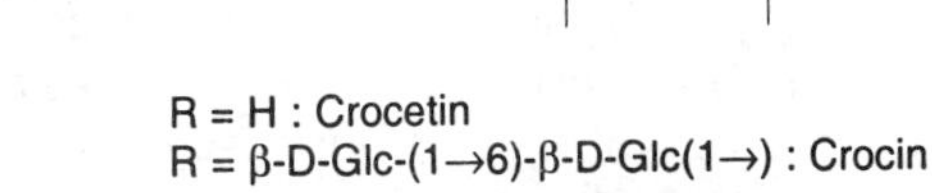

HOOC ... CO_2CH_3

ROOC ... COOR

R = H : Crocetin
R = β-D-Glc-(1→6)-β-D-Glc(1→) : Crocin

Fig. 23.3. Chemical constituents of *Bixa orellana*.

Natural bixin (*cis* double bond between 6 and 7) has been designated by several names as ordinary bixin, orelean bixin, *cis*-bixin, α-bixin, labile bixin, bixin-11 and lower melting bixin. It crystallizes as violet prisms and melts at 198°. In chloroform solution its absorption maxima are observed at 502, 471 and 446 mm. Bixin shows a high degree of thermostability and is relatively photostable. It is extremely sensitive to iodine, in light, to give all-*trans*-bixin.

On saponification of bixin the methyl ester group is hydrolysed and the resulting di-acid is called norbixin. Bixin and norbixin differ in solubility very much, and form the basis for oil soluble and water-soluble annatto colour, respectively.

On esterification the ethyl or methyl esters can be obtained. Ethyl bixin is used for colouring such as margarine, whereas, methyl bixin has poor tinctorial value. Natural methyl bixin has been obtained synthetically and shown to be identical with the methyl ester of natural bixin. Esters of bixin with higher alcohols like amyl, octyl, octadecyl and decyl have been prepared to be used as colouring agents.

Ishwarane, a tetracyclic sesquiterpene hydrocarbon has been isolated from the leaf oil of *Bixa orellana*. In addition to ishwarane, a few sesqueterpenes and monoterpenes are also reported. Tomentosic acid was isolated from the root of annatto tree. Three new flavone bisulphates have been found to occur in the leaves of *B. orellana* in addition to leucovanidin and ellagic acid. They have been identified as the τ-bisulphates of apigenin and luteolin and 8-bisulphate of hypolactin (1-OH luteolin).

Utilization

Bixin and norbixin are quite stable to pH changes, light exposures and oxidation reactions. They have good compatibility with food components. Annatto is generally employed in India for colouring butter and cheese. For the colouring of 1 kg of butter to ISI specifications, normally about one ml of the commercially available annatto extract in castor oil is sufficient. One litre of annatto colour in castor oil costs about Rs. 50. For colouring cheese dilute alkaline solution of annatto, consisting chiefly of sodium bixinate is used. In other countries annatto

or ethyl bixinate in oil medium are used for colouring margarine. It is also used for colouring citrus juices, concen-trates, drinks, Vienna sausages, candies and fish, especially salmon. A yellow, transparent water soluble ink, stable to heat, hydrogen peroxide and UV light has been prepared from the extracts of annatto. A 0.1% solution of bixin in ethanol has been used as an adsorption indicator in argentometric titrations. The end point is indicated by the precipitate acquiring a rose colour. Coloured coating materials have been made using annatto and cellulose acetate phthalate and used in coating tablets, pills and granules. Addition of annatto seed meal to the fodder of growing chickens has increased the flesh pigmentation. The vitamin A activity of annatto colour has been attributed to the presence of provitamin A in the petroleum ether soluble fraction.

MARIGOLD FLOWERS

Tagetes erecta (Asteraceae) is grown commercially in Mexico, Peru and Ecuador for extraction of xanthophyll pigments from the florets. There is an estimated world area of 8,00 ha given over to cultivation; each plant produces an average about 330 mg of xanthophylls having the same carbon skeletons as the carotenes. Lutein is 3,3'-dihydroxy-α-carotene. Xanthophylls are used commercially as an additive of chicken feed to give colour to egg yolks.

The common English garden marigold, *Calendula officinalis* is used to treat colds and cough.

Red beetroot

Powdered red beetroot, *Beta vulgaris* (Chenopo-

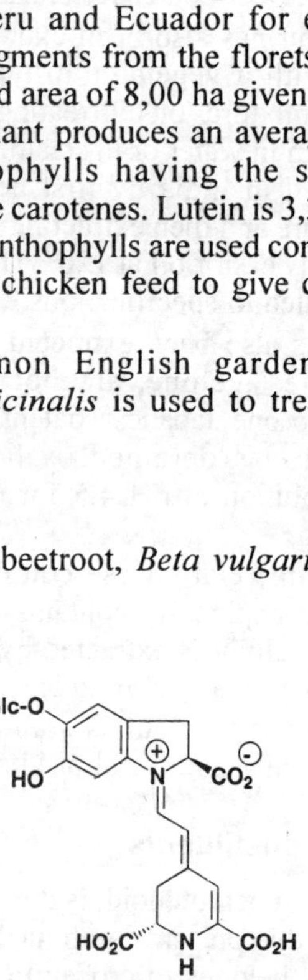

Fig. 23.4. Betanin.

diaceae), and the isolated red pigment betanin are widely used as a nontoxic food and pharmaceutical colourants. Betanin is a nitrogen-containing glycoside which on hydrolysis gives the aglycone betanidin and glucose.

Monascus

Monascus purpurea is a mould which is grown on cooked or autoclaved rice and then the whole dried and pulverized. It gives a food colourant used in Chinese cooking. Strains of mould have been selected to give various shades and that producing the dark red monascorubin is particularly important. With continuous fermentation it is important that the desired product is released to the medium. The red pigment serves as an edible, nontoxic substitute for expensive cochineal.

Red poppy petals

The dried petals of the field poppy or corn poppy, *Papaver rhoeas*, are used in the form of a syrup for colouring and sweetening liquid medicines. The petals contain anthocyanin pigments including the gentiobioside of cyanidin (mecocyanin) and alkaloids.

Red rose petals

The unexpanded petals of the Provence rose, *Rosa gallica*, are used for preparing the acid infusions of rose. The drug is mildly astringent. The infusions are used as a convenient vehicle for gargles containing alum or tannin. The petal extracts are unsuitable for prescribing with alkaline salts, due to the presence of the anthacyanin constituents.

Dyestuffs

Alkanna and henna contain naphthoquinone derivatives. Madder, the root of *Rubia tinctorum*

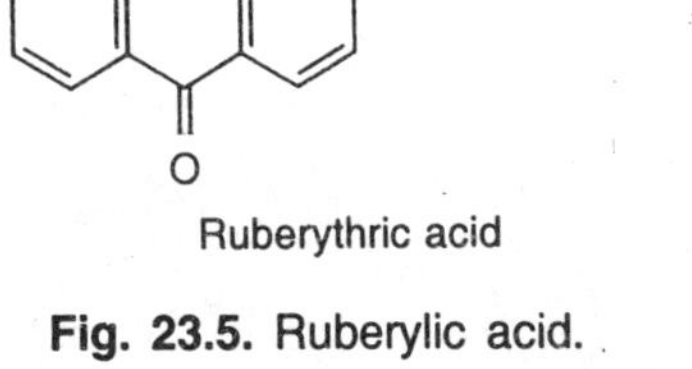

Ruberythric acid

Fig. 23.5. Ruberylic acid.

(Rubiaceae), grown in the area of Avignon, contains anthraquinone derivatives including ruberythric acid. On hydrolysis the latter yields primeverose and alizarin, the pigment responsible for Turkey red colour.

SWEETENING AGENTS

Our body's metabolism demands a continuous supply of its primary fuel, glucose. There are two forms of sugar in the food we eat, namely, naturally occurring sugars in fruits and dairy products and added sugars (white, brown or powdered sugar as well as corn syrup solids) in many processed foods. Sugar adds calories, which, if eaten more than required will cause weight gain. Weight gain increases the risk of getting heart disease, diabetes, high blood pressure or even some types of cancer. Also, if the body doesn't make enough insulin as in diabetes, then the sugar is increased in blood to unhealthy levels. The body breaks down sugar into the sugar you find in your blood (glucose). Unfortunately, there are no vitamins or minerals in sugar and so it is called as "empty" calorie. That is why it is the first food to be eliminated from a weight loss diet.

Sweetening agents to sucrose are used for medical purposes (e.g., for diabetics) and for diet improvement. Saccharin is the most widely used substitute. However, important natural products are:

Sorbitol

Sorbitol (D-glucitol), is a polyhedric alcohol (a hexitol) which was first isolated from mountain ash berries (*Sorbus aucuparia*, Rosaceae). It is prepared synthetically by the catalytic hydrogenation of glucose. Sorbitol solution (Sorbitol liquid) contains 70% of mainly sorbitol and is used as a sweetening agent and vehicle in elixirs, linctuses and mixtures.

Sorbitol is nearly half sweet as sucrose. It has humectant properties, is not metabolized rapidly and is not absorbed on oral ingestion. Therefore, it is used as an ingredient in toothpastes, chewing gums, in many dietetic products, and in conjugation with saccharin and other noncaloric sweetener in dietetic beverages. It acts as an osmotic laxative when taken in large amounts. A solution of hexitol combined with mannitol is used for urologic irrigation.

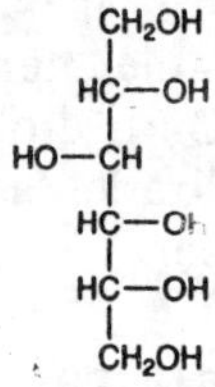

Fig. 23.6. Sorbitol.

Stevioside

Among ent-kaurane glycosides, the most important is stevioside which has properties about three-hundred times that of sucrose. It is obtained from *Stevia rebaudiana* (Asteraceae) growing in north-eastern Paraguay. The plant material (700-1000 tons) is processed annually by Brazil, Japan and other countries. Stevioside is used in soft drinks and food industries.

Stevia

Stevia is an herb that has been used as a sweetener in South America for hundreds of years and currently being heralded as a good substitute (not available in India). It is calorie-free, nontoxic and 100-300 times sweeter than sugar. Stevia can actually increase glucose tolerance and decrease blood sugar levels. Stevia is safe for use with children, is non-glycemic and is plaque-retardant (no cavities). The FDA has not approved Stevia as a sugar substitute, so it is sold only as a dietary supplement, probably due to pressure from the cola aspartame industry.

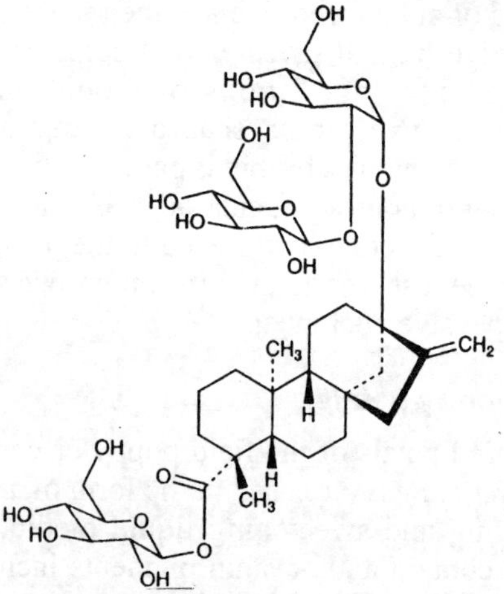

Fig. 23.7. Stevioside.

24

Fibres, Surgical Dressings and Sutures

Natural and artificial fibres are used in surgical dressings. The natural fibres are obtained from vegetable sources (e.g., Cotton, Flax, Hemp and Jute) or from animal sources (e.g., Wool and Silk). These fibres are made up of long chain molecules which may be a carbohydrate or a protein molecule. Some fibres, e.g., Nylon and Terylene, are synthetic fibres prepared from long chain molecules of polymers. Regenerated carbohydrate materials and chemically modified fibres are Viscose, Acetate Rayons, Alginate yarn and Oxidized Cellulose. Asbestos and glass are obtained from mineral sources.

A number of vegetable fibres have importance in pharmacy, particularly as components of surgical dressings and for the manufacture of artificial fibres and haemostatic dressings.

Fibres can be distinguished by chemical test and by studying their microscopic structures. Vegetable and regenerated carbohydrate materials are composed of cellulose units and respond to the following tests :

Tests of vegetable and regenerated carbohydrate fibres

1. With Molisch reagent they produce violet colour.
2. On heating with aqueous picric acid solution they are not stained permanently.
3. With chlor-zinc iodine or a mixture of iodine and sulphuric acid they yield blue colour.

4. On ignition as such or boiling with sodalime they do not produce foul smell.
5. Vegetable fibres are soluble in copper oxide ammonia solution (cuoxam) forming a blue colour.
6. On boiling with Millon's reagent they do not produce red colour.

Tests of animal fibres

Animal fibres are regenerated proteinous compounds containing peptide linkage. They show the following tests :
1. On ignition they produce disagreeable odour.
2. They are dissolved in 5% aqueous potassium hydroxide solution.
3. They respond positively with Millon's test.
4. They are stained permanently with picric acid.

Synthetic and mineral fibres give negative tests of vegetable and animal fibres. Glass fibres melt on heating and form beads. There is no effect of heat on asbestos fibres.

COTTON, RAW COTTON

Cotton consists of the epidermal trichomes of the seeds of *Gossypium herbaceum, G. barbadense* and other cultivated species of *Gossypium* (Malvaceae). The plants are shrubs or small tree. They bear three- to five-celled capsules containing numerous seeds. The USA produces about half of the world's cotton, other important sources being Egypt, India and South America.

The hairs of the different species vary in length or '*staple*'. The average fibre of which is under 25 mm long are called 'short staple' as in American variety; those between 25 and 30 mm 'medium staple' as in Brazilian, Peruvian and Indian varieties, and those from 30 to 40 mm 'long staple' as in Sea Island, up to 54.5 mm; Egyptian, 31-38 mm.

Preparation

The ripe capsules are collected, dried and subjected to a ginning process to separate the hairs from the seed. The gin is designed to pull the hairs through a narrow space. In ordinary American or Upland cotton the gin leaves the seeds with a coating of short hairs which are removed by a second type of gin known as a 'linter'. These short hairs are used for making the lower grades of cotton wool and rayons. The seeds are used for the preparation of cottonseed oil and cattle cake. Raw cotton contains various impurities, such as immature and broken seeds and fragments of leaf. These impurities are removed during the manufacture of yarn.

For spinning very fine yarns Sea Island cotton is used. Different machines are used for various types of yarn, which are known as *combed* and *carded*. The cotton-combine machine separates all the shorter fibres and a thread is spun consisting of long, well-paralleled, uniform fibres. The short fibres of *comber waste* are used for making the best grades of cotton wool. The carding machine uses fibres which are shorter and less uniform in length. The absence of combing is shown in the yarn by the irregular arrangement of the fibres.

Microscopy of unbleached cotton

Cotton consists of unicellular hairs appearing like empty, twisted fire-hoses. Their length is up to about 5 cm, diameter 9-24 µm. The number of twists varies from about 75 cm^{-1} in the Indian to 150 cm^{-1} in the Sea Island.

The apex is rounded and solid. The cotton is cylindrical when young but becomes flattened and twisted as it matures. The large lumen contains the remains of protoplasm. The cellulose wall of the hair is covered with a waxy cuticle which renders it non-absorbent. The cuticle may be stained with ruthenium red. Bleached cotton yarn and absorbent cotton wool are readily wetted by water.

Tests

1. On ignition, cotton burns with a flame, gives very little odour or fumes, does not produce a bead, and leaves a small white ash; distinction from acetate rayon, alginate yard, wool, silk and nylon.

2. Dried cotton is moisten with N/50 iodine and 80% w/w sulphuric acid is added. A blue colour is produced; distinction from acetate rayon, alginate yarn, jute, hemp, wool, silk and nylon.

3. With ammoniacal copper oxide solution, raw cotton dissolves with ballooning, leaving a few fragments of cuticle. Absorbent cotton dissolves completely with uniform swelling; distinction from acetate rayon, jute, wool and nylon.

4. In cold sulphuric acid (80% w/w) cotton dissolves; distinction from oxidized cellulose, jute, hemp and wool.

5. In cold sulphuric acid (60% w/w) cotton is insoluble; distinction from cellulose wadding and rayons.

6. In warm (40°C) hydrochloric acid it is insoluble; distinction from acetate rayon (also silk, nylon).

7. It is insoluble in 5% potassium hydroxide solution; distinction from oxidized cellulose, wool and silk.

8. Treat it with cold Shirlastain A for 1 min and wash out. It shows shades of blue, lilac or purple; distinction from viscose, acetate rayons, alginate yarn, wool, silk and nylon.

9. Treat it with cold Shirlastain C for 5 min and wash out; raw cotton gives a mauve to reddish-brown colour and absorbent cotton a pink one; distinction from flax, jute, hemp. The Shirlastains may be usefully applied to a small piece of the whole fabric under investigation to indicate the distribution of more than one type of yarn.

10. It does not give red stain with phloroglucinol and hydrochloric acid; distinction from jute, hemp and kapok.

11. It is insoluble in acetone distinction from acetate rayon.

ABSORBENT COTTON

Synonyms

Absorbent Wool; Purified Cotton; Kapas (Hindi).

Biological source

Absorbent cotton consists of epidermal hairs of the seeds of *Gossypium herbaceum* Linn. and other species of *Gossypium* like *G. hirsutum*, Linn., *G. arboreum* Linn. and *G. barbadense* Linn. which are freed from adhering impurities deprived of fatty matters, bleached and sterilized (Family : Malvaceae).

Habitat

Cotton is cultivated in Egypt, India, South America, USA, South Africa and Pakistan.

Preparation

The plants are shrubs or small trees which produce 3 to 5 celled capsules possessing numerous seeds. The capsules open on ripening along longitudinal sutures and a mass of white hair attached to the brownish seeds is visible. The cotton fibres are collected, dried and ginned to remove the hair from the seeds. The gin may be a roller or pneumatic type which is designed to pull the hair through a narrow space.

Cotton wool is mainly prepared from linters, card strips, card fly and comber waste. The comber waste of American and Egyptian cottons is preferred for best quality cotton wool. In this the fibres are reasonably long and twisted. They are suitable for producing a cotton wool having an average staple. It offers appreciable resistance when pulled and not shed a significant quality of dust when shaken gently.

Preparation

The comber waste is loosened by machinery and then heated with dilute caustic soda and soda ash solution at a pressure of 1-3 atmospheres for 10-15 h. This removes much of the fatty cuticle and produces the trichome wall absorbent. It is then well washed with water, bleached with dilute sodium hydrochlorite solution and treated with very dilute hydrochloric acid. After washing, it is dried to form a matted condition and is opened up by machines and then 'scutched'. In this way it is converted into a continuous sheet of fairly even thickness with the fibres loosened ready for the carding machine. The carding machine effects a combing operation and forms a thin continuous film of cotton wool. Several such films are superimposed on one another, interleaved with paper and packaged in rolls.

Tests

The tests are similar to that of cotton.

Structure of fibre

The cell wall of absorbent cotton consists of a primary and secondary wall. The formation of the former is modified to embrace the enormous longitudinal development of the cell, some thousands of times greater than the width. The microfibrils are unexpandable and are initially laid down in hoops around the fibre, restricting its lateral growth. Due to different orientation at the fibre end, longitudinal extension can take place. The original orientation is lost as the fibre matures due to development of pressure from successive layers of cellulose. Matrix polysaccharides and proteins derived from the Golgi apparatus are also present in the primary wall. The secondary wall, some 5-10 μm thick and consisting almost entirely of pure cellulose constitutes the main mass of the mature cotton fibre.

Chemical nature

Raw cotton consists of cellulose approximately 90%, moisture 7%, wax, fat, remains of protoplasm and ash.

Absorbent cotton is a very pure form of cellulose. The cellulose molecule is built up of glucose residues united by 1,4-β-glucosidic links. The wall of the cotton fibre, shows anisotropic properties. When swollen in water, the swelling is in a direction at right angles to the long axis with considerable tensile strength. It shows briefringenae in polarized light, value of the double refraction depending on the liquid in which the fibre is immersed. This phenomenon, characteristic of mixed bodies with rod-like structural elements, is known as in polarized light when oriented with its long axis parallel to the plane of polarization than when orientated with the long axis at right angles (dichroism). The fibre wall is built up of elongated structural units orientated in

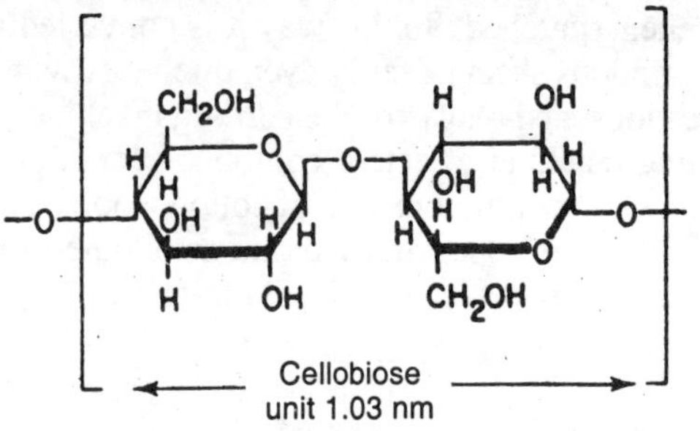

Cellobiose
unit 1.03 nm

Fig. 24.1. Cellobiose unit.

some definite manner (built up of repeating units 1.03 mm long) and orientated in a spiral manner, the spiral making an angle of 30° with the long axis of the fibre. The length of the repeating unit of structure corresponds to that of two glucose residues fully extended. This unit is the 'cellobiose unit', present in the polysaccharide molecule of cellulose.

The biosynthesis of cellulose in the cotton trichome involve UDP-glucose originating from sucrose.

The comber waste is loosened and heated with dilute sodium hydroxide solution and soda ash solution at 1-3 atmospheric pressure for 10-15 hours. Most of the fatty cuticle is removed and trichome wall becomes absorbent in this process. It is washed with water, decolourized with sodium hypochlorite solution and treated with dilute hydrochloric acid. The dried fibres are in matted conditions and opened up by machines. It is converted into a continuous flat sheet, packed and sterilized.

Characters

Absorbent cotton occurs as white, soft, fine hairy filament. Microscopically the filament consists of unicellular hair appearing like empty-twisted five-hoses, 2.5-5 cm in length, 9-24 μm in diameter. The number of twists varies from 75 per cm in Indian variety to 150 per cm in the Sea Island variety. The Cotton hair is cylindrical when young and becomes flattened and twisted on maturing. The Cotton is almost odourless and tasteless.

Purified cotton should be free from alkali, acid, fatty matter, dyes, and water-soluble substances. Such cotton consists almost exclusively of cellulose, a β-linked linear glucopyranosyl polymer. The β-linkage is not hydrolyzed by mammalian enzyme

systems, an important consideration in the application of many cellulose derivatives, but is hydrolyzed by cellulase, which is produced by many microorganisms, including the rumen microflora of herbivorous animals.

Chemical nature

Absorbent cotton consists of cellulose which is composed of glucose units linked by 1,4 β-linear glucoside bonds.

Uses

Absorbent cotton is used for surgical dressings. It serves for mechanical support to absorb blood, mucus and pus. It protects the wound from bacteria. Cotton is also used in textile industry; for manufacturing explosives, cellulose acetate, other cellulose derivatives like carbomethyl cellulose, cellulose acetate phthalate, ethyl cellulose, hydroxypropyl methyl cellulose, methyl cellulose, oxidized cellulose and pyroxilin.

Powdered cellulose is purified, mechanically disintegrated cellulose prepared by processing α-cellulose obtained as a pulp from fibrous plant materials. It exists in various grades and exhibits degrees of fineness ranging from a free-flowing dense powder to a coarse, fluffy, nonflowing material. It is used as a self-binding tablet diluent and disintegrating agent.

Microcrystalline cellulose is a purified, partially depolymerized cellulose prepared by treating α-cellulose, obtained as a pulp from fibrous plant material, with mineral acids. It is used as a diluent in the production of tablets.

Purified rayon is a fibrous form of bleached, regenerated cellulose. It is used as a surgical aid and may not contain more than 1.25% of titanium dioxide.

Gossypol, a dimeric sesquiterpene found in cotton tribe (Gossypiaceae), occurs as dextrorotatory gossypol with varying optical purity but an enantiomer (–) gossypol possessing irreversible antifertility activity in males in detected in excess only in one plant, *Gossypium barbadense*. Gossypol inhibits human sperm, has been renowned due to the discovery of its selective toxicity towards cancer cells.

JUTE

Synonyms

Gunny.

Biological source

Jute consists of the strands of phloem fibres obtained from the stem bark of *Corchorus capsularis* Linn., *C. olitorius* Linn. and other species of *Corchorus* (Family : Tilaceae).

Habitat

It is cultivated throughout the hotter parts of India in Bengal, Assam, Bihar and Orissa as well as in most tropical countries.

Jute is a rainy season crop. The maximum temperature during the crop season rarely exceeds 38°C. The seeds are sown from March to May. The crop is cultivated on alluvial soil. Jute seed is sown broadcast early from mid-February to mid-March. Germination takes place within 2 or 3 days. Jute plants respond quickly to early weeding, thinning and mulching. The plant harvests between June and September.

Preparation

Jute is an annual plant, 3-4 m in height. The straight stems are cut in July during flowering stage. The leaves are removed and the stems are submerged into water tank in bundles for retting. The bundles are covered with straw to protect them from direct sunlight which would make the fibres specky. After 3 weeks the bark from the wood and the strands of phloem fibres from the surrounding softer tissues are removed. The ends of stems are beaten with a mallet to separate the wood from the fibres. The fibres so obtained are cleaned by jerking them backwards and forwards on the surface of the water. They are hanged in the sun to dry and bleach for few days. The fibres are graded on the basis of length, colour and glossiness.

Characters

Jute is a yellowish-brown in colour, 1-3 m long and 30-140 μm in diameter. The individual fibres are 0.8-5 mm long and 10-25 μm in diameter. The apex is bluntly pointed, wall is without markings and lumen is varying in size. They give deep red colour with phloroglucinol, yellow with iodine and sulphuric acid and with chlor-zinc-iodine.

Chemical composition

Jute contains liganocellulose. The middle lamella is extensively lignified and is destroyed by oxidizing agent (a mixture of nitric acid and potassium chlorate).

Uses

Jute is used to prepare medicated tows, as a filtering and straining medium and to make gunny bags, yarns and ropes.

HEMP

Biological source

Hemp is prepared from the pericyclic fibres of the stem of *Cannabis sativa* (Fam. Cannabinaceae). Plant is grown for fibres in Russia, Italy, France and America. The fibres are prepared by retting process as in case of jute. The individual fibre is about 22 μm in diameter and 35-40 mm in length. The fibre ends are bluntly rounded, some ends are bifurcated like fork due to injuries to the stem. The lumen of the hemp fibre is large, uniform and flattened. The wall is thick with fine cross lines, some are intersecting. The fibres give slightly red colour with phloroglucinol, inner wall blue and middle lamella yellow with iodine and sulphuric acid and purple to yellow colour with chlor-zinc iodine. Hemp is used to manufacture rope, twine and sail-cloth.

FLAX

Biological source

Flax is the pericyclic fibres of the stem of *Linum usitatissimum* Linn. (Fam. Linaceae). Flax is prepared by the process of retting similar to jute. Flax fibres are non-lignified with sharply pointed ends, average length is 25-30 mm, diameter varies from 12-25 μm. Some fibres are up to 120 mm long and lumen is narrow. The fibres have good lustre and more tensile strength than cotton. The commercial fibres contain fine transverse injuries received during beating. The fibres of old plants are coarse and harsh in texture. Flax fibres give colourless or slight pink colour with phloroglucinol, blue or violet with iodine and sulphuric acid and purple to yellow with chlor-zinc iodine. Flax consists of pecto-cellulose. It is used as a filtering medium.

WOOL

Synonyms

Animal wool; Sheep's wool.

Biological source

Wool is obtained from the protective covering or fleece of the sheep, *Ovis aries* Linn (Family : Bovidae, order Ungulata).

Geographical source

Wool producing countries are Australia, Russia, Argentina, India and America.

Preparation

Wool obtained from the animal is spreaded on a frame covered with wire netting to separate it into wool of different sizes and qualities. Simul-taneously it is beaten over the netting to remove dust and dirt. The burrs and straw pieces are picked up. The wool is washed in tanks containing warm, soft, soapy water to remove wool greese. The wool is squeezed between rollers, dried and the fibres are mechanically loosened. Then it is carded and spun into yarns.

'Wool grease' from the washing process may be removed by mechanical means or by using organic solvents. Purified 'wool grease' is known as wool fat or anhydrous lanolin. It is employed in cosmetics and ointments.

Characters

Wool consists of elastic, lustrous and smooth hair. The hair are loosely fitted and slippery to touch. The outer most surface, cuticle, consists of imbricated, flattened, translucent epithelial scales. Wool is insoluble in warm hydrochloric acid and in cold concentrated sulphuric acid. Single wool fibre can resist breakage when subjected to weights of 15-30 g and when stretched as much as 25-30% of their lengths. Wool fibre has good to excellent affinity for dyestuffs. It may retain about 17% of moisture of its weight.

Wool fibre is deteriorated by ageing, larval attack such as by cloth moths and carpet beetles, exposure to sunlight and charing at 300°C. It does not continue to burn when removed from a flame. It has good resistance to dry-cleaning solvents, strong alkalies and high temperature.

From the washings of the scouring process 'wool grease' may be separated by mechanical means or by the use of organic solvents. When purified it is known as wool fat or anhydrous lanolin. Potassium salts may be recovered. After washing, the wool is dried, and the fibres are mechanically loosened, carded, and spun into yarn.

Microscopical

The hairs originate in deep hair follicles in the skin and the 'wool grease' is secreted by neighbouring sebaceous glands. Under the microscope, the fibres are seen to be covered with irregular masses of grease, the structure of the hair itself being indistinct. If raw wool is to be mounted for microscopical examination, it should be defatted by ether or chloroform, as it will not otherwise wet with water. Wool hairs are 2-50 cm long and usually 13-40 μm in diameter. As the fleeces are removed by shear-ing, the bases of the hairs are lacking, and tapering ends, known as 'lamb ends' are only found in wool from the first shearing. Three regions of the hair, known as the cuticle, cortex and medullar, and detected.

Cuticle

This consists of imbricated, flattened, translucent epithelial scales. The shape and arrangement of the scales varies in different breeds of sheep, edges being smooth and straight in some and serrated and wavy in others. The number of scales in a 100 μm length is constant, averaging about 9.7-12.1 μm in different wools. Such counts may be used to distinguish sheep's wool from angora wool.

Cortex

The cortex consists of elongated, fusiform cells coalesced into a horny mass in which scattered pigment cells are present.

Medulla

It consists of rounded or polyhedral cells contain-ing fatty matter or pigment and is best seen when its cells contain much air or pigment.

Tests

1. *Characteristic of animal fibres* : Wool resembles silk in its behaviour with picric acid, nitric acid and Millon's reagent. It is readily soluble in 5% potash.
2. *Characteristic of wool* :
   (a) Ammoniacal copper oxide solution causes separation of the scales; it also colours the fibres blue.
   (b) When lead acetate is added to a solution of wool in caustic soda, a black precipitate is formed owing to the high sulphur content (distinction from silk).
   (c) Wool is not appreciably soluble in warm hydrochloric acid (distinction from silk), or in cold concentrated sulphuric acid (distinction from cotton).

Chemical nature

Raw wool consists of wool fibres (31%), 'wool sweat' or 'suint' composed of potassium salts of fatty acids (32%), dirt and dust (25%) and wool grease (lanolin).

Wool fibres are composed of the protein keratin, which is more easily damaged in unfavourable conditions than the cellulose fibres. Keratin is rich in the amino acid cystine. A cystine bridge, joining adjacent polypeptide chains, can be represented as :

$$S—CH_2—CH(NH_2).COOH$$
$$|$$
$$S—CH_2—CH(NH_2).COOH$$

Fig. 24.2. Cystine.

The elasticity arises from a reversible intramolecular transformation of the fibre substance. The radiograph of the stretched fibre closely resembles that given by fibres, such as silk, with fully extended polypeptide chains. In this condition each amino acid residue is 0.34 nm long. This unstable form of keratin is known as β-keratin. The stable form, α-keratin, is contracted and the structural unit, corresponding to three amino acid residues, is 0.51 nm long. The relationship between the two forms can be represented as formulae. The elasticity is then visualized as being due to a reversible opening of the folds. α-Keratin leads to the formation of pseudo-diketo-piperazine rings. The R groups should be visualized as standing out perpendicular to the paper.

These polypeptide grids, flattened in β-keratin, can be represented as buckled in the stable α-keratin. In the building up of the fibre crystallites, the molecular grids are regarded as being orientated parallel to one another and to the long axis of the fibre by intermolecular attraction.

Stability of the protein is due to frequent primary valence cross-links (disulphide bonds) and secondary valence cross-links (hydrogen bonds) between neighbouring polypeptide chains.

Uses

Wool is used to prepare crepe bandages and dressings and as a medium for filtration and staining.

SILK

Biological source

Silk is obtained in the fibre form from the cocoons of *Bombyx mori* Linn. commonly known as silk worm or mulberry silk worm, and other species of *Bombyx* and of *Antheraea* such as *A. mylitta, A. assama, A. pernyi* and *A. yama-mai* (Order : Lepidoptera).

Geographical source

Silk is produced in China, Japan, India, Asia Minor, Italy, France and some other countries. Tie silk of *B. mori* forms the greater part of that used. Wild silks are produced by *Antheraea mylitta* (India), *A. assama* (India), *A. pernyi* (China) and *A. yamamai* (Japan).

Preparation

Cultivation of domesticated silk is called sericulture in which the care of the domesticated silk worm from the egg stage through completion of the cocoon, and also production of mulberry trees for worm food are involved. Before the silk worm passes from the larval or caterpillar to pupal (chrysalis) stage, it secretes an oval cocoon around itself. The cocoon is about 2-5 cm in length and consists of a filament up to 1200 m long. The thread is composed of two silk fibres joined together by a layer of silk glue known as sericin. Strands of semiliquid fibroin, produced by two glands in the insect, flow into a common exit-tube in the head, where they meet the secretion of silk glue produced by another pair of glands. The double fibre with its coating of sericin emerges from a spinneret in the head of the worm, coagulates and hardens on contact with the air and is spun into the cocoon by figure-of-eight movements of the head. If pupal or chrysalis are allowed to mature stage, the insect will escape damaging the cocoon. Therefore, the cocoon are collected at the chrysalis stage and heated at 60-80° for few hours or exposed to steam for a short period to kill the pupae. The cocoons are graded and kept in hot water to soften the silk glue and loosen the fibres. The ends of the fibres from 2-15 cocoons are woven into a single thread by twisting and reeling. Most raw silk is reeled from about five cocoons, and therefore, has 10 brins. Fibres containing less than six brins is very fine and cannot be used for commercial purposes. Silk is then usually scoured by treatment with hot soap solution to remove the sericin.

The double fibre in the coccon is called as a *bave* and its constituent fibres are known as *brins*. Silk containing sericin is called as raw silk. It is cleaned out by treatment with hot soap solution to remove sericin. This process is known as stripping or degumming. The degumming process leaves silk lustrous and semitransparent with a smooth surface. The silk is sometimes treated with a finishing substance, such as metallic salt, to increase its weight, density and to improve draping quality.

Characters

Silk is a continuous filament, 600-1200 m long. Silk fibres are soft, smooth and possess remarkable tensile strength. A silk filament can be stretched about 20% beyond its original length before breaking but does not immediately resume its original length when stretched more than 2%. Silk is soluble in ammonical copper oxide solu-tion, ammonical nickel oxide solution, concen-trated alkalies, and in concentrated hydrochloric acid. It is insoluble in water, alcohol, ether and dilute alkalies.

Microscopy

In fibres of raw silk mounted in water, the diameter of these is several times that of a single brin; the individual brins may be seen although difficult to count; and flakes of silk glue may be seen on the surface. If this raw silk is now boiled with soap solution or dilute sodium carbonate solution, the sericin completely dissolves.

The lack of cellular structure and the breadth of the brins are distinguishing characters of mulberry silk. Brins of mulberry silk measure 10-21 μm (mostly about 16 μm), whereas those of wild silks are 30-60 μm. The latter often show well-marked longitudinal striations.

Silk gives the general tests for animal fibres :

1. Silk is soluble in ammoniacal copper oxide solution. An alkaline solution of copper sulphate and glycerol of a certain strength is used for the separation of silk from wool and cotton.
2. Silk contains little or no sulphur and, therefore, gives no black precipitate with alkali and lead acetate solution (distinc-tion from wool).
3. Silk immediately dissolves in concentrated hydrochloric acid (distinction from wool).

The molecule has a chain-like structure, with a repeating unit 0.7 nm long. This repeating unit, as revealed by radiograph analysis, corresponds in length to that of two fully extended amino acid residues.

Chemical nature

Silk is consisted of the protein fibroin which on hydrolysis yields mainly glycine (44%), alanine (27%), serine (11%), tyrosine (5%) and other amino acids.

Uses

Silk is used for making ligatures and sieves.

REGENERATED FIBRES

Regenerated fibres are prepared from naturally occurring polysaccharides. These compounds are modified to yield a suitable fibre form. Viscose, cellulose acetate, oxidized cellulose and nitrocellulose are the regenerated fibres.

VISCOSE

Synonyms

Rayon; Regenerated cellulose.

Viscose is a viscous orange-red aqueous solution of sodium cellulose xanthogenate obtained by dissolving wood pulp cellulose in sodium hydroxide solution and treating with carbon disulphide.

The starting material is a cellulose prepared from coniferous wood (spruce), or scoured and bleached cotton linters. The wood is delignified similar to cellulose wadding. It reaches the rayon manufacturers as boards of white pulp, containing 80-90% of cellulose and some hemicellulose (mainly pentosans). The hemicellulose being alkali-soluble, are removed in the first stage of the process by steeping in sodium hydroxide solution. The excess alkaline liquor is pressed out and alkali-cellulose (sodium cellulosate) remains. This is dissolved by treatment with carbon disulphide and sodium hydroxide solution to give a viscous solution of sodium cellulose xanthate. After 'ripening' and filtering, the solution is forced through a spinneret, a jet with fine nozzles, immersed in a bath of dilute sulphuric acid and sodium sulphate, when the cellulose is regenerated as continuous filaments. These are drawn together as a yarn, which is twisted for strength, desulphurized by removing free sulphur with sodium sulphide, bleached, washed, dried and conditioned to a moisture content of 10%.

The viscose yarn may be left as such (i.e., *continuous filament-rayon*) for use as blouse fabrics, or it may be cut up to give *staple rayon* ('Fibro') of fixed length from 1 to 8 in. used in surgical dressings and many other fabrics are made to resemble cotton in dimensions. Suitable spinnerets are used to give a diameter of 15-20 μm and the fibre is cut into lengths usually of 4.8 cm. This staple can be processed on types of spinning and weaving machines used for cotton dressings or it may be left in a loose fibre form as *viscose rayon absorbent wool*.

Viscose rayon is a very pure form of cellulose. Its ash contains sulphur. The cellulose molecules of the original natural material are more separated from one another in the viscose solution than in the vegetable material and in the regenerated fibres are still less closely packed. The side-to-side aggregation of the long-chain mole-cules is different from that in natural celluloses. The size of the molecules is also reduced. Wood cellulose have molecules of

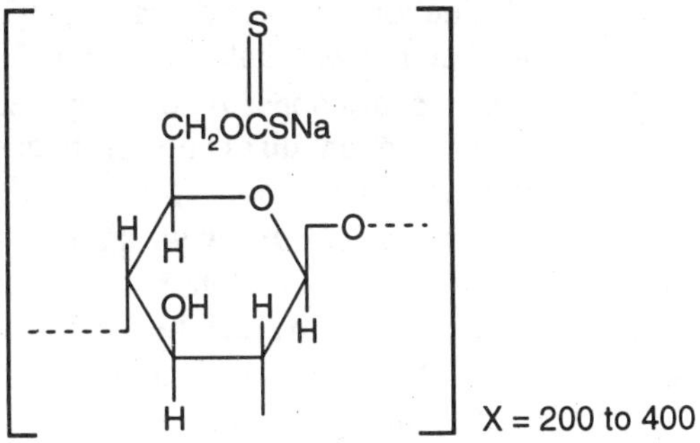

Fig. 24.3. Viscose.

the order of 9000 glucose residue units, while those of viscose rayon have only about 450.

Viscose rayon gauze and other rayon dressings show no loss of absorbency on storage.

Macroscopical characters

The rayon is a white, highly lustrous fibre. Its tensile strength varies from two-third to one- and-a-half times that of cotton. When wetted, it loses about 60% of its tensile strength. It has a proportionately greater loss than is found with cotton. The fabric is a water-repellent (e.g., cotton crepe bandage).

Microscopical characters

The fibres are solid and transparent and 15-20 μm in diameter. They have a slight twist, and show grooves along their length which are principally caused by the spinnerets being immersed in the regenerating solution (compare nylon). The grooves give a characteristic appearance to the transverse section. The ends of the fibres are abrupt and characteristic. The fibres are clearly seen in chloral hydrate solution or in lactophenol, but are almost invisible in cresol. They appear bright in polarized light with crossed Nicols.

Chemical tests

1. The fibres give the general tests for vegetable and regenerated carbohydrate fibres.
2. On ignition they behave like cotton; distinction from acetate rayon and alginate yarn, wool, silk, nylon and glass.
3. With N/50 iodine and sulphuric acid, 80%, they give a blue colour similar to that given by

cotton; distinction from acetate rayon, alginate yarn, jute, hemp, wool, silk and nylon.

4. With ammoniacal copper oxide they behave like absorbent cotton; distinction from acetate rayon, jute, wool and nylon.

5. Cold sulphuric acid, 60% w/w, dissolves the fibre; distinction from cotton, oxidized cellulose, alginate yarn, flax, jute, hemp and wool.

6. Warm (40°C) hydrochloric acid does not dissolve the fibre; distinction from acetate rayon, silk and nylon.

7. It is insoluble in boiling potassium hydroxide solution (5%); distinction from oxidized cellulose, wool and silk.

8. Shirlastain A produces a bright pink; distinction from cotton, oxidized cellulose, acetate, rayon, wool, silk and nylon.

9. Phloroglucinol and hydrochloric acid produce no red stain; distinction from jute, hemp and kapok.

10. The fibres, like cotton, are insoluble in acetone, formic acid 90% or phenol 90%; distinction from acetate rayon and nylon.

Delustring and dyeing of fibres

The appearance of rayon and other artificial fibres with a natural lustrous may be delustred by addition of the white pigment titanium oxide to the solution (e.g., viscose) or to the melt (e.g., nylon) before extrusion of the filaments. The pigment is evenly distributed inside each filament and delustring is permanent. These fibres may be similarly 'spun-dyed' by addition of an appropriate dye instead of the titanium oxide.

Matt viscose (*delustrated viscose rayon*) is normally used in the manufacture of surgical dressings. In general appearance these are very similar to those manufactured from cotton. The individual filaments have the appearance for the matt white colour and on microscopical examination the pigment particles, which appear black by transmitted light and are scattered throughout the filament. The amount of pigment is controlled by the ash value. Titanium is detected in the ash by dissolving in sulphuric acid, diluting and adding hydrogen peroxid, 3% when a yellow colour is produced.

Characters

Viscose is a white, highly lustrous, pure form of cellulose. The molecules contain 450 glucose residue units as compared to 9000 glucose units in wood cellulose. Tensile strength is from two-third to one-and-a-half times that of Cotton. Viscose fibres are solid, transparent, 15-20 μm in diameter, slightly twisted, and contain grooves. Fibre-ends are abrupt and peculiar. The fibres give general tests of vegetable fibres. They can be delustred by addition of white pigment titanium oxide to the solution before preparation of the yarns. The *delustred viscose rayon* or *matt viscose* is used to manufacture surgical dressings. The filaments are identical to Cotton filaments, but they are matted white. The amount of pigment is controlled by assaying ash value.

When viscose solution is allowed to pass through long narrow slits into a regenerating bath, sheets of Viscose are formed. These sheets are washed, bleached, treated with a glycerin solution and dried to produce cellophane. Cellophane is heat-sealable packing material and is also used as a dialysing membrane, as a protective dressing and as a substituent of oiled silk.

Uses

Viscose rayon is used to manufacture fabrics, surgical dressings, absorbent wool, enzyme and cellophane.

METHYLCELLULOSE

Synonyms

Cellulose methyl ether; Methocel, Cellothyl; Syncelose; Bagolax; Cethyplose; Cethytin; Cologel; Cellumeth; Hydrolose; Nicel; Tearisol; Tylose.

Methylcellulose is prepared from wood pulp or chemical cotton by treatment with alkali and methylation of the alkali cellulose with methyl chloride under pressure, to convert hydroxyl groups into methyl ether groups. The molecules containing two of the three hydroxyl methylated groups of the glucose residue units of the cellulose chain are considered of high quality.

Methylcellulose occurs as white, fibrous powder, odourless, tasteless; swells in water and forms a clear to opalescent, viscous, colloidal solution in cold water. It is insoluble in hot water, alcohol and ether. An aqueous solution is best prepared by dispersing the granules in hot water with stirring and chilling to +5°C. The solution is then stable at room temperature. The presence of inorganic salts increases the viscosity. The solubility is dependent upon the degree of substitution. Commercial methylcellulose has a methoxyl content of 29%. Clear film may be casted from the aqueous solution.

Uses

In pharmacy Methylcellulose is used to increase the viscosity and to stabilize lotions, suspensions, pastes, ophthalmic preparations and some ointments. In medicine it is used as a hydrophilic colloid, laxative in chronic constipation and to curb appetite in obese persons as it gives a feeling of fullness. It is also used as a substitute for water-soluble gums; to render paper grease proof, in adhesives, as thickening agent in cosmetics, as protective colloid in emulsions, as binder and stabilizer in foods and as a bulk producer in the formulation of dietetic foods.

Ethylcellulose is an ethyl ether of cellulose containing not less than 44% and not more than 51% of ethoxy groups. It is a free-flowing white powder. Ethylcellulose is a tablet binder and film coating.

Hydroxyethylcellulose is a hydroxyethyl ether of cellulose. It is available in varying degrees of substitution and is used as a thickening agent and as an ingredient in some formulations for artificial tears.

Hydroxypropylcellulose is a hydroxypropyl ether of cellulose. It contains not more than 80.5% of the hydroxypropyl groups. It is used as a stabilizer

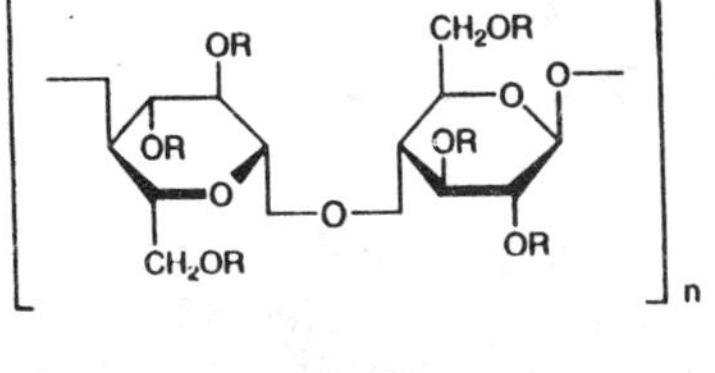

R is H, $-CH_2CH_3$, or $-CH_2CH_2OH$

Fig. 24.4. Cellulose ethyl hydroxylethyl ether.

and thickener in liquid preparations and as a binder and film coating in tablet formulations.

Hydroxypropyl methylcellulose is the propylene glycol ether of methylcellulose in which both hydroxypropyl and methyl groups are attached to the anhydroglucose rings of cellulose by ether linkages. A number of commercial products are available that differ somewhat in the composition of their ether substituents. The ether components of the products used medicinally and pharmaceutically fall in the following ranges : not less than 19% and not more than 30% of methoxy groups and not less than 4% and not more than 12% of hydroxypropyl groups. Hydroxypropyl methylcellulose occurs as a white, fibrous or granular powder. It is used as a suspending agent, a thickening agent, and a tablet excipient. Ophthalmic solution of this hydrophilic polymer are used as topical protectants or artificial tears for contact lenses.

Pyroxylin or *soluble gun* product is obtained by the action of a mixture of nitric and sulfuric acids on cotton. It is a mixture of cellulose nitrates. Pyroxylin is a pharmaceutic aid used in the preparation of collodion, flexible collodion and topical protectants.

Oxidized cellulose and *oxidized regenerated cellulose* are similar products that contain not more than 24% of carboxyl groups; they differ in that they contain not less than 16 or 18%, respectively, of carboxyl groups. They are usually available in the form of sterile pads, pledgets, and strips and are used as local hemostatics.

Cellulose acetate phthalate is a reaction product of phthalic anhydride and a partial acetate ester of cellulose. It contains not less than 19% and not more than 23.5% of acetyl groups and not less than 30% and not more than 36% of phthalyl groups. It is a free-flowing, white powder and is used for enteric coating of tablets. Various forms of *hydroxypropyl methylcellulose phthalate* are also used as tablet-coating agents.

Sodium carboxymethylcellulose is the sodium salt of a polycarboxymethyl ether of cellulose. It is a hygroscopic powder that is used as a suspend-ing agent, a thickening agent, a tablet excipient, and a bulk laxative. It is also used in varying proportions with microcrystalline cellulose to give suspending agents with different viscosities.

Carboxymethylcellulose and its sodium salt are used as bulking agents, usually combined with other drug substances, in products intended for appetite suppression.

CELLULOSE ACETATE

Synonyms

Acetate rayon; Partially acetylated cellulose.

Several acetates of cellulose are known, which differ from one another only in the degree of acetylation. In triacetates, not less than 92% of the hydroxyl groups are acetylated. In characterizing the degree of acetylation, per cent acetyl value and per cent combined acetic acid are used.

All cellulose acetates are obtained by treating cellulose with acetic anhydride at various temperatures for different length of time to produce amorphous white solid material in granular, flake or powder form from which fibres may be produced by extrusion. Acetate rayon is prepared by treating cotton linters or wood cellulose with acetic acid and acetic anhydride in the presence of sulphuric acid as a catalyst to yield acetone-insoluble fully acetylated cellulose (primary acetate). Primary acetylated group is hydrolyzed by addition of water and an acetone-soluble secondary acetate is produced. The acetone solution is forced through a spinneret into a warm air chamber. On evaporation of the solvent filament of Cellulose acetate rayon is obtained.

Characters

Cellulose acetate resembles with Viscose rayon in its appearance. Commercial products do not have sharp melting points. Solubility is affected by the acetyl value; the triacetate is insoluble in water, alcohol, ether, but soluble in glacial acetic acid. The penta acetate is insoluble in water, but soluble in alcohol. The filaments are highly lustrous, grooved and slightly twisted.

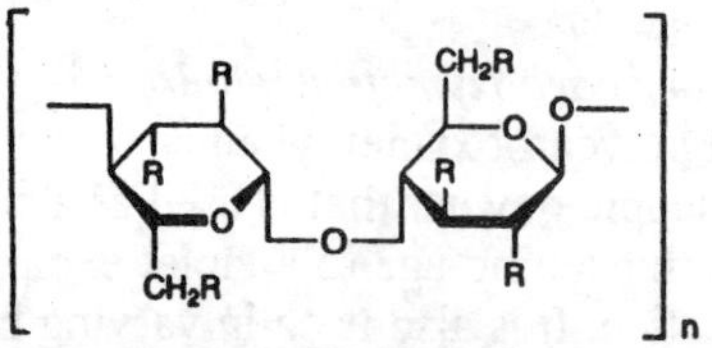

R = –OOCCH$_3$

Fig. 24.5. Cellulose triacetate.

Uses

Cellulose acetate rayon is used to manufacture rubber and celluloid substitutes, nonflammable photographic and cinema films, airplane dopes, varnishes and lacquers, filaments, phonograph records; water-proofing fabrics and rendering balloons gas-tight; sizing and finishing fabrics, coating skins, insulating electric wires; and tow for cigarette smoke filters. Acetate rayon is much less absorbent than viscose rayon. It is, therefore, unsuitable for manufacturing surgical dressings.

Carmellose Sodium (*sodium carboxymethyl-cellulose*) is an odourless and tasteless white hygroscopic powder or granules prepared by the action of monochloroacetic acid on alkali cellulose and removal of the byproduct salts. Substitution of hydroxyl groups by carboxymethyl groups occurs over a range depending on the conditions and the cellulose used. It is water-soluble, and a grade giving a medium viscosity contains 0.7 carboxymethyl groups per glucose residue units. It is insoluble in organic solvents. Its pharma-ceutical and medical uses are similar to those of methyl cellulose. As a laxative it is a useful antacid.

Pyroxylin (Cellulose nitrate)

Pyroxylin is prepared by the action of nitric and sulphuric acids on wood pulp or cotton linters that have been freed from fatty materials. When dry it is explosive and must be carefully stored, dampened with not less than 25% its weight of isopropyl alcohol or industrial methylated spirits. It is used for making Flexible Collodion BP.

Absorbable haemostatic dressings

Gelatin sponge, oxidized cellulose and alginate dressings are used to check bleeding and there is no need to remove them after the bleeding has been checked, since they are absorbed by the tissues.

OXIDIZED CELLULOSE

Synonyms

Absorable cellulose; Cellulosic acid; Poly-anhydro-glucuronic acid; Oxycel; Hemo-Pak.

It is a cellulose of varied carboxyl content retaining the fibrous structure. It is prepared by oxidizing cotton wool or gauze with nitrogen dioxide until the number of carboxylic groups formed by the oxidation of the primary alcohol groups of the glucose moieties of the cellulose molecules reaches 16-22 per cent. After reaction the cellulose molecule contains glucuronic acid residue units and some glucose residue units.

Characters

Oxidized cellulose is identical with the normal cotton in appearance. It has dull colour, a harsher texture, charred odour and a sour taste. It tends to disintegrate on handling and does not turn into pasty on chewing. The degree of oxidation is sufficiently high to make the product soluble in dilute alkaline solutions. It is insoluble in water or acidic solutions.

Tests

1. Oxidized cellulose does not give the tests for animal fibres and animal source-haemostatics.
2. On ignition it behaves like normal cotton.
3. With iodine and sulphuric acid or ammonical copper oxide solution it behaves like absorbent cotton.
4. It is slowly soluble in 80% sulphuric acid.
5. It is insoluble in warm hydrochloric acid.
6. It is soluble in the cold in 5% potassium hydroxide solution. Complete solubility in aqueous alkali is made the basis of a test for absence of unchanged cotton and foreign particles. The solution in alkali gives with excess acid a white flocculent precipitate.
7. It reduces Fehling's solution.
8. Shiriastain A gives a pale blue to mauve colour.
9. Shirlastain C gives a brown to olive green.

Uses

It is used as an absorbable haemostatic in surgery, but is incompatible with penicillin, delays bone repair and cannot be sterilized by heat. It is applied in chromatography.

ALGINATE FIBRES

Alginate fibres are composed of calcium alginate. An aqueous solution of sodium alginate is pumped through a spinneret which is immersed in a bath containing acidic calcium chloride solution. In the bath sodium cations are substituted with calcium cations and the insoluble calcium alginate is precipitated as continuous filaments. The filaments are collected, washed and dried for surgical purposes. The filaments are cut up to give stable form of length 1 to 8 inches for preparing calcium alginate wool or a fabric. Trace amounts of substances are added to the calcium alginate to inhibit mould and bacterial growth.

Alginate fibres are fairly lustrous and pale cream coloured. The fibres may be processed into absorbable, haemostatic dressings. They give general tests for vegetable fibres. They are soluble in ammonical copper nitrate and 5% sodium citrate solution.

Alginic acid is composed of polymers of both mannuronic and glucuronic acids. The properties of the two are variable and alginates of different origin have different compositions and properties. Kalostat haemostatic dressing is derived from the seaweed *Laminaria hyperborea* collected off the Norwegian coast and yields an alginate with a glucuronic-mannuronic ratio of 2 : 1. Other dressing is prepared from *Laminaria* and *Ascophyllum* species collected off the west coast of Scotland and gives an alginate with a glucuronic mannuronic acid ratio of about 1:2. On a wound surface the α-linkages of the glucuronic acid polymer are not easily broken so that fibre strength is retained and a strong gel is formed on contact with the wound exudate. A high ratio of mannuronic acid polymer (β-linkages) yields a product giving a weaker gel and less retention of fibre strength. The Kalostat dressing can be removed from the wound with forceps and Sorbsan is removed by irrigation with sodium citrate solution.

Calcium alginate fibres of commerce contain substantial traces of substances used to inhibit mould and bacterial growth in the sodium alginate spinning solution. Spinning lubricants such as lauryl or cetyl pyridinium bromide (antibacterial) are also applied to the filaments. These substances must not be used in the case of bacteriological swabs.

Before use as an absorbable haemostatic dressing some calcium alginate dressing must be immersed in sodium chloride to give a fibre of the calcium alginate covered by sodium alginate. The degree of conversion is conditioned to give the desired rate of absorption when in use; the greater the proportion of sodium alginate the faster the absorption rate.

Alginate filaments are composed of salts of the

long-chain molecules of alginic acid and there is little cross-linking between the chains in the fibre.

Appearance

These fibres are fairly lustrous with pale cream-colour which in microscopical appearance are very similar to those of viscose rayon, being solid grooved rods. The haemostatic dressing is almost tasteless and odourless and rather harsh to touch. The gauze is usually a knitted fabric. That with a fast rate of absorption when chewed readily assumes a pasty form like that of mashed potato. That with a slow rate of absorption remains smoothly coarser in the same time. They do not disintegrate easily on handling. First-aid dressings frequently embody an alginate gauze impregnated with a local anaesthetic.

Tests

These refer to calcium alginate fibre or the mixed sodium and calcium salt fibre. They give the general tests for vegetable and regenerated carbohydrate fibres.

1. The fibre burns in a flame and goes out when removed from flame.
2. With (N/50) iodine and sulphuric acid, a brownish-red colour is produced, the filaments swell and dissolve to leave a strand of insoluble alginic acid.
3. In ammoniacal copper nitrate solution they swell and dissolve.
4. The fibres are insoluble in 60% w/w sulphuric acid.
5. The fibres are insoluble in warm (40°C) hydrochloric acid.
6. The fibres are insoluble in boiling 5% KOH (swell and acquire a yellow tint).
7. The fibres are soluble in 5% sodium citrate solution.
8. Fibre, 0.1 g, boiled with 5 ml of water remains insoluble but dissolves when 1 ml 20% w/v sodium carbonate solution is added and boiled for 1 min. A white precipitate of calcium carbonate is formed, depending on the proportion of original calcium alginate pre-sent. When centrifuged and the clear supernatant acidified, a gelatinous precipitate of alginic acid is produced. The precipitate will give a purple

colour after solution in NaOH and addition of an acid solution of ferric sulphate.
9. Shirlastain A gives a reddish-brown colour.
10. Alginate haemostatic fibres are invisible in polarized light with crossed Nicols.

Uses

The alginate absorbable haemostatic dressings are non-toxic and nonirritant. They have advantages over oxidized cellulose, which include selective rate of absorption, sterilization (and resterilization) by autoclaving or dry heat and compatibility with antibiotics such as penicillin. They are used internally in neurosurgery, endural and dental surgery to be subsequently absorbed. Externally, they are used (e.g., for burns or sites from which skin grafts have been taken) to arrest bleeding and form a protective dressing which may be left or later removed in a manner appropriate to the type of dressing employed. Protective films of calcium alginate may also be used by painting the injured surface with sodium alginate solution and then spraying it with calcium chloride solution.

Calcium alginate wool as a swab for pathological work or bacterial examination of such things as food processing equipment and table-ware permits release of all the organisms by disintegration and solution of the swab in, for example, Ringer's solution containing sodium hexametaphosphate.

In fabrics the calcium alginate fibres would disintegrate in alkaline solutions (laundering), but this advantage is turned to a commercial virtue by the use of the yarn as a scaffolding thread to support yarns normally too fine to survive the weaving process. The scaffold is removed by an alkaline bath to leave a lightweight fabric.

Cellulose wadding

It is prepared from high-grade bleached sulphite wood pulp in the form of boards about 0.75 m square and 1 mm thick. These are packed in bales containing about 180 kg pulp. The pulp is put in a 'beater', to mix with about 20 times its weight of water and the mixture circulates between a power-driven roll and the bed-plate of the 'beater'. The effect of this is to break up the pulp into separate fibres. When this process is complete, the contents of the beater are mixed with a further quantity of water and then allowed to run in a steady flow on to the 'wire' of the paper machines. This 'wire' is a very fine wire gauze through which water runs, leaving a fine web of fibres on top of the 'wire'. This web is then dried and creped to give a thin, soft, absorbent sheet. About 30 of these thin sheets are laid together to form cellulose wadding.

When examined microscopically, chemical wood pulps or cellulose wadding show characteristic woody elements give lignin reaction (distinction from mechanical wood pulp). Tracheids with bordered pits and characteristic medullary ray cells are usually observed. The cellulose nature of the walls is shown by the blue colour obtained with iodine followed by 80% sulphuric acid and by their solubility in an ammoniacal solution of copper oxide.

Uses

Alginate fibres are used as absorbable haemostatic dressings; in neurosurgery, endaural and dental surgery; internally to arrest bleeding and form protective dressing for burns or sites from which skin grafts have been taken. Alginate fibres are compatible with antibiotics like penicillin. Calcium alginate wool is used as a swab for pathological work or bacterial study.

SYNTHETIC FIBRES

Synthetic fibres are produced by polycondensation of organic molecules which are more stronger than the natural fibres. Nylon, terylene, orlon and polyethylene are the polymers used as pharmaceutical aid.

NYLON

Synonyms

Caprolan; Enkalon; Grilon; Kabron; Mirlon; Perlon; Phrilon; Amilon.

Nylon is a manufactured fibre in which fibre forming substances are long-chain synthetic polyamide having recurring polyamide groups ($-CONH_2-$) as an integral part of the polymer chain. Nylon is usually prepared by condensing adipic acid with hexamethylene diamine. The molted polymer is pumped through a spinneret to produce filaments.

The filaments are smooth, solid cylinders, soften at 210° and melts at 223°; moisture regain is about 4%. Swelling is low. They are immune to microbiological attack; resistant to most organic chemicals, but dissolves in phenol, cresol and strong acids. They may be highly lustrous to dull white or coloured. On ignition the fibres melt and form a hard bead. They are soluble in 5 M hydrochloric acid, 90% formic acid, 90% phenol and insoluble in acetone. Chemically, nylon is represented as :

$$H-[NH (CH_2)_5 CO]_n OH; n = approx 200$$

Uses

Nylon is used to prepare filter cloth, sieves, non-absorbable sutures, nylon syringes, film, textile fibres, monofilament, tire cord, fishing lines and tow ropes.

TERYLENE (DACRON)

Terylene is a polyester fibre produced by condensating ethylene glycol with terephthalic acid. Its chemical formula may be represented as $H[OCH_2 CH_2 OOC C_6 H_4 CO]_n OH$. Terylene fibres are prepared by an identical process to that for nylon. On heating the fibres with phosphoric acid (90%) for 1 minute, it retain its form. This test is negative in case of nylon. Terylene is used in the same way as nylon.

ORLON

Synonyms

Polyacrylonitrile; Fiber A.

Orlon is obtained by polymerizing acrylonitrile. It is represented as $[CH_2 CH (CH)]_n$. It is a white fibre; sticks at 235°; ironing temperatures above 160° may cause yellowing; sp gr. is 1.17. Its inflammability is similar to that of rayon and cotton. Generally it has very good resistance to mineral acids; excellent resistance to common solvents, oils, greases, neutral salts, sunlight but it is degraded by strong alkalies. It resists attack by molds, mildew and insects. The 100% poly-acrylonitrile fibres are rarely used commercially due to difficulty in dyeing.

Orlon fibre is suitable for furnishing (awnings, tents, furniture), anode bags in electroplating, knitwear, rugs and dressings.

POLYETHYLENE

Synonyms

Polythene; Ethene homopolymer; Agilene; Alathon; Alkathene; Courlene; Lupolen; Platilon.

Polyethylene is prepared by polymerization of liquid ethylene at high temperature and under pressure. The polymer is a plastic solid of milky transparency, tough and flexible at room temperature, m.p. 85-110°.

It is a good electrical insulator. It burns but hardy supports combustion. It is stable to water, non-oxidizing acids and alkalies, alcohols, ethers, ketones and esters at ordinary temperature. It is attacked by oxidizing acids such as nitric acid, perchloric acid, free halogens, benzene, petroleum ether, gasoline and lubricating oils, aromatic and chlorinated hydrocarbons. It has flexibility over a wide range of temperature.

The polymer $[CH_2–CH_2]_n$ is transformed into filaments by melt spinning and heat sealable packing film by the similar process as adopted in nylon.

Uses

Polyethylene is used as laboratory tubing, in making protheses, electrical insulation; packing materials, kitchenwire; tank and pipe linings; paper coatings and textile. As fibres are resistant to acid, alkali and most solvents, they are used in filtering fabrics. An outstanding property of poly-ethylene, both as resin and filament, is its low specific gravity (0.92). A low softening point (110°) limits it application in wearing apparel uses.

SURGICAL DRESSINGS

A material used to protect a wound and to heal is called a surgical dressing. They serve various function for the injured site. They remove wound exudates from the site, prevent infection, give physical protection to the healing wound and mechanical support to the supporting tissues. A good quality of dressing should be durable, easy to handle, sterilized, formed from loose threads and fibres and it should not adhere to the granula-ting surface.

Surgical dressings are classified as :

1. **Primary wound dressings** : Primary wound dressings are applied over the wound surface to absorb pus, mucus and blood. They minimize maceration. Some dressings adhere to the wound surface and cause pain on removing them. Now nonadherent dressings are available such as petrolatum-impregnated gauge, viscose gauze impregnated with a bland, hydrophilic oil-in-water emulsion or an absorbent pad faced with a soft plastic film having openings.

2. **Absorbents** : Absorbent cotton is widely used to absorb wound secretions. Other absorbent materials are rayon wool, cotton wool, gauze pads, laparotomy sponges, sanitary napkins, disposable cleaners, eye pads, nursing pads and cotton tip applications. They are used in the shape of balls or pads.

3. **Bandages** : A bandage is a material which holds dressing at the required site, applies pressure or supports an injured part or checks haemorrhage. The bandages may be elastic or non-elastic in nature. Common gauze roller bandage and muslin bandage rolls are employed most frequently. Elastic bandages may be woven to form elastic bandage, crepe bandage and conforming bandage.

4. **Adhesive tapes** : Surgical adhesive tapes may be a rubber-based adhesive or an acrylate adhesive. Rubber adhesive tapes are cheap, superior and provide strength of backing. In case of operation or post-operation acrylate, adhesive tapes are used to reduce skin trauma.

5. **Protectives** : Protectives are employed to cover wet dressings, poultices and for retention of heat. They prevent the escape of moisture from the dressing. Some protectives are plastic sheeting, rubber sheeting, waxed or oil-coated papers and plastic-coated papers.

SUTURES AND LIGATURES

A surgical suture is a thread or sting used for sewing or stiching together tissues, muscles and tendons with the help of a needle. If these threads or fibres are used to tie a blood vessel to stop bleeding without the use of a needles, then they are digested in animal tissues, e.g., catgut, kangaroo tendon and synthetic polyesters. If the sutures are not absorbed in the body, they are called nonabsorbable sutures, e.g., Silk, Cotton, Nylon, Synthetic Polyester fibres and Stainless Steel wire. A good quality of suture should be well-sterilized, non-irritant; having well-mechanical strength, fine gauze and with minimum time of absorption.

Absorbable sutures

Surgical catgut

Catgut is a sterilized fibre or strand prepared from collagen of connective tissues obtained from healthy animals like sheep and cattle.

Preparation

The submucosal layer of small intestine of a freshly killed animal is used for the preparation of catgut. About 7.5 meter long intestine is cleaned and split longitudinally into ribbons. The inner most mucosa and two outer layers of submucosa, muscularis and serosal layers, are removed with the help of a machine leaving behind the submucosa. Up to six such ribbons are stretched, spun and dried to form a uniform strand. These fibres are polished to get smooth strings, gauzed for their diameter, cut into suitable lengths and sterilized by placing the catgut in glass tubes filled with anhydrous high-boiling liquids like toluene or xylene and then heating in an autoclave. Sterilization may be done by irradiating the suture by electron particles or by gamma rays from cobalt-60.

Kangaroo tendons, used in hernia and bone repairs, are prepared from the tails of kangaroo by the identical method adopted for the preparation of catgut. Chromicized surgical catguts are prepared by soaking the ribbons in solutions of chromium salts for tanning the tissues. These fibres are not affected by proteolytic enzymes in the body and they are not absorbed rapidly in the body.

Synthetic polyesters

The polymers obtained by condensation of cyclic derivatives of glycolic acid (glycolide) with cyclic derivatives of lactic acid (lacticide) are used to prepare synthetic absorbable sutures. These sutures have high tensile strength and degradated by hydrolysis and absorbed in the tissue.

Non-absorbable sutures

Non-absorbable sutures are not affected by the body fluid and remained unchange for a long period. They are removed after healing of the wounds. Silk, cotton, nylon and metallic sutures are classified as non-absorbable sutures.

Silk sutures

Silk sutures are prepared by spinning or twisting silk fibres into a single strand of varying diameters. The sutures are smooth and strong and braided by combining several twisted yarns into a compact mass. The strands are sterilized and boiled with water to soften them.

Cotton sutures

Cotton sutures have uniform size and recommended in critical parts where strength of the sutures is required for long time.

Nylon sutures

The microfilaments of nylon are braided into strands of required diameter. These sutures are strong, water resistant and used in skin and plastic surgery.

Linen suture

A linen suture is cheap, very strong under moist condition but not uniform in diameter.

Metallic sutures

Metallic wires of silver or stainless steel are used as surgical aid. These wires are available as monofilaments, twists and braids.

25

Pesticides

Pest control is a major problem in cultivation of plants throughout the world. A pesticide is any toxic substance used to kill animals or plants that cause economic damage to crop or ornamental plants or are hazardous to the health of domestic animals or humans.

Rodents damage stored food products in homes and in warehouses. Weeds interfere with the normal growth of crop and garden plants. Fungi grow on vegetable and fruit plants. Various types of insects destroy the crop and food articles.

All pesticides interfere with normal metabolic processes in the pest organisms and often are classified according to the type of organism they are intended to control, *viz*., fungicides, herbicides, insecticides, rodenticides, molluscacides, nematocides and fumigants. Methods of these pesticides employ similar toxic substances. The means of application, chemical nature, types of products, precautions to be taken, symptions of accidental poisoning and immediate means of treatment are part of knowledge which must be known to the distributors and customers. The manufacturer must provide the efficacy of the product, its safety toward human beings, crops, livestock, wildlife and the general environment. The pesticide should not be deposited as residue on food which causes such a hazard.

Types of pests

Rodents and anthropods are the most destructive animal pests. The plant pests include weeds and the fungi pathogenic to cultivated plants.

Rodents

Rodents are mammals like rat, mouse, rabbit and monkey, which have sharp gnashing incisor teeth. In some stores the crude drugs are often contaminated due to fecal pallets and hair from the fur of rats and mice. Rodents are responsible for transmitting diseases from which they are suffering. Biting of a rat causes rat-bite fever, an infectious disease caused by microorganisms. A large number of lice infected rodents transmit typhus fever, bubonic plague and rat leprosy. Rats carry ticks and mites which cause tularemia, Rocky Mountain spotted fever and undulant fever infections.

Arthropods

Arthropods are the insects, spiders, ticks, mites, and lice. Some of these cause discomfort only, while others cause fatal diseases. Insects represent the class of the phylum Arthropoda and according to their mouth parts they are divided into two morphologic groups :

1. biting and chewing, and
2. piercing and sucking.

The insects of the first category are dependent on the leaves and stems of plants. They are present in excess number in a cultivated field. Grass-hoppers and locusts destroy the crop during the developmental process and after maturity stage. Tomato horn worms and army worms cause destruction during larva or caterpiller stage.

Most of the insects possess a piercing-sucking modification of mouth parts with which they penetrate into the epidermal tissues of plant organs and suck the juice from the soft tissues. The examples are aphids (plant lice), San Jose scale, Chinch bugs, squash bugs, cabbage bugs and leaf-hoppers.

Cockroaches, termites, silverfish, cloth moths, carpet beetles, flies, bedbugs, fleas, and mosquitoes are house hold insects which have either chewing jaws or possess a piercing sucking mechanism. Mosquitoes and deerflies bite human beings and animals. The malarial mosquito expels some of its protozoan-laden saliva during penetration of the human epithelium. The microorganisms enter the blood stream when the long hollow tube, called probocis, contacts the capillaries to obtain the drop of blood. Malaria, yellow fever, sleeping sickness, dengue fever and other infectious diseases are spread by this process. The destruction of mosquitoes, flies, ticks and related arthropods stop spreading of these disastrous diseases for ever.

Piercing-sucking mouth parts are present in lice, fleas, mites, ticks and spiders. Rocky Mountain spotted fever is spread by the wood tick, *Dermacentor andersoni* and the dog tick, *D. variabilis*. The rat flea, *Xenopsylla cheopsis*, is responsible for the spread of endemic typhus fever and the body mouse, *Pediculis corporis*, causes typhus. Mites like *Sarcoptes scabiei* produce scabies. The hairy spiders bite can kill birds and small mammals. The black widow spider, *Latrodectus mactans*, bite is painful. A bacterium transmitted to human beings by the bite of a deer tick, *Ixodes ricinus*, causes lyme disease in USA which is an affliction of summer.

Weeds

Any undesirable plant is known as weed. A weed may be a dandelion in a lawn, a thistle plant (Gokhru) in a vegetable garden, or mustard in a clove field. Undesirable plants in gardens interfere in the growth of cultivated plants by consuming most of the available water contents and minerals of the soil. Weeds grow and flourish in the conditions of much sunshine, ample moisture and well-fertilized soil which are provided for cultivation of some ornamental plants and vegetables. If weeds are allowed to grow, they will soon acquire possession of the garden and gradually destroy the more dilicate, cultivated plants. Similarly, the quality of the field crops, specially grains, become poor due to the presence of weed seeds.

A considerable number of weeds are toxic in nature. Corn cockle, *Agostemma githago*, contains a cyanophore type of glycoside, and its seeds cause death when they are present in excessive quantities in wheat flour. A large number of plants give rise to allergic reactions in certain individuals. Once a person has been sensitized to a particular allergen, subsequent exposure to the materials produces an antigen-antibody reaction which results in the liberation of histamine or identical compounds causing allergic symptoms. Allergies are commonly asthma and dermatitis. Pollens of grasses like timothy (*Phleum pratense*), cocks foot (*Dactylis glomerata*) and perennial rye (*Lolium perenne*) as well as that of nettle (*Urtica dioica*), Plantain (*Plantogo* spp.) and ragweeds (*Ambrosia* spp.) are responsible for seasonal hay fever. A number of common moulds produce spores which cause rhinitis and asthma in sensitive individuals. *Rhus* spp. like *R. radicans* (poison ivy), *R. toxicodendron* (poison oak), *R. deversiloba* (Pacific poison oak) and *R. vernix* (poison elder) (fam. Anacardiaceae) contain contactant allergens which produce severe dermatitis associated with watery blisters. Sesquiterpene lactones from the species of Asteraceae, Lauraceae and Magnoliaceae and from the Liverwort *Frullania* (Fam. Jubulaceae) are a major class of compounds causing allergic contact dermatitis in human. The fruits and seeds of *Menispermum canadense* and *Datura stramonium* are poisonous when swallowed.

Some of the poisonous fungi when taken orally produce hallucinations. The examples are *Amanita, Psilocybe* and *Conocybe*. Certain cacti contain protoalkaloids, some of which have marked hallucinogenic properties.

Fungi parasitic on plants

Various type of fungi growing on plants produce many diseases such as wheat rust, white pine blister rust, Dutch elm disease, hollyhock rust, orange leaf rust of black berries and raspberries, asparagus rust and rose rust. Various fungicides and chemical agents are available for the control of fungus disease. Precaution is taken from the beginning of cultivation of a crop. The seeds should be freed of adhering fungus spores before being planted. It is treated with a suitable fungicide such as Thiram (tetramethyl-thiuram disulphide). Different type of windborne bacteria and fungi grow on tender shoots. They contaminate young seedlings and plants growing near these infected plants. In such cases, sprays or fungicidal dusts are applied to prevent germination of the parasite species.

Different types of microorganisms produce a number of plant diseases. Viral diseases are caused by tobacco mosaic and the bean mosaic. Bacteria are responsible for the diseases like carrot rot, 'fire blight' of pear and apple and the wilt of cucumber, squash and melon. Physymcetes cause 'damping off' fungus, downy mildew of grapes and 'late blight' of potatoes. The diseases such as powdery mildew of lilac, American chestnut blight and Dutch elm disease are produced by Ascomycetes. The micro-organisms Ascomycetes cause the corn smut, 'loose smut' of oats, wheat rust, apple rust and other rusts.

Methods of control of pests

The following methods are adopted for pest control.

Mechanical method

Mechanical methods include hand-picking, burning, trapping and pruning. Large caterpillers, *e.g.*, a large, green tomato hornworm larva, can be located rapidly and removed by hand. Weeds are removed by handpicking. The tent caterpillers gather on branches of trees and shrubs. By pruning or cutting out such branches is an effective measure. If the insect's tent is located near the trunk where cutting is difficult, then this part is burnt by a torch of burning oil-soaked rags at the end of a long pole. Burning helps in destruction of both animal pests removed by hand-picking or pruning.

For determining the spread of certain flying insects in an infected area, they are trapped by a pleasantly flavoured attractant placed in funnel-shaped containers. Anise oil, Rose oil or other attractants are mixed with sawdust and placed in glass containers over which a funnel-shaped entrance has been fitted. The insects fly or crawl through the opening into the jar. Japanese beetles, gypsy moth and codling moth are located by this method.

Special traps are used to catch larger field insects, rats and mice. Metal reinforcement corners on window frames and door sills are used to prevent the access of rodents to storage sheds. Modern concrete warehouses are helpful to control rodents. Window screens, electrified screens, specially coloured lights and other devices are also used for controlling insects.

Biological methods

Some animals or insects feed upon smaller forms which destroy the plants. Some insects have a short life cycle which parasitize larger insects. For examples, rabbits are helpful in destroying certain type of weeds. Cat, owls, kites and hawks are enemies of mice and rats. Insects are eaten by birds.

Certain flies and wasps lay eggs on the body of large destructive insects like slow-moving larvae. The eggs of the parasitic insects hatch rapidly into small larvae which consume the body tissues of the larger species. Ultimately, the larger forms die and the parasitized organism is deve-loped into cotton stage. It is emerged as an adult fly and begins the cycle once again.

Environmental methods

The environmental conditions surrounding the pest are changed either by removing its food supply or by interfering the completion of its life cycle. Mosquito larvae in water are killed by spreading a layer of oil.

Agricultural methods

A more select crop plant is developed that will resist attack by pests like fungus and bacterial attack. Plants can absorb sufficient organic phosphorus compounds through the roots and foliage to cause the death of insects eating the leaves. Crop rotation is another useful agricultural method. If the chief source of food of a particular insect is withheld for one or more seasons, insects are controlled dramatically. The development of varieties of winter wheat, grown when insect pests are inactive, is important. Grub stage of some insects is unearth by deep ploughing rather than shallow furrowing.

Chemical method

Chemicals are designated to be effective as rodenticide (against rats, mice and moles), insecticides (against various insects and arthropods), herbicides (against weeds and undesirable plants) and fungicides (against all types of fungi).

Particular chemical agents are used as poison baits, spray solutions, suspensions for spraying, aerosols, fumigants, residual poisons, stomach poisons and repellents. They may be inorganic, or organic compounds obtained from natural sources, or synthetic organic complexes.

Pest control by chemicals

The choice of chemicals is dependent on the type of pest. If the pest is a rat or mouse, the chemical used will differ according to the locating conditions of the pest. An insect pest may be a chewing or sucking type, a running or flying type, an indoor or outdoor type. Similarly, chemicals are selected properly to control weeds and parasitic fungi, herbicide or fungicide.

Rodenticides

Poisonous chemicals are put into poison baits to control rats and mice. The chemicals must be sufficiently toxic to kill in reasonably small amounts. A chemical known as Norbormide, is the most effective rodenticide. Norbormide consistently kills the laboratory rats but has no effect upon other test animals. The other most effective synthetic rodenticide is Warfarin, 3-(α-acetonylben-zyl)-4-hydroxycoumarin. It does not kill all rodents. Other chemicals are sodium fluoroacetate also known as 1080, 2-pivalyl-1-, 3-indandione or Pival, α-naphthyl-thiourea or ANTU, thallium sulphate, zinc phosphide, arsenic trioxide and barium carbonate. Precautions must be taken that animal pets and small children should not swallow any of these poisonous chemicals.

Two natural plant products used as rodenticides are Red Squill and strychnine. Red Squill and White Squill are both varieties of *Drimia maritima* (Fam. Liliaceae). The Red Squill has reddish-brown outer scales while deep purple inner ones are present in white variety. In addition to other cardio-active glycosides, the bulb of the Red Squill also contains the glucosides scilliro-side and scillirubroside. Unlike other mammals, rodents do not regurgitate the Squill bulb, and death follows convulsions and respiratory failure.

Salts of the alkaloid strychnine are used to control rodents. Such products are effective for small rodents, they are not commonly employed as rat poison. The toxicity of strychnine to other animals and its painful poisonous action do not make it a poison of choice.

Some fumigants have been used either to kill rodents or to drive them from their nesting place. These include calcium cyanide, methyl bromide, and carbon monoxide.

Insecticides

Insecticides are classified according to the life cycle of insects which they affect; e.g., *Ovicides*, against the egg stage; *Larvicides*, against the larvae, caterpillars, and maggots; *Muscicides*, against the house fly (*Mosca domestica*); *Pediculicides*, against the body louse (*Pediculus corporis*); and *Miticides* or *Scabicides*, against the scabies mite (*Sarcoptes scabiei*). Insecticides may be stomach poisons or contact poisons. They may be obtained from a natural source of synthesized by chemical reactions.

Systemic poisons

A systemic poison is ingested by the insect and distributed from the alimentary canal throughout its tissues.

Stomach poisoning chemicals are used to control chewing insects. The death of the insect is caused upon ingestion by interfering with respiratory system, depression of the nervous system, by over stimulation and consequent paralysis of the neuro-motor system or by some other mechanism. The poison is sprayed in the form of dust, solution and suspension over the area with the help of power-sprayers or by aeroplanes. The chewing insects consume the plants, the poison is taken into the stomach and is absorbed through the gastrointestinal tract. They remain effective till they are not washed away by rain or by sprinkling device or they are not readily oxidized to nontoxic forms.

Lead arsenate in acid or basic form, calcium arsenate, Paris green and arsenic trioxide are some important poisons. Calcium arsenate is used on cotton, tomatoes and potatoes. Use of calcium arsenate damages the leaves of many other plants. Paris green is a complex salt of copper and arsenic. In addtion to these, a number of phorphorus containing compounds have been synthesized as insecticides. For example, Schradan, (Octamethylpyrophosphoamide), Dementon, Methyl Demen-ton, Thimet and Di-Syston are the synthetic insecticides. They are readily absorbed through both the roots and the foliage of plants. They remain within the plants tissues and protect the plants against insects for a long time. These compounds are toxic to mammals and, therefore, are used to treat nonedible crops.

For household pests there are a number of stomach poisons for chewing insects. Cockroaches are killed by sodium fluoride and sodium fluorosilicate. The powdered chemical adhering to the antennae, leg bristles and other body hairs do not enter into the body until the insects clean themselves. During the cleaning process the poison is swallowed and then absorbed. If the powder is carried into the nesting places, other insects may be affected. Sodium arsenite or sodium arsenate in the form of sweetened baits or sodium fluoride as a dust are used to control the ants in the house.

Contact poisons

Contact poisons come into direct contact with the pests which are applied as dusts, sprays or aerosols. Insects gathering to the underside of leaves will not be effected if the poison is spread only at the upper side. Insects like flies and mosquitoes are effected only when they come into contact with the sprays or the atmosphere in the particular area is heavily saturated with the aerosol. Sometimes the insects develop resistance to the contact poison and then they are controlled with difficulty. Organic contact insecticides may be of natural origin or synthetic type. The important natural plant insecticides are white hellebore, sabadilla, rotenoids, rotenone, cinerins, pyrethrins, phyrethrum flowers, nicotine and its salts and powdered tobacco leaves.

The examples of synthetic insecticides are DDT, methoxychlor, TDE, benzene hexachloride and its isomer, lindane, chlordane, aldrin, dieldrin, heptachlor, toxaphene, the organic phosphorus insecticides such as parathion, malathion, and fluorophosphates and the organic nitrogen compounds.

Natural contact insecticides

Leaf tobacco

It consists of the cured and dried leaves of the Virginia tobacco plant, *Nicotiana tabacum* (Fam. Solanaceae). The genus *Nicotiana* is comprised of about 100 species. *Nicotiana tabacum* is a tall annual herb indigenous to tropical America and widely cultivated. The stem is simple, bearing large, pubescent, ovate, entire, decurrent leaves, the veins of which are prominent and hairy.

Nicotine (0.6-9%) is the characteristic alkaloid of the genus and is prepared commercially from waste material of the tobacco industry. A lesser amount of nornicotine and an aromatic compound, nicotianin or tobacco comphor are also present in the herb. The characteristic flavour is due to the nicotianin which is formed during the curing of the leaves. The roots of *N. tabacum* contain about eight pyridine alkaloids, including nicotine, nornicotine, anabasine and anatabine.

Nicotine is a pyridine-type alkaloid which is a pale yellow, oily liquid, very hygroscopic; turns brown on exposure to air or light; acrid burning taste; develops odour of pyridine; volatile with steam. It forms salts with almost any acid and double salt with many metals and acids. It is miscible with water below 60°C, very soluble in alcohol, chloroform, ether and petroleum ether. It is poisonous, being a local irritant and paralyzent.

Nicotine is used as insecticide and fumigant. As a contact poison, it is most effective as soap, *i.e.*, as the laurate, oleate, or naphthenate. As a stomach poison a combination with bentonite has come into use. Nicotine sulphate in a 40% solution (Black leaf 40) is quite toxic to aphids; if the solution is

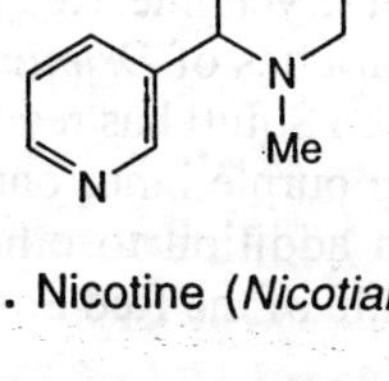

Fig. 25.1. Nicotine (*Nicotiana* spp.).

alkalised, the toxicity is increased. Soap solution decomposes the sulphate to the free alkaloid which is considerably more poisonous to the insects.

Nicotine is highly toxic. The symptoms include extreme nausea, vomiting, evacuation of bowel and bladder, mental confusion, twitching and convulsions. The base is readily absorbed through mucous membranes and intact skin, but the salts are not.

Commercial preparation of nicotine sulphate has been a popular insecticide, by its triple-action insecticidal property acting as stomach, contact and fumigant poison. As a free base it is more toxic to insects than as sulphate or hydrochloride. The range of insects subject to control by nicotine is very wide, although the alkaloid has been chiefly used against the minute soft bodied insects, i.e., aphids. It has been reported to be effective against white flies, red spider mites, leaf rollers, moths, fruit-tree borers, termites, cabbage butterfly larvae and sun lice. Basic nicotine is also used against house flies and rats and the lice that infest cattle and horses. Nicotine sulfate is used for combating apple wooly aphids (*Eriosoma lanigerum* Hausmann), a serious pest of apple, pear and crab apple in India and Pakistan; for fighting grape vine thrips (*Rhipiphorothrips cruentatus* Hood), a destructive pest of grape vine in India; for controlling mustard aphid (*Rhopalosiphum erysimi* Kaltenback), a serious pest attacking all cruciferous oil seeds like *toria, sarson, rye* and *taramira* (*Brassica* spp.); some minor pests like jute mealy bugs (*Phenacocus hirsutus* Cr.) and wheat aphid (*Macrosiphum miscanthi* Takahashi), generally as a spray solution containing 0.05% active ingredient.

One of the advantages of the insecticidal use of nicotine is its reported high margin of safety for plants, causing little or no damage to the foliage. Nicotine sulphate is safer, easier to handle and much less toxic to warm blooded animals as compared to synthetic pesticides. Because of high volatile nature of nicotine, insecticidal nicotine preparation leaves no appreciable residue on treated plants. The alkaloid disappears in relatively short time usually in minutes thus leaving no hazardous material on the marketable products. The above properties make nicotine preparation very ideal insecticide against the background of growing public concern over pesticide pollution.

Prospects of nicotine insecticide

On a worldwide scale 5,70,000 kg of nicotine sulphate and 6,75,000 kg of nicotine alkaloids are produced annually. Use of nicotine sharply declined from 1945 to 1955 after the advent of synthetic pesticides particularly Parathion which was actually developed for use as nicotine substitute. High degree of persistence, dose responsiveness at a much low concentration, comfortable handling and above all, its cost are some favourable points for the synthetic pesticide to win over the natural insecticides. Since 1955, however, the use of nicotine insecticide is slowly reviving and is showing a gradual increase in the present consumption pattern. This is probably due to awareness of pesticides residue problem associated with the synthetics in intensively cultivated areas. In India total production of nicotine sulphate during 1966-67 was 23,000 kg and in 1977-78 it was 89,756 kg. The total quantity exported was 17,200 kg in 1966-67 and 84,256 kg in 1977-78. Most of the indigenous nicotine sulphate is being exported to Japan, Switzerland, USA and Italy at an attractive price.

Existing manufacturing process of nitocine sulphate from tobacco waste involves mixing of tobacco waste with lime and extracting with water. Nicotine in the aqueous solution is further extracted with kerosene. The kerosene extract of nicotine is treated with sulphuric acid to obtain nicotine sulphate solution. The product is separated as a heavy layer and the denicotinized kerosene is recovered and recycled in the process. Extraction is usually a low efficiency process. Flue-cured Virginia Tobacco waste because of its low nicotine content, imposes further limitation to extraction efficiency thus forfeiting almost 50% of the existing raw material supply available in the organized marked of flue-cured tobacco trade circle. Further, kerosene is not an ideal solvent for nicotine extraction, since the distribution coefficient is very high: $C/C_1 = 1.11$ at 25°C when C is the concentration in the aqueous phase and C_1 is the concentration in the kerosene phase. Also kerosene being a petroleum based chemical, is usually in short supply and no longer a cheap solvent. Moreover, kerosene produces an undesirable odour in the final product which makes it unpleasant to handle and lacks consumer appeal.

In order to overcome some of these difficulties

in the existing process a new technology, ion-exchange recovery of nicotine from tobacco waste is being developed at the Central Tobacco Research Institute. In as much as alkaloids possess the property of forming the basic cation, they should be capable of being absorbed from dilute solutions on a cation exchanger. Adsorbed nicotine can be subsequently eluted with a suitable medium. The exchanger can be regenerated by washing with dilute mineral acid and can be reused over and over again.

Solubility in water is one of the reasons for the poor toxicity of nicotine sulphate; as hydrophilic molecules they have poor penetration through the insect cuticle or integument. Nicotine alkaloid when used as emulsion in a mineral oil base has almost twice the toxicity than when used alone.

PYRETHRUM FLOWERS
Synonyms

Pyrethrum Flower Heads, or Insect Flowers, Dalmation insect powder; Persian insect powder.

Biological source

These are the dried flower heads of *Chrysanthemum cinerariaefolium* or of *C. marschallii* (Fam. Asteraceae). Pyrethrum contains about 0.5% of total pyrethrins (Pyrethrin I and Pyrethrin II).

Pyrethrum flowers are collected from 2 to 6 years old plants by hand. They are dried and stored. The plant is widely grown in Kenya, Ecuador, Japan, Yugoslavia, east central Africa, Brazil and India.

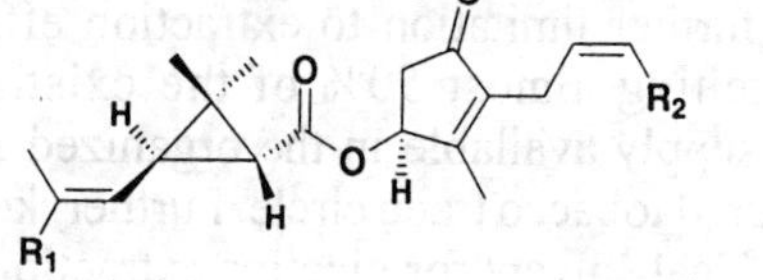

R_1 = CH_3 (pyrethric acid) : series I
R_1 = CO_2CH_3 (chrysanthemic acid) : series II
R_2 = CH–CH_2 : Pyrethrins I and II
R_2 = CH_3 : Cinerins I and II
R_2 = CH_2CH_3 : Jasmolins I and II

Fig. 25.2. General formula of pyrethrins.

The insecticidal activity of Pyrethrum arises from four esters, the pyrethrins I and II and the cinerins I and II. They are complex esters of chrysanthemum carboxylic acid and the mono-methyl ester of chrysanthemum dicarboxylic acid with pyrethrolones and cinerolones. The pyrethroids (or rethroids) are synthetic compounds of a similar structure of the pyrethrins themselves.

Kadethrin, an excellent knockdown insecticide, is prepared from resmethrin by addition of a thiolactone group to the acid side-chain.

Allethrin, tetramethrin, resmethrin, phenothrin and kadethrin are useful for the control of indoor pests (e.g., houseflies and mosquitoes) and stored-products pests, but they are not sufficiently stable in light and air for use in agriculture. Permethrin, the first photostable pyrethroid, is prepared by replacing the isobutenyl side-chain of phenothrin with a dichlorovinyl group. Introduction of an α-cyano substituent (only the *S* isomer is active) to the photostabilized pyrethroids enhances the insecticidal activity. One of the most potent

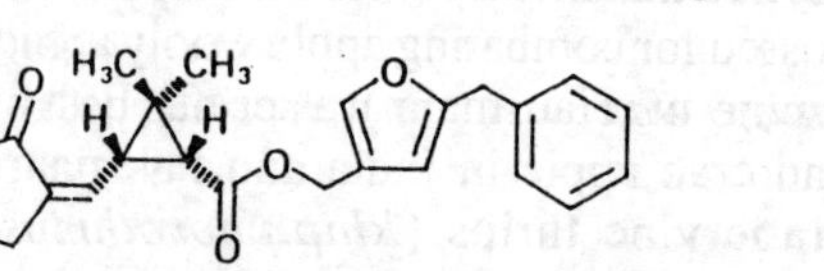

Kadethrin

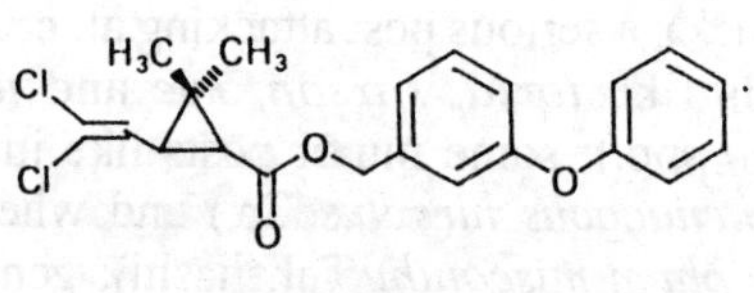

Permethrin

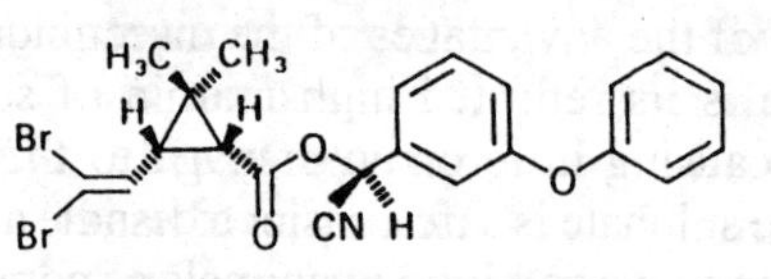

Decamethrin

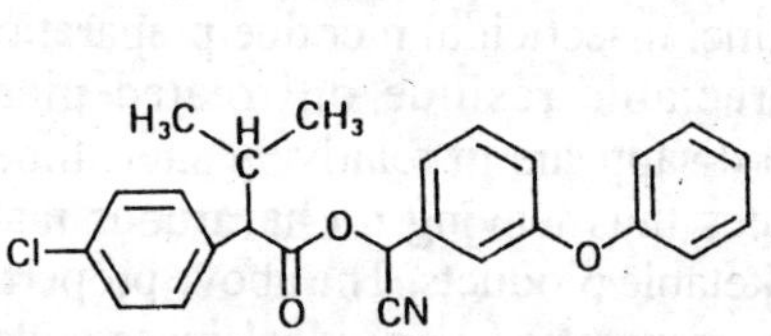

Fenvalerate

Fig. 25.3. Pyrethroids.

commercial pyrethroid insecticides (active at rates as low as 1 g ha^{-1}) is decamethrin.

Other insecticide has been produced from the structure-activity relationship studies of the rethrins is fenvalerate.

Uses of pyrethrum

Pyrethrum is used as an active ingredient of many insecticides and repellents. However, the concentration for using pyrethrum as repellent is 10 times lower than for insecticidal effects. Pyrethrum is mainly used for sanitary purposes in household and food shops. In closed rooms it serves against fleas, flies, bed bugs, ants, silverfish and mosquitoes. They are also used to combat ectoparasites of humans and animals, in post-harvest protection of grains, nuts, vegetables, fruits and processed food conservation and in food packing materials together with synergists. The treatment also prevents insect infestation in commercial dry fish. Before the introduction of synthetic insecticides, pyrethrins were also sold for use against cabbage loopers, cabbage moths and some other agricultural pests. But their high cost and low stability in sunlight have restricted their use in agriculture, and are at present commercially used in fumigant of young shoots and late pre-harvest application to combat some soil insects. In short, pyrethrins are highly toxic to a wide variety of insects and cause almost instantaneous paralysis among insects, but are least toxic to human beings. The oral toxicity is reported to vary between 200 to 1400 mg/kg of body weight. Although synthetic pyrethroids accounted for 30% of the world insecticide market in 1980 and continue to be widely used, there is still a demand for the natural pyrethrum. The present worldwide demand for pyrethrum flowers remains in excess of 25,000 tons annually and is satisfied by the estimated 150 million flowers still hand-harvested daily in natural stands and cultivated fields in Kenya, Tanzania and Ecuador.

The Pyrethrum flowers are a contact poison for insects. They are largely used in the form of powder, also as sprays in which the active principles are dissolved in kerosene or other organic solvent. It can cause severe allergic dermatitis and systemic allergic reactions. Large amounts may cause nausea,

vomiting, tonnitus, headaches and other CNS disturbances.

Derris and lonchocarpus

The roots of many species of *Derris* and *Lonchocarpus* (Fam. Papilionaceae) show insecticidal properties. Derris consists of the dried rhizome and roots of *Derris elliptica*, *D. malaccensis* and possibly other species. Lonchocarpus are the dried roots of *Lanchocarpus utilis*, *L. urucu* and some other species.

Derris is native of Malaya and cultivated there and in Burma, Thailand, Malaysia, Indonesia and the Philippine Islands. The genus Lonchocarpus is grown mainly in Mexico, Central and South America, England, Africa and Australia.

These roots contain rotenone (3-10%), deguelin, toxicarol, or tephrosin. Rotenone is a colourless

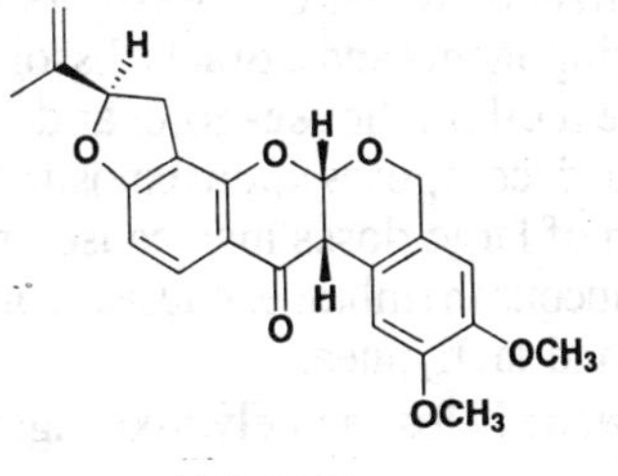

Rotenone

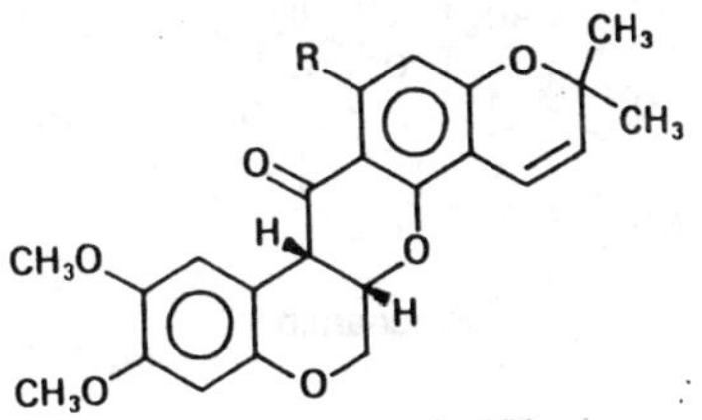

R = OH : Toxicarol
R = H : Deguelin

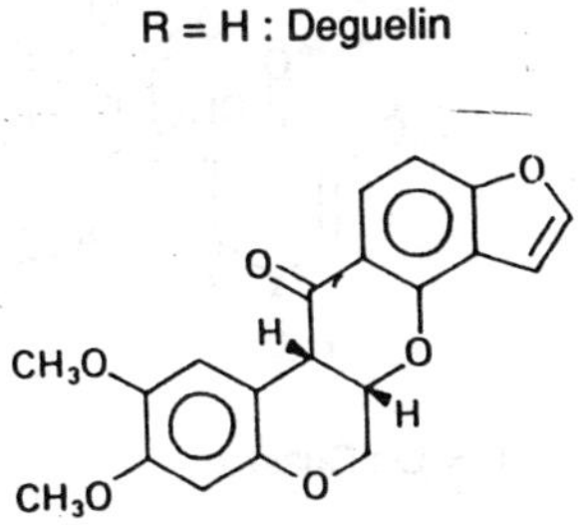

Elliptone

Fig. 25.4. Chemical constituents of Derris.

crystalline substance which is insoluble in water but soluble in many organic solvents. All these compounds show insecticidal properties. It is an insecticide which is widely used to control both chewing and sucking insects.

D. elliptica root also contains α-tubaic and β-tubaic acids; (−)-maackiain, (+)-maackiain, elliptone, deguelin, tephrosin; and 2,5-dihydroxymethyl-3,4-dihydroxypyrrolidine (in leaves). *D. malaccensis* also contains an isoflavone isomeric with toxicarol.

Derris and Lonchocarpus roots have been used as fish poisons. For dusting purposes the powdered root is finally ground and diluted with a suitable carrier (talc, clay) to a concentration of 1 per cent. For spray purposes the powdered roots may be mixed with water or preferably with organic solvents such as ethylene dichloride, trichloroethylene or chlorbenzene. Rotenone extracts with oil and emulsifying agents and extracts dissolved in paraffin oil are excellent house-hold and cattle sprays. Rotenone decomposes upon exposure. Inhalation or ingestion of large doses may cause problems in the of oral mucous membrane, nausea, vomiting, muscle tremors and tachypnea.

Rotenone is less acutely toxic against mammals than against fish and insects. Against insects, rotenone is active as a contact and stomach poison. It decreases oxygen uptake because it specifically inhibits the NADH-dependent dehydrogenase step of the mitochondrial respiratory chain. The rotenone insecticides are especially valuable for the control of leaf-chewing beetles and cater-pillars.

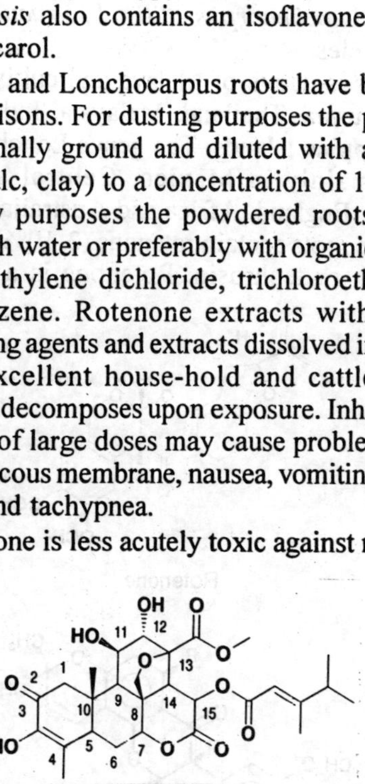

QUASSINOIDS

The woody parts of *Quassia amara* and *Picrasma excelsa* have been used to control sawflies and aphids, both as a contact and stomach poison.

The major insecticidal principle in the *Quassia* chips is the degraded (C_{20}) triterpenoid (decanor-triterpenoid) quassin. Another insecticidal compound isolated from *Q. amara* is neoquassin. Many related "quassinoids" have been isolated from other plants in the Simaroubaceae.

PHYTOALKALOIDS

Phytoalkaloids are basic plant compounds containing one or more heterocyclic nitrogen atoms. They are generally found in plants in the form of salts with organic acids. Over 6,000 phytoalkaloids are known and many of these exert actions upon animal nervous systems.

The toxicity of tobacco and *Veratrum* alkaloids to insects has long been known.

Veratrum alkaloids

Veratrum sabadilla Retz. and *V. album* (Liliaceae) have long been used as insecticides. The louscicidal properties of veratrum were recognized in the 16th century. Today, veratrum is used on a limited basis, mostly on citrus. The toxic principles include over 30 alkaloids, esters of polyol alka-mines with the ceveratrum nucleus. They are known collectively as veratrine. Commercial veratrine is predominantly a mixture of cevadine, veratridine, cevadilline, sabadine and cevine.

Cevadilla seed (or sabadilla) consists of the seeds of *Schoenocaulon officinale* (Fam. Liliaceae), a plant found from Mexico to Venezuela. The seeds are dark brown to black, sharply pointed and about 6 mm long. The seeds contain veratrine alkaloids (2-4%). The powdered seeds and preparations of 'Veratrine' are used as a dust or spray to control thrips and various true bugs which attack vegetables.

Bruceantin

R = O : Quassin

R = $\langle$ H / OH Neoquassin

Fig. 25.5. Quassinoids.

The *Veratrum* alkaloids are strong irritants to mucous membranes, and some are teratogenic.

Ryania alkaloids

The wood of some species of *Ryania*, a genus of tropical American shrubs and trees belonging to the Flacourtiaceae, has been used since the 1940s against the European cornborer, sugarcane borer and codling moth. The ground stemwood of *R. speciosa* is employed in a commercial insecticide formulation, marketed as Ryanex or Ryanicide. Although *Ryania* is a minor insecticide used on agricultural and garden pests, it has broader implications because of its efficacy and type of action. For example, *Ryania* is effective on some pests at less than 1 g equivalent ha^{-1}. It causes cessation of feeding and flaccid paralysis in insects owing to its poisoning of muscle.

The insecticidal principles of *Ryania* are ryanodine and 9,21-didehydroryanodine. Although ryanodine is structurally complex and highly toxic to mammals, its hydrolysis product ryanodol has low

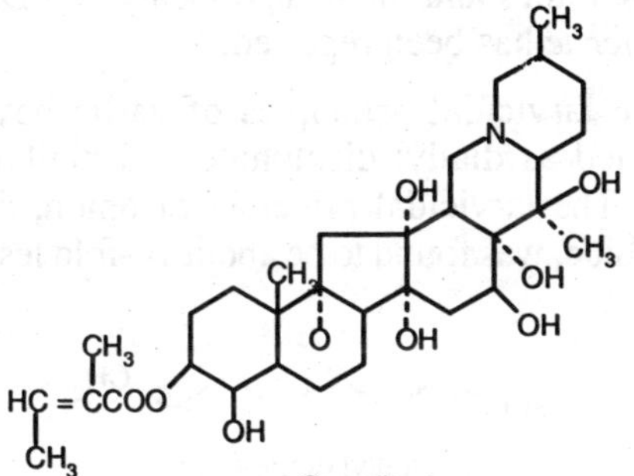

$R^1 = CH_3; R^2 = H; R^3 = -\overset{O}{\underset{}{C}}-$

Ryanodine

$R^1, R^2 = CH_2; R^3 = -\overset{O}{\underset{}{C}}-$

9,21-Didehydro-ryanodine

$R^1 = CH_3; R^2, R^3 = H$

Ryanodol

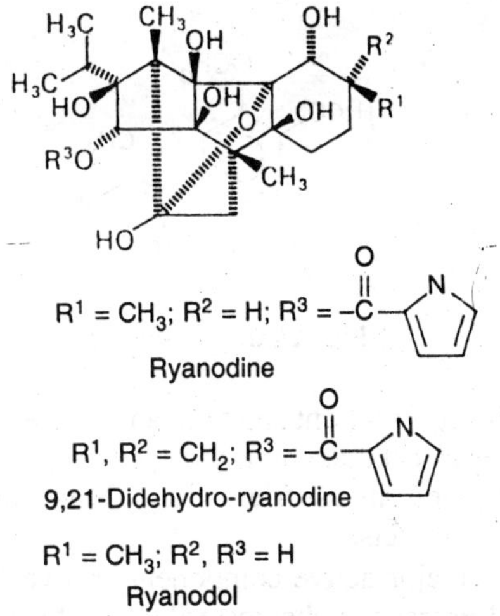

Fig. 25.7. Insecticidal principles of *Ryania*.

toxicity to mice and yet is a potent knockdown agent for insects.

It may be used as a dust made from a 40% extract. Due to its low toxicity, Ryania has no residue hazard.

Physostigmine

Physostigma venenosum (Papilionaceae) has long been known for the toxicity of its seeds. The toxic principle is the indole alkaloid physostigmine. Physostigmine reversibly inhibits acetylcholinesterase and can thereby prolong and exaggerate the effects of acetylcholine.

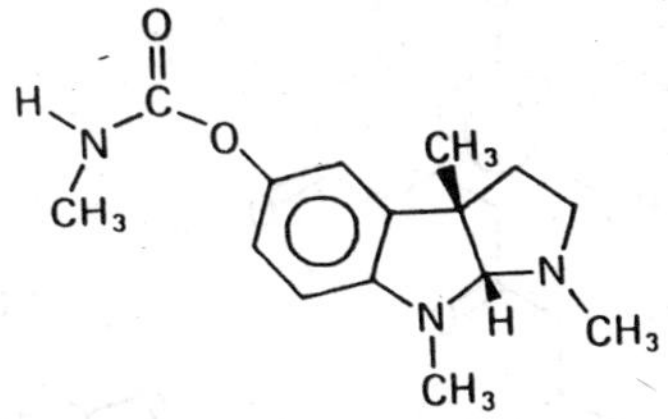

Cevadine

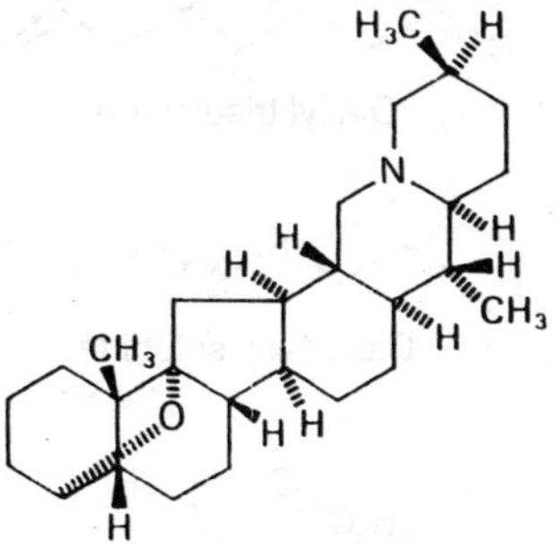

Veratriene

Fig. 25.6. Veratrum alkaloids.

Fig. 25.8. Physostigmine.

ACORUS

The roots of *Acorus calamus* L. (sweetflag) (Araceae) have long been used in India and Japan

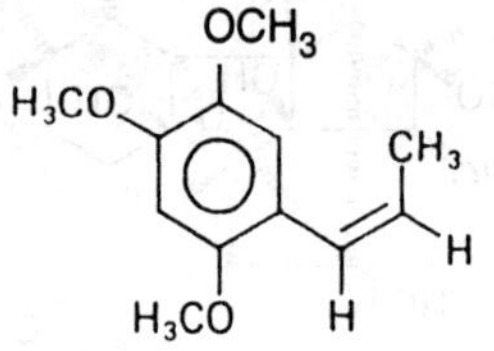

Fig. 25.9. *β-Asarone*

as an insect repellent and toxicant. The essential oil from the insecticidal roots is effective against moths, mosquitoes, houseflies, lice, fleas and stored products insects.

The major active component in sweetflag root oil is β-asarone, a chemosterilant for the red cotton bug *Dysdercus koenigii* and other species of insects. β-Asarone is a repellent for some other species of insects and an attractant for *Ceratitis capitata* (Mediterranean fruit fly).

MAMMAE

The leaves and seeds of *Mammea americana* L. (Clusiaceae) (mammyapple tree) have long been used in local insect control in the West Indies and tropical America. The leaves are used in a wrapping around garden plants to protect them against herbivorous insects. *Mammea* seeds (and other plant parts), when applied as a dust or a water suspension, are toxic or repellent to melonworms, fall armyworms, cockroaches, fleas, ticks, lice, mosquitoes and houseflies.

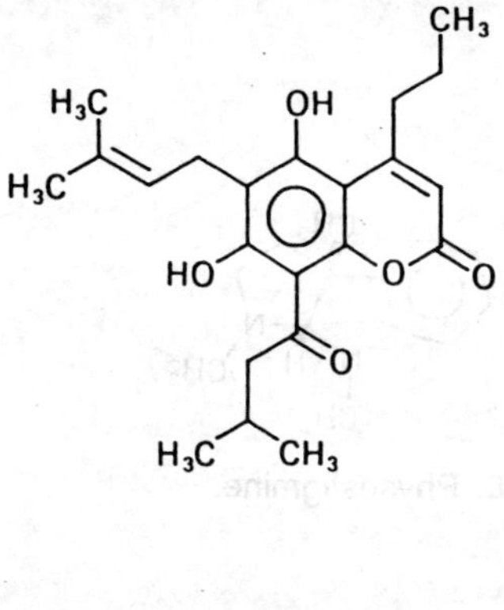

Mammein 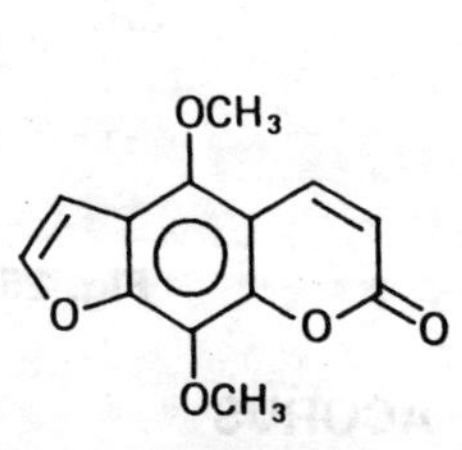   Isopimpinellin

Fig. 25.10. Coumarins of *Mammae americana.*

The compound responsible for the insecticidal activity of *M. americana* is mammein (4-*n*-propyl-5,7-dihydroxy-6-isopentenyl-8-iso-valeryl-coumarin). Several related insecticidal coumarins have been isolated from the same source. The insecticidal coumarins are uncouplers of oxidative phosphorylation.

Other insecticidal and insect-antifeedant coumarins have been isolated from other species of plants. For example, furanocoumarins, isolated from various plant species in the Rutaceae and Apiaceae were found to be active against insects. One of these coumarins, isopimpinellin, inhibits insect feeding and has been used in Japan to protect books from insects.

ALLIUM

Allium sativum L. (garlic) and *A. cepa* L. (onion) (Liliaceae) are among the oldest of all cultivated plants. Certain extracts of garlic and onions are antibacterial and antifungal, others antithrombotic. These extracts are also insecticidal. For example, the larvicidal property of garlic oil for five species of mosquitoes and the mango mealy bug *Drosicha mangiferae* has been reported.

The larvicidal principles of garlic have been identified as diallyl disulphide and diallyl trisulphide. The larvicidal principle of onion, dipropyl disulphide, was found to be about 10-fold less active

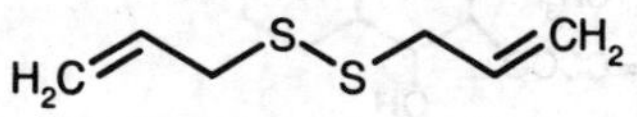

Diallyl disulphide

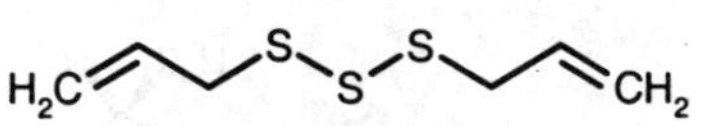

Diallyl trisulphide

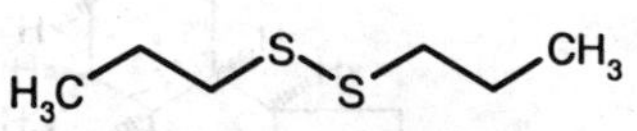

Dipropyl disulphide

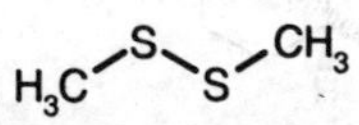

Dimethyl disulphide

Fig. 25.11. Chemical constituents of *Allium sativum.*

than diallyl disulphide against larvae of *Aedes aegypti* (L.) (yellow fever mosquito).

Garlic oil or its active principles, whether natural or synthetic, could possibly be used as mosquito larvicides.

TAGETES

Oil extracted from various parts of *Tagetes minuta* L. (Mexican marigold) (Asteraceae) is useful in the tropics as a blowfly dressing for livestock. Against mosquitoes, the oil is highly phototoxic, predominantly owing to the presence of α-terthi-enyl (2,2':5',2"-terthiophene). Its high level of activity may warrant its commercialization as a mosquito larvicide.

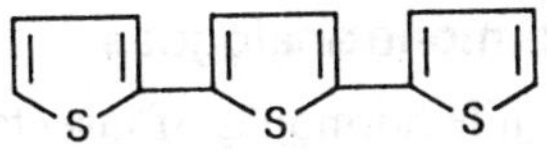

Fig. 25.12. α-Terthienyl.

HAPLOPHYTON

Three species of *Haplophyton* are known, all in the northern hemisphere. The leaves of these plants are insecticidal to cockroaches, flies, fleas, lice and mosquitoes. The leaves of *H. crooksii* (syn. *H. cimicidum*) (Apocynaceae) (Arizona or Mexican cockroach plant) have been used as insecticides. At

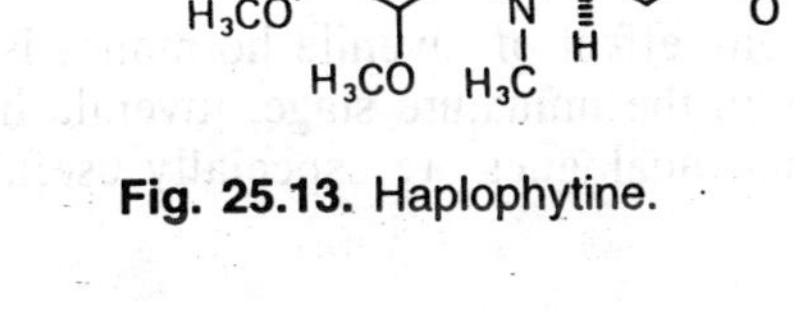

Fig. 25.13. Haplophytine.

least eight alkaloids have been isolated from *H. crooksii*, including the insecticidal haplophytine.

ANNONA

The genus *Annona* (family Annonaceae) is made up of more than 120 shrubs and trees, mostly in tropical areas, some of which yield important edible fruits (*e.g.*, soursop, cherimoya, custard apple). The seeds of various species of *Annona* have been used as insecticides and fish poisons. For example, the resins of seeds of *A. cherimola* and *A. squamosa* have been used against lice.

The insecticidal and insect-feeding-deterrent principles of *Annona* include aporphine-type alkaloids such as anonaine (or annonaine) and isoboldine.

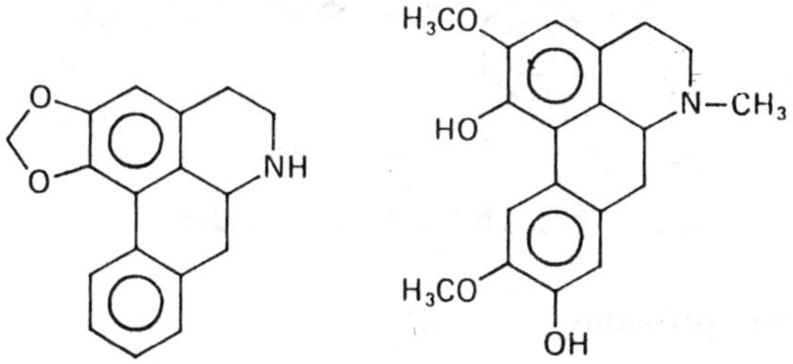

Anonaine   Isoboldine

Fig. 25.14. Alkaloids of Annona.

PLANT COMPOUNDS AS INSECTICIDES

(a) Isobutylamides

A number of isobutylamides, *N*-(2-methylpropyl) amides of polyunsaturated aliphatic straight-chain C_8 to C_{20} acids have been isolated from plants in the families Asteraceae, Piperaceae and Rutaceae. At least 28 of these compounds isolated from various species of *Heliopsis, Echinacea, Zanthoxylum, Anacyclus, Spilanthes, Fagara* and *Piper* possess insecticidal activity. For example, pellitorine, the most widely occurring isobutylamide known, is active against a number of species of insects. Other examples of insecticidal isobutylamides include affinin, guineensine, piperlonguminine and dihydropipercide.

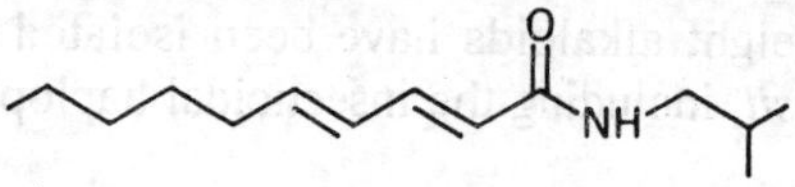

Pellitorine

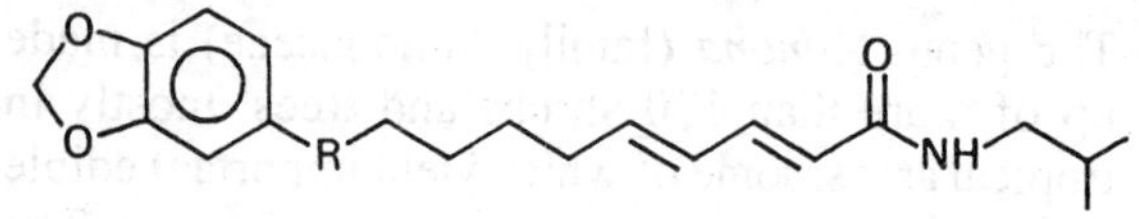

Affinin

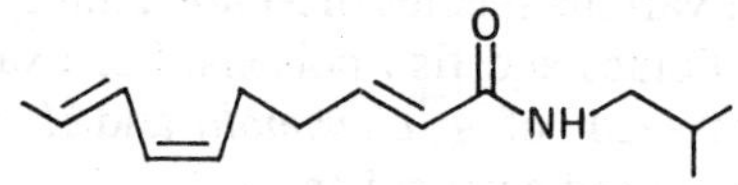

R = −CH$\overset{E}{=}$CH−CH$_2$CH$_2$−   Guineensine
R = −CH$\overset{E}{=}$CH−   Pipercide
R = −CH$_2$CH$_2$−   Dihydropipercide

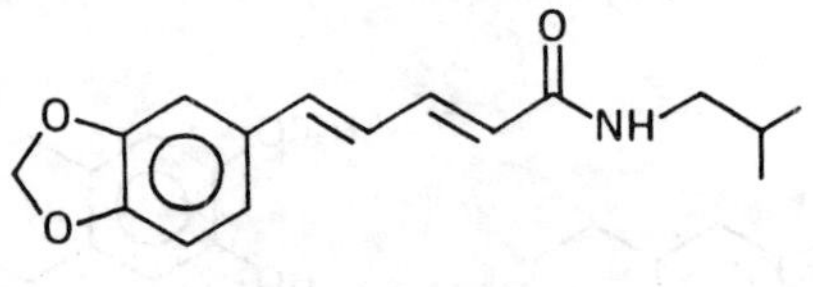

Piperlonguminine

Fig. 25.15. Isobutylamides.

Picrotoxinin

Picrotoxin is a mixture of heterocyclic lactones isolated from the seeds of *Anamirta cocculus* L. and other species in the plant family Menispermaceae. It is used to stun fish and to kill body lice. Picrotoxin has been used as an antidote for barbiturate poisoning. Picrotoxin is composed of the more potent picrotoxinin and the less potent picrotin. Picrotoxinin, a sesquiterpenoid epoxylactone, acts by blocking the γ-amino-butyric acid (GABA)-

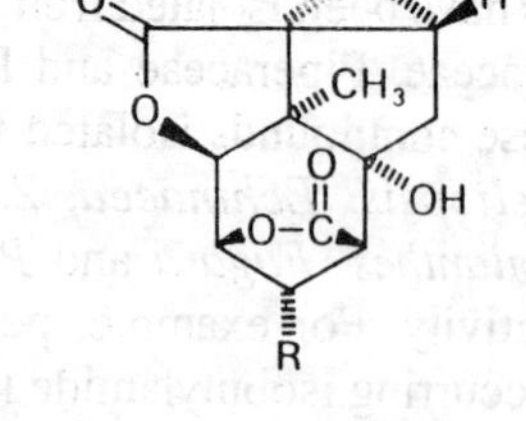

R = CH$_2$=CCH$_3$ Picrotoxinin
R = CH$_3$C(OH)CH$_3$ Picrotin

Fig. 25.16. Heterocyclic lactones.

regulated chloride ionophore in invertebrates and vertebrates.

The insecticidal activity of certain picrotoxinin analogs has led to the conclusion that the bridged bicyclic lactone skeleton and the isopro-penyl or isopropyl group (for steric bulkiness) are essential for insecticidal activity. The bridged bicyclic structures possessing two electronegative and one suitably positioned bulky sites are suited for binding to the picrotoxinin receptor.

PLANT COMPOUNDS AS INSECT-GROWTH REGULATORS

Plant compounds that regulate insect growth are slow-acting substances that specifically affect the growth and development of insects. These compounds include analogues and antagonists of two groups of endogenous insect hormones, namely the juvenile hormones and moulting hormones.

Juvenile-Hormone analogues

The five juvenile hormones of insects, all of which are epoxy methyl dodecadienoates (*e.g.*, juvenile hormones), are involved in the regulation of insect metamorphosis, reproduction, diapause and behaviour. These compounds act as "third-generation" pesticides (the second generation being conventional insecticides and the first generation being inorganic compounds. A few of these compounds are structural analogues of juvenile hormones. Examples include juvabione from *Abies balsamea* Mill. (balsam fir) (Pinaceae), juvocimenes (*e.g.*, juvocimene-1; from *Ocimum basilicum* L. (sweet basil) (Lamiaceae), echinolone from *Echinacea angustifolia* DC. (American coneflower) (Asteraceae) and farnesol, found in many plant oils.

Kinoprene (prop-2-ynyl (*E*), (*E*)-3,7,11-trimethyl-2,4-dodecadienoate) and methoprene (isopropyl (*E*), (*E*)-11-methoxy-3,7,11-trimethyl-2,4-dodecadienoate) have been registered in the United States for the control of mosquitoes, manure-breeding flies and stored-products pests.

Anti-juvenile-hormone compounds

Since one effect of juvenile hormones is to keep insects in the immature stage, juvenile hormones and their analogues are especially useful for the

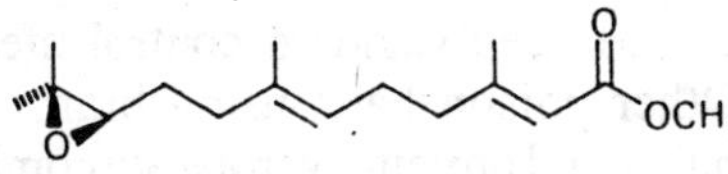

1. Epoxy methyl dodecadienoate
(Juvenile hormone 3)

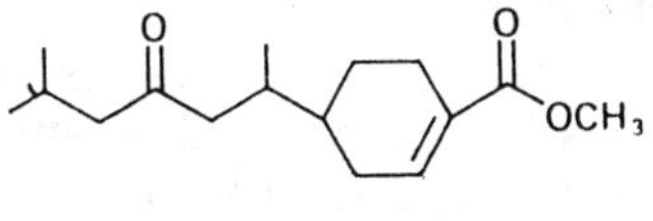

2. Juvabione

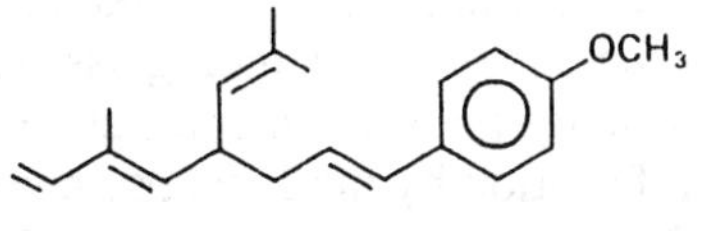

3. Juvocimene-1

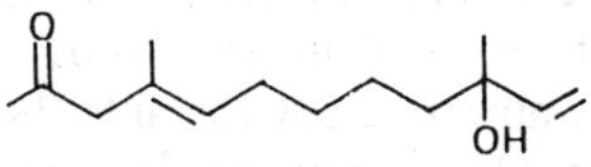

4. Echinolone

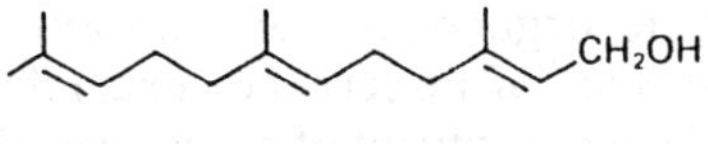

5. Farnesol

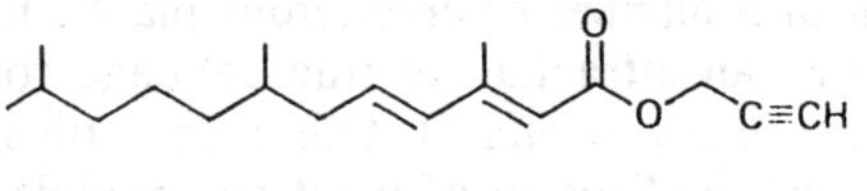

6. Kinoprene

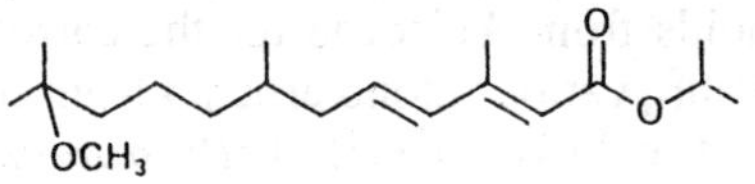

7. Methoprene

Fig. 25.17. Juvenile hormone analogues.

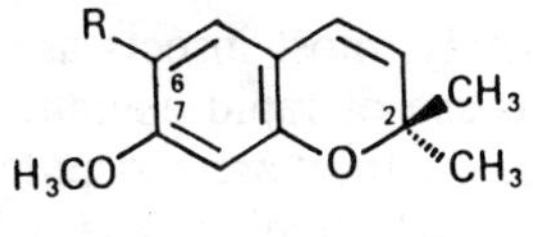

R = H   Precocene I
R = OCH_3 Precocene II
R = $COCH_3$ Encecalin

Fig. 25.18. Anti-juvenile hormone compounds.

promote metamorphosis to the adult stage. Compounds that can accomplish this include antijuvenile hormone compounds such as the precocenes I and II, chromenes isolated from the bedding plant *Ageratum houstonianum* Mill. Other insecticidal chromenes (*e.g.*, encecalin) have been isolated from other species of plants. Unfortunately, these compounds are highly effective only on a relatively few economically important species of insects, so their potential for commercialization may be limited.

Moulting-hormone analogues

The insect moulting hormones ecdysterone and ecdysone are involved in the moulting process, a requisite for normal growth in insects. Disruption of the normal titres of the moulting hormones can result in abnormalities and death. For example, *Pectinophora gossypiella* (Saunders) (pink bollworm) larvae fed ponasterone A, one of the many moulting-hormone analogues found in plants, were unable to complete the final stage of moulting (*i.e.*, ecdysis) and died in the pharate condition.

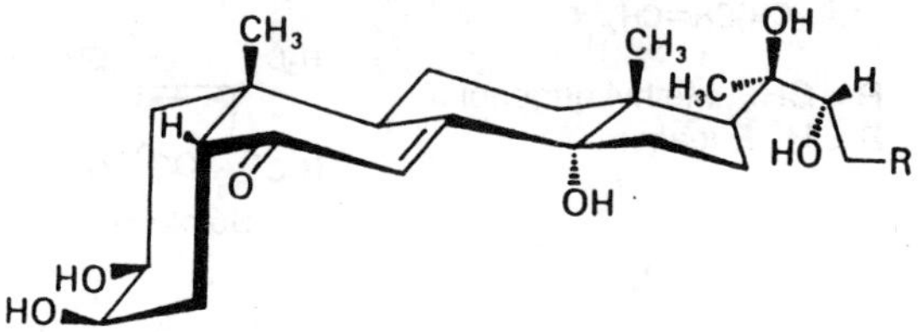

R = 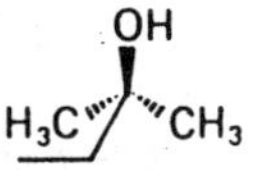   Ecdysterone,

R = 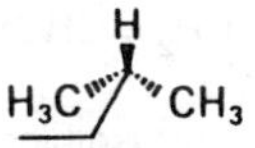   Ponasterone A

Fig. 25.19. Moulting hormone compounds.

control of insects that are economically important in their adult stage (*e.g.*, mosquitoes, fleas), but not for those insects that are economically important in their immature stages (*e.g.*, leaf-eating caterpillars). For the latter group of insects, it is desirable to

Unfortunately, most insects are unaffected by ingested (because of rapid excretion) or topically applied (because they are too polar to penetrate insect cuticle) ecdysteroids. The only commercial use of the moulting-hormone analogues in the sericultural industry is for the synchronization of cocoon spinning of silkworm colonies.

PLANT COMPOUNDS AS INSECT-BEHAVIOUR MODIFIERS

Attractants

Attractants are chemicals that cause insects to make oriented movement toward the source. Phytophagous insects use plant attractants to locate their food and to select sites to oviposit. Attractants are highly specific and normally active at very low concentrations.

Plant attractants have been used in insect control both to lure insects to traps or poison baits and to detect and monitor insect populations. Both food bait and pure compounds isolated from food bait have been used as insect attractants.

Poison baits (for example an infusion of bay and black hellebore in milk or sweet wine) have been used since classical times to kill flies and other insects. Poison baits for ants, incorporating syrup for sweet-eating species and fat for fat-eating species, have been standard control measures for years. Other poison baits using bran, mollasses, peanut butter and protein hydrolysate combined with suitable insecticides, have been used for the control of grasshoppers, cutworms, armyworms, crickets, earwigs and flies.

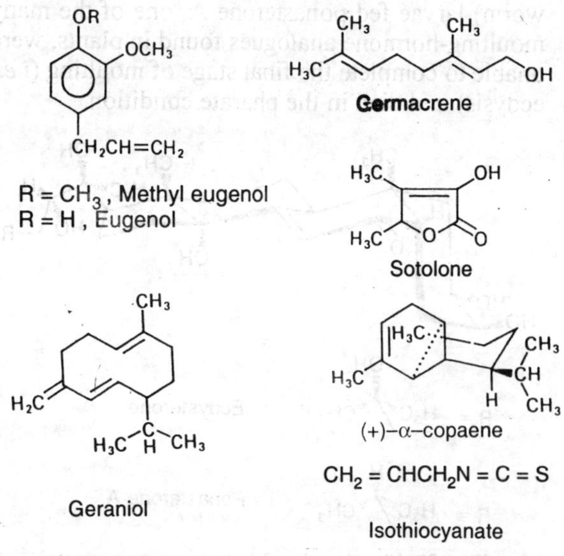

More recently, pure compounds isolated from food sources have been used as attractants. For example, methyl eugenol has been used to attract male oriental fruit flies *Dacus dorsalis* Hendel to toxic baits, and this compound remains the most effective lure for this insect. A mixture of geraniol (found in the oils of rose lemon grass) and eugenol (found in many plant sources), has been used to monitor infestation by the Japanese beetle *Popillia japonica* Newmann. A product (Beetle Trap Attack) incorporates floral lures (presumably containing eugenol or related phenolics) for Japanese beetles. Germacrene D mimics the cockroach sex pheromone, and as such attracts male cockroaches. Sotolone is an attractant for ants, houseflies, and cockroaches. (+)-α-Copaene, from angelica-seed oil and orange oil, is a potential attractant in population monitoring and control of the Mediterranean fruit fly, *C. capitata*.

Volatile organosulphur compounds attract certain species of insects. For example, dimethyl disulphide, a constituent of onion, was found to be a highly powerful lure for the black blowfly *Phormia regina* (Meig), and allyl isothiocyanate, a constituent of a number of cruciferous plants, has been used as an attractant to trap cabbage root flies (*Erioischia brassicae*). Other examples of the practical application of plant compounds for the trapping of insect pests include propyl mercaptan for the onion fly *Hylemya antiqua* (Meig), phenyl-propanoids from Apiaceae for the carrot fly *Psila rosae* Fabr., various monoterpenes from cotton-seed oil for the boll weevil *Anthonomus grandis* Boheman, and phenylacetaldehyde from *Araujia sericofera* Brot. for various Lepidoptera.

Several monoterpenes from the leaves of *Actinidia polygama* Miq. are attractant to male lacewings *Chrysopa septempunctata* Wesmael, a predator of thrips, aphids and scale insects.

R = CH₃ , Methyl eugenol
R = H , Eugenol

Germacrene

Sotolone

Geraniol

(+)-α-copaene

CH₂ = CHCH₂N = C = S

Isothiocyanate

Fig. 25.20. Insect attractants.

Repellents

Repellents are those substances which, as stimuli,

elicit avoiding reactions. Repellent chemicals prevent insect damage to plants or animals by rendering them unattractive, unpalatable or offensive. Certain plants have been used since antiquity as insect repellents. For example, gnats infesting damp gardens could be driven away by the fumes of burning galbanum resin, and a variety of insects could be kept away by burning garlic, cedar gum and various plants and roots.

The use of repellents has not generally been advantageous in the protection of agricultural crops from insects. To be effective, these chemi-cals need very thorough coverage over a large area, which is generally not feasible. An exception may be in home gardens, where the area involved is much smaller. In fact, a herbal repellent product is available for use against sucking and chewing insects. The Green Ban formulation contains eucalyptus oil, garlic, Dalmatian sage, *Hedera helix* L. and Norwegian kelp.

Natural plant compounds have been used more extensively to repel bloodsucking mosquitoes, flies, mites and ticks from skin and clothing. For example, oils of citronella, turpentine, pennyroyal, cedarwood, eucalyptus and wintergreen have long been used in insect-repellent formulations. Many other essential oils have been examined as repellents for mosquitoes, march flies and sand flies. Citronella

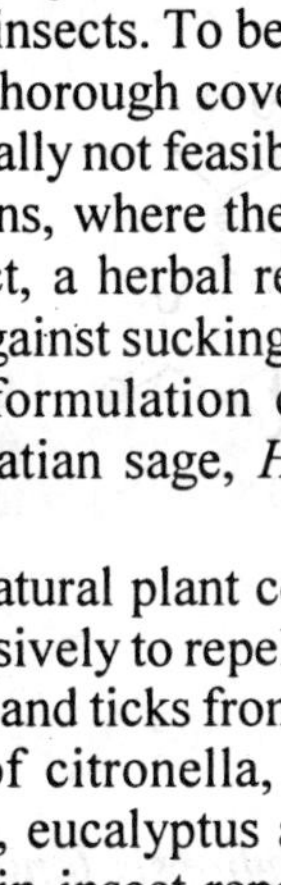

oil, from *Cymbopogon nardus* (Poa-ceae), containing citronellol and citronellal, as the principal repellents, is most widely used mosquito repellent. Today, citronella oil is marketed as a mosquito repellent in paraffin-based candles or coils.

Several pure plant compounds, including the monoterpenes citral and geraniol, have been found to be repellent to one or more species of insects. Seventeen species of insects were repelled by nepetalactone from the catnip plant *Nepeta cataria*. 1,8-Cincole, a monoterpenoid from certain essential oils isolated from plants in the families Asteraceae, Magnoliaceae and Rutaceae, has been found to be repellent to a number of species of insects. A product marketed as an insect repellent contains eucalyptus oil, a major source of 1,8-cineole, as its active ingredient. Green Ban, another repellent product, also contain eucalyptus oil.

Antifeedant

Antifeedants are substances that when tasted by insects, result either temporarily or permanently, depending upon potency, in the cessation of feeding. The existence of and potential for antifeedant compounds, both natural and synthetic, in practical insect control have been known for some time. For example, Bordeaux mixture (copper sulphate, hydrated lime and water), known for over 100 years, acts as a feeding deterrent to flea beetles, leaf hoppers and the potato psyllid (*Paratrioza cockerelli* (Sulc).

Several drimane sesquiterpenes, including warburganal and polygodial, that were shown to have potent activity against the African armyworm *Spodoptera exempta* (Walk.) have been synthesized. Some clerodane diterpenes, including clerodin and ajugarin I, found to be antifeedant for a number of species of insects, have been synthesized. A precise arrangement of the functional groups of the clerodane diterpenes, including the *trans*-epoxydiacetate and the furofuran or butenolide-containing side-chain, was found necessary for antifeedant activity.

One natural plant product is the limonoid azadirachtin. The antifeedant activity of azadirachtin is a slow-acting insecticide because it disrupts the hormonal balance in certain species of insects when ingested. In the laboratory, azadirachtin was found

R = CH₂OH   Citronellol
R = CHO   Citronellal

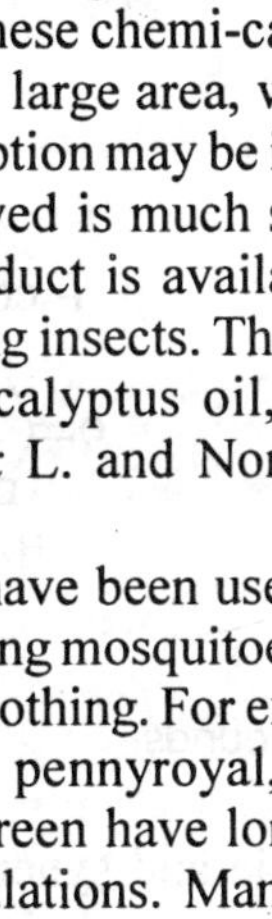

Citral

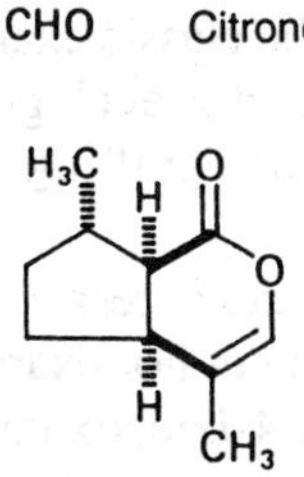

Nepetalactone

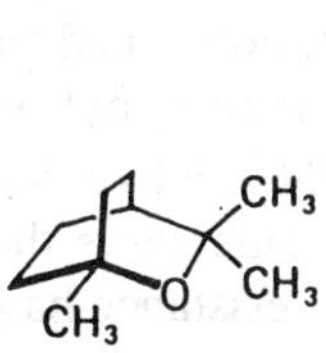

Cineole

Fig. 25.21. Insect repellents.

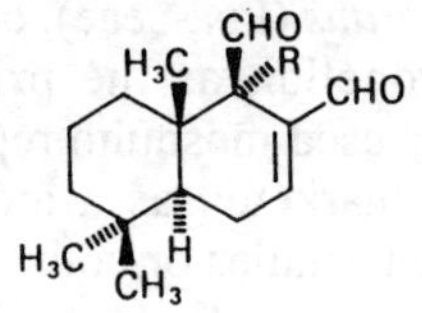

R = OH , Warburganal
R = H , Polygodial

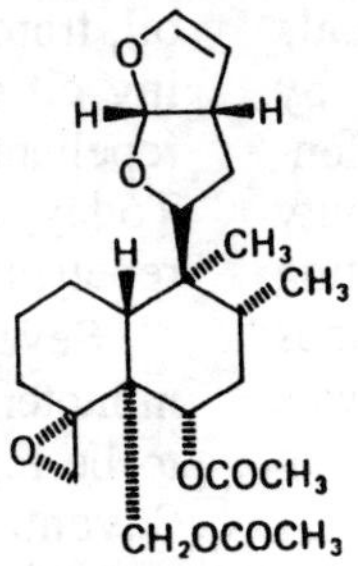

Clerodin

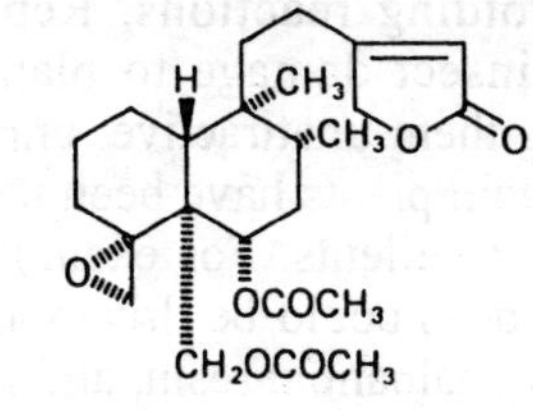

Ajugarin

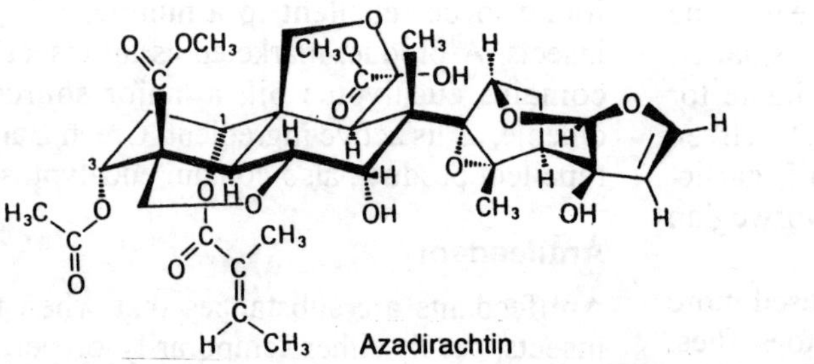

Azadirachtin

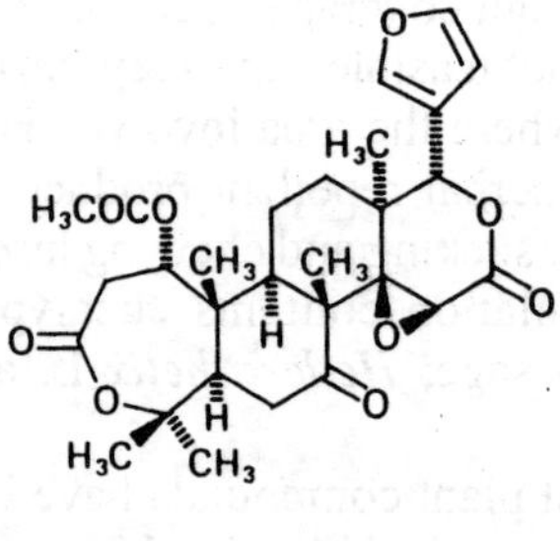

Nomilin

Fig. 25.22. Antifeedant compounds.

to act systemically in several crop plants and to be effective as a prophylactic from damage by several species of insects.

PLANT COMPOUNDS IN OTHER USES IN INSECT CONTROL

Synergists

The insecticidal effectiveness of certain insecticides (*e.g.*, pyrethrins and isobutylamides) can be enhanced by the addition of compounds called synergists or adjuvants, which may or may not be insecticidal in themselves. The most important synthetic synergist, piperonyl butoxide, and other related methylenedioxyphenyl or benzodioxole compounds, were developed from natural plant product prototypes. For example, sesamin found in the oil of sesame, *Sesamum indicum* L., has long been known to synergize pyrethrin. Sesamolin is another pyrethrin synergist from *S. indicum*.

Other synergists isolated from plants include myristicin, an insecticide and synergist from *Pastinaca sativa* L. (parsnips), and affinin, an

insecticide and synergist from *Heliopsis longipes*. These compounds inhibit mixed-function oxidase enzymes, thus slowing the detoxification of some insecticides.

Host-plant resistance

Another approach to insect control is to utilize the natural chemical defence of plants through the mechanism of host-plant resistance (HPR). HPR is the ability of a plant to reduce infestation or damage, or both, by an insect. The earliest documentation of HPR concerned the resistance of certain varieties of wheat to the Hessian fly, and the classic example of HPR concerned the resistance of French grapes to the grape phylloxera following grafting with American grape rootstock.

In some cases the plant chemicals responsible for the resistance have been isolated. For example, 2,4-dihydroxy-7-methoxy-2*H*-1,4-benzoxazin-3-one (DIMBOA) is a resistance factor in maize, *Zea mays* L. (Poaceae), for *Ostrinia nubilalis* (European corn borer). In *Lycopersicon hirsutum* f. *glabratum*

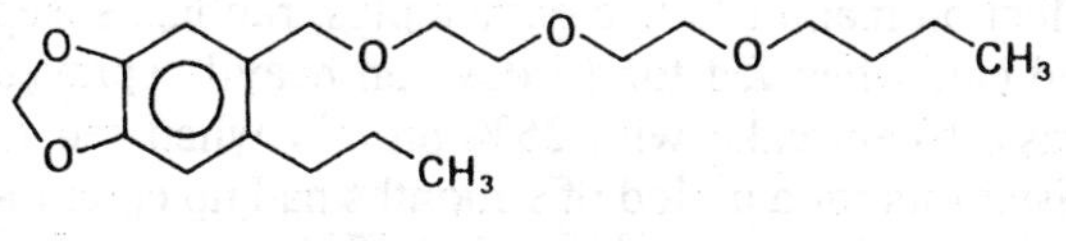

Piperonyl butoxide

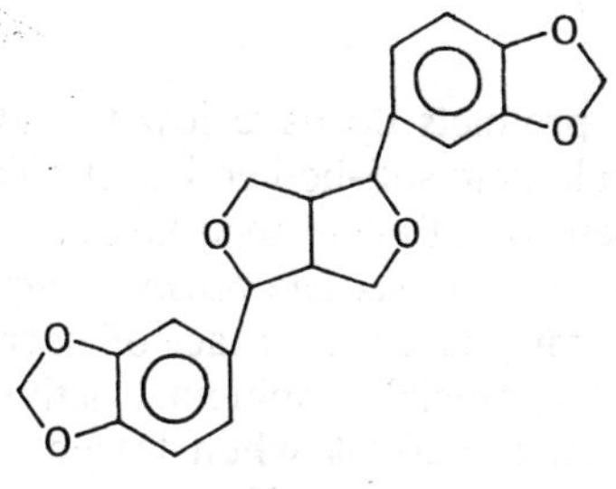

Sesamin

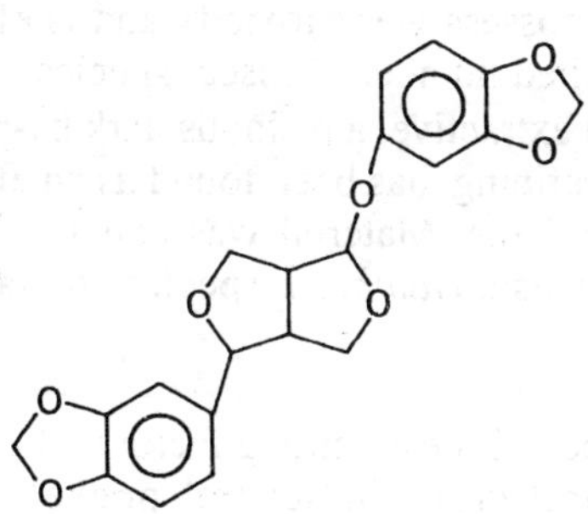

Sesamolin

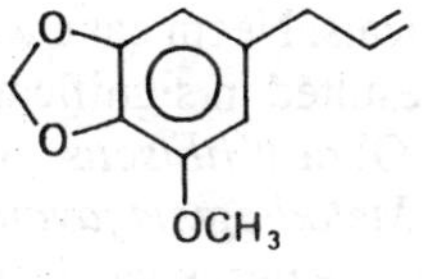

Myristicin

Fig. 25.23. Synergist compounds.

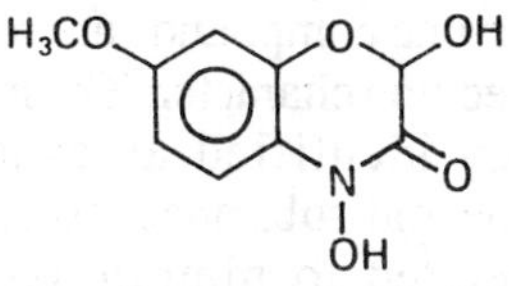

2,4-Dihydroxy-7-methoxy-2H-
1,4-benzoxazin-3-one (DIMBOA)

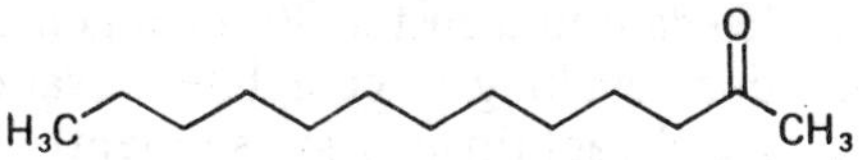

2-Tridecanone

Fig. 25.24. Host plant resistant compounds.

NEEM (*AZADIRACHTA INDICA* JUSS.) AS A SOURCE OF PEST CONTROL MATERIAL

Neem is one of the most valuable and yet least exploited of all tropical trees. It grows in arid regions, even nutrient deficient soil of India and Africa and is a fast growing source of fuel wood.

The dried neem leaves are mixed with grain for storage and with woollen clothes to protect them for ravages of insects. Water extract of leaves was used as contact poison on grubs of weevils infesting lucerne. Recent awareness about the hazards of persistent synthetic insecticides to our environment and their escalating costs have generated fresh interest and intensified research on insecticides of plant origin which are to a large extent, free from these limitations.

Neem has been found to possess several types of chemicals that could be exploited for pest management depending upon the nature of the pest.

Antifeedant

Satisfactory protection of stored wheat, maize, jowar, paddy and pulses over a period of 1 year has been achieved by mixing 1-2% neem kernel powder in grain, from several species of stored grain insects, viz., *Sitophilus arizae, Rhizopertha dominica, Trogoderma granarium, Tribolium castaneum* and *Collosobruchus chinensis.*

Extracts of neem seed inhibit feeding in some field pests like *Pieris brassicae* and *Chrotogonus trachypterous.* A 12% neem oil emulsion when sprayed paddy suppresses feeding deterrent and

C.M. Mull (Solanaceae), a wild species of tomato, the chemical factor responsible for resistance to several tomato pests is 2-tridecanone and related methyl ketones.

Another possible use of biologically active natural plant compounds in host plant resistance is the transfer of gene complexes associated with the biosynthesis of active compounds to plants of economic importance. For example, cowpeas are resistant to a variety of pests owing to the presence of natural plant proteins that inhibit the digestive enzyme trypsin.

interferes in the general metamorphosis of the hoppers. More than one compounds are responsible for imparting antifeeding character. The most active fraction has been identified as azadirachtin ($C_{35}H_{44}O_{16}$), a terpenoid substance. Its structure is biogenetically related to nimbin salanin and nimbolin B. Its yield was reported to be 0.75 g/kg neem seed. The compound has been evaluated as a strong antifeedant to locust at 40 micrograms/litre concentration resulting in complete cessation of feeding. Azadirachtin has subsequently been reported to be an effective antifeedant to *Plutella xylostella* and *Heliothis virescens*.

The other antifeedant chemicals identified are (i) miliantrol, a triterpenoid alcohol, and (ii) salanin. These compounds are less effective than azadirachtin. Neem cake was the richest source of the active ingredients, best extracted in ethanol. The extract was quite stable under high temperature conditions and temperature up to 100°C for 1 hour in no way impaired its efficacy. However, there is gradual drop degrade faster in cake than in seeds.

Oil free neem kernel's aqueous suspension showed antifeedant activity against locusts.

Attractant

Neem itself is attacked by several insects. At least 42 insect species have been recorded which feed on neem. Still strange at neem leaves are strong food attractants to adults of white grub and have been very successfully utilized for control of this pest.

Neem twigs with leaves are inserted in rows in the infested pockets around sun-set at the start of monsoon. At dusk large number of beetles collect on the twigs which are killed mechanically or chemically. The nature of the attractant is not known as yet.

Repellent

Neem contains several aromatic and odorescent principles which repel insects white ants (*Microtermes* sp.) and some species of ants do not like the neem scent and move away from the treated vicinity. Neem cake has been practically used in clearing termite infested areas in Madhya Pradesh. Neem oil is a strong deterrent to egg laying by potato tuber moth. A spray with extract of neem leaves at various concentrations had no repellent or toxic

effect on mammals like guinea pigs, rabbits, sheep and calf when fed for 15 days on heavily sprayed grass. Neem cake with 25% protein when fed to wistar rats for a period of 9 months had no carcinogenic activity during the period of observation.

Insecticide

Several neem products do have low to moderate toxicity particularly to soft-bodied insects. Toxicity of water suspension of neem seed kernel to *Aphis gossypii*, *Urentius echinus* and *Saisetia nigra* was reported. Non-fatty alcohol extract of neem seed cake possesses appreciable aphicidal activity, the LD_{50} value being 0.202% when tested against *Rhopalosiphum nymphae* L. However, the neem constituents possess weak toxicity and is effective against a limited number of insect species.

Neem oil extractive, a resinous dark by-product of neem oil refining, has been found as an effective mosquito larvicide. Material was equally toxic to insectivorous fish, *Gambusia* species and tadpole.

Nematicide

Nematodes constitute a limiting factor in the raising of agricultural crops in several pockets of the country. However, their control is extremely difficult due to the nature of the pest and prohibitive cost of nematicidal chemicals. Neem cake when applied @ 1800 kg/hectare resulted in significant reduction in the root galls of Okra (*Hibiscus esculentus*) and tomato caused by *Melodiogyne javonica*. Inhibitory effect on the larval emergence from the eggs of *Meloiodgyne incognita* and reduced egg-laying capacity of the females as a result of neem cake application are reported.

Application of N, P and K alone as fertilizers to soil results in marked increase of plant parasitic nematodes. But if applied in combination with neem, the population dwindles slowly and steadily. Water extract of neem cake was the most effective followed by Mahua, Karanj and Mustard. Nimbidin and thionimone (the bitter principles) efficiently killed the nematode and inhibited the larval growth. The neem cake is effective in managing nematode population.

Growth disruptor

Certain compounds interfere in the normal hormonal

balance of insects thereby causing disruption in normal growth. Such chemicals hold out promise in pest control. The seed extract prolonged the development and caused loss in the body weight of *Sitophallus oryzae*. The neem possesses growth disrupting activity. *Pieris* larvae fed for 48 h on foliage treated with neem products and subsequently reared on clean food, failed to develop to maturity and most of them died while moulting. Malformation in pupae and prolon-gation of pupal period up to 50 days as against 2 weeks in normal cases was observed. Eggs of *Trialeurodes* laid on the leaves of brussels sprouts sprayed with 1% seed suspension to the run-off point, either did not hatch or the larvae died in the egg shells partially hatched. Similarly eggs of *Stomoxys* incubated on filter paper moistened with 0.01% azadirachtin did not hatch the active ingredient of neem penetrated the egg shells and affected the developing embryo.

Mosquito larvae (*Culex fatigans*) when reared on medium containing 0.01-0.005% neem oil extractive failed to emerge as adults. About 40% died while trying to emerge out of the pupal shells. Metamorphic disturbances due to azadirachtin were recorded when applied to larvae of diamond back moth (*Plutella xylostella*), cabbage caterpillar (*Pieris brassicae*) and army worm (*Heliothis virescens*) at 0.025 mg per insect while at higher dosages 0.1 mg/larva, these died immediately. Similar effects have also been recorded on *Epilachna varivestris*, *Plutella maculipenis* and leat bug, *Piesma quardratum* and *Lymantria dispar*. Azadirachtin is structurally related to ecdyson of insects. The growth disturbances caused by it are attributed to the interference in normal hormonal balance of a particular insect.

Neem products may possess ecdyson-like growth disrupting properties. *Culex* and *Anopheles*, the vectors of malaria and *Musca*, the vector of cholera failed to reach maturity in the food media containing neem extracts. There might be some link between these findings and the general belief that the villages with preponderance of neem trees, have lower incidence of cholera and malaria. The berries of neem fall to the ground during monsoon and are carried by torrential rains to low lying areas, ponds and also over the rubbish heaps lying in the low lying areas which form the breeding sites for these vectors resulting in the reduction of vector population.

Inhibitor of pesticide degradation in soil

Pesticide degradation in soil is largely triggered by soil microorganisms. This deterioration, though a boon in the elimination of the persistent compounds, yet is a bottleneck in getting desired residual effectiveness of systemic soil insecticides.

Carbofuran protected the crop for some period, the ultimate yield would still be poor due to non-availability of nitrogen. Neem cake is known to reverse this process and is now an established nitrogen regulator. Therefore, while on one hand the neem cake prolongs the field life of carbofuran, on the other it increases the availability of nitrogen to the plant. This finding, in addition, provides a clue to develop insecticide granules with regulated release using antimicrobial agents, an entirely new approach.

Oviposition deterrent

A 2% kernel suspension in water was effective as a repellent and ovipositional deterrent for moths of tobacco caterpillar, *Spodoptera litura* (P). Oviposition deterrent activity of neem extractive against potato-tuber moth, *Phthorimea operculella* (PTM), is due to principles which are neither antifeedant nor repellent *per se*. Further the crude fraction provides complete deterrance to egglaying by the PTM and some species of mosquitoes. While in the case of mosquitoes egg laying is prevented only for 2-3 days, in the case of PTM, it is completely prevented for 7-9 days.

Systemic action

In young bean plants grown in soil treated with azadirachtin, damage by desert locust was negligible. Bean seedlings grown from seeds soaked in azadirachtin solutions were also protected against damage by desert locust adults for one week after germination.

Synergistic action

The neem extract had synergistic action in combination with custard apple (*Annona squamosa* L.) against pulse beetle (*Callosbruchus chinensis* Fab.), lesser grain borer (*Rhizopertha dominica* L.) and housefly (*Musca domestica nebulo* Fab.), Custard apple seed extract in combination with neem seed extract was half toxic against lesser grain borer and equitoxic as DDT to the housefly.

SYNTHETIC CONTACT INSECTICIDES

The synthetic organic insecticides are classified into four groups :

1. organic sulphur,
2. chlorinated hydrocarbons,
3. non-halogenated organic compounds, and
4. organophosphorus derivatives

Among the sulphur compounds are the carbamates, thiuram derivatives, mercaptans, thiazines, and organic thiocyanates (rhodanates). Sulphur is the traditional and ancient remedy for scabies. Tetraethylthiuram monosulphide, an organic sulphur compound, is as effective as sulphur.

Among halogenated organic compounds, naphthalene (moth flakes or moth balls) and para-dichlorobenzene (Dichloricide) are used as moth repellents.

A large number of chlorinated hydrocarbons have been employed as *contact poison*. These substances exert their lethal action after they have passed through the insect cuticle. Dicophane (DDT) is the best known of all chlorinated com-pounds. It is also known as chlorophenothane. Dicophane is also used for the eradiction of head lice. Important insecticides related to DDT are methoxychlor or TDE. These compounds may be degraded by living systems into less toxic meta-bolites. They remain unreacted for many years in soil and marine sediments and, therefore, present a continual threat to animal communities.

Gamma Benzene Hexachloride (Quellada), the γ-isomer of hexachlorocyclohexane, shows insecticidal properties. It has a strong, disagreeable odour and used as sprays for crop plants, animals and garden plants. It is also used to destroy head lice and to treat scabies. Aldrin, a chlorinated hydrocarbon insecticide, has been used to control grasshoppers. It is stable in alkaline condition. Its epoxy derivative, Dieldrin, shows identical action and retains a longer residual effect. Endrin is a stereoisomer of Dieldrin and exhibits excellent insect-killing effect. Chlordane insecticide is used to control insects in lawns, gardens and homes.

Pentachlorophenol, C_6Cl_5OH, protects lumber against termites and wood-rotting fungi when used as a 5% mixture in an organic suspension. Methyl bromide is an excellent fumigant for treating store products and green vegetables. In the form of solution methyl bromide is used as a soil sterilizant for the control of nematodes and certain insects. The simpler chlorinated hydrocarbons such as chloroform, paradichlorobenzene, carbon tetrachloride and trichloroethylene also have insecticidal activity and used as fumigants. The compounds like hydrocyanic acid gas and carbon disulphide hydrocarbons are toxic to man and animals and they should be kept well away from foodstuffs and animal feed.

Certain substituents on the benzene ring (C_2H_5-, CH_3O-, F-, Cl-, and Br-) increase the potency of these insecticides either by increasing the lipid solubility of the compounds or by improving the fit on the receptor surface. Other substituents (C_4H_9-, C_6H_8, NH_2-, NO_2-, -OH and COOH) reduce the potency. All the active compounds are very soluble in lipids and their molecular weights lie within the range 270 to 450.

Members of organophosphorus derivatives include the insecticides like tetraethylpyrophosphate (TEPP), parathion, chlorthion, diazinon, trichlorphon (dipterex) and octamethyl pyrophosphate (OMPA). These compounds are used both as contact poisons and as systemic poisons. A systemic poison is one that is ingested by the insect and distributed from the alimentary tract throughout its tissues. These poisons are applied to plants liable to attack by insects.

The organophosphorous insecticides form stable compounds with a number of esterases including cholinesterase. These insecticides are toxic to man and animals. They are being successfully employed in regions in which insects have developed resistance to the chlorinated hydrocarbons. Malathion (Carbofos; Prioderm) is extensively used as a dusting powder in cases of infestation with body lice.

Repellents

The natural product Citronella oil has been used as a mean of preventing insect attack. The synthetic products include dimethyl phthalate, Etho-hexadiol (Rutgers 612) and Butopyronoxyl. These com-

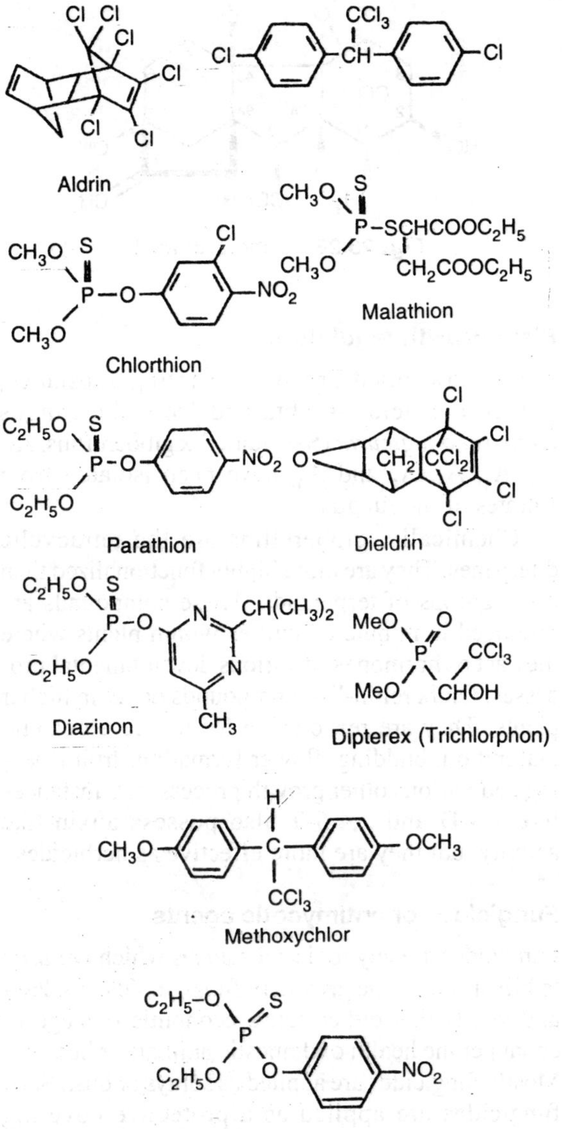

Aldrin

Chlorthion

Malathion

Parathion

Dieldrin

Diazinon

Dipterex (Trichlorphon)

Methoxychlor

Parathion

Fig. 25.25. Synthetic contact insecticides.

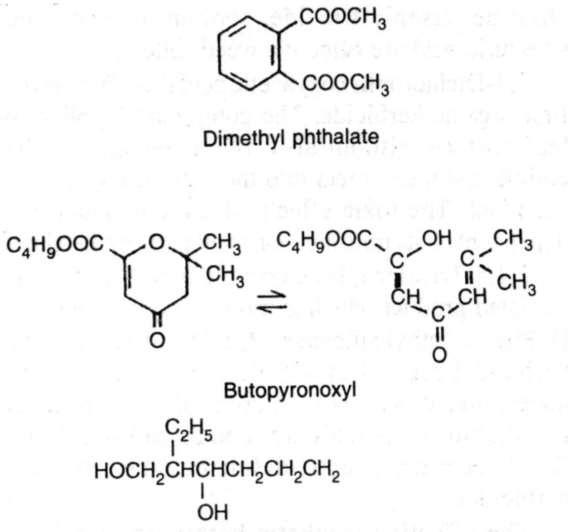

Dimethyl phthalate

Butopyronoxyl

Fig. 25.26. Dimethyl phthalate, butopyronoxyl and ethohexadiol.

pounds are mixed in Dimethyl phthalate in ratio of Dimethyl phthalate (6 parts), Ethohexadiol (2 parts) and Butopyronoxyl (2 parts), a synonym for this solution is 622 mixture. Diethyl-toluamide is another effective insect repellent.

Herbicides

Any agent, usually chemical, used for killing or inhibiting the growth of unwanted plants, are known as herbicides. They are classified as selective and nonselective depending upon their destructive properties. Selective herbicides eliminate undesirable species and produce some deleterious effect on the desired plants. Non-selective herbicides destroy all types of plant life.

Earlier sea salts, by-products of chemical industries, and various oils were used as weed-killers. Carbon disulphide, borax and arsenic trioxide are also used as weed killers. The herbicides are also divided as foliage applied and soil herbicides. Contact herbicides (*e.g.*, sulphuric acid, diquat, paraquat) kill only the plant organs. Translocated herbicides (*e.g.*, amitrole, picloram, 2, 4-D) are effective against roots or other organs to which they are transported from above ground. With respect to planting times, herbicides are also classified as preplant, pre-emergence, or post-emergence weed killers. Pre-plant herbicides may be applied to the soil or to weeds before crop planting.

Weeds and other vegetable grows along rail or road sides, highways, around buildings, vacant lands and playing grounds. They are killed by nonselective chemicals. Calcium cyanamide, potassium and sodium cyanides, ammonium thiocyanate, ammonium sulphamate, sodium chlorate, sodium chloride, arsenic trioxide, sodium arsenate and sulphuric acid are effective weed-killers.

2,4-Dichlorophenoxyacetic acid (2,4-D) was the first organic herbicide. The compound, applied to leaf surface without absorption, penetrates the cuticle and then enters into the vascular system of the plant. The toxic effects of the compound are dependent on its translocation to all parts of the plant.

2,4,5-Trichlorophenoxyacetic acid (2,4,5-T) is a related product which is more effective than 2,4-D. Phenoxyethyl sulphates, 2, 5-D and 3, 4-D have herbicidal properties identical to 2,4-D. Carbomates, urea derivatives, chlorinated acids, phenols and dinitro compounds are used as soil sterilizers, floral retarding agents, defoliants and selective herbicides.

The effective synthetic herbicides are 2, 2-dichloropropionic acid (Dalapon), 4-amino-3, 5, 6-trichloropicolinic acid (Tordon) and 3-amino-1, 2, 4-triazole (Aminotriazole). Dalapon is effective against grass-killer, whereas Tordon controls many woody species. Broadleaf weeds are perennial grasses and are controlled by amino-triazole.

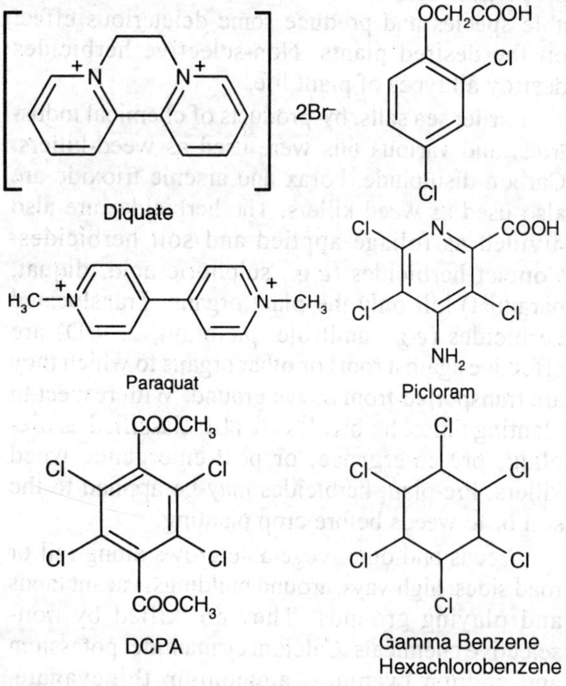

Fig. 25.27. Herbicidal compounds.

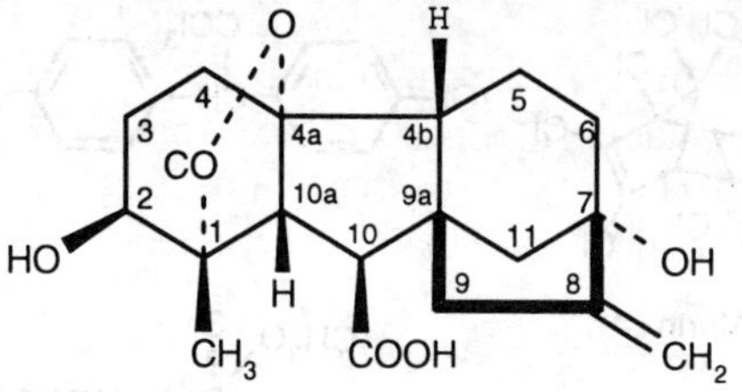

Fig. 25.28. Gibberellic acid.

Plant growth regulators

The natural plant growth-promoting substance, gibberellic acid, is obtained from the fungus *Gibberella fugikurai* (Sawada). Six gibberellins, A_1, A_2, A_3, A_4, A_7 and A_9, have been isolated from filtrates of the fungus.

Chemically, gibberellins are the tetracyclic diterpenes. They are more highly functionalized than other groups of terpenoids. These compounds are produced in minute quantities within plants where they act as hormones of various developmental processes. Gibberellin-like compounds occur in higher plants. They are responsible for the development, maturation, budding, flower formation, fruit ripening and various other growth processes. Substances like 2,4-D and 2,4,5-T also possess auxin-like activity, but they are more effective as herbicides.

Fungicides or antimycotic agents

Fungicides are any toxic substances which are used to kill or inhibit the growth of fungi, molds, mildews and yeasts that either cause economic damage or endanger the health of domestic animals or humans. Mostly fungicides are applied as sprays or dust. Seed fungicides are applied as a protective covering before germination. Systemic fungicides, or chemotherapeutants are applied to plants, where they become distributed throughout the tissue and act to eradicate existing disease or to protect against possible disease.

Protective fungicides are applied before the disease appears. They are used as sprays or dust to protect leaves and fruits and as seed disinfectants to eliminate the germination of spores simultaneously with seeds. Protectant agents are also used as wood preservatives to prevent dry rot and other fungus attacks on lumber. Eradicant fungicides are applied after the presence of fungi is observed. They kill by direct contact or else prevent the formation of spores. Thus, further spread of the fungus is inhibited.

A chemical combination of copper sulphate, lime and water is known as *Bordeaux mixture*. It is a protective fungicide. Sulphur is also used to control fungus disease. Lime-sulphur mixture is fungicide having both protective and eradicant properties. Its activity is due to calcium polysulphide which are very toxic to the fungus. Sulphur is mixed with nicotine, pyrethrum extracts and rotenone to get better result. The other useful fungicides are the thiocarbamates, especially the dimethylthiocarbamates and the ethylene bisthiocarbamates; mercury compounds, quaternary ammonium compounds, nitro and heterocyclic nitrogen compounds, antibiotics, chlorophenols and other phenols and formaldehyde.

Fumigant

Fumigant is any volatile, poisonous substance that is used to kill insects, nematodes and other animals or plants that damage stored foods or seeds, human dwellings, clothing and nursery stock. Soil fumigants are sprayed or spread over an area to be cultivated and are worked over an area to be cultivated and into the soil to control disease-causing fungi, nematodes and weeds.

Some chemically simpler chlorinated hydrocarbons such as chloroform, *p*-dichlorobenzene, carbon tetrachloride and trichloroethylene also have insecticidal activity and they are used as fumigants. They are applied in gaseous form or as an aerosol in enclosed spaces such as rooms, cupboards and boxes. These chlorinated hydrocarbons are highly dangerous to man and they must be used with care.

Index